Diagnostic Imaging in Polytrauma Patients

Vittorio Miele • Margherita Trinci
Editors

Diagnostic Imaging in Polytrauma Patients

Springer

Editors
Vittorio Miele
Department of Radiology
Careggi University Hospital
Florence
Italy

Margherita Trinci
Dept of Emergency Radiology
S. Camillo Hospital
Rome
Italy

ISBN 978-3-319-62053-4 ISBN 978-3-319-62054-1 (eBook)
https://doi.org/10.1007/978-3-319-62054-1

Library of Congress Control Number: 2017958549

Printed on acid-free paper

This Springer imprint is published by Springer Nature
The registered company is Springer International Publishing AG
The registered company address is: Gewerbestrasse 11, 6330 Cham, Switzerland

Dedicated to our parents, Antonio and Anna, Maurizio and Margherita

Foreword

According to the statistics, polytrauma is worldwide the fourth leading cause of death in general and the leading cause of death under the age of 40. The exponential growth of the "trauma culture" over the recent years has been driven forward by a significant technological advancement imposed by the digital explosion. This, in connection with an increasing use of multidetector computed tomography (MDCT), has led to the demand for a systematic imaging protocol to be followed in a still more complex pathology. The massive public interest in the main causes of death such as tumors, cardiovascular diseases, and brain diseases has been accompanied by a growing attention focused on the field of polytrauma.

The operators' training is mainly pragmatic and experimental. They dedicate less time to writing and publishing scientific papers than to practical work and are progressively being confronted with saving strategies in events which were up to a few years ago classified as irreversible.

This evolution has led to a growing demand for texts, which integrate the vast knowledge that different competent specialists have accumulated in the field of emergency imaging. What is required is a text presenting a holistic vision acquired by those who work with polytrauma patients every day. These specialists are well aware of the priorities, the existence of pitfalls in apparently simple cases, and the need for an immediate, definitive decision.

Who could be better equipped for such a challenging task than Vittorio Miele and Margherita Trinci after their successful publication of *Imaging Trauma and Polytrauma in Pediatric Patients* and *Imaging Non-traumatic Abdominal Emergencies in Pediatric Patients*.

Vittorio and Margherita have worked with some of the most qualified specialists sharing their daily tasks in the emergency rooms of the largest hospital in Rome, San Camillo, and in one of the most important academic centers for teaching and care, the Careggi University Hospital of Florence. They have dedicated themselves to emergency medicine, exchanging knowledge also with other specialists in the field through correspondence and conferences over the last 10 years.

The original version of this book was revised and Foreword is included in front matter in this version.

I have personally met the editors and several of the authors both as a colleague and as a patient or a relative of others in need of care. And I am well aware that the publication of this book requires great theoretical and practical skills that the authors have managed to put down on paper—a task which is not always easy.

The result of these efforts is a complex and complete edition of *Diagnostic Imaging in Polytrauma Patients*. In 25 chapters this volume provides the practical and theoretical framework of an issue, which implies not only great technical and scientific responsibilities but also a great emotional and media impact.

In every Emergency Department, this volume will certainly be of great use to specialists who must make an instant diagnosis by interpreting images obtained in polytrauma patients. They know that an immediate response must be provided to what has happened from head to toe—like life in the trenches. They can leave their patients with a smile or with regret, knowing that all possible attempts were made. Just like those who have produced this text which I am sure will be present in the bookcase of every radiologist to be consulted daily or to be studied for further cultural education.

Corrado Bibbolino
National Union of the Radiological Area (SNR),
Rome, Italy

Contents

Contributors

Ciro Acampora Department of Radiology, A.O.R.N. A. Cardarelli, Naples, Italy

Manlio Acquafresca Department of Radiology, Careggi University Hospital, Florence, Italy

Gloria Addeo Department of Radiology, Careggi University Hospital, Florence, Italy

Simone Agostini Department of Radiology, Careggi University Hospital, Florence, Italy

Giulia Angelini Department of Diagnostic and Interventional Radiology, University of Pisa, Pisa, Italy

Salvatore Alessio Angileri Diagnostic and Interventional Radiology Department, San Paolo Hospital, University of Milan, Milan, Italy

Giacomo Aringhieri Department of Diagnostic and Interventional Radiology, University of Pisa, Pisa, Italy

Lina Bartolini Department of Radiology, Careggi University Hospital, Florence, Italy

Eva Berardi Department of Radiology, S. Andrea Hospital, Sapienza University, Rome, Italy

Elena Bertelli Department of Radiology, Careggi University Hospital, Florence, Italy

Alessandra Bindi Department of Radiology, Careggi University Hospital, Florence, Italy

Luigi Bonasera Department of Radiology, Careggi University Hospital, Florence, Italy

Marta Brandani Department of Radiology, Careggi University Hospital, Florence, Italy

Luca Brunese Department of Medicine and Health Sciences, University of Molise, Campobasso, Italy

Grazia Loretta Buquicchio Department of Emergency Radiology, S. Camillo Hospital, Rome, Italy

Giovanna Calabrese Department of Emergency Radiology, S. Camillo Hospital, Rome, Italy

Raffaella Capasso Department of Medicine and Health Sciences, University of Molise, Campobasso, Italy

Ferdinando Caranci Department of Medicine and Health Sciences, University of Molise, Campobasso, Italy

Gianpaolo Carrafiello Diagnostic and Interventional Radiology Department, San Paolo Hospital, Università degli Studi di Milano, Milan, Italy

Alessandro Castellani Department of Radiology, Careggi University Hospital, Florence, Italy

Valentina Caturano Department of Emergency Radiology, S. Camillo Hospital, Rome, Italy

Edoardo Cavigli Department of Radiology, Careggi University Hospital, Florence, Italy

Alfonso Cerase, M.D. UOC Neuroimmagini e Neurointerventistica, Dipartimento Scienze Neurologiche e Neurosensoriali, Azienda Ospedaliera Universitaria Senese, Policlinico "Santa Maria alle Scotte", Siena, Italy

Andrea Coppola Unit of Radiology, Insubria University, Varese, Italy

Diletta Cozzi Department of Radiology, Careggi University Hospital, Florence, Italy

Matteo Crippa Vascular Surgery Department, San Paolo Hospital, Università degli Studi di Milano, Milan, Italy

Gavina Cuneo Department of Emergency Radiology, S. Camillo Hospital, Rome, Italy

Giuseppe D'Amico Department of Radiology, Careggi University Hospital, Florence, Italy

Ginevra Danti Department of Radiology, Careggi University Hospital, Florence, Italy

Riccardo Ferrari Department of Emergency Radiology, S. Camillo Hospital, Rome, Italy

Chiara Floridi Diagnostic and Interventional Radiology Department, Fatebenefratelli Hospital, Milan, Italy

Sonia Fulciniti Department of Radiology, A.O.R.N. A. Cardarelli, Naples, Italy

Nicola Gagliardi Department of Radiology, A.O.R.N. A. Cardarelli, Naples, Italy

Michele Galluzzo, M.D. Department of Emergency Radiology, S. Camillo Hospital, Rome, Italy

Giovanni Maria Garbarino Department of Surgery, S. Andrea Hospital, Sapienza University, Rome, Italy

Francesco Gaudino Department of Emergency Radiology, S. Camillo Hospital, Rome, Italy

Stefano Giannecchini Department of Emergency Radiology, S. Camillo Hospital, Rome, Italy

Roberto Grassi Department of Radiology, Second University of Naples, Naples, Italy

Giulia Grazzini Department of Radiology, Careggi University Hospital, Florence, Italy

Federico Greco Department of Emergency Radiology, S. Camillo Hospital, Rome, Italy

Franco Guida Department of Radiology, "Pineta Grande" Hospital, Castel Volturno (CE), Italy

Francesca Iacobellis Department of Radiology, "Pineta Grande" Hospital, Castel Volturno (CE), Italy

Department of Radiology, Second University of Naples, Naples, Italy

Stefania Ianniello, M.D. Department of Emergency Radiology, S. Camillo Hospital, Rome, Italy

Anna Maria Ierardi Diagnostic and Interventional Radiology Department, San Paolo Hospital, University of Milan, Milan, Italy

Veronica Iodice Department of Diagnostic and Interventional Radiology, University of Pisa, Pisa, Italy

Ettore Laccetti Department of Radiology, "Pineta Grande" Hospital, Castel Volturno (CE), Italy

Monica Marina Lanzetta Department of Radiology, Careggi University Hospital, Florence, Italy

Antonio Leone Istituto di Radiologia, Università Cattolica del Sacro Cuore, Fondazione Policlinico Universitario "Agostino Gemelli", Rome, Italy

Giorgio Loreni Department of Interventional Radiology, Sandro Pertini Hospital, Rome, Italy

Silvia Lorenzi Department of Diagnostic and Interventional Radiology, University of Pisa, Pisa, Italy

Silvia Lucarini, M.D., Ph.D. Department of Radiology, Careggi University Hospital, Florence, Italy

Natalie Lucchina Unit of Radiology, Insubria University, Varese, Italy

Nicola Maggialetti Department of Medicine and Health Sciences, University of Molise, Campobasso, Italy

Alessia De Marco Department of Medicine and Health Sciences, University of Molise, Campobasso, Italy

Maria Gabriella Merola Department of Emergency Radiology, S. Camillo Hospital, Rome, Italy

Vittorio Miele Department of Radiology, Careggi University Hospital, Florence, Italy

Francesco Morelli Postgraduation School in Radiodiagnostics, Diagnostic and Interventional Radiology Department, San Paolo Hospital, Università degli Studi di Milano, Milan, Italy

Chiara Moroni, M.D. Department of Radiology, Careggi University Hospital, Florence, Italy

Mario Moroni, M.D. Department of Radiology, Careggi University Hospital, Florence, Italy

Barbara Mugellini Department of Diagnostic and Interventional Radiology, University of Pisa, Pisa, Italy

Peiman Nazerian Department of Emergency Medicine, Careggi University Hospital, Florence, Italy

Riccardo Palliola Department of Emergency Radiology, S. Camillo Hospital, Rome, Italy

Francesca Pancrazi Department of Diagnostic and Interventional Radiology, University of Pisa, Pisa, Italy

Francesca Patella Postgraduation School in Radiodiagnostics, Diagnostic and Interventional Radiology Department, San Paolo Hospital, Università degli Studi di Milano, Milan, Italy

Filippo Pesapane Postgraduation School in Radiodiagnostics, Diagnostic and Interventional Radiology Department, San Paolo Hospital, Università degli Studi di Milano, Milan, Italy

Filippo Piacentino Unit of Radiology, Insubria University, Varese, Italy

Claudia Lucia Piccolo, M.D. Department of Medicine and Health Sciences, University of Molise, Campobasso, Italy

Matteo Pignatelli Department of Emergency Radiology, S. Camillo Hospital, Rome, Italy

Antonio Pinto Department of Radiology, A.O.R.N. A. Cardarelli, Naples, Italy

Caterina Pizzi Department of Emergency Radiology, S. Camillo Hospital, Rome, Italy

Silvia Pradella Department of Radiology, Careggi University Hospital, Florence, Italy

Mariagrazia Ramunno Department of Emergency Radiology, S. Camillo Hospital, Rome, Italy

Claudio Raspanti Department of Interventional Radiology, Careggi University Hospital, Florence, Italy

Marco Rastelli Department of Interventional Radiology, Sandro Pertini Hospital, Rome, Italy

Carmelo Rende Department of Emergency Radiology, S. Camillo Hospital, Rome, Italy

Federica Romano Department of Radiology, "Pineta Grande" Hospital, Castel Volturno (CE), Italy

Luigia Romano Department of Radiology, A.O.R.N. A. Cardarelli, Naples, Italy

Piercarlo Rossi Department of Diagnostic and Interventional Radiology, University of Pisa, Pisa, Italy

Andrea Sacrini Diagnostic and Interventional Radiology Department, San Paolo Hospital, University of Milan, Milan, Italy

Valeria Saracco Department of Emergency Radiology, S. Camillo Hospital, Rome, Italy

Mariano Scaglione, M.D. Department of Radiology, "Pineta Grande" Hospital, Castel Volturno (CE), Italy

Sunderland Royal Hospital, NHS Trust, Sunderland, UK

Germano Scevola Department of Interventional Radiology, Sandro Pertini Hospital, Rome, Italy

Serena Schipani Department of Medicine and Health Sciences, University of Molise, Campobasso, Italy

Alessandra Scionti Department of Diagnostic and Interventional Radiology, University of Pisa, Pisa, Italy

Massimo Silva Department of Radiology, A.O.R.N. A. Cardarelli, Naples, Italy

Antonia Sorbo Department of Radiology, "Pineta Grande" Hospital, Castel Volturno (CE), Italy

Alessandro Stasolla, M.D. Diagnostic and Interventional Neuroradiology, S. Camillo Hospital, Rome, Italy

Michele Tonerini Department of Emergency Radiology, Cisanello University Hospital, Pisa, Italy

Caterina Maria Trinci Department of Emergency Radiology, S. Camillo Hospital, Rome, Italy

Margherita Trinci, M.D. Department of Emergency Radiology, S. Camillo Hospital, Rome, Italy

Viola Valentini, M.D. Department of Emergency Radiology, S. Camillo Hospital, Rome, Italy

Giovanni Battista Verrone Department of Radiology, Careggi University Hospital, Florence, Italy

Marcello Zappia Department of Medicine and Health Sciences, University of Molise, Campobasso, Italy

Giuseppe Zocco Department of Emergency Radiology, Cisanello University Hospital, Pisa, Italy

1 Management of Polytrauma Patients

Vittorio Miele, Gloria Addeo, Diletta Cozzi, Ginevra Danti, Luigi Bonasera, Margherita Trinci, and Roberto Grassi

1.1 Introduction

Trauma is the leading cause of death in people under 45 years old [1], the third most common cause of death in patients aged between 45 and 54 years, and the fifth most common cause of death overall [2]. Approximately 5.8 million people die each year worldwide as a result of injuries (15,000 people die every day), and estimates predict injury deaths to become one of the top 20 leading causes of death in the world by 2030 [1]. Approximately a quarter of the 5.8 million deaths that are referred to as unintentional injuries are from road traffic injuries. Other main causes of death are the result of suicide, homicide, falls, drowning, burns, poisoning, and war [1]. Road traffic injuries represent a significant proportion of worldwide unintentional injury deaths. In 2015, accidents were the fourth leading cause of death in the USA and the leading cause of death for those aged 1–44 although car safety and driver awareness of the use of safety devices have continuously improved. Nearly 200,000 people die from injury each year, which is one person every 3 min [3].

Because injuries usually occur in young healthy individuals (road traffic injuries are the leading cause of death for those aged between 15 and 29 years), they result in potentially life-long disability, significant psychological trauma, and subsequent financial loss [4]. Unintentional injuries were responsible for more than 138 million disability-adjusted life-years lost in 2004, while those from road traffic account for approximately one-third of unintentional injury disability-adjusted life-years in all regions [5]. More than 90% of deaths that result from injury occur in low- and middle-income countries. Comparing high-income countries (North America and Europe) with low-income countries (Africa and Southeast Asia), the mortality rate of unintentional injury deaths is double for low-income countries (65 vs. 35 per 100,000 people), and the rate of life-years disability-adjusted is triple for low-income countries (2398 vs. 774 per 100,000) [4].

V. Miele (✉) • G. Addeo • D. Cozzi • G. Danti
L. Bonasera
Department of Radiology, Careggi University Hospital, L.go G. A. Brambilla 3, 50134 Florence, Italy
e-mail: vmiele@sirm.org

M. Trinci
Department of Emergency Radiology, S. Camillo Hospital, Rome, Italy

R. Grassi
Department of Radiology, Second University of Naples, Piazza Miraglia, Naples, Italy

V. Miele, M. Trinci (eds.), *Diagnostic Imaging in Polytrauma Patients*,
https://doi.org/10.1007/978-3-319-62054-1_1

People with poorer economic backgrounds have higher rates of death from injury and nonfatal injuries; this is due to, among other things, the poorer access to quality emergency trauma care and rehabilitation services. To minimize the effects of injuries, it is necessary to organize a national or regional multidisciplinary trauma system that includes trauma prevention, prehospital care, and improved hospital structures, care, and rehabilitation. The cost for the national medical system in medical care and lost productivity from traumatic injury is astronomical if one includes other nonmedical costs that stem from short-term or permanent disabilities that may result in continuing restrictions on their physical functioning, psychosocial consequences, or reduced quality of life. Road accidents are also a major cause of hospitalization and access to emergency care and can cause severe traumatic disability, such as paraplegia, quadriplegia, and intracranial trauma. Additional expenses resulting from unintentional injuries that occur in high- (87.5%) versus low-income countries (12.5%) is estimated to be 518 billion US dollars [6]. In the case of children, the cost in terms of future job disability and impaired quality of life amounted to 17,000 per child for a total of 347 billion dollars per year [7].

In Italy, over 7000 and 250,000 people died or were injured, respectively, in road accidents or were victims of accidents at work, home, or while partaking in sport events. Trauma is the third cause of death in Italy and the first in young people under 40 years of age; also, it greatly contributes to the number of permanently disabled people. In 2013, the number of road accidents resulting in deaths or injuries in Italy was 181,227; this included 3385 deaths (deaths within 30 days) and 257,421 injured persons [8]. In 2004, road accidents caused less than 1.5% of the annual deaths. More than 40% of deaths included young people between 15 and 24 years, constituting by far the leading cause of death in this age group; therefore, trauma is responsible for extremely serious consequences in terms of human and social costs [9].

1.2 Trauma Definition

Major trauma is defined as a traumatically induced structural injury and/or physiological disruption of a body function determined by an external dynamic force that causes single or multiple life-threatening lesions immediately after an event. Under this aspect, trauma should be considered itself a "vector-borne disease," whose means of transmission is a motor vehicle, firearm, or another blunt object, and which is followed by an admission to an emergency department to formulate a course and treatment.

A major trauma (or polytrauma) is defined when the injury severity score (ISS) is greater than 15; this threshold was first described by Boyd et al. in 1987 as being predictive of 10% mortality [10]. Injury mortality, which was originally described with a trimodal distribution, is now more accurately described as bimodal, since deaths presenting in the immediate and early hospital stages with the advancements in prehospital care, early resuscitation, and critical care have produced near elimination of the late deaths that occur after days or weeks due to sepsis and multiple organ failure.

Immediate deaths, which account for about 60% of all injury-related deaths, are mainly due to non-salvageable injuries, like the rupture of the heart or vessels, and occur immediately after trauma (<1 h), while early deaths account for around 30% and occur during the first 6 h of injury and are due to evolving conditions like hemorrhagic injuries of abdominal organs or expanding intracranial mass lesions [11].

Early deaths are commonly considered preventable given that organization of assistance of trauma patients is optimized at both on-scene and within the hospital by implementing technical and nontechnical skills at various levels.

1.2.1 Emergency and Trauma Care System

The aphorism "*Time is life: the smaller the delay until patients'* admission at the ER, the better the prognosis indeed" summarizes the relationship between shortened prehospital time and improved survival of the traumatized patient well [12]. These authors extensively demonstrated that helicopter medical services are superior to ground medical transportation by referencing historical wars. As a matter of fact, a 52% reduction in the mortality rate was observed in trauma patients treated at the site of injury and transported to the trauma center by air medical transport when compared with standard prehospital management services [12].

The adequacy of initial management of patients from the scene of injury and definitive care are factors that determine prognosis and remote outcome in traumatic events. The term "*golden hour,*" which is ubiquitous in emergency situations, refers to a time period lasting for 1 h or less, during which there is the highest likelihood that prompt medical treatment will prevent death [13]. However, the literal meaning of the term does not imply that survival rates drop off after 60 min. Some use the term to refer to the core principle of rapid intervention in trauma cases rather than the narrow meaning of a critical 1-h time period. It is well established that the patient's chances of survival are greatest if they receive care—both intra- and extra-hospital care—by narrowing the critical time within a short period after a severe injury.

So, if a successful and definite diagnosis and therapeutic evaluation is done within the first hour after trauma (i.e., in the golden hour), the polytrauma patient's chances for survival significantly increase. Thus, therapeutic procedures and diagnostic evaluation must be performed as soon as possible and simultaneously by a multidisciplinary team (trauma team) made up of different professional specialists and technicians who are all dedicated to the patient's management [14].

Effective emergency and trauma care systems—from first aid at the scene of the injury to operating theater trauma surgery—are key factors that affect the success of healthcare facilities in preventing avoidable mortality and morbidity during mass casualty incidents [15]. Building up trauma centers and services to manage with most serious traumas and deliver specialist facilities relatively quickly must therefore be a priority.

Evidence during the last two decades has shown that rapid patient triage followed by transportation to a designated trauma center is associated with a significant reduction in mortality after severe injury compared with transport to a non-trauma center [16, 17]. During initial evaluation, an accurate and timely diagnosis of bleeding and other important injuries is essential to plan and prioritize therapy [18].

For a significant reduction in the number of fatal wounds in a geographical area, it is necessary to develop an integrated system of care. A trauma care system is an organized and coordinated effort to deliver the full spectrum of care to an injured patient from the time of the injury to transport to an acute care facility, and to rehabilitative care. A trauma care system consists of three major providers—pre-hospital, acute care, and rehabilitation—that, when closely integrated, ensure a continuum of care [19] (Fig. 1.1).

1.2.2 Prehospital Care: Triage

Emergency medical services provide out-of-hospital medical care and transport patients to hospitals for extended evaluations by the diagnostic structure. Patients receiving prehospital care have a lower in-hospital mortality compared to those directly managed in the hospital and a reduced length of stay, considerably less than might be expected with; they also experience possible cost savings and reduced risks of long-term disabling sequelae. However, specific situations,

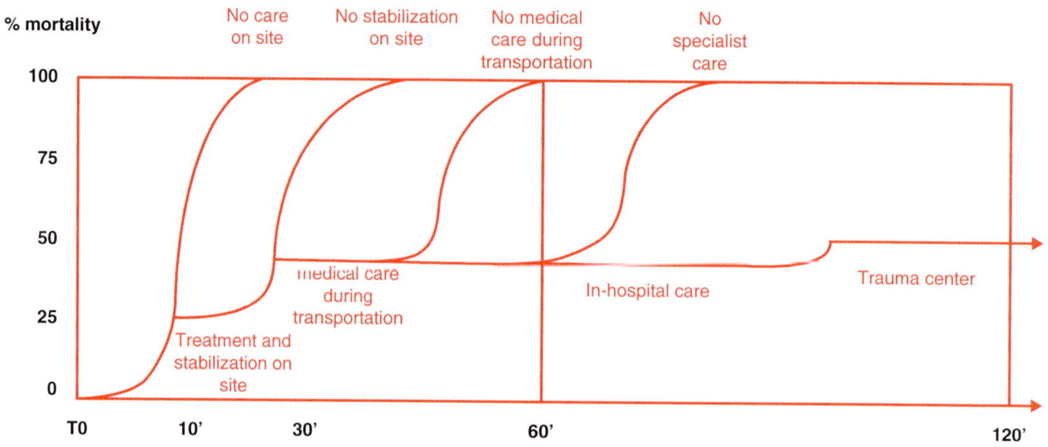

Fig. 1.1 Timely healthcare and best chance of survival. An early continuing healthcare significantly increases the probability of survival in patients with polytrauma. Mortality rates tend to decrease monotonically with life-saving primary care at the accident scene by rapid transfer to the most appropriate hospital for the definitive care. Treatment as early as 1 h or shorter after the traumatic event, especially first aid—prehospital care—platinum 10 min—can help reduce preventable deaths

particularly in the case of inefficiency of emergency department services—mainly in the phase of management and diagnostic classification at the hospital with patients receiving a standard of care that was less than good practice—increased the proportion of preventable trauma deaths.

So, when clinical teams and facilities (e.g., hospital, community, primary care) are organized to meet best practice clinical guidelines and standard services within the trauma system, each patient's mortality could be significantly reduced [20]. The golden rule would mean that if the right team in a dedicated major trauma center with an efficient organization treats the patient, significant outcome benefits for patients with major trauma will be obtained.

Therefore, the quality of the emergency management system (EMS) as well as response times is critical to life-saving practices. To meet the growing demand of emergency medical services and prevent early deaths, it is crucial for care providers to calibrate and reduce transport time. Once an emergency call is received, the dispatch center identifies the urgency of the call, and on the basis of urgency, the center makes decisions on whether an ambulance or helicopter needs to be dispatched. This depends mainly on the distance to the site of the accident, the accessibility of the site to motor vehicles, traffic intensity, and the right hospital that is able to manage the identified injuries. European health systems provide treatment at the site of the incident, and healthcare professionals are able to correctly apply the principles of patient trauma stabilization and triage procedures and to continue care during transport aboard a land or air ambulance.

The initial assessment is indicated in the guidelines of the advanced trauma life support [ATLS] approach outlined by the American College; the ATLS is a training program for medical providers in the management of acute trauma cases. Nowadays, ATLS is widely accepted as the standard of care for initial assessment and treatment in trauma center.

It suggests to first treat the greatest threat to life. Prehospital trauma care is addressed immediately according to the ABCDE scheme, focusing on the following steps, A: Airway management; B: Breathing, ventilation, and oxygenation; C: circulation and external bleeding control; D: disability, immobilization of the spine, disability, or neurological status; and E: exposure or undressing of the patient while also protecting from hypothermia. There are conflicting views about the most suitable procedure to follow at the scene of the injury—for example, to start with a consistent, high-quality patient care at the accident site or to transfer the injured patient without delay to the trauma unit.

This dualism has had consequences in different countries.

Out-of-hospital care concepts such as "*scoop and run*" (rapid transport to hospital), "*stay and play*" (treatment and stabilization on site), or "*load, go, and play*" (charge quickly and stabilize the patient during the transport) have been compared in recent decades. The "*stay and play*" relief model, which is currently applied in European countries for closed traumas, predicts the presence of medical and paramedic figures aboard.

Staff administering Advanced Life Support (ALS) at the site of trauma results in an average trip time to the hospital of about 18.5 min. In the "*scoop and run*" procedure, where only Basic Life Support (BLS) is provided, emergency trips average 5 min less than the "*stay and play*" procedure [21].

A study undertaken to investigate changes in prehospital care for patients with severe traumatic brain injury demonstrated that the overall mortality rate did not change for the historic BLS cohort (average time on scene 7.5 min) with respect to the current ALS cohort (about four times as long as in the historic cohort) [22]. Regardless of the procedure followed in the rescue of the patient, the best common practice is to carry out life-saving operations on site as quickly as possible and to transport the patient to the most appropriate center in the shortest possible time.

In addition to the aforementioned golden hour, which indicates the importance of early relief and treatment during the first hour after the traumatic event, special attention is paid to the first "*platinum 10 minutes*" in which the causes of preventable deaths (e.g., airway obstruction, hemorrhagic shock) easily lead to death. The first "*platinum 10 minutes*" becomes important to make the golden hour effective and should be distributed as follows to make it fruitful: assessment of the victim and primary survey, 1 min; resuscitation and stabilization, 5 min; and immobilization and transport to nearby hospital, 4 min [23].

This philosophy has been likely borrowed from the military, as many battlefield fatalities occur within the first minutes post injury. Seriously injured patients should have no more than 10 min of scene-time stabilization by emergency medical personnel prior to transport to definitive care at a trauma center [24]. Two possible errors can lead to negative potential consequences at the scene of the rescue that is under- and over-triage of the patient's injury.

Triage protocols were developed by an expert panel and indicate that over-triage is safer than under-triage because if the patient does not require care in a higher level trauma and is unnecessarily transported to such a center, this causes an overutilization of financial and human resources and can lead to overcrowding of the trauma center [25]. Over-triage rates vary in the approximate range 25–50% and may be able to be reduced while maintaining low under-triage rates [26].

Based on presenting signs and symptoms, the protocols recommend patients to one of four alternatives: (1) ambulance transport to an emergency department (ED); (2) transport to an ED by alternative means; (3) referral to a primary care provider (PCP) within 24 h; or (4) treatment at the scene only [27].

According to the "Guidelines for Field Triage of Injured Patients" published by the Centers for Disease Control and Prevention (CDC, 2011), if any of the following alterations that fall into four categories (physiologic, anatomic, mechanism-of-injury, and special considerations) are identified, it is recommended to transport the patient to a facility that provides the highest level of care within the defined trauma system [28, 29]:

Physiologic Criteria

- Glasgow Coma Scale <13
- SBP of <90 mmHg
- Respiratory rate of <10 or >29 breaths per minute (<20 in infant aged <1 year) or need for ventilation support

Anatomic Criteria

- All penetrating injuries to head, neck, torso, and extremities proximal to the elbow or knee
- Chest wall instability or deformity (e.g., flail chest)
- Two or more proximal long-bone fractures
- Crushed, degloved, mangled, or pulseless extremity
- Amputation proximal to the wrist or ankle
- Pelvic fractures
- Open or depressed skull fractures
- Paralysis

Mechanism of Injury

- Falls
  - Adults: >20 ft (one story = 10 ft)
  - Children: >10 ft or two to three times the height of the child
- High-risk auto crash
  - Intrusion, including roof: >12 in. occupant site; >18 in. any site
  - Ejection (partial or complete) from automobile
  - Death in same passenger compartment
  - Vehicle telemetry data consistent with a high risk for injury
- Automobile versus pedestrian/bicyclist thrown, run over, or with significant (>20 mph) impact
- Motorcycle crash >20 mph

Special considerations: EMS personnel must determine whether persons who have not met physiologic, anatomic, or mechanism steps have underlying conditions or comorbid factors that place them at higher risk of injury or that aid in identifying the seriously injured patient.

- Older adults
  - Risk for injury/death increases after age 55 years
  - SBP <110 might represent shock after age 65 years
  - Low-impact mechanisms (e.g., ground-level falls) might result in severe injury
- Children
  - Should be triaged preferentially to pediatric capable trauma centers
- Anticoagulants and bleeding disorders
  - Patients with head injury are at high risk for rapid deterioration
- Burns
  - Without other trauma mechanism: triage to burn facility
  - With trauma mechanism: triage to trauma center
- Pregnancy >20 weeks
- EMS provider judgment

The ideal triage system will direct patients to the appropriate health services for their needs. Updated ambulance technology can speed up response times and improve emergency communications using high-tech wireless networks and making it possible to relay critical patient data to headquarters in real time. Nowadays, there are new apps that allow ambulance personnel to transmit key information to the trauma center, including vital signs and, more importantly, photos or video of the patient's wounds; thus, the trauma center is able to make the necessary preparations for the patient's arrival [30].

EMS service technologies are emerging that provide more options for healthcare providers and make patients' lives better during ambulance transport. Boarded personnel are able to communicate via secure instant messaging with the center to obtain information regarding, for example, traffic and other obstacles; this helps to gain precious minutes when transporting patients to the trauma center.

1.3 Trauma Network

Trauma centers are specially designed to care for the most critically injured patients. New trauma centers are placed geographically with good motorway access, given that the prompt treatment of polytrauma patients by a specialized team has a higher probability of favorable outcomes. Stakeholders and healthcare planners should therefore consider this factor in the development of trauma systems [31]. In a research work comparing the availability of hospital facilities to urban and rural communities, rural communities were found to have higher risk than urban communities because they have less access to trauma centers.

The ACS-COT (Optimal Care of the Injured Patient, by the American College of Surgeons Committee) trauma center classification scheme (Level I through Level IV) is intended to assist communities in their trauma system development [32]. ACS oversees designation of trauma centers in various levels according to hospital resources and educational and research commitments. These categories may vary from state to state and are typically outlined through legislative or regulatory authorities. The different levels (i.e., Level I, II, III, IV, or V) refer to the kinds of resources available in a trauma center and the number of patients that are admitted yearly.

Level I trauma center is a comprehensive regional resource that is a tertiary care facility that is central to the trauma system. In this center, total care for every aspect of injury—from prevention through rehabilitation—is supplied, including educational and research branches.

Level II trauma centers are also able to provide complete treatment for trauma patients, but they do not have educational and research programs. Level III centers have the stabilization and initial resuscitation measures for major trauma patients. Level IV centers assure initial care and have well-functioning protocols for rapid transfer of the patients [33, 34]. Generally, the regional emergency service is organized in specialist centers of excellence (major trauma center [MTC] or "*hub*") located in the regional capitals, which are equipped and staffed to provide care for patients suffering from major traumatic injuries.

An MTC must admit at least 1200 trauma patients yearly or have 240 admissions with an injury severity score of more than 15; they also must be equipped with specialist medical and nursing care. MTCs are directly connected with peripherals, radially diffused, trauma units ("*spokes*") that no longer have to provide major trauma care but still play an essential role in less severely injured patients in whom transfer to an MTC may result in worse outcome.

Despite the longer transport times this entails, triage of major trauma patients to an MTC results in a 30% decrease in mortality in the first 48 h compared with transport to a non-MTC, which may be the closest medical facility [17]. This happened because the key point is not the time to reach a hospital but the efficiency of the final treatment [i.e., interventional radiology (IR) or surgery]. MTC trauma services run 24/7 for diagnostic and interventional services and provide 24/7 whole-body computed tomography (WBCT) by experienced personnel together with the image interpretation as well as 24/7 access for IR services for emergency bleeding control.

1.3.1 Inhospital Care: Primary and Secondary Survey

It is undeniable that application of time-dependent EMS interventions (e.g., airway obstruction, respiratory arrest, external hemorrhage at a compressible site) has potential positive effects on outcomes for most trauma patients. However, it is also plausible that the "golden hour" is primarily dependent on the timeliness of hospital-based interventions (i.e., initiation of definitive care after arrival at an ED) rather than out-of-hospital care [35].

The ATLS method establishes priorities in emergency trauma care by dividing the assessment of each patient's trauma into a primary and secondary survey. The radiologist plays a key role in the early diagnosis of possible life-threatening injuries in the trauma room for defining focused treatments (primary survey) and then in the identification and definition of prognostic scores to assist in stratification of patients in clinical management (secondary survey).

1.3.1.1 The Trauma Resuscitation Team

Once the patient arrives to the hospital, the trauma team takes charge of the patient from the ambulance crew and the traumatized patient is transferred to a trauma room. The trauma resuscitation team consists of physicians, nurses, and allied health personnel, and they are all dedicated to managing the patient. Typically, trauma centers have a single level of trauma, while others may have two or three that are specifically defined in policy and monitored through the trauma quality-assurance process. The size and composition of the team may vary with hospital size, the severity of injury, and the corresponding level of trauma team activation.

A high-level response to a severely injured patient usually consists of a team with the following professionals: general surgeon, emergency physician, anesthetist, radiologist, laboratory technician, radiology technologist, and critical care nurse. The main tasks of the trauma team are the maintenance and improvement of vital functions, diagnosis and early treatment of lesions, and execution of emergency procedures. Major trauma, covering various organs and districts, is certainly the disorder/disease for which a multidisciplinary approach could provide a significant outcome. All levels are based specifically on the hospital resources available to the trauma patient as well as the patient's physiological status. Hospital staff may rely on a report from EMS about the life-threatening injuries identified by the rescue team aboard the ambulance by application of the systematic ATLS primary survey protocol to confirm previously detected vital sign changes.

Therefore, the first step is the activation of the trauma team and to provide immediate resuscitation to the seriously injured trauma patient using hospital resources. In this way, the trauma leader continuously reevaluates the prior ATLS findings since the patient's condition may change (e.g., deteriorate) rapidly. Usually, when a polytrauma patient is identified, the trauma team activates all resources within 15 min of notification.

Each trauma center acts according to internal protocols clearly documented by a "trauma team activation policy" with defined roles and responsibilities for each component. These protocols are subjected to continuous improvements to meet the needs of the plurality of cases encountered. Since there are a variety of hospitals at different organizational levels, no definitive list of trauma team activation criteria exists that is safely employed at all facilities. Each ED that treats polytrauma patients should develop an internal protocol for appropriate multidisciplinary team mobilization on the basis of the internal human and facility-based resources.

In Level I and II trauma centers, the highest level of activation requires the response of the full trauma team within 15 min of arrival of the patient; this includes a surgeon, emergency physician, trauma-trained nurses, imaging department team support, laboratory team support, and respiratory team support.

1.3.1.2 Primary Survey

Historically, the standard of care for trauma patients (i.e., the advanced trauma life support [ATLS] approach) outlined by the American College of Surgeons [36] indicates the guidelines for a reliable evaluation of traumatized patients. The protocol states to identify the most immediate life-threatening conditions and adopt the measures for minimizing the potential risk. The objectives of the initial evaluation of the trauma patient are as follows: (1) to rapidly identify life-threatening injuries, (2) to initiate adequate supportive therapy, and (3) to efficiently organize either definitive therapy or transfer to a facility that provides definitive therapy.

In the primary survey, the sequence and timing of the resuscitation procedures are identified by successive phases following the order A–B–C–D–E (airways–breathing–circulation–disability–exposure/environment). The initial assessment and the arrangement in the primary survey and resuscitation phases can and should be rapid (5–10 min).

A (Airway): Airways and Cervical Spine Protection

The first priority is airway patency by determining the ability of air to pass unobstructed into the lungs. An acute airway obstruction is the leading cause of death in trauma patients. Maxillofacial trauma, neck trauma, and laryngeal trauma are the most common causes of airway dysfunction. As obstruction may partially or totally prevent air from getting into the lungs, and consequent clinical signs ranging from stridor, dysphonia, wheezes, or high respiratory rates together with an altered state of consciousness (e.g., restlessness, stupor, coma) can be a consequence of a respiratory tract obstruction. The most common cause of airway obstruction in the unconscious patient is the hypotonic tongue, but foreign body upper airway obstruction, secretions in the airway, soft tissue damage, and respiratory tract irritation are all potential causes of an obstructed airway. The most basic airway maneuvers are the chin lift and jaw thrust. In a patient who has not been cleared of a cervical spine injury, these maneuvers must be done without significant neck extension. Once the basic maneuvers have been performed, the oral cavity is carefully cleaned, by aspiration of foreign bodies and liquids using electric vacuum suction, which hinders vomit and worsening of the situation. Immobilization of the cervical spine must be instituted until a complete clinical and radiological evaluation has excluded injury (Fig. 1.2).

Oropharyngeal and nasopharyngeal airway devices can provide temporary return of airway patency in an unconscious patient until the airway is definitely secured though intubation. Tracheal intubation is indicated for airway protection (GCS < 9; severe maxillofacial fractures; laryngeal or tracheal injury; evolving airway loss with neck hematoma or inhalation injury) and as a conduit for ventilation (apnea, respiratory distress—tachypnea >30, hypoxia/hypercarbia) [37].

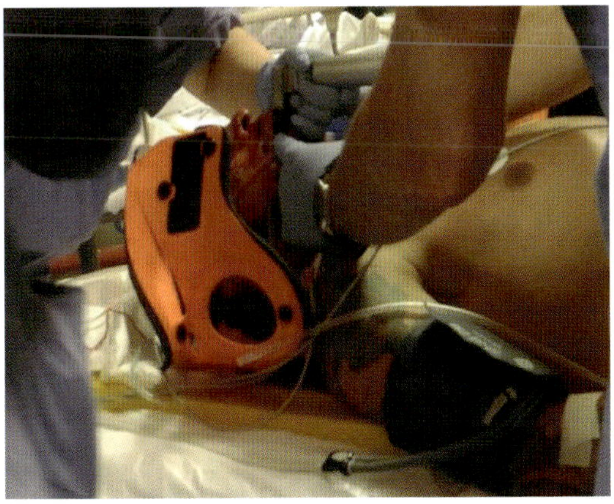

Fig. 1.2 Immobilization of the cervical spine and maneuvers to ensure the patency of the airway

B (Breathing): Ventilation and Oxygenation

A consequential step is the immediate evaluation of the patient's ability to ventilate and oxygenate. A thorough physical examination of the chest should be performed quickly after the initial assessment to rule out possible tension pneumothorax, massive hemorrhage, flail chest, and cardiac tamponade, which are all life-threatening conditions. According to the ATLS, the patient's chest should be exposed to adequately assess chest wall excursion, then auscultation should be performed to assure gas flow in the lungs; then, percussion should be performed to exclude the presence of air or blood in the chest, and finally visual inspection and palpation may detect injuries to the chest wall that may compromise ventilation. A pulse oximeter can be applied to evaluate the efficiency of breathing, and if needed provide supplemental oxygen with bag-valve mask unit or tracheal intubation. In the case of flail chest/severe pulmonary contusion, pneumothorax, or hemothorax, re-expansion of alveolar volume can be obtained by performing endotracheal intubation, mechanical ventilation using a thoracentesis needle, or tube thoracostomy.

C (Circulation): Circulation and Hemorrhage Control

For the hemorrhagic shock in the injured patient who is unresponsive to the usual measures of resuscitation, pericardiocentesis treatment is applied during the primary survey. Circulation is initially assessed by simple observation of the patient, then the peculiar stress and hypovolemia response is taken into account; moreover, the traumatized patient, to compensate for a significant hemorrhage, releases a significant amount of catecholamine and increases cardiac contractility, which increases the heart rate and the systemic resistance. As blood loss progresses, mental status deteriorates, heart rate increases, blood pressure falls, and oliguria is apparent [38]. The estimated blood loss, using vital signs proposed by ATLS to manage the best resuscitation strategy, classifies the state of shock into four classes, according to the blood loss, pulse rate, and pulse pressure [39].

The patient whose persistent vital sign evaluation suggests hypotension is at significant risk for loss of 30–40% of blood volume on presentation and often leads to imminent cardiac arrest. Rapid and accurate assessment of the patient's hemodynamic status based on clinical and hemodynamic criteria is assessed by a combination of parameters: cardiovascular (blood pressure, pulse, pulse pressure); pulmonary (oxygen saturation via pulse oximetry, respiratory rate); skin appearance (color, temperature, capillary refill); CNS (consciousness level); renal-urine output (normal 0.5 cc/kg/h in adults, 1.0 cc/kg/h in children, 2.0 cc/kg/h in neonates).

The estimated blood loss using vital signs proposed by ATLS to manage the best resuscitation strategy classifies the state of shock into four classes according to the blood loss, pulse rate, and pulse pressure [39]:

- Class I: Blood Loss <15% (<750 mL); Pulse rate < 100, normal BP, normal Pulse/Pressure;
- Class II: Blood Loss 15–30% (750–1500 mL); P = 100–120, normal BP, decreased PP;
- Class III: Blood Loss 30–40% (1500–2000 mL); P = 120–140, decreased BP, decreased PP;
- Class IV: Blood Loss >40% (>2000 mL); P > 140, decreased BP, decreased PP.

It is important to note that with the increase of blood loss, particularly when quantification of the loss amount is not feasible (e.g., trauma and occult bleeding), the vital signs that are used to guide fluid replacement in trauma patients with hypovolemic shock due to hemorrhage are not altered. In fact, in Class II, when faced with a circulating blood volume reduction of up to 30%, patients may display blood pressure values that are quite normal but with altered pulse and pulse pressure values. Patients only exhibit tachypnea, tachycardia (HR > 120), decrease in systolic BP, delayed capillary refill, decreased urine output, and a change in mental status for Class III hemorrhages, which are characterized by 30–40% blood loss (1500–2000 mL). For each class, ATLS allocates therapeutic recommendations for example, either the replacement of intravenous fluids (class I–IV) or the administration of blood products (class III–IV) [39].

It is always required to identify the presence of any source of external bleeding with a systemic approach by applying direct pressure; in the presence of uncontrolled bleeding from limbs, pneumatic tourniquets should be immediately used. All polytraumatized patients should be connected to a multi-parameter monitor in order to have a continuous reassessment of the respiratory and circulatory parameters. Two large-bore intravenous lines should be obtained to replace fluids and deliver medications. In case of hypovolemic shock, the infusion plan involves the administration of 250–500 mL warmed boluses; often, a total of 2–3 L of IV fluids is necessary, which will then need to be followed by blood transfusion bolus if hemodynamic stability is not achieved. The positive response to therapy leads to a substantial improvement of vital signs manifested through blood pressure, tachycardia, CNS-mental status normalization, urine output, and organ perfusion improvement [40].

A shock condition in traumatized patients is attributed to hemorrhage until proven otherwise; in relation to the context, of course, different and concurrent causes should be assessed: bleeding from the thorax (massive hemothorax, vascular injury, penetrating cardiac injury); abdomen (solid-organ injury [liver, spleen, or kidney], major vessel injury, or mesenteric bleeding); retroperitoneum (pelvic fracture); long bone fractures (e.g., femur); and also myocardial dysfunction after contusion due to thoracic trauma, or medullary impairment with neurogenic shock (hypotension without increase of heart rate or vasoconstriction) due to head and neck injuries.

D (Disability): Neurological Assessment

A brief neurologic exam is carried out to assess whether a serious head or spinal cord injury exists. This assesses the patient's level of consciousness, papillary size, and reaction and possible lateralizing signs. The level of consciousness is classified according to the Glasgow coma scale (GCS) or the AVPU score. The GCS evaluates the severity of head injury by classifying three different aspects of behavioral response to external stimulation: eye opening; motoric reaction; and verbal response. The score ranges from 3 to 15, where a score of 15 represents a patient's eyes spontaneously opening, obeying commands, and being normally oriented. The worst score is 3 points.

A decreased GCS can be caused by a focal brain injury (i.e., an epidural hematoma, a subdural hematoma, or a cerebral contusion) and by diffuse brain injuries ranging from a mild contusion to diffuse axonal injury [41]. The pupils are also examined for size, symmetry, and reactiveness to light, the spinal cord is assessed for injury by observing the spontaneous movement of the extremities and spontaneous respiratory effort. Oxygenation, ventilation, perfusion, drugs, alcohol, and hypoglycemia may all also affect the level of consciousness. Patients should be reevaluated frequently at regular intervals, as deterioration can occur rapidly, and often patients can be lucid following a significant head injury before worsening.

E (Exposure): Exposure and Thermal Protection

Trauma patients should be completely undressed for a thorough physical examination. Soon after, they should be protected from thermal dispersion. Then, the trauma patient is treated prophylactically with the administration of warmed intravenous fluids, blankets, heat lamps, and warmed air-circulating blankets as needed.

Formulation of the Patient's Severity Index

At the end of the qualitative and quantitative assessment of all phases summarized with the acronym ABCDE, the patient's chance of survival is calculated according to the injury severity score (ISS), which correlates the mortality, morbidity, and hospitalization time after trauma with a number varying between 0 and 75. A major trauma (or polytrauma) is described by an ISS index greater than 15 [42]. In addition to the ISS, many trauma score systems have been developed and used. For instance, the revised trauma score (RTS) [43] is the most widely used although its calculation is too complicated for easy use in the ES [44].

According to the ATLS indications, imaging is helpful during the primary survey, but the use should neither stop nor delay life-saving maneuvers. The inherent instability of the trauma patient in this setting provides a requirement for rapid imaging and accurate, timely interpretation. It is especially relevant because evaluation by history and clinical examination alone has been shown to result in misdiagnosis in 20–50% of patients with blunt polytrauma [45]. A common concept in trauma management that early intervention leads to improved outcomes is that of the "golden hour" [36]. Since its inception, the advanced trauma life support (ATLS) program has been adopted in over 60 countries and has repeatedly undergone important changes. Throughout these revisions, the role of medical imaging has evolved. The current iteration of the program includes, after the "ABCDE" of the primary survey, descriptions of a trauma series (plain film radiographs of the cervical spine, chest, and pelvis), a focused assessment with sonography for trauma (E-FAST) examination, and the selective use of MDCT. The secondary survey is essentially a head-to-toe examination with completion of the history and reassessment of progress and vital signs.

Flowchart of Diagnostic Imaging

The diagnostic procedure to be used varies according to the patient's hemodynamic condition. An "unstable" patient is one with blood pressure < 90 mmHg and heart rate > 120 bpm, with evidence of skin vasoconstriction (cool, clammy, decreased capillary refill), altered level of consciousness, and/or shortness of breath [46]. In particular, in the case of hemodynamically stable patients (blood pressure > 90 mmHg, pulse < 120/min) or patients stabilized after primary resuscitation, full-body CT scan remains the gold standard in the evaluation of injured patients because it allows a detailed view of the body. In contrast, for hemodynamically unstable patients (blood pressure < 90 mmHg, pulse rate > 120/

min), the time-consuming TC scan is not suggested; instead, it is suggested to use X-ray and US during the primary survey [47, 48].

X-rays and ultrasonography provide an initial diagnosis of conditions that can endanger the patient during the diagnostic phase, and in this scenario, the radiologist plays a key role at the emergency setting to provide a first effective diagnostic confirmation of potentially life-threatening clinical situations [49].

During maneuvering, resuscitators are beside the patient who is lying supine, making all the maneuvers to stabilize the patient and carrying out imaging tests such as chest X-ray (CXR) with an AP view, cervical spine X-ray with an LL view, pelvis X-ray with an AP view, and E-FAST scan (extended focused assessment with sonography for trauma). Subsequently, as mentioned above, the hemodynamically stabilized patient undergoes a TC exam that obtains a complete evaluation of all of the body parts (Fig. 1.3).

Emergency Radiology During the Primary Survey

Radiology is the key component of the trauma center, which is a determining factor for the diagnosis and subsequent treatment of trauma injuries, and therefore radiologists are a part of the trauma team. In dedicated trauma services in large hospitals, the team leader of the emergency radiology (ED) directs the evaluation and resuscitation in cooperation with general and orthopedic surgeons, physicians, radiologists, and anesthetists of the ED staff. Neurosurgeons interventions, when significant central nervous system injury is present, can be life saving. A well-integrated team should include all medical professionals involved in the patient's care in addition to the radiologist. Often trauma patients are unconscious and uncooperative with medical staff, and this hampers the correct interpretation of the injury mechanism within the right context of the trauma event. This does not properly address the physician and radiologist toward the best-suited technique and protocol for the patient considering the technological resources available to the ED. So, radiologists undergo a significant amount of formal education to provide their expertise to the emergency staff in cooperation with other specialists to improve the quality of patient management.

Logistics of the ED put the patient at the center of the scenario; specialists in the emergency room surround the patient (Fig. 1.4). In this context, the role of the radiologist is of primary importance because he is the only specialist that

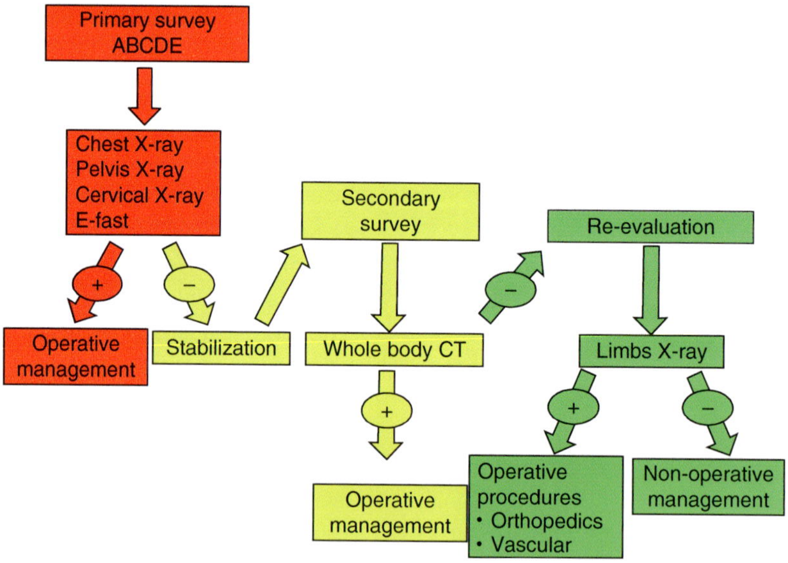

Fig. 1.3 Outline of the current algorithm for the assessment and management of polytraumatized patients

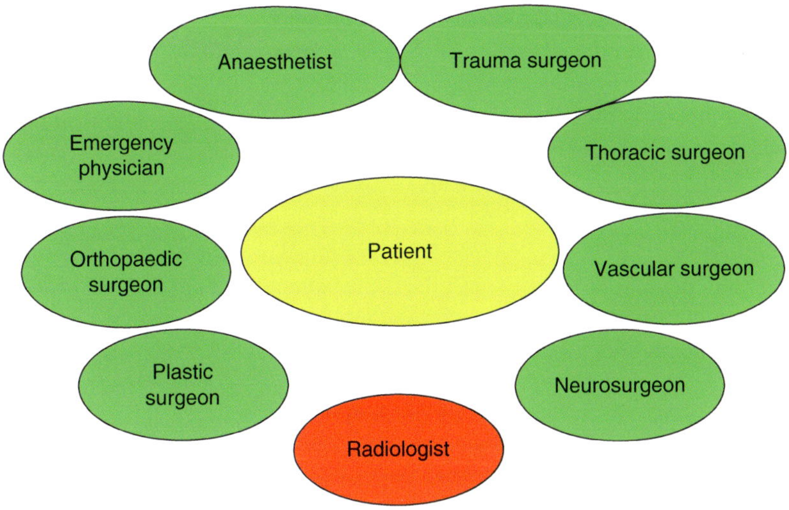

Fig. 1.4 The use of multidisciplinary in-hospital polytrauma teams within an Emergency and Admission Department in a context of concrete and complete collaboration improves patient outcomes

has a full understanding of the final product (the images) and the knowledge of technical equipment and imaging techniques.

Radiology can no longer be viewed as an "add-on" to ED. Indeed, there is no case of urgency or a few cases that are not followed by an imaging act. Emergency radiology is distinguished mostly by the adaptation to any clinical patient's situation, and the radiological response can oftentimes be the most effective, most specific, fastest, and least expensive.

Imaging services therefore must be as rigorous as the other specialties involved in the ED, and they should have the same human resources as other medical services. The powerful informatics systems introduced in the medical arena have allowed to rapidly solving complex health problems and are dependent on the development, for the main part, of the social and political interaction skills of the developer. Therefore, before being a hardware problem, the radiological emergency is a human-based problem.

The clinical radiologist orients and adapts the radiological prescription under its responsibility by an immediate interpretation, and intervening eventually on therapeutics (interventional radiologist). Efficient and optimized care is realized with the cooperation of team members that contribute to the patient's health. Therefore, each qualified "professional" that is directly involved in the diagnostic and therapeutic management will discuss with the radiologist the choice of explorations according to the patient's problem. Efficient patient management requires communication between team members and the radiologist. Each team member supports the patient-centered care to the best of his or her ability.

In order to minimize delay and transport, lifesaving maneuvers need to be performed without stopping resuscitation—this may even require bringing mobile diagnostic apparatus to the patient's bedside. From the emergency room, the patient is transported to the operating block in the shortest possible time; therefore, the CT room must be located within the emergency care area.

Chest X-Ray (CXR)

The plain anteroposterior chest radiograph remains the standard initial exam for the evaluation of the polytraumatized patient in the emergency room. Because of the inaccuracy of clinical signs, important thoracic problems that require possible intervention can be identified using a chest X-ray.

In cases of hemodynamic instability, the presence of respiratory failure (hypoxemia and dyspnea), or after pleural decompression or pleural drainage insertion, an ordinary chest X-ray is recommended. In all cases of blunt trauma, the patient must have a chest X-ray in the supine position in the resuscitation room since unstable spinal fractures have not been ruled out at this stage. In penetrating trauma (penetrating injuries), both from firearms and stab wounds, a chest X-ray should be taken preferably with the patient seated upright to increase the sensitivity for detecting small hemothorax, pneumothorax, or diaphragm injury.

Cervical Spine X-Ray

Cervical spine injuries are the most dreaded among all spinal injuries because of the potential serious neurological sequelae. Significant cervical spine injury is very unlikely in the case of trauma if the patient has normal mental status without neck pain, tenderness on neck palpation, neurologic signs, or symptoms referable to the neck (such as numbness or weakness in the extremities), other distracting injuries, and history of loss of consciousness [50]. However, the radiological series for excluding a cervical spine fracture requires a posteroanterior view, a lateral view, and an odontoid view. The lateral view must include seven cervical vertebrae as well as the C7-T1 interspace, allowing visualization of the alignment of C7 and T1.

According to current evidence, CT imaging of the cervical spine in polytrauma patients has replaced plain film imaging due to its greater sensitivity.

Pelvis X-Ray

Pelvic fractures resulting from motor vehicle accidents and also from falls from heights are very complex, as they imply high-energy trauma that disrupt the solid pelvic ring. These fractures are rarely isolated and are often associated with life-threatening complications such as bleeding (arterial, venous, and cancellous bone).

Up to 60% of mortality rates likely related to significant differences in fracture types have been reported [51]. Hemodynamic instability and multiple organ failure as direct consequences of pelvic hemorrhage have been identified as the primary causes of death following pelvic fracture [52]. In the prehospital exam, signs and symptoms of pelvic injury include deformity, bruising, or swelling over the bony prominences, pubis, perineum, and/or scrotum. Leg-length discrepancy or rotational deformity of a lower limb (without fracture in that extremity) may also appear. Wounds over the pelvis or bleeding from the patient's rectum, vagina, or urethra may indicate an open pelvic fracture. Neurological abnormalities may also rarely be present in the lower limbs after a pelvic fracture [53]. Screening radiographs of the pelvis are recommended when the mechanism of injury or the degree of hemodynamic instability indicates the possibility of a pelvic fracture. According to the mechanism and severity, pelvic fractures are classified into three main patterns of injuries: anteroposterior compression, lateral compression, and vertical shear [54].

Anterior posterior compression is secondary to a direct or indirect force in an AP direction leading to diastasis of the symphysis pubis with or without obvious diastasis of the sacroiliac joint or fracture of the iliac bone. AP compression injuries cause an increased pelvic volume with any resulting hemorrhage that is unlikely to spontaneously tamponade. Pelvic wrapping therefore should be a priority in early management [55]. The AP projection, recommended by the ATLS program performed during the primary survey provides a large amount of information about the mechanism of injury. In the anterior, the AP projection can identify the presence and extent of the diastasis of symphysis pubis and/or the fracture of the obturator ring. In the posterior, the AP projection recognizes the presence and extent of dislocation of the injured side of the pelvis, dislocations of the sacroiliac joint, or fractures of L5 transverse apophysis. However, this type of projection does not help to evaluate the real dimension of the injury, especially its posterior component [56].

Lateral compression is a lateral compression force that causes rotation of the pelvis inwards, leading to fractures in the sacroiliac region and pubic rami. The lateral fractures are the most common type of pelvic fractures that are mainly associated (88% of cases) to the sacral fractures [54]. In lateral fractures, there is a reduction of the pelvic volume with hemorrhage that is more likely to spontaneously tamponade.

Vertical shear is an axial shear force that disrupts the iliac or sacroiliac junction and is combined with cephalic displacement of the fracture component from the main pelvis. In vertical shear injuries, the hemipelvis is shifted cranially, and fractures are vertically and rotationally unstable. There is a high rate of associated injuries to the torso and spine and a high rate of hemodynamic instability [55].

Other projections that can add more information are the following: the oblique outlet view, performed with patient in supine position; caudal-cranial inclination of 30° of the incidental beam centering on the pubis is useful in quantifying the cranial dislocation of the injured hemipelvis; and the oblique inlet view, which is performed with patient in supine position, caudal-cranial inclination of 30° of the incidental beam centering on the umbilicus is useful in documenting the posterior sacroiliac joint dislocation or pubic branches dislocation on AP view or the inward/outward rotation of the pelvis [56].

Focused Assessment with Sonography for Trauma (FAST) and Extended to Thorax-FAST (E-FAST)

Ultrasound (US) is an important adjunct to the primary survey of polytraumatized patients and has replaced diagnostic peritoneal washing or sometimes laparotomy in the resuscitation room because it is noninvasive, repeatable, safe, nonirradiating, inexpensive, and quick to perform [57]. There are no absolute contraindications against its use except in cases where the patient may require immediate surgery. However, before transferring the patient to the operating room for emergency laparotomy, it may be necessary to exclude pericardial tamponade or pneumothorax.

In the trauma setting, the FAST and E-FAST examinations are usually performed in hypotensive and hemodynamically unstable patients because they help to determine whether immediate surgery is needed before the patient undergoes a CT evaluation [58] (Fig. 1.5).

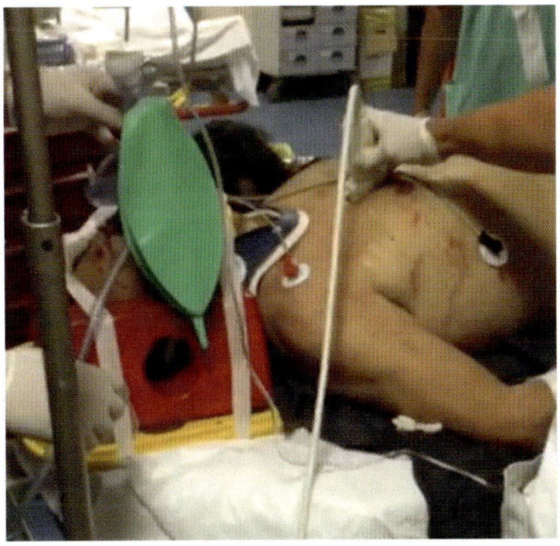

Fig. 1.5 The extended FAST examination (e-FAST) during the primary survey is essential for the exclusion of pneumothorax and pericardial tamponade in unstable patient

In patients with major trauma, the first-line abdominal US examination is generally performed with a FAST protocol (i.e., focused assessment with sonography for trauma), which aims to identify a free-fluid effusion within the peritoneal cavity or pericardial sac through the ultrasound exploration of four regions (subxiphoid region, right and left hypochondriac regions, pelvic cavity). The FAST scan is performed at bedside in the ER; it is usually performed with a portable machine using a lower frequency transducer, such as a 3.5–5 MHz convex array [59]. Although the effectiveness of the FAST scan to detect free intra-peritoneal fluid has been reported by many studies, the sensitivity of the FAST examination as a diagnostic test for therapeutic laparotomy accounts for only 75% (while confounded by multiple variables); similarly, its positive predictive value was only 37.3% [59]. In another review, a positive FAST exam was found to vary in the 24.2–56.3% range for penetrating trauma, while the diagnostic modality was highly specific (94.1–100.0%) but not very sensitive (28.1–100%) [60]. If the free abdominal effusion is considered as the only diagnostic finding, the rate of false negatives may further increase, since too-early scans might miss significant releases of intra-peritoneal fluid, requiring more time to accumulate [61]. Even if it is claimed that ultrasound can detect as little as 100 mL of free intra-peritoneal fluid, for a negative response it is necessary to observe the patient for at least 4–6 h and, if indicated, repeat the FAST scan or conduct a CT scan [62]. Some clinicians incorporate inferior vena cava (IVC) evaluation into the FAST examination to help determine the patient's volume status and fluid responsiveness [63].

Ultrasound may also be technically limited in the traumatized patient due to bowel gas, obesity, subcutaneous emphysema, or patient positioning. Other limitations to FAST assessments include its poor sensitivity in detecting the hemoretroperitoneum, parenchymal traumatic injuries, and almost bowel and mesenteric injuries detection; the latter two are both diagnosable with a CT scan.

Although FAST has a high specificity, false-positive results can be encountered in patients with a history of ascites or inflammatory processes in the abdomen or pelvis or even ovarian cyst rupture.

The Consensus Conference recommends that hemodynamically unstable patients with positive FAST examination should generally be followed by a laparotomy, while a search for extra-abdominal sources of hemorrhage should follow a negative exam [64].

In hemodynamically stable patients, a positive FAST result should be followed by a TC exam to better define the nature of the injuries. For negative FAST scan cases, a period of monitoring for at least 6 h, serial FAST scans, or further investigations (e.g., CT scan or peritoneal lavage) are recommended.

In many trauma centers, the use of the FAST technique is extended to the thorax (Extended-FAST) for the detection of hemothorax and pneumothorax, including the presence of hemopericardium (whose evaluation is already performed with a FAST scan) through the execution of some standard scanning with a convex and linear probe (transducer) [58]. Thoracic ultrasound (e-FAST) is defined as a rapid and accurate first-line bedside diagnostic modality for the diagnosis of pneumothorax in unstable patients with major chest trauma during the primary survey in the emergency room [58].

The diagnostic performance of ultrasound is high (i.e., 77% sensitivity, 99.8% specificity, 98.5% positive predictive value, 97% negative predictive value, and 97.2% accuracy). This sensitivity value is statistically significantly higher than that of supine chest radiograph (approximately 50%, as reported in the literature). According to anti-gravity laws, PNX air in the pleural space tends to accumulate in the least-dependent part of the chest [65, 66]. When the patient lies in the supine position, the area of interest corresponds to the anterior and inferior part of the chest on both sides of the thorax, which is approximately the third–fourth intercostal space between the parasternal and the mid-clavicle lines [67, 68]. The probe should be placed in the intercostal acoustic window of the located area.

The parietal pleura appears as a thin echogenic horizontal line located between and below two adjacent ribs. Sometimes, it is necessary to scan more intercostal spaces by moving the probe laterally and inferiorly in order to evaluate the extension of PNX or to confirm the diagnosis. Sonographic signs that can help in the diagnosis of a pneumothorax are the absence of lung sliding (the visualization of lung sliding has a 100% negative predictive value), lung pulse, loss of B lines, and identification of the lung point (100% specificity) [69].

Patients in physiologic extremis and suspected of having PTXs on physical examination should undergo immediate tube or needle thoracostomy without awaiting imaging studies [70] (Fig. 1.6). The limitations in the evaluation for pneumothorax include main-stem bronchus intubation, severe chronic obstructive pulmonary disease, or other lung pathology that inhibit adequate visualization of lung sliding, and small apical or localized pneumothoraces may not be visualized [63].

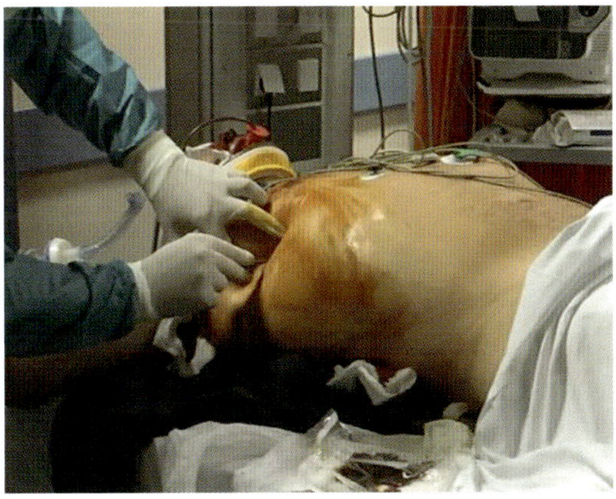

Fig. 1.6 The use of the e-Fast protocol allows to place as promptly as possible a pleural drainage in a patient with pneumothorax and subcutaneous emphysema

Contrast-Enhanced Ultrasound (CEUS)

Ultrasonography has in recent years found new application areas through the use of contrast enhancement based on microbubbles [48]. This method has many advantages mainly due to the fact that avoiding ionizing radiation represents a safe tool—particularly in selected series, including pediatric patients and females of reproductive age [71].

Its application for children is still considered off-label, and it is allowed only after the parents (or legal guardians) have been adequately informed and given their specific consent. CEUS also exhibits an advantage compared to contrast-enhanced MRI and CT because it can be used in patients with renal failure or allergy [72]. The CEUS technique can be carried out in a variety of scenarios, including bedside, operating room, and trauma suite [71]. Also, compared to other techniques, it is not expensive. There is still debate for how to integrate CEUS in the trauma patient workup [73, 74].

Although it is considered to be more sensitive and accurate than baseline US and almost as sensitive as CT in the identification and characterization of solid-organ lesions in blunt abdominal trauma, the CEUS use in the primary survey is limited by several factors such as the lack of panoramic view, typical of CT, and, like conventional US imaging, insensitivity in depicting diaphragmatic rupture, bowel, or mesenteric traumatic injuries [75]. Moreover, CEUS is strongly operator dependent, requiring dedicated contrast agent-specific software, and it takes a long time to be performed [76]. An excellent correlation was found between the size of the traumatic injury (as shown at CT) and the related CEUS findings with respect to hepatic traumatic injuries, advocating its employment as a first-line examination in mild blunt abdominal trauma and in pediatric patients and leaving CT as the gold standard for polytrauma and major trauma [74].

Nowadays, contrast-enhanced ultrasound (CEUS) has an important role in the follow-up of conservatively treated traumatic injuries of the abdominal parenchymal organs (liver, spleen, and kidneys) or as a first-line examination in low-energy or mild isolated abdominal trauma [76, 77]. It can integrate conventional US imaging in the triage of hemodynamically stable patients, in particular with low-energy abdominal trauma; also, it can be routinely used as a completion of a US FAST examination to scan severe trauma patients in the assessment of solid-organ injuries [78]. This happens especially when the use of CT exposes patients to excessive radiation dose. In some departments, protocols for the follow-up of blunt abdominal trauma that are conservatively treated include a CEUS at 24 and 72 h after trauma as well as CEUS and MRI after 1 month [79].

CEUS cannot replace abdominal CT, but it represents a noninvasive and repeatable imaging tool that is capable of providing a reliable assessment of trauma severity and expediting the patient's treatment [71].

1.3.1.3 Secondary Survey

Once any life-threatening problems have been identified using diagnostic procedures during the primary survey, hemodynamic stability is re-established through a series of therapeutic maneuvers (plasma expanders, fluid recovery, drainages). The effectiveness of vital organs are then maintained, and the secondary survey identifies other injuries with the definitive treatment.

To this end, in accordance with the ATLS protocol, a comprehensive head-to-toe physical assessment is carried out to detect other significant but not immediately life-threatening injuries that were not detected or managed during the initial assessment and resuscitation.

A brief medical history of the patient is obtained according to the procedure summarized in the acronym SAMPLE (S—Signs/symptoms, A—Allergies, M—Medications, P—Pertinent past medical history, L—Last oral intake, E—Events leading to disease or injury) and a reassessment of all vital signs (pulse, respirations, skin signs, pupils, and blood pressure). Heart tones and peripheral pulses are also checked. If any clinical deterioration is detected during monitoring of the vital signs, the primary survey must be repeated immediately and measures must be taken to rectify the problem.

The head-to-toe examination takes no more than 2–3 min and identifies and urgently treats lacerations, bruising, swellings, bleedings, discolorations, bone protrusions, tamponading bleeding, and splinting fractures.

At this stage, the role of trauma radiology, essentially based on the use of CT, is important to depict life-threatening diagnoses, properly determine the stage, help the medical team to suggest treatment options, debate prognosis, and take the prognostic scores that can dictate a surgical or conservative treatment. Finally, CT scanning remains the gold standard in terms of radiological assessment for diagnosing abdominal injuries during the secondary survey for both hemodynamically stable patients and patients stabilized after primary resuscitation.

Radiology in the Secondary Survey

Whole-Body Computed Tomography (WBCT) in Trauma

Current scanners are capable of rendering submillimeter resolution images of the entire body in a matter of seconds [80]. Among the long list of advantages derived from MSCT technology for obtaining useful imaging information, we enucleate three: (a) shorter scan time, (b) extended scan range, and (c) improved longitudinal resolution, particularly when 3D post-processing is part of the clinical protocol. The ability to acquire volume data also paved the way for the development of three-dimensional (3D) image processing techniques, such as multiplanar reformation (MPR), maximum intensity projection, surface-shaded display, and volume-rendering techniques, which have become a vital component of medical imaging today. CT has become an especially vital component of patient evaluation in the ED and is helped by the increased diffuse use of picture archiving and communication systems (PACSs), teleradiology, and voice recognition software, which facilitate all the rapid image dissemination and interpretation [80–83]. CT is well suited for the ED: it provides rapid, minimally invasive, high-resolution imaging that can quickly direct patients toward further treatment. Factors that might limit the growth of CT use include cost-containment efforts [84], intervention to improve evidence-based guideline adherence [85], and concerns regarding radiation exposure [86].

WBCT is a sensitive and comprehensive tool for the diagnosis of a wide range of traumatic injuries, especially in the severely injured patient [87–91].

Contrary to selectively performing CT scans on one or more body regions, a WBCT scan comprises a CT of the head without intravenous contrast, cervical spine (acquired before, or following, intravenous contrast), and chest, abdomen, and pelvis following intravenous contrast. In the largest systematic review and meta-analysis that determined the odds of mortality in trauma patients, patients who underwent a WBCT scan were less likely to have a fatal outcome compared to those who received selective CT.

Indications for WBCT in Trauma

What Is Major Trauma?

A crucial step for major trauma care is the accurate identification of trauma patients—both for rapid transport to Major Trauma Centers and for triaging patients for WBCT.

A threshold criterion ISS >15 is routinely assumed to describe the severity of trauma, calculate the probability of survival, and evaluate trauma care of patients [92] in order to appropriately match the CT trauma protocol to major trauma victims [93–96]. For the ISS calculation, a physician who is experienced in trauma care management and radiological diagnostics determines the abbreviated injury scale (AIS), which is an anatomical scoring system. The body is divided into six regions: head, face, chest, abdomen, extremities, and external. The ISS score is the sum of the squares of the highest AIS grade in each of the three most severely injured body regions. Injuries are ranked on a scale of 1–6, where 1 is minor, and 6 represents a fatal injury. The three most injured body regions have their AIS squared and added together to produce the ISS score.

The ISS score takes values from 0 to 75. If an injury is assigned an AIS score of 6 (unsurvivable injury), the ISS score is automatically assigned to 75 [92]. An analysis of >1 million US trauma patients (between 2002 and 2006) showed that anatomic and physiological parameters only have a sensitivity of 56% for detecting patients with an ISS score >15; this highlights the importance of using a combination of criteria-physiological, anatomical, and mechanism of injury to identify severely injured patients with occult or compensated injuries [97]. The mechanism of injury information, which is ascertained during the prehospital survey, is routinely provided during patient handover to ED staff. However, the mechanism alone has a low sensitivity as an indicator of serious injury, resulting in an over-triage rate of up to 75% [98].

A prospective observational study of hemodynamically stable trauma patients with unremarkable examination and physiological parameters who underwent WBCT screening based on mechanism of injury alone (including automobile vs. pedestrian injury with the pedestrian thrown more than 10 ft) discovered that 19% of patients had their management changed on the basis of the CT findings, resulting in eight laparotomies in patients with normal findings on abdominal examinations [88]. Most of the unexpected findings were thoracic, but they were also intracranial, cervical spine, and abdominal, which suggests the need of WBCT. There is no consensus and no validated clinical prediction rule that defines clear-cut criteria for WBCT following trauma or indicates patients in whom WBCT can be safely omitted. Broadly, criteria for performing a WBCT include the mechanism of injury, injury location or pattern, initial vital signs (before resuscitation), or a combination of these [99].

According to the standardized trauma concept, all patients have initial resuscitation and then are subjected to a scoring system (triage rule) to decide further diagnostics. If only one parameter in one of the three categories is positive, serious injuries in one or more organ systems are suspected, and the CT trauma protocol will be initiated [92].

During the initial resuscitation of blunt trauma patients, time and accuracy of diagnoses are essential for planning further therapy. According to the ATLS handbook, "CT is a time consuming procedure that should be used only in patients with no hemodynamic abnormalities" [39]. The handbook states that conventional diagnosis is performed first, e.g., chest radiography (CXR) and focused abdominal sonography in trauma (FAST), followed by selective use of computed tomography (CT) of specific body regions, if indicated.

Patients who are ABC unstable first undergo immediate CXR and FAST.

After stabilization, they undergo a total-body CT if possible or go to the operating room (Fig. 1.7). CT is increasingly used in the trauma bay: a standard ATLS plain radiograph trauma series (lateral c-spine, supine chest radiograph, and pelvis) contributes with only 2 mSv to the trauma patient's radiation dose burden versus 10–20 mSv for a WBCT [100, 101].

CT is highly sensitive in detecting several injuries, since up to 76% of pneumothoraces and other significant chest complications detected on CT are occult on supine plain chest radiography; this questions its value if CT is immediately available for use in the ED [102, 103]. In a prospective study over a 7-year period, a direct comparison was made between polytrauma patients utilizing ATLS guidelines and standard trauma radiographs (AP chest, lateral C-spine, and AP pelvis) versus patients utilizing a whole-body helical MDCT protocol (CT brain, C-spine, thorax, abdomen, and pelvis). The study concluded that CT allows

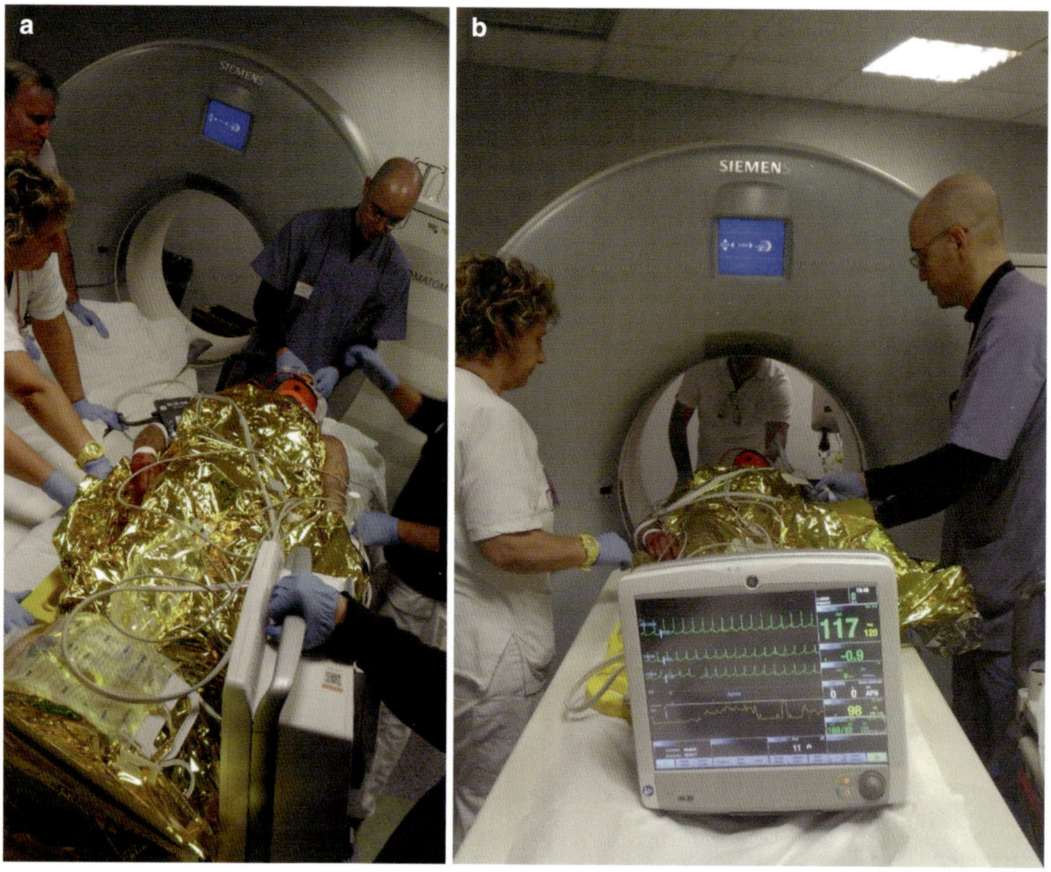

Fig. 1.7 (**a**, **b**) A whole-body CT should be taken during the secondary survey, only after stabilization of the patient's condition with continuous monitoring of the vital signs and cardiac status

the detection of a significant number of injuries not found by clinical assessment and plain radiography (19 missed cervical spine fractures and 36 pneumothoraces missed on radiography but identified via CT) [87].

Other authors reported that thoracic CT is highly sensitive in detecting thoracic injuries after blunt chest trauma and is superior to routine chest X-ray in visualizing lung contusions, pneumothorax, and hemothorax [102]. Furthermore, MDCT has a far superior sensitivity (99%) in detecting cervical fractures compared to cervical spine plain film (52%) [104], especially for the evaluation of the traumatized spine in delineating extension of fracture fragments into the spine canal [105].

MDCT plays an important role for the cervical spine, especially in intubated patients, where the craniocervical junction and the lower cervical spine is often difficult to evaluate [106, 107].

Finally, MSCT could replace plain radiography in the primary modality for the diagnosis of thoracolumbar spine fractures in severe trauma patients [108, 109].

Arm Positioning and Imaging Quality

The multipass CT acquisition technique involves separate CT phases of different body regions. Typically, this approach involves a non-contrast CT of the head and cervical spine during which the arms are long on the hips; then, a single helical acquisition is performed or as separate arterial and venous phases following intravenous contrast of the chest, abdomen, and pelvis with the arms positioned behind the head. The shift of the upper limbs with the consequent repositioning of intravenous lines and ventilation tubing results in lengthening the total examination time from 4 to 8 min [110].

In the single-pass technique, there is a single acquisition of a non-contrast CT scan of the head followed by a single helical acquisition of the neck, chest, abdomen, and pelvis without repositioning the upper extremities after contrast injection. Various studies have been carried out to evaluate the effect of limb positioning on radiation dose and image quality.

Nowadays, modern CT scanners use automated exposure control that modulates the tube current based on photon attenuation derived from the topograms or during the helical acquisition [111]. The presence of the limbs in the scan field results in an upmodulation of the current in the tube with a greater radiation emission. When the arms were placed behind the head, the highest image quality of the thoraco-abdominal district was associated with the lowest radiation dose with respect to the positioning the arms along the hips [112].

A novel technique in which subjects crossed their upper extremities and rested them on a pillow placed across their chest has been suggested [113]. A comparison of the arms-up and arms-down positions confirmed that the arms-up position was associated with the lowest radiation dose (approximately 25% lower) and highest image quality and that the arms-down position significantly improved when the arms were placed across the chest compared with the standard arms-down position. As this technique avoids the need of repositioning the arms and life-support tubing between passes, the approach is currently used for trauma patients.

Contrast Injection Protocols

At trauma centers, protocols (whose choice depends on the equipment available), staff experience, and guidelines traditionally suggest the use of a non-contrast CT followed by a contrast-enhanced CT. In other centers, a direct scan of the head, which is crucial to detecting bleeding, eliminates chest and pelvic irradiation because the unenhanced CT scan is not very sensitive in diagnosing organ lesions.

However, the preliminary acquisition of a non-enhanced phase is recommended as a routine procedure in order to detect detached bone fragments, especially as a result of fractures of chest or pubic bones. The lack of a direct CT imaging makes it difficult for observers to distinguish an intense bone calcification from an arterial active extravasation of the intravenous contrast medium, requiring multiple scans to obtain diagnostic certainty.

1.4 Contrast Administration

Nonionic contrast agents with a high iodine concentration (320–400 mg I/mL) are the most common contrast media used for computed tomography scanning. The dose of the contrast medium (CM) is administered according to the patient's body weight [(mL/kg body weight: 80–100 mL (<60 Kg); 100–120 mL (<80 Kg); 120–140 mL (>80 Kg)] by intravenous injection in the antecubital vein at a flow rate (typically 4 mL/s) using a dual-head power injector, immediately followed by a saline flush (40–50 mL) with a rate of injection of 4 mL/s. Higher CM flow rates increased arterial enhancement. According to the different individual cardiac output or local vascular pathology (stenosis, aneurysm), CT angiography is done using a bolus-tracking technique with an automatic triggering threshold of 100 HU ROI (region of interest) in the descending thoracic aorta [114].

Contrast injection causes CIN (contrast-induced nephropathy) in 11% of cases and severe CIN in 1% [115]. Trauma patients may have an increased risk of nephrotoxicity due to the compromised hemodynamic status (hypotension and bleeding) and time-consuming measurement of kidney function, which may delay life-saving maneuvers. In light of these considerations, we believe that the administration of contrast media, although risky, provides benefits in terms of survival over the likelihood of a possible nephropathy. Therefore, it is good practice to perform adequate hydration of the patient after undergoing a CT scan.

1.4.1 Precontrast Phase

A cranial CT scan acquisition starts from the vertex to the base of skull including the cervical vertebrae without intravenous contrast medium [116]. The initial images should be analyzed at the CT console parallel to the positioning of the arms along the body. A slice thickness of 3–4 mm is used for the parenchyma evaluation and 1–2 mm for the assessment of the bony structures. Sagittal and coronal multiplanar reconstructions (MPRs) are obtained using the bone window using a distance of 2 mm and thickness of 2 mm. In all cases, the lateral scanogram should be enlarged as many fractures can be identified, particularly their possible crossing of the medial meningeal artery or of a venous sinus. An unenhanced CT scan has a crucial role in the hyperacute phase of traumatic brain injury as it provides to demonstrate intra- and extra-axial hematomas and parenchymal injury [117].

Chest abdomen, pelvis, and spinal column CT acquisition starts at the middle of the seventh cervical spinal column and ends at the proximal femur. The arms are positioned over the head. Lung parenchyma, soft tissue, and bone window images are reconstructed using a 5-mm slice thickness. A precontrast phase CT of the thorax, abdomen, and pelvis is indicated to detect pneumothorax, hemothorax, and hemoperitoneum and to differentiate them from a fluid-corpuscular collection of other density (bile, intestinal content). It is also used for the identification of the sentinel clot sign and for the identification of small bone fragments, especially in the thoracic cage and pelvic bones.

1.4.2 Contrast Phase

Many studies have reported an increased use of post-contrast CT since it is considered to be more sensitive than angiography in the detection of active bleeding; its sensitivity ranges from 87 to 95%, and its negative predictive values range from 93 to 98% [118–121]. There are several contrast-enhanced CT protocols, which differ in the number of phases, bolus times, and injection times.

An arterial phase of the thorax is preferred for the detection and characterization of blunt thoracic great vessel injury; the lowest radiation and contrast dose is preferred [122] to search for pseudo-aneurysms, arteriovenous fistula, and active arterial bleeding in the spleen [123, 124]. For pseudo-aneurysms, the routine use of arterial phase CT becomes necessary due to the fact that the venous phase is neither sensitive nor specific if directly acquired to detect pseudo-aneurysms that may have become isointense to surrounding splenic parenchyma on delayed phase images.

1.4.3 Arterial Phase

Using the bolus tracking with a 100 HU ROI at the level of descending thoracic aorta, a caudal-cranial scan direction acquisition from the pubic symphysis to the jugular fossa is preferred. With a minimum scan delay of 7 s, the injection of contrast medium is already complete when the thoracic inlet is reached. This reduces artifacts from in-flowing contrast medium, and the aorta and the supra-aortic vessels are maximally enhanced. If possible, the scans should be obtained while the patients hold their breath or, if tolerable, when the ventilator is kept in inspiration in order to reduce motion artifacts. Images are reconstructed using soft tissue, bone, and lung windows.

A slice thickness of 1 mm is recommended for CT angiography. CT angiography has been shown to be an accurate diagnostic tool in assessing traumatic aortic injury [125]. Its use is recommended to study epiaortic vessels, thoraco-abdominal aorta, and parenchymal vessels in order to detect non-contained and contained vascular injuries (e.g., post-traumatic dissections, spasm, hematomas, devascularization of organs, or parts of organs) and differentiate vascular lesions (e.g., pseudo-aneurysms, arteriovenous fistula) from actively bleeding lesions and defining the presence and the extent of bleeding in relation to progressive increase of the area of extravasation [126].

1.4.4 Venus or Portal Phase

Thirty-five seconds after the beginning of the arterial phase (about 70 s after the beginning of the injection), the CT acquisition in the portal phase starts with a cranial-caudal scan direction acquisition from the diaphragm to the pubic symphysis; this is performed carefully to include both the proximal part of the femurs. All images are observed in the soft tissue, bone, and also lung parenchyma windows using a 5-mm slice thickness; the latter provides sensitive proof of free intra-abdominal air [117]. Also, sagittal and coronal MPRs are obtained using the bone and soft tissue windows.

The venous phase is required to evaluate extension and characteristics of solid-organ lesions, ranging from small contusion to a parenchymal hematoma or lacerations. It is also important to evaluate any venous supply of hematoma or to better demonstrate the distribution of a contrast material leakage from the blood vessels that have already been detected in the arterial phase; it is possible to extend the study to the chest if there are significant alterations in the enhanced scan or in the arterial phase (e.g., thoracic wall hematoma or parenchymal lacerations).

1.4.5 Delayed or Excretory Phase

A delayed phase is often required to differentiate active bleeding from an iodinated urine extravasation and to detect the exact topographical location of extravasation iodinated urine from intrarenal urinary tracts, the ureters, and the bladder. Depending on the lesions found in the previous analysis, the CT acquisition starts with a cranial-caudal scan direction from the diaphragm to the pubic symphysis in the delay range 3 to 8–10 min from the beginning of the portal phase. Images are reconstructed using soft tissue with a slice thickness of 5 mm.

These delayed images are helpful in several different scenarios. In acute injury to kidneys or ureters, delayed imaging often helps to identify or further characterize injury to the collecting system or ureters. Secondly, in soft tissue organ injuries, we use delayed imaging for definitive characterization of hyper-attenuating foci (contrast blush) seen on early acquisitions. This includes differentiating active arterial extravasation of contrast from vascular injury such as pseudoaneurysm or arteriovenous fistula. This differentiation may also be useful in mesenteric, muscular, or other areas of potential arterial injury. An additional benefit in patients with acute hemorrhage is the added information of an image at a second moment in time. Given the delay of 5 min, subjective determination of any increase in the area of hemorrhage may be a potential indication of the rate of bleeding [127].

Bladder injuries usually occur in patients with severe blunt trauma found to have sustained pelvic fractures. CT cystography, in which the bladder is filled in a retrograde flush with 350 mL of dilute (3–5%) contrast via a bladder catheter, is a powerful diagnostic adjunct tool, especially in equivocal cases.

The distinction between intra- and extraperitoneal bladder rupture is crucially important, since intra-peritoneal ruptures require surgical repair, while the latter are usually treated with conservative catheter drainage [128].

1.5 Postprocessing

Given the current trend of performing immediate TBCT scans for detecting injuries from the head to the pelvis, a number of images not less than 1000 are obtained which increase to about 4000 for the angiographic acquisition of the extremities. There are several reconstruction techniques that use these axial images to visualize volume forms. These techniques include multiplanar visualization, maximum intensity projection, and 3D volume rendering [127].

1.5.1 Multiplanar Reformations

The multiplanar reconstruction (MPR) method provides 2D sectional images in all axial, coronal, and sagittal planes perpendicular to the original axial plane; this method is particularly useful in the study of tortuous structures such as vessels [129, 130]. Thanks to the fact that these sections overlap, spiral/helical CT has greatly improved the quality of the MPRs by eliminating the stair-step artifacts, which often occur with the conventional slice-by-slice CT.

Multislice CT has further improved the quality of MPRs as it allows isotropic imaging in which the image quality of the reconstructed MPR is equivalent to that of the original axial image. In the polytrauma patient, subtle fractures, especially those involving the pelvic region and oriented in the axial plane, are better seen on MPR images or 3D volume-rendered images. Complex injuries can be better demonstrated with 3D volume-rendered images, and complicated spatial information about the relative positions of fracture fragments can be easily demonstrated to the orthopedic surgeons. Including these techniques of reconstruction in routine pelvic imaging protocols can change management in a significant number of cases. Such visualization techniques provide more intuitive information that optimizes, on one hand, the high amount of acquired images and, on the other hand, the coronal and sagittal reconstruction, which is condensed on fewer images and which permit a faster and more easily comprehensible communication with clinical colleagues.

1.5.1.1 Three-Dimensional Reformation

The introduction of multidetector computed tomography (MDCT) brought tremendous advantages by providing a thinner slice thickness in a reduced amount of time as well as isotropic voxel data, which contribute to the unprecedented quality of 3D reformats. Specialized 3D reconstruction techniques allow the visualization of anatomical details that would otherwise not be visible using axial reconstructions alone and provide visualization of the vessel flow [126] and complex bone fractures, which require specific techniques such as maximum intensity projection (MIP), minimum intensity projection (MinIP), surface-shaded volume rendering (SS-VRT), and virtual endoscopy [131].

MIP reconstruction emphasizes the voxels with maximum intensity and is mainly used to show contrasted vessels in CT angiography (CTA) and MR angiography (MRA), but it is also used in PET examination to provide clear views of lesions [132]. SS-VRT typically exploits real-time user manipulation of view perspectives and virtual light sources to zoom in and highlight minute anatomical details, which is particularly useful in bone fractures. It is also particularly helpful in documenting more extensive lesions, such as multiple rib fractures or complex fractures with multiple dislocated fragments as may be seen in maxillofacial trauma or even distal limb fractures [133]. 3D reconstruction techniques for examining volumetric data works well and also improves the speed of interpretation, recognition, and description of life-threatening injuries through the use of a software package that is directly incorporated into the PACS workstations [131].

CT scan imaging of traumatic injuries that affect multiple organs and structures are extensively dealt with in the following chapters.

1.5.1.2 Secondary Survey: Upper and Lower Limbs X-Rays: Limbs

The most common mechanisms that produce major trauma of the extremities are open fractures, crush injuries, and major soft tissue injuries, which often mask more serious internal injuries and are mainly due to road traffic accidents, falls, assaults, and sports injuries with lower limbs. Limb traumas may exhibit varying degrees of involvement and severity that vary from simple neurovascularly intact fractures to cramped extremity or traumatic amputation. A severe crush injury can result in a serious limb-threatening injury that includes complex open fractures and/or dislocations, vascular lesions, mangled extremity, traumatic amputation, compartment syndrome, or neurological lesions. Depending on the injury pattern, there may be several life-threatening injuries. Penetrating trauma with the lesion involvement of the brachial, femoral, or popliteal arteries can induce massive bleeding.

The traumatic involvement of both the axillary and proximal femoral arteries, which are vessels that are not directly compressible because they are positioned under the clavicle and the inguinal canal, respectively, is considered as trauma to the torso and require immediate surgical intervention. Open fractures, associated with the concomitant disruption of overlying tissue and skin involve a high risk of infection and consequently a greater chance of limb loss [134]. A crush injury, defined as a direct injury that results from a crush, can afford crush syndrome, which expresses as muscle cell damage resulting from pressure or crushing [135]. A crush injury or crush syndrome may occur as a result of natural disasters or any other situation resulting in the compression between two hard surfaces, or they can occur due to severe brief pressure, such as when a limb is run over by a heavy vehicle and the limb is then freed and reperfused. These conditions result in impaired blood flow to the extremity, resulting in ischemia and potential necrosis of tissue distal to the injury collapse.

A compartment syndrome should be suspected when there is a long bone fracture, because any subsequent hemorrhage and/or hematoma causes a pressure increase within the compartment formed by muscles, vessels, and nerves covered by an inelastic fascia, and, if prolonged, determines ischemia and necrosis. All of these injury patterns can be associated with nerve lesions, so that it becomes important to proceed with a complete neurologic examination for pulses, peripheral warmth, paresthesia, and paralysis. In any case, a general examination of the limbs should carefully inspect for deformity, presence of an open wound, degree of soft tissue involvement, contamination, active bleeding, and wounds, especially if in proximity to an artery, as well as palpation for the crepitus, pulsatile hematoma, palpable thrill, and swelling. Radiological examinations are performed if one or more fractures, presence of foreign bodies, skeletal deficits, and/or subcutaneous emphysema is suspected.

Most emergency radiology departments perform orthogonal views in frontal (i.e., anteroposterior or posteroanterior) and lateral projections for the long bones. Since one projection is most commonly performed to detect a fracture/dislocation, it is essential to take at least two images including the joints above or below the fracture site to adequately inspect the degree of deformity. Fractures to the shoulder, scapula, clavicle (especially the middle third), and proximal humerus are often the consequence of a direct blow to the area from a fall, collision, or motor vehicle accident and may especially impact elderly patients.

The standard radiographic examination of the shoulder should provide, in addition to the standard AP projection (anterior–posterior), one or more apical oblique projections (APEX) that are helpful in the convenient setting of acute traumas and in fracture and dislocation visualization [136, 137].

A traumatic forearm and elbow injury is another common site of the upper-extremity musculoskeletal injuries, especially in children [138]. The minimal radiographic series includes anteroposterior (AP) and lateral images, while an oblique radial head-capitellum view can help detect subtle fractures by removing osseous overlap of the radial head and coronoid [139].

Among the fractures of the forearm and the wrist, the distal radial growth plate is a common site of injury among adolescents, while a fracture of the distal radius with a dorsal displacement of the distal fragment (Colles fracture) is very common in the elderly. An anteroposterior and a lateral projection should be performed to detect fractures and fragment displacement.

Pelvic fractures that have already been treated in the primary survey section are frequently associated with femur fractures. Femoral shaft fractures occur at any age, and their pattern can be transverse, oblique, spiral, streaked, or greenstick and equally in the upper, middle, and lower third of the shaft. Proximal and distal femur fractures, however, occur more in high-speed traumas in young, while low-energy trauma occur in the elderly because of osteoporosis. Given that hip and tibial shafts and ligamentous disruptions of the knee are frequently associated with fractures of the patella, a radiograph should include the hip and knee joints [140]. The radiographic series includes anteroposterior (AP) and lateral images. One of the most feared complications of the femoral head fracture with nutrient and capsular vessel lesion is avascular necrosis, which is associated in many cases with both displaced and nondisplaced fractures. If the X-rays are negative but there is clinical suspicion, a CT should be performed with its excellent spatial resolution and multiplanar capability, because this is useful for demonstrating fractures; alternatively, an MRI should be considered [141].

The numerous different fractures and fracture dislocations of the ankle are diagnosed via X-ray on anteroposterior and lateral projections centered over the joint. This concerns the particular cases of spiral fractures of the distal fibula and fractures of the posterior lip of the distal tibia that is often best seen on the lateral view [142]. In addition to fractures, any subluxation or dislocation can be deduced from the apparent diastasis of the distal tibiofibular joint and displacement of the talus.

1.5.2 Open Issues Associated with the CT Use in Polytrauma Patients

1.5.2.1 WBCT Radiation Dose

One of the major concerns against the use of WBCT as a diagnostic test is the exposure to unnecessary radiation risk. However, the evidence does not support this concern in the case of polytrauma patients who require a balanced judgment regarding the risk/benefit balance to undergo a CT scan. The dose of exposure for a single WBCT changes in the 14–22.7 mSv range according to the scanning protocol, the scanner type, and the patient size and positioning. Usually, when a responsive patient is informed that they need a CT scan, the natural compliance to undergoing CT imaging did not significantly change, the natural unwillingness significantly changed undergoing CT imaging, although the patient becomes more willing to consider other imaging options if equally effective [143].

Although 1.5–2% of cancers may eventually be caused by the ionizing radiation used in CT [144], we believe that the potential risks of exposure to ionizing radiation during the radiological examination supported by a clinical suspect justify the potential clinical benefits. From this perspective, all members of the radiology team cooperate to ensure safety and protection through an effective communication in order to keep the radiation dose as low as possible. Reducing or preferably eliminating unnecessary or inappropriate procedures is the most effective means to decrease radiation associated with imaging. There are several ways to reduce the CT radiation dose. As discussed in the previous paragraphs, the arm positions impact organ doses during CT scans: a patient having raised arms received smaller doses to organs located within the chest, abdomen, or pelvis when compared with the patient having lower arms. Considering the use of tube current modulation (TCM), the patient with lowered arms may receive 50% higher radiation dose to most of the organs because of the increased tube current. Modern machines have internal modulators that regulate the radiation emission according to the patient-specific characteristics. The use of dual source CT (DSCT) may further decrease the administered dose due to the different delivery of the voltage tube to different body regions; this helps to capture the images faster, and the 3D images can be rebuilt. Future efforts should seek techniques to reduce CT dosage without compromising the diagnostic information of the radiological technique.

1.5.2.2 Early WBCT in Trauma

Although level 1 evidence of survival benefit for early WBCT is lacking, several retrospective studies have shown an association between total-body CT scanning and survival in patients with trauma [145–150]. A decrease in the absolute mortality and an increase in the probability of survival in patients with polytrauma (ISS $\geq$ 16) who had received a total-body CT scan compared with a non-total-body CT scan has been reported [151, 152]. In contrast, REACT-2, a multicenter randomized controlled trial, concluded that no difference was found between the mortality of the two groups [153]. However, total-body CT did shorten the median time to finish the diagnostic workup as well as the median time to diagnosis, abbreviating the time between a patient's arrival to the ED and the initiation of life-saving procedures.

In an analysis of registry data, with the use of TBCT, the average time from trauma room admission to CT was significantly lower with respect to non-TBCT given [151]. The same research group also found significant differences in time from the admission in the ED to the operating room. Time to reach a definitive diagnosis was also shorter for the TBCT scan than the conventional protocol utilizing CR, FAST, and radiographic imaging supplemented with selective CT [154–156].

After the results of REACT-2, it is still unclear whether conventional radiographs may be used in the safe treatment of polytrauma patients or should be supplanted by TBCT as the sole means of investigation. TBCT scanning is increasingly used in trauma assessment. Many centers use TBCT as their only radiological tool, while many others use it in addition to conventional radiographs. In our opinion, a regional trauma center must be equipped with all of the equipment needed to carry out the investigation. Many trauma centers that have a WB-MSCT scanner available in the resuscitation room should undergo a severely injured patient who is presumed to have multiple organ damage. In order to obtain a complete picture of the patient and to issue a rapid, accurate, and complete diagnosis, the initial use of WBCT should be mandatory. Instead of the arrival of a patient with penetrating injury such as a stab or gunshot wound that requires immediate surgical intervention, the initial X-ray diagnosis of the chest and pelvis along with a simultaneous FAST should be simultaneously performed with life-saving procedures, such as chest-tube insertion, thoracotomy, and cardiopulmonary resuscitation. Therefore, the ability to perform X-ray imaging is essential in the resuscitation room, even in the presence of a CT scanner. Here, after stabilization, a definite diagnosis can be conducted by WB-MSCT [157].

1.5.2.3 Innovation

Starting from a patient's arrival to the ED to operative and intensive care, the major time constraints are the transfer to the CT scanner (45%), time for scanning (35%), and data acquisition, manipulation, and interpretation (20%) [158]. These factors can preclude the use of CT scanning for hemodynamically unstable patients. This group of severely injured patients might potentially benefit the most from early CT scanning during the "golden hour." Advantages of WBCT are earlier diagnosis and targeted, priority orientated treatment planning. Also, the integration of multiple imaging modalities into a single system in one room minimizes patient transfers and can save almost 15 min [159]. Minimizing the transfer time of admitted patients from the emergency room to the CT suite can optimize workflow, especially in situations of true mass casualty incidents. Conventionally, an average of 15 min is required for basic radiological diagnosis (sonography, cervical spine, thorax, and pelvis), even in tightly structured programs. Next, the time needed for diagnosis and patient relocation for CT causes unnecessary delays as well as additional risks associated with transferring traumatized patients. Therefore, CTs have been positioned close to the ED to save as much time as possible. Ideally, conventional radiology equipment along with angiography and MR suites should also be located close to the ED [48, 83]. An optimal solution is to install the CT suite next to the resuscitation bay. This also offers a "parking option" if the scanner is already in use.

The term "focused assessment with computed tomography in trauma" (FACTT) was introduced for whole-body computed tomography during the primary trauma survey [160]. The term emphasizes to first focus on the search for life-threatening injuries, then on the need for damage control surgery, and third on other injuries and surgery. A prerequisite for applying FACTT is an accessible MSCT scanner that is either situated in or close to the trauma room. Trauma workflow first provides the management of respiratory problems (Airway, Breathing) to detect causes of bleeding (Circulation) or intracranial pathologies (Disability).

After controlling respiratory problems and obvious external bleedings, WBCT is performed in order to detect relevant internal bleeding in the chest, abdomen/pelvis, or intracranial pathology. The first images on the CT console enable the trauma team to "look into the patient" and search for life-threatening problems and injuries that require emergency procedures and operations, such as chest-tube insertion, thoracotomy, laparotomy, pelvic C-clamp, or CT-guided aortic balloon occlusion [160]. After life-threatening conditions are managed or excluded, a secondary survey supported by multiplanar reconstruction (MPR) is carried out. The observed mortality rate was significantly lower than the expected mortality rate [157], and WBCT examinations are increasingly used. In Germany, WBCT is used almost as much as CT. Nowadays, CT, in most hospitals, is very close to the ED and is located in the trauma bay or less than 1 min away [161]. A retrospective multicenter cohort study showed that the closer the CT is located to the trauma room, the better the probability of survival of severely injured patients [162]. For distances greater than 50 m, distances had a significant negative effect on the outcome. If new emergency departments are planned or rebuilt, the CT scanner should be placed preferably in the trauma room for logistic reasons.

A further improvement was introduced for the shock room resuscitation. A moveable, multislice computed tomography (MSCT) scanner was placed in this room that is able to scan patients during the initial trauma resuscitation phase without patient transfers. By this means, a complete diagnostic trauma workup was made possible within the shock room [163]. Moreover, resuscitation can be simultaneously performed while obtaining critical imaging information with the CT scanner. The new trauma workflow concept, as proposed by Ping et al. (2008), combines a moveable multislice CT scanner, a conventional X-ray installation, and a multifunctional extended carbon-fiber radiolucent patient table with a sliding carbon-fiber patient treatment board. The multislice CT scanner is placed on rails to enable the CT scanner to move between two-mirrored traumas rooms separated by radiation-shielded sliding doors. With this construction, the patient can be initially evaluated on one end of the tabletop (e.g., ATLS procedures, conventional X-ray imaging), and, subsequently, the patient treatment board can be transferred over the tabletop toward the CT gantry side. Then, the latter slides over the patient using its rails. The construction of both scanning rooms has the option of scanning the patient with the feet entering the gantry first, thereby reducing the need to reposition IV lines and monitors before scanning. The multifunctional extended carbon-fiber tabletop has eliminated the need for patient transfers onto trolleys until the patient leaves the trauma resuscitation room after all imaging has been completed; this ultimately prevents further falls.

References

1. World Health Organization. Injuries and violence: the facts. 2010. http://www.who.int/violence_injury_prevention/key_facts/en/. Accessed 16 June 2014.
2. Heron M. Deaths: leading causes for 2010. National vital statistics reports. Vol. 62, no. 6. Hyattsville: National Center for Health Statistics; 2013.
3. Centers for Disease Control and Prevention, National Center for Injury Prevention and Control. Web-based Injury Statistics Query and Reporting System (WISQARS) Fatal Injury Data. 2016.
4. Chandran A, Hyder AA, Peek-Asa C. The global burden of unintentional injuries and an agenda for progress. Epidemiol Rev. 2010;32:110–20. doi:10.1093/epirev/mxq009. Epub 22 Jun 2010.
5. World Health Organization. The Global burden of disease: 2004 update. Geneva: World Health Organization; 2008.
6. Jacobs G, Aeron-Thomas A, Astrop A. Estimating global road fatalities. Crowthorne: Transport Research Laboratory (TLR Report 445); 2000.
7. Danseco ER, Miller TR, Spicer RS. Incidence and costs of 1987-1994 childhood injuries: demographic breakdowns. Pediatrics. 2000;105:E27. doi:10.1542/peds.105.2.e27.
8. Road accidents in Italy, Year 2013. ISTAT. Published 4 Nov 2014.
9. Taggi F, Giustini M, Dosi G, et al. I "veri" dati sanitari della sicurezza stradale in Italia: mortalità, invalidità, ricoveri, accessi al pronto soccorso, costi. In: Taggi F, editor. Aspetti sanitari della sicurezza stradale. Roma: Istituto Superiore di Sanità, Ministero delle Infrastrutture e dei Trasporti; 2003. p. 83–7.
10. Boyd CR, Tolson MA, Copes WS. Evaluating trauma care: the TRISS method. J Trauma. 1987;27:370–8.
11. Gunst M, Ghaemmaghami V, Gruszecki A, et al. Changing epidemiology of trauma deaths leads to a bimodal distribution. Proc (Bayl Univ Med Cent). 2010;23:349–54.
12. Wintermark M, Poletti PA, Becker CD, et al. Traumatic injuries: organization and ergonomics of imaging in the emergency environment. Eur Radiol. 2002;12:959–68. doi:10.1007/s00330-002-1385-3.

13. Lerner EB, Moscati RM. The golden hour: scientific fact or medical "urban legend"? Acad Emerg Med. 2001;8:758–60. doi:10.1111/j.1553-2712.2001.tb00201.x.
14. Philipp MO, Kubin K, Hörmann M, Metz VM. Radiological emergency room management with emphasis on multidetector-row CT. Eur J Radiol. 2003;48:2–4.
15. World Health Organization. Mass Casualty Management Systems: strategies and guidelines for building health sector capacity. Geneva: World Health Organization; 2007.
16. MacKenzie EJ, Rivara FP, Jurkovich GJ, et al. A national evaluation of the effect of trauma-center care on mortality. N Engl J Med. 2006;354:366–78. doi:10.1056/NEJMsa052049.
17. Haas B, Stukel TA, Gomez D, et al. The mortality benefit of direct trauma center transport in a regional trauma system: a population-based analysis. J Trauma Acute Care Surg. 2012;72:1510–5; discussion: 1515–7. doi:10.1097/TA.0b013e318252510a.
18. Gunn ML, Kool DR, Lehnert BE. Improving outcomes in the patient with polytrauma: a review of the role of whole-body computed tomography. Radiol Clin N Am. 2015;53:639–56, vii. doi:10.1016/j.rcl.2015.02.006.
19. Committee on Injury Prevention and Control, Institute of Medicine. Overview of trauma care systems. In: Bonnie RJ, Fulco CE, Liverman CT, editors. Reducing the burden of injury: advancing prevention and treatment. Washington, DC: National Academies Press (US); 1999. p. 139–41.
20. Norton K, Longley M, Ponton M with assistance from Simpson A and Kimani S. The best configuration of hospital services for Wales: a review of the evidence. Welsh Institute for Health and Social Care, University of Glamorgan; 2012. p. 43.
21. Taran S. The scoop and run method of pre-clinical care for trauma victims. Mcgill J Med. 2009;12:73.
22. Aubuchon MMF, Hemmes B, Poeze M, et al. Prehospital care in patients with severe traumatic brain injury: does the level of prehospital care influence mortality? Eur J Trauma Emerg Surg. 2013;39:35–41. doi:10.1007/s00068-012-0218-6.
23. http://speciality.medicaldialogues.in/initial-management-of-severe-trauma-standard-treatment-guidelines/
24. Battlefield Advanced Trauma Life Support (BATLS). J R Army Med Corps. 2000;146:110–4. doi:10.1136/jramc-146-02-12. http://jramc.bmj.com/ on August 12, 2017, Published by group.bmj.com
25. Committee on Trauma American College of Surgeons. Chapter 3: Prehospital trauma care. In: Resources for the optimal care of the injured patient. Chicago: American College of Surgeons; 2014.
26. Cone D, Benson R, Schmidt T. Field triage system: methodologies from the literature. Prehosp Emerg Care. 2004;8:130–7. doi:10.1080/312703004222.
27. Schmidt T, Atcheson R, Federiuk C, et al. Evaluation of protocols allowing emergency medical technicians to determine need for treatment and transport. Acad Emerg Med. 2000;7:663–9. doi:10.1111/j.1553-2712.2000.tb02041.x.
28. Sasser SM, Hunt RC, Faul M, et al. Guidelines for field triage of injured patients: recommendations of the National Expert Panel on Field Triage, 2011. MMWR Recomm Rep. 2012;61(RR-1):1–20.
29. McCoy CE, Chakravarthy B, Lotfipour S. Guidelines for field triage of injured patients: in conjunction with the morbidity and mortality weekly report published by the Center for Disease Control and Prevention. West J Emerg Med. 2013;14:69–76. doi:10.5811/westjem.2013.1.15981.
30. Pulsara. https://www.pulsara.com/time
31. Hsia R, Shen YC. Possible geographical barriers to trauma center access for vulnerable patients in the United States: an analysis of urban and rural communities. Arch Surg. 2011;146:46–52. doi:10.1001/archsurg.2010.299.
32. American College of Surgeons Committee on Trauma (ACS-COT). Document regional trauma systems: optimal elements, integration, and assessment—systems consultation guide. 2008.
33. Ciesla DJ, Kerwin AJ, Tepas JJ III. Chapter 4: Trauma systems, triage, and transport. In: Moore EE, Feliciano DV, Mattox KL, editors. Trauma. 4th ed. New York: McGraw-Hill; 2000.
34. Hoff WS, Schwab CW. Trauma system development in North America. Clin Orthop Relat Res. 2004;422:17–22.
35. Newgard CD, Schmicker RH, Hedges JR, et al. Emergency medical services intervals and survival in trauma: assessment of the "golden hour" in a North American prospective cohort. Ann Emerg Med. 2010;55:235–46. doi:10.1016/j.annemergmed.2009.07.024. Epub 23 Sept 2009.
36. American College of Surgeons Committee on Trauma. Advanced trauma life support for doctors. Chicago: American College of Surgeons; 2012.
37. ATLS Algorithms, Pocket ICU Management. https://anesth.unboundmedicine.com/anesthesia//pview/Pocket-ICU-Management/534159/all/ATLS%20 Algorithms
38. American College of Surgeons. Advanced trauma life support program for physicians. 9th ed. Chicago: American College of Surgeons; 2012.
39. Committee on Trauma, American College of Surgeons. Advanced trauma life support for doctors–student course manual. 8th ed. Chicago: American College of Surgeons; 2008.
40. Craniomaxillofacial trauma. An issue of atlas of the oral and maxillofacial surgery clinics. E-Book. In: Bitonti DA, editor. Elsevier Health Sciences; 5 Apr 2013.
41. Kool DR, Blickman JG. Advanced trauma life support®. ABCDE from a radiological point of view. Emerg Radiol. 2007;14:135–41. doi:10.1007/s10140-007-0633-x.
42. Baker SP, O'Neill B, Haddon W Jr, Long WB. The injury severity score: a method for describing patients with multiple injuries and evaluating emergency care. J Trauma. 1974;14:187–96.

43. Champion HR, Sacco WJ, Copes WS, et al. A revision of the trauma score. J Trauma. 1989;29:623–9.
44. Kondo Y, Abe T, Kohshi K, et al. Revised trauma scoring system to predict in-hospital mortality in the emergency department: Glasgow Coma Scale, Age, and Systolic Blood Pressure score. Crit Care. 2011;15:R191. Published online 10 Aug 2011. doi:10.1186/cc10348.
45. Nguyen D, Platon A, Shanmuganathan K, et al. Evaluation of a single-pass continuous whole-body 16-MDCT protocol for patients with polytrauma. AJR Am J Roentgenol. 2009;192:3–10. doi:10.2214/AJR.07.3702.
46. Committee of Trauma of ACS. Advanced Trauma Life Support (ATLS) student manual. 9th ed. Chicago: ACS; 2012.
47. Miele V, Piccolo CL, Trinci M, et al. Diagnostic imaging of blunt abdominal trauma in pediatric patients. Radiol Med. 2016;121:409–30. doi:10.1007/s11547-016-0637-2. Epub 13 Apr 2016.
48. Miele V, Andreoli C, Grassi R. The management of emergency radiology: key facts. Eur J Radiol. 2006;59:311–4. Epub 27 Jun 2006.
49. Saltzherr TP, Jin PH, Bakker FC, et al. An evaluation of a Shockroom located CT scanner: a randomized study of early assessment by CT scanning in trauma patients in the bi-located trauma center North-West Netherlands (REACT trial). BMC Emerg Med. 2008;8:10. doi:10.1186/1471-227X-8-10.
50. Graber MA, Kathol M. Cervical spine radiographs in the trauma patient. Am Fam Physician. 1999;59:331–42.
51. Eastridge BJ, Starr A, Minei JP, et al. The importance of fracture pattern in guiding therapeutic decision-making in patients with hemorrhagic shock and pelvic ring disruptions. J Trauma. 2002;53:446–50; discussion 450–1.
52. Smith W, Williams A, Agudelo J, et al. Early predictors of mortality in hemodynamically unstable pelvis fractures. J Orthop Trauma. 2007;21:31–7. doi:10.1097/BOT.0b013e31802ea951.
53. Lee C, Porter K. The prehospital management of pelvic fractures. Emerg Med J. 2007;24:130–3. doi:10.1136/emj.2006.041384.
54. Young JW, Burgess AR, Brumback RJ, Poka A. Pelvic fractures: value of plain radiography in early assessment and management. Radiology. 1986;160:445–51. doi:10.1148/radiology.160.2.372612.
55. Slater SJ, Barron DA. Pelvic fractures-a guide to classification and management. Eur J Radiol. 2010;74:16–23. doi:10.1016/j.ejrad.2010.01.025.
56. Miele V, Di Giampietro I, Giannecchini S, et al. Pediatric polytrauma management. In: Miele V, Trinci M, editors. Imaging trauma and polytrauma in pediatric patients. Cham: Springer International Publishing; 2015. p. 1–28.
57. Poletti PA, Wintermark M, Schnyder P, Becker CD. Traumatic injuries: role of imaging in the management of the polytrauma victim (conservative expectation). Eur Radiol. 2002;12:969–78. doi:10.1007/s00330-002-1353-y. Epub 15 Mar 2002.
58. Ianniello S, Di Giacomo V, Sessa B, et al. First-line sonographic diagnosis of pneumothorax in unstable major trauma: accuracy of e-FAST and comparison with multidetector computed tomography. Radiol Med. 2014;119:674–80. doi:10.1007/s11547-014-0384-1. Epub 28 Jan 2014.
59. Moylan M, Newgart C, Ma J, et al. Association between a positive ED FAST examination and therapeutic laparotomy in normotensive blunt trauma patients. J Emerg Med. 2007;33:265–71. doi:10.1016/j.jemermed.2007.02.030. Epub 5 Jul 2007.
60. Quinn AC, Sinert R. What is the utility of the Focused Assessment with Sonography in Trauma (FAST) exam in penetrating torso trauma? Injury. 2011;42:482–7. doi:10.1016/j.injury.2010.07.249.
61. Miele V, Di Giampietro I, Ianniello S, et al. Diagnostic imaging in pediatric polytrauma management. Radiol Med. 2015;120:33–49. doi:10.1007/s11547-014-0469-x. Epub 7 Nov 2014.
62. Goldberg GG. Evaluation of ascites by ultrasound. Radiology. 1970;96:217–21.
63. AIUM Practice parameters for the performance of the focused assessment with sonography for trauma (FAST) examination 2014. http://www.aium.org/resources/guidelines/ fast.pdf
64. Scalea TM, Rodriguez A, Chiu WC, et al. Focused assessment with sonography for trauma (FAST): results from an international consensus conference. J Trauma. 1999;46:466–72.
65. Soldati G, Testa A, Pignataro G, et al. The ultrasonographic deep sulcus sign in traumatic pneumothorax. Ultrasound Med Biol. 2006;32:1157–63. doi:10.1016/j.ultrasmedbio.2006.04.006.
66. Ball CG, Kirkpatrick AW, Laupland KB, et al. Factors related to the failure of radiographic recognition of occult posttraumatic pneumothoraces. Am J Surg. 2005;189:541–6; discussion 546. doi:10.1016/j.amjsurg.2005.01.018.
67. Tocino IM, Miller MH, Fairfax WR. Distribution of pneumothorax in the supine and semi-recumbent critically ill adult. AJR Am J Roentgenol. 1985;144:901–5. doi:10.2214/ajr.144.5.901.
68. Volpicelli G. Sonographic diagnosis of pneumothorax. Intensive Care Med. 2011;37:224–32. doi:10.1007/s00134-010-2079-y. Epub 20 Nov 2010.
69. Lichtenstein DA, Mezière G, Biderman P, Gepner A. The "lung point": an ultrasound sign specific to pneumothorax. Intensive Care Med. 2000;26:1434–40.
70. American College of Surgeons Committee on Trauma. Advanced trauma life support (ATLS) for physicians. 7th ed. Chicago: American College of Surgeons; 1997.
71. Pinto F, Valentino M, Romanini L, et al. The role of CEUS in the assessment of haemodynamically stable patients with blunt abdominal trauma. Radiol Med.

2015;120:3–11. doi:10.1007/s11547-014-0455-3. Epub 21 Aug 2014.
72. Miele V, Piccolo CL, Galluzzo M, et al. Contrast enhanced ultrasound (CEUS) in blunt abdominal trauma. Br J Radiol. 2016;89:20150823. doi:10.1259/bjr.20150823. Epub 8 Jan 2016.
73. Poletti PA, Platon A, Becker CD, et al. Blunt abdominal trauma: does the use of a second-generation sonographic contrast agent help to detect solid organ injuries? AJR Am J Roentgenol. 2004;183:1293–301. doi:10.2214/ajr.183.5.1831293.
74. Miele V, Buffa V, Stasolla A, et al. Contrast enhanced ultrasound with second generation contrast agent in traumatic liver lesions. Radiol Med. 2004;108:82–91.
75. Menichini G, Sessa B, Trinci M, et al. Accuracy of contrast enhanced ultrasound (CEUS) in the identification and characterization of traumatic solid organ lesions in children: a retrospective comparison with baseline US and CE MDCT. Radiol Med. 2015;120:989–1001. doi:10.1007/s11547-015-0535-z. Epub 31 Mar 2015.
76. Regine G, Atzori M, Buffa V, et al. Second-generation sonographic contrast agents in the evaluation of renal trauma. Radiol Med. 2007;112:581–7. Epub 11 Jun 2007.
77. Sessa B, Trinci M, Ianniello S, et al. Blunt abdominal trauma: role of Contrast-Enhanced Ultrasound in the detection and staging of abdominal traumatic lesions compared with US and CE-MDCT. Radiol Med. 2015;120:180–9. doi:10.1007/s11547-014-0425-9. Epub 25 Jun 2014.
78. Pinto F, Miele V, Scaglione M, et al. The use of contrast-enhanced ultrasound in blunt abdominal trauma: advantages and limitations. Acta Radiol. 2014;55:776–84. doi:10.1177/0284185113505517. Epub 23 Sep 2013.
79. Miele V, Piccolo CL, Sessa B, et al. Comparison between MRI and CEUS in the follow-up of patients with blunt abdominal trauma managed conservatively. Radiol Med. 2016;121:27–37. doi:10.1007/s11547-015-0578-1. Epub 8 Aug 2015.
80. Flohr TG, Schaller S, Stierstorfer K, et al. Multi-detector row CT systems and image reconstruction techniques. Radiology. 2005;235:756–73. doi:10.1148/radiol.2353040037. Epub 15 Apr 2005.
81. Broder J, Warshauer DM. Increasing utilization of computed tomography in the adult emergency department, 2000-2005. Emerg Radiol. 2006;13:25–30. doi:10.1007/s10140-006-0493-9. Epub 10 Aug 2006.
82. Griffey RT, Ledbetter S, Khorasani R. Changes in thoracolumbar computed tomography and radiography utilization among trauma patients after deployment of multidetector computed tomography in the emergency department. J Trauma. 2007;62:1153–6. doi:10.1097/01.ta.0000200818.58534.5a.
83. Miele V, Di Giampietro I. Diagnostic imaging in emergency. Salute Soc. 2014;(2EN):127–38. doi:10.3280/SES2014-002010EN.
84. Iglehart JK. Health insurers and medical imaging policy—a work in progress. N Engl J Med. 2009;360:1030–7. doi:10.1056/NEJMhpr0808703.
85. Vartanians VM, Sistrom CL, Weilburg JB, et al. Increasing the appropriateness of outpatient imaging: effects of a barrier to ordering low-yield examinations. Radiology. 2010;255:842–9. doi:10.1148/radiol.10091228.
86. Smith-Bindman R, Lipson J, Marcus R, et al. Radiation dose associated with common computed tomography examinations and the associated lifetime attributable risk of cancer. Arch Intern Med. 2009;169:2078–86. doi:10.1001/archinternmed.2009.427.
87. Sampson MA, Colquhoun KB, Hennessy NL. Computed tomography whole body imaging in multi-trauma: 7 years experience. Clin Radiol. 2006;61:365–9. doi:10.1016/j.crad.2005.12.009.
88. Salim A, Sangthong B, Martin M, et al. Whole body imaging in blunt multisystem trauma patients without obvious signs of injury: results of a prospective study. Arch Surg. 2006;141:468–73; discussion 473–5. doi:10.1001/archsurg.141.5.468.
89. Gupta M, Schriger DL, Hiatt JR, et al. Selective use of computed tomography compared with routine whole body imaging in patients with blunt trauma. Ann Emerg Med. 2011;58:407–16.e15. doi:10.1016/j.annemergmed.2011.06.003. Epub 3 Sep 2011.
90. Stengel D, Ottersbach C, Matthes G, et al. Accuracy of single-pass whole-body computed tomography for detection of injuries in patients with major blunt trauma. CMAJ. 2012;184:869–76. doi:10.1503/cmaj.111420. Epub 5 Mar 2012.
91. Deunk J, Brink M, Dekker HM, et al. Routine versus selective multidetector-row computed tomography (MDCT) in blunt trauma patients: level of agreement on the influence of additional findings on management. J Trauma. 2009;67:1080–6. doi:10.1097/TA.0b013e318189371d.
92. Nast-Kolb D, Waydhas C, Kanz KG, Schweiberer L. [An algorithm for management of shock in polytrauma]. Unfallchirurg. 1994;97:292–302.
93. Copes WS, Champion HR, Sacco WJ, et al. The injury severity score revisited. J Trauma. 1988;28:69–77.
94. Esposito TJ, Offner PJ, Jurkovich GJ, et al. Do prehospital trauma center triage criteria identify major trauma victims? Arch Surg. 1995;130:171–6.
95. Stalp M, Koch C, Ruchholtz S, et al. Standardized outcome evaluation after blunt multiple injuries by scoring systems: a clinical follow-up investigation 2 years after injury. J Trauma. 2002;52:1160–8.
96. Stewart TC, Lane PL, Stefanits T. An evaluation of patient outcomes before and after trauma center designation using trauma and injury severity score analysis. J Trauma. 1995;39:1036–40.
97. Brown JB, Stassen NA, Bankey PE, et al. Mechanism of injury and special consideration criteria still matter: an evaluation of the National Trauma Triage Protocol. J Trauma. 2011;70:38–44; discussion 44–5. doi:10.1097/TA.0b013e3182077ea8.

98. Boyle MJ. Is mechanism of injury alone in the prehospital setting a predictor of major trauma—a review of the literature. J Trauma Manag Outcomes. 2007;1:4. doi:10.1186/1752-2897-1-4.
99. Asha S, Curtis KA, Grant N, et al. Comparison of radiation exposure of trauma patients from diagnostic radiology procedures before and after the introduction of a panscan protocol. Emerg Med Australas. 2012;24:43–51. doi:10.1111/j.1742--6723.2011.01504.x. Epub 7 Dec 2011.
100. Brenner DJ, Elliston CD. Estimated radiation risks potentially associated with full-body CT screening. Radiology. 2004;232:735–8. Epub 23 Jul 2004.
101. Kim PK, Gracias VH, Maidment AD, et al. Cumulative radiation dose caused by radiologic studies in critically ill trauma patients. J Trauma. 2004;57:510–4.
102. Trupka A, Waydhas C, Hallfeldt KK, et al. Value of thoracic computed tomography in the first assessment of severely injured patients with blunt chest trauma: results of a prospective study. J Trauma. 1997;43:405–11; discussion 411–2.
103. Brar MS, Bains I, Brunet G, et al. Occult pneumothoraces truly occult or simply missed: redux. J Trauma. 2010;69:1335–7. doi:10.1097/TA.0b013e3181f6f525.
104. Holmes JF, Akkinepalli R. Computed tomography versus plain radiography to screen for cervical spine injury: a meta-analysis. J Trauma. 2005;58:902–5.
105. Watura R, Cobby M, Taylor J. Multislice CT in imaging of trauma of the spine, pelvis and complex foot injuries. Br J Radiol. 2004;77 Spec No 1:S46–63.
106. Schenarts PJ, Diaz J, Kaiser C, Carrillo Y, et al. Prospective comparison of admission computed tomographic scan and plain films of the upper cervical spine in trauma patients with altered mental status. J Trauma. 2001;51:663–8; discussion 668–9.
107. Jelly LM, Evans DR, Easty MJ, et al. Radiography versus spiral CT in the evaluation of cervicothoracic junction injuries in polytrauma patients who have undergone intubation. Radiographics. 2000;20 Spec No:S251–9; discussion S260–2.
108. Wintermark M, Mouhsine E, Theumann N, et al. Thoracolumbar spine fractures in patients who have sustained severe trauma: depiction with multi-detector row CT. Radiology. 2003;227:681–9. doi:10.1148/radiol.2273020592. Epub 17 Apr 2003.
109. Brown CV, Antevil JL, Sise MJ, et al. Spiral computed tomography for the diagnosis of cervical, thoracic, and lumbar spine fractures: its time has come. J Trauma. 2005;58:890–5; discussion 895–6.
110. Beenen LF, Sierink JC, Kolkman S, et al. Split bolus technique in polytrauma: a prospective study on scan protocols for trauma analysis. Acta Radiol. 2015;56:873–80. doi:10.1177/0284185114539319. Epub 17 Jul 2014.
111. Gunn ML, Kohr JR. State of the art: technologies for computed tomography dose reduction. Emerg Radiol. 2010;17:209–18. doi:10.1007/s10140-009-0850-6. Epub 20 Nov 2009.
112. Brink M, de Lange F, Oostveen LJ, et al. Arm raising at exposure-controlled multidetector trauma CT of thoracoabdominal region: higher image quality, lower radiation dose. Radiology. 2008;249:661–70. doi:10.1148/radiol.2492080169.
113. Karlo C, Gnannt R, Frauenfelder T, et al. Whole-body CT in polytrauma patients: effect of arm positioning on thoracic and abdominal image quality. Emerg Radiol. 2011;18:285–93. doi:10.1007/s10140-011-0948-5. Epub 7 Apr 2011.
114. Cademartiri F, Mollet NR, van der Lugt A, et al. Intravenous contrast material administration at helical 16-detector row CT coronary angiography: effect of iodine concentration on vascular attenuation. Radiology. 2005;236:661–5. doi:10.1148/radiol.2362040468.
115. Mitchell AM, Jones AE, Tumlin JA, Kline JA. Incidence of contrast induced nephropathy after contrast-enhanced computed tomography in the outpatient setting. Clin J Am Soc Nephrol. 2010;5:4–9. doi:10.2215/CJN.05200709. Epub 3 Dec 2009.
116. Eichler K, Marzi I, Wyen H, et al. Multidetector computed tomography (MDCT): simple CT protocol for trauma patient. Clin Imaging. 2015;39:110–5. doi:10.1016/j.clinimag.2014.09.011. Epub 16 Oct 2014.
117. Linsenmaier U, Krötz M, Häuser H, et al. Whole-body computed tomography in polytrauma: techniques and management. Eur Radiol. 2002;12:1728–40. doi:10.1007/s00330-001-1225-x. Epub 13 Dec 2001.
118. Marmery H, Shanmuganathan K, Mirvis SE, et al. Correlation of multidetector CT findings with splenic arteriography and surgery: prospective study in 392 patients. J Am Coll Surg. 2008;206:685–93. doi:10.1016/j.jamcollsurg.2007.11.024. Epub 11 Feb 2008.
119. Maturen KE, Adusumilli S, Blane CE, et al. Contrast enhanced CT accurately detects hemorrhage in torso trauma: direct comparison with angiography. J Trauma. 2007;62:740–5. doi:10.1097/01.ta.0000235508.11442.a8.
120. Hamilton JD, Kumaravel M, Censullo ML, et al. Multidetector CT evaluation of active extravasation in blunt abdominal and pelvic trauma patients. Radiographics. 2008;28:1603–16. doi:10.1148/rg.286085522.
121. Anderson SW, Lucey BC, Rhea JT, et al. 64 MDCT in multiple trauma patients: imaging manifestations and clinical implications of active extravasation. Emerg Radiol. 2007;14:151–9. doi:10.1007/s10140-007-0600-6. Epub 5 May 2007.
122. Gunn ML. Imaging of aortic and branch vessel trauma. Radiol Clin N Am. 2012;50:85–103. doi:10.1016/j.rcl.2011.08.002. Epub 22 Oct 2011.
123. Atluri S, Richard HM 3rd, Shanmuganathan K. Optimizing multidetector CT for visualization of splenic vascular injury. Validation by splenic arteriography in blunt abdominal trauma patients. Emerg

Radiol. 2011;18:307–12. doi:10.1007/s10140-011-0961-8. Epub 26 May 2011.
124. Boscak AR, Shanmuganathan K, Mirvis SE, et al. Optimizing trauma multidetector CT protocol for blunt splenic injury: need for arterial and portal venous phase scans. Radiology. 2013;268:79–88. doi:10.1148/radiol.13121370. Epub 28 Feb 2013.
125. Melton SM, Kerby JD, McGiffin D, et al. The evolution of chest computed tomography for the definitive diagnosis of blunt aortic injury: a single-center experience. J Trauma. 2004;56:243–50. doi:10.1097/01.TA.0000111751.84052.24.
126. Regine G, Stasolla A, Miele V. Multidetector computed tomography of the renal arteries in vascular emergencies. Eur J Radiol. 2007;64:83–91. Epub 27 Jul 2007.
127. Anderson SW, Lucey BC, Varghese JC, Soto JA. Sixty-four multi-detector row computed tomography in multitrauma patient imaging: early experience. Curr Probl Diagn Radiol. 2006;35:188–98. doi:10.1067/j.cpradiol.2006.06.004.
128. Quagliano PV, Delair SM, Malhotra AK. Diagnosis of blunt bladder injury: a prospective comparative study of computed tomographic cystography and conventional retrograde cystography. J Trauma. 2006;61:410–21; discussion 421–2. doi:10.1097/01.ta.0000229940.36556.bf.
129. Lucey BC, Stuhlfaut JW, Hochberg AR, et al. Evaluation of blunt abdominal trauma using PACS-based 2D and 3D MDCT reformations of the lumbar spine and pelvis. AJR Am J Roentgenol. 2005;185:1435–40. doi:10.2214/AJR.04.1396.
130. Falchi M, Rollandi GA. CT of pelvic fractures. Eur J Radiol. 2004;50:96–105. doi:10.1016/j.ejrad.2003.11.019.
131. Perandini S, Faccioli N, Zaccarella A, Re T, Mucelli RP. The diagnostic contribution of CT volumetric rendering techniques in routine practice. Indian J Radiol Imaging. 2010;20:92–7. doi:10.4103/0971-3026.63043.
132. Shreiber R. 3-D reconstruction in radiology. http://www.carestream.es/3dRecon_whitePaper.pdf
133. Pretorius ES, Fishman EK. Spiral CT and three-dimensional CT of musculoskeletal pathology. Emergency room applications. Radiol Clin North Am. 1999;37:953–74, vi.
134. Major extremity trauma module. PAH Department of Emergency Medicine Major Extremity Trauma Revised 2016.
135. Consensus Meeting on Crush Injury and Crush Syndrome, Faculty of Pre-Hospital Care of the Royal College of Surgeons of Edinburgh, May 2001.
136. Kornguth PJ, Salazar AM. The apical oblique view of the shoulder: its usefulness in acute trauma. AJR Am J Roentgenol. 1987;149:113–6. doi:10.2214/ajr.149.1.113.
137. Garth WP Jr, Slappey CE, Ochs CW. Roentgenographic demonstration of instability of the shoulder: the apical oblique projection. A technical note. J Bone Joint Surg Am. 1984;66:1450–3.
138. Piccolo CL, Galluzzo M, Trinci M, et al. Upper limbs trauma in pediatrics. Semin Musculoskelet Radiol. 2017;21:167–74. doi:10.1055/s-0037-1602416.
139. Greenspan A, Norman A. Radial head-capitellum view: an expanded imaging approach to elbow injury. Radiology. 1987;164:272–4.
140. Piccolo CL, Galluzzo M, Trinci M, et al. Lower limbs trauma in pediatrics. Semin Musculoskelet Radiol. 2017;21:175–83. doi:10.1055/s-0037-1602417.
141. Piccolo CL, Galluzzo M, Ianniello S, et al. Pediatric musculoskeletal injuries: role of ultrasound and magnetic resonance imaging. Musculoskelet Surg. 2017;101(Suppl 1):85–102. doi:10.1007/s12306-017-0452-5.
142. Mark Davies A, Pettersson H. Fractures of the ankle. In: Ostensen H, Pettersson H, editors. The WHO manual of diagnostic imaging. Radiographic anatomy and interpretation of the musculoskeletal system. Geneva: World Health Organization; 2002.
143. Harvey JJ, West ATH. The right scan, for the right patient, at the right time: the reorganization of major trauma service provision in England and its implications for radiologists. Clin Radiol. 2013;68:871–86. doi:10.1016/j.crad.2013.01.006. Epub 1 Mar 2013.
144. Brenner DJ, Hall EJ. Computed tomography—an increasing source of radiation exposure. N Engl J Med. 2007;357:2277–84.
145. Sierink JC, Saltzherr TP, Reitsma JB, et al. Systematic review and meta-analysis of immediate total-body computed tomography compared with selective radiological imaging of injured patients. Br J Surg. 2012;99(Suppl 1):52–8. doi:10.1002/bjs.7760.
146. Healy DA, Hegarty A, Feeley I, et al. Systematic review and meta-analysis of routine total body CT compared with selective CT in trauma patients. Emerg Med J. 2014;31:101–8. doi:10.1136/emermed-2012-201892. Epub 12 Jan 2013.
147. Van Vugt R, Kool DR, Deunk J, Edwards MJ. Effects on mortality, treatment, and time management as a result of routine use of total body computed tomography in blunt high-energy trauma patients. J Trauma Acute Care Surg. 2012;72:553–9. doi:10.1097/TA.0b013e31822dd93b.
148. Caputo ND, Stahmer C, Lim G, Shah K. Whole body computed tomographic scanning leads to better survival as opposed to selective scanning in trauma patients: a systematic review and meta-analysis. J Trauma Acute Care Surg. 2014;77:534–9. doi:10.1097/TA.0000000000000414.
149. Surendran A, Mori A, Varma DK, Gruen RL. Systematic review of the benefits and harms of whole-body computed tomography in the early management of multitrauma patients: are we getting the whole picture? J Trauma Acute Care Surg. 2014;76:1122–30. doi:10.1097/TA.0000000000000178.

150. Jiang L, Ma Y, Jiang S, et al. Comparison of whole-body computed tomography vs selective radiological imaging on outcomes in major trauma patients: a meta-analysis. Scand J Trauma Resusc Emerg Med. 2014;22:54. doi:10.1186/s13049-014-0054-2.
151. Huber-Wagner S, Lefering R, Qvick LM, et al. Effect of whole-body CT during trauma resuscitation on survival: a retrospective, multicentre study. Lancet. 2009;373:1455–61. doi:10.1016/S0140-6736 (09) 60232-4. Epub 25 Mar 2009.
152. Huber-Wagner S, Biberthaler P, Haberle S, et al. Whole-body CT in haemodynamically unstable severely injured patients—a retrospective, multicentre study. PLoS One. 2013;8(7):e68880. doi:10.1371/journal.pone.0068880. Print 2013.
153. Sierink JC, Treskes K, Edwards MJ, et al. Immediate total-body CT scanning versus conventional imaging and selective CT scanning in patients with severe trauma (REACT-2): a randomised controlled trial. Lancet. 2016;388(10045):673–83. doi:10.1016/S0140-6736(16)30932-1. Epub 28 Jun 2016.
154. Wurmb TE, Quaisser C, Balling H, et al. Whole-body multislice computed tomography (MSCT) improves trauma care in patients requiring surgery after multiple trauma. Emerg Med J. 2011;28:300–4.
155. Wurmb T, Balling H, Frühwald P, et al. [Polytrauma management in a period of change: time analysis of new strategies for emergency room treatment]. Unfallchirurg. 2009;112:390–9.
156. Wurmb TE, Frühwald P, Hopfner W, et al. Whole-body multislice computed tomography as the first line diagnostic tool in patients with multiple injuries: the focus on time. J Trauma. 2009;66:658–65.
157. Topp T, Lefering R, Lopez CL, et al. Radiologic diagnostic procedures in severely injured patients—is only whole-body multislice computed tomography the answer? Int J Emerg Med. 2015;8:3. doi:10.1186/s12245-015-0053-8. eCollection 2015.
158. Nicolaou S, Eftekhari A, Sedlic T, Hou DJ, Mudri MJ, Aldrich J, Louis L. The utilization of dual source CT in imaging of polytrauma. Eur J Radiol. 2008;68:398–408.
159. Hauser H, Bohndorf K, Ruter A. [Traumatologic emergency in the shock department. Analysis of the spectrum and temporal aspects of diagnostic imaging]. Unfallchirurg. 1998;101:129–36.
160. Kanz KG, Paul AO, Lefering R, et al. Trauma management incorporating focused assessment with computed tomography in trauma (FACTT)—potential effect on survival. J Trauma Manag Outcomes. 2010;4:4. doi:10.1186/1752-2897-4-4.
161. Rouger M. Organisation and logistics crucial to imaging in emergencies—daily news from Europe's leading imaging congress. ECR TODAY; 2013. Saturday 9 Mar 2013.
162. Huber-Wagner S, Mand C, Ruchholtz S, et al. Effect of the localisation of the CT scanner during trauma resuscitation on survival—a retrospective, multicentre study. Injury. 2014;45(Suppl 3):S76–82. doi:10.1016/j.injury.2014.08.022.
163. Fung Kon Jin PH, Goslings JC, Ponsen KJ, et al. Assessment of a new trauma workflow concept implementing a sliding CT scanner in the trauma room: the effect on workup times. J Trauma Inj Infect Crit Care. 2008;64:1320–6.

Traumatic Injuries: Mechanisms of Lesions

2

Federica Romano, Francesca Iacobellis, Franco Guida, Ettore Laccetti, Antonia Sorbo, Roberto Grassi, and Mariano Scaglione

2.1 Introduction

Trauma is the result of the transfer of kinetic energy to the body from an outside force [1].

It is well known that consequences of each trauma are strongly related to the mechanisms of injury.

From a general point of view, two main categories of traumatic injuries can be identified: blunt trauma and penetrating trauma. Both these mechanisms may cause different lesions according to direction of forces, strength, and predisposing factors too (age, habitus, presence or absence of physical restraint devices) (Table 2.1).

A rapid overview of the situation to establish a tailored appropriate therapeutic strategy is mandatory, as survival rate after trauma is influenced by the preclinical and clinical trauma management within the first hour after an injury, known as "the golden hour" [2].

Notoriously clinical evaluation of patients who suffered high-energy trauma may be unreliable [3].

Physical examination of those patients is indeed often insidious as they may show multiple concomitant injuries, thereby diverting the responding "physician's" attention, or because of an altered state of consciousness due to drug or alcohol intoxication.

In this context, as a member of the trauma team, the radiologist has the major role of promptly recognizing (or to exclude) critical injuries requiring immediate treatment and also identifying the mechanisms of injury that may suggest subtle associated lesions that could be easily overlooked (Fig. 2.1) [4]. Actually, MDCT

F. Romano • F. Guida • E. Laccetti • A. Sorbo
Department of Radiology, "Pineta Grande" Hospital, Via Domitiana Km 30.000, 81030 Castel Volturno (CE), Italy

F. Iacobellis
Department of Radiology, "Pineta Grande" Hospital, Via Domitiana Km 30.000, 81030 Castel Volturno (CE), Italy

Department of Radiology, Second University of Naples, Piazza Miraglia 2, 80138 Naples, Italy

R. Grassi
Department of Radiology, Second University of Naples, Piazza Miraglia 2, 80138 Naples, Italy

M. Scaglione, M.D. (✉)
Department of Radiology, "Pineta Grande" Hospital, Via Domitiana Km 30.000, 81030 Castel Volturno (CE), Italy

Department of Radiology, Sunderland Royal Hospital, NHS Trust, Kayll Road, Sunderland SR4 7TP, UK
e-mail: scaglionefun@gmail.com

V. Miele, M. Trinci (eds.), *Diagnostic Imaging in Polytrauma Patients*,
https://doi.org/10.1007/978-3-319-62054-1_2

Table 2.1 Trauma mechanisms

Trauma	Main etiology	Mechanism		Main injuries
Blunt	Motor vehicle collision (MVC) fall from height	Direct impact	Direct-impact forces transmitted along the trajectory of the "force vector"	Extremity injuries, head and thoracoabdominal parietal and parenchymal injuries
		Compression	Collision of the tissues with a fixed object	Thoracic injuries (flail chest, tracheobronchial tree injuries), abdominal parenchymal (spleen, liver injuries) and pelvic injuries
		Acceleration/deceleration	Stretching of the organ at the fixed points of attachment	Vessel, mesenteric, tracheobronchial tree injuries
		Combined compression and deceleration (airbag/seat belt injuries)		Sternal fractures, spinal trauma, bowel and mesenteric injuries
Penetrating	Stab wound Gunshot wound	Tissue disruption	Direct injury to a focal area with tissue penetration	Depend on the involved anatomical region
Blast	Improvised explosive devices (IEDs)	Barotrauma	High-pressure blast wave followed by sudden drop in pressure	Lung contusions, mesenteric and bowel injuries
		Penetrating trauma		Depend on the involved anatomical region
		Combined blunt and penetrating		Bone fractures, as well as visceral injuries and closed head injuries
		Thermal and inhalation injuries	Thermal and chemical exposure of the respiratory mucosa	Respiratory mucosa and lung injuries

has revolutionized the management of trauma patients, representing the most useful screening tool to quickly assess injuries [1, 2, 5].

Modern technologies allow fast evaluation of traumatic injuries with the maximum concentration of time, which has a great impact on the results in terms of resuscitation and safety [6, 7].

This chapter will discuss the most common mechanisms of injuries and related imaging findings, focusing on the importance for radiologists to look for anatomic sites at risk of lesion according to direction of forces with the aim to individuate expected but also unexpected injuries.

2.2 Mechanisms of Lesions

Forensic medicine distinguishes two main transfers of kinetic energy, blunt or penetrating traumas (Table 2.1) [1]. Blunt trauma is considered as an injury in which tissues are not penetrated by external objects; it occurs most frequently in the context of road traffic accidents and is classified according to whether the primary mechanism of injury is related to a compression or deceleration forces [8] (Fig. 2.1).

As this trauma is usually the result of motor vehicle crushes (MVCs), it is the most frequent cause in the western countries

Conversely, penetrating injuries result from an object entering the body and sometimes exiting the body, causing damage along its path (Table 2.1) [1].

Commonly the object penetrates the fascia and injures underlying structures resulting in "open" injuries (Fig. 2.2).

Penetrating trauma involves a disruption of the skin and underlying tissues in a small, focused area (Fig. 2.2).

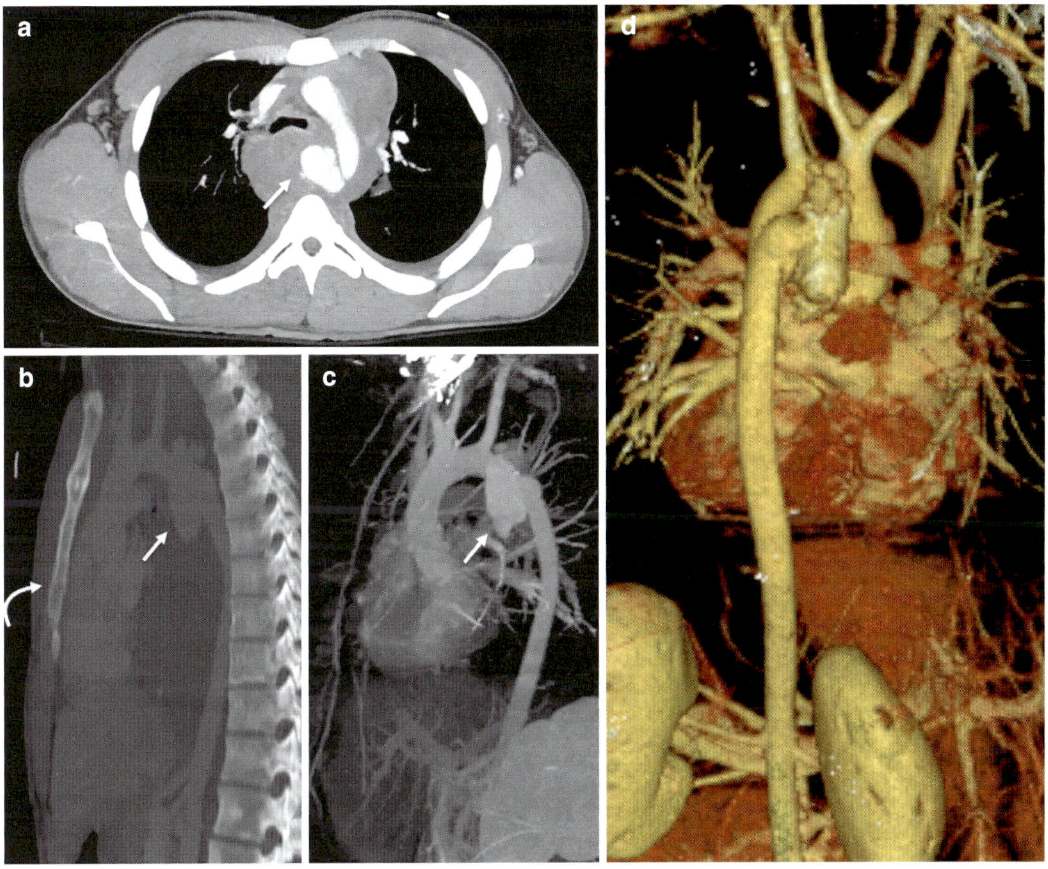

Fig. 2.1 Contrast-enhanced MDCT shows a large traumatic pseudoaneurysm of the descending thoracic aorta (**a**, *arrows*) with typical location and morphology (**a–c** *straight arrows*) with a large mediastinal hematoma displacing and compressing the carina, in a patient after high-energy blunt trauma. Note also a sternal fracture (**b**, *curved arrow*)

The severity of a stab wound depends on the area involved, depth of penetration, blade length, and angle of penetration.

Firearms are the primary mechanism resulting in penetrating trauma.

One point to consider is that every penetrating event results in open injuries, but not all open injuries are caused by penetrating mechanisms. For example, an open fracture from motor vehicle collision (MVC) is by definition a blunt trauma in which bone fragments become secondarily exposed by an indirect mechanism, due to the high energy of the trauma (Fig. 2.3).

Nowadays a particular mechanism of trauma is injury resulting by the use of improvised explosive devices (IEDs) such as the ones encountered in terrorist attacks. As the terrorism represents a matter of big concern in modern countries, radiologists working in a trauma center have to be aware of "blast injury patterns". Recent evidence emerged from the victims of Boston marathon bombing has underlined the role of imaging in the evaluation of foreign bodies and skeletal trauma in blast injuries [9].

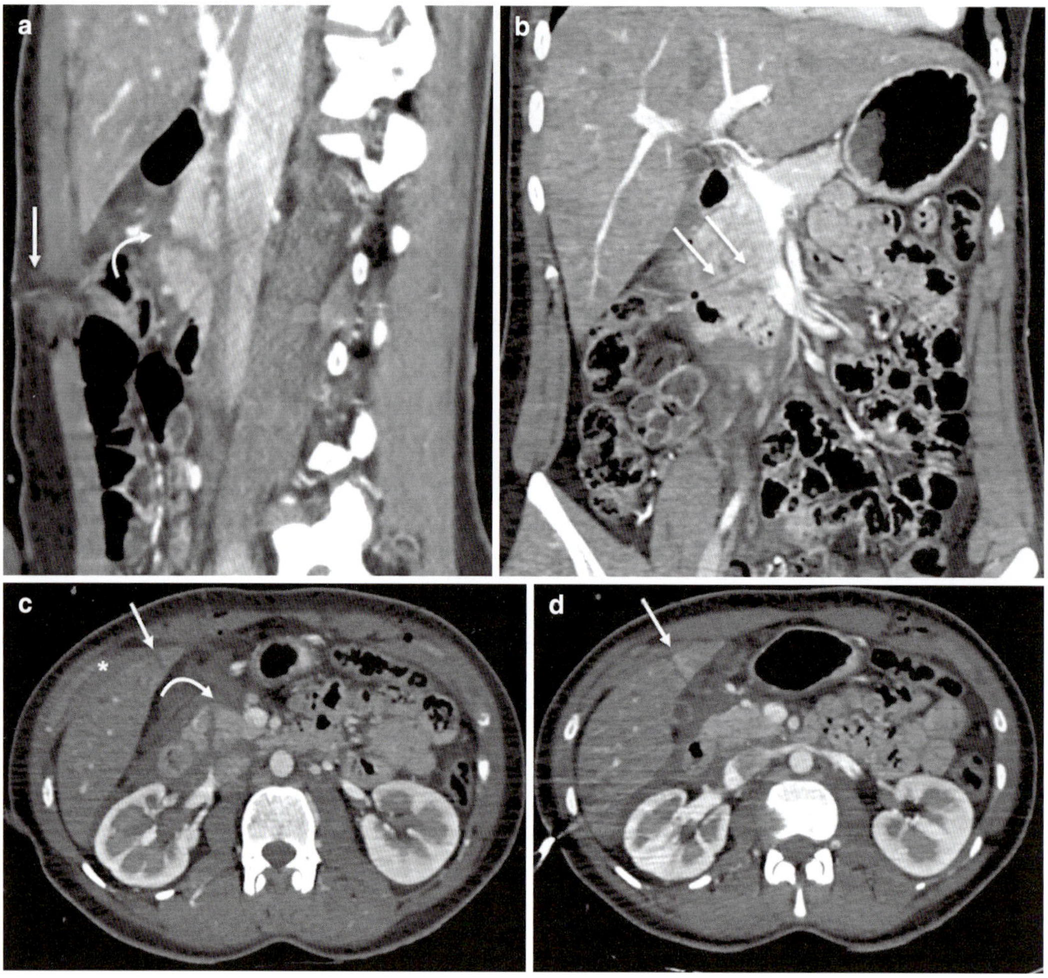

Fig. 2.2 Contrast-enhanced MDCT in sagittal (**a**), coronal (**b**), and axial (**c, d**) views showing the entry point of a penetrating trauma (**a**, *straight arrow*) involving the uncinate process of the pancreas (**a**, *curved arrow*; **b**, *straight arrows*) and the fifth liver segment (**c**, **d**, *arrows*) with hemoperitoneum (**c**, *asterisk*)

2.3 Imaging

MDCT represents "the cornerstone" of the decision-making process in polytrauma patients, and the emergency radiologist is the leader of this process, who must be present in CT room 24/7 to provide a continuous coverage [2, 4]. Nowadays, modern CT scanners allow enhanced image resolution with a marked reduction of the time needed for scanning, thereby allowing examination of the whole body within a few minutes. Motion artifacts can be minimized with this shorter acquisition time. Moreover the location of CT scanner next to the emergency unit allows rapid examination even in patients with some degree of hemodynamic instability [4, 10]. Wurmb et al. demonstrated in their study that direct whole-body CT accelerated diagnostic interval from a median of 70 to 23 min and decision-making process interval from 82 to 47 min [4, 11].

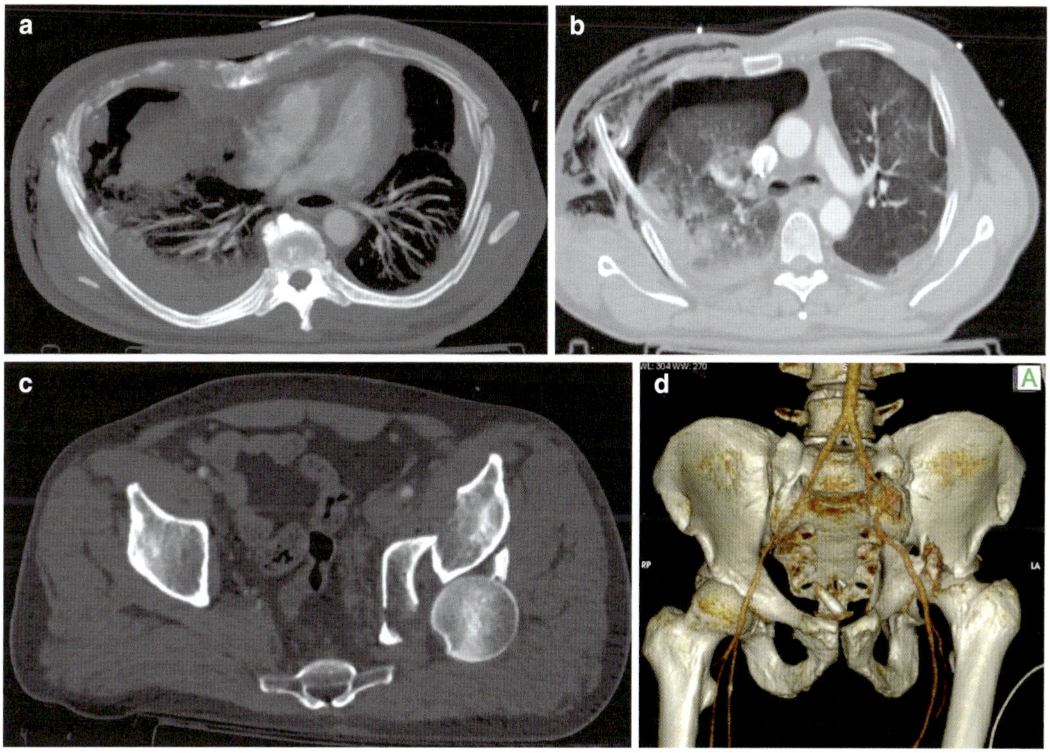

Fig. 2.3 Contrast-enhanced MDCT and MIP reconstruction in the axial plane (**a**) showing multiple displaced rib fractures in more than one-point "flail chest." Pulmonary window in the axial plane (**b**) shows multiple lung contusions, hemothorax, pneumothorax, and subcutaneous emphysema. Multifragmentary fracture of the acetabulum (**c**) with displacement of the femoral head (**c, d**)

As mentioned above, clinical examination is often unreliable, as patients may be unconsciousness due to the trauma or due to altered mental status; thus hollow visceral or vessel injuries may be easily overlooked in the presence, for example, of multiple bone fractures, differing time to treatment with life and cost consumption.

2.4 Blunt Trauma

As previously mentioned blunt trauma represents the most frequent mechanism of injury in modern countries [1]. It recognizes two major situations: motor vehicle collisions (MVCs) and falls.

2.5 MVC

Motor vehicle collisions are the leading cause of trauma death in all age groups from 1 to 65 years [1].

The injuries produced from MVC strongly depend from the energy of the impact, the direction of the forces, and also the presence of restraint devices. Frontal collision determines a moving forward of the occupant, if unrestrained, as long as the patient impacts the stationary vehicle chassis. Often the first site of the impact is represented by the extremities, resulting in arm and leg fractures; then injuries may occur to the head and spine, also because of torsional forces. Conversely in lateral collisions, the victim is moved away from the side

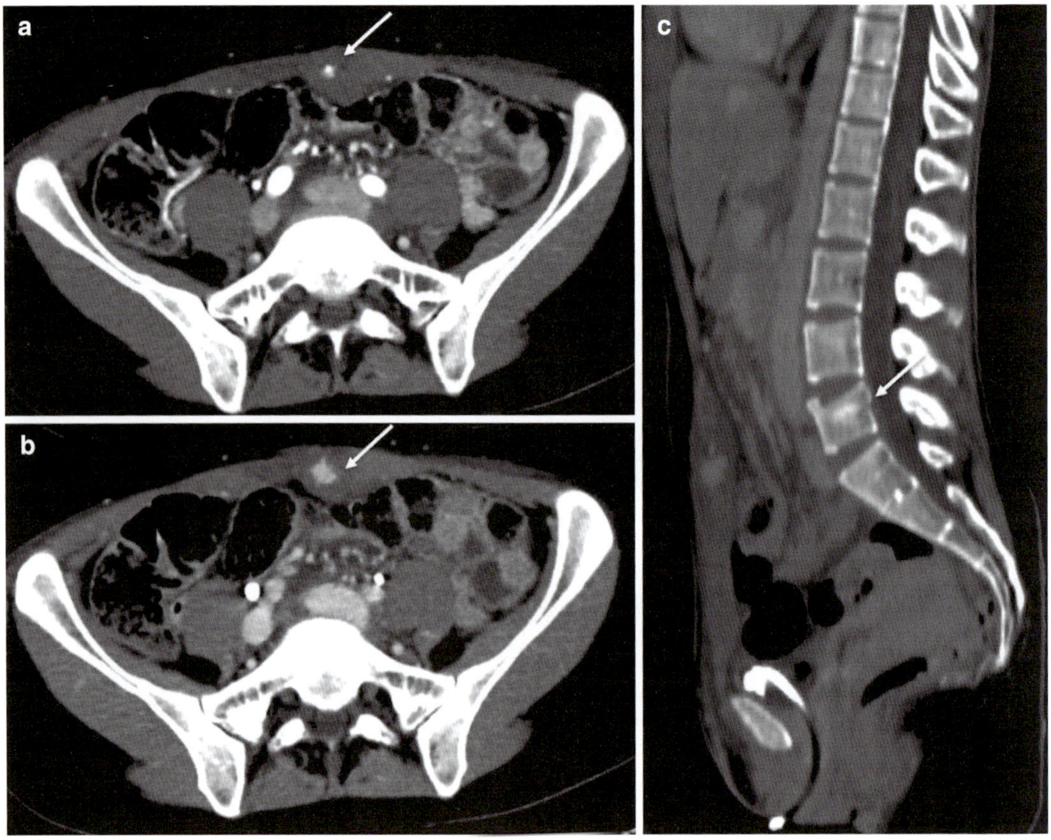

Fig. 2.4 Contrast-enhanced CT in the arterial phase in axial (**a**, **b**) and sagittal planes (**c**) after a seat belt injury. Note a spot of active bleeding (**a**, **b** *arrows*) within the anterior abdominal wall and a fracture of the fifth lumbar vertebra (**c**, *arrow*) along the same force vector

of the vehicle; it determines more often compressive pelvic and thoracoabdominal injuries. With the wide use of restraint devices (i.e., airbags, seat belts), there has been in last years a drastic reduction of both morbidity and mortality from crashes but a corresponding increase in the number of injuries attributable to these devices [12].

Airbags are responsible of injuries to upper extremities, the face, and the neck; corneal abrasions; and cervical hyperflexion injuries if the victim is seated too close to the restraint.

Seat belt injuries may vary from simple chest and/or abdominal abrasion at the site of seat belt contact to sternal fractures, spinal trauma (Fig. 2.4), and injuries to the bowel and mesentery (Figs. 2.5 and 2.6) [13].

It is a well-known issue that motorcyclists are at substantially higher risk of dying from crashes than car occupants.

Globally, motorcyclists account for nearly a quarter of all road traffic deaths (WHO 2015). In 2014, in the United States, motorcyclists accounted for less than 1% of person per miles traveled but more than 13% of the total mortality from motor vehicle crashes [14]. Most of the injuries are to the head, so these are often critical injuries, as in the final ground impact deceleration/acceleration mechanisms are strongly involved.

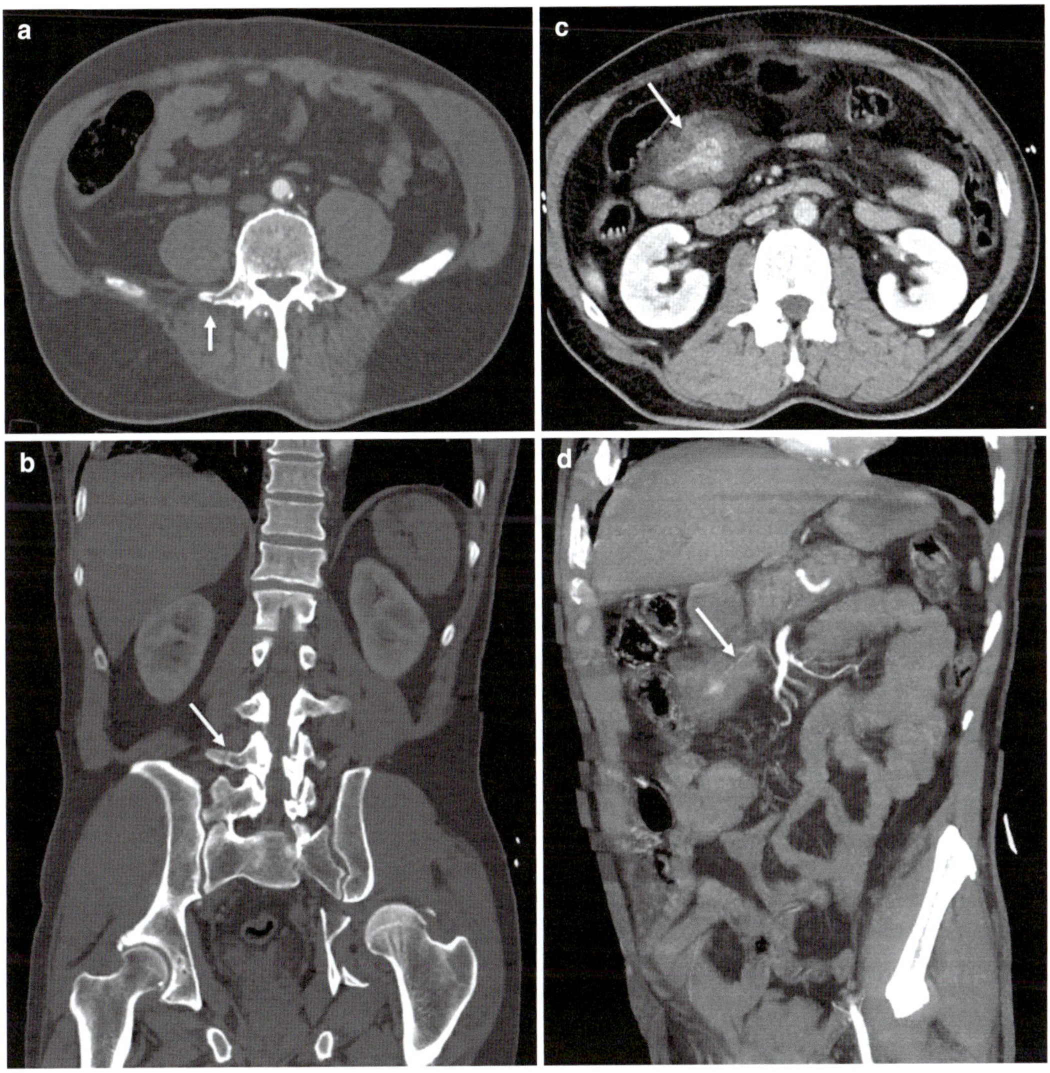

Fig. 2.5 Contrast-enhanced MDCT in arterial phase in axial (**a**, **c**), coronal (**b**), and oblique views (**d**) after a seat belt injury. Note the lumbar transverse process fracture (**a**, *arrow*) and a pooling of active bleeding in the mesentery (**c**, **d** *arrows*)

2.6 Falls

Falls represent one of the most common mechanisms of trauma across all age groups, varying from simple ground-level falls to falls from significant height, the latter resulting in severe injuries [1].

Simple ground-level falls often do not require any diagnostic imaging, but may be dangerous in the elderly, as the bones are more fragile, and bone injuries, as lumbar, femoral, and radial fractures, as well as subdural hematomas are quite common. Injuries from falls from significant heights may be intentional or not (work-related accidents); almost all these patients show multiple lesions, and the musculoskeletal system is often involved [1, 15]. Falls from a height result in an axial load, and injury patterns depend on several factors: the height of the fall, the landing position of the victim, the surface of the

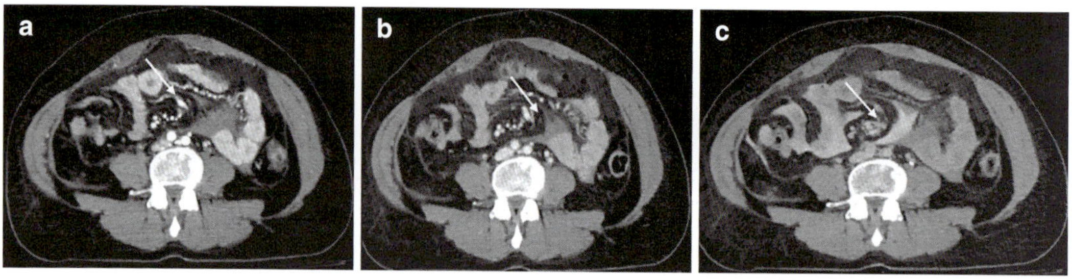

Fig. 2.6 Multiphasic contrast-enhanced MDCT in a seat belt injury shows increasing amount of active mesenteric bleeding in the arterial (**a**), venous (**b**), and late phases (**c**)

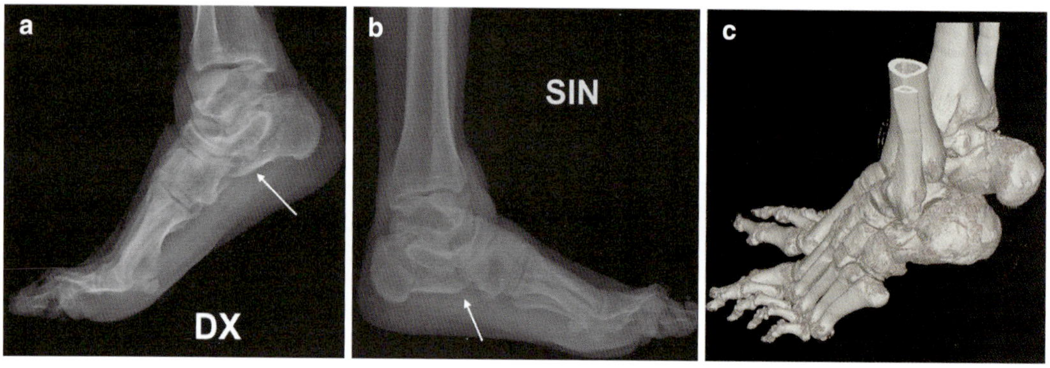

Fig. 2.7 Plain film views (**a**, **b**) and CT volume rendering (**c**) of bilateral calcaneal fractures (**a**, **b**, *arrow*) due to a fall from height

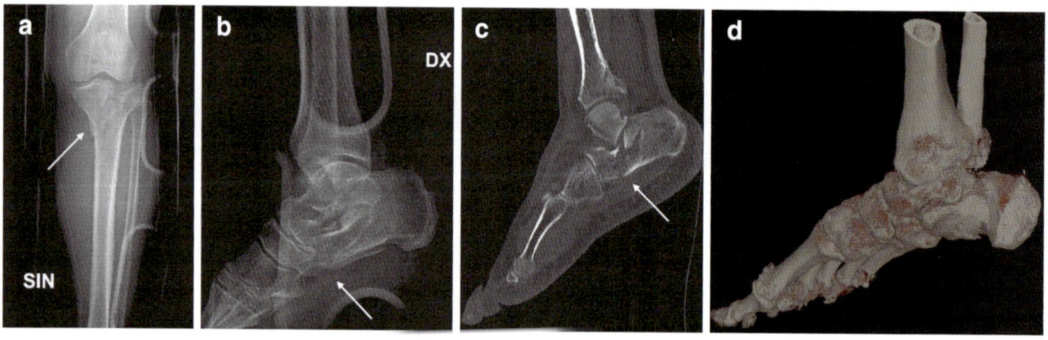

Fig. 2.8 Plain film views (**a**, **b**), CT in sagittal plane (**c**), and volume rendering CT (**d**) of a proximal tibia (**a**, *arrow*) and astragalo-calcaneal fractures (**b**, **c**, *arrows* and **d**) due to a fall from height

impact, as well as age and comorbidities of the patient. For example, landing on the feet can result in calcaneus and long bone fractures (Figs. 2.7 and 2.8), with secondary involvement of the lumbar and thoracic spine as the kinetic energy travels up the body [1].

The American College of Surgeons recommend that patients injured in falls from heights greater than 20 ft need to be taken to a trauma center, as the height is a factor exponentially related to the energy produced, resulting in life-threatening injuries [15].

2.7 Mechanisms of Blunt Trauma

Blunt trauma resulting injuries essentially depends from changes in pressure and shear forces produced by three main mechanisms [16–19]: (a) direct-impact, (b) compression, and (c) rapid acceleration/deceleration injuries (Table 2.1) [2].

2.7.1 Direct Impact

Direct-impact injuries are generally considered less dangerous, resulting, more often, in minor injuries, such as rubbings, ecchymosis, and/or hematomas that sometimes do not even require any imaging evaluation. In some cases, however, direct-impact injuries resulting from a motor vehicle accident, fall, or a direct blow from a moving object can lead to localized wall injuries, such as fractures of the skull, ribs, and sternum and sternoclavicular joint dislocation. Depending on the high kinetic energy, direct-impact forces may be transmitted through the body to the deeper tissues and organs, such as the brain, lungs, heart, liver, and spleen along the trajectory of the "force vector." In these cases, for example, a direct blow to the chest wall may cause significant vascular injuries requiring immediate treatment, even in the absence of skeleton fractures. Therefore, according to the energy delivered by the injury, a direct impact may evolve into a compression mechanism, as internal organs may be secondarily involved by compression/shearing forces. An example of direct injury is extra-axial brain hematoma (epidural, subdural, and subarachnoid/intraventricular) and intra-axial injury (cortical contusion, intracerebral hematoma) (Figs. 2.9 and 2.10). In blunt brain injuries, cortical contusion may occur when the brain is pushed against the irregular inner surfaces of the skull at the time of impact at the coup site or, more commonly, at the opposite site. This last is produced by the impact of the moving brain to a fixed point, and it is more dangerous when the blow occurs to the occiput, due to the irregular surfaces of the anterior and central skull base, with characteristic

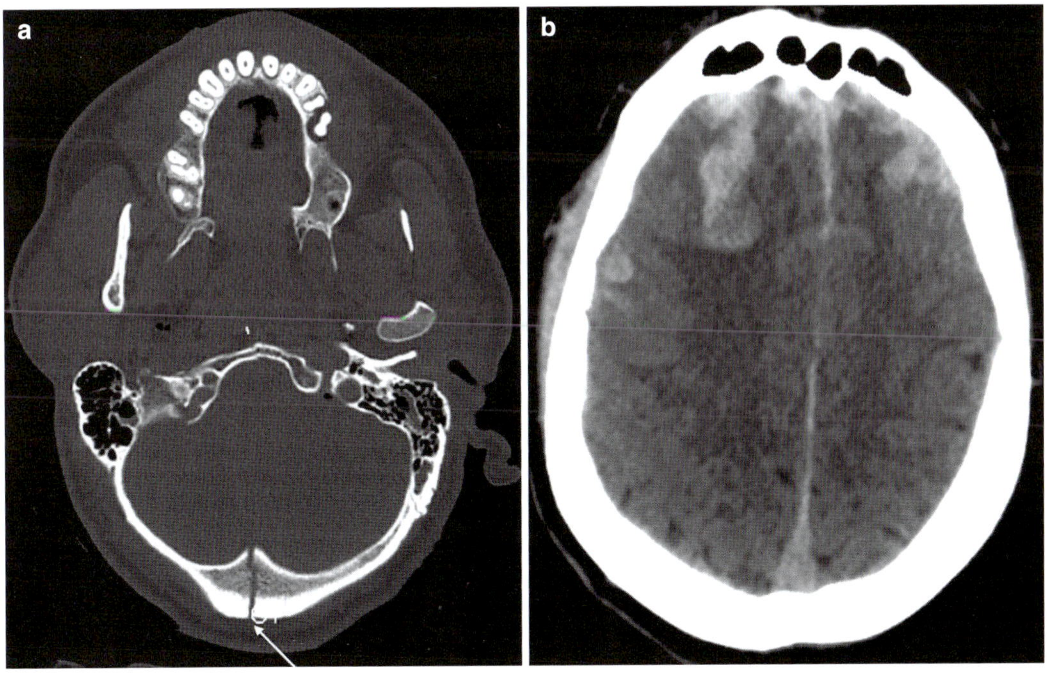

Fig. 2.9 MDCT scan in a patient underwent a direct trauma to the skull. Note the occipital fracture (**a**) in the site of the direct impact and the typical hemorrhagic contusions in the opposite site (frontal lobe) (**b**)

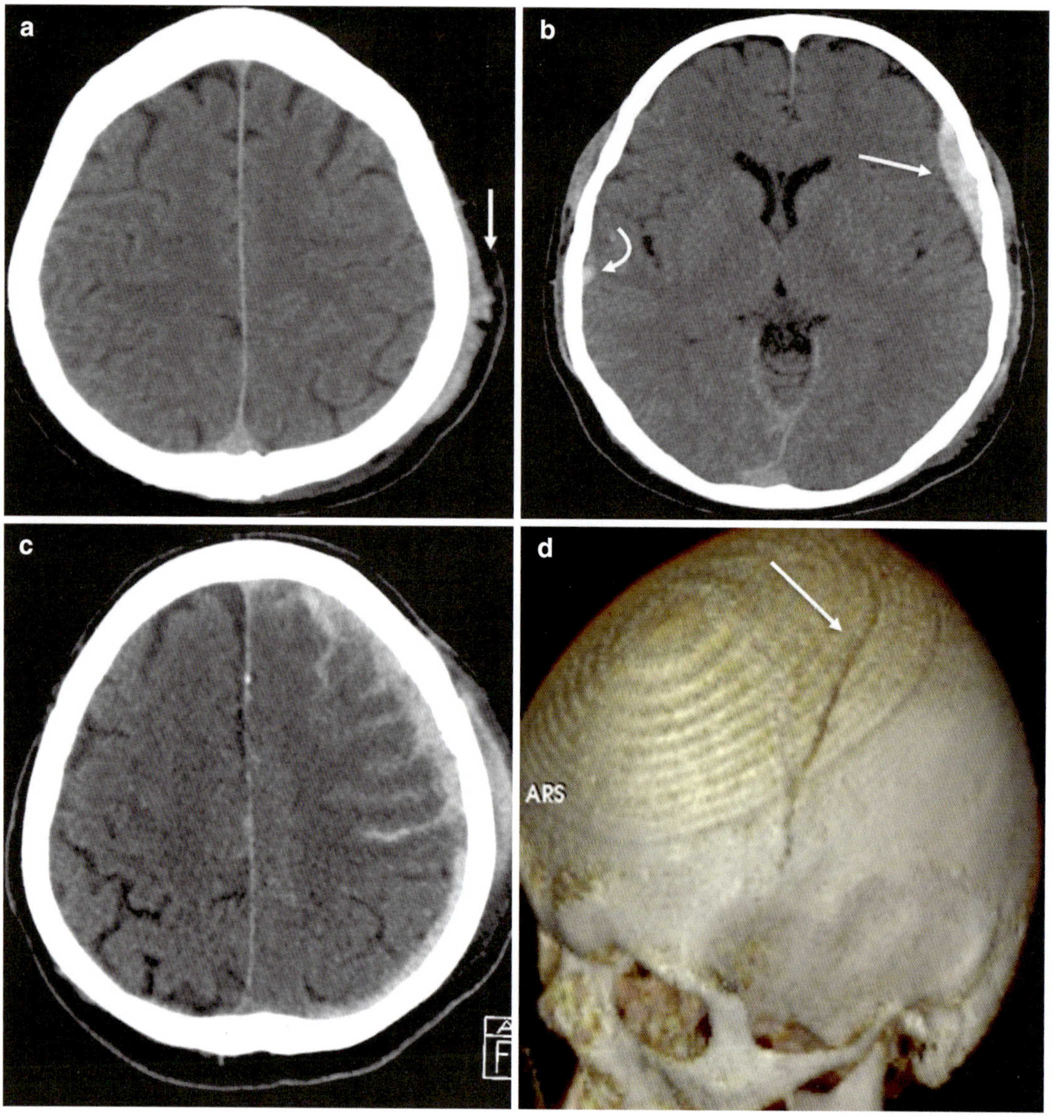

Fig. 2.10 MDCT scan in axial planes (**a**–**c**) and volume rendering (**d**) in a patient underwent a direct head trauma. There is a subgaleal (**a**, *arrow*) and epidural hematomas (**b**, *straight arrow*) in the site of impact and brain contusion on the opposite site (**b**, *curved arrow*). Note also a subarachnoid hemorrhage on the left side (**c**). Finally, volume rendering image demonstrates the parietal fracture (**d**, *arrow*)

hemorrhagic contusions seen in the inferior frontal and temporal lobes (Fig. 2.9) [20]. In the acute setting, a direct trauma to the skull, especially in elderly patients, requires a non-contrast CT scan, which represents the modality of choice, as it promptly allows depiction of intracranial traumatic lesions.

2.7.2 Compression Mechanisms

Compression injuries result from strike of the tissues to a fixed object like the chest/abdominal wall or spine, leading to organ rupture, contusion, or hemorrhage. These injuries may follow a direct impact or may be the result of a deceleration injury.

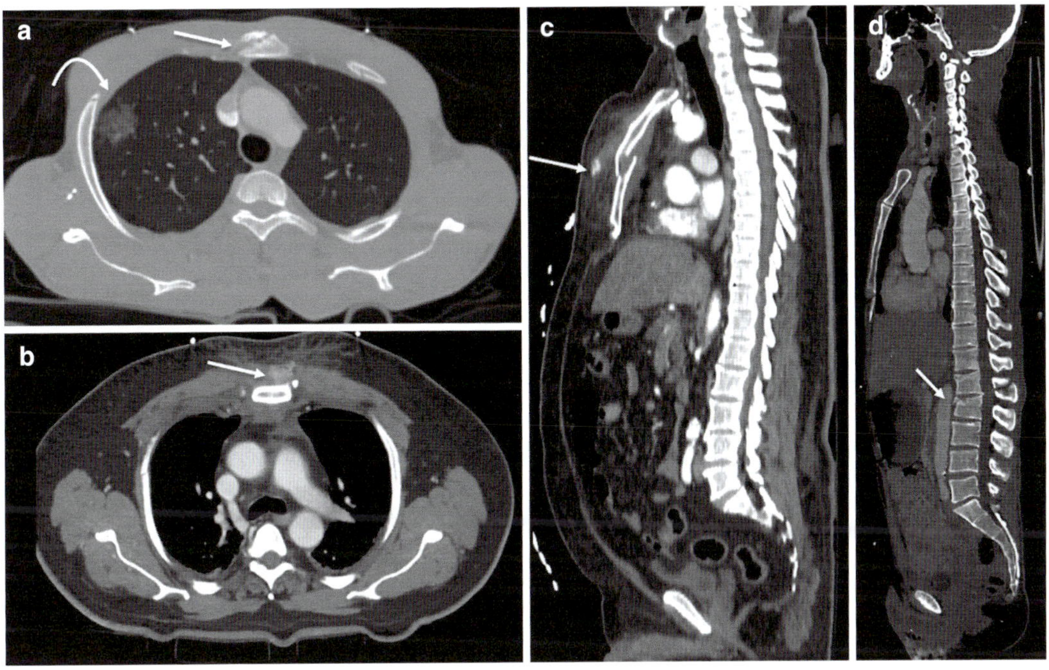

Fig. 2.11 Contrast-enhanced MDCT scan in a deceleration injury with thoracic compression and compression-distraction injury of the lumbar spine. There is a sternal fracture (**a**, *straight arrow*) with an adjacent active bleeding (**b**, **c**, *straight arrows*), rib fracture with pulmonary contusion (**a**, *curved arrow*), and fractures of the L2 body vertebra (**d**, *arrow*) and L1 spinous process (**d**)

Chest wall deformities are fairly common, as a result of compressive forces directed latero-laterally, *right-sided thoracic injuries* or *left-sided thoracic injuries*, and anteroposteriorly, *midline thoracic injuries*, which typically involve the sternum or the spine.

Of importance is the "flail chest" which involves three or more consecutive rib fractures in two or more sites and produces a free-floating, unstable segment of the chest wall [2, 27].

Thoracic compression may frequently cause lung parenchyma (contusion and laceration) (Fig. 2.11) and pleura (pneumothorax and hemothorax) injuries.

Furthermore, relatively uncommon but potentially life-threatening injuries include fractures, lacerations, and disruptions of the tracheobronchial tree and the diaphragm. Airway injuries constitute only a small fraction of admission to trauma centers, as many patients die before their arrival to the hospital. Rapid anteroposterior compression of the chest may cause lateral traction on the lungs and tearing of the bronchus from the fixed carina, with consequent rupture of the tracheobronchial tree [2, 21].

Rupture may also occur in the presence of an abrupt increase in pressure against a closed glottis or after compression of the trachea between the sternum and spinal column. Involvement of vital structures, as the heart and great vessels, represents the leading cause of death in compression injuries with a direct compression of the heart to the sternum and spine. The right ventricle is more often involved, as it is anterior and retrosternal. The heart can also be secondarily involved in the presence of delayed traumatic diaphragmatic hernias that can produce a cardiac tamponade by compression of the left ventricle due to direct herniation of abdominal contents into the pericardial sac or into the pleural space [22]. It is important to note that compression chest injuries may not be necessarily confined to

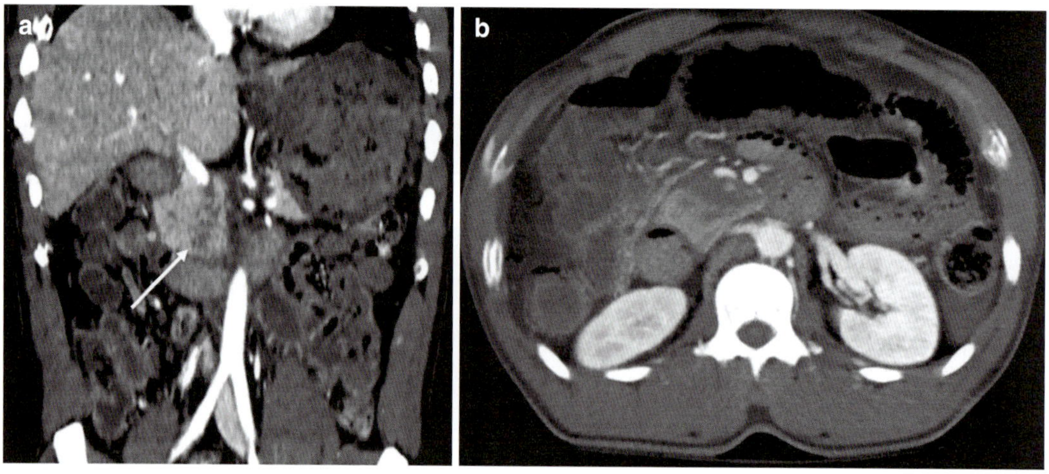

Fig. 2.12 Contrast-enhanced MDCT scan after a motor vehicle accident in coronal (**a**) and axial (**b**) views. Note a fracture of the pancreatic uncinate process (**a**, *arrow*)

the chest but also involve the homolateral abdominal side—*right- and left-sided thoracoabdominal injury*—causing abdominal solid-organ and/or very serious vessel injuries. Considerable forces are needed to injure directly the abdominal viscera [3]. Compression of the abdominal viscera occurs in the presence of a direct blow or of a direct compression against a fixed object (e.g., compression of the upper abdomen between vehicle chassis and spine) [8]. In order of frequency, the spleen represents the most commonly injured abdominal organ, followed by the liver, kidneys, small bowel and/or mesentery, bladder, colon/rectum, diaphragm, pancreas (Fig. 2.12), and major vessels [3]. Spleen trauma accounts indeed 40% of abdominal organ injuries; compression mechanisms may lead to minor injuries as contusions or lacerations and to critical lesions as shattered spleen (Figs. 2.13, 2.14, and 2.15). The spleen is quite commonly involved in the presence of left lower rib fractures (9–12 ribs). Conversely right lower rib fractures are often associated with liver injuries. The liver represents the second most frequently injured abdominal organ in blunt trauma, with a prevalence of liver injury between 1 and 8% [3]. As for the spleen, compression mechanisms may cause different traumatic liver injuries, from contusion to lacerations, with or without vascular and biliary involvement. Vascular injuries are more frequently related to deceleration mechanisms, as further described below. Abdominal compression mechanisms may also produce hollow viscus organ injuries. Despite bowel and mesenteric injuries are quite rare, representing only 4–15% of blunt abdominal trauma, they may carry devastating effects if missed. Even a short delay in diagnosis can result indeed in high morbidity and morbidity, these lesions are usually overlooked unless the clinical picture is highly suggestive, and in this context imaging has a pivotal role (Figs. 2.5 and 2.6). It is well known that delay in diagnosis and treatment of the hollow viscus injuries (HVI) results in early peritonitis and hemodynamic instability with increased mortality and morbidity. Hollow viscus injuries tend to occur secondary to three major mechanisms: a sudden increase in intra-abdominal pressure, direct compression of the viscera between the anterior abdominal wall and the vertebral columns, and secondary to shear forces resulting in pedicle injuries (in deceleration trauma).

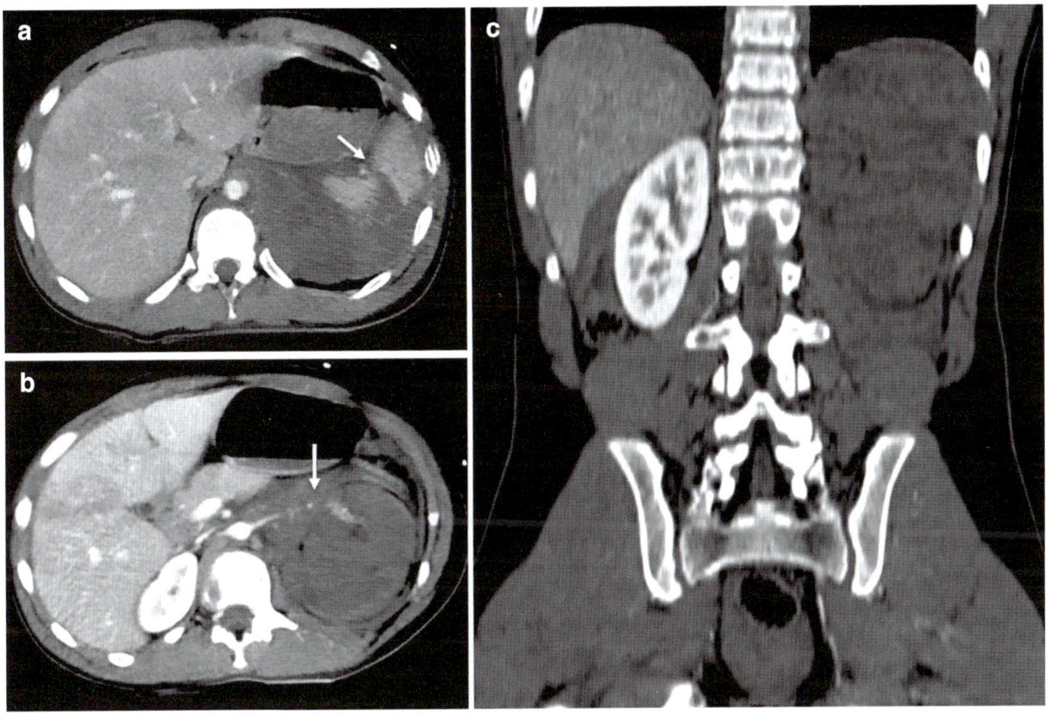

Fig. 2.13 Contrast-enhanced MDCT scan after a motor vehicle accident. There is a spleen fracture (**a**, *arrow*) and a transection of the left renal artery (**b**, *arrow*) with active bleeding and devascularization of the left kidney, anteriorly displaced (**c**). MPR in coronal view gives an optimal depiction of the above mentioned CT findings

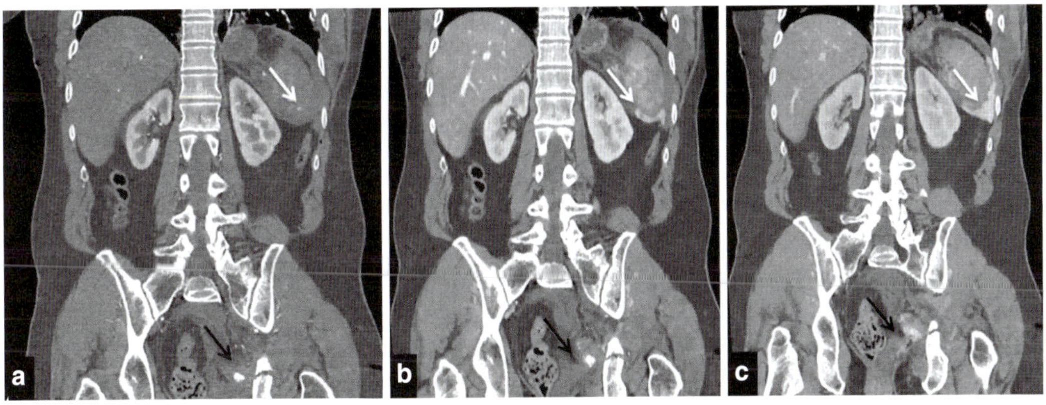

Fig. 2.14 Multiphasic MDCT scan in a patient with spleen fracture. Note the increasing arterial active bleeding (**a–c**, *arrows*) in two sites (i.e., around the spleen (*white arrows*) and in the left obturator space next to pelvic fracture (*black arrows*))

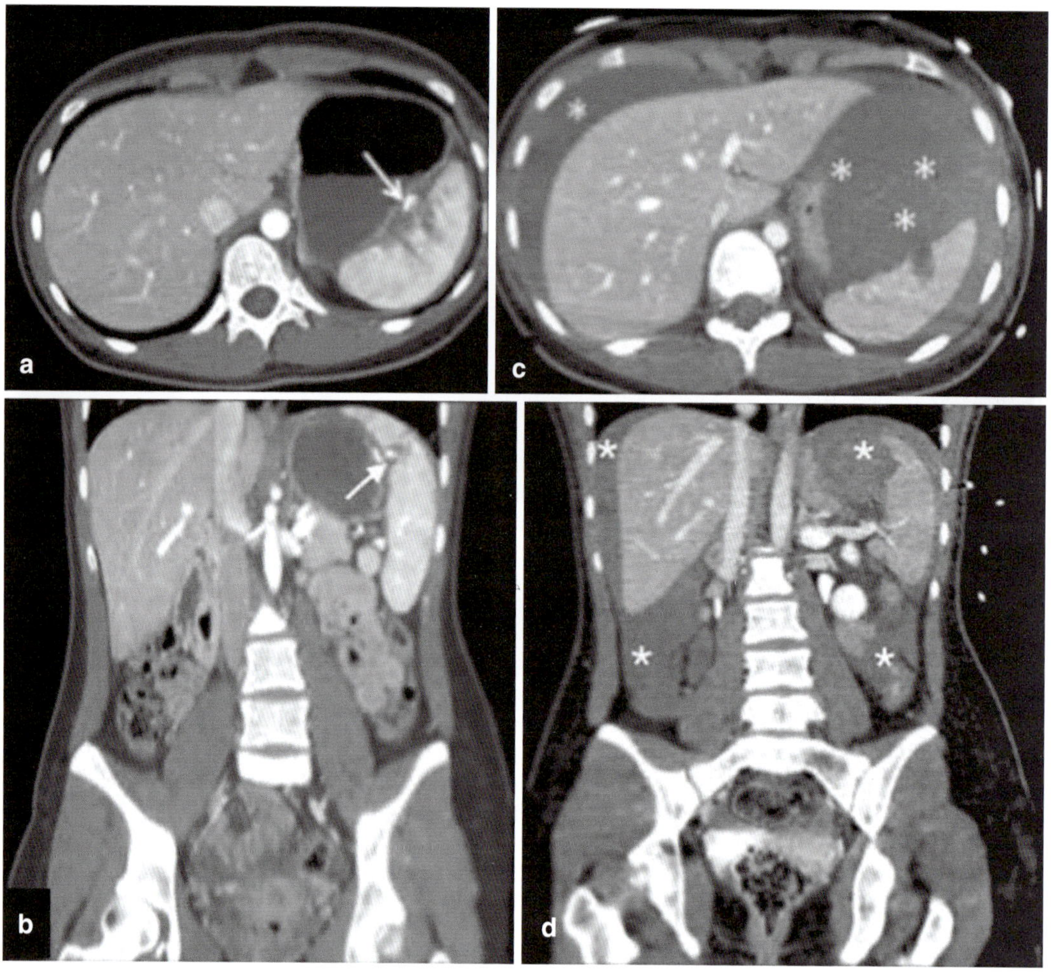

Fig. 2.15 Contrast-enhanced MDCT scan in a patient with splenic injury. At admission, there is a spot of active bleeding in axial (**a**, *arrow*) and coronal views (**b**, *arrow*) which was conservatively managed. After 6 h, the patient becomes hemodynamically unstable and therefore was immediately taken to the CT suite. Follow-up CT shows a large perisplenic hematoma with free hemoperitoneum (**c**, **d** *asterisks*)

Restraint devices as seat belts may produce mesenteric/bowel tears and contusions, as an abrupt increase of intra-abdominal pressure may cause deformation of hollow organs resulting in an increase intraluminal pressure that may lead to rupture of the intestinal wall, if overfilled. Thus, in patients presenting with possible seat belt injury, meticulous analysis of MDCT for signs of bowel and mesenteric trauma is required. In thoracolumbar trauma seat belt injuries represent a classical example of compression-distraction mechanism; they may determine characteristic horizontal fractures involving the anterior and posterior elements of the lumbar spine, frequently at L2 or L3 levels (Fig. 2.4). Other causes of spine compression injuries are falls from height, where axial loading or lateral flexion produces a visible loss of vertebral body height or disruption of the vertebral endplate (Fig. 2.16) [23]. Because of its retroperitoneal location, the pancreas is a very rare site at risk of injury in blunt abdominal trauma. However in the presence of severe anteroposterior compression, this organ may be secondly involved to impact against the spinal column, in connection with seat belt injuries, handlebar compression trauma, as well as deceleration injuries [24]. High compression forces in anteroposterior direction as in latero-lateral

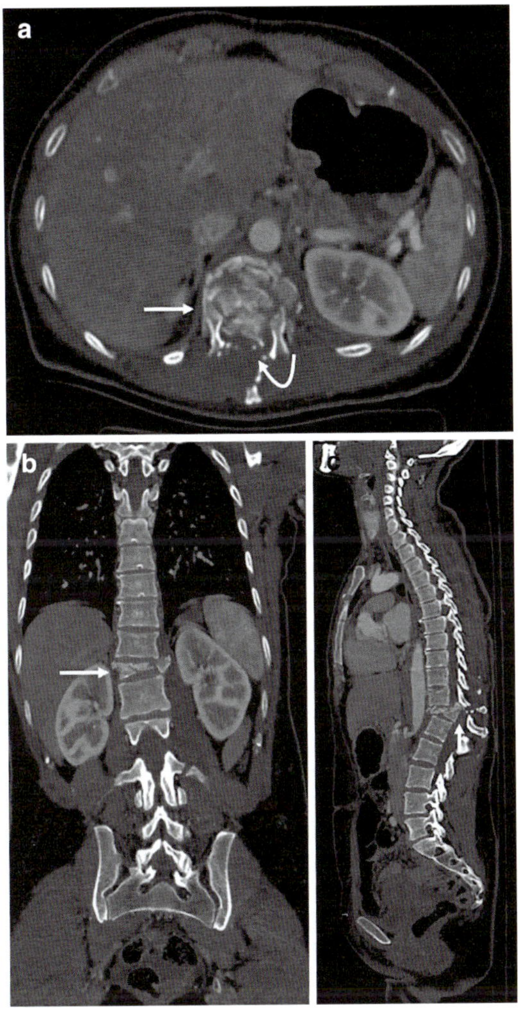

Fig. 2.16 Contrast-enhanced MDCT scan of a patient who underwent spine compression injury. Axial view (**a**) shows disruption of the vertebral body with height loss (**b**, coronal view, *arrow*) and posterior displacement of the lumbar spine (**c**, sagittal view, *arrow*)

direction are responsible for severe pelvic ring fractures (Fig. 2.3). Pelvic ring fractures are a common consequence of motor vehicle accidents or falls from heights. CT with multiplanar reformatted imaging (MPR) allows diagnosis, classification, and surgical planning of these complex fractures. In addition CT angiography is essential to detect active bleeding from injured bones, vessels, or soft tissues, as these lesions may cause significant hemorrhage, and it is mandatory for the radiologist to promptly recognize the source of blood loss [25].

2.7.3 Acceleration/Deceleration Mechanisms

Acceleration/deceleration injuries are the most common and lethal injuries in our part of the world. This mechanism is responsible for major head injuries, tracheobronchial tree injuries, aortic lesions, diaphragmatic ruptures, and mesenteric injuries. Rapid deceleration produces stretching and linear shearing at interfaces between fixed and mobile parts in the body, for example, at the gastrointestinal tract between mobile parts of bowel loops and their mesenteric attachments or avulsion of vascular pedicles with massive hemorrhage [2, 26]. Diffuse axonal injury (DAI) represents a dramatic consequence of shearing forces from deceleration injury; in this case a high-speed motor vehicle crash or prolonged head shaking leads to shearing and straining of the axonal cytoskeleton due to sustained acceleration/deceleration. Damage to the neurons occurs not only at the moment of the trauma but also in the hours, days, and years following the accident, due to Wallerian-type degeneration and progressive neuronal loss [20]. Blunt aortic injuries follow closely behind head injury as a cause of death after blunt trauma. Falls from heights and MVCs involving a pedestrian are other recognized causes. In these cases the mechanisms of injury are rapid deceleration, production of shearing forces, and direct luminal compression against points of fixation (especially at the ligamentum arteriosum). Many of these patients die from vessel rupture and rapid exsanguination at the scene of the injury or before reaching definitive care. Given that disruption of the aorta requires high-force trauma, other injuries are often present in the lung (contusions), pleura (hemothorax and pneumothorax), diaphragm, bones, and spines. Predictor markers of a possible aortic traumatic injury are fractures of the first and second ribs, even though patients with thoracic aortic injury may also not present any scratch or abrasion [5, 27]. Wilson et al. [28], as do many others, believe that traumatic aortic injuries must be suspected in all patients who have been involved in a motor vehicle accident in which speeds exceed 30 miles/h.

Before the advent of CT, this diagnosis was rarely made in the acute clinical setting. MDCT is the best diagnostic tool to quickly and accurately evaluate the aorta allowing not only to diagnose or rule out aortic injuries but also to show appropriate grade of injuries that correlates to the need of urgent treatment. This is of particular importance in the acute setting because these patients usually have more than one problem to solve at the same time: stabilizing the patient before taking any treatment may be the key to a successful outcome. Acceleration/deceleration mechanisms are fairly associated to cervical spine injuries, as this segment, with its wide range of motion and its relatively lack of supporting structures, is particularly susceptible to those mechanisms of trauma, resulting in lesions of the bone, ligaments, and soft tissues (Fig. 2.17) [29]. As previously mentioned in blunt abdominal injuries, deceleration/acceleration mechanisms produce lesions to solid organs in their points of attachment, for example, if the blunt force comes from the front to the upper right abdomen, the liver may be propelled in an anteroposterior direction; in this context, as the vena cava is relatively fixed, the liver lacerates along Cantlie's line. Conversely if the blunt force comes from the front to left upper abdomen, the left lobe of the liver is pushed backward, and the laceration is produced to the left of the falciform ligament. The hepatic veins and the portal veins or hepatic bile ducts may be avulsed in deep lacerations of this pattern of injury. Avulsion of vascular pedicles, due to shear forces, represents a critical lesion, as it leads to secondary devascularization of the supplied organ and massive hemorrhage. In the abdomen shearing forces may also disrupt ureteropelvic junction or ureterovesical junction that represents the only fixation points of the ureters; in this case laceration of the ureter and extravasation of contrast media can be easily detected on CT delayed scans [30].

2.8 Penetrating Injuries

Penetrating injuries result from an object entering the body and sometimes exiting the body along a defined trajectory (Table 2.1) [1]. It recognizes two major origins: stab and gunshot wounds. The velocity, size of the implement, direction of entry,

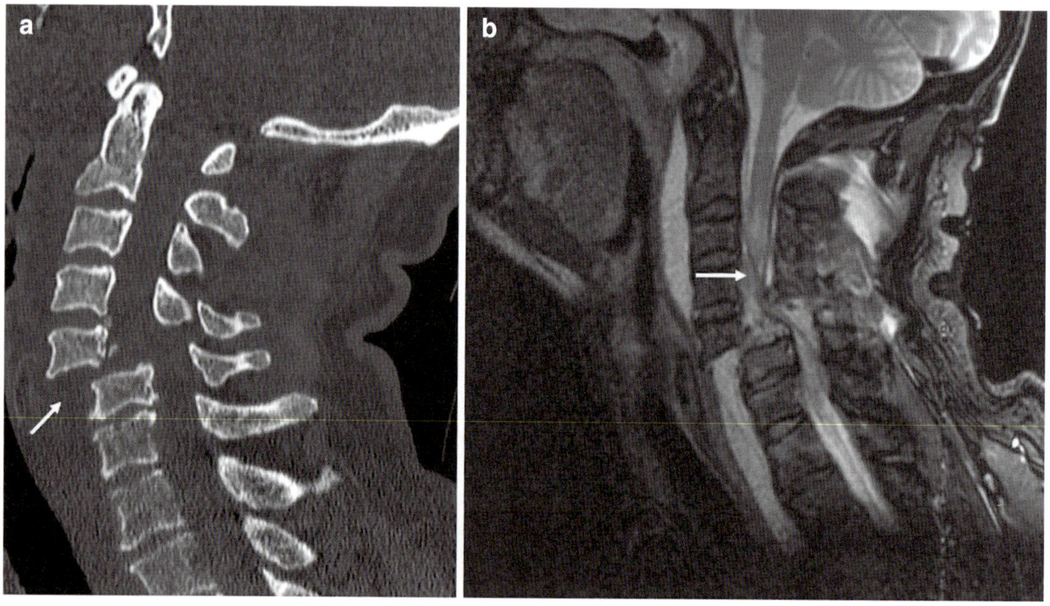

Fig. 2.17 CT scan (**a**) and MR in sagittal views (**b**) in a patient with a severe cervical spine injury (**a**, *arrow*) and spinal cord transection (**b**, *arrow*)

and above all the trajectory determine the lesions produced. As this mechanism of trauma always leads to open injuries, penetrating injuries are often associated with a non-sterile condition, with increased risk of bacterial growth that may require secondary surgical debridement.

2.9 Stab Wound

Stab wound victims usually present minor injuries that may benefit from nonoperative management. In these circumstances the radiologist has the role to exclude the presence of critical injuries that may be overlooked during clinical local wound examination. Local wound exploration may be indeed unreliable in obese patients or in back and flank injuries, as well as for long or obliquely oriented wounds. In this context CT allows identification of subtle internal lesions, providing a focused time-saving approach used to triage patients for surgery or expectant management [31]. Identification of wound track is important with imaging because it permits to select the anatomic sites at risk of lesion, as they are directly correlated with the trajectory of the knife. With the advances in imaging and introduction of multi-detector CT, path of the penetrating injuries is easier to identify thanks to multiplanar reformatted images (MPR) and volume rendering (VR) (Fig. 2.18). As a consequence, a dedicated technique has been reached manipulating isotropic data during post-processing analysis. This technique, defined as CT trajectography (CTT), allows a trajectory analysis marking the point of entry and rotating the cut planes on orthogonal planes to visualize the wound track in profile, in a double-oblique orientation. This technique seems to be more accurate in the presence of gunshot wounds compared with stab wounds, as lesion produced from stab wounds may be harder to see. Therefore, the radiologist has to look for indirect signs of knife wound tracks, depicting small discontinuous foci of gas on thin section images; however, migration of soft tissue emphysema along the body wall can hide the real track. Usually stab wound injuries involve the abdomen in the region of the flank, the epigastric region, the intercostal region, and the back. Approximately 50% of stab wounds to the anterior abdomen and 85% of stab wounds to the posterior abdomen may be safely managed without surgery [32]. Life-threatening injuries involve more frequently the left thoracic region, as a knife wound may damage the hearth and major vessels, with the hemomediastinum, hemothorax, and/or pneumothorax. In the abdomen the liver represents the most injured organ, followed by the small bowel and the colon. Lacerations, hematomas, and active extravasation are the most frequent lesions detected. Signs of small bowel injuries can be very difficult to recognize as a sign like pneumoperitoneum, that is, a significant specific predictor of significant small bowel lesions in blunt traumas in penetrating injuries is unremarkable, as free air can enter the peritoneal cavity by the knife wound or because there is a direct communication of the peritoneum with the outside air. The most common CT finding of intraperitoneal injury is free fluid, seen in 85% of patients, with an accuracy of

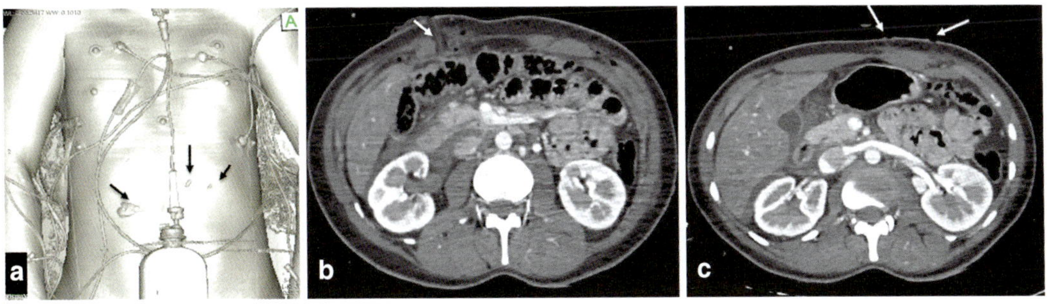

Fig. 2.18 Contrast-enhanced MDCT scan after a penetrating trauma. (**a**) Volume rendering image shows multiple holes in the skin from a knife (**a**, *arrows*). Axial scans (**b**, **c**) show inner tracts of the wounds (*arrows*)

CT evaluation next to 99% [31]. Lozano et al. [32] recommend a triple-contrast CT protocol in the presence of penetrating trauma, by using oral, intravenous, and rectal contrast in stable patients. However, this triple-contrast protocol is time-consuming and also presents some risks for aspiration of the contrast material.

2.10 Gunshot Wounds

Gunshot wounds are recognized as a specific mechanism of injury known as the "blast" effect. The bullet produces a cavitation within the tissues, a permanent hole, that typically measures between 0.5 and 2 cm; the surrounding tissue stretched and deformed by the bullet constitutes the temporary cavity, whose size is function of the velocity of the bullet and the elasticity of the tissues involved. The damage entity is indeed inversely related to tissue elasticity and directly correlated to the amount of energy dissipated [1, 30] (Fig. 2.19). Bullets may exit from the body or be retained (Fig. 2.20), with exit wounds usually larger than entrance wounds. Different studies have reported the high accuracy of CT for determining the bullet trajectory, peritoneal involvement, and visceral injuries in selected patients with gunshot wounds to the torso [8]. Bullet may follow an oblique path crossing different body regions, producing multiple lesions that need to be promptly recognized with imaging. It is mandatory for radiologists to depict the "nonlinear" trajectories and possible fragmentation of the bullet within the body that may result in effects on tissues remote to the tract. While less than one-third of knife wounds require surgical repair [33], gunshot wounds are responsible of internal wounds in over 80–90%, and in 75% of cases, more than one organ is injured [31]. As previously described wounding potential is inversely related to tissue elasticity, so dense tissues as the renal parenchyma, liver, spleen, and bones exhibit greater degrees of tissue destruction and fragmentation [34]. Delayed CT phases are often necessary to rule out lesions to ureters and bladder. Obviously the most dangerous injuries are those associated with transmediastinal gunshot wounds, with possible involvement of the heart and major vessels. Clearly gunshot wounds are often intentional resulting in critical lesion. In the past victims of transmediastinal injuries, when stable, were studied with panendoscopy, esophagogram, and echocardiography, with time and cost consumption. CT allows quick identification of injuries, defining the trajectory of the bullet, to avoid useless and invasive additional procedures. The most common transabdominal gunshot wounds involve the liver and bowel; retroperitoneal colonic segments may also be injured. CT provides excellent depiction of those injuries. If the bullet follows a transpelvic trajectory, a careful imaging evaluation of the rectum, bladder, and prostate should be taken, as in the past, the alternatives were time- and cost-consuming techniques like proctosigmoidoscopy and conventional cystography, in conjunction with digital rectal examination, but they were of limited accuracy in an unprepared bowel [8].

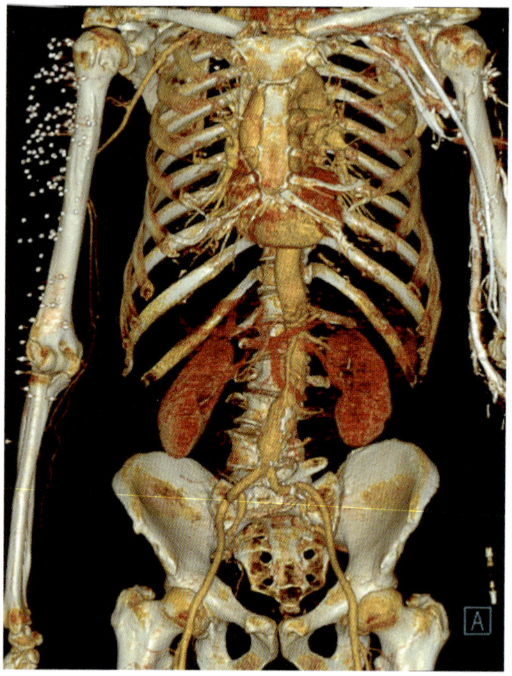

Fig. 2.19 Volume rendering image of a patient with multiple gunshot wounds on the right upper limb

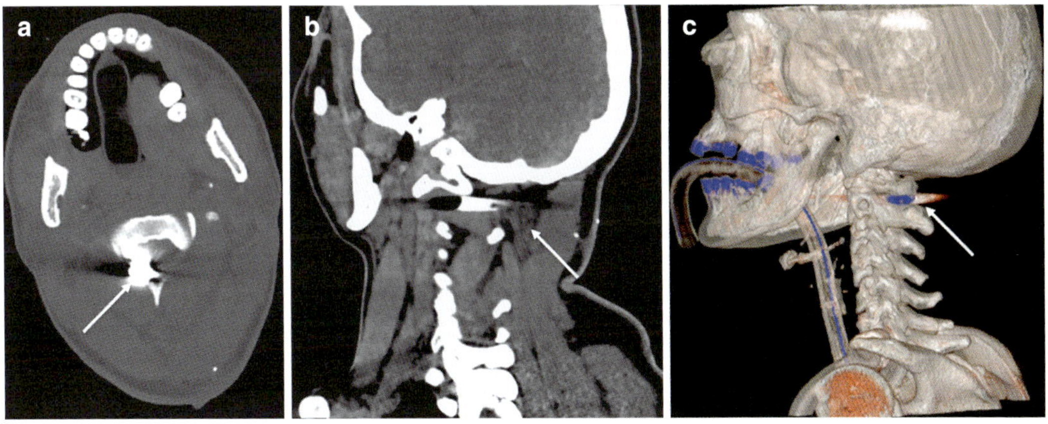

Fig. 2.20 CT scan of a patient with a bullet retained within C1–C2 space (**a**, **b**, *arrows*). Volume rendering image gives a exact identification of the retained bullet (**c**, *arrow*)

2.11 Blast Injuries

Nowadays radiologist should be aware of the mechanism of injury and the spectrum of lesions produced by improvised explosive devices (IEDs) as the ones encountered in terrorist attacks (Table 2.1). Ajay K et al. have recently published a work about imaging findings emerged from the victims of Boston marathon bombing [9]. The authors classify injuries produced by IED in four categories as primary, secondary, tertiary, and quaternary injuries. Primary injuries are caused by barotrauma, determined by the high-pressure blast wave and the subsequent sudden drop in pressure. The mechanisms of primary blast injuries are compression and shearing of tissues as the wave crosses the body and causes lesions to gas or fluid-filled structures as the ear, the lungs, and the bowel, as well as the brain. Lungs are involved because the combination of increased pressure and sudden decrease causes disruption of interalveolar septa, alveolar hemorrhage, and rupture. CT shows lung contusions, ground glass opacities, pneumothorax/hemothorax, as well as systemic air embolism caused by traumatic alveolar-venous fistulas [35]. Typically injuries are more severe at interfaces as between the lung and mediastinum, at the costophrenic angles, and at the intercostal spaces. Clinically victims will present cough, dyspnea, and hypoxia, known as "blast lung syndrome" [36]. Blast bowel injuries occur as a consequence of sudden compression in the positive pressure phase, followed by sudden expansion in the negative pressure phase of fluid-filled cavity, with associated shearing forces. Imaging shows bowel intramural hematoma, with possible pneumoperitoneum due to secondary perforation as stretching of mesenteric vessels with consequent mesenteric ischemia. Blast bowel syndrome is characterized by nausea, vomiting, melena, hematemesis, and peritonitis [9]. While for primary blast injuries the main mechanism can be attributable to a blunt mechanism, for secondary injuries the mechanism can be led to penetrating lesions. IEDs usually contain debris such as rocks, glass, screws, as well as bullets with the aim to increase the lethality of the devices, so secondary blast injuries are caused by the penetration of the debris thrown out from the bomb. These injuries can lead to critical injuries, if it involves the brain, the heart, or major vessels as minimal superficial injuries confined in soft tissues. Imaging is useful to detect fragments retained within the body and their relation to neurovascular structures and to depict subtle internal injuries in selected patients that may be missed. Tertiary blast injuries are caused by a combined mechanism (blunt and penetrating) and are the result of the crash of the victim against surrounding cars, walls, or fences. These injuries generally involve musculoskeletal segments, with bone fractures, as well as visceral injuries and closed head injuries. CT findings are usually similar to those encountered with victims of MVC and falls. Quaternary blast injuries are caused by thermal and inhalation injuries. Imaging plays a little role in this category of injuries.

Nowadays radiologists working in big cities have to be aware of lesion caused by IEDs as terrorism represents a matter of big concern, so knowing mechanism of lesion can be useful to understand findings in these particular categories of victims.

Conclusions

MDCT has revolutionized the management of polytraumatized patients. Victims of major injuries are often unconscious or may present multiple traumas; therefore, clinical evaluation may be unreliable. In this context radiologist plays the major role to quickly assess/rule out critical injuries and to guide the most tailored and timely management. Dedicated protocols and post-processing algorithms may allow definition of trajectories of penetrating lesions as well as depiction of subtle unexpected injuries related to specific mechanisms of trauma, such as contrecoup brain lesions in closed head injuries, spine fractures due to axial load forces, or vascular complications caused by shear forces before they become clinically evident. Knowledge of the mechanisms of injury means to know what to exclude/look for and how to do it, with the maximum concentration of time. Saving time by addressing victims to tailored management means saving lives. Imaging findings can make the difference between life, death, or serious disability. Hence, the patient's life is in the radiologist's hands (and eyes!) because important management decisions are taken on the basis of his report.

References

1. Bell L. Chapter 1: Mechanisms of injury. In: Nayduch D, editor. Nurse to nurse: trauma care. New York: McGraw-Hill Medical; 2009. Softcover; isbn:978-0-07-159677-0. p. 1–31.
2. Scaglione M, Pinto A, Pedrosa I, Sparano A, Romano L. Multi-detector row computed tomography and blunt chest trauma. Eur J Radiol. 2008;65(3):377–88.
3. Soto JA, Anderson SW. Multidetector CT of blunt abdominal trauma. Radiology. 2012;265(3):678–93.
4. Schueller G, Scaglione M, Linsenmaier U, Schueller-Weidekamm C, Andreoli C, De Vargas Macciucca M, Gualdi G. The key role of the radiologist in the management of polytrauma patients: indications for MDCT imaging in emergency radiology. Radiol Med. 2015;120:641–54.
5. Iacobellis F, Ierardi AM, Mazzei MA, Magenta Biasina A, Carrafiello G, Nicola R, Scaglione M. Dual-phase CT for the assessment of acute vascular injuries in high-energy blunt trauma: the imaging findings and management implications. Br J Radiol. 2016;89(1061):20150952.
6. Scaglione M. The use of ultrasound versus CT in the triage of blunt abdominal trauma: the European perspective. Emerg Radiol. 2004;10:296–8.
7. Hauser HMA, Bohndorf K. Acute multiple trauma: analysis of the spectrum of radiologic workup and time requirement. Emerg Radiol. 1998;5:84–91.
8. Elias DA, Lewis D, Meacock Khan LM, Bew D. Mechanisms of injury and CT findings in bowel and mesenteric trauma. Clin Radiol. 2014;69:639–47.
9. Singh AK, Ditkofsky NG, York JD, Abujudeh HH, Avery LA, Brunner JF, Sodickson AD, Lev MH. Blast injuries: from improvised explosive device blasts to the Boston Marathon bombing. RadioGraphics. 2016;36:295–307.
10. Matthes G, Stengel D, Seifert J, Rademacher G, Mutze S, Ekkernkamp A. Blunt liver injuries in polytrauma: results from a cohort study with the regular use of whole-body helical computed tomography. World J Surg. 2003;27:1124–30.
11. Wurmb TE, Frühwald P, Hopfner W, Keil T, Kredel M, Brederlau J, Roewer N, Kuhnigk H. Whole-body multislice computed tomography as the first line diagnostic tool in patients with multiple injuries: the focus on time. J Trauma. 2009;66:658–65.
12. Wallis LA, Greaves I. Injuries associated with airbag deployment. Emerg Med J. 2002;19:490–3.
13. Greingor JWL, Lazarus S. Chest and abdominal injuries caused by seat belt. South Med J. 2006;99(4):534–5.
14. Puac-Polanco V, Keyes KM, Li G. Mortality from motorcycle crashes: the baby-boomer cohort effect. Inj Epidemiol. 2016;3(1):19.
15. Auñón-Martín I, Doussoux PC, Baltasar JL, Polentinos-Castro E, Mazzini JP, Erasun CR. Correlation between pattern and mechanism of injury of free fall. Strategies Trauma Limb Reconstr. 2012;7:141–5.
16. Westaby S, Brayley N. ABC of major trauma. Thoracic trauma. BMJ. 1990;300:1639–43.
17. Brainard BJ, Slauterbeck J, Benjamin JB, et al. Injury profiles in pedestrian motor vehicle trauma. Ann Emerg Med. 1989;18:881–3.

18. Besson A, Saegesser F. A colour atlas of chest trauma and associated injuries. London: Wolfe Medical Publications Ltd. Part 1 and 2; 1982–1983.
19. Wintermark M, Schnyder P. Introduction to blunt trauma of the chest. In: Schnyder P, Wintermark M, editors. Radiology of blunt trauma of the chest. Berlin: Springer; 2000. p. 1–7.
20. Kim JJ, Gean AD. Imaging for the diagnosis and management of traumatic brain injury. Neurotherapeutics. 2011;8(1):39–53.
21. Scaglione M, Ronza R, Rossi C, Martino MT, Iacobellis F, Grassi R, Vaidya S. Acute tracheobronchial injuries. Medical Radiology. Springer; 2016. p. 1–11.
22. Co SJ, Yong-Hing CJ, Galea-Soler S, Ruzsics B, Schoepf UJ, Ajlan A, Farand P, Nicolaou S. Role of imaging in penetrating and blunt traumatic injury to the heart. RadioGraphics. 2011;31(4):E101–15.
23. Khurana B, Sheehan SE, Sodickson A, Bono CM, Harris MB. Traumatic thoracolumbar spine injuries: what the spine surgeon wants to know. RadioGraphics. 2013;33:2031–46.
24. Linsenmaier U, Wirth S, Reiser M, Körner M. Diagnosis and classification of pancreatic and duodenal injuries in emergency radiology. RadioGraphics. 2008;28:1591–601.
25. Pinto A, Niola R, Tortora G, Ponticiello G, Russo G, Di Nuzzo L, Gagliardi N, Scaglione M, Merola S, Stavolo C, Maglione F, Romano L. Role of multidetector-row CT in assessing the source of arterial haemorrhage in patients with pelvic vascular trauma. Comparison with angiography. Radiol Med. 2010;115(4):648–67.
26. Scaglione M, Pinto A, Pinto F, Romano L, Ragozzino A, Grassi R. Role of contrast-enhanced helical CT in the evaluation of acute thoracic aortic injuries after blunt chest trauma. Eur Radiol. 2001;11(12):2444–8.
27. Iacobellis F, Iadevito I, Ierardi AM, Carrafiello G, Perillo F, Nicola R, Scaglione M. Imaging assessment of thoracic cage injuries. Semin Musculoskelet Radiol. 2017;21(3):303–14.
28. Wilson RF, Arbulu A, Bassett JS, Walt AJ. Acute mediastinal widening following blunt chest trauma. Arch Surg. 1972;104:551–9.
29. Stabler A, Eck J, Penning R, Milz SP, Bartl R, Resnick D, Reiser M. Cervical spine: postmortem assessment of accident injuries—comparison of radiographic, MR imaging, anatomic, and pathologic findings. Radiology. 2001;221:340–6.
30. Alonso RC, Nacenta SB, Martinez PD, Sanchez Guerrero A, Garcia C. Fuentes kidney in danger: CT findings of blunt and penetrating renal trauma. RadioGraphics. 2009;29:2033–53.
31. Dreizin D, Munera F. Multidetector CT for penetrating torso trauma: state of the art. Radiology. 2015;277(2):338–55.
32. Lozano JD, Munera F, Anderson SW, Soto JA, Menias CO, Caban KM. Penetrating wounds to the torso: evaluation with triple-contrast multidetector CT. RadioGraphics. 2013;33:341–59.
33. Biffl WL, Moore EE. Management guidelines for penetrating abdominal trauma. Curr Opin Crit Care. 2010;16(6):609–61.
34. Lamb CM, Garner JP. Selective non-operative management of civilian gunshot wounds to the abdomen: a systematic review of the evidence. Injury. 2014;45(4):659–66.
35. Horrocks CL. Blast injuries: biophysics, pathophysiology and management principles. J R Army Med Corps. 2001;147(1):28–40.
36. Ritenour AE, Baskin TW. Primary blast injury: update on diagnosis and treatment. Crit Care Med. 2008;36(7 Suppl):S311–7.

Head Injuries

3

Claudia Lucia Piccolo, Alessia De Marco,
Nicola Maggialetti, Marcello Zappia,
Raffaella Capasso, Serena Schipani,
Ferdinando Caranci, and Luca Brunese

3.1 Introduction

Traumatic brain injuries (TBIs) are the leading cause of mortality and morbidity in patients younger than 40 years, affecting 1.7 million people every year in the USA. They are responsible for one-third of all injury-related deaths, whereas patients who survive may develop severe debilitating long-term sequelae [1–3].

They consist of a wide spectrum of diseases, defined as a whole as an "alteration in brain function, or other evidence of brain pathology, caused by an external force." The causes may vary depending on patient's age: abuse traumas are most commonly observed in infants, while traumatic and sports related injuries are seen in toddlers and children. Motor vehicle accidents involve most commonly young adults, whereas the elderly population is more prone to accidental falls [4–9].

TBIs are clinically divided into minor, mild, moderate, and severe traumas by using the Glasgow Coma Scale (GCS), the most commonly used grading scale to evaluate the entity of head injuries within the first 48 h, which aims to provide a uniform approach to the clinical assessment of patients involved in acute head traumas. GCS is the sum of three components which are eye opening, motor response, and verbal response; a minor trauma has a GCS = 15; mild, GCS > 13; moderate, GCS 9–12; and severe, GCS < 8.

An additional TBI clinical classification is provided by the Brain Injury Interdisciplinary Special Interest Group of the American Congress of Rehabilitation Medicine, based on the loss of consciousness, loss of memory for events occurred immediately before or after trauma, changes in mental status, and focal neurologic deficits. According to this classification, a mild trauma is defined as a physiologically disruption of brain functions, evaluated by the presence of one of the previous described criteria; additional findings are no abnormalities on computed tomography (CT) scan, GCS > 12, no surgical lesions, and length of hospital recovery less than 48 h. Moderate trauma is defined as a GCS of 9–12, hospital recovery of at least 48 h, surgical intracranial lesions, and positive CT scan findings. Severe traumas are evident at the moment of clinical presentation.

C.L. Piccolo, M.D. (✉) • A. De Marco
N. Maggialetti • M. Zappia • R. Capasso • S. Schipani
F. Caranci • L. Brunese
Department of Medicine and Health Sciences, University of Molise, Contrada Tappino, Campobasso, Italy
e-mail: clapiccolo@libero.it

V. Miele, M. Trinci (eds.), *Diagnostic Imaging in Polytrauma Patients*,
https://doi.org/10.1007/978-3-319-62054-1_3

Chronologically, TBIs are divided into primary (injuries occurring at the time of impact) and secondary lesions (lesions occurring after the initial injury, i.e., cerebral herniation, swelling, ischemia, infection, hydrocephalus), resulting from complication of physiological response to injury. Secondary injuries are potentially preventable by stabilizing the patient, by monitoring vital parameters, and, in some cases, by performing decompressive hemicraniectomy [10–14].

Other classifications are based on the mechanism of injury (open or blunt trauma) and on the location, dividing them into intra-axial lesions (cortical contusions, diffuse axonal injury, intracerebral hematoma) and extra-axial lesions (subdural, epidural, subarachnoid, and intraventricular hematomas).

Given these data, it is easy to understand the significative role of imaging in this clinical setting, since its goals are to identify treatable lesions, assist to prevent secondary damage, and provide prognostic information.

In this chapter we aim to review the most commonly encountered and severe brain injuries and their complications.

3.2 Imaging Techniques

CT without contrast media injection is the imaging technique of choice to assess acute TBI because it is rapidly available, fast, compatible with life-support devices, and really sensitive to detect neurosurgical emergencies; in fact, basing on CT findings, the physician can decide how to manage the patient, if surgically or medically [15, 16].

A relatively recent cost-effectiveness study showed that the liberal use of CT in this field is justified because the possible consequences of undiagnosed brain injury are unacceptable. A further study showed that an early CT scan is a feasible and cost-saving management procedure [17, 18].

Several decisional algorithms have been proposed to assess the best clinical management of head traumas; one study proposes to quickly perform CT scan for patients with a GCS < 13; another study proposes an algorithm based on three risk categories (low, moderate, and high risk), advocating the use of CT scan for the latter one and close observations for the other groups, reserving CT for patients exhibiting clinical deterioration [19, 20].

Several decision rules about the use of CT scans in patients with minor trauma have been proposed, and the most well known are the New Orleans Criteria and the Canadian CT Head Rules [21–23].

The first one proposes CT for patients older than 60 years, with headache, vomiting, short-term memory defect, or injury above the level of the clavicles. The Canadian CT Head Rule decision rules indicate CT for medium-risk patients (retrograde amnesia more than 30 min in duration and a severe mechanism of injury) and high-risk patients (GCS < 15 after 2 h from the injury, suspected skull fractures, vomiting, and at least 65 years of age).

CT scan is characterized by some drawbacks, because, while it is able to detect acute hemorrhages and hemorrhagic contusions, some parenchymal injuries are difficult to detect, such as diffuse axonal injury, brainstem injury, and deep gray matter trauma. Although their misdiagnosis may not impair the treatment, their detection can be helpful to better understand unexplained neurological deficits.

In a trauma setting, images must be reviewed with brain, subdural, and bone windows. Bone window helps to assess skull fractures; the images are then reconstructed in multiple planes to increase the accuracy of interpretation and avoid misses (Fig. 3.1).

The use of contrast media is reserved to evaluate the vascular structures at submillimeter resolution. It should be performed using a rapid contrast bolus injection with vessel tracking; the classic imaging parameters are a slice thickness of 1.25 mm with a 0.625-mm overlap and a bolus

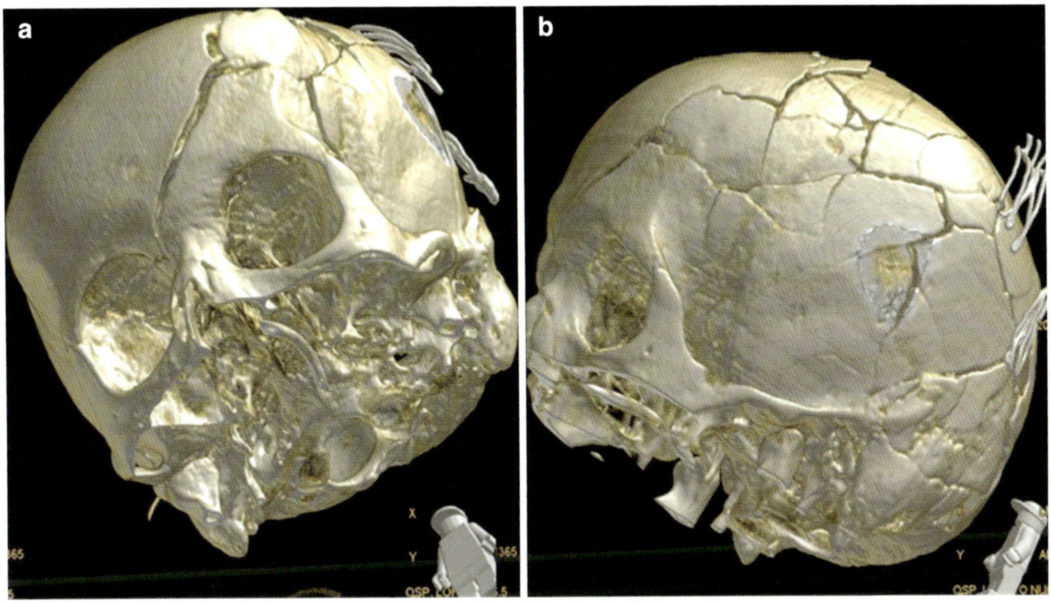

Fig. 3.1 (**a**, **b**) Three-dimensional CT reconstructions. Comminute cranial vault fracture, well delineated on 3D reconstructions

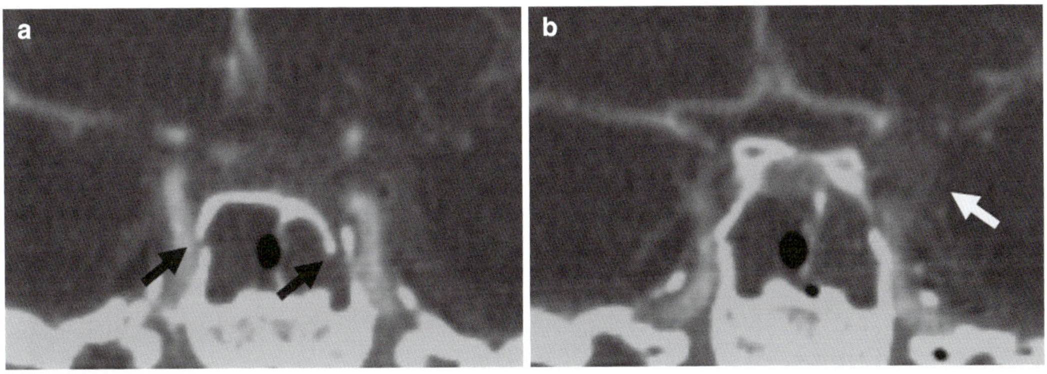

Fig. 3.2 (**a**, **b**) CT angiography (coronal reconstructions). Presence of bilateral sphenoid fractures (*black arrows*); the left internal carotid artery is interrupted at the supraclinoid segment from dissection, associated with a small hemorrhagic collection (*white arrows*)

injection rate between 3 and 4 mL/s. Its use is required when a vascular injury is suspected, such as pseudoaneurysm, carotid–cavernous fistula, laceration–extravasation, and dissection. It is performed in cases of penetrating head injury or skull base fractures traversing the carotid canal or a venous sinus also (Fig. 3.2). When these findings are positive, a catheter angiography must be performed to confirm and to treat the vascular injuries [24–28].

In some diagnostic dilemma not resolved by CT scans, magnetic resonance imaging (MRI) can serve as a problem-solving tool, since, owing to its higher contrast resolution for soft tissues, it is by far more capable than CT to detect all the stages of the hemorrhage, diffuse axonal injury, small subdural collections (the only indicator of child abuse), and ischemia.

Nevertheless, MRI has some downsides in the emergency settings, owing to long imaging times, incompatibility of many medical devices, insensitivity to acute subarachnoid hemorrhage, and excessive sensitivity to patient's motion. The key sequences are fluid-attenuated inversion recovery (FLAIR), gradient-recalled echo (GRE) or better susceptibility-weighted images (SWIs), and diffusion-weighted imaging (DWI). FLAIR is a T2-weighted sequence with suppression of the cerebrospinal fluid, improving detection of lesions in periventricular regions and cerebral cortex; it is very sensitive to cortical contusions, diffuse axonal damage, and subarachnoid hemorrhage. GRE sequences are particularly sensitive to blood breakdown products and can easily depict small areas of micro-hemorrhage not visible on CT. The blood products result in areas of signal loss because of the alteration of local magnetic susceptibility. This sequence is particularly indicated to evaluate subacute and chronic TBI, since hemosiderin can persist indefinitely. SWI is the most sensitive sequence for evaluating petechial hemorrhage (Fig. 3.3); this is a high-spatial-resolution three-dimensional gradient echo technique involving phase post-processing that enhances the paramagnetic properties blood products. By using this sequence, a mask is created to enhance the phase difference between susceptibility artifacts and surrounding tissue, and the contrast-to-noise ratio is optimized by increasing the mask and magnitude images; the phase images are sensitive to regions of local alteration of the magnetic field caused by some substances, such as hemorrhage, iron, and so on. SWI is three to six times more sensitive than GRE to detect hemorrhagic diffuse axonal injuries. A potential drawback of this sequence is the signal loss within the veins because of the magnetic properties of the intravascular deoxygenated hemoglobin and the resultant phase differences with adjacent tissues; to avoid misinterpretation and to minimize partial volume effects, it is auspicable to adjust the thickness of the minimal intensity projection to the brain size [29–36].

DWI is the sequence of choice when an acute diffuse axonal injury (Fig. 3.4) or ischemia is suspected. DWI is based on the random motion of water molecules (Brownian motion), which is affected by the intrinsic speed of water displacement based on tissue properties and type (gray matter, white matter, cerebrospinal fluid). In the nervous system, water diffusion is impeded by cell membranes, myelin sheaths, proteins, and all the subcompartment structures within the living nervous cell; therefore water diffusion is faster in the extracellular than in the intracellular space. When water molecules move from the extracellular space to the intracellular one, the overall diffusion is restricted; this restriction correlates with cytotoxic edema, allowing the early election of ischemia [37, 38].

Diffusion tensor imaging (DTI) is sensitive to the spatial orientation of water diffusion and allows the virtual reconstruction of axonal networks within the brain by observing restricted water diffusion; in healthy white matter, there is a greater diffusion along the long axis of the axonal bundles rather than the radial ones. The concept behind DTI is that water diffusion in the white matter tracts occurs in one direction rather than randomly, which is called anisotropy. The key indices of DTI are fractional anisotropy (FA) and ADC. FA is sensitive to changes in white matter integrity providing information about the degree of white matter damage; therefore, in the presence of an acute TBI in which a huge damage of white matter occurs, FA values are expected to be very low.

On the other hand, ADC correlates with the average magnitude of water movement in a voxel; so, it increases in the presence of vasogenic edema and decreases with cytotoxic edema and when diffusion is impeded by injured swollen cells [39–41].

Magnetic resonance spectroscopy (MRS) evaluates noninvasively brain chemical environment, revealing posttraumatic neurometabolite abnormalities when conventional neuroimaging is normal. The most common brain metabolites measured are sensitive to hypoxia, neuronal injury, inflammation, and energy dysfunction;

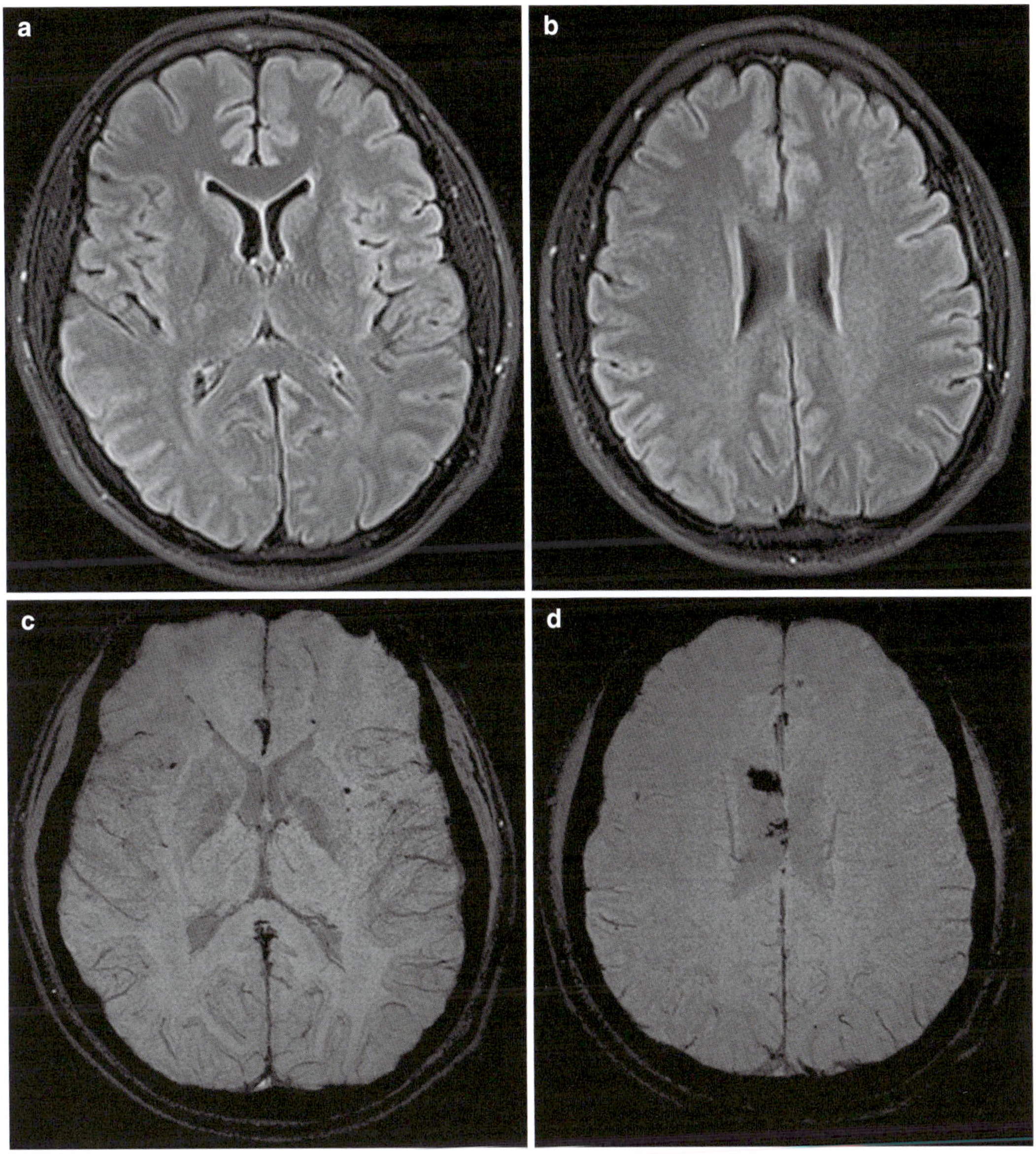

Fig. 3.3 (**a**, **b**) FLAIR axial sections; (**c**, **d**) SWI axial sections. Presence of small hemorrhagic foci in the right portion of the corpus callosum, the bilateral external capsulae, and the left fronto-mesial region due to axonal damage (**c**, **d**), not identifiable on FLAIR (**a**, **b**)

they include *N*-acetylaspartate (NAA), creatine (Cr), choline (Cho), glutamate (Glu), lactate, and myoinositol. Basically, a reduction of NAA (indicating either neuronal loss or neuronal/mitochondrial dysfunction) occurs as a dynamic process after TBI: it remains low in patients with poor prognosis and returns normal in patients with good outcomes.

Cho is a marker for membrane synthesis or repair, inflammation, or demyelination and is typically increased in TBI.

Several studies performed on the brain of injured patients found a great increase in Cho levels and decrease in NAA levels, indicating membrane disruption and increased cell membranes turnover on one hand and a permanent neuro-

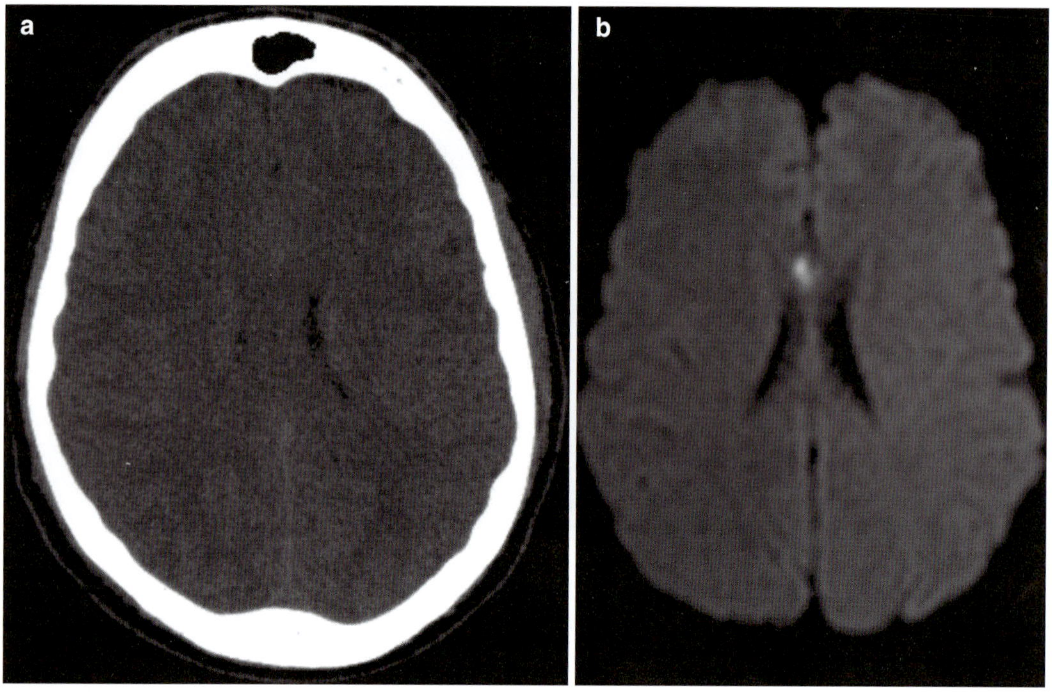

Fig. 3.4 (**a**) CT scan; (**b**) DWI on axial plane. Presence of a restricted diffusion focal area located in the right portion of the corpus callosum, not identifiable on CT

axonal damage or reversible axonal dysfunction on the other hand, respectively [42–47]. Cr is a marker for intact brain metabolism, and an increased Cr level may be an expression of repair mechanism associated with increased mitochondrial function in areas of injury. After a TBI an alteration of levels of Glu, the brain's major neurotransmitter, as well as an increase in lactate may be observed.

Cr peak is the most stable index in a wide spectrum of conditions, so allowing a ratio with the other metabolites.

3.3 Extra-axial Injuries

3.3.1 Fractures

A close examination of the scalp should be one of the first steps to perform while interpreting a trauma head CT, since the identification of a soft tissue lesion helps to identify the coup site, which must be carefully inspected to recognize any underlying skull fracture, a soft tissue laceration, and the eventual presence of foreign bodies.

The three main types of fractures are the linear (the most common), depressed, and basal fractures. The linear one is the less commonly associated with parenchymal injuries, although it has a high clinical impact when involving bones close to the vascular structures. Therefore, temporal bone fractures are more prone to injure the middle meningeal artery, with a following arterial epidural hematoma, while occipital ones can damage venous sinuses, with a venous epidural hematoma.

On axial plane they can be easily missed, and a close examination of the "scout" may help to recognize them.

Depressed fractures are more often associated with brain injuries, and they are usually surgically explored to evaluate a potential dural tear, to remove some fragments, and to reduce the risk of infections.

Basal fractures are the most dangerous from a prognostic point of view, since they can be complicated by injuries to the cranial nerves and vessels of the base of the skull (the petrous and cavernous portions of the internal carotid artery (ICA), the transverse and sigmoid sinuses).

Temporal bone fractures can be classified as "longitudinal" versus "transverse" with respect to the long axis of the petrous temporal bone or as "otic capsule sparing" versus "otic capsule involving" fractures. Longitudinal TBF is the most commonly (95%) encountered and is often associated with a fracture extending to the squamosal portion of the temporal bone. It typically spares the otic capsule but may involve the ossicles, resulting in conductive hearing loss. It is usually associated with facial paresis due to the facial nerve injury.

Transverse fracture is much less common and results from an occipital impact. It is more prone to injure the otic capsule, resulting in sensorineural hearing loss and/or facial nerve injury.

Independently from this classification, many fractures, mixed or obliquely oriented, can be identified, thanks to the new multislice techniques and the possibility to reconstruct them on multiple planes [48–51].

3.3.2 Vascular Injuries

Blunt cerebrovascular injuries (BCVIs) include carotid and vertebral artery injuries, occurring in the setting of either generalized multitrauma or direct craniocervical trauma.

Some recent studies report a prevalence ranging from 1.1 to 1.6% among all blunt traumas, while among severely injured patients, the prevalence may be as high as 2.7%. The morbidity and mortality associated with vascular injuries are usually attributed to cerebral or cerebellar infarction. Blunt carotid artery injuries are associated with morbidity and mortality rates of 32%–67% and 17%–38%, respectively. The morbidity rate for blunt vertebral artery injuries is 14–24%, and the mortality rate is 8–18%. Considering only BCVI-specific deaths, the mortality rate for untreated BCVI ranges from 25 to 38% [52–55].

Several studies advocate an early treatment to prevent or limit the infarction development after a vascular injury; however, some authors prefer to adopt a nonoperative management with anticoagulants or antiplatelet therapy. In selected patients the endovascular treatment can be performed [56, 57].

The gold standard examination to diagnose a vascular injury is the four-vessel digital subtraction angiography, which is characterized by some drawbacks, being invasive and associated with some rare complication such as stroke. On the other hand, CT scans with contrast media injection are widely accepted because of its rapidity, safety, and noninvasivity.

The mechanism responsible for cerebrovascular injury seems to be related with the longitudinal stretching of the artery beyond its mechanical limits, with partial or complete loss of mural integrity; vertebral artery injuries occur when spinal subluxation or dislocation stretches the relatively fixed vertebral artery over the adjacent bone structures, or against the dural margins in cases of craniocervical junction injury [58]. Displacement of bone fragments from fractures of the skull base or cervical spine can lead to direct injury to the carotid (Fig. 3.2) or vertebral arteries, respectively. An ICA injury may occur also with a strong hyperflexion of the head or a posterior displacement of mandible fragments, crushing the ICA between the mandible and the spine [59–61] (Fig. 3.5).

In the acute setting, a vascular damage is suspected in the presence of fixed lateralizing or central neurologic deficits that are incongruent with the results of brain imaging or when imaging signs of unexplained cerebral or cerebellar ischemic stroke are present.

Additional clinical signs include active hemorrhage from the mouth, nose, ears, or open wounds, an expanding neck hematoma, cervical bruit in a patient younger than 50 years, transient ischemic attack or amaurosis fugax, pulsatile tinnitus, and Horner syndrome.

Signs and symptoms suggestive of posttraumatic carotid cavernous fistula include orbital pain; pulsatile exophthalmos; chemosis; proptosis; palsies of cranial nerves III, IV, or VI; and blurred vision.

It is a shared opinion that patients with clinical or imaging evidence of severe craniofacial or

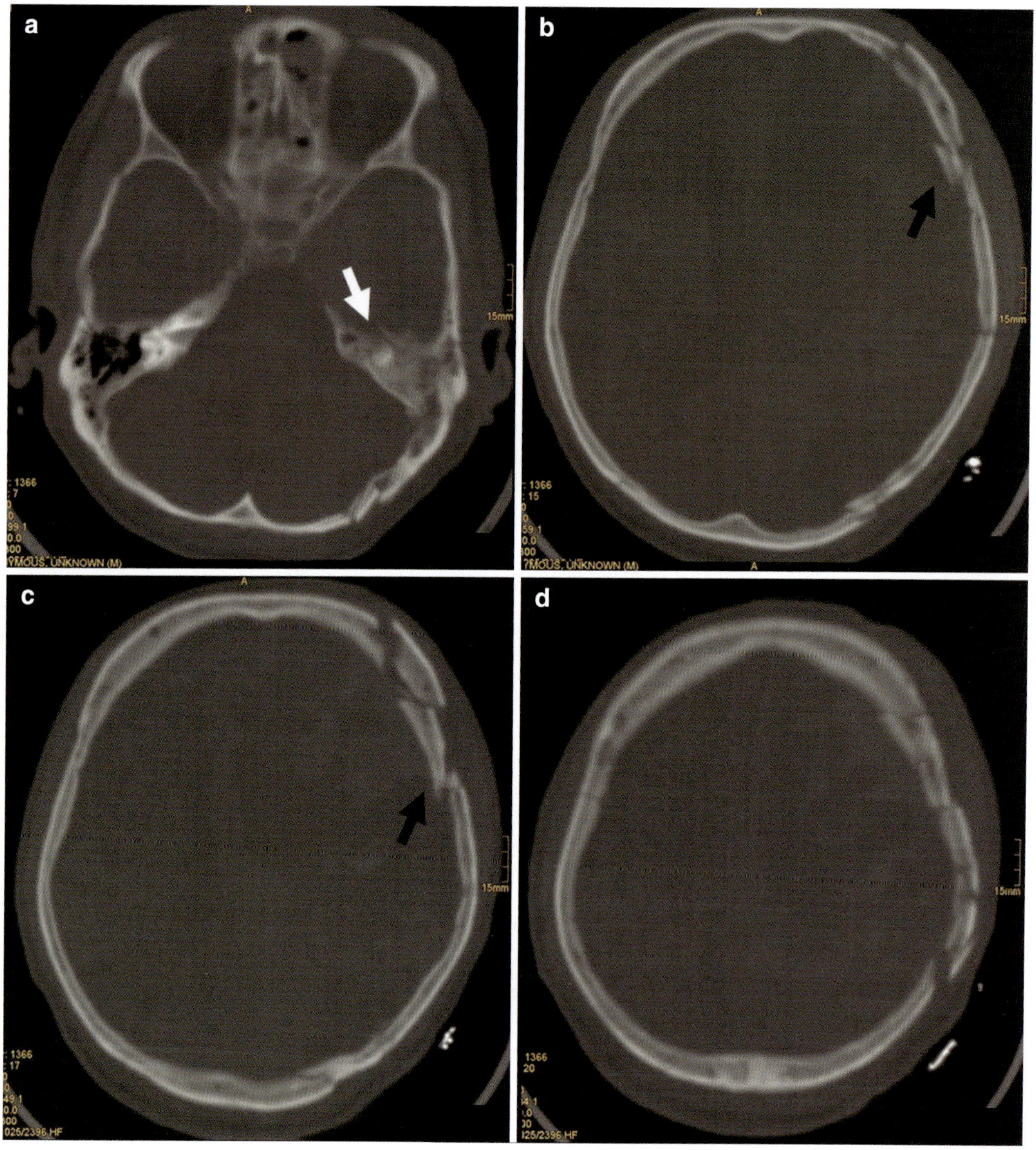

Fig. 3.5 (**a–d**) CT scan. Presence of comminuted fractures in the left occipital and frontal regions with depressed bone fragments (*black arrows*); a longitudinal left temporal fracture is associated (*white arrow*)

neck trauma are considered to suffer from brain vascular injury. In fact some studies reported that central skull base fractures and those involving the carotid canal are risk factors for blunt carotid artery injury and that severe facial fractures (Le Fort II and III injuries) and diffuse axonal injury have been identified as independent risk factors for carotid artery injury.

Several studies have identified cervical spine injuries as predictors of blunt vertebral artery injury, especially those involving C1–C3, the transverse foramen or other lateral vertebral elements, and subluxation–dislocation [62]. The so-called Denver criteria group together the most common risk factors for vascular injuries, including Le Fort II or III facial fractures, basilar skull fractures involving the carotid canal, diffuse axonal injury with a Glasgow Coma Scale score under 6, cervical spine fracture patterns that involve C1–C3, cervical spine fracture extending into a transverse foramen, cervical spine subluxation, and near hanging with anoxic brain injury. In addition, a major chest trauma (injury scale score > 3) has also been associated with vascular injuries [63, 64].

The subtypes of traumatic cerebrovascular injury can range from minimal intimal injury, raised intimal flap, separation of the intima from the media resulting in dissection, and medial and adventitial perforation with the consequent pseudoaneurysm to complete vascular transection or occlusion. *The minimal intimal injuries* appear as areas of luminal irregularity best appreciated on multiplanar or three-dimensional reformatted images.

Raised intimal flaps appear as linear intraluminal filling defects rising from the arterial wall [64, 65].

Dissection with intramural hematoma can either be focal or involve a long arterial segment. The hematoma causes mural thickening which may be eccentric or circumferential. Luminal narrowing may be minimal to nearly occlusive and is usually eccentric [66–70].

ICA dissection occurs more commonly in the cervical and petrous segments of the artery, and it is highly suspected in the presence of a skull base fracture near the carotid canal. Also the distal cervical vertebral artery is very prone to dissection in blunt trauma. An interesting study reported that 35% of patients with a carotid canal fracture were found at angiography to have an ICA dissection, but 40% of the patients with an ICA dissection did not have a carotid canal fracture.

The diagnosis can be performed using CT angiography, MR imaging or MR angiography, and catheter angiography. The advances in multidetector CT have made this technique a first-line tool to assess a neurovascular injury, showing mural irregularity, narrowing, or occlusion. On MR imaging, the most common finding is a crescent hyperintensity (representative of intramural hematoma) around the lumen of the dissected vessel. Unenhanced T1-weighted images using fat saturation technique and proton density and T2-weighted images are particularly sensitive for detecting the intramural hematoma associated with arterial dissection (Fig. 3.6).

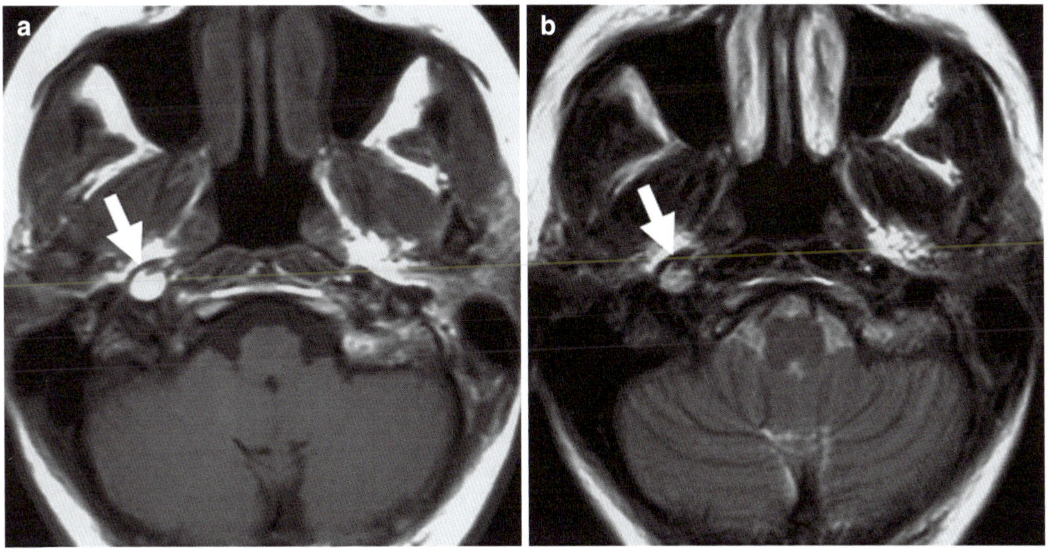

Fig. 3.6 (**a**) T1-weighted axial section; (**b**) T2-weighted axial section; (**c**, **d**) 3D TOF MR angiography (MIP reconstructions). Internal carotid artery dissection demonstrated by the presence of a hyperintense intramural hematoma with eccentric narrowed lumen (*arrows*). MR angiography confirms the ICA occlusion after the carotid bifurcation (*arrow*), with the flow of the terminal branches sustained by the circle of Willis

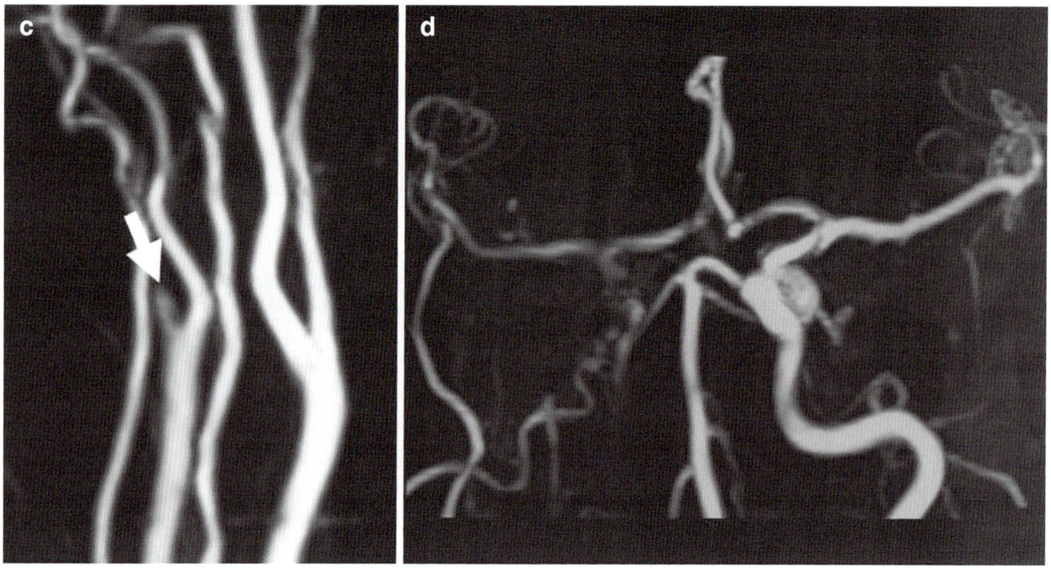

Fig. 3.6 (continued)

Vertebral artery dissections are more commonly extracranial in location because of the close proximity to the adjacent bone as the artery courses through the vertebral artery canal or along the sides of the C1–C2 vertebral body complex.

Pseudoaneurysms are characterized by eccentric outpouchings of contrast media from the arterial lumen with an intact adventitia, which provides a little support, being thus more prone to rupture.

On imaging their appearance varies from minimal contour abnormality to large, irregular, and saccular, with a wide neck. At times, a pseudoaneurysm can narrow the native arterial lumen, with potentially significant compromise of arterial flow (Fig. 3.7). At MRI, in the absence of thrombosis or turbulent flow, the pseudoaneurysm appears as a round area of signal void on both T1- and T2-weighted images [64, 71].

Active hemorrhage appears as an irregular collection of extravascular contrast material that surrounds the parent vessel, although the exact site of arterial transection may be impossible to identify.

The *traumatic arteriovenous fistula* (AVF) appears when laceration of an artery occurs adjacent to a vein, resulting in communication between the two systems [72].

The archetypal traumatic arteriovenous fistula is the carotid cavernous fistula (CCF), which results from a laceration of the ICA with direct communication to the cavernous sinus. It usually occurs in the presence of skull base fractures involving the carotid canal. Symptoms often develop in a delayed fashion, days to weeks after the initial trauma; therefore, these injuries can pass misdiagnosed [73–77].

Clinical findings of CCF include proptosis, chemosis, and ophthalmoplegia, with vision loss and facial pain variably present. The cross-sectional imaging findings of a CCF include early venous enhancement during the arterial phase, enlargement of the involved draining veins (i.e., a dilated superior ophthalmic vein-normal diameter < 4 mm), retrobulbar fat stranding, enlarged extraocular muscles, and proptosis, findings that reflect venous engorgement resulting from increased venous outflow from the intracranial circulation.

On conventional catheter angiography, there is an abnormal early filling of the cavernous sinus during the arterial phase and early venous outflow to the superior ophthalmic vein, inferior petrosal sinus, and/or contralateral cavernous sinus [78].

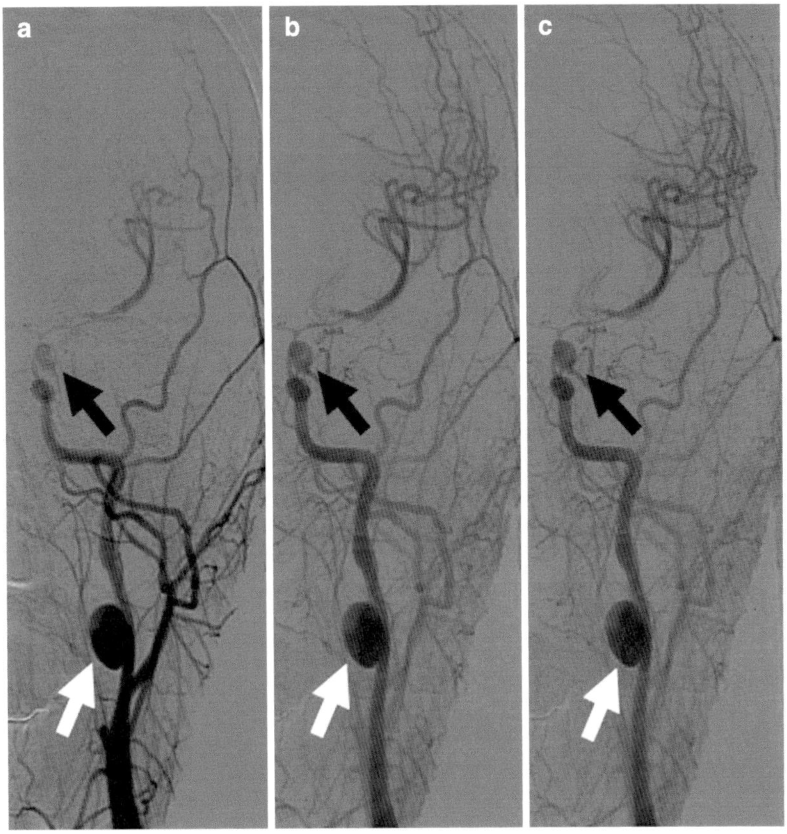

Fig. 3.7 Common carotid artery digital angiography (anteroposterior view). Presence of an extracranial ICA pseudoaneurysm (*white arrows*), associated with another syphon pseudoaneurysm and narrowing of the arterial lumen, involving the homolateral terminal branches (*black arrows*)

A traumatic AVF can also result from laceration of the middle meningeal artery with fistulous communication to the middle meningeal veins.

In addition to these traumatic AVFs that may present acutely, venous thrombosis in the setting of head trauma can lead to formation of indirect, generally lower flow dural AVFs in a delayed fashion.

3.3.3 Epidural Hematoma

Epidural hematoma (EH) is usually arterial in its origin and represents a hemorrhagic collection within the inner table of the skull and the outer dural layer. It usually results from a skull fracture, often a temporal fracture, which strips away the dura from the inner table, and injures the middle meningeal artery, with consequent filling of the newly formed epidural space. Being the dura tightly adherent to the skull at cranial suture lines, the EH does not typically cross the cranial sutures (with an exception at the level of the sagittal suture, since dura does not cover the suture due to the presence of the superior sagittal sinus).

The majority of cases occur at the coup site with an underlying fracture being identifiable in the 90% of cases.

The loss of consciousness is often immediate, although many patients may experience the so-called lucent interval, during which time the EH expands until it can impact the patient's level of consciousness.

EH is a neurosurgical emergency requiring immediate evacuation since it causes mass effect symptoms with shift of the midline structures, compression of the lateral ventricle and subfalcine herniation, and sometimes uncal herniation. Small EHs can be managed conservatively.

Venous EHs can also occur, associated with skull fractures, manifesting typically infratentorially or within the anterior aspect of the middle cranial fossa, after injuries to the transverse/sigmoid

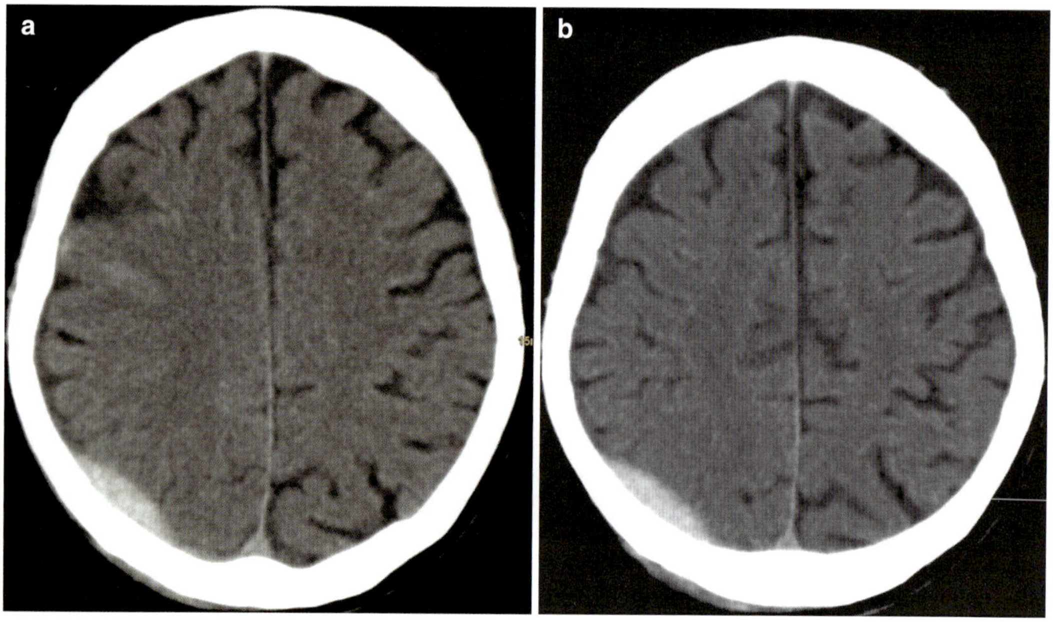

Fig. 3.8 (**a**, **b**) CT scan. Epidural hematoma: presence of a well-defined biconvex, hyperdense, extra-axial collection in the right parietal region

sinuses or the sphenoparietal sinus, respectively; EHs located in the anterior aspect of the middle cranial fossa have a better prognosis.

On non-contrast CT it appears as a well-defined biconvex, hyperdense, extra-axial collection not crossing sutures (Fig. 3.8). Occasionally, an acute EH may contain heterogeneous foci which appear hypodense at imaging (Fig. 3.9), indicating active extravasation of fresh unclotted blood (swirl sign); these lesions have a worse prognosis as they are more prone to further enlargement than the homogeneous EH, requiring thus an immediate surgical management [79–82].

Other CT findings associated with an adverse outcome are thickness greater than 1.5 cm, volume greater than 30 mL, location within the lateral aspect of the middle cranial fossa, and midline shift greater than 5 mm.

A rapidly expanding EH can occur also after a decompressive craniectomy, maybe because of the removal of the tamponade effect on a previous extra-axial collection. Some studies suggest performing a postoperative CT scan in patients with a skull fracture remote from the planned craniotomy or a small collection not surgical in nature, remote from the craniectomy.

Chronic EHs show low density and peripheral enhancement and they might be concave [83, 84].

3.3.4 Subdural Hematoma

Subdural hematoma (SDH) is usually venous in its origin and represents a hemorrhagic collection within the space between the inner meningeal layer of the dura and the arachnoid. Acute SDHs result from a significant head injury causing the disruption of the bridging cortical veins. They can be found both in the coup and in the contrecoup side, the latter one being more common.

They usually occur along the cerebral convexities, the falx cerebri, and the tentorium cerebelli; they can cross the suture lines but not the dural reflections, such as the falx and tentorium.

They can also occur in patients without a history of head trauma, such as elderly patients, those ones on anticoagulant therapy and hemodialysis, and thrombocytopenic patients; thus the symptoms may be very subtle and remain undiscovered for days and weeks until it enters the subacute or chronic stage.

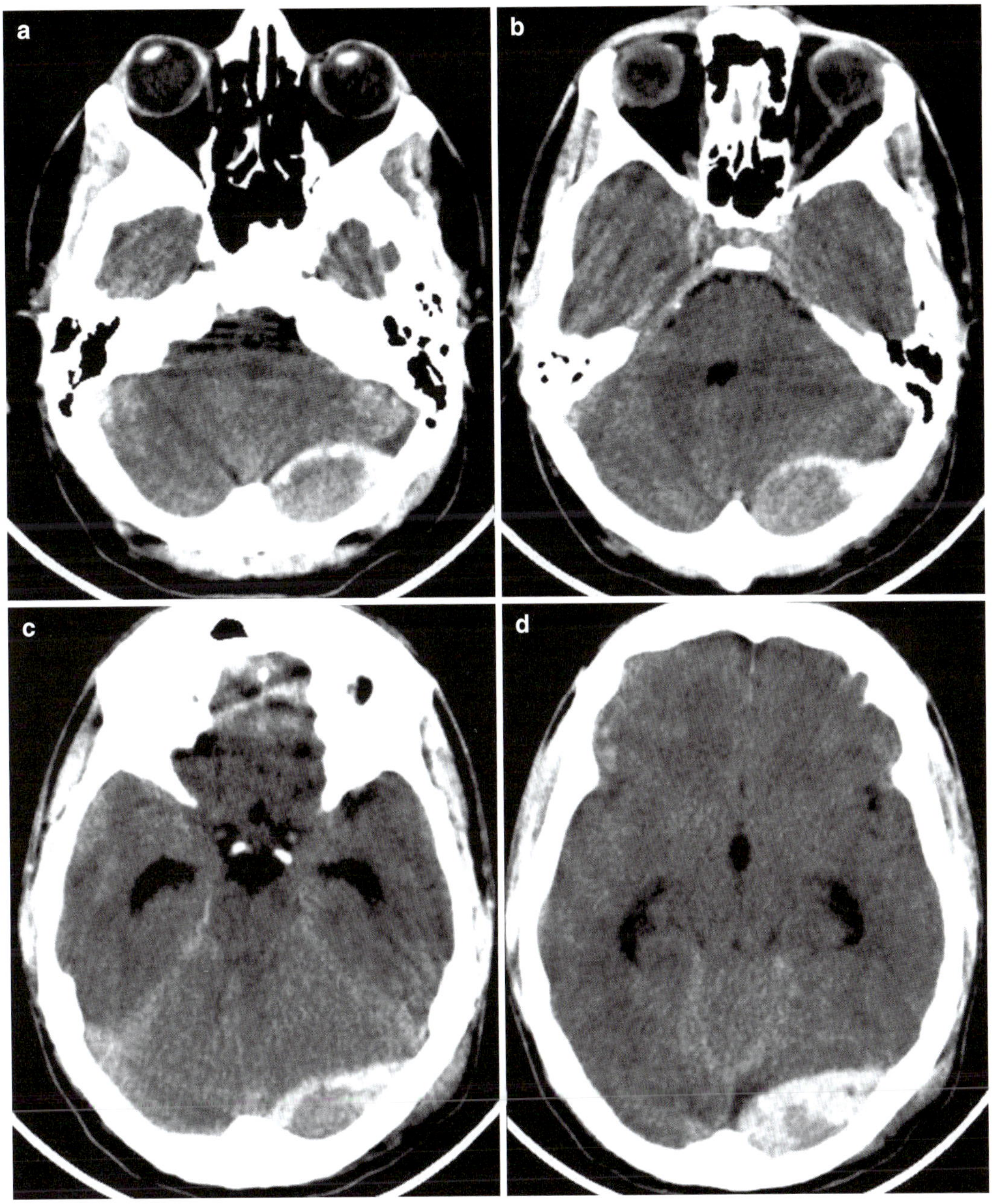

Fig. 3.9 (**a–d**) CT scan. Epidural hematoma of venous origin: presence of a left retrocerebellar biconvex, extra-axial collection, inhomogeneously hyperdense due to the presence of fresh unclotted blood. The fourth ventricle and the aqueduct of Sylvius are compressed, with supratentorial hydrocephalus

Infratentorial SDHs are rare in adults and are more commonly seen in neonates secondary to perinatal injury [69, 83, 85–88].

They can be divided into three stages, namely, acute, subacute, and chronic, with their own distinct imaging features.

Acute SDH is usually a crescentic, hyperdense extra-axial collection on CT. In some specific conditions, they may be iso- or hypodense due to an underlying anemia or have a mixed density because of active bleeding in the hyperacute setting: in these cases the hypodense areas correspond to the

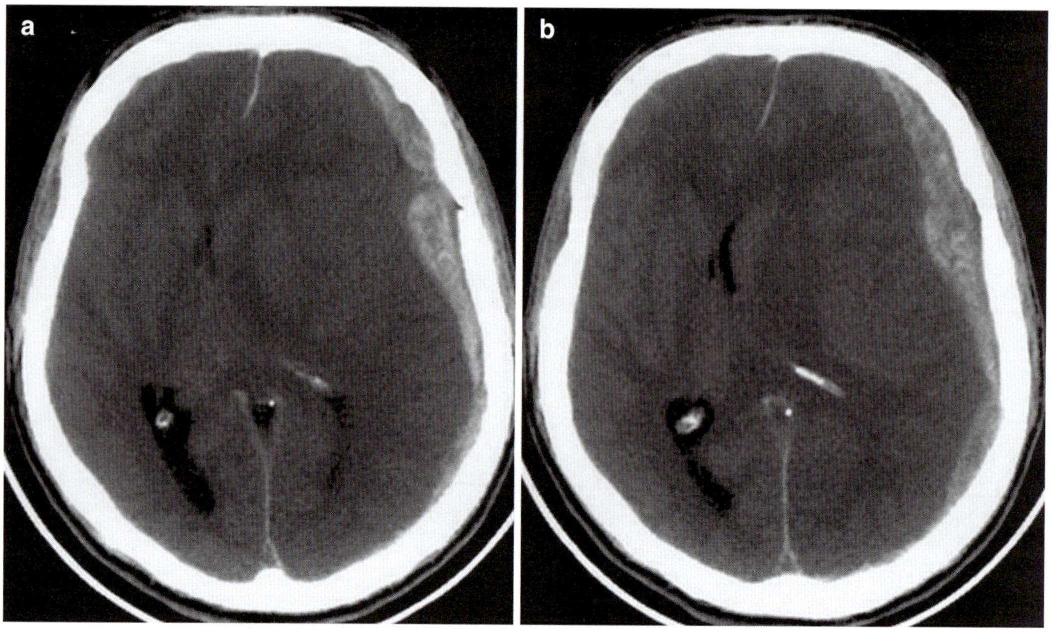

Fig. 3.10 (**a**, **b**) CT scan. Acute subdural hematoma: presence of a hyperdense extra-axial collection in the left frontotemporal region, associated with subfalcine herniation; it has a mixed density because of unclotted blood, and a somewhat crescentic/lentiform shape

unclotted blood. Alternatively, a preexisting chronic SDH or an arachnoid tear can show a mixed density due to rebleeding, resulting in a mixture of blood with CSF. These "atypical" acute SDHs may be lentiform (biconvex) rather than crescentic in shape, likely secondary to adhesions in the subdural space, as a typical epidural hematoma (Fig. 3.10). Small SDHs may be overlooked on traditional CT "brain windows," because of the high convexity location, beam hardening artifacts, or narrow window settings; an additional wider "subdural window" (width 200; level 70) should be used in all trauma patients to detect these small SDHs, helping to differentiate between bone and hemorrhage.

SDHs occurring at the falx cerebri appear as hyperdense collection between the two hemispheres. The thin SDHs over the tentorium can be very difficult to recognize because of volume averaging effect with the brain, so that thinner axial CT slices, or coronal ones, may help to identify them.

As for as their management, because acute SDHs can rapidly enlarge, they often require surgical intervention; on the contrary small acute SDHs that remain static in size over few days after the trauma are not surgically treated.

Subacute (1–3 weeks) SDHs usually appear isodense to the gray matter on CT, making it difficult to be recognized on CT; possible imaging clues include the so-called abnormally thick cortex, a medial displacement of the gray–white junction from the inner table, white matter buckling, midline shift, compression of the ipsilateral ventricle, and sulcal effacement.

As mentioned before, in the elderly, most SDHs are discovered in the subacute–chronic stage because of the subtle clinical presentation; in particular, brain atrophy seems to play a central role in developing of these lesions, since as the distance between the cortex and the dura increases, small veins extending from the cortex to the dura (the "bridging" veins) become stretched and can be disrupted by violent head motions even in the absence of a high-energy head trauma. SDHs can slowly increase over a few weeks or months, because of repeated small hemorrhages, producing a subdural collection composed of blood products of different stages (Fig. 3.11), often having a thick proteinaceous consistency.

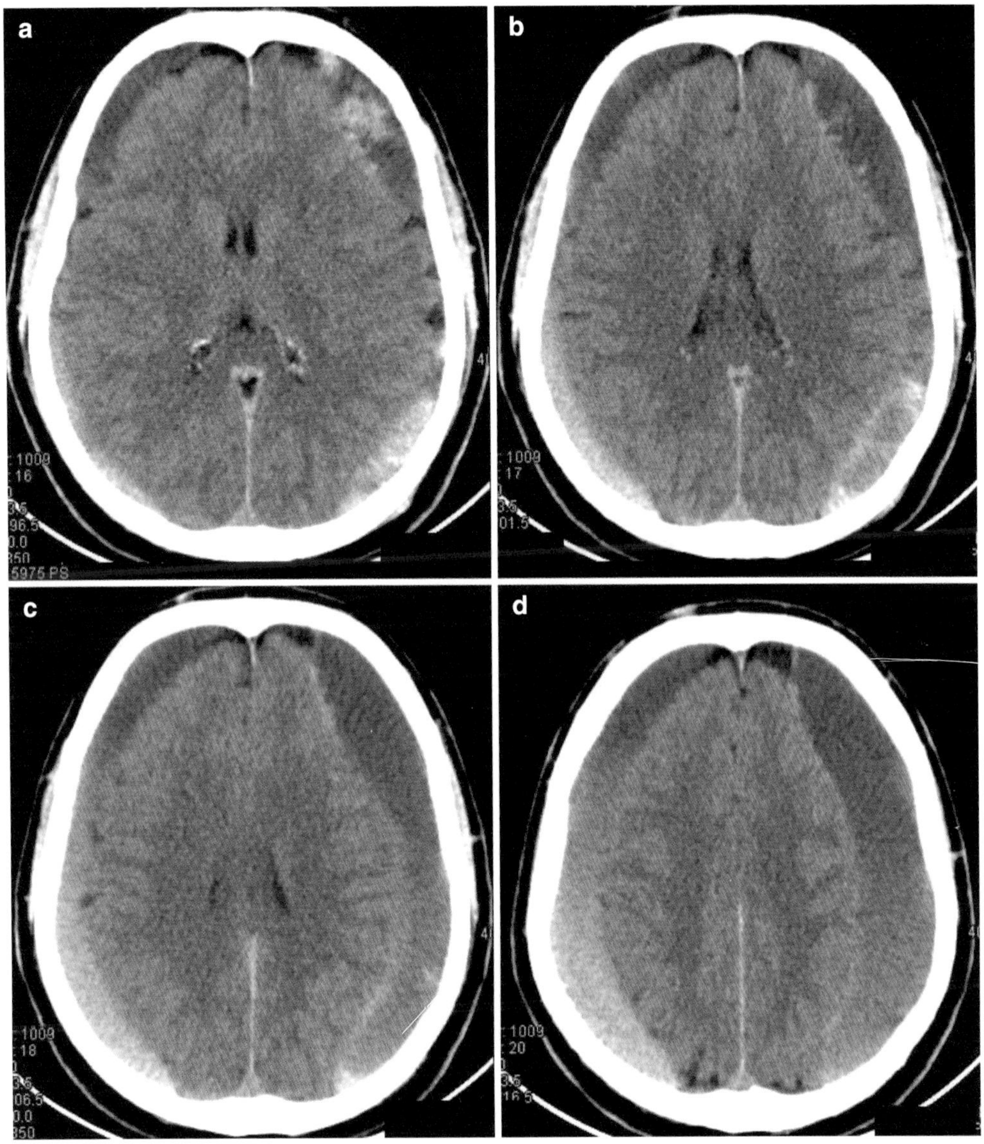

Fig. 3.11 (a–d) CT scan. Subacute–chronic subdural hematomas: bilateral subdural collections composed of blood products in different stages deriving from repeated hemorrhages

Chronic SDHs (>3 weeks) appear as homogeneous hypodense crescentic collection; when a rebleeding occurs, a bilayered appearance may result, with a hypodense layer (the chronic hemorrhage) in the less dependent position and the hyperdense component (the acute hemorrhage) in the dependent position (Fig. 3.12). In this phase multiple adhesions and membranes within the collection can be observed, giving the appearance of multicompartment collection.

MR imaging is more sensitive than CT in the detection of small SDHs and tentorial and interhemispheric SDHs; in addition, MR can easily stage the disease according to the blood signal intensity changes over the time. In the first few days, blood is in the stage of intracellular deoxyhemoglobin; the SDH will be isointense to gray matter on T1-weighted images and hypointense on T2-weighted images. After a few days, being blood in the stage of intracellular

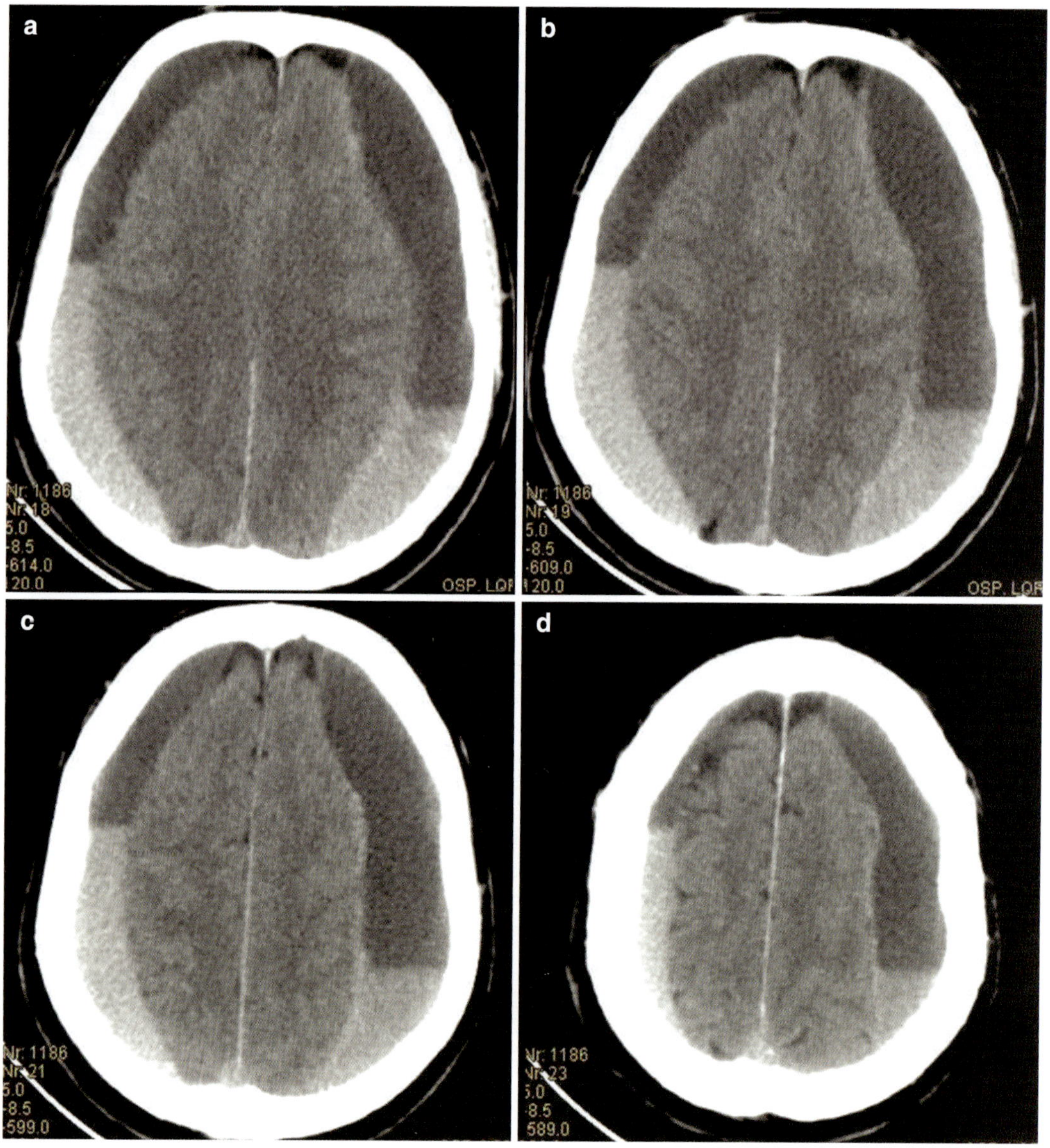

Fig. 3.12 (**a–d**) CT scan. Chronic subdural hematomas: bilateral bilayered crescentic collections, with a hypodense component (the chronic hemorrhage) in the less dependent position and the hyperdense component (the acute hemorrhage) in the dependent position

methemoglobin, SDHs become hyperintense on T1-weighted images. After the first week, with lysis of red blood cells and production of extracellular methemoglobin, SDHs become hyperintense on both T1- and T2-weighted images, a finding that can persist for many months, associated with hypointense components on T2*-weighted images (Fig. 3.13) [32, 33, 35].

3.3.5 Subarachnoid Hemorrhage

Subarachnoid hemorrhage (SAH) results from injury to the small, bridging, cortical vessels on the pia and arachnoid that cross the subarachnoid space, from extension of interventricular hemorrhage via the fourth ventricular outlet foramina, or from contiguous extension of an intracerebral contusion/hematoma into the subarachnoid space.

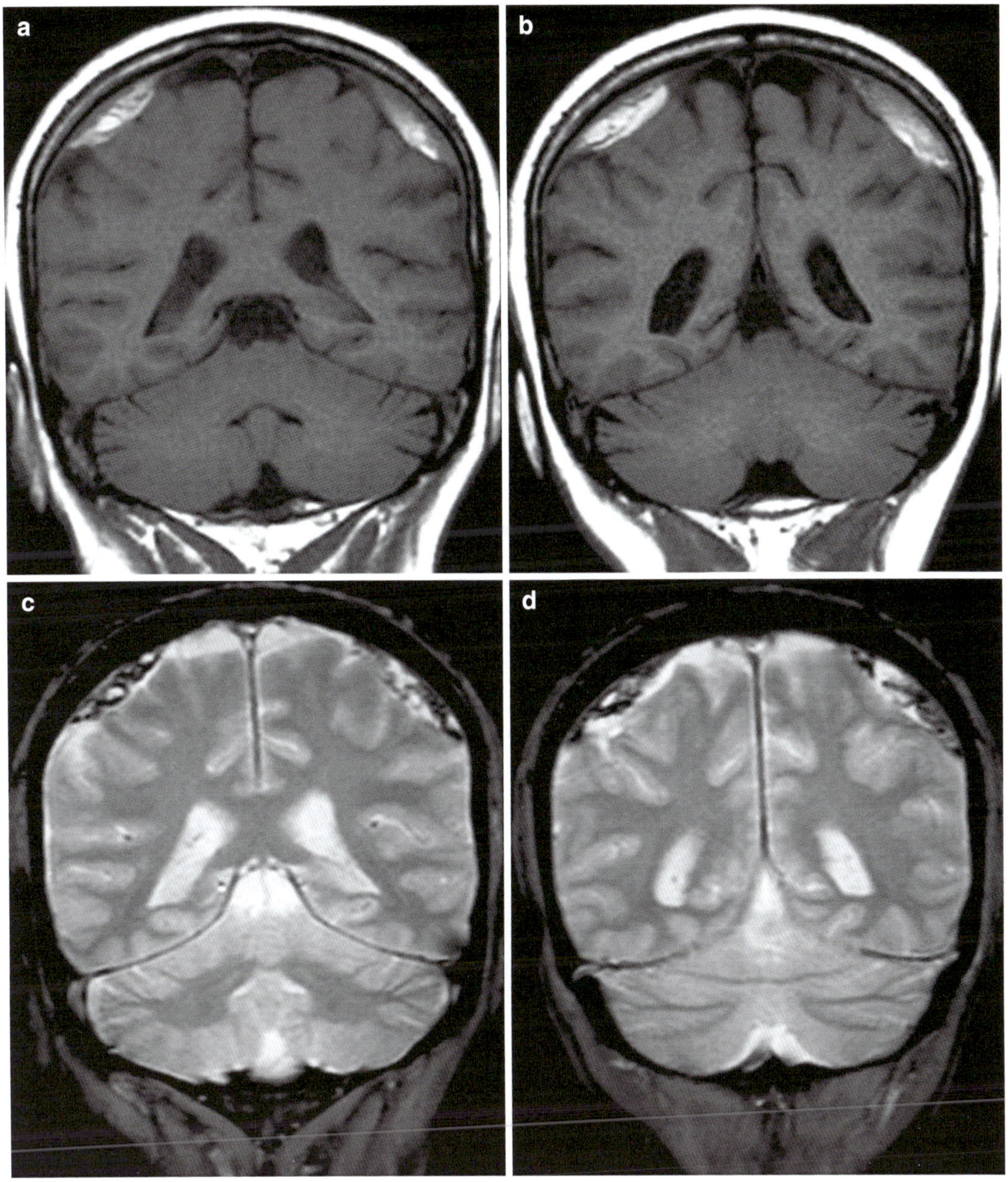

Fig. 3.13 (a, b) T1-weighted coronal sections; (c, d) T2*-weighted coronal sections. Subacute–chronic subdural hematomas: bilateral subdural collections hyperintense on T1-weighted images, with hypointense components on T2*-weighted images

The most common locations are the convexity, the fissures (contrecoup Sylvian fissure), and the basal cisterns [69, 89–91].

Aneurysmal SAHs can be differentiated from the traumatic ones basing on the distribution of the hemorrhage [92]; in fact while the aneurysmal SAHs are more centrally located, involving the suprasellar, interpeduncular, and prepontine cisterns, the latter have a peripheral distribution. On CT they appear as hyperdensity within the subarachnoid space (Fig. 3.14); occasionally, effacement of the sulci, secondary to the presence

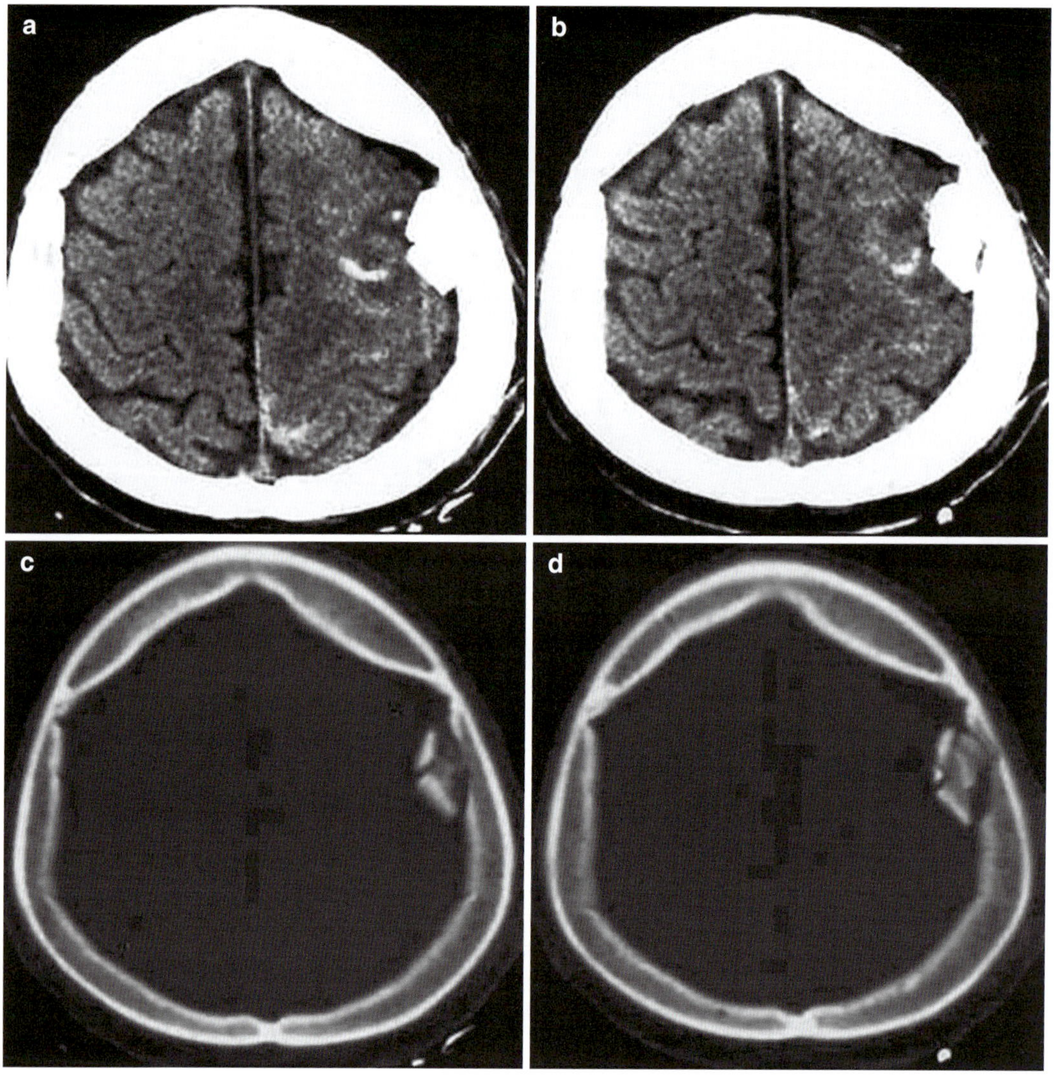

Fig. 3.14 (**a–d**) CT scan. Subarachnoid hemorrhage: presence of linear hyperdensities within the left frontoparietal subarachnoid spaces, associated with a contiguous depressed fracture

of intrasulcal SAH, can be the only indicator of SAH.

It is important to differentiate SAH from the "pseudo-SAH," which is a phenomenon observed in the setting of acute TBI, characterized by diffuse brain swelling and downward transtentorial herniation. It consists of an increased density in the subarachnoid spaces caused by its contraction due to a decrease in the amount of CSF in that space and/or engorgement of small pial vessels by low-density cerebral edema (Fig. 3.15).

3.3.6 Intraventricular Hemorrhage

Intraventricular hemorrhage (IVH) can result from tearing of subependymal veins along the surface of the ventricles, from contiguous extension of a parenchymal hematoma into the ventricular system, from retrograde flow of SAH into the ventricles, or from a direct penetrating injury. Isolated IVH hemorrhage is rare, as it is usually associated with SAH and contusions [69, 90, 93].

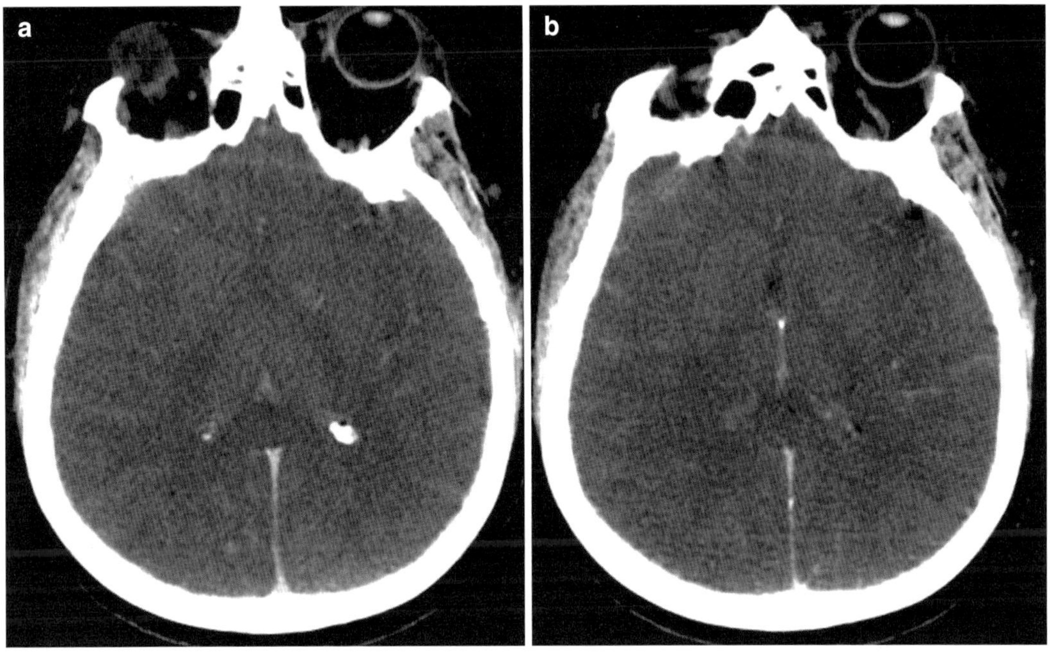

Fig. 3.15 (a, b) CT scan. Pseudo-subarachnoid hemorrhage: increased density in the subarachnoid spaces caused by diffuse brain swelling with consequent decrease of CSF and engorgement of small pial vessels

The typical aspect is a fluid–fluid level layering dependently within the occipital horns or as an intraventricular clot. Patients with IVH are at risk for developing noncommunicating hydrocephalus secondary to the obstruction of the aqueduct from ependymal adhesions and scarring.

3.4 Intra-axial Injuries

3.4.1 Parenchymal Injuries

Parenchymal injuries can be divided into four categories. The first two categories, contusion and diffuse axonal injury, are more common than the last two, brainstem injury and deep gray matter injury, which have a worse prognosis.

3.4.2 Cortical Contusions

Cortical contusions occur in up to 43% of patients with blunt head injuries. They consist of bruises and lacerations of the brain, covered by the dura, occur on gyral surfaces, and can extend into the white matter. Brain contusions can be classified as fracture contusions, coup contusions, and/or contrecoup contusions. Fracture contusions occur at a site of direct impact, usually beneath a depressed skull fracture. The coup contusions occur when the brain strokes the skull at the site of an externally applied force and is not necessarily associated with a fracture. Contrecoup contusion is found at an opposite point (180°) from the site of impact, where the brain strikes the inner table of the skull; a classic example of the contrecoup contusion is the injury of the anterior and inferior orbitofrontal and temporal lobes from an occipital impact [69, 94, 95].

At imaging they are wedge-shaped with the base on the cortical surface and the tip pointed toward the center of the brain. Contrecoup lesions are usually a little bit larger than coup lesions.

About one-half of acute contusions are hemorrhagic, and they usually appear as rounded-shaped or oval hyperdense foci at gyral surfaces, surrounded by edema. A characteristic

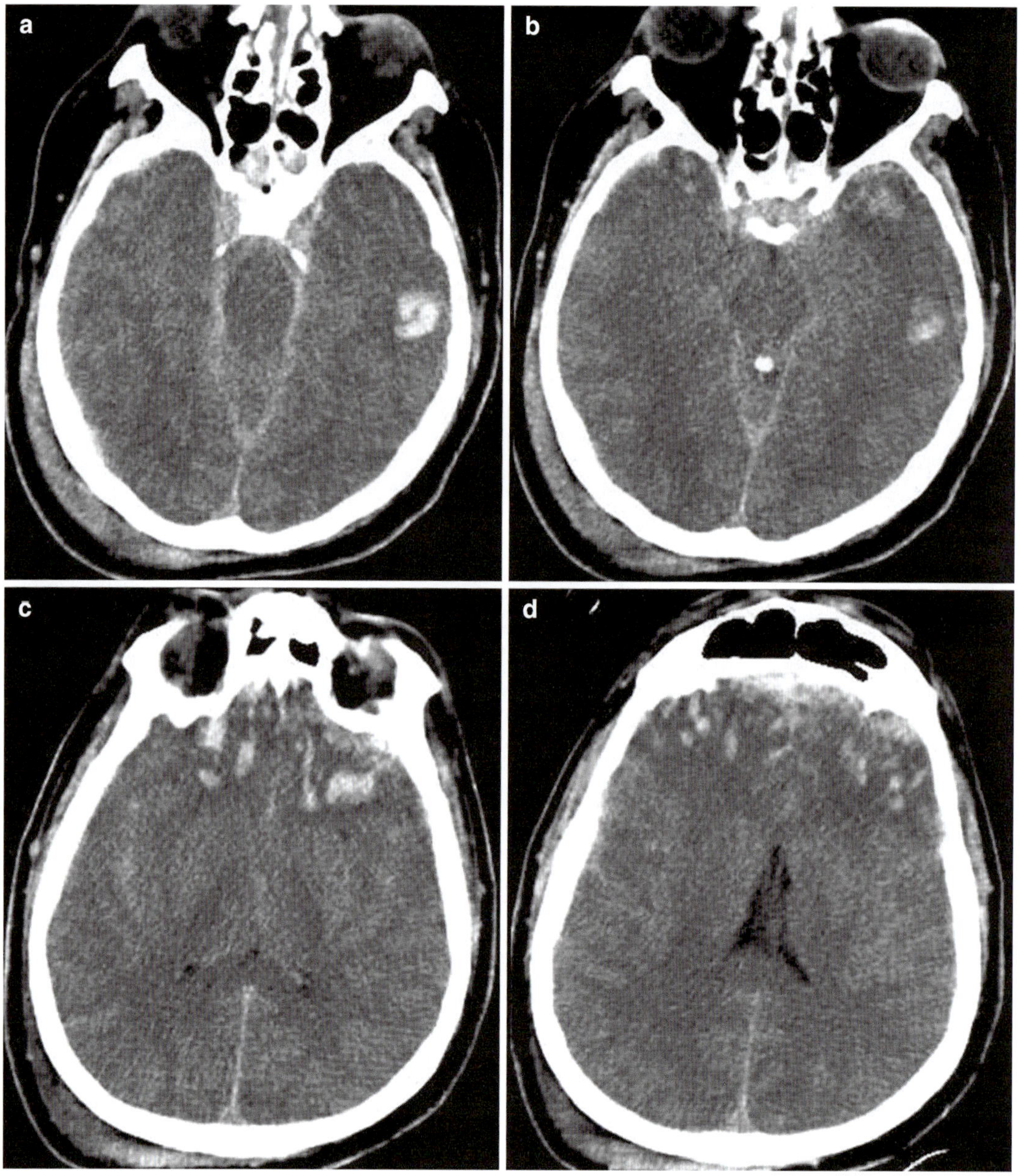

Fig. 3.16 (a–d) CT scan. Hemorrhagic contusion: rounded-shaped and oval hyperdense foci at gyral surfaces of the frontal and temporal lobes, surrounded by edema

"salt-and-pepper" pattern of mixed hypodense and hyperdense areas becomes more evident after the first week from the trauma (Fig. 3.16). In some severe cases, the whole temporal lobe may be contused, resulting in the so-called burst lobe.

Nonhemorrhagic contusions may be difficult to detect on CT; some days after trauma, they can be recognizable since they become more conspicuous developing a hypodense appearance (Fig. 3.17). Delayed hemorrhage can be seen within initially nonhemorrhagic lesions a few days after trauma (Fig. 3.18).

Four to six weeks after trauma, contusions become less conspicuous on CT examination, as hemorrhage and edema resolve, leaving a region of encephalomalacia as the unique evidence of trauma [30].

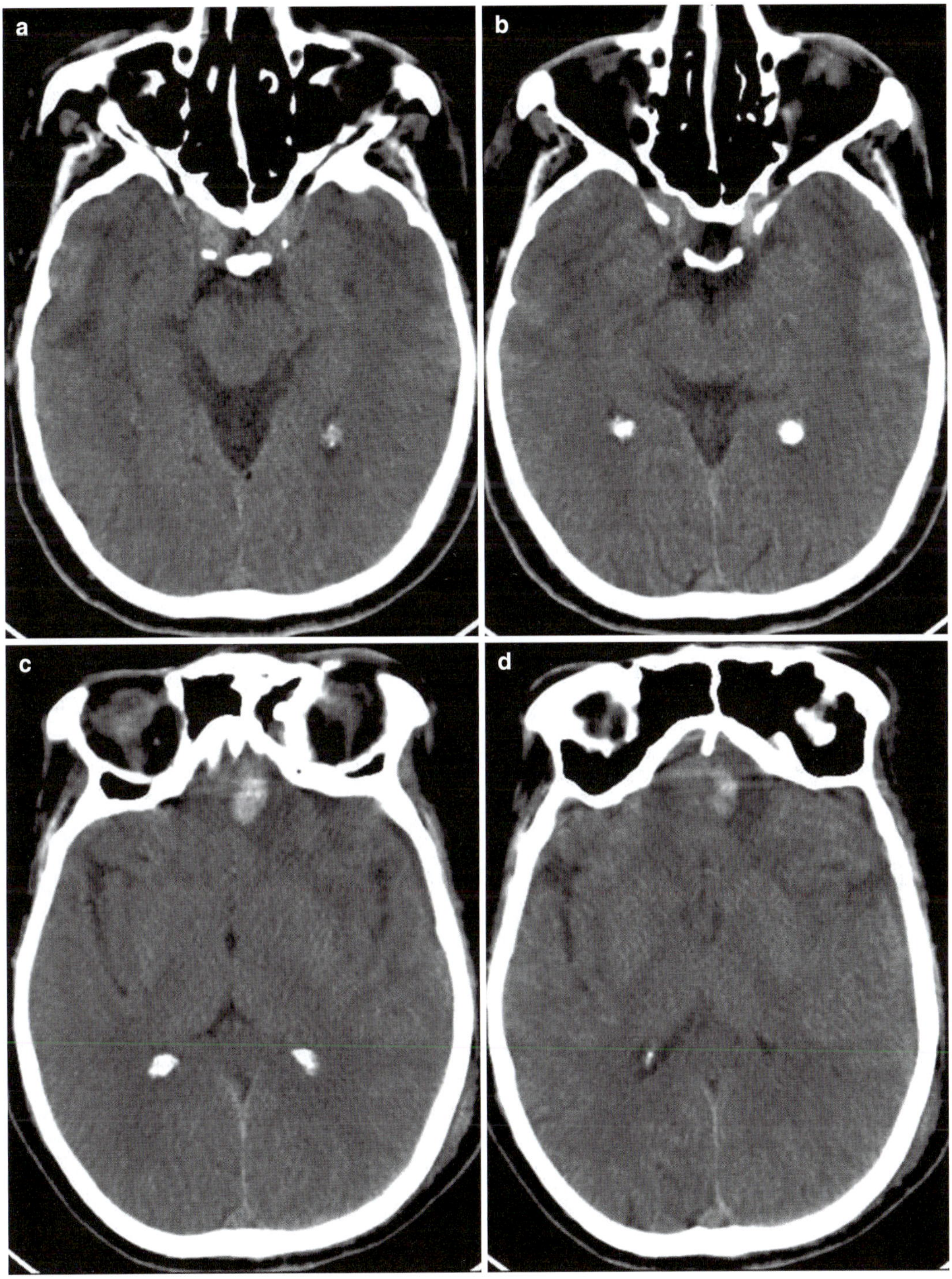

Fig. 3.17 (**a–d**) CT scan. Nonhemorrhagic contusions in the temporal lobes, with a hypodense appearance, associated with a hemorrhagic lesion in the left fronto-basal region

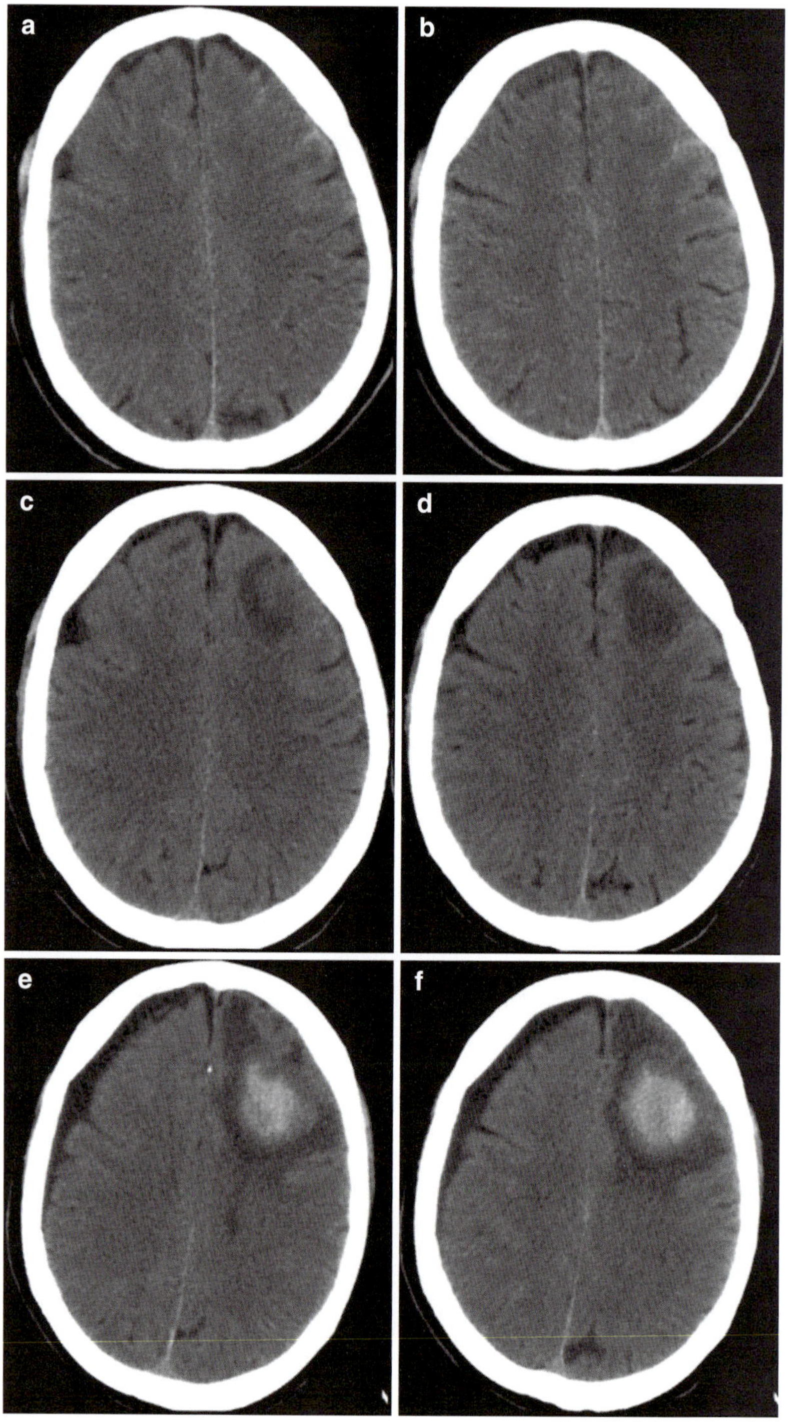

Fig. 3.18 (**a**–**f**) CT scan. Presence of linear hyperdensities, from subarachnoid hemorrhage, within the left frontal subarachnoid spaces (**a**, **b**); presence of a nonhemorrhagic contusion in the left frontal lobe 2 days after trauma (**c**, **d**); delayed hemorrhage within the initially nonhemorrhagic lesion 6 days after trauma (**e**, **f**)

Contusions are more easily detectable and appear more conspicuous on MR than on CT, especially when they involve the gyral crests over the convexity and skull base, where beam hardening artifact limits CT. Nonhemorrhagic contusions appear hypointense on T1-weighted and hyperintense on T2-weighted images [30, 83].

MR imaging is more sensitive to the presence of parenchymal hemorrhage than CT. As demonstrated by several authors, nonhemorrhagic contusions on CT often have hemorrhagic components on MR imaging, especially when using a GRE sequence, and the products of hemorrhage can be detected by MR imaging for many months after trauma.

An acute hemorrhagic contusion has a central dark signal (deoxyhemoglobin) with surrounding hyperintense edematous cortical tissue on T2-weighted images. After 2 days, the subacute contusion develops increasing vasogenic edema, and deoxyhemoglobin evolves into intracellular methemoglobin, resulting in T1 hyperintensity.

The subacute contusion and hematoma often demonstrate ring enhancement following intravenous contrast administration.

Chronic contusion appears as a focal, wedge-shaped, peripheral area of encephalomalacia, often lined with hemosiderin, resulting in the characteristic dark T2 signal intensity seen on GRE and SWI sequences [69, 96].

3.4.3 Diffuse Axonal Injury

Diffuse axonal injury (DAI) is one of the most common types of primary neuronal injury in patients with severe head trauma and the most common cause of significant morbidity and mortality after head trauma, causing immediate and sustained loss of consciousness. It is characterized by a widespread disruption of axons occurring at the time of an acceleration or deceleration injury.

Histologically DAI is characterized by axonal damage in the parasagittal white matter and gray–white matter junctions of the cerebral cortex and in the corpus callosum and brainstem.

The clinical manifestations depend on the severity of the injury and can vary from mild symptoms to coma. The identification of DAI-related white matter lesions is critical, as they are thought to be responsible for the majority of TBI cognitive deficits. Unfortunately, DAI is often underdiagnosed with conventional imaging techniques.

They can be hemorrhagic or nonhemorrhagic with the former being sometimes identifiable on CT scan, where focal punctate regions of high density surrounded by a collar of low-density edema may be observed.

Nonhemorrhagic lesions are very difficult to be detected on CT [97] and are more conspicuous on MR, where they appear hypointense on T1-weighted images and hyperintense on T2-weighted images. Hemorrhagic DAI lesions have various signal intensities corresponding to the age of the blood products and are hypointense on T2*-weighted images [98–102] (Fig. 3.19). Patients with a discrepancy between the clinical status and their CT findings should undergo MR imaging, because of its increased sensitivity to white matter and brainstem injury.

The most common locations of TAI are the lobar gray–white matter junction, the corpus callosum, and the dorsolateral midbrain: these locations correspond to the classic "shear injury triad." The location of TAI tends to correlate with the severity of the trauma; specifically, mild DAI (grade I) involves only the gray–white junction of the lobar white matter, commonly the parasagittal regions of the frontal lobes, and periventricular regions of the temporal lobes. Moderate DAI (grade II) involves the corpus callosum, particularly the posterior body and splenium, in addition to the lobar white matter. In severe DAI (grade III), the dorsolateral midbrain, in addition to the lobar white matter and corpus callosum, is involved. Other areas include the fornices, capsules, periventricular white matter, and superior cerebellar peduncles.

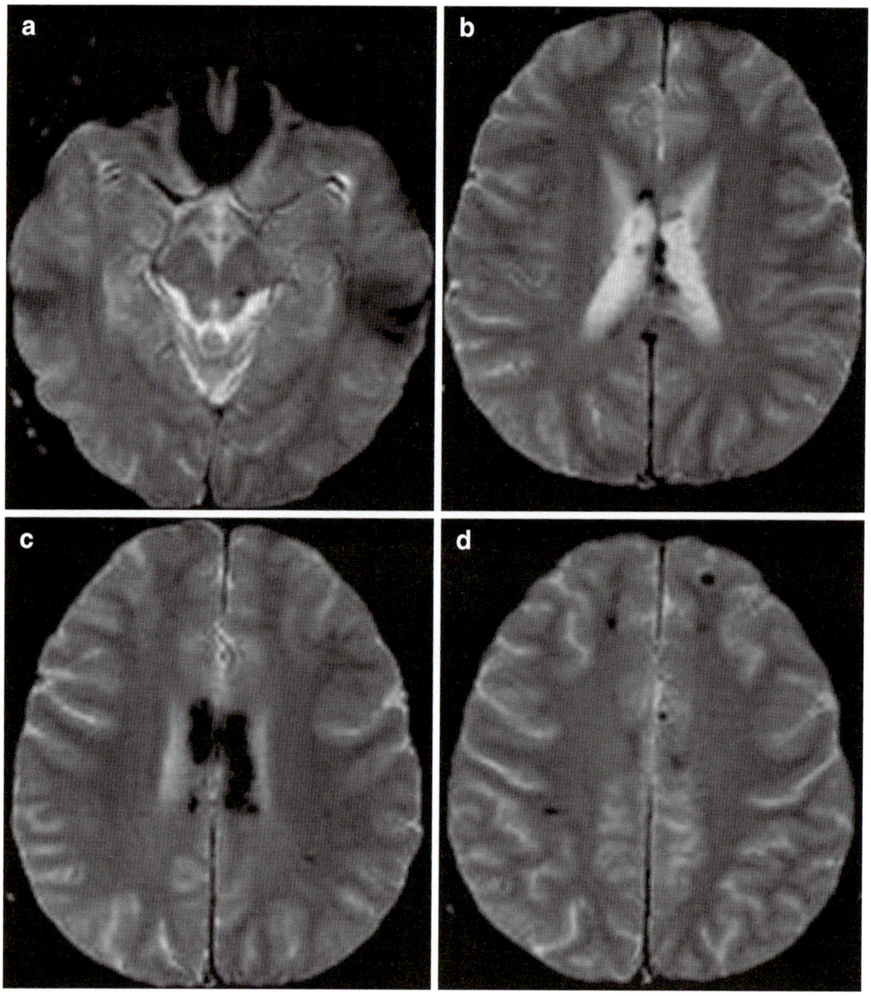

Fig. 3.19 (**a**–**d**) T2*-weighted axial sections. Diffuse axonal injury: presence of multiple, small hypointense foci located within the lobar gray–white matter junction (**d**), the corpus callosum (**b**, **c**), and the dorsolateral midbrain (**a**), corresponding to the classic "shear injury triad"

3.4.4 Brainstem Injury

Brainstem injuries are classified as primary or secondary according to whether they occur as the immediate result of the trauma or delayed in onset. Primary brainstem injury is the result of the direct impact of the brainstem with the tentorium; they usually occur along with DAI and deep gray matter injuries, and they are usually located in the posterolateral aspect of the pons, in the periaqueductal region. They can be hemorrhagic or nonhemorrhagic, being the latter ones more difficult to be detected on CT [103–105].

Secondary injuries usually appear in the ventral part of the brainstem, and they include the so-called Duret hemorrhage, occurring in the setting of abrupt and prolonged downward herniation which leads to stretching and rupture of the perforating vessels of the brainstem, causing punctuate hemorrhages, and compression of the midbrain by uncal herniation resulting in a lateral translation of the brainstem, causing the contralateral cerebral peduncle to be compressed against the tentorial edge, leading to the "Kernohan notch." This phenomenon is responsible for the false-localizing sign resulting in ipsilateral motor weakness and ischemic injury.

The compression responsible for the Duret hemorrhages can cause a severe compromising of the respiratory centers, leading to death.

As mentioned before, these lesions may be nonhemorrhagic also, being more difficult to be evaluated by means of CT scans; in these cases MR is much more feasible because of the better contrast resolution and the absence of artifacts, helping to predict the outcomes, since the recognition of bilateral pontine injuries has a poor prognosis.

3.4.5 Deep Gray Matter Injury

Injury in the thalamus and basal ganglia is a rare manifestation of TBI, accounting for about 5% of parenchymal traumatic lesions. These lesions are associated with severe neurological impairment and poor outcomes [106]. They can be hemorrhagic, appearing on CT as small foci of hyperdensity in the basal ganglia, possibly because of the disruption of small perforating blood vessels. The lesions are generally associated with a low initial GCS score [83, 103, 107].

Nonhemorrhagic lesions appear as hypodense regions of variable size within the basal ganglia and thalamus.

Both of these forms are much more conspicuous on MR, especially by applying the SWI sequences [108].

3.5 Secondary Lesions

Most secondary injuries are represented by an increased intracranial pressure and cerebral herniations. They occur in the early posttraumatic period. CT and MR allow to easily distinguish these lesions from the late sequelae of a brain injury, such as hydrocephalus, pneumocephalus, cerebrospinal fluid leak, infections [109], and encephalomalacia.

The most important lesions which can be a real danger for patient's life are cerebral edema and brain herniation. [110, 111]

3.5.1 Cerebral Edema

Cerebral edema may occur because of either an increase of cerebral blood volume or an increase of tissue fluid content, as a response to direct focal injury, such as contusion or DAI [6, 83, 112].

Regardless of the type of fluid accumulation (blood or fluid), the imaging effects are the same, such as effacement of sulci, suprasellar and quadrigeminal plate cistern, and compression of the ventricular system. On CT brain edema appears as focal or diffuse areas of low attenuation with loss of normal gray–white differentiation. In cases of severe, diffuse cerebral edema, the brain becomes very low in attenuation and dura and circulating blood in the cranial vasculature appears hyperdense on CT "pseudo-subarachnoid hemorrhage"; the so-called white cerebellum sign is characterized by relatively hyperdense cerebellum with respect to edematous cerebral hemispheres.

Another visible sign is that on MRI brain edema is noted as areas of high signal intensity on FLAIR and T2-weighted sequences [113]. In addition, DWI may detect subtle areas of cytotoxic edema when they are not still visible on the other sequences, as seen in acute stroke.

3.5.2 Brain Herniation

Cerebral herniations represent a mechanical displacement of the brain through or across one compartment to another, secondary to a mass effect, as occurs in cases of hematoma or cerebral edema.

The types of brain herniation recognized are subfalcine herniation, transtentorial herniation (descending and rarely ascending due to upward herniation of the cerebellum), uncal herniation (or temporal lobe herniation), and tonsillar herniation, when cerebellar tonsils are forced through the foramen magnum. All types of herniation are a serious sign of cerebral injury accompanied by displacement of blood vessels and nerves.

The subfalcine herniation occurs when the cingulate gyrus is displaced across the midline under the falx, between the supratentorial compartments, and anterior cerebral artery is displaced resulting in secondary ischemia and infarction. On imaging the ipsilateral cingulate gyrus is pushed down and under the midline falx, compressing the contralateral gyrus, along with depression of the ipsilateral corpus callous with elevation/compression of the contralateral one. If posteriorly located, these herniations may compress the internal cerebral veins, Galen vein and the deep subependymal veins, with an increasing of ICP.

The transtentorial herniation can be ascending or descending. The ascending form, less common than the descending one, is caused by an increased pressure in the posterior fossa pushing the cerebellum upward, through the tentorial incisura. On CT images the signs may be very subtle [114] and changes can often be bilateral and symmetric; imaging features are the "spinning top" appearance of the midbrain, caused by the bilateral compression of the posterior aspects of the midbrain by the posterior fossa, narrowing the ambient cisterns. A prolonged herniation causes effacement of the quadrigeminal cistern, displacing the midbrain anteriorly against the clivus; over time mass effect causes occlusion of the cerebral aqueduct and, finally, hydrocephalus. Rapidly expanding lesions clinically present with compressions symptoms such as respiratory failure, coma, and death.

Descending transtentorial herniation is a very serious consequence of brain injury. It occurs when the cerebral structures are forced through the incisura of the tentorium. The structures involved are the uncus, parahippocampal gyrus, perimesencephalic cistern, posterior cerebral artery, mesencephalon, and the third cranial nerve. On imaging it can be recognized by a dilatation of the contralateral ventricular system, compression of the basal cisterns, and midline shifts of the brain parenchyma.

Uncal herniation is characterized by a medially and inferiorly displacement of the uncus over the edge of the tentorium into the suprasellar cistern. On imaging one can observe the effacement of the classic "star" configuration of the suprasellar cistern on the same side of the herniation. One or both the cerebral peduncles are compressed and the midbrain results rotated or tilted. Clinically it can be observed contralateral hemiparesis and blown pupil due to compression of the ipsilateral cerebral peduncle and on the third cranial nerve.

Tonsillar herniation occurs when cerebellar tonsils are pushed through the foramen magnum; this form is usually associated with an ascending transtentorial herniation. It may cause compression of the posterior inferior cerebellar arteries, with cerebellar infarction, compression of the forth ventricle with hydrocephalus, and compression of brainstem with respiratory failure, coma, and death.

References

1. Marion DW. Evidenced-based guidelines for traumatic brain injuries. Prog Neurol Surg. 2006;19:171–96.
2. Menon DK, Schwab K, Wright DW, et al. Position statement: definition of traumatic brain injury. Arch Phys Med Rehabil. 2010;91(11):1637–40. doi:10.1016/j.apmr.2010.05.017.
3. Readnower RD, Chavko M, Adeeb S, Conroy MD, Pauly JR, Mccarron MR, Sullivan PG. Increase in blood-brain barrier permeability, oxidative stress, and activated microglia in a rat model of blast-induced traumatic brain injury. J Neurosci Res. 2010;88(16):3530–9. doi:10.1002/jnr.22510. Epub 29 Sep 2010.
4. Corrigan JD, Selassie AW, Orman JA. The epidemiology of traumatic brain injury. J Head Trauma Rehabil. 2010;25:72–80. doi:10.1097/HTR.0b013e3181ccc8b4.
5. Hyder AA, Wunderlich CA, Puvanachandra P, Gururaj G, Kobusingye OC. The impact of traumatic brain injuries: a global perspective. NeuroRehabilitation. 2007;22:341–53.
6. Much CA, Talbott JF, Gean A. Imaging evaluation of acute traumatic brain injury. Neurosurg Clin N Am. 2016;27:409–39. doi:10.1016/j.nec.2016.05.011. Epub 10 Aug 2016
7. Miele V, Di Giampietro I, Ianniello S, Pinto F, Trinci M. Diagnostic imaging in pediatric polytrauma management. Radiol Med. 2015;120:33–49. doi:10.1007/s11547-014-0469-x.
8. Miele V, Di Giampietro I. Diagnostic imaging in emergency. Salute Soc. 2014;2EN:127–38. doi:10.3280/SES2014-002010EN.
9. Miele V, Piccolo CL, Trinci M, Galluzzo M, Ianniello S, Brunese L. Diagnostic imaging of blunt abdominal trauma in pediatric patients. Radiol Med. 2016;121:409–30. doi:10.1007/s11547-016-0637-2.
10. Teasdale G, Jennett B. Assessment of coma and impaired consciousness. A practical scale. Lancet. 1974;2:81–4.

11. Haddad SH, Arabi YM. Critical care management of severe traumatic brain injury in adults. Scand J Trauma Resusc Emerg Med. 2012;20:12–27. doi:10.1186/1757-7241-20-12.
12. Ruff R. Two decades of advances in understanding of mild traumatic brain injury. J Head Trauma Rehabil. 2005;20:5–18.
13. Stiver SI, Manley GT. Prehospital management of traumatic brain injury. Neurosurg Focus. 2008;25:E5. doi:10.3171/FOC.2008.25.10.E5.
14. Davis PC. Head trauma. AJNR Am J Neuroradiol. 2007;28:1619–21.
15. Ro YS, Shin SD, Holmes JF, et al. Comparison of clinical performance of cranial computed tomography rules in patients with minor head injury: a multicenter prospective study. Acad Emerg Med. 2011;18(6):597–604. doi:10.1111/j.1553-2712.2011.01094.x.
16. Mower WR, Hoffmann JR, Herbert M, Wolfson AB, Pollack CV Jr, Zucker MI, Nexus II Investigators. Developing a decision instrument to guide computed tomographic imaging of blunt head injury patients. J Trauma. 2005;59(4):954–9.
17. Stein SC, Burnett MG, Glick HA. Indications for CT scanning in mild traumatic brain injury: a cost-effectiveness study. J Trauma. 2006;61:558–66.
18. Ingebrigtsen T, Romner B. Routine early CT-scan is cost saving after minor head injury. Acta Neurol Scand. 1996;93:207–10.
19. Servadei F, Ciucci G, Loroni L, Cuscini M, Piola C, Arista A. Diagnosis and management of minor head trauma: a regional multicenter approach in Italy. J Trauma. 1995;39:696–701.
20. de Bruïne FT, Spilt A, Van Erkel AR, Van Buchem MA. Choosing radiological modalities in patients with head trauma. Emerg Radiol. 1999;6:327–9.
21. Haydel MJ, Preston CA, Mills TJ, Luber S, Blaudeau E, DeBlieux PM. Indications for computed tomography in patients with minor head injury. N Engl J Med. 2000;343:100–5.
22. Stiell IG, Wells GA, Vandemheen K, et al. The Canadian CT Head Rule for patients with minor head injury. Lancet. 2001;357:1391–6.
23. Haydel M. Clinical decision instruments for CT scanning in minor head injury. JAMA. 2005;294(12):1551–3.
24. Biffl WL, Egglin T, Benedetto B, Gibbs F, Cijoffi WG. Sixteen-slice competed tomographic angiography is a reliable non-invasive screening test for clinical significant blunt cerebrovascular injuries. J Trauma. 2006;60(4):745–51.
25. Enterline DS, Kapoor G. A practical approach to CT angiography of the neck and brain. Tech Vasc Interv Radiol. 2006;9(4):192–204.
26. Berne JD, Reuland KS, Villarreal DH, McGovern TM, Rowe SA, Norwood SH. Sixteen-slice multi-detector computed tomographic angiography improves the accuracy of screening for blunt cerebrovascular injury. J Trauma. 2006;60(6):1204–9.
27. Schneidereit NP, Simons R, Nicolaou S, et al. Utility of screening for blunt vascular neck injuries with computed tomographic angiography. J Trauma. 2006;60(1):209–15.
28. Biffl WL, Ray CE, Moore EE, et al. Treatment related outcomes from blunt cerebrovascular injuries: importance of routine follow-up arteriography. Ann Surg. 2002;235(5):699–706.
29. Woodcock RJ Jr, Short J, Do HM, Jensen ME, Kallmes DF. Imaging of acute subarachnoid hemorrhage with a fluid attenuated inversion recovery sequence in an animal model: comparison with non-contrast enhanced CT. AJNR Am J Neuroradiol. 2001;22:1698–703.
30. Gentry LR, Godersky JC, Thompson B. MR imaging of head trauma: review of the distribution and radiopathologic features of traumatic lesions. AJR Am J Roentgenol. 1988;150:663–72.
31. Yanagawa Y, Tsushima Y, Tokumaru A, et al. A quantitative analysis of head injury using T2-weighted gradient-echo imaging. J Trauma. 2000;49:272–7.
32. Messori A, Polonara G, Mabiglia C, Salvolini U. Is haemosiderin visible indefinitely on gradient-echo MRI following traumatic intracerebral haemorrhage? Neuroradiology. 2003;45(12):881–6. Epub 25 Oct 2003.
33. Miele V, Piccolo CL, Sessa B, Trinci M, Galluzzo M. Comparison between MRI and CEUS in the follow-up of patients with blunt abdominal trauma managed conservatively. Radiol Med. 2016;121:27–37. doi:10.1007/s11547-015-0578-1. Epub 8 Aug 2015.
34. Haacke EM, Xu Y, Cheng YC, Reichenbach JR. Susceptibility weighted imaging (SWI). Magn Reson Med. 2004;52:612–8.
35. Babikian T, Freier MC, Tong KA, et al. Susceptibility weighted imaging: neuropsychologic outcome and pediatric head injury. Pediatr Neurol. 2005;33:184–94.
36. Wu Z, Li S, Lei J, An D, Haacke EM. Evaluation of traumatic subarachnoid hemorrhage using susceptibility weighted imaging. AJNR Am J Neuroradiol. 2010;31:1302–10. doi:10.3174/ajnr.A2022. Epub 25 Feb 2010.
37. Liu AY, Maldjian JA, Bagley LJ, Sinson GP, Grossman RI. Traumatic brain injury: diffusion-weighted MR imaging findings. AJNR Am J Neuroradiol. 1999;20:1636–41.
38. Huisman TA, Sorensen AG, Hergan K, Gonzalez RG, Schaefer PW. Diffusion-weighted imaging for the evaluation of diffuse axonal injury in closed head injury. J Comput Assist Tomogr. 2003;27:5–11.
39. Mori S, van Zijl PC. Fiber tracking: principles and strategies. A technical review. NMR Biomed. 2002;15:468–80.
40. Shimony JS, McKinstry RC, Akbudak E, et al. (1999) Quantitative diffusion-tensor anisotropy brain MR imaging: normative human data and anatomic analysis. Radiology. 212:770–784.

41. Arfanakis K, Haughton VM, Carew JD, Rogers BP, Dempsey RJ, Meyerand ME. Diffusion tensor MR imaging in diffuse axonal injury. AJNR Am J Neuroradiol. 2002;23:794–802.
42. Muccio CF, Di Blasi A, Esposito G, Brunese L, D'Arco F, Caranci F. Perfusion and spectroscopy magnetic resonance imaging in a case of lymphocytic vasculitis mimicking brain tumor. Pol J Radiol. 2013;78(3):66–9. doi:10.12659/PJR.884011. issn:1733-134X.
43. Gasparovic C, Yeo R, Mannell M, et al. Neurometabolite concentrations in gray and white matter in mild traumatic brain injury: an 1H-Magnetic Resonance Spectroscopy Study. J Neurotrauma. 2009;26(10):1635–43. doi:10.1089/neu.2009-0896.
44. Danielsen ER, Christensen PB, Arlien-Soborg P, Thomsen C. Axonal recovery after severe traumatic brain injury demonstrated in vivo by 1H MR spectroscopy. Neuroradiology. 2003;45:722–4. Epub 27 Aug 2003.
45. Govind V, Gold S, Kaliannan K. Whole-brain proton MR spectroscopic imaging of mild-to-moderate traumatic brain injury and correlation with neuropsychological deficits. J Neurotrauma. 2010;27:483–96. doi:10.1089/neu.2009.1159.
46. Cohen BA, Inglese M, Rusinek H, Babb JS, Grossman RI, Gonen O. Proton MR spectroscopy and MRI-volumetry in mild traumatic brain injury. AJNR Am J Neuroradiol. 2007;28:907–13.
47. Castillo M. Whole-brain N-acetyl-aspartate: a marker of the severity of mild head trauma. AJNR Am J Neuroradiol. 2007;28:914–5.
48. Little SC, Kesser BW. Radiographic classification of temporal bone fractures: clinical predictability using a new system. Arch Otolaryngol Head Neck Surg. 2006;132:1300–4.
49. Cannon CR, Jahrsdoerfer RA. Temporal bone fractures: review of 90 cases. Arch Otolaryngol. 1983;109:285–8.
50. Dahiya R, Keller JD, Litofsky NS, Bankey PE, Bonassar LJ, Megerian CA. Temporal bone fractures: otic capsule sparing versus otic capsule violating clinical and radiographic considerations. J Trauma. 1999;47:1079–83.
51. Zayas JO, Feliciano YZ, Hadley CR, Gomez AA, Vidal JA. Temporal bone trauma and the role of multidetector CT in the emergency department. Radiographics. 2011;31:1741–55. doi:10.1148/rg.316115506.
52. Davis JW, Holbrook TL, Hoyt DB, Mackersie RC, Field TO Jr, Shackford SR. Blunt carotid artery dissection: incidence, associated injuries, screening, and treatment. J Trauma. 1990;30(12):1514–7.
53. Biffl WL, Moore EE, Offner PJ, Burch JM. Blunt carotid and vertebral arterial injuries. World J Surg. 2001;25(8):1036–43.
54. Biffl WL, Moore EE, Ryu RK, et al. The unrecognized epidemic of blunt carotid arterial injuries: early diagnosis improves neurologic outcome. Ann Surg. 1998;228(4):462–70.
55. Carrillo EH, Osborne DL, Spain DA, Miller FB, Senler SO, Richardson JD. Blunt carotid artery injuries: difficulties with the diagnosis prior to neurologic event. J Trauma. 1999;46(6):1120–5.
56. Fabian TC, Patton JH Jr, Croce MA, Minard G, Kudsk KA, Pritchard FE. Blunt carotid injury: importance of early diagnosis and anticoagulant therapy. Ann Surg. 1996;223(5):513–25.
57. Miller PR, Fabian TC, Bee TK, et al. Blunt cerebrovascular injuries: diagnosis and treatment. J Trauma. 2001;51(2):279–86.
58. Caranci F, Napoli M, Cirillo M, Briganti G, Brunese L, Briganti F. Basilar artery hypoplasia. Neuroradiol J. 2012;25(6):739–43. issn:1971–4009.
59. Mulloy JP, Flick PA, Gold RE. Blunt carotid injury: a review. Radiology. 1998;207(3):571–85.
60. Cothren CC, Moore EE. Blunt cerebrovascular injuries. Clinics. 2005;60(6):489–96. Epub 12 Dec 2005.
61. Stemper BD, Yoganandan N, Sinson GP, Gennarelli TA, Stineman MR, Pintar FA. Biomechanical characterization of internal layer subfailure in blunt arterial injury. Ann Biomed Eng. 2007;35(2):285–91.
62. Caranci F, Briganti F, La Porta M, Antinolfi G, Cesarano E, Fonio P, Brunese L, Coppolino F. Magnetic resonance imaging in brachial plexus injury. Musculoskelet Surg. 2013;97(Suppl 2):181–90. doi:10.1007/s12306-013-0281-0. issn:2035–5106.
63. McKevitt EC, Kirkpatrick AW, Vertesi L, Granger R, Simons RK. Identifying patients at risk for intracranial and extracranial blunt carotid injuries. Am J Surg. 2002;183(5):566–70. Epub 7 Dec 2006.
64. Sliker CW. Blunt cerebrovascular injuries: imaging with multidetector CT angiography. Radiographics. 2008;28:1689–710. doi:10.1148/rg.286085521.
65. Biffl WL, Moore EE, Offner PJ, Brega KE, Franciose RJ, Burch JM. Blunt carotid arterial injuries: implications of a new grading scale. J Trauma. 1999;47(5):845–53.
66. Núñez DB Jr, Torres-León M, Múnera F. Vascular injuries of the neck and thoracic inlet: helical CT angiographic correlation. Radiographics. 2004;24(4):1087–98.
67. Staller B, Múnera F, Sanchez A, Núñez DB Jr. Helical and multislice CTA following penetrating trauma to the subclavian and axillary arteries (pictorial essay). Emerg Radiol. 2005;11(6):336–41. Epub 14 Jun 2005.
68. Stallmeyer MJ, Morales RE, Flanders AE. Imaging of traumatic neurovascular injury. Radiol Clin North Am. 2006;44(1):13–39.
69. Provenzale JM. Dissection of the internal carotid and vertebral arteries: imaging features. AJR Am J Roentgenol. 1995;165:1099–104.
70. Leclerc X, Godefroy O, Salhi A, Lucas C, Leys D, Pruvo JP. Helical CT for the diagnosis of extracranial internal carotid artery dissection. Stroke. 1996;27(3):461–6.
71. Coldwell DM, Novak Z, Ryu RK, et al. Treatment of posttraumatic internal carotid arterial pseu-

doaneurysm with endovascular stents. J Trauma. 2000;48(3):470–2.
72. Briganti F, Tedeschi E, Leone G, Marseglia M, Cicala D, Giamundo M, Napoli M, Caranci F. Endovascular treatment of vertebro-vertebral arteriovenous fistula. A report of three cases and literature review. Neuroradiol J. 2013;26(3):339–46. issn:1971–4009.
73. Coskun O, Hamon M, Catroux G, Gosme L, Courtheoux P, Theron J. Carotid-cavernous fistulas: diagnosis with spiral CT angiography. AJNR Am J Neuroradiol. 2000;21:712–6.
74. Anderson K, Collie DA, Capewell A. CT angiographic appearances of carotid-cavernous fistula. Clin Radiol. 2001;56(6):514–6.
75. Stanton DC, Kempers KG, Hendler BH, Cutilli BJ, Hurst RW. Posttraumatic carotid-cavernous sinus fistula. J Craniomaxillofac Trauma. 1999;5:39–44.
76. Kumbhat S, LeBlang SD, Falcone S. CT-choroidal effusions as a sign of carotid cavernous. AJNR Am J Neuroradiol. 2000;21(4):779–80.
77. Chen CC, Chang PC, Shy CG, Chen WS, Hung HC. CT angiography and MR angiography in the evaluation of carotid cavernous sinus fistula prior to embolization: a comparison of techniques. AJNR Am J Neuroradiol. 2005;26:2349–56.
78. Briganti F, Caranci F, Leone G, Napoli M, Cicala D, Briganti G, Tranfa F, Bonavolontà G. Endovascular occlusion of dural cavernous fistulas through a superior ophthalmic vein approach. Neuroradiol J. 2013;26(5): 565–72. issn:1971–4009.
79. Zimmerman RA, Bilaniuk LT. Computed tomographic staging of traumatic epidural bleeding. Radiology. 1982;144:809–12.
80. Subramanian SK, Roszler MH, Gaudy B, Michael DB. Significance of computed tomography mixed density in traumatic extra-axial hemorrhage. Neurol Res. 2002;24:125–8.
81. Pruthi N, Balasubramaniam A, Chandramouli BA, et al. Mixed-density extradural hematomas on computed tomography-prognostic significance. Surg Neurol. 2009;71:202–6. doi:10.1016/j.surneu.2007.10.032. Epub 6 Mar 2008.
82. Al-Nakshabandi NA. The swirl sign. Radiology. 2001;218(2):433.
83. Gean AD, Fischbein NJ, Purcel DD, Aiken AH, Manley GT, Stiver SI. Benign anterior temporal epidural hematoma: indolent lesion with a characteristic CT imaging appearance after blunt head trauma. Radiology. 2010;257(1):212–8. doi:10.1148/radiol.10092075. Epub 16 Aug 2010.
84. Milo R, Razon N, Schiffer J. Delayed epidural hematoma. A review. Acta Neurochir. 1987;84(1–2):13–23.
85. Smith WP Jr, Batnitzky S, Rengachary SS. Acute isodense subdural hematomas: a problem in anemic patients. AJR Am J Roentgenol. 1981;136:543–6.
86. Young RJ, Destian S. Imaging of traumatic intracranial hemorrhage. Neuroimaging Clin N Am. 2002;12:189–204.
87. Keeney SE, Adcock EW, McArdle CB. Prospective observations of 100 high-risk neonates by high-field (1.5 Tesla) magnetic resonance imaging of the central nervous system: I. Intraventricular and extracerebral lesions. Pediatrics. 1991;87:421–30.
88. Kubal WS. Updated imaging of traumatic brain injury. Radiol Clin N Am. 2012;50(1):15–41. doi:10.1016/j.rcl.2011.08.010.
89. Wiesmann M, Mayer TE, Yousry I, Medele R, Hamann GF, Bruckmann H. Detection of hyperacute subarachnoid hemorrhage of the brain by using magnetic resonance imaging. J Neurosurg. 2002;96:684–9.
90. Given CA 2nd, Burdette JH, Elster AD, Williams DW 3rd. Pseudo-subarachnoid hemorrhage: a potential imaging pitfall associated with diffuse cerebral edema. AJNR Am J Neuroradiol. 2003;24:254–6.
91. Greene KA, Marciano FF, Johnson BA, Jacobowitz R, Spetzler RF, Harrington TR. Impact of traumatic subarachnoid hemorrhage on outcome in nonpenetrating head injury. Part I: a proposed computerized tomography grading scale. J Neurosurg. 1995;83:445–52.
92. Briganti F, Napoli M, Leone G, Marseglia M, Mariniello G, Caranci F, Tortora F, Maiuri F. Treatment of intracranial aneurysms by flow diverter devices: long-term results from a single center. Eur J Radiol. 2014;83(9):1683–90. doi:10.1016/j.ejrad.2014.05.029. issn:0720-048X.
93. LeRoux PD, Haglund MM, Newell DW, Grady MS, Winn HR. Intraventricular hemorrhage in blunt head trauma: an analysis of 43 cases. Neurosurgery. 1992;3:678–84; discussion: 684–5.
94. Braun M, Cordoliani YS, Dosch JC. Head and brain injuries. Place of imaging. Ann Fr Anesth Reanim. 2000;19:296–8.
95. Hoelper BM, Reinert MM, Zauner A, Doppenberg E, Bullock R. rCBF in hemorrhagic, non-hemorrhagic and mixed contusions after severe head injury and its effect on perilesional cerebral blood flow. Acta Neurochir Suppl. 2000;76:21–5.
96. Gentry LR, Godersky JC, Thompson B, Dunn VD. Prospective comparative study of intermediate-field MR and CT in the evaluation of close head trauma. AJR Am J Roentgenol. 1988;150(3):673–82.
97. Caranci F, Tedeschi E, Leone G, Reginelli A, Gatta G, Pinto A, Squillaci E, Briganti F, Brunese L. Errors in neuroradiology. Radiol Med. 2015;120(9):795–801. doi:10.1007/s11547-015-0564-7.
98. Adams JH, Graham DI, Murray LS, Scott G. Diffuse axonal injury due to nonmissile head injury in humans: an analysis of 45 cases. Ann Neurol. 1982;12:557–63.
99. Chang MC, Jang SH. Corpus callosum injury in patients with diffuse axonal injury: a diffusion tensor imaging study. NeuroRehabilitation. 2010;26(4):339–45. doi:10.3233/NRE-2010-0571.
100. Meythaler JM, Peduzzi JD, Eleftheriou E, Novack TA. Current concepts: diffuse axonal injury-associated traumatic brain injury. Arch Phys Med Rehabil. 2001;82:1461–71.
101. Mittl RL, Grossman RI, Hiehle JF, et al. Prevalence of MR evidence of diffuse axonal injury in patients

with mild head injury and normal head CT findings. AJNR Am J Neuroradiol. 1994;15:1583–9.
102. Kinoshita T, Moritani T, Hiwatashi A, et al. Conspicuity of diffuse axonal injury lesions on diffusion-weighted MR imaging. Eur J Radiol. 2005;56:5–11.
103. Gentry LR, Thompson B, Godersky JC. Trauma to the corpus callosum: MR features. AJNR Am J Neuroradiol. 1988;9:1129–38.
104. Gentry LR, Godersky JC, Thompson B. Traumatic brainstem injury: MR imaging. Radiology. 1989;171:177–87.
105. Firsching R, Woischneck D, Klein S, Ludwig K, Dohring W. Brain stem lesions after head injury. Neurol Res. 2002;24:145–6.
106. Cirillo M, Caranci F, Tortora F, Corvino F, Pezzullo F, Conforti R, Cirillo S. Structural neuroimaging in dementia. J Alzheimers Dis. 2012;29(Suppl 1):16–9. doi:10.3233/JAD-2012-129000.
107. Kou Z, Wu Z, Tong KA, et al. The role of advanced MR imaging findings as biomarkers of traumatic brain injury. J Head Trauma Rehabil. 2010;25(4):267–82. doi:10.1097/HTR.0b013e3181e54793.
108. Versaci F, Trivisonno A, Olivieri C, Caranci F, Brunese L, Prati F. Late renal artery stenosis after renal denervation: is it the tip of the iceberg? Int J Cardiol. 2014;172:e507–8. doi:10.1016/j.ijcard.2014.01.018.
109. Muccio CF, Caranci F, D'Arco F, Cerase A, De Lipsis L, Esposito G, Tedeschi E, Andreula C. Magnetic Resonance features of pyogenic brain abscesses and differential diagnosis using morphological and functional imaging studies: a pictorial essay. J Neuroradiol. 2014;41(3):153–67. doi:10.1016/j.neurad.2014.05.004. issn:0150–9861.
110. Hammoud DA, Wasserman BA. Diffuse axonal injuries: pathophysiology and imaging. Neuroimaging Clin N Am. 2002;12:205–16.
111. Pinto A, Brunese L, Pinto F, Reali R, Daniele S, Romano L. The concept of error and malpractice in radiology. Semin Ultrasound CT MR. 2012;33:275–9. doi:10.1053/j.sult.2012.01.009.
112. Zimmerman RA, Bilanuik LT, Buce D, Dolinskas C, Obrist W, Kuhl D. Computed tomography of pediatric head trauma: acute general swelling. Radiology. 1978;126:403–8.
113. Battipaglia G, Avilia S, Morelli E, Caranci F, Perna F, Camera A. Posterior reversible encephalopathy syndrome (PRES) during induction chemotherapy for acute myeloblastic leukemia (AML). Ann Hematol. 2012;91(8):1327–8. doi:10.1007/s00277-011-1398-6.
114. Laine FJ, Shedden AI, Dunn MM, Ghatak NR. Acquired intracranial herniation: MR findings. AJR Am J Roentgenol. 1995;165:967–73.

Maxillofacial Injuries

4

Alessandro Stasolla

4.1 Radiologists and Facial Trauma

The face is a complex three-dimensional anatomic region involved in special senses, cosmetics and personal identity, whose even minor injury may be associated with significant damage.

During acute trauma assessment, the radiologist is often the primary specialist interpreting facial injuries, therefore assuming a special clinical responsibility. Indeed, even if facial injuries are almost always clinically obvious, soft tissue swelling, limited patient cooperation and polytrauma can present a significant challenge to the physical examination.

Apart from the diagnosis of fractures themselves, radiologists should try to anticipate the *complications* of the trauma, therefore facilitating the clinical approach. Indeed maxillofacial injuries are heterogeneous conditions that may:

- Be *immediately life-threatening* when they affect the airway (e.g. flail mandible) or cause vascular lesions
- Lead to early *loss of vision*, sometimes avoidable with expedite surgery
- Lead to *delayed life-threatening* complications (e.g. meningitis from CSF leak)
- Impair major *functions* such as mastication
- Severely affect patient *cosmetics* (e.g. nasal fractures)
- Be a cause of *chronic pain* and/or *late infections* (e.g. retained foreign body)

Provided that the airway is secured and vascular injuries are expeditiously excluded on contrast-enhanced images (post-contrast imaging of the face is recommended), tension orbit and globe injury are the diagnostic priority of facial imaging. *Which is the benefit in detecting a hairlike fracture of the maxillary sinus wall, if you miss signs of impending loss of vision?*

4.2 General Features of Facial Fractures

The epidemiology of maxillofacial fractures is variable, depending on the geographical area and socioeconomic differences. Common causes

A. Stasolla, M.D.
Diagnostic and Interventional Neuroradiology, S. Camillo Hospital, Rome, Italy
e-mail: alestaso@tiscali.it

V. Miele, M. Trinci (eds.), *Diagnostic Imaging in Polytrauma Patients*,
https://doi.org/10.1007/978-3-319-62054-1_4

of facial fractures are road traffic accidents (RTAs), assaults, falls, sports and work injuries. In Europe there has been a recent decreasing trend in maxillofacial trauma; furthermore cases due to assaults and falls nowadays outnumber those due to RTAs [1]. With the progressive ageing of the population, road and work legislation are thought to be responsible for this change [1]. The most frequently observed fractures are mandibular fractures, orbital-zygomatic-maxillary (OZM) fractures (24%), orbital fractures (16%), nasal fractures (9%), Le Fort fractures (5%), frontal sinus fractures (3%) and naso-orbital-ethmoidal (NOE) fractures (1%). Condylar fractures are the most commonly observed mandibular fracture, accounting for the 34% [1]. It should be noted that in children relatively minor traumas can cause buckled or "greenstick" (i.e. mandibular fractures, trapdoor fractures of the orbital floor).

The so-called facial buttresses are the thickest bone structures providing support to the facial skeleton; therefore repair of injured buttresses is the key to surgically restore shape and function of the face. The facial skeleton is indeed formed by a series of vertical and relatively frail horizontal struts, the former being the paired *nasomaxillary*, *zygomaticomaxillary* and *pterygomaxillary buttress* and unpaired *frontoethmoidal-vomerine buttress* and the latter being the *superior alveolar ridges*, *palate* and *inferior orbital rims*.

Surgical treatment of maxillofacial fractures is aimed to restore function and cosmetics, preventing complications. Surgery is generally performed within a week after the trauma; sometimes, however, it needs to be delayed either for general reasons or due to the occurrence of life-threatening injuries [2]. Unstable fracture fragments have to be fixed to stable structures; open reduction is most often accomplished by internal fixation with miniplates and miniscrews. Nasal haemorrhages may require anterior and posterior nasal packing, manual reduction of fractures, surgical ligation or catheter embolization of external carotid artery branches.

Up to 50–70% of patients with facial trauma are reported with concomitant injuries; cervical spine injuries can be seen in 4–10%, and 18–45% of patients with a facial fracture may have an associated head injury [3]; therefore radiologists should carefully look associated findings in the field of view of CT scans.

4.3 Imaging of Facial Trauma

Plain films should no longer play a significant role in evaluating facial trauma. Computed tomography (CT) with bone and soft tissue algorithms and coronal and sagittal multiplanar reformations (MPR) is the standard for diagnosing maxillofacial injuries. Thin sections are mandatory (≤1.25 mm).

Fracture identification should rely entirely on this data set. Soft tissue images should not be overlooked, e.g. orbital content is inaccurately depicted on bone algorithm images; furthermore skin and soft tissue modifications, particularly when clinical information are scant and dynamics of the trauma are unknown to the radiologist, can direct the imager to the fractures and associated injuries. Volume-rendering (VR) three-dimensional CT post-processing may be helpful for a fast understanding of complex pattern of fracture and fragment displacement; however, radiologists should not rely on these beautiful images for fracture detection (Fig. 4.1): as a matter of fact, VR imaging can easily miss maxillary, orbital, sphenoidal and especially ethmoidal fractures [4]. *CT angiography* can show vascular complications including leaks, dissections, aneurysms and occlusion, and its use should be stressed in the daily practice. Cone beam volume computed tomography (*CBVCT*) may be useful in detecting isolated fractures as a low-dose technique but cannot depict soft tissue injuries. Magnetic resonance (MR) imaging is used occasionally to assess the optic nerve. Plain films

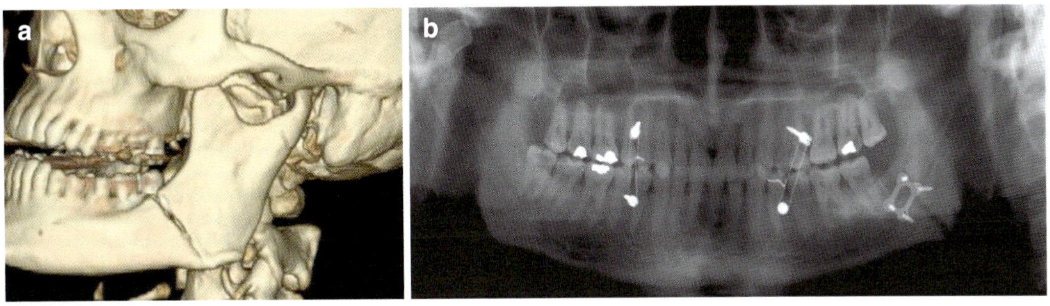

Fig. 4.1 Volume rendering (VR) should not be overemphasized as a screening tool to diagnose facial fractures. In that case, the left non-displaced condylar fracture, barely demonstrated on VR, is an easy diagnosis on panoramic radiography. Note bilateral intermaxillary fixation, left side mandibular angle fracture treated with screws and a displaced right extracapsular condylar fracture

have still a role as *panoramic imaging* for mandibular injuries (Fig. 4.1) and *dental images* for teeth and alveolar fractures. As X-ray examination of nasal fracture gives a much too high number of false positive and false negative results, its use has been discouraged [5].

The *clear sinus sign*, i.e. the absence on CT scans of sinus fluid or opacification to exclude fractures involving the sinus walls, can be used for a rapid triage of facial fractures. Generally speaking, fractures through sinus walls tear mucosal vessels producing haemorrhage; thus, in the acute phase, the absence of free fluid in a sinus cavity is an evidence against the hypothesis of a fracture. As the floor of the orbit is the roof of the maxillary sinus, the medial orbital wall is the lamina papyracea, and the orbital roof is the floor of the supraorbital ethmoidal cells or the frontal sinus; fractures may cause blood levels in these sinuses. The clear sinus sign is reliable to exclude injuries requiring surgical intervention, identifying severe facial ZMC and orbital and sinus fractures. However, it should be stressed that 10% of complex facial fractures may not have associated sinus opacification (Fig. 4.2); furthermore *nasal bone and mandibular fractures cannot be ruled out at all* [6].

A note about the CT appearance of *foreign bodies* is mandatory before offering a systematic approach to facial fractures. Metallic foreign bodies are easy to find with CT, while glass, plastic, wood and vegetable matter have a variable density and may be overlooked. As a general rule, *any density with a highly geometric shape is likely a foreign body* [7]; blood and gas may be a clue to the presence of a possible foreign body. When a wooden foreign body is suspected, CT evaluation with −500 HU level and 1000–2000 HU width is recommended, given the aspected density in the range of +20 to −600 HU [7]. Apart from the special harm of foreign bodies into the orbit, delayed consequences of an overlooked, retained foreign body in other soft tissues of the face (e.g. pain, suppurative infection, tetanus) cannot be underestimated.

4.4 Orbital Fractures

Orbital fractures may rarely require emergency orbital surgery, as most of the fractures can be addressed with close observation or can be repaired after several weeks [8]. However, provided that the airway is secured and vascular injuries are excluded, orbital trauma should be *addressed at the beginning of the reporting process*, as a comprehensive ophthalmic clinical evaluation is usually limited in the acute polytrauma setting, especially in the unconscious patient. Therefore, the radiologist is often the primary specialist calling for *globe injuries and tensive orbit*.

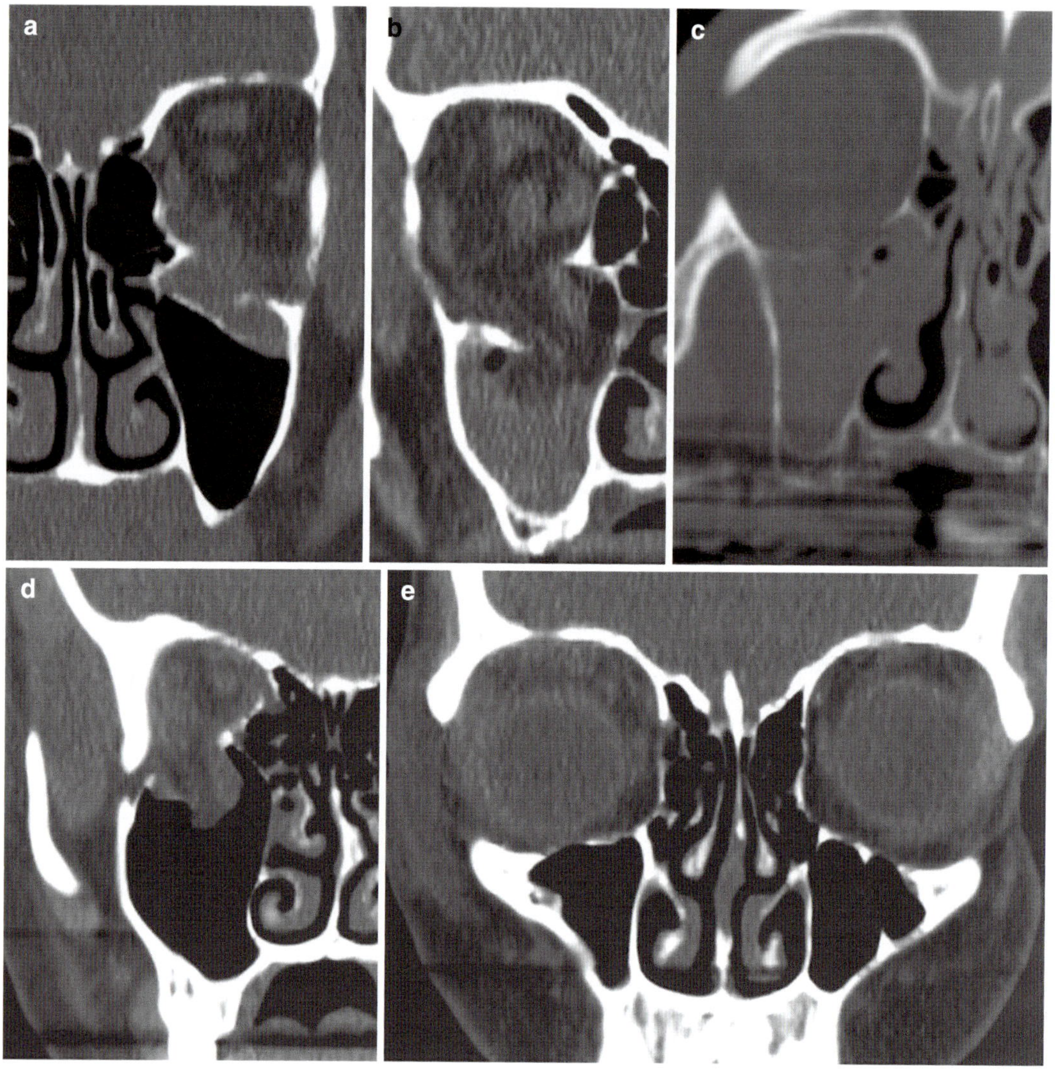

Fig. 4.2 Orbital floor "blow-out" fractures on parade. (**a**) Displaced fracture with subperiosteal haematoma and rounding of the inferior rectus muscle. Note the lack of haemosinus and, therefore, a false negative clear sinus sign. (**b**) Displaced fracture with large herniation of fat and inferior rectus muscle. (**c**) Displaced fracture with complete haemorrhagic opacification of the maxillary sinus. (**d**) Displaced fracture with herniation orbital content and hypoglobus (**e**), again with a false negative clear sinus sign

Systematic approaches can be used in the setting of a busy emergency workflow; general radiologists taking patient responsibility "from head to toe" and even neuroradiologists having little clinical interest in head-neck imaging may take advantage from some mnemonics such as "BALPINE"—*bones*, *anterior chamber*, *lens*, *posterior globe structures*, *intraconal orbit*, *neurovascular structures* and *extraocular muscles/extraconal orbit* [9].

While the absence of an orbital fracture doesn't rule out a globe injury, an eye which is intact on CT scan is likely not to have a penetrating injury, and immediate surgical intervention is probably not required [10].

Evaluation of the globe (Figs. 4.3 and 4.4) should include width of anterior chamber (decreased in corneal lacerations or anterior displacement of the lens, increased in globe ruptures), lens position (dislocation) and density

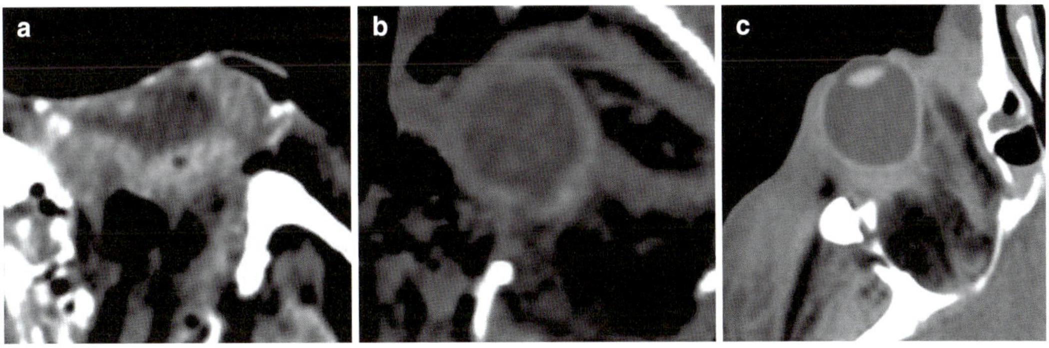

Fig. 4.3 "Flat tyre" appearance (**a**) and abnormal contour of the globe (**b**), suggesting an open globe injury. Both the eyes had eventually to be enucleated. Posterior "tenting" of the globe, secondary to posttraumatic haematoma and tension orbit (**c**)

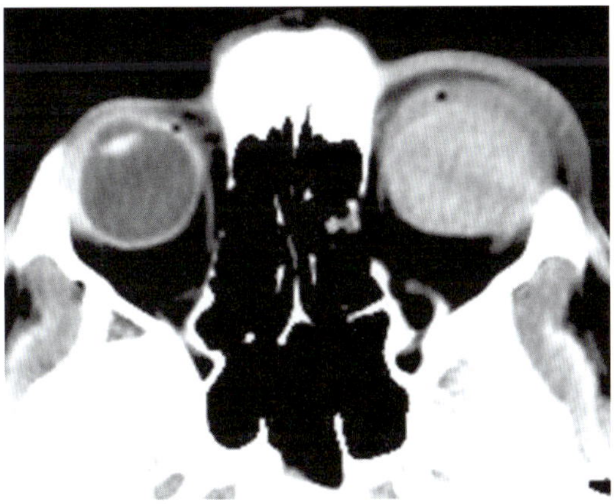

Fig. 4.4 Young firework casualty with a massive vitreous haemorrhage. Homogeneous hyperattenuation in the posterior segment of the globe and periorbital soft tissue swelling. The anterior segment is obscured

(acute traumatic cataract, hypoattenuating compared with the nonaffected side), posterior chamber haemorrhage, globe deformity, intraocular air and foreign bodies (vide infra). CT provided an overall accuracy of 81% in the diagnosis of globe rupture [11]. Reference to the ophthalmologic examinations is in any case pivotal to avoid misinterpretations in case of previous ocular surgery, e.g. intraocular haemorrhage as seen on CT confused with surgical changes (Fig. 4.5).

After an orbital trauma, *tension orbit* (Figs. 4.3c, 4.6 and 4.7) can be defined as a threat to vision because of the presence of an acute and exceeding increase of orbital content (blood, air, bone, foreign bodies) stretching the optic nerve [12]. The anterior displacement of the eye (proptosis), caused by the mass effect, stretches the optic nerve, thus compromising its vascular supply and ultimately leads to ischaemic optic neuropathy. The procession of CT changes in tension orbit is described by Mancuso and Verbist [12]: (1) space-occupying process within the orbit; (2) proptosis; (3) full extended, stretched optic nerve, entirely visible all in one plane of section; and (4) optic nerve diameter diminished due to the stretching. At point 4 tension orbit is incipient, and a potential emergency surgical decompression may be warranted. By the next point, a loss of visual acuity can be predicted with near certainty: (5) posterior globe assuming a cone-shaped or tented appearance and (6) continued worsening of previous points, mainly the tenting of the globe. Even when "incipient", direct communication with the clinical team is mandatory for the radiologist.

Orbital fractures can be isolated or associated with other midfacial fractures (e.g. Le Fort II and III, NOE, ZMC fractures). A solitary non-displaced fracture of an orbital wall usually doesn't require any treatment. Displaced wall fractures may have a blow-in or a blow-out pattern.

The *orbital apex*, formed by the superior orbital fissure and optic canal, is the crossroad between the orbit and the intracranial structures. Fracture of this area can be associated with optic nerve impingement and intraorbital haematoma. Given the little room available in that area, even

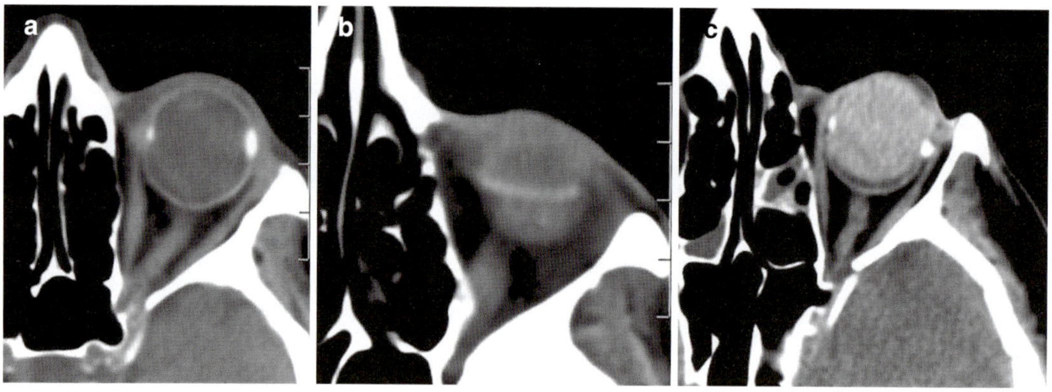

Fig. 4.5 Radiologist should familiarize with materials used to treat retinal detachment, including gas, scleral bands and silicon oil (**a–c**). Note the hyperattenuating silicon oil in the posterior segment of the globe, mimicking haemorrhage

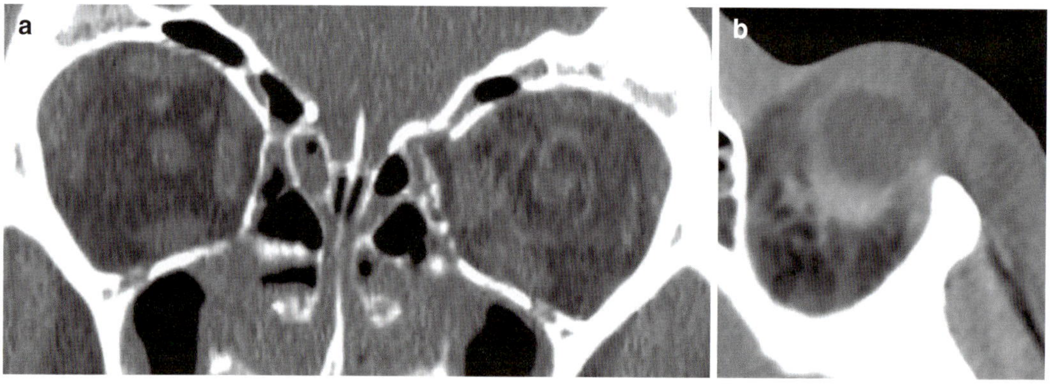

Fig. 4.6 Despite the absence of significant displaced fractures, intraconal and retrobulbar haematoma should induce a prompt clinical evaluation for tension orbit

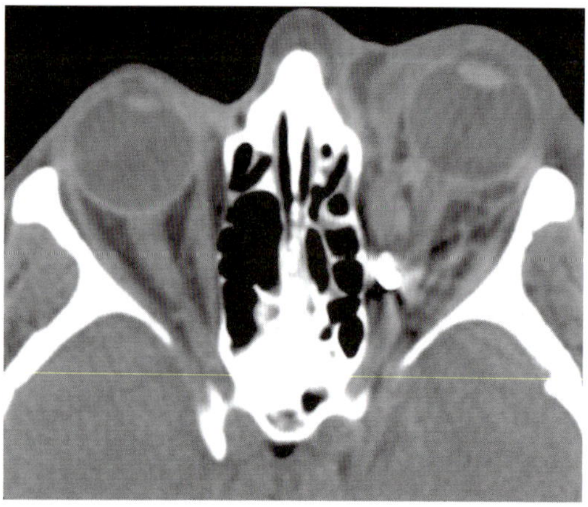

Fig. 4.7 An extraocular metallic foreign body is seen in the region of the medial rectus muscle, along the path of the optic nerve. Note the extra- and intraconal haematoma tracking along the nerve, which appears stretched, with evident proptosis

small injuries can be extremely dangerous to the optic nerve: extremely careful inspection and reporting are therefore de rigueur (Fig. 4.8).

Blow-out fractures (Figs. 4.2 and 4.9) are among the most common orbital fractures. They are produced by a direct impact on the orbit causing a sudden increase in intraorbital pressure. This leads most commonly to a fracture of the medial wall and/or the *orbital floor*. It should be noted that non-traumatic dehiscence of lamina papyracea can be found in 6.5% of population [13]. Medial and inferior rectus muscles can be trapped in the fracture, leading to restriction of gaze and diplopia. Indirect signs of blow-out fractures are orbital emphysema (from communication with adjacent air-containing sinuses), fat and/or extraocular muscle projecting as a soft tissue mass into the maxillary or ethmoidal sinuses and fluid (blood) in the sinuses. Extraocular muscles may appear swollen and round, as a result of contusive damage and lack of soft tissue support.

In children a characteristic orbital floor blow-out fracture is the so-called trapdoor fracture, a greenstick fracture in which prolapsed orbital tissues may be entrapped on the maxillary sinus side of the orbital floor. These features may be easily overlooked at imaging [14].

Fracture of the *orbital roof* occurs in the adult population, although they are more common in children. It is often frequently associated with frontal sinus and skull base fractures, dural tears, intracranial haemorrhage and brain injuries. Direct blows to the forehead may cause inward displacement fractures of the orbital roof: these so-called blow-in fractures (Fig. 4.10) may be associated to globe injuries, and displaced bone fragments may impinge and damage the optic nerve. Prior to age 7, the frontal sinus is not pneumatized, and frontal hits can fracture the orbital roof in isolation [15]. Apart from the classic cases above-mentioned, "blow-in" and "blow-out" patterns may variably affect the orbital walls (Fig. 4.11).

The optic nerve is vulnerable to shearing effects that may lead to *traumatic optic neuropathy*. The risk of traumatic optic neuropathy may be predicted by the presence of intraconal haematoma (the best predictor), intraconal emphysema, optic canal fracture, haematoma along the poste-

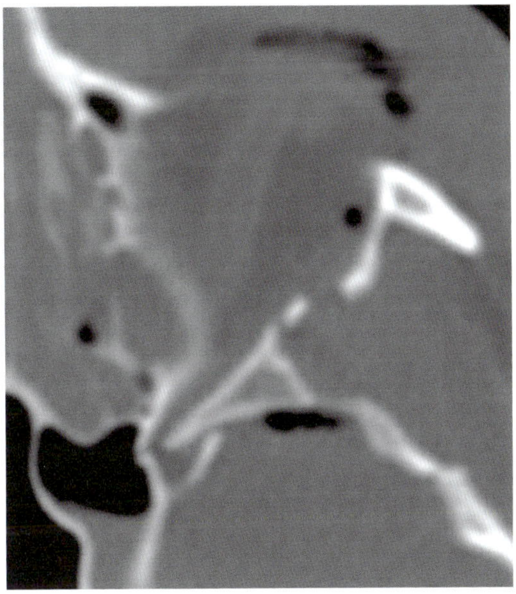

Fig. 4.8 Bone impingement of the superior orbital fissure. Such a detail may be overlooked in the bone disaster of a big facial crash but can be responsible for ptosis, proptosis, ophthalmoplegia, fixation and dilatation of the pupil, anaesthesia of the upper eyelid and forehead

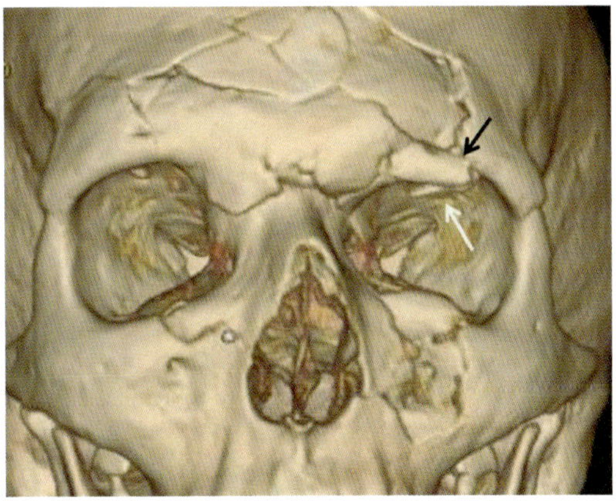

Fig. 4.10 Left superior orbital rim fracture (*black arrow*) with "blow-in" of the roof (*white arrow*) in the setting of a complex midfacial fracture involving the frontal bone. Note the reduction in the vertical dimension of the left orbit

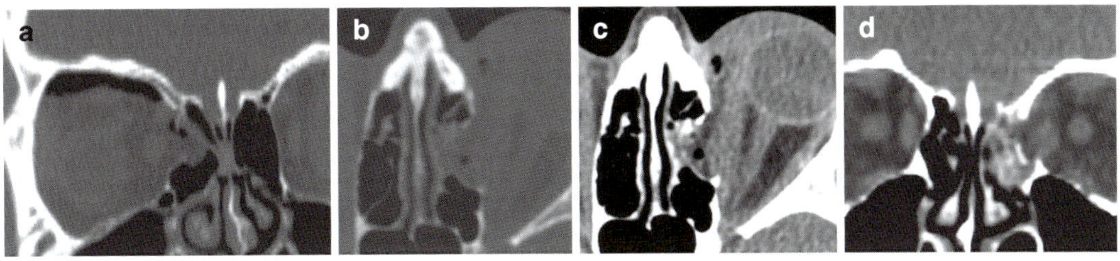

Fig. 4.9 Medial orbital wall blow-out fractures: note the variable amount of orbital emphysema and the swollen medial rectus muscle

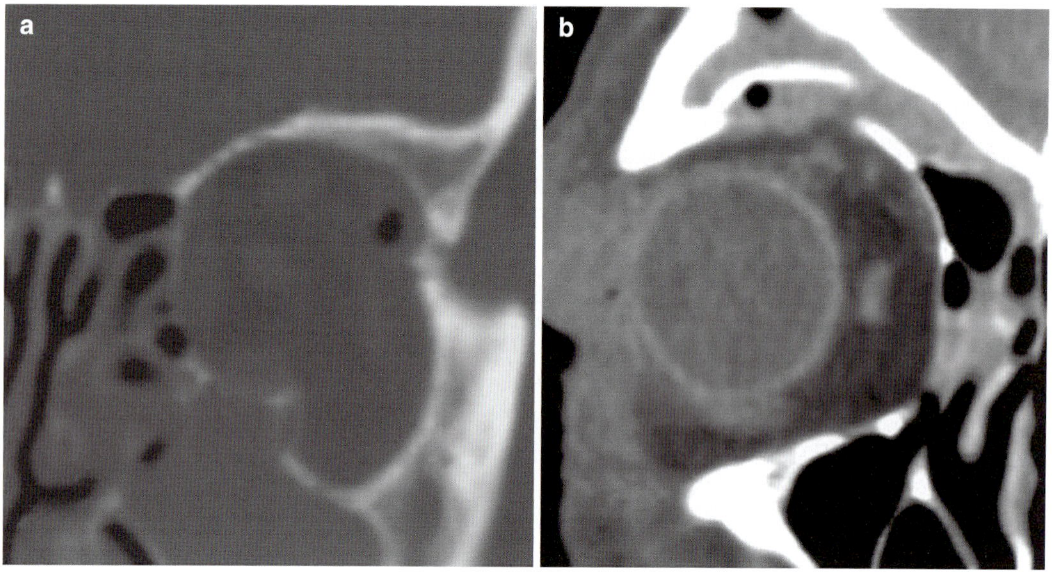

Fig. 4.11 Although less usual than the counterparts, "blow-in" patterns may affect the floor (**a**) and "blow-out" the roof (**b**) of the orbit. Note orbital emphysema in both cases and quite extensive subperiosteal haematoma in (**b**), continuing in the frontal sinus

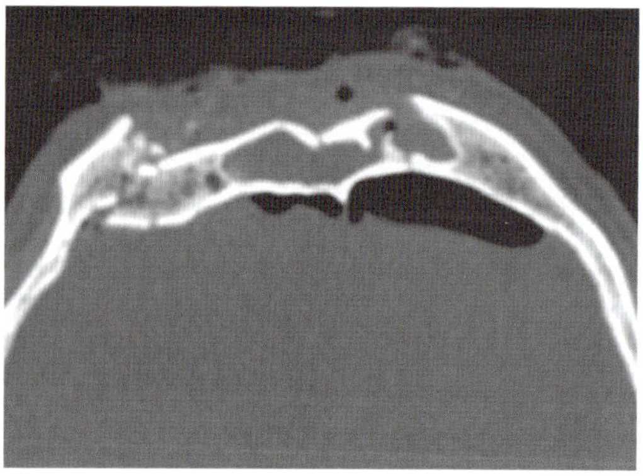

Fig. 4.12 Comminuted and displaced fracture of the anterior and posterior walls of the frontal sinus with associated opacification of the sinus and pneumocephalus, suggesting a dural tear

rior globe and extraconal haematoma. In these cases early ophthalmologic consultation is recommended [16].

The orbit should be also screened for dilation of the ophthalmic veins, as a sign of traumatic carotid-cavernous fistula.

4.5 Frontal Sinus Fractures

Frontal sinus fractures can lead to significant complications such as *meningitis*, *encephalitis*, *intracranial abscesses*, *osteomyelitis* and *mucoceles*. Posterior table involvement and the presence of pneumocephalus should be noted, suggesting an associated dural tear (Fig. 4.12). Nasofrontal outflow tract injury and obstruction are to be stressed [17]. As already stated, prior to age 7, the frontal sinus is not pneumatized, and frontal hits often fracture the orbital roof in isolation [15].

4.6 Midfacial Fractures

4.6.1 Nasal Bone Fractures

The nasal bones are the commonest fractured bones of the face (Fig. 4.13). Most of nasal fractures occur within the lower and thinner portion of the bones, in the transverse plane, while nor-

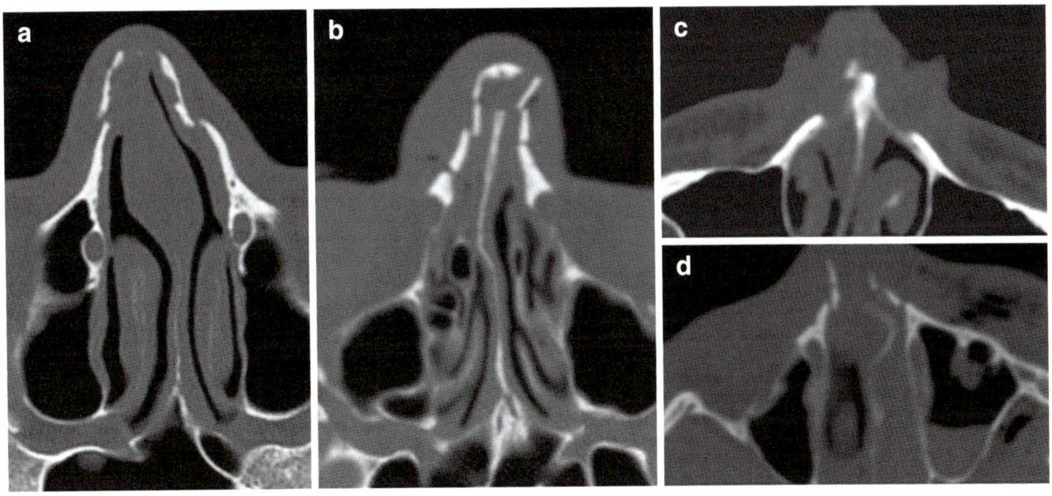

Fig. 4.13 Nasal fractures may heal by fibrosis; the lack (**a**) or the presence (**b**) of soft tissue injury suggests, respectively, an old and an acute fracture. Clinical examination is however pivotal for a correct diagnosis. Anterior nasal spine fractures (**c**) should not be overlooked, as this maxillary structure has a role in the nasal shape. Nasal septum fractures (**d**) can evolve with septal haematoma and abscess

mal sutures and nasociliary grooves are longitudinally oriented and do not cross the midline, as fractures can. Plain films of nasal bone fractures have high rates of false positive and false negative findings and are inadequate for an accurate diagnosis of nasal bone fractures. Old nasal fractures heal by ossification in only 50% of cases, whereas the remaining heal more or less by fibrosis connecting the fragments, and thus the old fractures are visible on CT/X-rays for the rest of the patient's life [18]. Fracture and focal thickening of the nasal septum should be carefully reported, as they may lead to haematoma, necrosis, infection, abscess and eventually airflow obstruction or nasal saddling. The anterior nasal spine is an often overlooked structure; however, it is involved in the cosmetics of the lower nose. Although treatment usually consists of a simple closed reduction, incorrect diagnoses and inadequate reductions can cause secondary deformity. Additional operation like corrective rhinoplasty or septoplasty could be needed later [19].

4.6.2 Naso-Orbital-Ethmoidal Fractures

Naso-orbital-ethmoidal (NOE) fractures involve the central upper midface and are distinguished from nasal fractures by posterior disruption of the medial canthal region, the ethmoids and the medial orbital walls. By definition, NOE fractures include damage to the ethmoidal sinus and walls (Fig. 4.14).

NOE fractures can be also thought as a "telescoping" injury of nasal bones, posteriorly displaced into the ethmoidal sinuses involving commonly the frontal bones. Telecanthus, i.e. increased distance between the medial canthi of the eyes, is a typical finding. The status of the medial canthal insertion onto the lacrimal fossa (so-called central fragment) is the key factor in grading of NOE fractures. According to the Markowitz and Manson system [20], in type I (Fig. 4.14), the fractured piece is large, and the medial canthal insertion around the lacrimal fossa is intact. In type II,

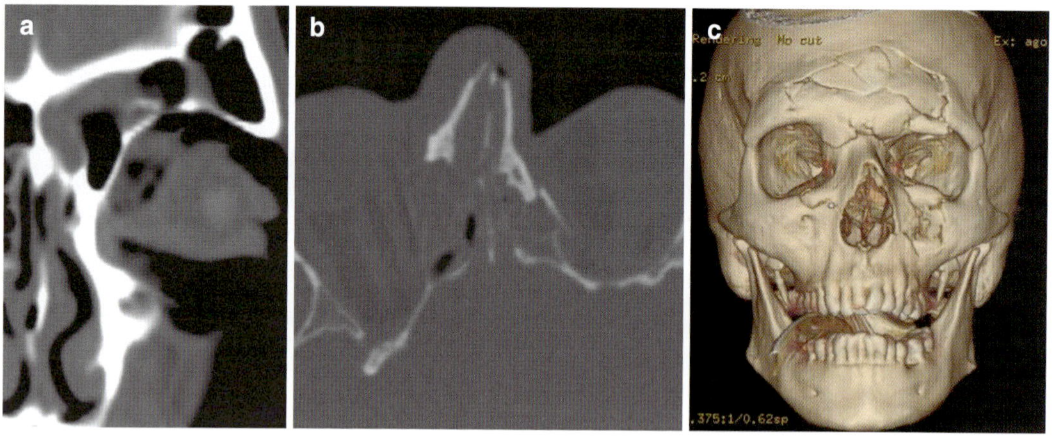

Fig. 4.14 (**a**) Osseous insertion of the medial canthal ligament. The NOE fractures are categorized on the morphology of that area, referred to as the "central fragment". (**b**, **c**) Bilateral naso-orbital-ethmoidal (NOE) fracture associated with frontal sinus fracture. The fractures involve the nasomaxillary buttresses of the facial skeleton; these are Markowitz type I fractures, with a single large NOE fragment bearing the medial canthal tendon

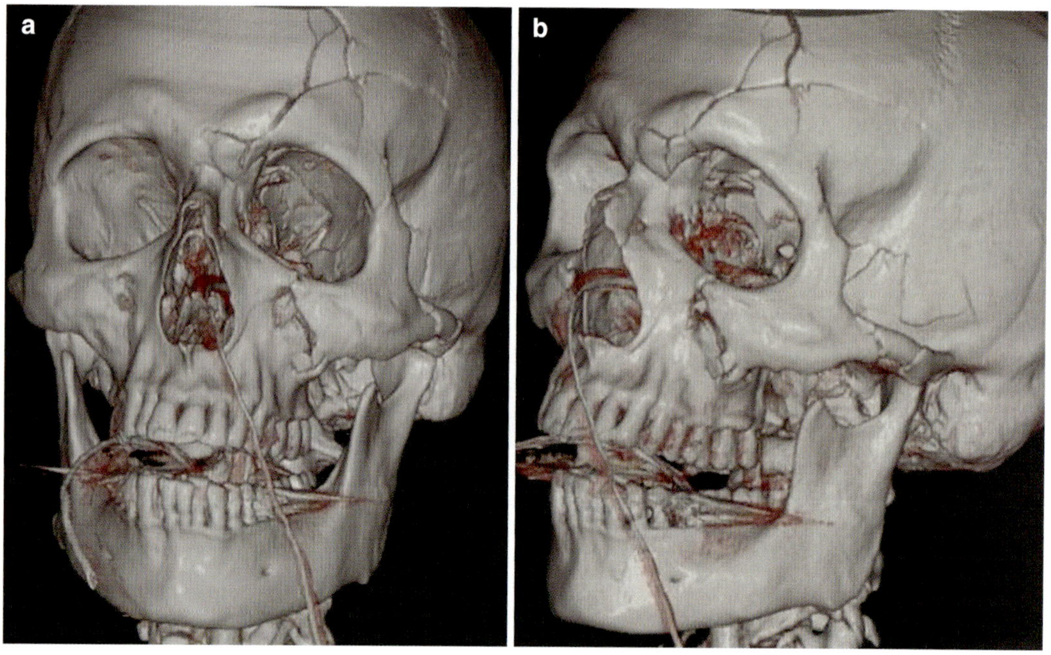

Fig. 4.15 Unilateral left NOE type II or III fracture, with comminution of the central fragment

there is comminution of the buttress and the canthus is attached to a small bone fragment (Fig. 4.15). The type III pattern cannot be diagnosed with imaging. Injury to the frontal sinus outflow tract should be noted, as it may lead to obstruction and late frontal mucocele development [21].

4.6.3 Zygomatic Fractures

The zygoma is the most anteriorly projected bone in the facial skeletal structure, making it prone to injury from any blow to the anterolateral midface. Zygomatic fractures are also known as a zygomaticomaxillary complex

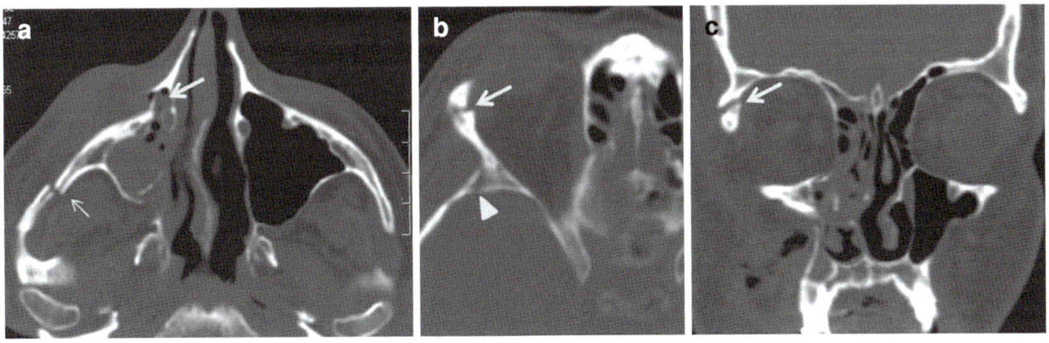

Fig. 4.16 Zygomaticomaxillary complex (ZMC) fracture: (**a**) zygomaticomaxillary (*small arrow*) and zygomaticotemporal fractures (*arrow*). (**b** and **c**) Non-displaced zygomaticofrontal suture fracture (*white arrow*). There is also a fracture of the sphenosquamosal suture (*arrowhead*, **b**)

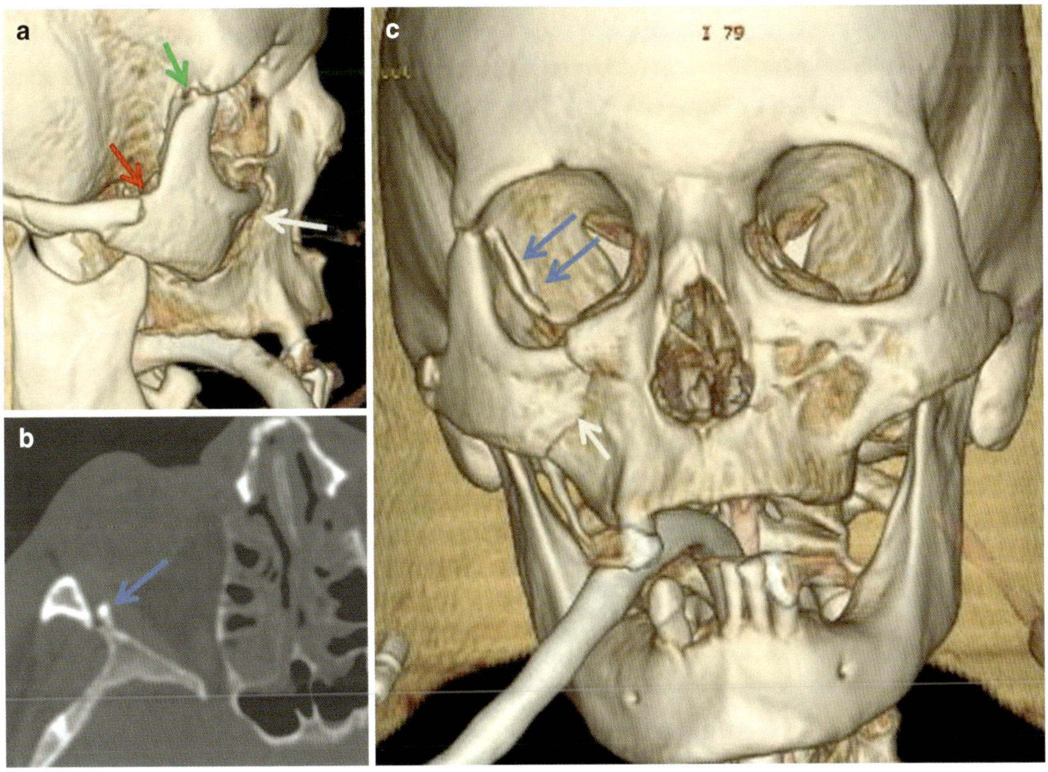

Fig. 4.17 (**a**) Impaction of the malar prominence (*white arrow*), with non-displaced zygomaticofrontal (*green arrow*) and zygomaticotemporal suture (*red arrow*) fractures, (**b**, **c**) zygomatic-sphenoidal fracture with minimal rotational displacement (*blue arrow*)

(ZMC); tripod, tetrapod or quadripod fracture; trimalar fracture; or malar fracture. They result from direct blows to the malar eminence. As the zygoma is articulated with the frontal bone, the maxillary bone, the temporal bone, and the sphenoid bone and gives a contribution to the orbital floor, ZMC fractures involve (1) the zygomatic arch, (2) inferior orbital rim and floor, (3) lateral orbital rim and (4) maxillary sinus walls. The sphenozygomatic junction is also fractured and may be associated to a significant displacement (Figs. 4.16 and 4.17).

Zygomatic arch fractures may occur in isolation and may impinge on the temporalis muscle or the coronoid process of the mandible, damaging the mastication.

4.6.4 Isolated Posterior Maxillary Wall Fractures

Isolated posterior maxillary wall fractures (Fig. 4.18) are associated with ipsilateral mandibular fractures. As it is considered as an effect of a puncture to the posterior maxillary wall by the anteriorly displaced coronoid process, that kind of fracture should prompt further investigation of the mandible and possibly the TMJ to exclude concomitant injury [22].

4.6.5 Le Fort Fractures

The Le Fort system is a useful and widely accepted method for classifying midfacial fractures: Le Fort I pattern is the so-called palatofacial disjunction, Le Fort II *midfacial disjunction* and Le Fort III *craniofacial disjunction*. Apart from the above-mentioned pattern of fracture, knowledge of Le Fort fractures is helpful to the radiologist by increasing the detection rate of distributed injuries in which one traumatic finding leads to a focused search for related injuries [22].

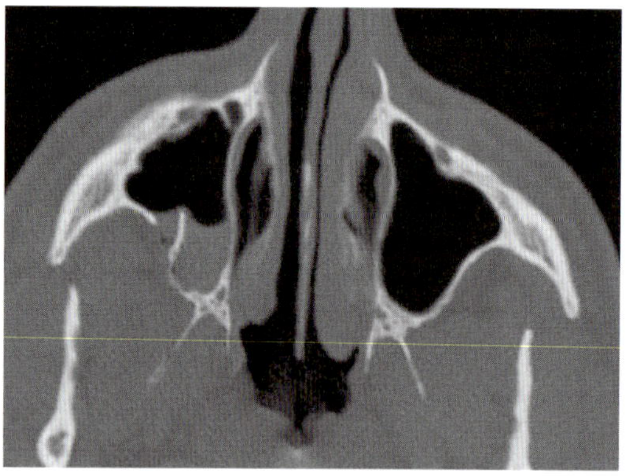

Fig. 4.18 Isolated posterior maxillary wall fractures should prompt further investigation to exclude concomitant TMJ injury

Furthermore, radiologists, if unaware of these patterns, may create a litany of fractures without clinical context, whereas an appropriate categorization helps the surgeon in determining the treatment plan, surgical access, incisions, expected treatment outcomes and prognostication [23]. Finally, using a common language may enhance the dialogue that takes place between the radiology service and the clinical service; otherwise the surgical services should be induced to review imaging independently of the radiologist [24].

To diagnose Le Fort fractures, a sequential examination of the facial bones should be performed one side at a time, starting at the pterygoid processes, as, by definition, all Le Fort fractures involve the pterygoid [23, 25]. Thereafter, fractures unique to a particular Le Fort level should be specifically sought. The easiest place to start is at the zygomatic arches (for Le Fort III), then the inferior orbital rims (for Le Fort II) and then the pyriform aperture (for Le Fort I) (Figs. 4.19 and 4.20). The mandible and zygomatic bone fractures (tripod or malar complex injury) should then be evaluated, as they were found to be common associations with Le Fort injuries [25].

Any combination is possible among the pattern on each side of the face. Furthermore, facial trauma often produces complex forces with facial fracture patterns not conforming to "classic" Le Fort patterns. Given the frequent recognition of unexpected associated fractures, describing in detail the fractures is recommended apart from categorizing the injuries into the Le Fort system.

High-energy injuries involving the entire midface, mandible and calvarium are sometimes referred to as "panfacial" fractures.

4.7 Mandibular Fractures

The mandible is one of the most frequently injured bones, fractured in isolation or in association with midfacial injures, particularly Le Fort fractures. As a consequence of its "ring-shaped" structure, mandible and temporomandibular joint (TMJ) fractures are often multiple or accompanied by

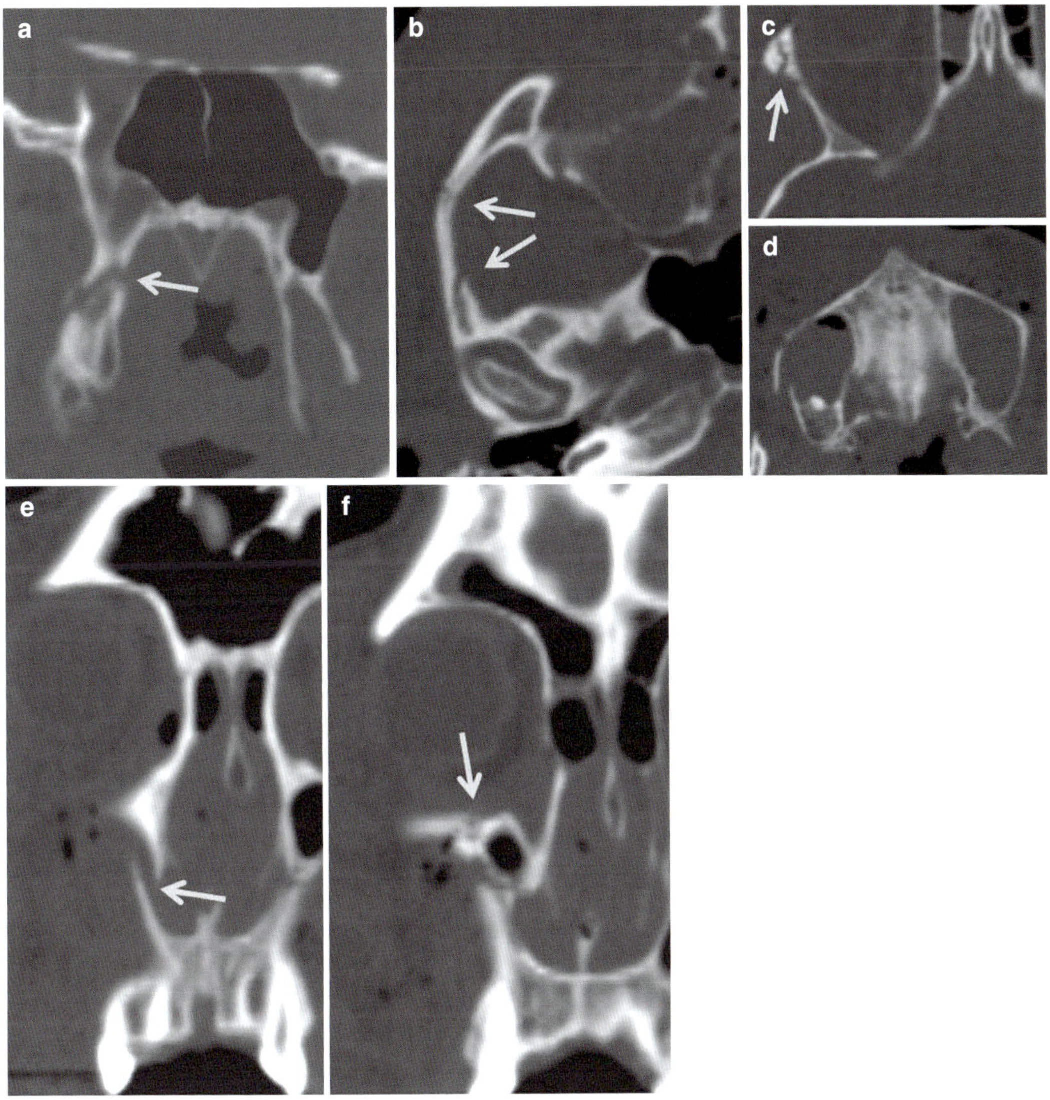

Fig. 4.19 (**a**) Pterygoid process fracture, suggesting a Le Fort fracture. (**b**) Zygomatic arch fracture, unique to Le Fort III. Fracture of frontal-zygomatic suture (**c**) is also typical of that pattern, while fractures of the maxillary sinus walls (**d**) are less specific of this pattern. Coronal reformations show fractures involving the anterolateral margin of nasal fossa (**e**) and inferior orbital rim (**f**) that are, respectively, unique to Le Fort I and II patterns. Diagnosis: right Le Fort I + II + III fractures

TMJ dislocation; bilateral injuries are frequent (Fig. 4.21). The trauma team should be alerted to forms of *flail mandible*, including trifocal (parasymphyseal and bicondylar), bilateral angle and bilateral body fractures, any of which may lead to airway compromise [26].

In children solitary mandibular fractures are the commonest, with frequent involvement of the condylar and subcondylar areas [15].

The body, ramus and angle of the mandible are frequently involved (Figs. 4.22 and 4.23). *Symphyseal* fractures are within the central incisors; *parasymphyseal* fractures are within the canines.

The report should mention inferior alveolar nerve, foramen or canal involvement and presence or absence of teeth in line of fracture [27].

Condylar fractures can be classified as condylar head (intracapsular), condylar neck

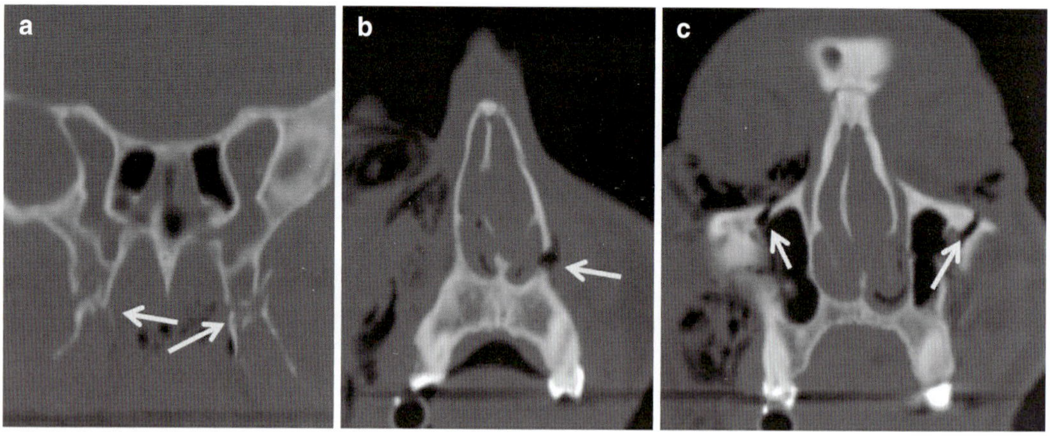

Fig. 4.20 (**a**) Bilateral pterygoid process fractures, suggesting bilateral Le Fort fracture. (**b**) On the left there is fracture of the anterolateral margin of nasal fossa, unique to Le Fort I pattern. (**c**) Bilateral fracture of the inferior orbital rim unique to Le Fort II pattern. Diagnosis: right Le Fort II, left Le Fort I + II fractures

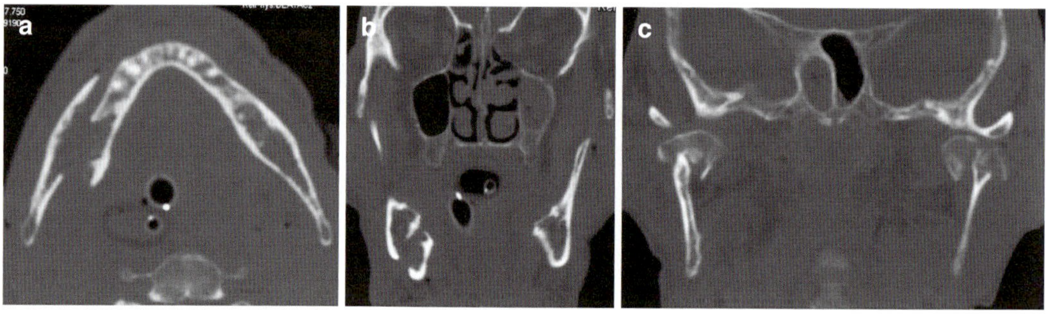

Fig. 4.21 CT scans showing a displaced longitudinal disruption of the right mandibular body (**a**, **b**) associated with bilateral condylar fractures (**c**)

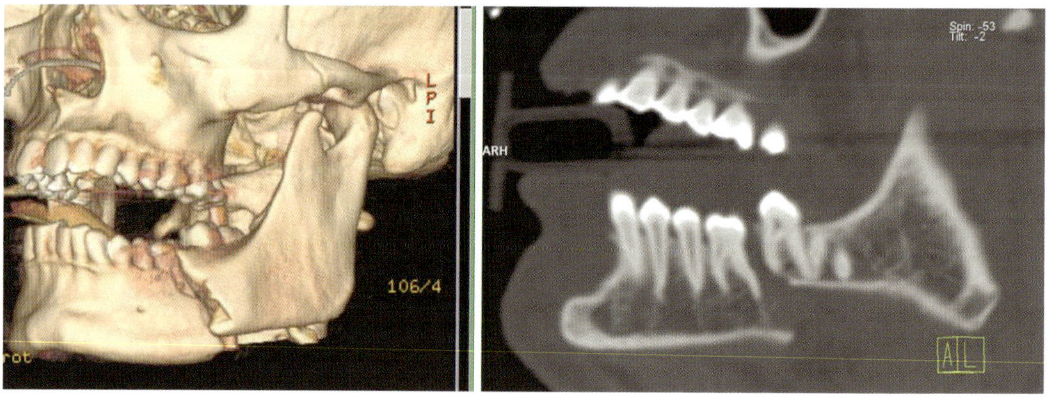

Fig. 4.22 A displaced fracture through the body of the mandible that has not interrupted the tooth root

(extracapsular) or subcondylar [28] (Fig. 4.24). The degree of condylar displacement has been categorized into four classes: (1) non-displaced, (2) deviation at the fracture line, (3) displacement (condylar fragment not in contact with the distal fragment but condyle still in the glenoid fossa) and (4) dislocation (condyle dislocated from the glenoid fossa) [29]. Complications of condylar fractures are impaired occlusal function, deviation of the mandible, internal derangements of the TMJ and ankylosis of the joint. Radiologists reporting brain CT scan for "head injuries" are recommended to look for an "empty" glenoid fossa as a sign of unexpected condylar displaced fracture (Fig. 4.25).

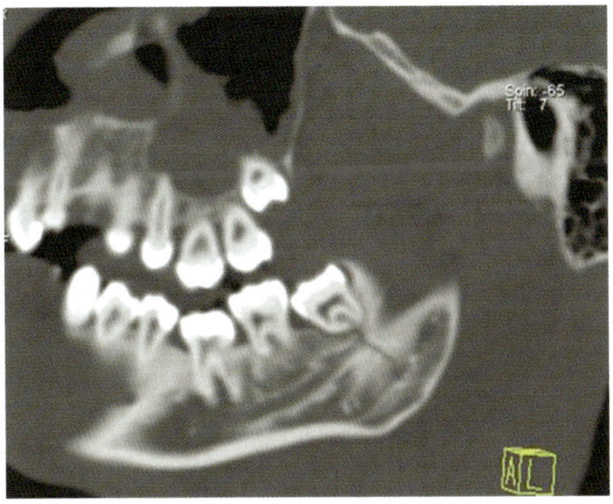

Fig. 4.23 CT sagittal reformation showing a linear non-displaced fracture of the mandibular angle, entering the last molar tooth socket

Dentoalveolar fractures are uncommon; isolated dentoalveolar fractures are commonest among children. The teeth may be fractured at the crown or at the root. A fracture through the root may be an indication for extraction. Fractured, extruded or grossly displaced primary teeth should be extracted (Fig. 4.26). All fractures involving the dentoalveolar structures should be considered open fractures. Further investigations (e.g. careful scrutiny of neck CT or chest X-ray) are indicated if teeth are absent and cannot be located or the patient is obtunded to rule out aspiration or swallowing [30] (Fig. 4.27).

4.8 Final Thoughts from the Diagnostic Forefront

- Radiologist is often the primary specialist interpreting facial injuries, therefore assuming a special clinical responsibility.
- Reporting by shortcuts as 3D VR images or clear sinus sign should be avoided: unfortunately all

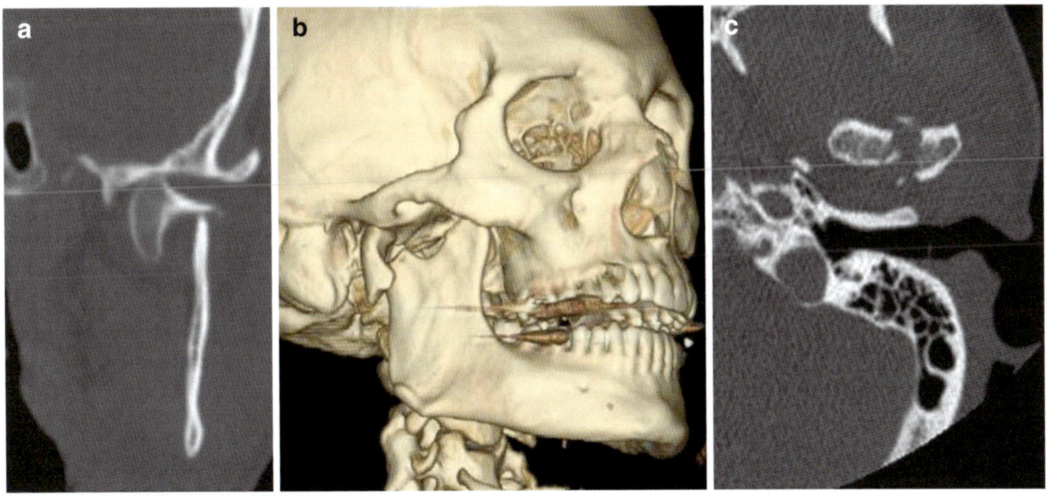

Fig. 4.24 Patterns of mandibular condyle fractures. Condylar neck displaced fractures (**a**, **b**). Comminuted intracapsular fracture of the condylar head dislocated from the temporomandibular joint fossa (**c**)

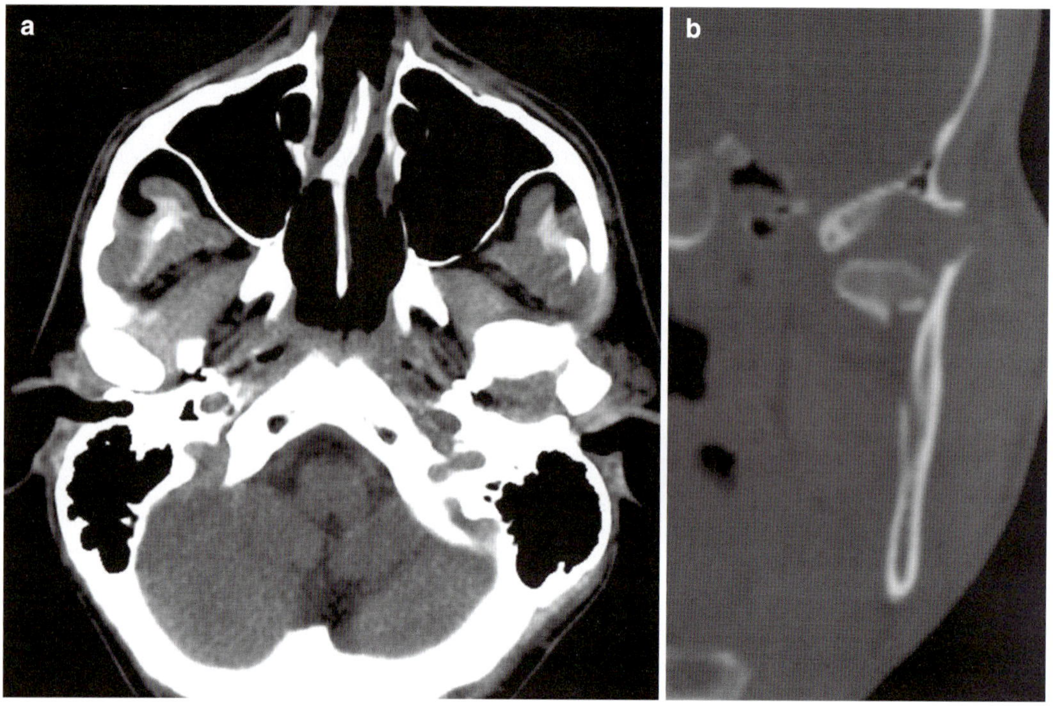

Fig. 4.25 Mandibular condyle should be always given attention on brain CT scan. In that case the radiologist noted displacement of the left condyle (**a**) and completed the examination with maxillofacial CT (**b**) that confirmed diagnosis of a displaced fracture

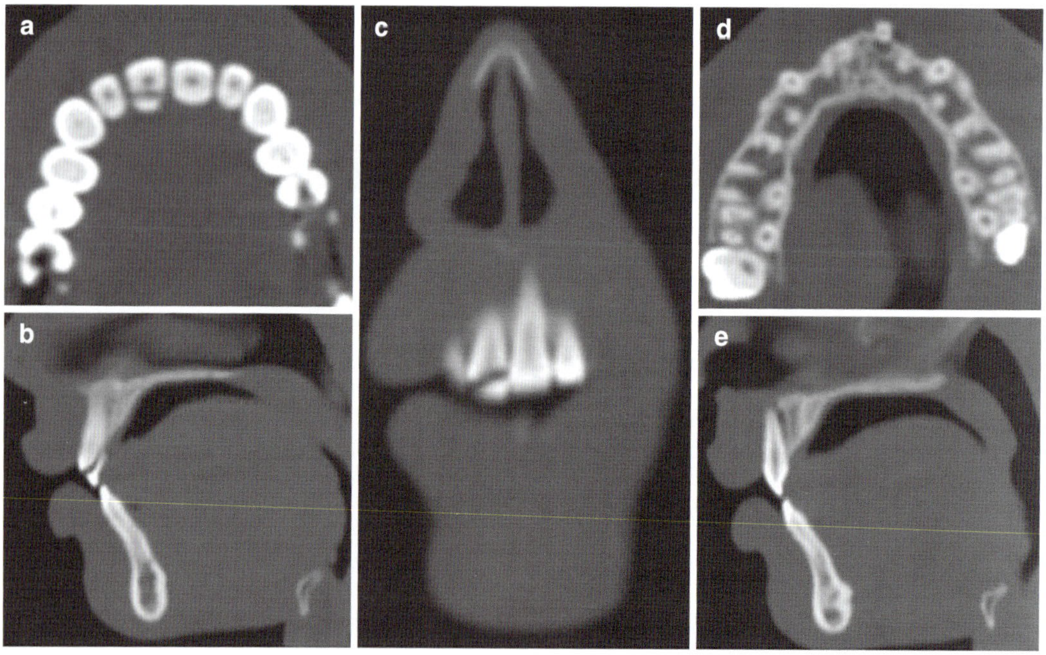

Fig. 4.26 Right upper central incisor injury: crown facture (**a**–**c**) and root dislodgement (**d**, **e**) from the alveolus

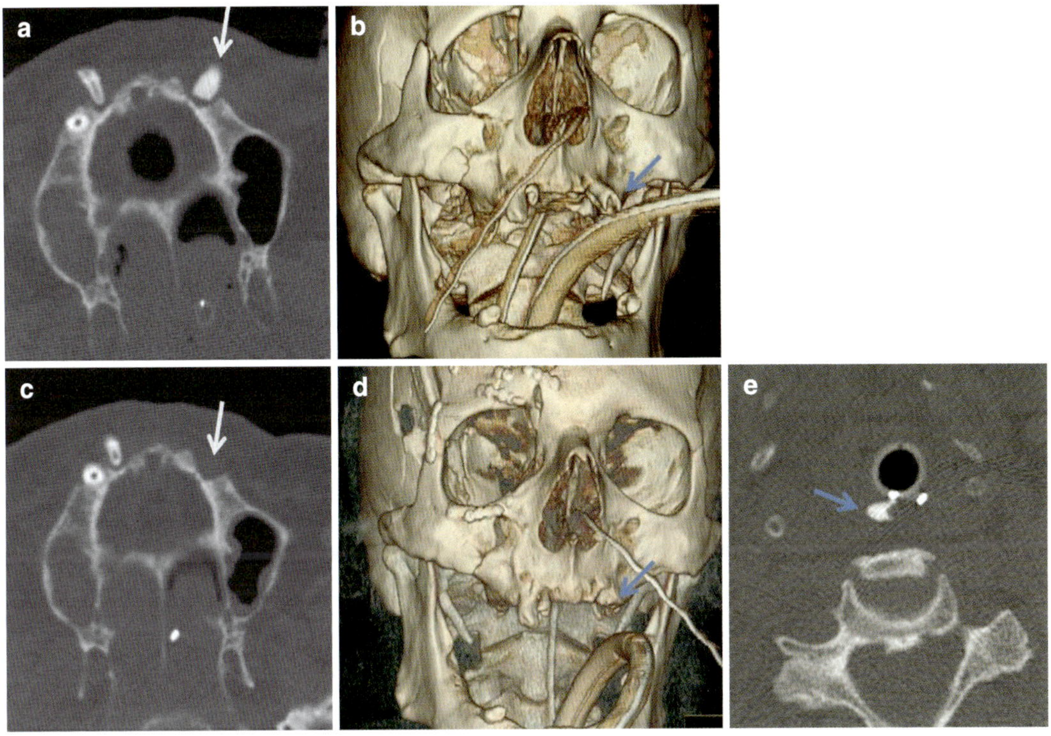

Fig. 4.27 CT scans of a patient before (**a**, **b**) and after (**c**, **d**) multiple facial fractures fixation, showing a missing teeth (*arrow*). In these cases a careful search for a swallowed or as in (**e**) aspirated teeth is mandatory

the axial, coronal and sagittal images have to be evaluated.

- Bone algorithm images do not suffice.
- Look at the brain and cervical spine while reporting the face.
- An early and active search for tension orbit and globe injuries is mandatory; if you find them, shout and dial the phone number to alert the whole clinical team: you are part of it!

References

1. Boffano P, Roccia F, Zavattero E, et al. European Maxillofacial Trauma (EURMAT) project: a multicentre and prospective study. J Craniomaxillofac Surg. 2015;43:62–70.
2. Pagnoni M, Marenco M, Ramieri V, Terenzi V, Bartoli D, Amodeo G, Mazzoli A, Iannetti G. Late treatment of orbital fractures: a new analysis for surgical planning. Acta Otorhinolaryngol Ital. 2014;34:439–45.
3. Anuja KA, Ranzer MJ, Cohen MN. Clinical assessment of the trauma patient. In: Taub PJ, et al., editors. Ferraro's fundamentals of maxillofacial surgery. New York: Springer; 2015.
4. Du H, Zhang Y, Chen Y, Zhao T. [Clinical application of multiplanar reconstruction and volume rendering with 64-slice spiral CT in the complex midfacial fracture]. Lin Chung Er Bi Yan Hou Tou Jing Wai Ke Za Zhi. 2009;23(4):160–2.
5. Illum P. Legal aspects in nasal fractures. Rhinology. 1991;29(4):263–6.
6. Grechushkin V, Boroda K, Chaudhry A, et al. Reevaluating the utility of maxillary sinus opacification as a screening tool for facial bone fracture a decade after its original analysis. Cureus. 2016;8(2):e487. doi:10.7759/cureus.487.
7. Maroldi R, Sala F. La diagnostica per immagini nella patologia traumatica maxillo-facciale. In: Rotondo A, editor. Odontoiatria. Diagnostica per immagini. Idelson Gnocchi, Napoli, 2008.
8. Banta J. Ocular trauma. 1st ed. Philadelphia: Saunders; 2007.
9. Betts AM, O'Brien WT, Davies BW, et al. A systematic approach to CT evaluation of orbital trauma. Emerg Radiol. 2014;21:511.
10. Chaudhary R, Upendran M, Campion N, Yeung A, Blanch R, Morgan-Warren P, Gibb I, Nelson T, Scott R. The role of computerised tomography in

predicting visual outcome in ocular trauma patients. Eye. 2015;29:867–71.
11. Yuan WH, Hsu HC, Cheng HC, Guo WY, Teng MM, Chen SJ, Lin TC. CT of globe rupture: analysis and frequency of findings. AJR Am J Roentgenol. 2014;202(5):1100–7.
12. Mancuso AA, Verbist BM. Tension orbit and its acute threat to vision. In: Mancuso AA, Hanafee WN, editors. Head and neck radiology. Philadelphia: Wolters Kluwer Health/Lippincott Williams & Wilkins; 2011.
13. Han MH, Chang KH, Min YG, Choi WS, Yeon KM, Han MC. Nontraumatic prolapse of the orbital contents into the ethmoid sinus: evaluation with screening sinus CT. Am J Otolaryngol. 1996;17(3):184–9.
14. Alcalá-Galiano A, Arribas-García IJ, Martín-Pérez MA, Romance A, Montalvo-Moreno JJ, Juncos JM. Pediatric facial fractures: children are not just small adults. Radiographics. 2008;28:441–61.
15. Clopton D, Mukherjee S, Christophel JJ, Wintermark M, Raghavan P. Head and neck trauma. In: Raghavan P, et al., editors. Manual of head and neck imaging. Berlin: Springer; 2014.
16. Bodanapally UK, Van der Byl G, Shanmuganathan K, Katzman L, Geraymovych E, Saksobhavivat N, Mirvis SE, Sudini KR, Krejza J, Shin RK. Traumatic optic neuropathy prediction after blunt facial trauma: derivation of a risk score based on facial CT findings at admission. Radiology. 2014;272(3):824–31.
17. Bush K, Huikeshoven M, Wong N. Nasofrontal outflow tract visibility in computed tomography imaging of frontal sinus fractures. Craniomaxillofac Trauma Reconstr. 2013;6:237–40.
18. Hong HS, Cha JG, Paik SH, Park SJ, Park JS, Kim DH, Lee HK. High-resolution sonography for nasal fracture in children. Am J Roentgenol. 2007;188(1):W86–92.
19. Gharehdaghi J, Samadi Rad B, Samani VG, Kolahi F, Zonoozian AK, Marashian SM. Comparison of Physical Examination and Conventional Radiography in Diagnosis of Nasal Fracture. Indian J Otolaryngol Head Neck Surg. 2013;65(Suppl 2):S304–307.
20. Markowitz BL, Manson PN, Sargent L, et al. Management of the medial canthal tendon in nasoethmoid orbital fractures: the importance of the central fragment in classification and treatment. Plast Reconstr Surg. 1991;87(5):843–53.
21. Hopper RA, Salemy S, Sze RW. Diagnosis of Midface Fractures with CT: what the surgeon needs to know. Radiographics. 2006;26:783–93.
22. Simonds JS, Whitlow CT, Chen MYM, Williams DW III. Isolated fractures of the posterior maxillary sinus: CT appearance and proposed mechanism. AJNR Am J Neuroradiol. 2011;32:468–70.
23. Magagula S, Hardcastle T. Defining current facial fracture patterns in a quaternary institution following high-velocity blunt trauma. S Afr J Rad. 2016;20(1):1–6.
24. Ludi EK, Rohatgi S, Zygmont ME, Khosa F, Hanna TN. Do radiologists and surgeons speak the same language? A retrospective review of facial trauma. AJR Am J Roentgenol. 2016;207:1–7.
25. Rhea JT. Novelline RA how to simplify the CT diagnosis of Le Fort fractures. AJR Am J Roentgenol. 2005;184(5):1700–5.
26. Dreizin D, Nam AJ, Tirada N, Levin MD, Stein DM, Bodanapally UK, Mirvis SE, Munera F. Multidetector CT of mandibular fractures, reductions, and complications: a clinically relevant primer for the radiologist. Radiographics. 2016;36(5):1539–64.
27. Hagopian T, Parelli J, Tran L, et al. A retrospective analysis of mandibular trauma radiology dictations. Oral Radiol. 2015;31:36.
28. Silvennoinen U, Iizuka T, Lindqvist C, Oikarinen K. Different patterns of condylar fractures: an analysis of 382 patients in a 3-year period. J Oral Maxillofac Surg. 1992;50(10):1032–7.
29. MacLennan WD. Consideration of 180 cases of typical fractures of the mandibular condylar process. Br J Plast Surg. 1952;5:122.
30. Hoffman W, Taub PJ. Dentoalveolar fractures. In: Taub PJ, et al., editors. Ferraro's fundamentals of maxillofacial surgery. New York: Springer; 2015.

Spine Trauma

5

Alfonso Cerase and Antonio Leone

Spine trauma is an extremely complex event, whose effects and related choice of time of treatment and appropriate treatment is classically based on the evidence of the lesions, anatomic landmarks, and mechanisms of injury at diagnostic imaging. Patient's prognosis depends on the type of lesions of the spine, spinal cord, and nerve roots, and their early management. For instance, early removal of a bone fragment displaced into the spinal canal and early spinal stabilization can stop the chain of neurolesive events that otherwise would result in further progression or chronicity of the neurological damage.

This chapter will review epidemiology of spinal trauma, indications to different diagnostic imaging techniques, spinal functional anatomy, and diagnostic imaging findings which have to be searched in a patient with spinal trauma, in order to adopt a pattern-based approach for efficient imaging interpretation and communication with physicians involved in spinal trauma.

5.1 Epidemiology

In large trauma centers, the annual frequency of spinal fractures ranges from 6 to 23% and that of spinal cord injury from 5 to 22% [35, 38]. The influence of spinal trauma on patient's social and financial well-being is often more significant than that of other traumatic injuries since they may have the poorest functional outcomes and the lowest rates of return to work among all major organ system injuries. In USA [2, 21] and Canada [37], the annual incidence of spinal cord injury resulting in permanent paralysis or neurological deficit is ~40 and ~35 cases per million persons, respectively.

In developed countries, traffic accidents are the first cause of spinal trauma and spinal cord injuries trauma, followed by accidental falls in workplace and during sport, and violence assaults. The higher incidence is in males, mainly in the age group between the second and fourth decade. Spinal injury in children is rare,

A. Cerase, M.D. (✉)
UOC Neuroimmagini e Neurointerventistica, Dipartimento Scienze Neurologiche e Neurosensoriali, Azienda Ospedaliera Universitaria Senese, Policlinico "Santa Maria alle Scotte", Viale Mario Bracci, 16, 53100 Siena, Italy
e-mail: alfonso.cerase@ao-siena.toscana.it; alfonsocerase@gmail.com

A. Leone, M.D.
Istituto di Radiologia, Università Cattolica del Sacro Cuore, Fondazione Policlinico Universitario "Agostino Gemelli", Largo Agostino Gemelli, 1, 00168 Rome, Italy
e-mail: antonio.leone1@unicatt.it

V. Miele, M. Trinci (eds.), *Diagnostic Imaging in Polytrauma Patients*,
https://doi.org/10.1007/978-3-319-62054-1_5

associated with a high prevalence of spinal cord injury, particularly in the age group of 8 years and under [27].

Spinal injuries include vertebral fractures (which may involve the vertebral body, laminae, and pedicles, as well as the spinous, articular, and transverse processes), subluxations (which involve joints and ligaments injuries, also without bony injury), and dislocations (which typically involve the facets, but also the vertebral bodies or osseous fragments in more severe injuries). Lumbar spine is the most common region of spinal fractures, accounting for about half of fractures, followed by cervical and/or thoracic spines (each segment accounting for 20–30%, according to different results in different series), while sacrum is the site of about 2% of fractures [38, 57]. The first lumbar vertebra is the most commonly injured, followed by the adjacent vertebrae. The spinal segments more exposed to traumatic injuries are those physiologically provided by high mobility, such as the cervical spine and the thoracolumbar junction. Notably, the thoracolumbar junction is a transition zone between a spinal segment in kyphosis and quite rigid (the thoracic spine, moreover bounded in its movements by the ribs) and one in lordosis and very mobile (lumbar spine), as well as between a segment in which the prevailing intervertebral motion is the rotation (thoracic spine) and one in which prevails the flexion-extension (lumbar spine).

Up to 20% patients have multiple fractures involving different areas of the spine [38, 45], most frequently of the lumbar and thoracic spines, followed by thoracic and cervical spines, and then by all the other possible associations [57]. The prevalence of multilevel fractures in pediatric patients is up to 7.4% [27]. Up to 79% patients may have associated head injuries; conversely, 24% of patients with head injuries may have spinal injury [27, 38].

The worst prognosis and highest medical costs result from cervical spine injury, while lumbar spine injury is the most curable. Notably, acute cervical trauma may result in the most serious and catastrophic traumatic injury of the spinal cord, because of biomechanical predisposing features such as small size of the vertebrae, less massive muscle support, need to support the head with a lever arm not always favorable. This results in about 20% of deaths in road accidents.

5.2 Diagnostic Imaging

Diagnostic imaging plays an essential role in the management of patients with spinal trauma since continuous technological evolution has resulted in the availability of radiography, computed tomography (CT), and magnetic resonance imaging (MRI), which show both the spinal "containing," i.e., bone, discs, ligaments, and joints, and the spinal "content," i.e., meninges, subarachnoid space, nerve roots, and spinal cord. It has also been proposed the use of ultrasound for the study of the posterior ligamentous complex of the thoracolumbar spine. Thus, diagnostic imaging may show lesions, injury mechanisms, residual stability, and provide support for prognosis of spinal cord injury, as well as allows the follow-up of complications of spinal trauma and its treatment, and the evaluation of outcome [4, 6, 7, 9, 12, 15, 16, 19, 20, 24, 26, 28, 31, 34, 39, 42, 47].

5.2.1 Radiography

Radiography remains the most easily accessible examination and simple to perform, with a sufficient direct view of osseous structure and lesions, including vertebral fractures (Fig. 5.1), dislocation, and subluxation. When performed by a correct and rigorous technique, including adequate positioning and views (anteroposterior, lateral, open-mouth, swimmer, bending), when possible to perform, radiography may also show indirect signs of discal, ligamentous, and joints injuries, possibly providing a general diagnostic interpretation, by demonstrating the

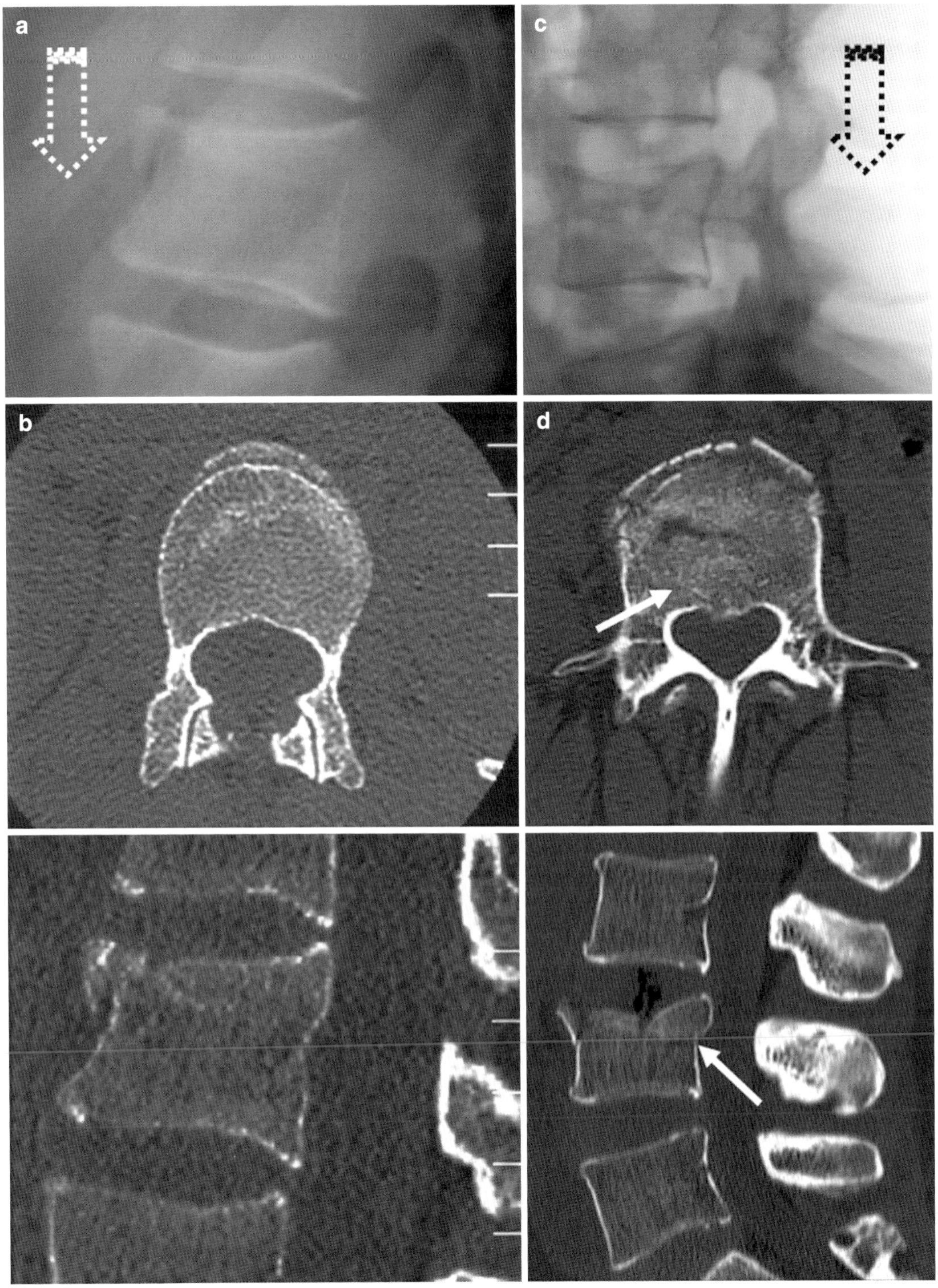

Fig. 5.1 Lumbar and thoracic fractures by axial loading injury mechanism (*dashed open arrows*): potential and limitation of radiography (two different patients). In both patients, radiographs (**a**, **c**) clearly show the reduction in height of the vertebral body, resulting from the axial loading injury mechanism. Source axial and 2-D reformatted sagittal CT images (**b**, **d**) did not show fracture line extending to posterior somatic wall in one patient, (**a**, **b**)while in the other one (**c**, **d**) clearly show that the fracture line involves the posterior somatic wall (*solid arrows*), thus reclassifying the L4 fracture as a burst one

overall alignment, including areas of kyphosis or lordosis, changes in disc height, or changes to the interspinous distances [4, 6, 23, 24]. For instance, a simple lateral view of the cervical spine (Fig. 5.2) allows to:

- Assess the continuity and regularity of four longitudinal lines, almost parallel to each other and convex anteriorly. The anterior vertebral or marginal line passes along the anterior margin of the vertebral body, the posterior vertebral or marginal line passes along the posterior margin of the vertebral body, the spinolaminar line passes along the anterior margin or the base of the spinous processes at the junction with the laminae, and the posterior spinous line passes along the tips of the spinous processes. The discontinuity of one of these lines is an expression of abnormal spinal motion in the sagittal plane.
- Suspect an underlying, generally previously not known, condition of cervical stenosis, through the evaluation of the anteroposterior diameter of the spinal canal (distance between posterior vertebral line and spinolaminar one) and/or the Torg-Pavlov ratio, i.e., between anteroposterior diameter of the spinal canal and vertebral body, lower than 0.8.
- Assess the height of intervertebral, interarticular, and interpinous spaces, as well as the thickness of prevertebral tissues whose increase is the sign of anterior longitudinal ligament lesion.
- Be the easiest way to perform dynamic studies (flexion, extension, lateral bending), for the evaluation of spinal stability. Dynamic studies avoid overlook of discal, ligamentous, and joints injuries potentially dangerous for the spinal stability and myeloradicular function. In cervical distorsive trauma, lateral radiographs in maximum flexion allows to demonstrate the abnormal increase of the interspinous space, as well as the increase of the interapophyseal articular range of motion or properly the dislocation, even if modest, of a vertebral body, such as indirect signs of possible discoligamentous or joints injury. Certainly, dynamic studies must be conducted in an absolutely safe state, in relation to the patient's clinical conditions.

However, despite its diagnostic potential, technical limitations of radiography in depicting the highly complex anatomy of the spine are well known, above all in the craniocervical junction, cervicothoracic junction (Fig. 5.3), and thoracic spine, as well as in the presence of associated spinal diseases, mostly in elderly patients (Fig. 5.3). Notably, studies have shown that radiography has only 30–60% sensitivity in evaluating fractures and ligamentous injuries [18, 30, 44]. The rate of missed cervical spine injuries by conventional radiography is high: in a retrospective evaluation of 800 patients with polytrauma, CT identified fractures with a sensitivity of 98.5%, compared with a sensitivity of 43% for radiography [34]. Clear visualization of the cervicothoracic junction is mandatory as a fracture of C7 (Figs. 5.3 and 5.4) or a fracture or dislocation of C7-T1 (Fig. 5.5) accounts for nearly 17% of cervical spine injuries [14]. This explains the frequent need of CT (Figs. 5.3, 5.4, and 5.5) and/or MRI (Fig. 5.5). In pediatric patients, diagnostic imaging of spinal injury, especially the cervical one, remains a difficult issue. Clinical assessment is essential, and it has been proposed to use radiography more selectively, i.e., by a single lateral view. However, since every effort should be made to rule out a potentially devastating injury, doubtful cases need to be followed by cross-sectional imaging [50].

Thus, radiography is indicated in conscious adult patients, without radiculo-medullary symptoms, but still at risk of spinal injury after a low-energy trauma. On the other side, radiography should not be used as a first-line diagnostic procedure in adult patients unconscious, or with radiculo-medullary symptoms, after major trauma, who represent indications to CT and/or MRI.

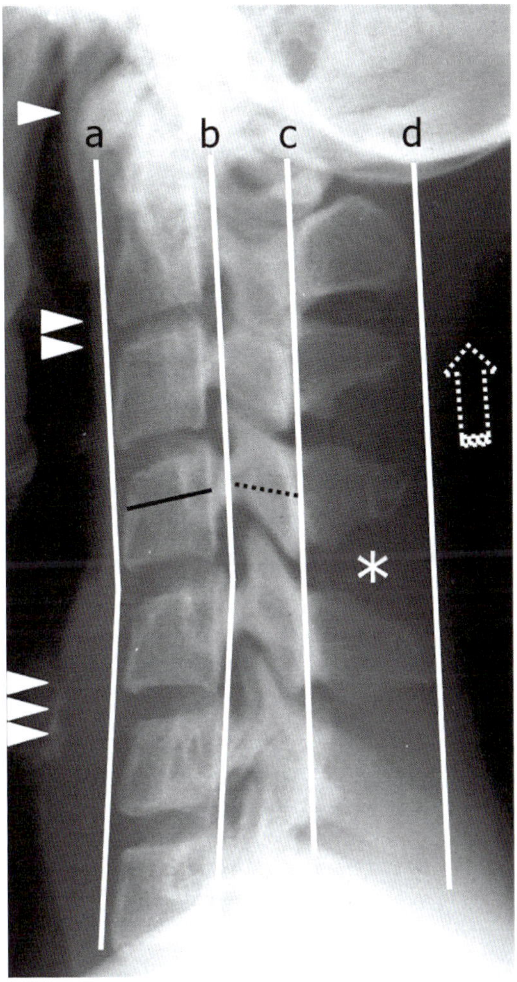

Fig. 5.2 Cervical spine ligamentous injury by anterior flexion distraction injury mechanism: potential of radiography. Lateral view of the cervical spine shows anteriorly concave with fulcrum at C4-C5 level anterior vertebral or marginal (**a**) and posterior vertebral or marginal (**b**) lines, straight spinolaminar (**c**) and posterior spinous (**d**) lines, as well as the increase of the C4-C5 interarticular and interpinous (*asterisk*) spaces, from anterior flexion distraction injury mechanism (*dashed open arrow*). The low ratio between anteroposterior diameters of the spinal canal (*dashed line*) and vertebral body (*continuous line*), i.e., the Torg-Pavlov ratio, indicating a congenital stenosis of the cervical spinal canal. Intervertebral spaces are normally symmetric. Prevertebral soft tissues, i.e., nasopharyngeal (*single arrowhead*), retropharyngeal (*double arrowhead*), and pretracheal (*triple arrowhead*) spaces, are normal. These findings required prompt CT scan (*not shown*) for complete evaluation of posttraumatic scenario

5.2.2 Computed Tomography

CT is significantly superior to radiography in terms of sensitivity, specificity, and diagnostic accuracy (Figs. 5.1 and 5.3). Axial, multiplanar 2D-, and 3D-reformatted CT images are the optimal tools to show the more complex anatomic regions of the spine, such as craniocervical (Fig. 5.6), cervicothoracic, and thoracolumbar junctions, as well as the classical anatomical model of the "three columns" of Denis [5] of the thoracic and lumbar spine (Fig. 5.7a), as well as the anatomic model of the "four columns" of the subaxial cervical spine (Fig. 5.7b) for the Cervical Spine Injury Severity Score [33]. CT may confirm the diagnosis of compression fracture at radiography or reclassify the lesion as a burst fracture (Fig. 5.1), with possible impact on the management plan. Similarly, only CT defines with certainty the fracture lines involving bone and joint components of the lateral arches (Figs. 5.3 and 5.4). Surely, CT is the best technique for the recognition of vertebral bony portions and fragments (Fig. 5.8), as well air or gas, which may not be recognized or wrongly interpreted as bone by MRI. Notably, also thanks to multislice technique and providing the most accurate assessment of the fine anatomy of the osseous spine, CT allows the identification of indirect signs of discoligamentous or capsular injury, sometimes hardly recognizable in lateral view radiographs, although CT analysis of the soft tissues is less accurate than that directly provided by MRI (Figs. 5.8, 5.9, 5.10, and 5.11) [9, 16, 20]. These reasons explain why CT is now considered the first-line procedure in polytrauma patients who however require CT of the head, chest, abdomen, and pelvis to rule out intracranial and visceral injuries.

Furthermore, thanks to technological progress and the availability of multislice CT scanners, a further advantage is the possibility of performing CT angiography (CTA) of cervicocranial arteries in patients with associated risk

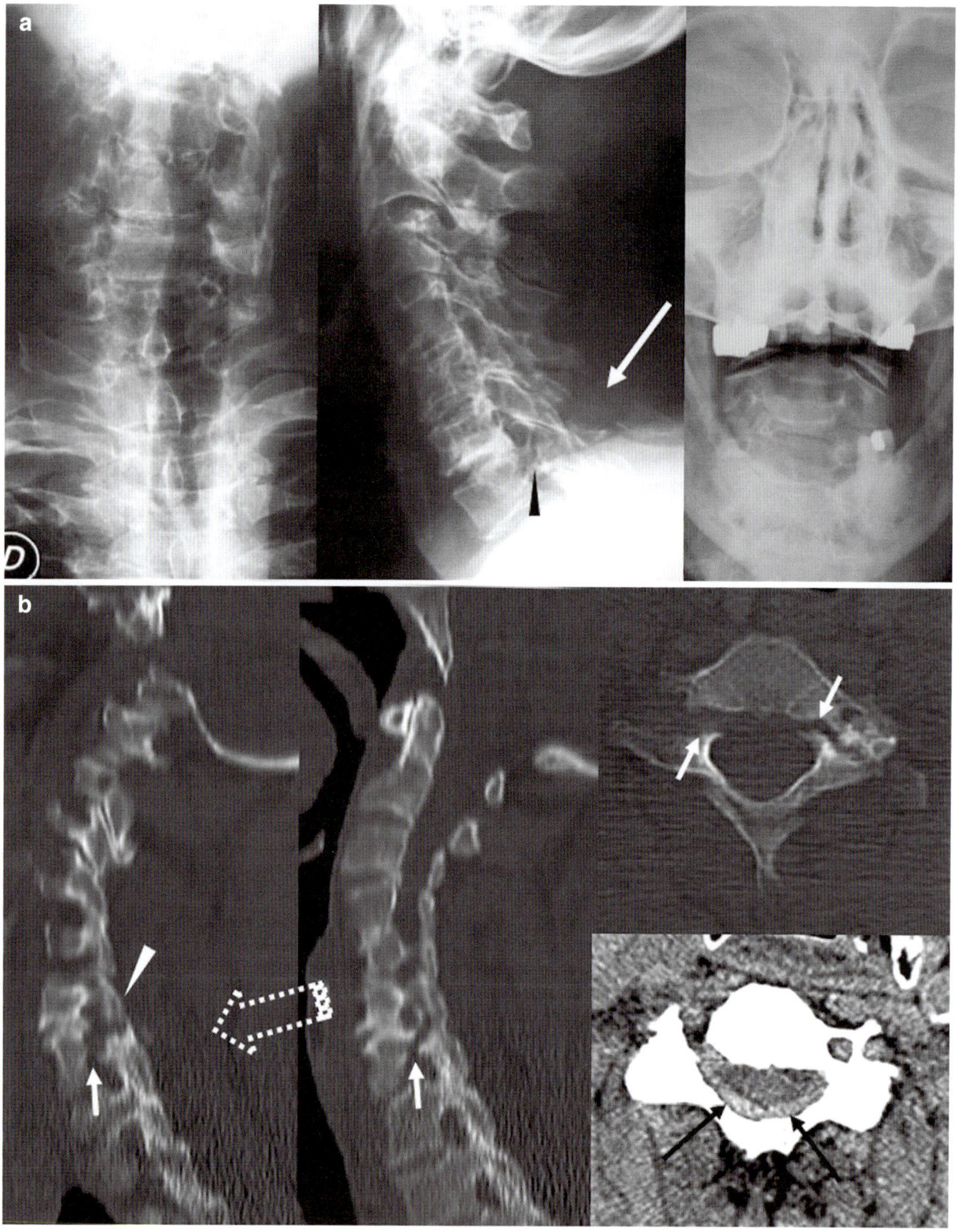

Fig. 5.3 C6 and C7 fracture dislocation and subluxation by translational injury mechanism in an elderly patient with degenerative spinal disease: potential and limitation of radiography. Anteroposterior, lateral, and open-mouth views (**a**) show an avulsion fracture of the C6 spinous process (*long white arrow*) and a fracture line in the peduncular area of C7 (*arrowhead*). Only right- and left-side 2D-reformatted sagittal and source axial CT images (**b**) allow the identification of both C7 pedicles fracture lines (*short white arrows*), and C6-C7 facet joints right dislocation (*white arrowhead*) and left subluxation from translational injury mechanism (*dashed open arrow*). Note also a thin posterior epidural hematoma (*black arrows*). MRI (*not shown*) did not add further significant information

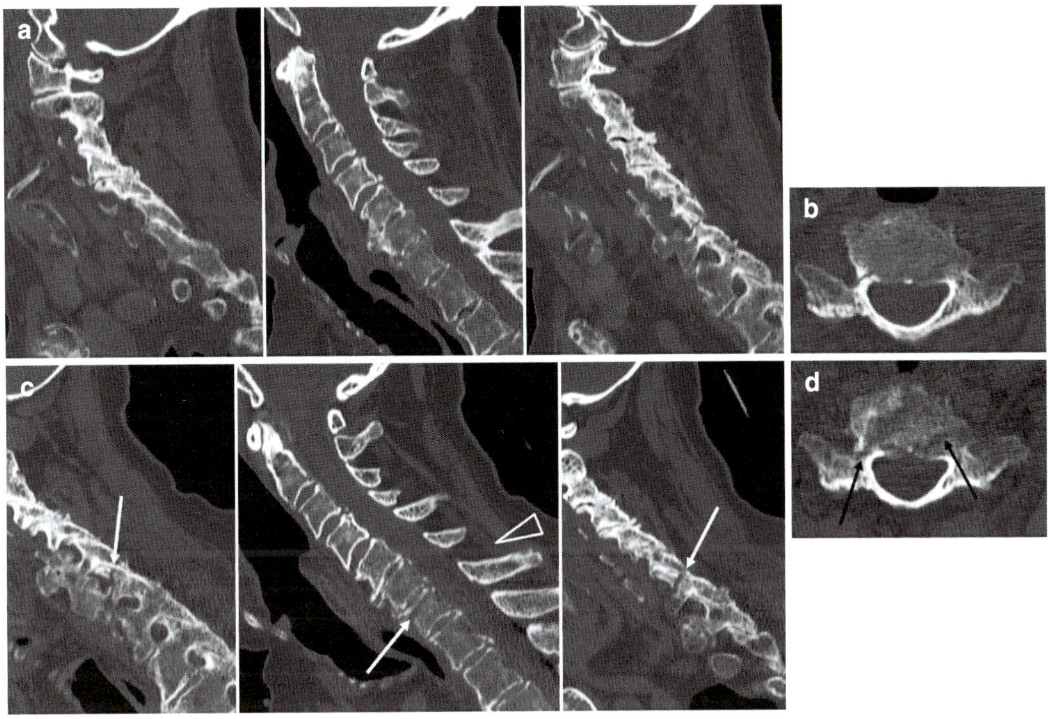

Fig. 5.4 C7 fracture: nonconsecutive right to left 2D-reformatted sagittal (**a**) and source axial (**b**) CT images at admission show thin fracture lines in both the posterior hemiarches and in the posterior third of the vertebral body; C6-C7 interspinous space is not clearly enlarged. Despite appropriate immobilization, 10 days later similar CT images (**c**, **d**) show clear-cut diastasis of the bony fragments in both the C7 vertebral body (*black arrows*) and the posterior hemiarches (*white arrows*) incipient kyphosis and C6-C7 interspinous space enlargement (*arrowhead*)

of blunt cerebrovascular injury [1, 3, 13, 36, 49]. An Italian study performed by a 16-slice CTA showed that blunt cerebrovascular injury occurred in more than 3% of 1153 patients admitted as multi-trauma, i.e., with two or more injuries (of which at least one life-threatening or Injury Severity Score ≥ 16) and/or high-speed trauma or fall from an height > 3 m [1]. Fractures, dislocations, and subluxation of the craniocervical junction and the cervical spine are among the conditions at risk (Figs. 5.10, 5.12, 5.13, and 5.14), including fractures of the transverse processes with involvement of the transverse foramen where the vertebral artery passes (Fig. 5.13). Other risk factors include injuries from high-energy trauma, such as LeFort fractures, fracture of the first rib and of the sternum, as well as associated signs of neck trauma suggesting hanging as the mechanism of injury. Catheter digital subtraction angiography is still considered the "gold standard" technique; however, it is relatively invasive, has a significant cost, requires specific resources, and is not always available. In the screening evaluation at the time of admission for trauma, it has to be replaced by modern-scanners multislice CTA [36]. CTA may be performed by a "whole body" or a sequential technique on the basis of institutional experience: always it has to include the aortic arch and cover the intracranial arterial vessels [1, 49].

Additionally, iodine contrast medium intrathecal injection, i.e., myelography completed by high-resolution CT myelography, may be still

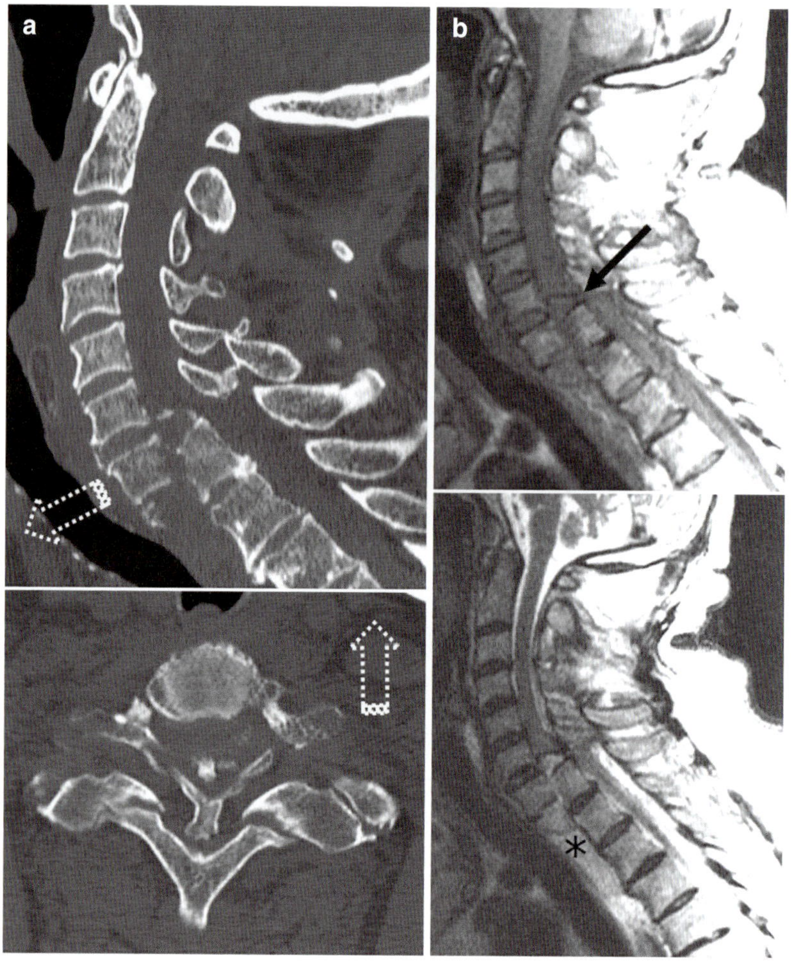

Fig. 5.5 C7-T1 severe fracture-dislocation and spinal cord transection: 2D-reformatted sagittal and source axial CT images (**a**), and T1- and T2-weighted sagittal MR images (**b**). CT clearly shows the bilateral interfacetal dislocation resulting from translational injury (*dashed open arrow*). Despite poor quality due to cervical collar and spinal longboard, MRI shows a spinal cord divided into a cranial and caudal portion (*solid arrow*). At C7-T1 level, the disconnection of flavum, interspinous, and supraspinous ligaments are obviously evident. *Asterisk* indicates a hemorrhagic prevertebral collection resulting from anterior longitudinal ligament tear

advocated for a more detailed evaluation of post-traumatic nerve root avulsions, especially in brachial plexus injuries, providing a support to somatosensory evoked potentials in prognosis and surgical exploration planning, especially when high-resolution MRI including MR myelography is contraindicated or provides uncertain findings [43, 60].

Finally, various potential pitfalls may mimic or mask spinal injuries at multislice CT [19], including anatomical and developmental variants resulting from failure of fusion or segmentation, vascular channels (Fig. 5.15), intervertebral discs, motion-related and beam-hardening artifacts, and non-traumatic or underlying conditions. The (neuro)radiologist has to be familial with such possibilities.

5.2.3 Magnetic Resonance Imaging

MRI is the only imaging procedure providing a direct study of the spinal cord and spinal root. Thus, it is indicated in patients with spinal cord symptoms and signs and in those with discrepancy between findings at radiography and/or CT and neurological clinical status [12, 15, 31, 39, 47].

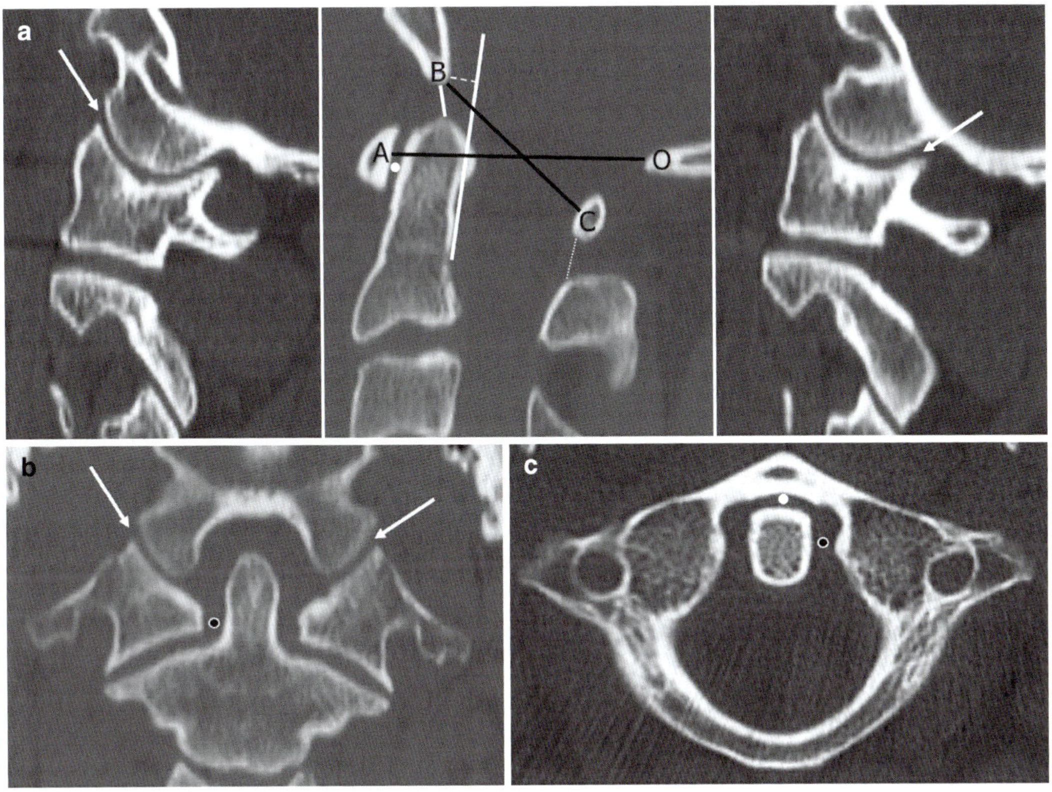

Fig. 5.6 Potential of CT in depicting the normal anatomy of the craniocervical junction: nonconsecutive right to left 2D-reformatted sagittal (**a**), 2D-reformatted coronal (**b**), and source axial (**c**) CT images. *Long arrows* indicate normal relationship of the joints between occipital condyles and C1 lateral masses, i.e., the occipitoatlantal joints, which show close apposition and almost equidistant space along their extent. 2D-reformatted midsagittal image shows the atlantodental (*white dots*) and basion-dens (*continuous short line*) spaces, the posterior axial line (*continuous long line*), the basion to posterior axial line distance (*dashed line*), and the C1–C2 interspinous distance (*dotted line*). *Black dots* indicate laterodental spaces. Powers ratio measures the relationship between the foramen magnum and the atlas, by the ratio between the lines from the basion (*B*) to the posterior spinolaminar line of the atlas (*C*) and the line between the anterior arch of the atlas (*A*) and the opisthion (*O*) in the midsagittal plane, i.e., *BC*/*AO*. The McGregor line (*not shown*), i.e., a modification of the Chamberlain line, connects the posterior edge of the hard palate to the most caudal point of the occipital curve. When the odontoid process lies more than 4.5 mm above the McGregor line, this is defined basilar invagination

High contrast resolution of MRI, especially in short tau inversion recovery (STIR) and fat-suppressed T2-weighted images, results in the further advantages of direct identification of posttraumatic bone edema, as well as intervertebral discs, ligaments, and joints lesions, even with normal findings at radiography or CT.

MRI examination should always include:

- T1-weighted sagittal images, for anatomical details and sensitivity in the identification of a possible spinal hematoma (Figs. 5.5, 5.8, 5.9, 5.10, 5.11, and 5.15)
- T2-weighted sagittal images, for the evaluation of the spinal cord (Figs. 5.5, 5.8, 5.9, 5.10, 5.11, 5.15, and 5.16);
- STIR or fat-suppressed T2-weighted sagittal images (Figs. 5.10, 5.11, 5.16, 5.17, 5.18, and 5.19), for a better evidence of bone edema and soft tissues damage
- T2- or T2*-weighted axial images to confirm spinal cord injury since in sagittal planes arti-

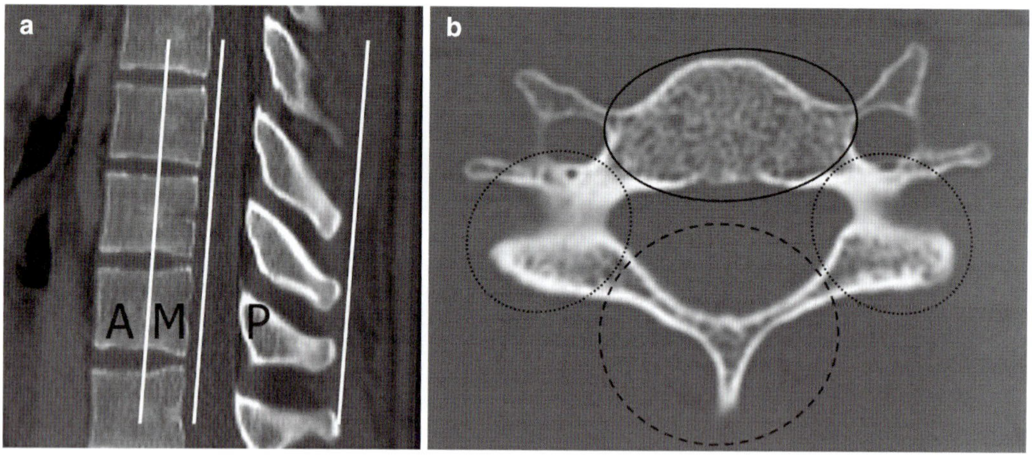

Fig. 5.7 Potential of CT images in depicting the "three-column" model of Denis of the thoracic and lumbar spine (**a**), and the "four-column" model of the cervical spine (**b**). In the thoracic spine (**a**), a 2D-reformatted sagittal CT image shows the anterior column (*A*) formed by the anterior longitudinal ligament and the anterior (two-thirds) of the vertebral body and intervertebral disc, the middle column (*M*) formed by the posterior (one-third) of the vertebral body and intervertebral disc and posterior longitudinal ligament, and the posterior column (*P*) formed by the structures which are posterior to the posterior longitudinal ligament including pedicles, laminae, articular processes and facet joints, flavum ligaments, i.e., neural arch and interconnecting ligaments. In the cervical spine (**b**), a source axial CT image shows the anterior column (*continuous circle*) formed by the vertebral body, intervertebral disc, anterior and posterior longitudinal ligaments, the lateral columns (*dotted circles*), i.e., the pillars, formed by the pedicles, superior and inferior facets, lateral mass, and facet joints, and the posterior column (*dashed circle*) formed by the flavum ligament flavum, lamina, spinous processes, and nuchal ligaments, i.e., infraspinous, supraspinous, and nuchae ligaments

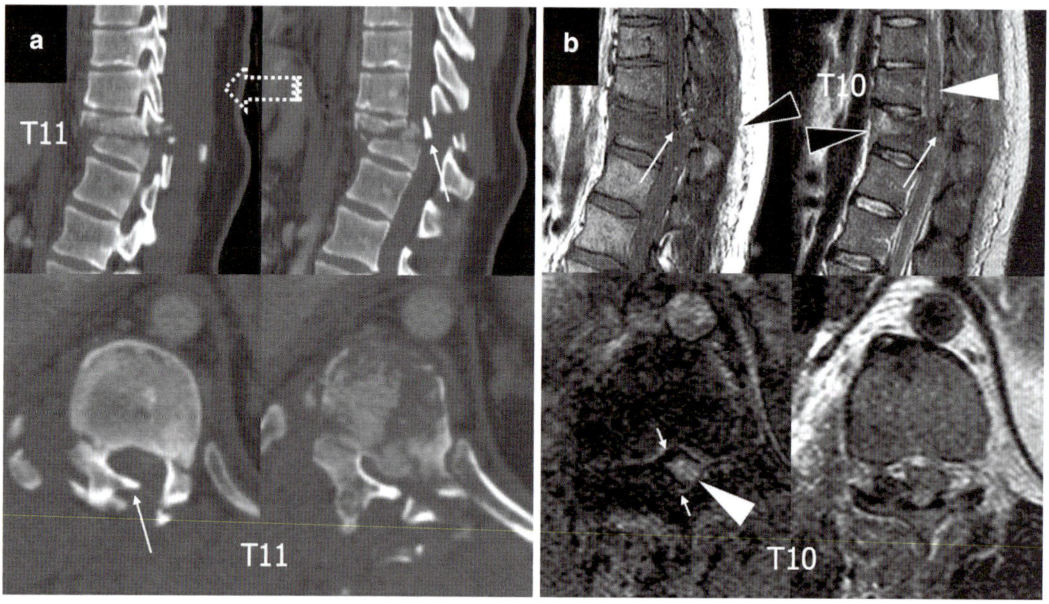

Fig. 5.8 T11 translational injury (*dashed arrow*): nonconsecutive 2D-reformatted sagittal and T11 source axial CT images (**a**), T1- and T2-weighted sagittal and nonconsecutive T2*- and T2-weighted T10 axial MR images (**b**). CT better depicts the osseous fractures and the displacements of T11 fragments, most notably of its right superior facet (*long white arrows*) with low signal intensity on both T1- and T2-weighted sagittal MR images. On the other hand, at T10 level the T2* low signal intensity on the surface of the spinal cord (*short white arrows*) results from hemorrhage and not from bone fragments; at the same level, *white arrowhead* shows spinal cord edema. *Black arrowheads* show tears of anterior longitudinal ligament, T10-T11 flavum ligament and adjacent portion of supraspinous ligament

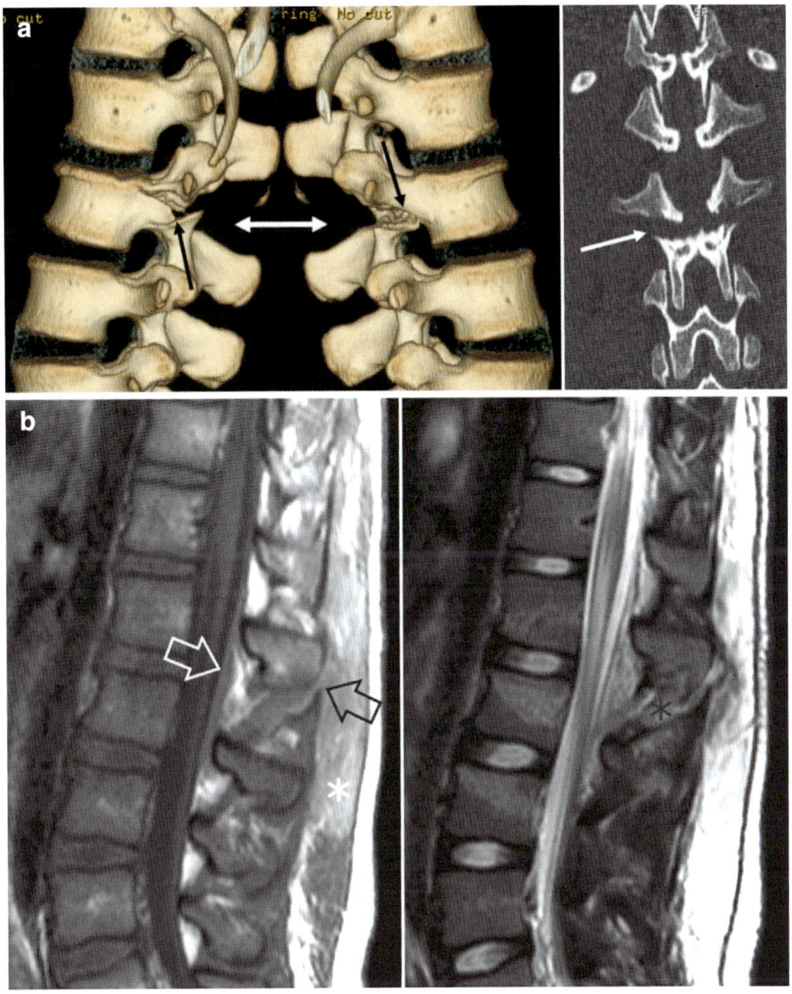

Fig. 5.9 L2 Flexion distraction fracture (Chance fracture): 3D-reformatted right and left oblique and 2D-reformatted coronal CT images (**a**), and T1- and T2-weighted sagittal MR images (**b**). CT clearly shows the fractures lines of both L2 pedicles (*black and white arrows*), and the increase of interspinous processes (*double arrow*) indicating L2-L3 interspinous ligament injury. At L2-L3 level, MRI better depicts hemorrhage in the interspinous ligament (*black asterisk*), as well as the complete tear of supraspinous ligament (*black arrowhead*), with associated large hemorrhagic collection in the subfascial space (*white asterisk*). Note also a subtle posterior subdural hematoma (*white arrowhead*) and bone edema in L2 and L3 vertebral bodies

factual images can "overlap" to the spinal cord (Figs. 5.8, 5.10, and 5.18);

- T2*-weighted sagittal or axial (Figs. 5.8, 5.10, and 5.18) images, for the best demonstration of hematomyelia compared to T2-weighted images, since they allow a more satisfactory conspicuity of areas with low signal intensity within a larger abnormal T2 area.

Furthermore, in the evaluation of the neurological damage, a significant advantage of MRI is to study neural roots (Fig. 5.19) and plexi, limiting the need for radiography and CT myelography. Root avulsions and lesions of the neural pockets possibly resulting in pseudomeningocele may be shown already in the acute phase, especially by high-resolution 3D T2-weighted "myelographic" sequences. However, when necessary, the complete MR study of a plexus is generally performed on a later stage (generally after 1 month from the trauma) since it requires complete patient's immobility, absorption of possible posttraumatic hemorrhage, and finally possible surgical therapeutic options (nerve reconstruction) are not performed in the acute phase but generally in 2–3 months

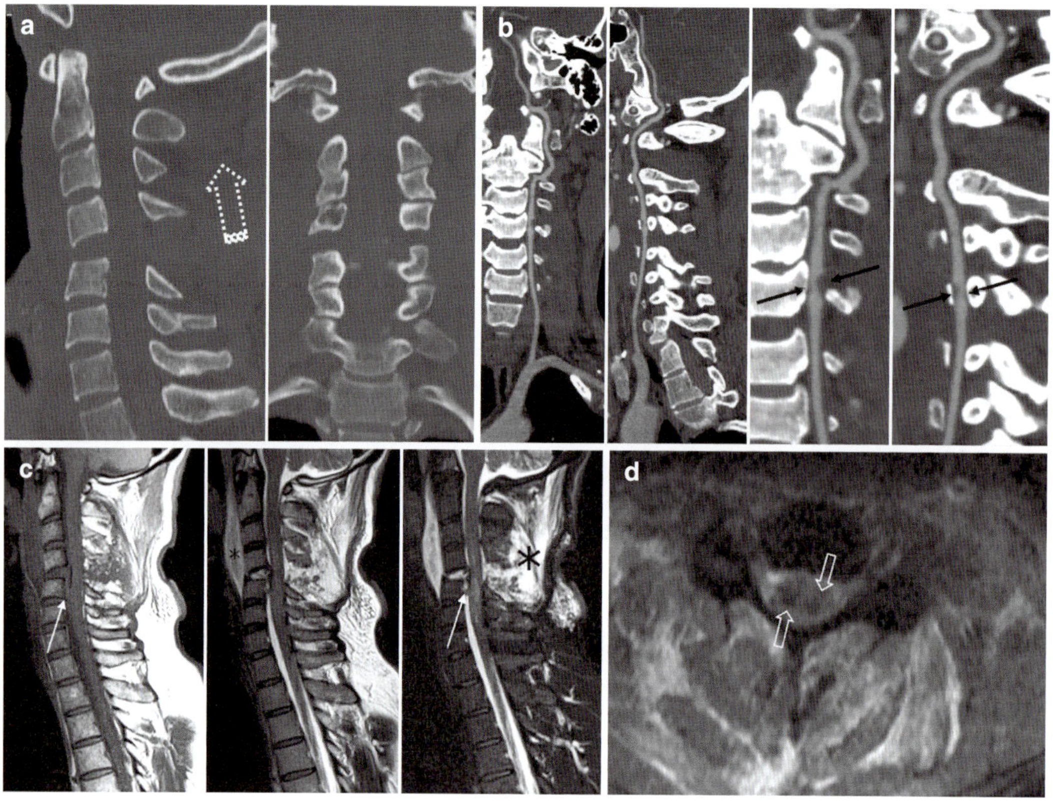

Fig. 5.10 C4-C5 flexion distraction injury complicated by left vertebral artery dissection and hematomyelia: 2D-reformatted sagittal and coronal CT images (**a**), coronal and sagittal CT angiography images including magnification (**b**), T1- and T2-weighted, and STIR sagittal (**c**), and T2*-weighted axial (**d**) MR images. At C4-C5 level, the distraction injury mechanism (*open dashed arrow*) resulting in pure discal and ligamentous damage is clearly evident. CTA shows intimal flap (*black arrows*) of the left vertebral artery. MRI better shows an acute posttraumatic C4-C5 posterior disc herniation (*long white arrows*) directly depicts tear of anterior longitudinal, and interspinous ligaments resulting in prevertebral (*small asterisk*) and paravertebral (*large asterisk*) hemorrhagic collections. At C5-C6 level, MRI shows also an inhomogeneous centromedullary spinal cord area of prevalent T2 high signal intensity with portions of T2* low signal intensity (*solid open arrows*), such as hematomyelia in edema/contusion. Still note that there are no bony lesions

from trauma. In addition to "myelographic" images for assessing the integrity of roots and neural pockets, the study should include STIR or fat-suppressed T2-weighted images to rule out or show damage of the plexus elements. Intravenous paramagnetic contrast medium may be useful to demonstrate the damage of the blood–neural barrier in the subacute and chronic phase.

Additionally, MR imaging is superior to CT in the evaluation of bone edema, disc and ligaments injury. Recently, it has been advocated as appropriate to include STIR or fat-suppressed T2-weighted sagittal images of a spinal segment wider than the area of the posttraumatic injury (Figs. 5.11 and 5.16), and possibly of the whole spine. This is to rule out other spinal lesions

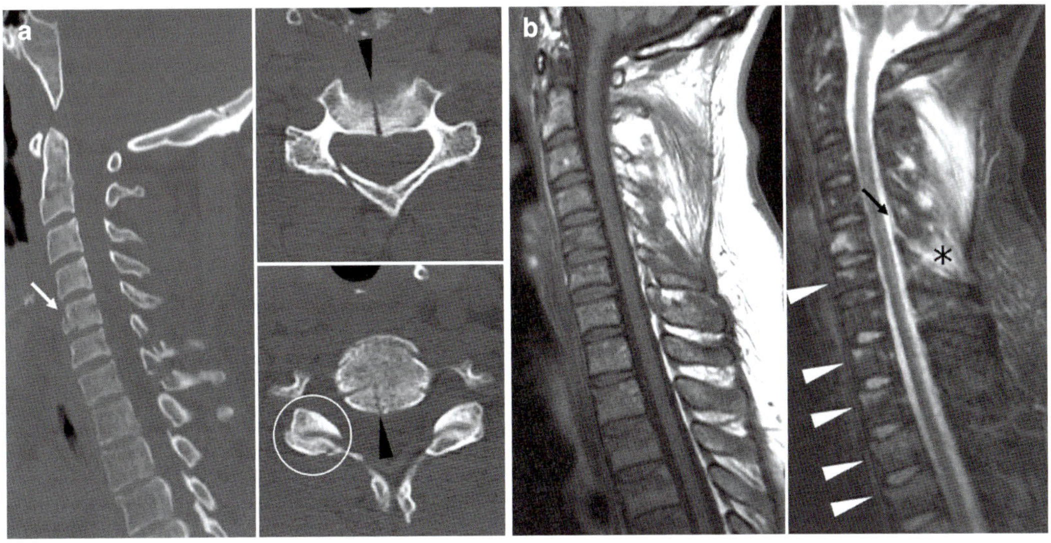

Fig. 5.11 C5 teardrop split fracture by flexion distraction and compression injury mechanisms: 2D-reformatted sagittal and nonconsecutive source axial CT images (**a**), and T1-weighted and STIR sagittal MR images (**b**). Fracture lines involve the C5 anterior lower body (*white arrow*), as well as both superior and inferior endplates (*black arrowheads*), i.e., a split fracture, with involvement of the posterior wall. MRI clearly depicts tear of the flavum (*black arrow*) and interspinous (*asterisk*) ligaments, as well as bone edema in the vertebral bodies of C6, T1, T2, and T3 (*white arrowheads*), some of which show reduction in height. Note also the incipient subluxation of right C5-C6 facet joint, as well as a subtle fracture of the ipsilateral C6 superior articular process (*white circle*)

which, although generally of no great clinical relevance, can be important for overall clinical prognosis and surgical planning [38, 45, 57]. Supraspinous ligament injury may be diagnosed by the discontinuity or nonvisualization of its black stripe of low signal intensity on T1- and/or T2-weighted sagittal images (Figs. 5.8, 5.9, 5.10, and 5.18), i.e., a sign which may be advocated also for flavum ligament injury (Figs. 5.8, 5.10, 5.11, 5.17, and 5.18). Interspinous ligament injury may be diagnosed by high signal intensity on STIR and fat-suppressed T2-weighted images (Figs. 5.9 and 5.17), consistent with hematoma [16], despite this evidence does not mean its certain disruption (Fig. 5.10). Surgical exploration remains the standard reference for the identification of the ligamentous damage. Thus, abnormal T2 signal intensity seen in the capsules or ligaments with normal bone relationships results in an "indeterminate" score in TLICS and SLIC classification systems [52, 53]. Nevertheless, diagnostic imaging aimed to the specific lesional situation seems to facilitate the most appropriate therapeutic choice.

Finally, in the acute phase, certainly the quality of MR studies may be reduced by the presence of cervical collar or spinal longboard (Fig. 5.4).

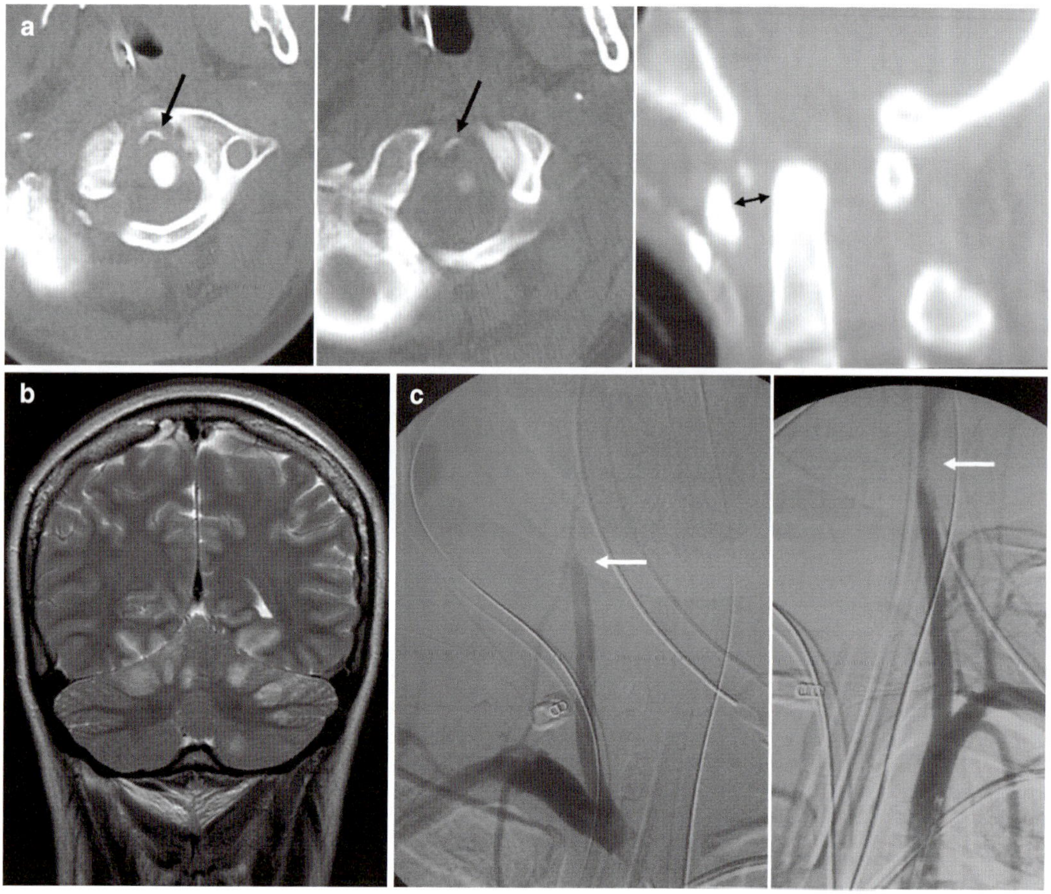

Fig. 5.12 Fracture subluxation of the craniocervical junction complicated by bilateral vertebral artery dissection in pre-CTA era: source axial and 2D-reformatted sagittal CT images (**a**), T2-weighted coronal MR image of the head (**b**) and digital subtraction angiography anteroposterior view (**c**). At admission, CT showed type III left occipital condyle fracture from ipsilateral alar ligament avulsion (*black arrows*). One day later, the patient underwent abrupt worsening of her neurological conditions, and MRI showed signs of ischemia in both infra- and supratentorial posterior circulation. Angiography showed right vertebral artery occlusion and left vertebral artery stenosis (*white arrows*), both signs consistent with arterial dissection

5.3 Anatomy, Function, and Stability

Two adjacent vertebrae and the corresponding interconnected soft tissue are the simplest and principal functional motion segment of the spine, i.e., the *functional spinal unit*. Stability is strongly correlated with the integrity of discal, joint, and ligamentous structures supporting bony elements.

In the craniocervical junction, occipital condyles, atlas, and axis are provided by a number of ligamentous and articular structures including the transverse ligament of the atlas and the apical ligament (which both form the so-called cruciform ligament), the alar ligaments, the tectorial membrane which blend with the posterior longitudinal ligament, and the atlanto-odontoid, occipitoatlantal, and atlantoaxial joints.

In the subaxial cervical spine and in the thoracolumbar spine, the functional spine unit is formed by an anterior and a posterior portion. The anterior portion includes the two aligned vertebral bodies, the interposed intervertebral disc

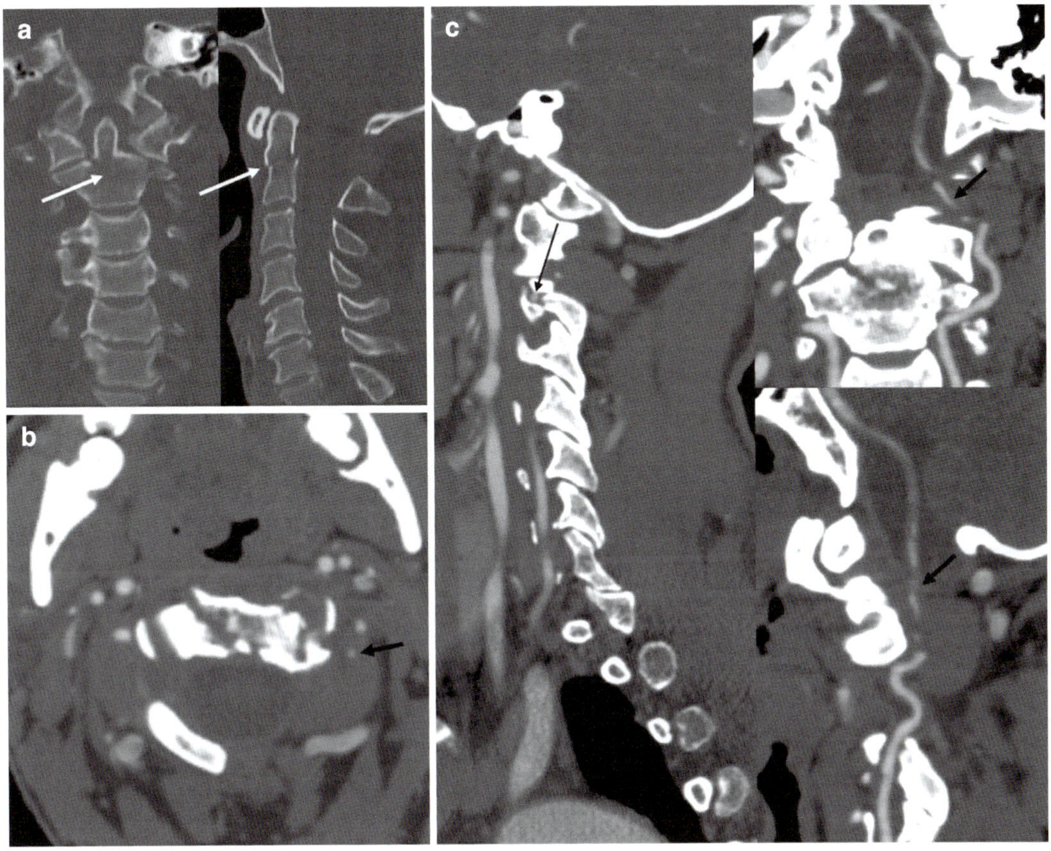

Fig. 5.13 Fracture of C2 odontoid process (type III or "low") and mass complicated by vertebral artery dissection: 2D-coronal and sagittal unenhanced CT (**a**), source axial (**b**), and 2D-reformatted sagittal and coronal CT angiography (**c**) images show the axis fracture (*white arrows*), the impingement of a fragment of its left lateral mass on the left vertebral artery (*long black arrow*), and left vertebral artery irregularity and stenosis (*short black arrows*)

containing a central hydrated nucleus pulposus and a peripheral annulus fibrosus, and the anterior and posterior longitudinal ligaments. The anterior longitudinal ligament is a strong band of variable thickness and width running the entire length of the spine from the skull base to the sacrum, connecting the anterior vertebral body to the anterior annulus fibrosus. The posterior longitudinal ligament is a strong band, spanning from the body of the axis to the posterior surface of the sacrum, connecting the posterior vertebral body to the posterior annulus fibrosus, forming the anterior wall of the vertebral canal, and superiorly blending with the tectorial membrane. The anterior portion primarily supports axial, or compressive, loading, which is resisted by vertebral bodies and intervertebral disc, which directs forces circumferential towards anterior and posterior ligaments.

The posterior portion includes the vertebral arches, flavum ligaments, facet joints, interspinous and supraspinous ligaments. Flavum ligaments connect the laminae of the adjacent vertebrae and keeps them aligned. Facet joints are posterior portions of the laminae and are the primary elements allowing spinal movements on the basis of their morphology in the cervical, thoracic, and lumbar segments. In the cervical spine, the upward and superomedial inclination of superior articular facets allows free flexion and

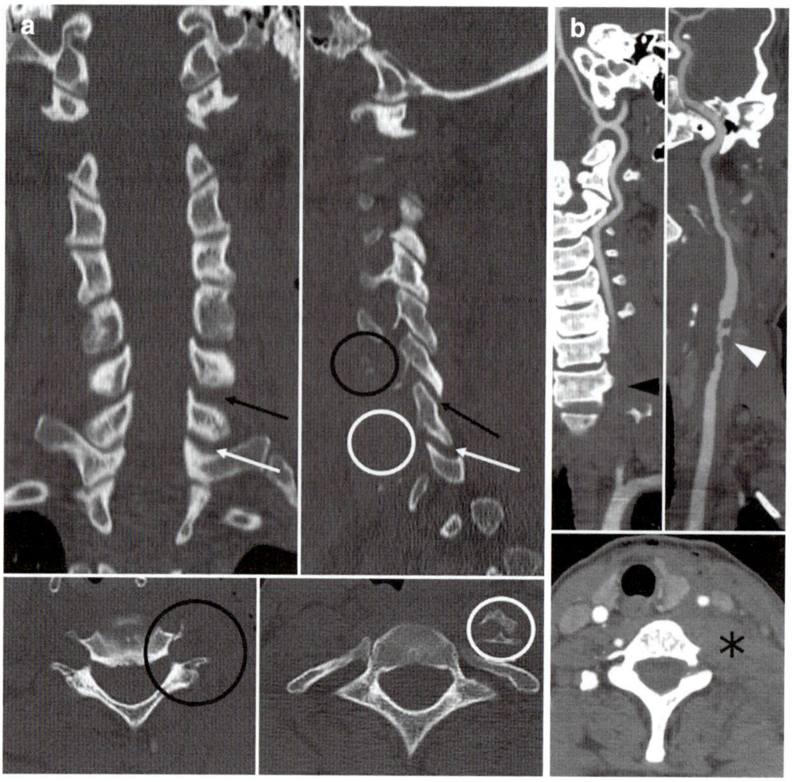

Fig. 5.14 C6 left mass fracture-dislocation and C7 left mass fracture associated with C6-C7 and C7-T1 subluxation from extension distraction injury, complicated by carotid artery dissection: 2D-reformatted coronal and sagittal, and nonconsecutive source axial CT images (**a**), and 2D-reformatted coronal and sagittal, and source axial CT angiography images (**b**). CT images show fracture-dislocation of left C6 mass (*black circle*) and fracture of left C7 (*white circle*) mass, as well as C6-C7 (*black arrows*) and C7-T1 (*white arrows*) facet joint subluxation. CTA shows intimal injury and thrombus in the left internal carotid artery (*white arrowhead*). Note also occlusion of the proximal V2 segment of the left vertebral artery (*black arrowhead*) associated with hematoma in the left longissimus muscles and anterior scalenus muscles region (*asterisk*)

extension, as well as combination of lateral flexion and rotation. In the thoracic spine, superior articular facets are oriented in the coronal plan, face posteriorly, and are directed a little superolaterally, resulting in free lateral rotation and minimized flexion and extension. In the lumbar spine, superior articular facets are oriented in a sagittal oblique plan and face posteromedially, resulting in a wider range of extension than flexion, while rotation is minimized. Interspinous ligament is a weak and thin membrane connecting the adjacent spinous processes. Supraspinous ligament is a strong cordlike ligament connecting the tips of the spinous processes from C7 to the sacrum. The posterior portion of the functional spinal unit primarily supports movements of the spine, including flexion, extension, and rotation, resisting excessive tensile forces possibly resulting also in translational injuries.

Spinal stability is defined as the ability of the spine to prevent progressive deformity and neurologic injury by maintaining relationships between vertebrae and limiting reciprocal displacements in the different positions, under the action of physiological loading and normal range of movements: this may result only from the whole integrity of vertebrae, intervertebral discs, joints, ligaments, muscles, and neural control [4, 23, 24, 58, 59].

A posttraumatic spinal lesion is considered stable when it can be reduced with external maneuvers and maintained reduced with external means

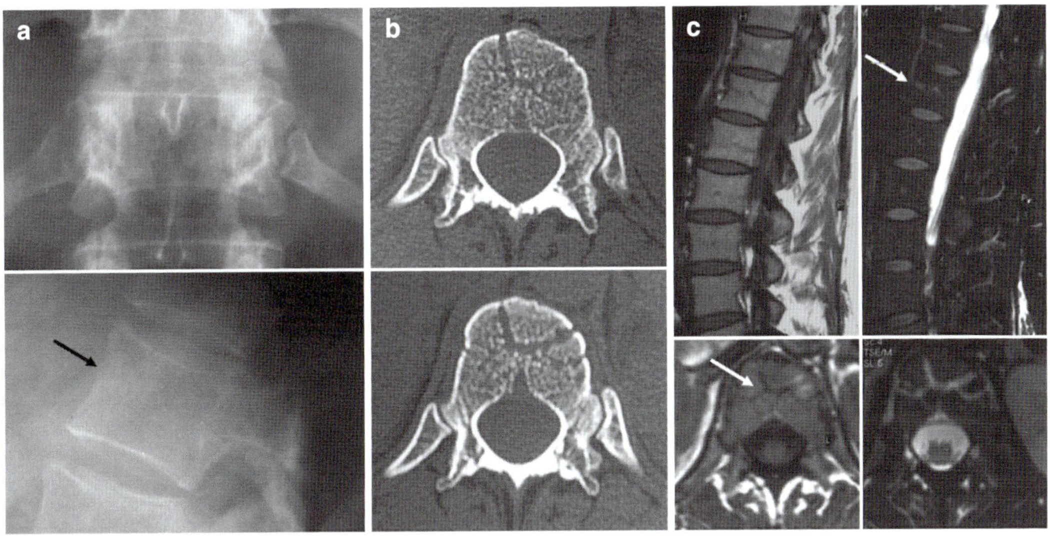

Fig. 5.15 Basivertebral veins: anteroposterior and lateral radiographic views (**a**), consecutive axial CT images (**b**), and T1-weighted and fat-suppressed T2-weighted sagittal and axial MR images (**c**). Radiography shows a subtle radiolucency (*black arrow*) along the anterior wall of T12 vertebral body: this finding was considered suspicious for fracture after a skiing fall. CT clearly depicts the vertebral body basivertebral veins which course horizontally receiving tributaries from numerous small venous channels, through many openings in the anterior and lateral surfaces of the vertebral body, then draining into the anterior internal vertebral plexus in the middle of the posterior vertebral body. MRI confirms this finding, i.e., its morphology (*white arrows*) associated with T1 low and T2 high signal intensity. Furthermore, MRI does not show bone edema

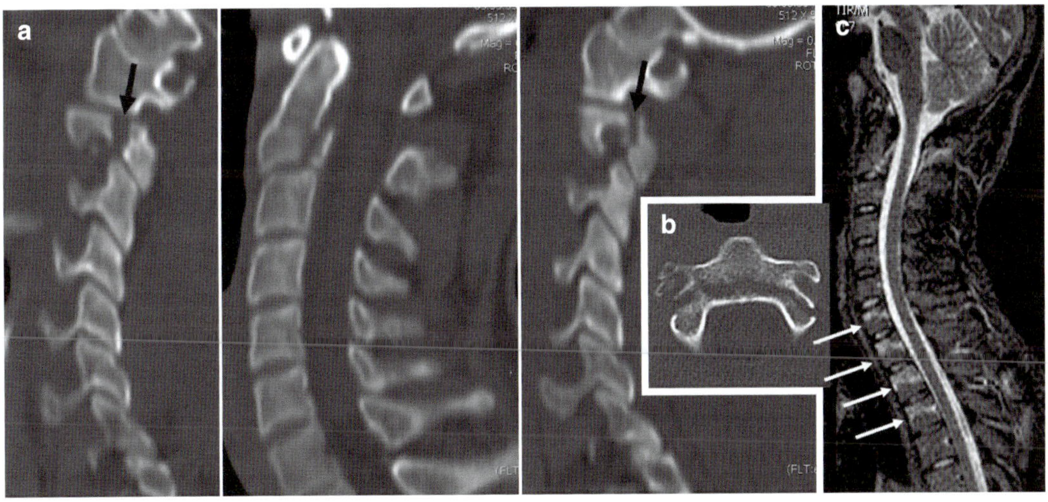

Fig. 5.16 C2 atypical traumatic spondylolisthesis in multiple vertebral injuries: nonconsecutive right to left 2D-reformatted sagittal (**a**) and source axial (**b**) CT images, and STIR sagittal MR image (**c**). The fracture line involving both axis pedicles and axis body (*black arrows*) is well depicted. MRI shows posttraumatic bone edema in the C7, T1, T2, and T3 vertebral bodies

(casts, corsets) till to healing, and unstable when it cannot be reduced by external maneuvers nor it can be maintained reduced by external elements until the healing. Therefore, an unstable posttraumatic spinal lesion requires surgery to restore the stability. However, the differentiation between

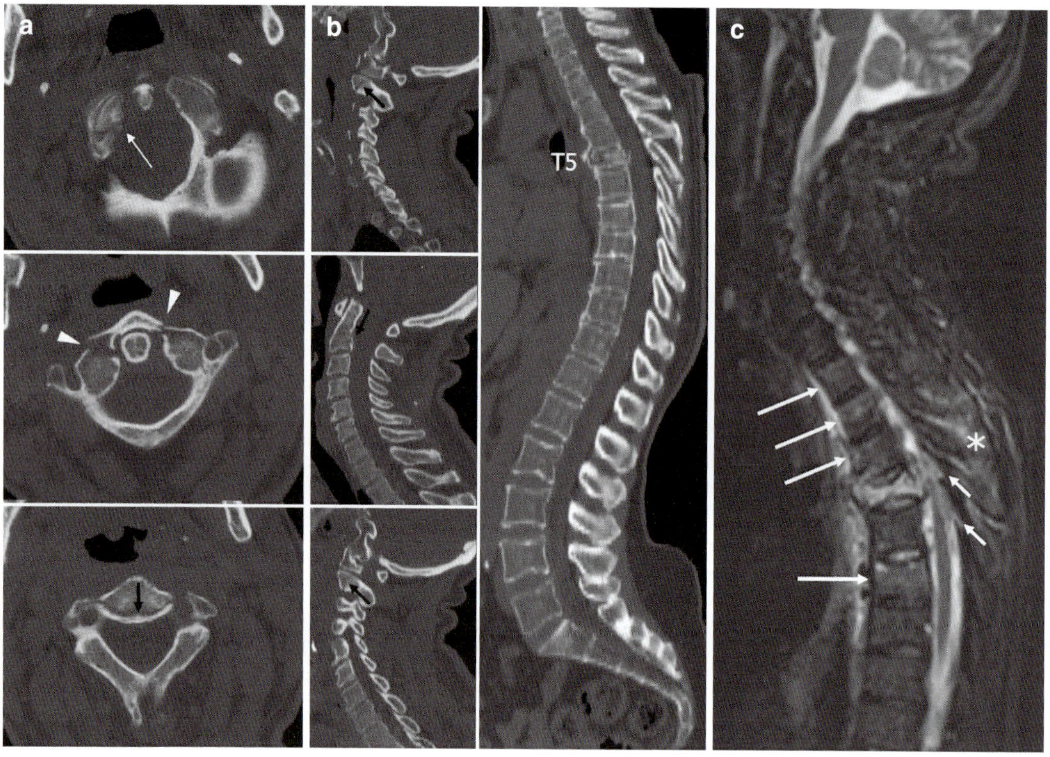

Fig. 5.17 Multiple fractures of the craniocervical junction and thoracic spine: nonconsecutive source axial (**a**), right to left 2D-reformatted sagittal, and midsagittal (**b**) CT, and STIR sagittal MRI (**c**) images. In the craniocervical junction, CT shows a type I right occipital condyle fracture (*thin long white arrow*), a type II atlas fracture (*white arrowheads*), and an atypical traumatic spondylolisthesis of the axis (*black arrow*) of the posterior third of the body of the atlas. Note also the burst fracture of T5, the edema (*thick long white arrows*) in the T2, T3, T4, and T7 vertebral bodies, the interruption of T5-T6 and T6-T7 ligamenta flava (*short white arrows*), as well as signal alteration in T3 to T6 interspinous ligaments (*asterisk*)

stable and unstable lesions is still under discussion, and there are no stability or instability criteria universally accepted, even for the specific anatomical and functional characteristics of spinal segments. This resulted in the development of many classification systems guiding clinical and surgical treatment, historically based on anatomic structures and injury mechanisms (axial loading or compression/burst, distraction in flexion or extension, translation/rotation, seat belt injury) determined through analysis of osseous components and their relationships [5, 17, 25, 29, 33, 42, 46, 52, 53].

For instance, for a long time the evaluation of thoracolumbar fractures has been performed on the *Denis three-column model classification system* (Fig. 5.5), which was based on morphology from compression, burst, seat belt, and fracture dislocation injury mechanisms [5]. Fractures of articular, transverse, and spinous processes, and pars articularis were considered minor fractures. This classification system introduced and highlighted the involvement of the posterior vertebral body and intervertebral disc and the posterior longitudinal ligament, i.e., the "middle column," whose lesions (Fig. 5.4) were defined to render the spine mechanically unstable and preferably requiring surgery. However, it has been demonstrated that "two-column" "unstable" injuries can also be successfully treated nonsurgically, if the posterior ligamentous complex is intact [29]. Notably, the anatomical models of the columns are not free from criticism since the columns do

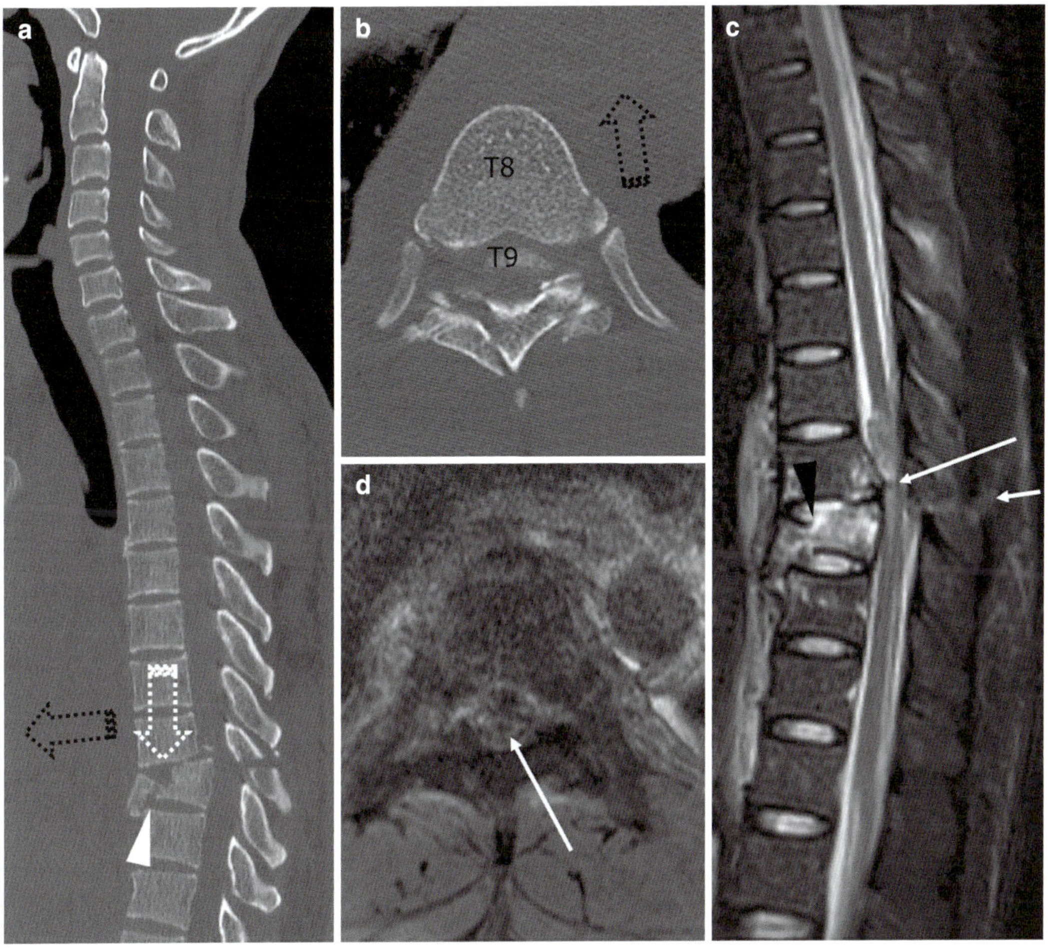

Fig. 5.18 T9 split fracture by a mixed compression (*white dashed open arrow*) and translation (*black dashed open arrow*) injury mechanisms: 2D-reformatted midsagittal (**a**) and source axial CT (**b**), and fat-sat T2-weighted sagittal (**c**) and T2*-weighted axial (**d**) MR images. *Solid arrowheads* indicate the involvement of both endplates, i.e., a split fracture. *Short white arrow* indicates tears of supraspinous ligament at T8 T9 level and T8-T9 ligamentum flavum, as well as injury to T8-T9 ligamentum flavum. *White long arrow* indicates hematomyelia. The spinal cord is highly compressed and distorted

not represent anatomical or functional biomechanical realities.

A more accurate classification system of fractures of the thoracolumbar spine based on mechanism of injury was then proposed by Magerl et al. in 1994 and also called AO (*Arbeitsgemeinschaft für Osteosynthesefragen or Association for Osteosynthesis*) classification system [25]. The three main lesional mechanisms give the name to the three main groups of the lesion, i.e., compression, distraction, and translation/rotation. On the basis of fracture location, morphology, osseous or ligamentous disruption, and direction of displacement, each of these three groups is divided into three other and each of the resulting nine subgroups is further divided, for a total of 53 subtypes. The main principle was that fractures represent a continuum of progressively increasing injury severity and instability groups from A to C, resulting in an increasing likelihood of the need for surgery. AO system introduced and highlighted the role of injuries to soft tissues, namely the posterior ligamentous complex. Nevertheless, the complexity of this classification resulted in a certain degree of limited interobserver disagreement, providing poor prognostic data, and thus resulting in a limited use. Additionally, these classification systems did not provide information on the patient's neurologic status, which is the other basis guiding surgical intervention. Notably, most classification systems lacked an overall assessment of the stability of the spine which has to include a comprehensive assessment of injury mechanism (as expression of immediate mechanical stability), ligamentous injury (as expression of long-term mechanical stability), and neurological status (as expression of clinical stability).

To overcome some of these limitations, in the first decade of 2000s, thoracolumbar injury classification and severity score system, or TLICS [52] and the subaxial cervical spine injury classification system, or SLIC [53] have been proposed for the management and treatment options of fractures of the thoracolumbar and subaxial cervical spine, respectively. These classification systems identified three major characteristics resulting in a weighted score critical to clinical decision-making: (1) injury morphology as determined by the pattern of spinal column disruption on available imaging studies, (2) integrity of the posterior ligamentous complex, or "posterior tensioning band" formed by flavum ligament, facet capsule, interspinous and supraspinous ligaments in the thoracolumbar spine, and of the discoligamentous complex formed by the anterior longitudinal ligament, intervertebral disc, and posterior longitudinal ligament anteriorly, flavum ligament, facet capsule, interspinous and supraspinous ligaments posteriorly in the subaxial cervical spine, and (3) neurologic status of the patient.

More recently, a new comprehensive modified AO spine fracture classification systems have been proposed [54, 55], taking the best of the Magerl, TLICS, and SLIC systems, and scoring fracture morphology, neurologic status, and relevant site- and patient-specific modifiers for therapeutic decisions.

5.4 Patterns of Injuries

The results of a spinal trauma depend upon its injury mechanism and the capacity of resistance and resilience of normal bony, discal, joint, and ligamentous structures.

5.4.1 Injury Mechanisms

The knowledge of axial loading, distraction, and translational/rotational mechanisms of injury is crucial to understand the morphological features of vertebral fractures and to recognize their radiological signs. Each mechanism has typical features, however a combination of the three primary morphologies is relatively frequent and results in more complex fracture patterns of spine failure. For instance, a severe rotational injury may be associated with a burst fracture, which would be best described as a rotation burst fracture. Similarly, a distraction injury may be associated with a compression and a translation component, resulting in the best description of a distraction translation compression injury.

Axial loading is the injury mechanism where the energy is transferred along the spine by the movement of a vertebral body against the one below and pressure increase along the circumference of the intervertebral disc. Diagnostic imaging shows a loss of height through a portion, i.e., the endplate, or the entire vertebra. Axial compression fracture prevails in the anterior column of Denis, with buckling of the anterior wall of the vertebra and possible kyphosis (Fig. 5.1a). Involvement of the posterior somatic vertebral body wall (Fig. 5.1b) or of three columns of Denis results in the so-called axial burst fracture, with various degrees of somatic fragments retropulsion in the more severe forms. Associated forces may result in flexion compression or burst, i.e., the so-called teardrop injury of the subaxial cervical spine (Fig. 5.11), flexion compression or burst with distraction of posterior elements, lateral compression, or lateral burst injury mechanism, as well as in associated translation (Fig. 5.15) and/or rotation.

AO spine classification system defines axial loading injury mechanism as Group A and includes:

- No bony injury or minor injury such as an isolated lamina fracture or spinous process fracture (A0); compression fracture involving a single endplate without involvement of the posterior wall of the vertebral body (A1); coronal split or pincer fracture involving both endplates without involvement of the posterior wall of the vertebral body (A2); burst fracture involving a single endplate with involvement of the posterior vertebral wall (A3); burst fracture or sagittal split involving both endplates (A4) in the subaxial cervical spine [55].
- Minor, nonstructural fractures, i.e., fractures which do not compromise the structural integrity of the spinal column such as transverse process or spinous process fractures (A0); wedge-compression fracture, i.e., fracture of a single endplate without involvement of the posterior wall of the vertebral body (A1); split fracture, i.e., fracture of both endplates without involvement of the posterior wall of the vertebral body (A2); incomplete burst fracture, i.e., fracture with any involvement of the posterior wall and only a single endplate fractured. (A3); complete burst fracture, i.e., fracture with any involvement of the posterior wall and both endplates (A4) in the thoracolumbar spine. In A3 and A4 fractures, vertical fracture of the lamina is usually present and does not constitute a tension band failure [54].

Distraction is the injury mechanism where the energy transmission determines the displacement of a vertebral body from the underlying along the sagittal plane, leaving a space in between. Distraction injuries are less common than compressive ones. In hyperflexion, the anterior column of Denis is compressed and the posterior one is distracted (Figs. 5.2 and 5.9), while the opposite occurs in hyperextension which disrupts the anterior longitudinal ligament and widens the anterior disc space (Fig. 5.19). This can occur through a circumferentially disruption of anterior and posterior ligaments, through anterior and posterior bony elements, or a combination of both. Thus, distraction signifies a greater degree of anatomic disruption and potential instability.

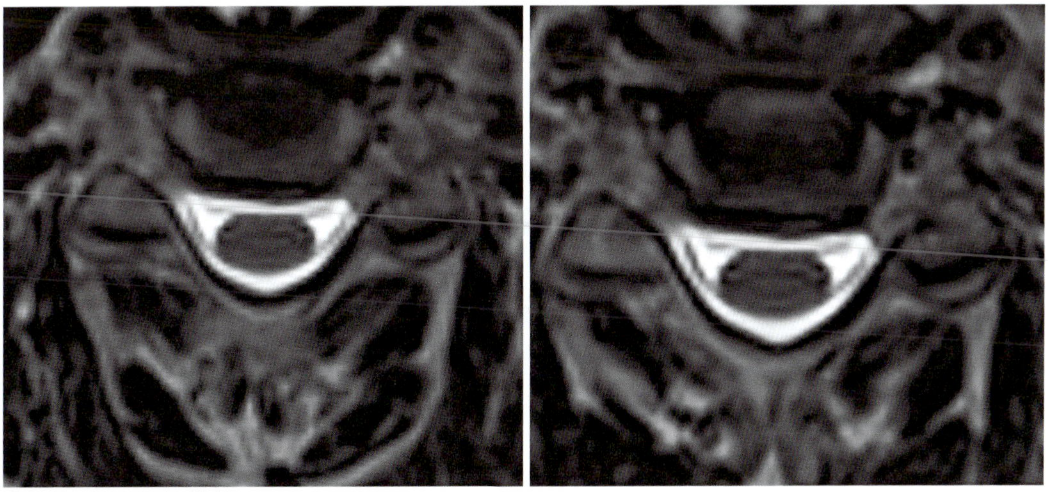

Fig. 5.19 Potential for MRI in depicting nerve roots: nonconsecutive 2D-reformatted axial images from high-resolution 3D-TSE T2-weighted images. At C4-C5 (*left image*) and C5-C6 (*right image*), anterior and posterior nerve roots are clearly evident

Diagnostic imaging shows disconnection between a cranial and a caudal portion of the spine through the disc space or through the facet joints, such as that seen in facet subluxation or dislocation without fracture and translation/rotation. Hyperflexion injury may also be associated with concomitant axial loading injury of the vertebral body. Hyperextension injury may also be associated with concomitant compression across the posterior elements resulting in posterior element fractures or spinal cord compression through inward buckling of the ligamentum flavum.

Translational/rotational forces may be associated.

AO spine classification system defines distraction injury mechanism as Group B and includes:

- Posterior tension band bony injury, i.e., physical separation through fractured bony structures only (B1); posterior tension band bony, capsuloligamentous, and ligamentous injury, i.e., complete disruption of the posterior capsuloligamentous or bony capsuloligamentous structures together with a vertebral body, disc, and/or facet injury (B2); and anterior tension band injury, i.e., physical disruption or separation of the anterior structures (bone/disc) with tethering of the posterior element (B3) in the subaxial cervical spine [55].
- Transosseous tension band disruption, i.e., the so-called classical Chance fracture, i.e., monosegmental pure osseous failure of the posterior tension band (B1); posterior tension band disruption, i.e., bony and/or ligamentous failure of the posterior tension band together with a Type A fracture (which should be classified separately) (B2), and hyperextension, i.e., injury through the disc or vertebral body leading to a hyperextended position of the spinal column (B3) in the thoracolumbar spine [54]. In the thoracolumbar spine, B3 fractures are commonly seen in ankylotic disorders (Fig. 5.20). Anterior structures, especially the anterior longitudinal ligament, are ruptured but there is a posterior hinge preventing further displacement.

Translation/rotation is the injury mechanism where the energy transmission determines the displacement of a vertebral body from the one below along the axial plane (Fig. 5.21). If the

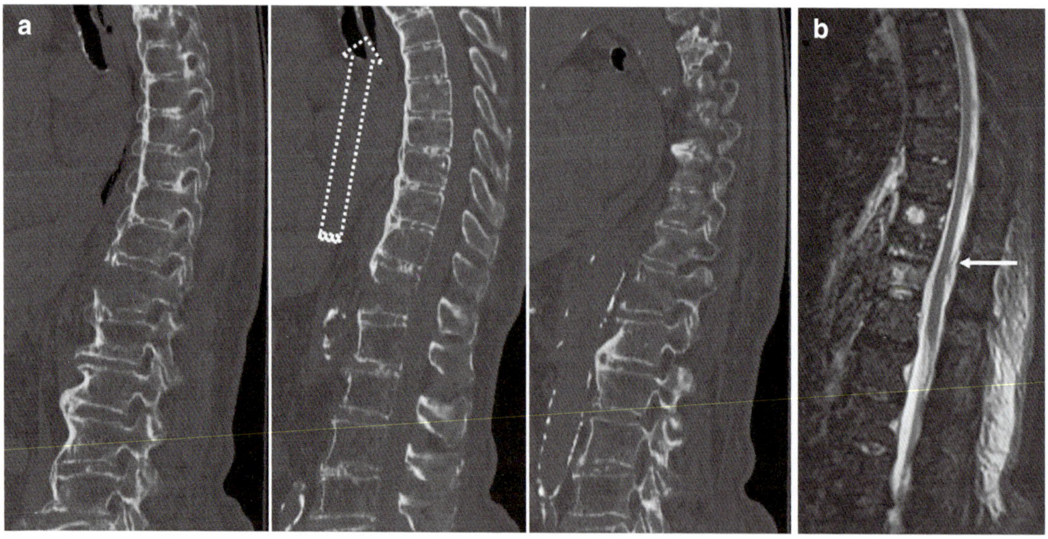

Fig. 5.20 T12 fracture by extension distraction mechanism injury in ankylosing spondylitis: nonconsecutive right to left 2D-reformatted sagittal CT images (**a**) and STIR sagittal MR image (**b**). *Dashed open arrow* shows the extension distraction mechanism injury, without involvement of the pedicles. MRI shows a small posterior epidural hematoma (*arrow*)

facet joint(s) is(are) intact but dislocated (unilaterally or bilaterally), the term dislocation can be interchanged. Diagnostic imaging shows an anteroposterior/posteroanterior to lateral horizontal displacement of one part of the spine with respect to the other in the axial plan. For instance, facet jump or abnormal alignment of the pedicles above and below the level of the injury indicate a translational/rotational injury. These signs have to be searched on all the three imaging plans and may be evidenced on either static or dynamic (abnormal displacement exceeding normal physiologic ranges) imaging.

Associated axial loading may result in translation/rotation compression or burst, unilateral or bilateral facet dislocation compression or burst.

AO spine classification system defines translation/rotation mechanism as Group C and includes:

- Translational injury in any axis-displacement or translation of one vertebral body relative to another in any direction in the subaxial cervical spine [55]
- Displacement or dislocation in the thoracolumbar spine [54]

5.4.2 Facet Joints

In the subaxial cervical spine, injuries involving the facet joints or lateral masses may result from lateral compressive forces and/or a distractive mechanism of injury. This results in Group F in the AO spine classification system for the subaxial cervical spine [55], including nondisplaced facet fracture with fragment <1 cm in height, <40% of lateral mass (F1), facet fracture with fragment >1 cm, > 40% lateral mass, or displaced (F2), floating lateral mass (F3), pathologic subluxation or perched/dislocated facet (F4), and bilateral injury (BL).

5.4.3 Discal, Joints, and Ligamentous Injuries

The integrity assessment of these structures relies on the measurements and angulations obtained by radiography and CT [4, 23, 24, 42, 58, 59] and can be supported significantly by MRI [16, 42]. Identification and description of injury to such ligamentous discoligamentous and joint damage help in the therapeutic choice.

In TLICS and SLIC classification systems [52, 53], diagnostic imaging has to indicate if the structure is intact, the findings are "undetermined" (when it is not possible to define with certainty the presence of the damage), or if the structure is certainly damaged. In both scoring systems, there is inherent overlap since abnormal bone relationships described in the morphology score are absolute indicators of discal, joints, or ligamentous injury. Notably, distraction injuries are scored 3 on the basis of morphology and receive other 2 points for discal and/or ligamentous injury, therefore requiring surgery. Although an indeterminate score was meant to be used infrequently, it has been reported in up to 30% of cases. For instance, an indeterminate score may be given when isolated interspinous widening is seen at CT since interspinous ligament is the weakest support structure, and its integrity plays a small role in overall stability, as well as when bone relationships are normal but abnormal T2 signal intensity is seen in the capsules or ligaments at MRI.

5.5 Associated Conditions

In daily clinical evaluation, regardless of any classification scheme the choice of treatment cannot ignore the careful evaluation of specific associated conditions or properly confounding variables, such as age or systemic diseases including obesity and osteopenia. The prediction versus surgical and nonsurgical management is still under evaluation, due to some inherent limitations. For instance, patients may be affected by degenerative osteoarthritis (Fig. 5.3), diffuse idiopathic skeletal hyperostosis and ossification of posterior longitudinal ligament, ankylosing spondylitis (Fig. 5.20), or rheumatoid arthritis that may alter surgical planning or lead to unnecessary surgery. Furthermore, it is increasingly frequent the occurrence of a trauma—even minor—deter-

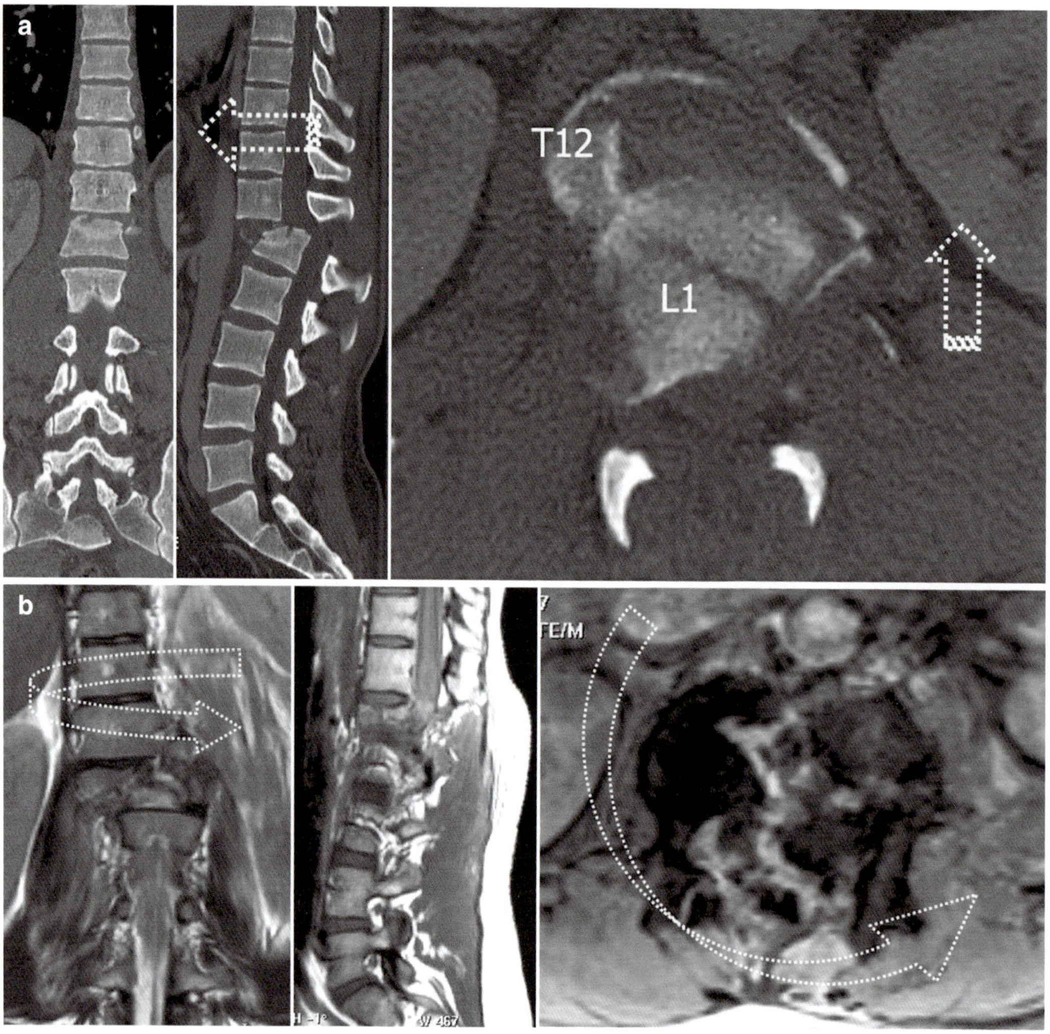

Fig. 5.21 Translational (**a**) and rotational (**b**) injury mechanisms in two different patients with fractures of L1: 2D-reformatted coronal and sagittal, and source axial CT images (**a**), T1-weighted sagittal, T2-weighted coronal and T2*-weighted axial MRI images (**b**). *Linear dashed open arrow* indicates the anterior translation of the spine above the fracture level. *Curvilinear dotted open arrow* indicates the rotation leading to the spinal destruction

mining spinal cord injury because of a predisposing cervical spine degenerative or mixed constitutional/degenerative stenosis of which the patient was not aware. Some of these variables are important for designating those injuries with stable injuries from a bony standpoint for which ligamentous insufficiency may help to determine whether operative stabilization has to be considered. TLICS was the first comprehensive injury grading scale to consider these variables (defined as *qualifiers)* to be added to morphologic and neurologic status into a system capable of guiding injury management [52].

AO spine classification systems include the following confounding variables in Group M, i.e., *modifiers* (Group M):

– Posterior capsuloligamentous complex injury without complete disruption (M1), vertebral artery abnormality (M2), critical disc herniation (M3), stiffening/metabolic bone disease, i.e., diffuse idiopathic skeletal hyperostosis, ankylosing spondylitis, ossification of posterior longitudinal ligament, and ossification of the

ligamentum flavum (M4) in the subaxial cervical spine [55]
- Fractures with an indeterminate injury to the tension band based on spinal imaging with or without MRI (M1), and patient-specific comorbidity (i.e., ankylosing spondylitis or burns affecting the skin overlying the injured spine) which might argue either for or against surgery for patients with relative surgical indications (M2), in the thoracolumbar spine [54]

5.6 Neurological Status

Patient's neurologic status, i.e., degree of spinal cord and root nerves injury, is of great importance as a critical indicator for prognosis and treatment reccomendation. The severity of spinal cord injury is usually assessed by the American Spinal Injury Association (ASIA) Impairment Scale (AIS) which is a clinician-administered scale based on the Frankel scale. Grade A defines complete spinal cord injury (no motor or sensory function preserved in sacral segments S4-S5), grades B (sensory, but not motor function preserved below the neurologic level and includes sacral segments S4-S5), C (motor function preserved below the neurologic level, and more than half of key muscles below the neurologic level have muscle grade < 3), and D (motor function preserved below the neurologic level, and at least half of key muscles below the neurologic level have muscle grade ≥ 3) define incomplete spinal cord injury, and grade E (motor and sensory functions are normal) defines spinal trauma without spinal cord injury. In TLICS and SLIC classification systems [52, 53], incomplete spinal cord injury, incomplete conus medullaris injury, and cauda equina syndrome are assigned the highest score, since patients with these type of injury may receive greater potential benefit from surgical decompression than patients with no initial neurologic injury or with complete spinal cord or conus medullaris injuries. In the AO spine classification systems [54, 55], the neurological status is then clinically defined as intact (N0), transiently deficitary (N1), radiculopathy (N2), incomplete spinal cord injury (N3), complete spinal cord injury (N4), unknown for sedation or coma (NX), with a "plus" for ongoing cord compression in setting of incomplete neurologic deficit or nerve injury in cervical spinal cord injury.

5.6.1 Diagnostic Imaging

Clinical neurologic status cannot be directly determined by diagnostic imaging. However, CT clearly shows the vertebral fractures, bone fragments, and spinal canal occupation, and MRI may show spinal cord and/or nerve root injury. Notably, severe kyphotic deformities, higher canal occupation by bony fragments, higher spinal cord compression, larger lesion length, spinal cord hemorrhage, and/or swelling are associated with poor initial neurological status and recovery. Qualitative and quantitative parameters measured at diagnostic imaging have a significant role in predicting initial severity of neurological status and outcome [42, 48]. In the acute setting, MRI is an excellent modality to evaluate the spinal cord, and its findings are significant and useful in the prediction of neurological outcome [48].

5.6.2 Clearance of the Cervical Spine

After blunt trauma, airway protection and cervical spine immobilization are the first steps required by the Advanced Trauma Life Support protocol developed by the American College of Surgeons Committee on Trauma. Unstable cervical spine injuries possibly resulting in neurologic injury or death has to be considered present until proven otherwise. Thus, cervical spine injury has to be ruled out, or "cleared," in order to safely remove cervical spine precautions, i.e., the collar. Early removal of cervical spine collar results in a reduced frequency of complications, fewer days of mechanical ventilation, and a short stay in the intensive care unit, while the rate of secondary neurologic injury is extremely high in cases of missed or delayed diagnoses.

Asymptomatic, stable, and alert (i.e., Glasgow Coma Scale Score-GCS: 15) adult patients require radiography when a clinical evaluation results in concern for a cervical spine injury. The Canadian C-spine rule and the

National Emergency X-Radiography Utilization Study (NEXUS) have become the standard of care, resulting in a negative predictive value for fractures, 100% and 99.8%, respectively. Canadian C-spine rule requires (1) age <65 years, (2) no dangerous mechanism (such as fall from height of >3 ft, i.e., 90 cm, axial loading injury to the head, i.e., diving, motor vehicle high speed, i.e., >110 km/h, rollover, ejection, motorized recreational vehicles, bicycle struck or collision), (3) no paresthesias, (4) low-risk factor allowing safe assessment of range of motion (simple rear-end motor vehicle collision, sitting position in emergency department, ambulatory at any time, delayed onset of neck pain, absence of midline cervical spine tenderness), and (5) the ability for neck rotation of 45° left and right. Canadian C-Spine rule is not applicable in the presence of age <16 years, GCS <15, non-trauma cases, unstable vital signs, acute paralysis, known vertebral diseases, previous cervical spine surgery, and pregnancy. According to NEXUS criteria, cervical spine radiography is indicated for patients with neck trauma unless they meet all of the following criteria: no posterior midline cervical spine tenderness, no evidence of intoxication, a normal level of alertness, i.e., a GCS: 15, no focal neurologic deficit, no painful distracting injuries. Thus, on the other side, all the patients with a presumptive significant injury mechanism and meeting the Centers for Disease and Control and Prevention criteria from trauma team alert presenting at a Level I trauma center have to undergo CT [11]. The American College of Radiology currently recommends cervical spine CT for patients with positive findings at radiography.

Patients may be obtunded by trauma itself, as well as by analgesia or sedation, thus their neurological symptoms and signs may be masked. Notably, a Scottish population-based study demonstrated associated cervical spine injuries in ~5.3% of head injury patients [8], and about one-third of polytrauma patients have a closed head injury, a finding that increases the risk of cervical spine injury by 8.5% [9]. American College of Radiology recommends screening CT as the standard of care for initial screening of obtunded polytrauma patients. Higher diagnostic accuracy of CT clearly counterbalances the increased estimated lifetime cancer risk and monetary cost in both low- and high-risk patients of all ages [51]. Obtunded patients with negative findings at screening cervical spine CT may undergo early discontinuation of cervical spine precautions. Notably, despite the higher sensitivity of MRI for spinal and spinal cord lesions, evidence from both large studies and meta-analyses demonstrated that MRI also has a false-positive rate. Isolated signal abnormalities without bone injury or abnormal alignment are generally of uncertain importance although may result in unnecessary spinal immobilization. Few patients have positive MRI findings requiring a change in the management or develop evidence of delayed instability. The need for MRI is liberal and depends upon patient's clinical condition [9, 11, 28].

5.6.3 Absence of Diagnostic Imaging Alterations

The acronym SCIWORA, i.e., spinal cord injury without radiographic alterations, was first defined in children with signs of acute traumatic myelopathy in the absence of spinal column findings on radiography and/or CT, most probably related to traumatic cervical spine motion beyond the normal physiological range but not until the risk of fracture, and injury to the spinal cord by contusion or ischemia from temporary occlusion of vertebral arteries then returning to their original position. Availability of MRI showed that approximately two-thirds of patients with SCIWORA have demonstrable injury to the spinal cord, soft tissue components of the spinal column or vertebral body endplate, likely explaining a posttraumatic concussion syndrome. This results in the proposed acronyms of SCIWORET, SCIWOCTET, i.e., spinal cord injury without radiography or CT evidence of trauma. Notably, physicians and (neuro)radiologists involved in trauma patients have to know that patients with blunt trauma and transient neurologic symptoms, even if resolved at the time of initial evaluation and/or admission, may have injury to the spinal cord and/or spine, despite a normal physical examination and normal spine radiographs and/or CT, thus requiring MRI [10].

5.7 Diagnostic Imaging Findings

In this section, diagnostic imaging findings of spinal trauma will be discussed by site, i.e., craniocervical junction, subaxial cervical spine, thoracolumbar spine, and spinal cord and nerve roots.

5.7.1 Craniocervical Junction

Occipital condyle fractures should not be considered uncommon, occurring possibly in as many as 16% of patients with craniocervical injury [9, 22]. They should be suspected in all patients sustaining high-energy trauma to the head and/or neck involving components of either axial compression, lateral bending, axial rotation, or direct blow, regardless of the clinical condition and physical examination results. The great potential of these fractures for long-term morbidity due to pain and limited motion, serious neurologic deficits, or even death explains the need for an accurate diagnosis. According to Anderson and Montesano classification system [9, 22],

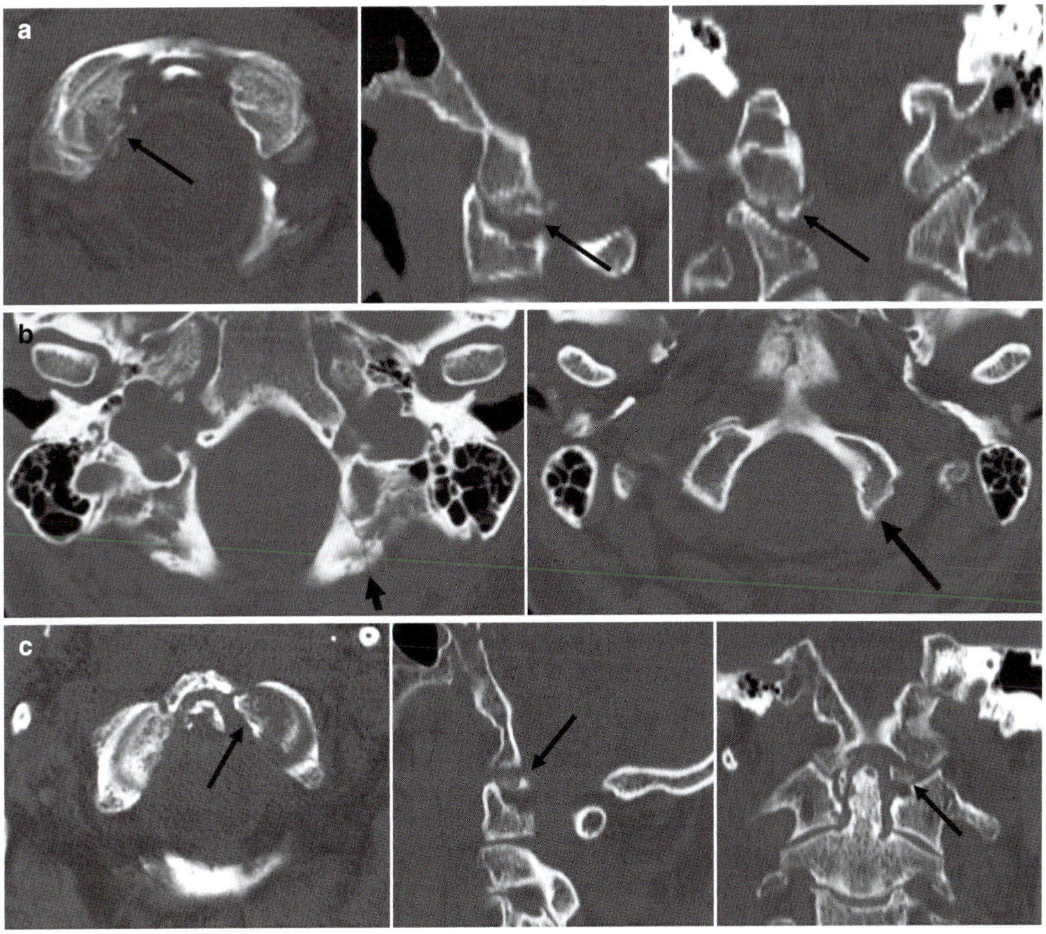

Fig. 5.22 Occipital condyle fractures types I (**a**), II (**b**), and III (**c**): source axial and 2D-reformatted sagittal and coronal (**a, c**) and nonconsecutive source axial (**b**) CT images. *Black arrows* indicate the fracture lines

occipital condyle fractures are classified into types I, II, and III. Type I (Figs. 5.17 and 5.22) is an impaction-type fracture resulting in a comminution of the occipital condyle, with or without minimal fragment displacement, most likely resulting from axial loading of the skull onto the atlas, similar to a Jefferson fracture of the atlas, with or without lateral bending. It is considered stable since the tectorial membrane and contralateral alar ligament are intact; however, bilateral lesions may be unstable. Type II (Figs. 5.17 and 5.22) is part of a more extensive basioccipital fracture, involving one or both occipital condyles, resulting from direct blow to the skull. An intact tectorial membrane and alar ligaments preserve stability. Type III (Figs. 5.17 and 5.22) is an avulsion type of fracture near the alar ligament resulting in medial fragment displacement from the inferomedial aspect of the occipital condyle into the foramen magnum. The mechanism of injury is forced rotation, usually combined with lateral bending. Contralateral alar ligament and tectorial membrane may be stressed and "loaded", resulting in a partial tear or complete disruption. Thus, type III is considered a potentially unstable injury.

Atlas fractures include type I involving posterior arches (considered stable), type II involving the anterior arch (considered stable) (Fig. 5.17), type III including bilateral posterior arch with bilateral or single unilateral anterior arch (i.e., the classic "Jefferson burst" fracture, whose stability depends on the integrity of transverse ligament), type IV involving a lateral mass (considered stable), and type V which is transversely oriented through the anterior arch from avulsion of longus colli muscle or atlantoaxial ligament (considered stable), according to the classification system of Jefferson modified by Gehweiler et al. [9]. The typical Jefferson burst fracture of the atlas results from an axial loading force transmitted from the top of the skull, through the occipital condyles, to the lateral masses of the atlas, which will be displaced laterally. The classic form consists of the fracture of all four vertebral atlas emiarches (Fig. 5.23). Transverse ligament of the atlas may remain intact or be damaged partially or completely; the complete injury can cause an anterior or lateral atloaxial dislocation. Fracture of the anterior vertebral emiarches may result in an increase in thickness of the prevertebral soft tissue due to hematoma and lesion of the anterior longitudinal ligament. Isolated fractures of posterior arch including laminar fractures, and avulsion fracture of the anterior arch result from distraction injury mechanism.

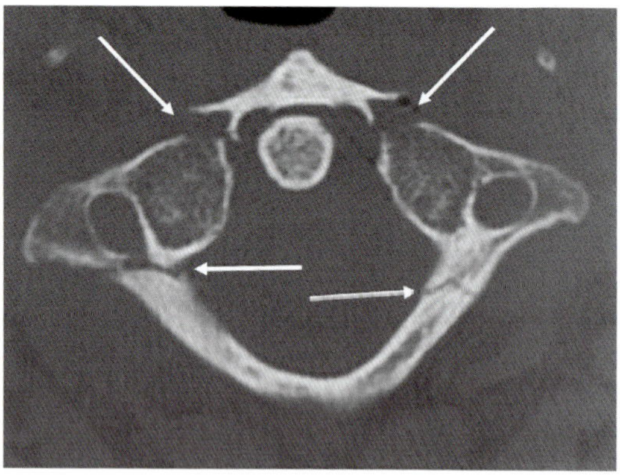

Fig. 5.23 Typical Jefferson fracture of the atlas: source axial CT image. *Arrows* indicate four line fractures of both anterior and posterior arches

Axis fractures include fractures of the odontoid process, the so-called hangman fracture, and teardrop fracture of the body.

Fractures of the odontoid process (Fig. 5.24) may result from multiple injury mechanism, including hyperflexion, hyperextension, and lateral bending or combination of these forces. They can be comminuted, but typically consist of a simple fracture with variable displacement of the cranial fragment, whose dislocation extent is correlated with nonunion. The injury mechanism can be recognized depending on localization, front or posterior, of the cranial fragment. They are, in most cases, isolated but may be associated with other fractures, such as the fracture of atlas posterior arch or C2 traumatic spondylolisthesis and the teardrop fracture by hypertension. Depending on fracture location, they have been classified into types I (through the dens apex from alar ligament avulsion), II (through the dens-base junction), and III (fracture involving C2 vertebral body), according to Anderson and D'Alonzo classification system [9]. However, it has been demonstrated that type I is rare and

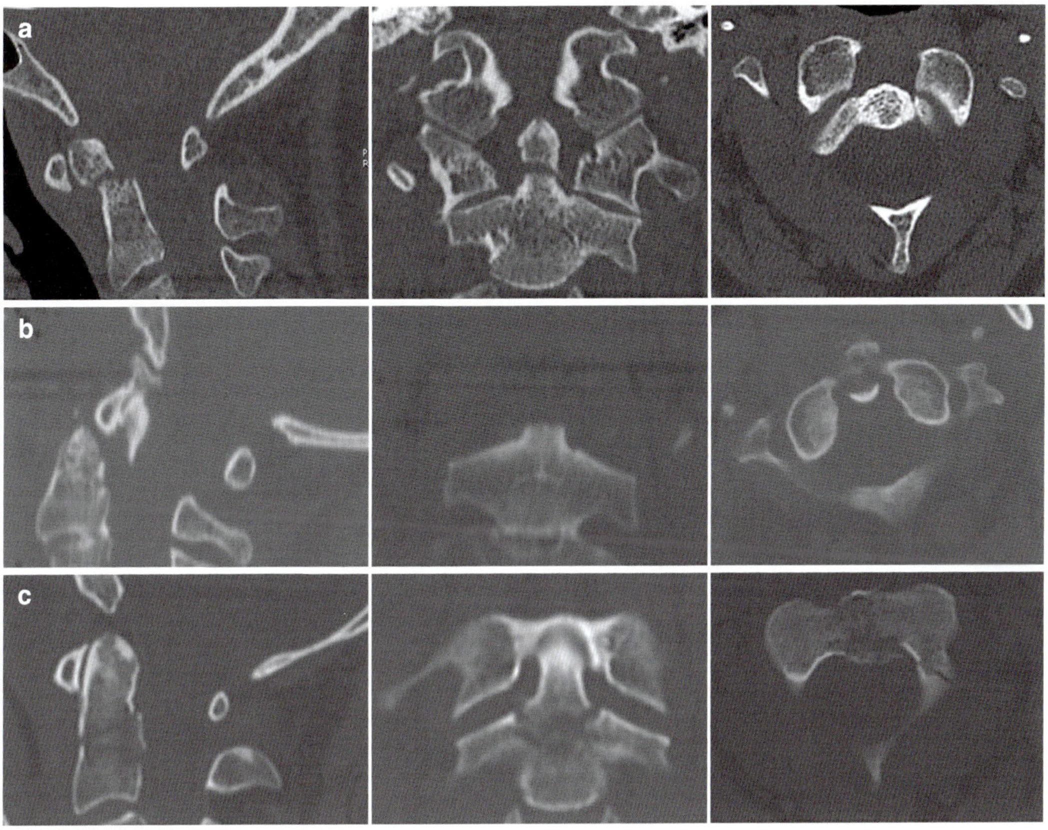

Fig. 5.24 Fractures of the odontoid process: 2D-reformatted sagittal and coronal, and source axial CT images of flexion (**a**) and extension (**b**) "high," and "low" (**c**) fractures

doesn't deserve a specific designation. Therefore, it has been proposed to classify odontoid fractures in "high", corresponding to types I and II, and "low", corresponding to type III (Fig. 5.24). In the "high" fractures, the involved dens portion is essentially represented by poorly vascularized cortical bone: thus, nonunion is very frequent, reaching most 100% if the posterior displacement of the cranial fragment is >0.5 cm. Dens apex avulsion is generally stable. Fracture at the dens-base junction may lead to atlantoaxial instability since the fragment and the atlas constitute a single unit. In the "low" fractures, the rim fracture extends to the cranial portion of C2 body, i.e., predominantly well-vascularized spongy bone; thus, the fracture consolidates in the vast majority of cases. Nevertheless, even the "low" fractures are considered mechanically unstable because dens, atlas, and occiput move as a single unit. Obviously, fractures' fragments may compromise spinal canal.

"Hangman" fracture of the axis is a bilateral fracture involving the thin portion of articular process located between the upper and lower facet joints, i.e., the interarticularis isthmus of axis. Many authors prefer the definition of traumatic spondylolisthesis. Most commonly this occur during a car crash, especially with no seat belt, when the chin can slam against the steering wheel, dashboard, or windshield, causing hyperextension, such as in hanging. Neurological deficits occur in <30% of patients because of the favorable ratio between the volume occupied by the spinal cord and the width of central spinal canal at C2 level. These fractures are classified into type I or hairline fracture (where extension is followed by compression, resulting in anterior displacement of C2 over C3 <2 mm, without angulation between opposed vertebral endplates of C2 and C3, considered stable), types II and IIa (where extension and axial compression are followed by hyperflexion and/or distraction, resulting in anterior displacement of C2 on C3 >2 mm and angulation between the opposite endplates of C2 and C3 >11°, or severe angulation without displacement, respectively; type II and IIa are considered variably stable), and type III (where extension is followed by flexion distraction injury mechanism resulting in uni- or bilateral interfacetal dislocation, considered unstable), according to Effendi et al. classification system modified by Levine and Edwards [9].

The term atypical traumatic spondylolisthesis means a variant in which one of the two fractures (unilateral atypical) or both (bilateral atypical) affect the posterior margin of C2 vertebral body (Fig. 5.16); if the atypical fracture is bilateral, a posterior fragment of C2 body can migrate into the spinal canal and compress the spinal cord.

"Teardrop" fracture of the body of the axis is the most frequent, and located along the lower front edge of the vertebral body, generally affecting the elderly patients with osteopenia or degenerative disease of the spine. A small somatic fragment results from hyperextension causing distraction of the anterior longitudinal ligament. This fracture is considered unstable in extension, since the anterior longitudinal ligament is detached from C2 body, but stable in flexion for the integrity of facet joints and discoligamentous complex, unless other lesions are associated.

Occipitocervical dissociation, including occipitoatlantal and atlantoaxial dissociation (Fig. 5.25), and *atlantoaxial rotational dissociation* may also affect craniocervical junction.

Occipitocervical dissociation may be incomplete (subluxation) or complete (dislocation). The traumatic energy, which exceeds the physiological tolerance of the ligaments that extend between occiput and atlas, and between occiput and axis, involves first of all the destruction of the ligamentous structures (Fig. 5.24). Occipitoatlantal dissociation is generally a fatal injury easily recognizable with only lateral radiographs of the cervical spine. Subluxation is less common, difficult to recognize with radiography and generally without neurological deficits. Powers ratio (Fig. 5.6) is a measurement of the relationship of the foramen magnum to the atlas, used in the diagnosis of occipitoatlantal dissociation. Normal values are <1 at radiography and <0.9 at CT. A ratio >1 leads to the suspect of the anterior occipitoatlantal dissociation. Because of technical limitations of radiography, including magnification, measurements would be made by multidetector CT [40] (Fig. 5.25).

Atlantoaxial rotational dissociation, i.e., subluxation and dislocation, is a rare lesion, with no clear mechanism of injury, from a traumatic event resulting in incomplete (subluxation) or full (dislocation) destruction of lateral atlantoaxial joints. The rotation of the atlas around the dens significantly reduces the space between the anterior arch of the atlas and the dens and causes the dislocation of the atlas joint masses ahead (on one side) and back (the other side) compared to dens and articular masses of axis. Atlantoaxial rotational dissociation include types I (rotatory fixation in normal physiologic range, <48°–52° left or right, where dens acts as a pivot, alar and transverse ligaments are intact, and is variably stable), II (where transverse ligament is injured, the center of rotation shifts to a lateral mass, and atlas is anteriorly displaced <5 mm, considered unstable), III (where transverse and alar ligaments are injured, similar to type II but at last is anteriorly displaced >5 mm, considered unstable), IV (where odontoid process is injured, with atlas posteriorly displaced, considered unstable), according to Fielding and Hawkins classification system [9]. A possible atlantoaxial rotational subluxation remains a difficult differential diagnosis, i.e., a simple functional condition rather than the clear-cut result of an anatomical damage.

The distance between the anterior arch of the atlas and the dens (normal value <3 mm in adults and <7 mm in children who show physiological ligamentous laxity) increases in anterior atlantoaxial subluxation with anatomical and/or func-

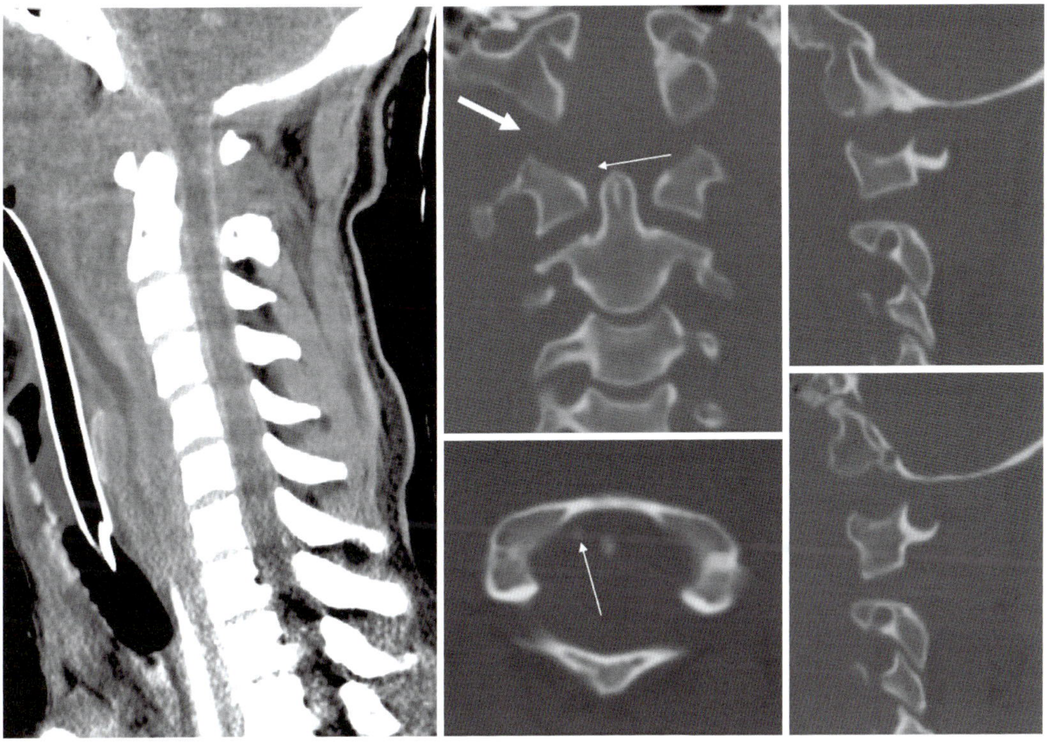

Fig. 5.25 Occipitoatlantal and atlantoaxial dissociations: 2D-reformatted midsagittal and coronal, source axial, and 2D-reformatted right and left sagittal CT images. Occipitoatlantal (*thick arrow*) is greatly more severe than atlantoaxial dislocation. Note the massive prevertebral hematoma and the intraspinale peridural hemorrhagic collection. Note also a tiny avulsion bone fragment (*thin arrow*) from the anterior arch of the atlas, indicating tear of the transverse ligament of the atlas

tional damage of the transverse ligament of the atlas.

A cranial displacement >2 mm of the apex of the dens compared to the line of McGregor is expression of a vertical atlantoaxial subluxation. Lateral dislocation >7 mm of one or both of the lateral masses of the atlas with respect to the underlying body of axis is the expression of a lateral subluxation due to complete damage of the transverse ligament of the atlas.

5.7.2 Subaxial Cervical Spine

In the subaxial cervical spine, the most severe lesional mechanism is the translation/rotation, followed by distraction, burst fracture, and compression. Translation and/or rotation is generally associated with distraction mechanisms in hyperflexion or in hyperextension.

Translation/rotation fractures may be associated with hyperflexion (interfacetal unilateral and bilateral dislocation, fracture-dislocation) or hyperextension (pedicle-laminar fracture).

Bilateral interfacetal dislocation presents typical findings of the lesion of the posterior ligamentous complex, the intervertebral disc, and often the anterior longitudinal ligament, with dislocation of the vertebral inferior articular processes that goes over the upper articular processes of the vertebra below, going to be wedged in the underlying root canals. Bilateral interfacetal dislocation often results in spinal cord injury and is always highly unstable because of widespread ligamentous damage (Figs. 5.3 and 5.5). It is the only cervical traumatic injury that may result in anterior displacement of the vertebral body more than half of anteroposterior diameter of the underlying soma.

Fracture-dislocation is an injury where a rotational force vector that involves the dislocation of an interapophyseal joint, while the contralateral acts as a fulcrum. From the side of the dislocation, the inferior articular process spinal goes over the superior one of the underlying vertebra and goes to wedge itself into the root canal below. The latter finding, in the absence of fractures of the articular processes, causes the "blocking" of the vertebra and allows the lesion to be mechanically stable, even in the presence of a lesion of the posterior ligamentous complex. In general, however, it is not a pure dislocation, but a fracture-dislocation (fracture of an articular process) resulting in loss of structural bone integrity and, therefore, instability. The vertebral body is not only rotated to the right or left, it is also displaced forward, but this location never goes beyond the half of the vertebra below. Furthermore, since a mechanism of hyperflexion is also present, the interspinous distance will increase for the destruction of the posterior ligamentous complex.

Pedicle-laminar fractures consist of the fracture of the pedicle and ipsilateral lamina, from a prevalent hyperextension injury mechanism followed by rotation. The corresponding joint mass becomes a free fragment. Three types are unilateral and characterized by an increasing degree of rotation of the articular mass and, therefore, of instability. A fourth type is bilateral, characterized by interfacetal dislocation from the side of the pedicle-laminar fracture and by the fracture of the contralateral articular mass, and unstable. The practical importance of recognizing the lesional mechanism as hyperextension, i.e., not considering these fractures as by hyperflexion, is that immobilization in extension or traction reproduce the mechanism of injury. Anterior translation of a vertebral body associated with pedicle-laminar fracture, the rotation, and the possible comminuted fracture of a joint mass should suggest a fracture by hyperextension-rotation.

Distraction injuries (Fig. 5.2) include "clay shoveler's," and "teardrop" fracture, both in hyperflexion.

"Clay shoveler's fracture" or "of diggers" owes its name to the fact that has been observed for the first time in coal miners. It represents an avulsion fracture of the spinous process of C7, C6 (Fig. 5.3), and T1, in decreasing order of incidence. It is the result of an abrupt flexion of the head and neck that causes, after the stretching of the posterior ligamentous complex, the fracture of the proximal portion of the spinous process. It is typically considered stable, but may be associated with more complex fractures, and possibly require CT and/or MRI (Fig. 5.3).

"Teardrop" fracture by hyperflexion (Fig. 5.11) is the most destructive cervical fracture among those compatible with life. The high traumatic energy in flexion involves the separation of a bone fragment along the anterior-inferior margin of the vertebral body and the intracanal migration of the remaining body with lesion of the anterior longitudinal ligament, the posterior one, and intervertebral disc. In addition, the traumatic energy acting on the posterior column may result in injury of the posterior ligamentous complex (increased interspinous distance in the lateral radiographs or in 2D-reformatted sagittal CT images), complete or incomplete uni- or bilateral interfacetal subluxation or dislocation. Teardrop fracture by hyperflexion, therefore, is a highly unstable lesion.

Furthermore, distraction injury mechanism by hyperflexion may result in a highly destructive potential and bad neurological prognosis, despite associated only with minor fractures of the articular masses (Fig. 5.10) or resulting in isolated discal, joints, and ligamentous injury (Fig. 5.14).

Axial loading fractures show the characteristic finding of a comminuted fracture of the vertebral body, with the cervical spine that appears more straight or in extension. Therefore, it lacks the attitude of the cervical spine in flexion seen in the "teardrop" fractures by hyperflexion, and there are no signs of posterior distraction such as increasing of the interspinous distance. Because of the consequent pressure increase, "burst" with more or less significant migration of the fragments occurs. Somatic posterior fragment then migrates into the central spinal canal, causing a more or less significant compression of the ventral surface of the spinal cord.

5.7.3 Thoracolumbar Spine

In the thoracolumbar spine, the most serious mechanism of injury is distraction, followed by translation/rotation and axial loading (simple, with lateral angulation >15° and burst).

Distraction fractures are more often in flexion. More frequently, they result from a car accident where a passenger with a seat belt is pushed forward by the force of the trauma, by hyperflexion with rotation center in the anterior abdominal wall. Generally, the posterior and medium columns of Denis suffer a huge distraction, while the anterior column is compressed. This may result in the involvement of single vertebra, or bone-ligament involvement of many. In the so-called Chance fracture, the fracture line, with horizontal course, goes through the spinous process, the laminae and the pedicles up to the posterior third of the vertebral body; for its horizontal course, the fracture line might not be seen in the axial CT images and thus requires attention to 2D-reformatted multiplanar and 3D-reconstructed images (Fig. 5.9). When the injury is also ligamentous, destruction of interspinous and supraspinous ligaments, dislocation of interfacetal joints, and destruction of the posterior longitudinal ligament are evident.

The less frequent fractures in extension generally occur in ankylosing spondylitis (Fig. 5.20).

Translation and/or rotation fractures are characterized by the dislocation of a vertebral body compared to the adjacent one in the axial plane. They can lead to a severe damage of the spinal cord. Fractures/dislocations by multiple mechanisms generally involve all three columns of Denis and, therefore, are highly unstable (Figs. 5.8, 5.18, and 5.21).

Axial loading fractures represent almost 50% of all thoracolumbar fractures. They are the consequence of a predominant axial force, possibly associated with hyperflexion, with the traumatic energy that spreads along the spine. In compression fracture, the involvement of the only anterior column of Denis results in a "wedge" morphology with a posterior base, resulting in a stable fracture (Fig. 5.1a). Burst fractures result from a higher traumatic energy, with involvement of the middle columns or of all three columns of Denis. Therefore, they are generally unstable and characterized by migration of vertebral fragments (Figs. 5.1b and 5.17). Associated more or less severe neurological deficits are frequent.

5.7.4 Discs, Joints, and Ligaments of the Subaxial Cervical Spine and Thoracolumbar Spine

The following signs have been proposed for subaxial cervical spine and thoracolumbar spine posttraumatic instability resulting from joints and ligamentous injury [4, 23, 24, 40, 41, 56, 58, 59]:

- Anterior, posterior, or lateral luxation, or dislocation greater than 2 mm by all or a major portion of a vertebra (displacement).
- An increase in the distance between the laminae or spinous processes greater than 2 mm at contiguous levels (wide interlaminar or interspinous space).
- An increase in width, malalignment, or loss of contact between contiguous facets, i.e., overlapping <50% or diastasis >2 mm of joint space (wide facet joints).
- Any fracture, rotation, displacement, angulation, or absence of the posterior margin of the vertebral body (disrupted posterior vertebral body line).
- An increase in the interpedicular distance of more than 2 mm at contiguous levels (wide vertebral canal).
- Kyphotic deformity resulting in angular displacements >11° between adjacent vertebrae, as measured by Cobb angle (the angulation or sagittal rotation criterion).
- Thickening of cervical spine prevertebral soft tissues. In adulthood, upper limits are 8.5 mm at C1, 6 mm at C2, 7 mm at C3, 18 mm at C6, and 18 mm at C7 levels [41]. In childhood, upper limits in patients 0–2 years old, 3–6 years old, 7–10 years old, and 11–15 years old at C2 and C6 levels are 7.6, 8.4, 6.8, and 6.8 mm, and 9.0, 9.8, 12.1, and 14.5, respectively; for all age groups the highest variability is at C3 and C4 [56].

MRI has the ability to directly identify the disc, joints, and ligamentous structures and the possibility to demonstrate ligaments interruptions/tears or edema/hematoma, by the correct integration of T1- and fat-suppressed T2-weighted, and STIR images. The finding may be of certain integrity or interruption (Figs. 5.9, 5.10, 5.11, 5.17, and 5.18), but may remain "undetermined," and surgical exploration remains the standard reference. Whether suspected or indeterminate injuries can still result in progressive instability is still a matter of discussion and debate about the adjuvant role of MRI; nevertheless, MRI seems to facilitate the most appropriate therapeutic choice.

5.7.5 Spinal Cord and Nerve Root Injuries

The main advantage of MRI is to allow direct identification of the spinal cord injuries [12, 15, 31, 39, 47] which Ramon et al. [39] have classified into the following six patterns:

- 0: normal findings at MRI.
- I: hemorrhage, or hematomyelia. It appears as an area of low signal intensity on T2- or T2*-weighted images, however as an isolated pattern is a rare occurrence. More often, it presents in the context of a contusion, which then appears more inhomogeneous for areas of low T2 and T2* signal intensity (Figs. 5.10 and 5.18). Then, lesion evolution is characterized by the classical evolution of hemoglobin metabolites. Hematomyelia constitutes a negative prognostic factor due to the cascade of biochemical events induced by micro-hemorrhages in the gray matter. Notably, a bleeding larger than 10 mm is generally correlated with complete neurological damage, with little chance of recovery.
- II: edema, which appears as an area of substantially homogeneous variable high signal intensity on T2-weighted images for intracellular and interstitial edema (Fig. 5.8), with possible spinal cord bulge.
- III: contusion, which appears as mixed central signal on T2-weighted images with peripheral high signal intensity; hematomyelia may be associated (Figs. 5.10 and 5.18).
- IV: compression, which appears as a less or more obliteration of the subarachoid space surrounding the spinal cord, and a variable alteration of its morphology (Figs. 5.8, 5.10, and 5.18), possibly preventing detection of signal alterations including hematomyelia; the percentage of spinal canal compromise may be calculated by the following formula: $(1-x/y) \times 100$ where x = spinal canal midsagittal diameter at the injury level, and y = mean midsagittal diameter of the spinal canal one segment above and one segment below the injury level [32].
- V: transection or laceration, which appears as a partial or complete discontinuity of the spinal cord in the sagittal images (Fig. 5.5), obviously resulting in deterioration of the prognosis.

The central portion (gray matter) of the spinal cord is the most common site of the lesions, i.e., patterns I, II, and III. The level is generally the point of greater mechanical impact; signal alteration extent correlates with the degree of initial neurological deficit.

The primary lesion determined directly from the trauma is followed by minor alterations to a cascade of biochemical events, worsened by hematomyelia, leading to neurolysis with propagation of the damage in cranio-caudal direction and the surrounding white matter.

Nerve root avulsions and pseudomeningoceles may be seen by high-resolution 3D "myelographic" sequences.

Additionally, MRI is the method of choice for intraspinal hematoma (Figs. 5.9 and 5.20), superior to CT, since it allows its detection and differential diagnosis, shows its location and extent, and the degree of spinal cord and cauda equina compression. However, in some cases MRI fails to show the exact location of hematoma, i.e., the subdural or epidural space, which may be disclosed only at surgery. This occurs more frequently in poor quality exam obtained with cervical collar or spinal longboard. Epidural hematoma generally results from a lesion of the venous plexus or epidural veins rather than epidural arteries; more frequently, it appears as an area with biconvex morphology with tapered cranial and caudal ends (Fig. 5.20). Anteriorly, it does not extend over the median line (i.e., the sign of the tent), due to the close adhesion of the dura to the posterior longitudinal ligament, while posteriorly can exceed the midline due to the absence of adhesion of the dura to the vertebral arch (Fig. 5.3). Subdural hematoma results from rupture of subarachnoid or subdural space veins: morphology is most often circular or semicircular rather than biconvex in the axial images, and linear in the sagittal ones (Fig. 5.20). Epidural hematoma pushes the dura within the spinal canal, while subdural hematoma is contained within the dura. Posttraumatic intraspinal subarachnoid hemorrhage is uncommon. The search for intraspinal hemorrhage justifies the use of T2*-weighted images in the MRI protocol for spinal trauma.

Normal spinal cord and spinal cord edema are generally associated with more favorable neurological outcome. Spinal cord contusion shows lesser neurological recovery, when compared to edema. Spinal cord hemorrhage, mean spinal canal compromise, mean spinal cord compression, and spinal cord lesion length are higher in patients presenting with ASIA A impairment scale injury and generally associated with the poorest prognostic value in spine injury.

Decreasing trends towards ASIA E impairment scale injury at admission and neurological recovery is generally associated with lower mean spinal canal compromise and spinal cord compression, and lesion length [26].

5.8 Extra-Spinal Findings

In polytrauma patients with spinal trauma, morbidity and mortality may result from extra-spinal clinically relevant injuries associated to the spinal ones. Despite the frequent concomitant evaluation by "whole body" CT including head, neck, thorax, abdomen, and pelvis, some findings may be overlooked. For instance, CT limited to the cervical spine may overlook lesions of only partially imaged skull and facial bones (such as pneumocephalus or air–fluid levels in the paranasal sinuses), prevertebral hematomas narrowing the aerodigestive tract, laryngeal cartilages fractures, foreign bodies within the airway, sternal fractures (which may be associated with clinically significant mediastinal hematomas), and rib fractures which may be the sign of an underlying pneumothorax or a factor risk for cerebrovascular injury [1, 3, 13, 19, 36, 49].

5.9 Outcomes and Complications

Radiography and CT are essential for evaluating the consolidation of bone fractures and spinal stability. MRI is the technique of choice to assess the results of the spinal cord damage. A few weeks after the trauma, spinal cord edema is reabsorbed, necrotic tissue and hemoglobin degradation products are removed by macrophages, with evolution in a glial reaction and possible subsequent residual cavitation. Notably, the final findings of spinal trauma are represented by gliosis, myelomalacia, spinal cord medullary cysts, syringomyelia, and/or medullary atrophy. Gliosis and myelomalacia show T2 high signal intensity and variable T1 low signal intensity (greater in myelomalacia), with poorly defined margins and irregular shape, possibly associated with atrophy. Myelomalacia is more frequent in the cervical spine and can extend up to four metamers. Spinal cord cyst and syringomyelia are the results of the coalescence of microcysts in a tissue with myelomalacia. The cysts are formed generally in the point of maximum compression at the time of the trauma; they have round or oval shape, with a maximum diameter less than 2 cm. They are well demarcated of comparable signal to that of the cerebrospinal fluid; it is possible that the wall is made of glial cells. Pathogenesis of syringomyelia is still not well known although it seems to be correlated with hematomyelia in acute phase. Subsequent colliquative necrosis would form a cavity also for the CSF and/or interstitial fluid inflow from the ependymal central canal or from the CSF perimedullary spaces through the interstitial perivascular spaces of Virchow-Robin. According to another hypothesis, even syringomyelia is derived from the coalescence of microcysts. The cyst is stable over time, while the syringomyelia is generally a condition in evolution (both at MRI and clinically). In some cases, the progression of syringomyelia, with increased swelling, occurs many years after the trauma and determines a late worsening especially of pain and spasticity. The spinal cord atrophy occurs with reduction of the diameters of the involved cord, and increased perimedullary CSF space. Other possible outcomes include subarachnoid adhesions—which can cause attraction and fixation of the spinal cord—and arachnoid cysts, usually single, most often in the dorsal spine, which can lead to spinal cord compression.

Conclusions

Images and information provided by modern diagnostic imaging allows the (neuro)radiologist an overall assessment of spinal content and spinal containing. The anatomical and functional complexity requires proper "readiness" in dealing with spinal trauma.

(Neuro)radiologist should use the key components of the SLICS and TLICS and AOS to analyze, evaluate, and report osseous, discal, joint, and ligamentous lesions, as well as the mechanism of injury. Following the algorithm proposed by AOS classification systems, the first step for a morphologic classification should be the search for displacement or dislocation which indicates a translation/rotational injury mechanism. In the absence of translation/rotation injury, the second step should be the search for discoligamentous complex injury in the subaxial cervical spine and posterior tension band injury in the thoracolumbar spine which both indicate a distraction injury mechanism. In the absence of translation/rotation and distraction injury mechanisms, the third step is to evaluate and characterize vertebral body and arches fractures in order to characterize the axial loading injury mechanism.

Radiography and, above all, CT provide the great majority of the information useful for this purpose. MRI can provide additional data on the state of the discoligamentous and capsular structures, thus being able to contribute to better definition of the stability of the spine. Of course, MRI is mandatory in all the cases of neurological compromise or discrepancy between clinical and CT findings. The report must specify the type of bone, joints, ligamentous, spinal cord, and nerve root damage, for its prognostic implications. Best results come from the knowledge of anatomy, biomechanics, and clinical features, which only allow when and how to proceed to CT and/or MRI, of course according to the framework conditions in which the (neuro)radiologist operates.

Acknowledgements The authors thank Carolina Bongini, MD, Department of Medical, Surgical and Neurological Sciences, Section of Diagnostic Imaging, University of Siena, Siena, Italy, for her help in the preparation of the manuscript.

References

1. Bonatti M, Vezzali N, Ferro F, Manfredi R, Oberhofer N, Bonatti G. Blunt cerebrovascular injury: diagnosis at whole-body MDCT for multi-trauma. Insights Imaging. 2013;4:347–55.
2. Bracken MB, Freeman DH Jr, Hellenbrand K. Incidence of acute traumatic hospitalized spinal cord injury in the United States, 1970-1977. Am J Epidemiol. 1981;113:615–22.
3. Bromberg WJ, Collier BC, Diebel LN, Dwyer KM, Holevar MR, Jacobs DG, Kurek SJ, Schreiber MA, Shapiro ML, Vogel TR. Blunt cerebrovascular injury practice management guidelines: the Eastern Association for the Surgery of Trauma. J Trauma. 2010;68:471–7.
4. Daffner RH, Deeb ZL, Goldberg AL, Kandabarow A, Rothfus WE. The radiologic assessment of post-traumatic vertebral stability. Skelet Radiol. 1990;19:103–8.
5. Denis F. The three column spine and its significance in the classification of acute thoracolumbar spinal injuries. Spine. 1983;8:817–31.
6. Dosch JC, Moser T, Dupuis MG, Dietemann JL. [How to read radiography of the traumatic spine?]. J Radiol. 2007;88(5 Pt 2):802–16. French.
7. Dosch J, Moser T, Dietemann J. Imaging of acute spinal injury. J Radiol. 2010;91(9 Pt 2):998–1009.

8. Drainer EK, Graham CA, Munro PT. Blunt cervical spine injuries in Scotland 1995-2000. Injury. 2003;34:330–3.
9. Dreizin D, Letzing M, Sliker CW, Chokshi FH, Bodanapally U, Mirvis SE, Quencer RM, Munera F. Multidetector CT of blunt cervical spine trauma in adults. Radiographics. 2014;34:1842–65.
10. Dreizin D, Kim W, Kim JS, Boscak AR, Bodanapally UK, Munera F, Stein DM. Will the real SCIWORA please stand up? Exploring clinicoradiologic mismatch in closed spinal cord injuries. AJR Am J Roentgenol. 2015;05:853–60.
11. Duane TM, Young AJ, Vanguri P, Wolfe LG, Katzen J, Han J, Mayglothling J, Whelan JF, Aboutanos MB, Ivatury RR, Malhotra AK. Defining the cervical spine clearance algorithm: a single-institution prospective study of more than 9,000 patients. J Trauma Acute Care Surg. 2016;81:541–7.
12. Flanders AE, Schaefer DM, Doan HT, Mishkin MM, Gonzalez CF, Northrup BE. Acute cervical spine trauma: correlation of MR imaging findings with degree of neurologic deficit. Radiology. 1990;177:25–33.
13. Geddes AE, Burlew CC, Wagenaar AE, Biffl WL, Johnson JL, Pieracci FM, Campion EM, Moore EE. Expanded screening criteria for blunt cerebrovascular injury: a bigger impact than anticipated. Am J Surg. 2016;212:1167–74.
14. Goldberg W, Mueller C, Panacek E, Tigges S, Hoffman JR, Mower WR. Distribution and patterns of blunt traumatic cervical spine injury. Ann Emerg Med. 2001;38:17–21.
15. Gupta R, Mittal P, Sandhu P, Saggar K, Gupta K. Correlation of qualitative and quantitative MRI parameters with neurological status: a prospective study on patients with spinal trauma. J Clin Diagn Res. 2014;8:RC13–7.
16. Haba H, Taneichi H, Kotani Y, Terae S, Abe S, Yoshikawa H, Abumi K, Minami A, Kaneda K. Diagnostic accuracy of magnetic resonance imaging for detecting posterior ligamentous complex injury associated with thoracic and lumbar fractures. J Neurosurg. 2003;99(1 Suppl):20–6.
17. Holdsworth F. Fractures, dislocations, and fracture dislocations of the spine. J Bone Joint Surg Am. 1970;52:1534–51.
18. Jones C, Jazayeri F. Evolving standards of practice for cervical spine imaging in trauma: a retrospective review. Australas Radiol. 2007;51:420–42.
19. Khoo JN, Chong le R, Chan EH, Poh AC. Pitfalls in multidetector computed tomography imaging of traumatic spinal injuries. Emerg Radiol. 2011;18:551–62.
20. Khurana B, Sheehan SE, Sodickson A, Bono CM, Harris MB. Traumatic thoracolumbar spine injuries: what the spine surgeon wants to know. Radiographics. 2013;33:2031–46.
21. Lasfargues JE, Custis D, Morrone F, Carswell J, Nguyen T. A model for estimating spinal cord injury prevalence in the United States. Paraplegia. 1995;33:62–8.
22. Leone A, Cerase A, Colosimo C, Lauro L, Puca A, Marano P. Occipital condylar fractures: a review. Radiology. 2000;216:635–44.
23. Leone A, Guglielmi G, Cassar-Pullicino VN, Bonomo L. Lumbar intervertebral instability: a review. Radiology. 2007;245:62–77.
24. Leone A, Arrigucci U, Cerase A. Patologia traumatica vertebromidollare. In: Colosimo C, editor. Neuroradiologia. I Edizione. Milano: LSWR; 2013. p. 281–96.
25. Magerl F, Aebi M, Gertzbein SD, Harms J, Nazarian S. A comprehensive classification of thoracic and lumbar injuries. Eur Spine J. 1994;3:184–201.
26. Magu S, Singh D, Yadav RK, Bala M. Evaluation of traumatic spine by magnetic resonance imaging and correlation with neurological recovery. Asian Spine J. 2015;9:748–56.
27. Martin BW, Dykes E, Lecky FE. Patterns and risks in spinal trauma. Arch Dis Child. 2004;89:860–5.
28. Mascarenhas D, Dreizin D, Bodanapally UK, Stein DM. Parsing the utility of CT and MRI in the subaxial cervical spine injury classification (SLIC) System: is CT SLIC enough? AJR Am J Roentgenol. 2016;206:1292–7.
29. McAfee PC, Yuan HA, Fredrickson BE, Lubicky JP. The value of computed tomography in thoracolumbar fractures: an analysis of one hundred consecutive cases and a new classification. J Bone Joint Surg Am. 1983;65:461–73.
30. McCulloch PT, France J, Jones DL, Krantz W, Nguyen TP, Chambers C, Dorchak J, Mucha P. Helical computed tomography alone compared with plain radiographs with adjunct computed tomography to evaluate the cervical spine after high-energy trauma. J Bone Joint Surg Am. 2005;87:2388–94.
31. Miyanji F, Furlan JC, Aarabi B, Arnold PM, Fehlings MG. Acute cervical traumatic spinal cord injury: MR imaging findings correlated with neurologic outcome-prospective study with 100 consecutive patients. Radiology. 2007;243:820–7.
32. Mohanty SP, Bhat NS, Abraham R, Ishwara Keerthi C. Neurological deficit and canal compromise in thoracolumbar and lumbar burst fractures. J Orthop Surg (Hong Kong). 2008;16:20–3.
33. Moore TA, Vaccaro AR, Anderson PA. Classification of lower cervical spine injuries. Spine (Phila Pa 1976). 2006;31(11 Suppl):S37–43; discussion S61.
34. Nuñez DB Jr, Ahmad AA, Coin CG, LeBlang S, Becerra JL, Henry R, Lentz K, Quencer RM. Clearing the cervical spine in multiple trauma victims: a time effective protocol using helical computed tomography. Emerg Radiol. 1994;1:273–8.
35. Oliver M, Inaba K, Tang A, Branco BC, Barmparas G, Schnüriger B, Lustenberger T, Demetriades D. The changing epidemiology of spinal trauma: a 13-year review from a Level I trauma centre. Injury. 2012;43:1296–300.
36. Paulus EM, Fabian TC, Savage SA, Zarzaur BL, Botta V, Dutton W, Croce MA. Blunt cerebrovascular injury screening with 64-channel multidetector com-

puted tomography: more slices finally cut it. J Trauma Acute Care Surg. 2014;76:279–83; discussion 284–5.
37. Pickett GE, Campos-Benitez M, Keller JL, Duggal N. Epidemiology of traumatic spinal cord injury in Canada. Spine (Phila Pa 1976). 2006;31:799–805.
38. Pirouzmand F. Epidemiological trends of spine and spinal cord injuries in the largest Canadian adult trauma center from 1986 to 2006. J Neurosurg Spine. 2010;12:131–40.
39. Ramon S, Dominguez R, Ramirez L, Paraira M, Olona M, Castello T, Garcia Fernandez L. Clinical and magnetic resonance imaging correlation in acute spinal cord injury. Spinal Cord. 1997;35:664–73.
40. Rojas CA, Bertozzi JC, Martinez CR, Whitlow J. Reassessment of the craniocervical junction: normal values on CT. AJNR Am J Neuroradiol. 2007;28:1819–23.
41. Rojas CA, Vermess D, Bertozzi JC, Whitlow J, Guidi C, Martinez CR. Normal thickness and appearance of the prevertebral soft tissues on multidetector CT. AJNR Am J Neuroradiol. 2009;30:136–41.
42. Ruiz Santiago F, Tomás Muñoz P, Moya Sánchez E, Revelles Paniza M, Martínez Martínez A, Pérez Abela AL. Classifying thoracolumbar fractures: role of quantitative imaging. Quant Imaging Med Surg. 2016;6:772–84.
43. Sakellariou VI, Badilas NK, Mazis GA, Stavropoulos NA, Kotoulas HK, Kyriakopoulos S, Tagkalegkas I, Sofianos IP. Brachial plexus injuries in adults: evaluation and diagnostic approach. ISRN Orthop. 2014;2014:1–9. doi:10.1155/2014/726103.
44. Schenarts PJ, Diaz J, Kaiser C, Carrillo Y, Eddy V, Morris JA Jr. Prospective comparison of admission computed tomographic scan and plain films of the upper cervical spine in trauma patients with altered mental status. J Trauma. 2001;51:663–8; discussion 668–9.
45. Seçer M, Alagöz F, Uçkun O, Karakoyun OD, Ulutaş MÖ, Polat Ö, Dağlıoğlu E, Dalgıç A, Belen D. Multilevel noncontiguous spinal fractures: surgical approach towards clinical characteristics. Asian Spine J. 2015;9:889–94.
46. Sethi MK, Schoenfeld AJ, Bono CM, Harris MB. The evolution of thoracolumbar injury classification systems. Spine J. 2009;9:780–8.
47. Shimada K, Tokioka T. Sequential MR studies of cervical cord injury: correlation with neurological damage and clinical outcome. Spinal Cord. 1999;37:410–5.
48. Singh R, Kumar RR, Setia N, Magu S. A prospective study of neurological outcome in relation to findings of imaging modalities in acute spinal cord injury. Asian J Neurosurg. 2015;10:181–9.
49. Sliker CW. Blunt cerebrovascular injuries: imaging with multidetector CT angiography. Radiographics. 2008;28:1689–708; discussion 1709–10.
50. Smart PJ, Hardy PJ, Buckley DM, Somers JM, Broderick NJ, Halliday KE, Williams L. Cervical spine injuries to children under 11: should we use radiography more selectively in their initial assessment? Emerg Med J. 2003;20:225–7.
51. Theocharopoulos NC, Chatzakis G, Damilakis J. Is radiography justified for the evaluation of patients presenting with cervical spine trauma? Med Phys. 2009;36:4461–70.
52. Vaccaro AR, Lehman RA Jr, Hurlbert RJ, Anderson PA, Harris M, Hedlund R, Harrop J, Dvorak M, Wood K, Fehlings MG, Fisher C, Zeiller SC, Anderson DG, Bono CM, Stock GH, Brown AK, Kuklo T, Oner FC. A new classification of thoracolumbar injuries: the importance of injury morphology, the integrity of the posterior ligamentous complex, and neurologic status. Spine (Phila Pa 1976). 2005;30:2325–33.
53. Vaccaro AR, Hulbert RJ, Patel AA, Fisher C, Dvorak M, Lehman RA Jr, Anderson P, Harrop J, Oner FC, Arnold P, Fehlings M, Hedlund R, Madrazo I, Rechtine G, Aarabi B, Shainline M, Spine Trauma Study Group. The subaxial cervical spine injury classification system: a novel approach to recognize the importance of morphology, neurology, and integrity of the disco-ligamentous complex. Spine (Phila Pa 1976). 2007;32:2365–74.
54. Vaccaro AR, Oner C, Kepler CK, Dvorak M, Schnake K, Bellabarba C, Reinhold M, Aarabi B, Kandziora F, Chapman J, Shanmuganathan R, Fehlings M, Vialle L, AOSpine Spinal Cord Injury & Trauma Knowledge Forum. AOSpine thoracolumbar spine injury classification system: fracture description, neurological status, and key modifiers. Spine (Phila Pa 1976). 2013;38:2028–37.
55. Vaccaro AR, Koerner JD, Radcliff KE, Oner FC, Reinhold M, Schnake KJ, Kandziora F, Fehlings MG, Dvorak MF, Aarabi B, Rajasekaran S, Schroeder GD, Kepler CK, Vialle LR. AOSpine subaxial cervical spine injury classification system. Eur Spine J. 2016;25:2173–84.
56. Vermess D, Rojas CA, Shaheen F, Roy P, Martinez CR. Normal pediatric prevertebral soft-tissue thickness on MDCT. AJR Am J Roentgenol. 2012;199: W130–3.
57. Wang H, Zhang Y, Xiang Q, Wang X, Li C, Xiong H, Zhou Y. Epidemiology of traumatic spinal fractures: experience from medical university-affiliated hospitals in Chongqing, China, 2001-2010. J Neurosurg Spine. 2012;17:459–68.
58. White AA 3rd, Panjabi MM. The clinical biomechanics of the occipitoatlantoaxial complex. Orthop Clin North Am. 1978;9:867–78.
59. White AA 3rd, Panjabi MM. The basic kinematics of the human spine. A review of past and current knowledge. Spine (Phila Pa 1976). 1978;3:12–20.
60. Yoshikawa T, Hayashi N, Yamamoto S, Tajiri Y, Yoshioka N, Masumoto T, Mori H, Abe O, Aoki S, Ohtomo K. Brachial plexus injury: clinical manifestations, conventional imaging findings, and the latest imaging techniques. Radiographics. 2006;26(Suppl 1): S133–43.

6 Neck Vascular Lesions

Riccardo Ferrari, Michele Galluzzo, Stefania Ianniello, Caterina Pizzi, Margherita Trinci, and Vittorio Miele

6.1 Introduction

Neck injuries are often a challenge for emergency radiologists because this small part of the body contains so many important anatomical structures, such as the epi-aortic arterial vessels, cervical vertebrae, and spinal cord.

Misdiagnosis of vascular neck injuries is very often a dramatic mistake because the neck vessels are important for cerebral vascularization. An error in the description of the interruption of cerebral blood flow can cause a huge cerebral ischemia with a high rate of morbidity and mortality.

Vascular lesions can be caused by penetrating or blunt trauma: these two mechanisms have a different etiopathology and could produce a different type of lesion. Thus, recognition by emergency radiologists of all the types of lesions is very important.

6.2 Anatomy of the Epi-aortic Vessels

The epi-aortic vessels arise directly from the aortic arch; from right to left the first branch is the brachiocephalic trunk, then the common left carotid and the left subclavian artery. The right common carotid artery arises from a bifurcation of the brachiocephalic trunk (the right subclavian artery is the other branch). The left common carotid artery arises directly from the aortic arch. The left and right common carotid arteries do not give off any branches in the neck, passing laterally to the trachea and inferiorly to the sternocleidomastoid muscles.

Around the level of the C4 vertebra, the common carotid arteries split into external and internal carotid arteries in an area called the carotid triangle. Before this bifurcation, the common carotid arteries are slightly dilated in an area called the carotid sinus, where important blood pressure baroreceptors are located.

The external carotid artery gives blood to the areas of the neck and head that are external of

R. Ferrari (✉) • M. Galluzzo • S. Ianniello • C. Pizzi
M. Trinci
Department of Emergency Radiology,
S. Camillo Hospital, Rome, Italy
e-mail: ferraririccardo@gmail.com

V. Miele
Department of Radiology, Careggi University
Hospital, Florence, Italy

V. Miele, M. Trinci (eds.), *Diagnostic Imaging in Polytrauma Patients*,
https://doi.org/10.1007/978-3-319-62054-1_6

the cranium. It arises from the common carotid arteries, passes posterior to the ramus of the mandible, and ends in the parotid gland, dividing into the superficial temporal artery and the maxillary artery. The external carotid artery gives off six branches: superior thyroid artery, lingual artery, facial artery, ascending pharyngeal artery, occipital artery, and posterior auricular artery.

The deep structures of the face are mainly supplied by the maxillary artery; the superficial structures of the face are mainly supplied by the facial and superficial temporal arteries.

The internal carotid arteries supply the brain, eyes, and forehead, entering the skull within the carotid canal in the petrous part of the temporal bone. The internal carotid artery does not supply any structures in the neck.

The vertebral arteries arise directly from the subclavian arteries. They run in the foramen transversarium inside the transverse processes of the cervical vertebrae. The vertebral arteries enter into the skull through the foramen magnum and converge, giving off the basilar arteries, which supply the posterior part of the brain. The vertebral arteries do not give off any branches in the neck. Branches of the subclavian arteries are the main supply for the neck [1].

6.3 Penetration Trauma: Perforating and Cutting

Perforating and cutting lesions to the neck are typically inflicted by the penetration of sharp objects or gunshots. The percentage of vascular injuries is surprising lower than expected (only 25–33% described in the literature). Classification of penetrating neck wounds is obtained by dividing the neck into three different anatomical zones. The site of the injury is clinically evaluated at admission to separate patients who need direct surgical exploration from patients for whom a computed tomography (CT) angiography scan is needed.

Even if this classification is no longer mandatory in many important emergency centers (that is, in the presence of a stable condition, one prefers to obtain a diagnostic CT scan before exploration), this knowledge is important for radiologists to correctly communicate with clinicians.

Starting from the bottom, the three zones are described as follows.

Zone I: From the sternal notch, clavicles to cricoid cartilage. There is an overlap with the thoracic inlet and superior mediastinum in the inferior part. Many important structures are located in this part of the neck, such as the innominate artery, brachiocephalic veins, segments of the subclavian arteries and veins, the common carotid and vertebral arteries, and the esophagus, trachea, and thyroid. Damage in this zone could require the attention of both thoracic and general surgeons: an exact description of the pathology can help with better and more precise surgical planning.

Zone II: From the cricoid cartilage to the angle of the mandible. This second zone includes the common, internal, and external carotid arteries and jugular veins, and the larynx, upper esophagus, and pharynx. This zone allows a safer surgical approach, and patients with lesions in this zone are usually directly sent to exploratory surgery; also, now many centers prefer to send patients (if hemodynamically stable) to CT angiography for a noninvasive approach.

Zone III: From the angle of the mandible to the base of the skull. Included in this zone are the internal carotid and vertebral arteries, external carotid artery branches, internal jugular vein, and pharynx. Many of the vital structures in this region are poorly accessible to the surgeon because of their proximity to the skull base.

We have mentioned that only 25% to 33% of penetrating injuries of the neck result in arterial injury. Among penetrating arterial injuries of the neck, 80% involve the carotid arteries and 43% involve the vertebral arteries. Carotid artery injuries have a particularly poor prognosis, causing stroke in 15% of patients and death in 22%. Vessel damage may consist of partial or total wall damage. Radiological signs of arterial injuries include occlusion, free blood extravasation, contained extravasation that results in a pseudo-aneurysm, intimal flap, dissection, or arteriovenous fistula.

Penetrating venous injuries are seen in 16% to 18% of patients with penetrating neck trauma. A recent review in the literature assesses the superiority of CT angiography to surgical exploration in the evaluation of venous lesions [2–5].

6.4 Blunt Trauma: Direct or Distraction

Blunt neck trauma can have direct or distraction causes. The majority of the injuries are caused by motor vehicle accidents; minor causes include falls, chiropractic error, trauma from an intra-oral object (babies), and fracture of the basicranium and transverse process of cervical vertebrae (with involvement of the vertebral arteries) [6].

The most frequent pathological mechanism of injury is the stretch of the arterial vessels between the third and fourth cervical vertebral soma; this site in the neck has the possibility of major mobility excursion, and the mechanism of rapid flexo-extension and rotation can involve both carotid and vertebral arteries.

Blunt trauma of the neck has a low rate of associated vascular injuries (0.67–1.1%), which has justified a more conservative approach in the past, but the possibility of tragic consequences in the case of misdiagnosed traumatic injury has led the scientific community to include as mandatory the study of the neck arterial vessels in traumatized patients, especially in high-energy impacts. Morbidity rates of 40–80% and mortality rates of 5–40% are described in cases of neck arterial vessel lesions in victims of blunt trauma. The Denver criteria modified from the Eastern Association of Surgery and Trauma substantially assessed that patients who suffer a high-energy trauma, patients with GCS < 8, and patients with complex fractures of the skull and cervical spine should also be investigated for supraaortic injuries.

Partial or complete occlusion of arterial vessels after blunt trauma is reported in the literature with the same percentage as penetrating trauma (33%). Radiological signs of occlusion are narrowing of the lumen, no enhancement of the vessel after contrast administration, and luminal irregularity [7–11].

6.5 Imaging Techniques and Findings

The epi-aortic arterial vessels can be investigated with different technologies, from US performed directly in a red room, to CT examination, to magnetic resonance (MR) and angiography procedures that could also be part of surgical repair with stenting.

In the management of trauma patients we perform a focused assessment with sonography (FAST) thoracic and abdominal US scan directly in the emergency red room to investigate the presence of blood and fluid in the abdominal or pleural cavity and pneumothorax; if hemodynamically stable with no evidence of blood in the peritoneum, the patient undergoes a total-body CT scan [12]. In this workflow we prefer to use US in the very first evaluation and to study the epi-aortic vessels with CT for its high sensitivity and fast scanning.

Magnetic resonance (MR) evaluation has some advantages in term of radiation exposure and the possibility of obtaining images without administration of contrast media, but it is not feasible in a monitored or intubated patient because of the presence of high magnetic fields and the long scanning times. MR exams could be used in follow-up to reduce patient X-ray exposure. Diffusion-weighted sequences are mandatory in the study of cerebral parenchyma and to evaluate the very early ischemic suffering of cerebral cells.

Arterial vessel pathology includes occlusion, wall vessel rupture, pseudo-aneurysm, intimal flap, dissection, and arteriovenous fistula. The mechanism of the stretching of an artery causes an intimal lesion and rupture of the vasa vasorum, resulting in an intramural hematoma that can be evolved in dissection; the dissection usually evolves cranially in the same direction as blood flow. In consequence of dissection and the intramural hematoma, compression of the real lumen and dilatation of the arterial diameter occur. When the lesion extends to the adventitia, blood pressure causes the formation of a pseudo-aneurysm.

Extracranial carotid dissection, in most cases, spares the carotid bifurcation as well as the intracranial part of the internal carotid [13–16].

6.5.1 Color Doppler Ultrasound

A high-frequency linear transducer should be used to investigate the common internal carotids, the bifurcation, and the external and internal carotid arteries bilaterally.

A fresh mural hematoma is visible as a hypoechoic thickening of the wall. The presence of hyperechoic plaque with some posterior cancellation of the US signal suggests calcified plaque, which is typical of chronic atherosclerosis and tends to exclude acute pathology. The intimal flap is well depicted by US and Doppler signal; thus, dissection of the proximal part of the carotid arteries could be missed because of the impossibility of reaching it even with a low-frequency transducer. The possibility of evaluating the vertebral arteries is very difficult in an emergency setting with US examination.

Increased Doppler velocity is linked with different grades of stenosis of the arterial vessel with peak systolic velocity (PSV) less than 125 cm/s, meaning normal flow even with evidence of atherosclerotic plaque that could be estimated in less than 50%; PSV from 125 to 230 cm/s means that the stenosis is evaluated as 50% to 69%; and PSV <230 cm/s means that stenosis is evaluated as greater than 70%.

Many pitfalls could cause underestimation or overestimation of peak velocity and thus the stenosis: redundancy of the internal carotid artery, fibromuscular dysplasia, vasospasm, and malformation could affect both blood flow and velocity peak [17].

6.5.2 CT Angiography

CT angiography is the gold standard in a patient with high-energy traumatization after a FAST US performed directly in the red code emergency room. Stable patients without signs of intraperitoneal blood at the FAST US exam are sent for CT evaluation, which should be performed before and after intravenous injection of iodine contrast media.

In addition to the percentage of neck vascular injuries in polytrauma patients being reported as very low (0.6–1.1%), the sedated condition of many of the patients does not allow us to understand the changing of neurological status in the case of misdiagnosis of carotid artery or vertebral artery lesions, and the consequences are very often dramatic.

CT has a high sensitivity and specificity for epi-aortic vessel lesions and can depict well the lumen and vessel wall irregularities. The use of a correct scanning protocol combined with the right use of contrast media and the post-processing visualization algorithm allow perfect and easy evaluation of the neck vessels [18–21].

6.5.2.1 Protocol of Study

The epi-aortic arteries present a very high blood flow that allows the use of the "fast protocol." Before describing the scan protocol parameters, it is important to present a brief reminder about the characteristics of arterial enhancement in CT angiography.

Arterial enhancement follows a peak–plateau dynamic and depends on several factors (Fig. 6.1):

1. The iodine rate per second influences the declivity of the ascendant part of the curve. The correct iodine rate per second described in the literature to obtain a correct enhancement is 1.8–2.0 g I/s.
2. The cardiac ejection fraction determinates the peak of the curve.
3. The amount of contrast media influences the plateau of the curve.

Of these factors, the only one that can be modified by the radiologist is the iodine rate per second,

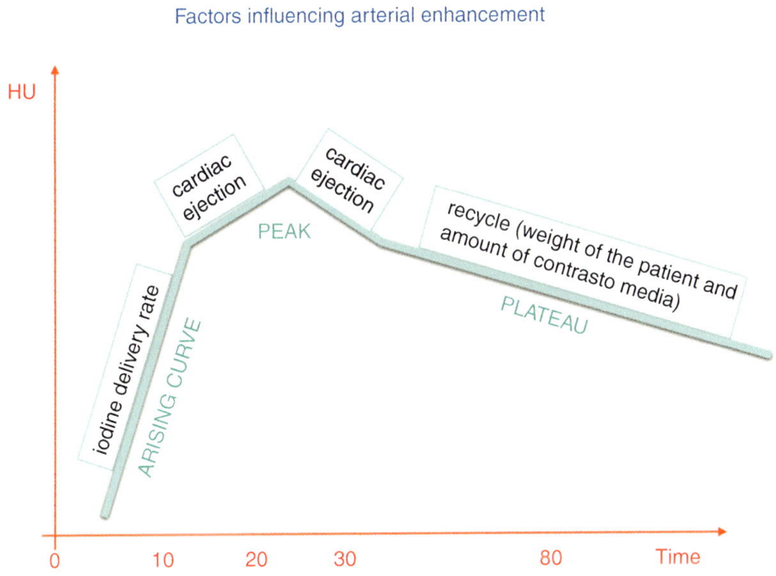

Fig. 6.1 Scheme of the curve of enhancement in the arterial district: description of factors that influenced the different steps

which depends on the injection flow and the iodine concentration of the contrast media.

For example, to obtain the correct iodine rate per second inside the arterial vessels (1.8 g/s–2.0 g/s), we could use a 370-mg iodine contrast at 5 ml/s ($5 \times 0.37 = 1.85$ g I/s) or a 400-mg I at 4.5 ml/s ($4.6 \times 0.4 = 1.84$ g I/s); by moving these two parameters we can obtain the same arterial enhancement with different contrast media concentrations.

CT angiography for epi-aortic vessels in trauma cases constitutes a pre-contrast phase, mandatory to delineate recent bleeding, an arterial phase, and a venous phase for late venous bleeding. A pre-contrast brain scan is mandatory to better delineate the presence of parenchymatous hemorrhage.

The scout view has to delineate the aortic arch where the bolus tracking should be positioned. Minimum delay from the peak of 100 HU inside the aortic arch is preferred.

The scan could be managed in a caudo-cranial direction from the aortic arch to the brain, and next a cranio-caudal full-body scan in late arterial phase must be performed to evaluate the parenchymatous organs. The pitch parameter should be set as fast as possible; rotation time should be the lowest possible to correctly scan a narrow window time using a very high contrast administration flow.

Table 6.1 Technical multi-detector computed tomography (CT) parameters

Technical parameter	
Pitch	Maximum possible
Gantry rotation	0.5 s
Collimation	0.6 mm
Trigger-scan delay	5 s
Bolus tracking	At the level of aortic arch
Scan direction	Caudo-cranial
Multi-phase scan	Pre-contrast, arterial, and venous phase
Kv	100
mA	Variable with modulation

The use of a low-kilovolt setting [100 or 80 KV, depending on body mass index (BMI)] allows a better delineation of high-density structures as the X-ray spectrum created is less penetrating and tends to stop better on high-density structures, in particular on vessels full of iodine contrast media.

The use of milliampere (mA) modulation and an iterative reconstruction algorithm are mandatory to reduce patient exposure, especially for young patients (Table 6.1). In cases of polytrauma patients and high-energy impacts, it is mandatory to comprehend the study of the neck vessels in the total body scan.

Use of the right scan protocol and the choice of the right concentration (g/s) of iodine contrast allow very easy diagnosis of lesions. Automatic or manual reconstruction with the multiplanar reconstruction algorithm, oblique reformation along the vessel axis, and maximum intensity projections (MIP) and volume-rendering (VR) reconstructions allow the easiest recognition of the lesions and better communication with the clinician or surgeon for the right surgical or medical choice and programming [21–23].

6.5.2.2 CT Signs of Pathology

Intraluminal dissection and hematoma of the vessel wall should be visible on unenhanced CT as a "crescent moon" hyperdensity. In many cases the carotid dissection spares the carotid bifurcation and the intracranial part.

The use of an arterial and portal phase scan after the administration of contrast media is mandatory to evaluate the false and real lumen; the real lumen is usually thinner and will be enhanced sooner.

Carotid dissection is characterized by narrowing of the lumen, the intimal flap, which is very well depicted when the right contrast enhancement is achieved (Figs. 6.2, 6.3, and 6.4).

Vertebral arterial dissections are very well depicted with CT angiography. Chen et al. (2004) reported a sensitivity of 100% and specificity of 98%. In CT angiography of the vertebral arteries, the finding of an intimal flap is less common than in the carotid artery with a prevalence of wall hematoma. Potential artifacts in the study of vertebral arteries could be the presence of bone artifacts at the level of the skull base or dental implant artifacts.

Venous injuries are less common in blunt trauma. The most frequent evidence is the presence of a thrombus inside the jugular vein that appears as a hypodense tissue inside the hyperdense contrast (Fig. 6.5).

6.5.3 MR Angiography

Magnetic resonance (MR) imaging is very difficult to be used suitably for a trauma patient. The high magnetic field and long acquisition times make the continuous monitoring of life parameters quite impossible without the presence of nonmagnetic life support equipment. Other disadvantages of the MR exam are the impossibility of evaluating pulmonary parenchyma and of evaluating many districts in a short time as CT can do.

The advantage of MR exams are that patients are not exposed to ionizing radiation, an advantage when many follow-ups are necessary, especially in young patients (Fig. 6.6). The possibility of evaluating cellular cerebral parenchyma suffering in a very early stage with the use of diffusion-weighted imaging should be an option when clinical evaluation is not possible [24].

6.5.3.1 Protocol of Study

The angiographic study of epi-aortic vessels with MR could be done with time-of-flight (TOF) sequences without the administration of contrast media or with phase-contrast and contrast enhancement sequences after the administration of gadolinium-based contrast media. The TOF sequences have less spatial resolution than MR angiography post-contrast sequences, but TOF sequences allow a larger scanning volume in a small scanning time. The TOF sequences for their technical characteristics could create some artifacts when blood flow is not linear. The post-contrast angiographic sequences on the other hand could suffer from some artifacts such as segmental blurring or signal intensity loss in the vertebral artery, especially in a young patient where the blood flow is particularly fast. These artifacts (feathering artifacts) are caused by rapidly changing signal intensity in small vascular structures around the vertebral artery during sampling the central part of the K-space. These artifacts could mimic stenosis or dissection of the vertebral artery.

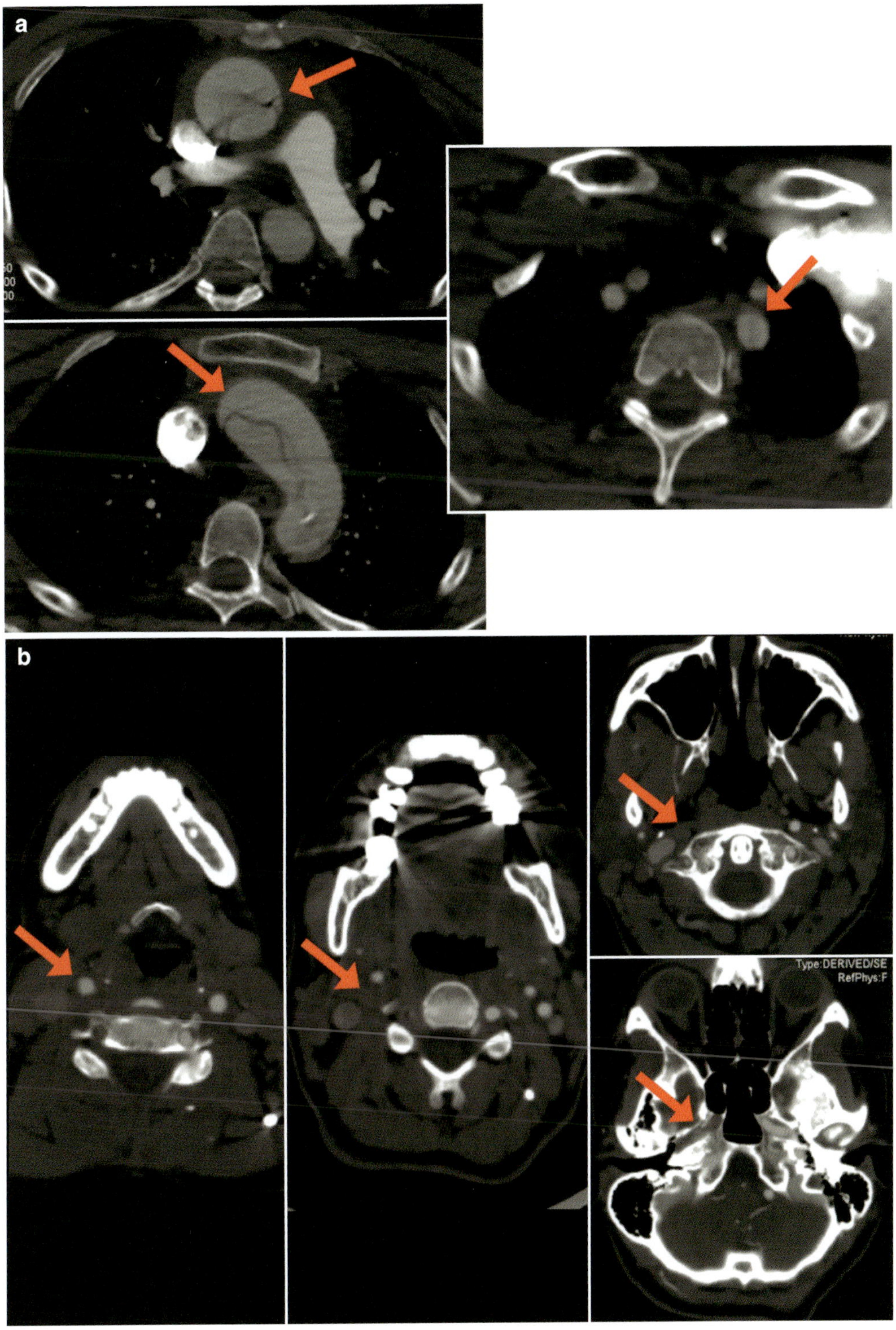

Fig. 6.2 Axial contrast enhancement computed tomography (CT) images of aortic arch dissection after a motor vehicle accident (**a**). The dissection seems not to involve the origin of common carotid arteries, but there is dissection and occlusion of the internal carotid arteries bilaterally (**b**). (**c**) Tridimensional maximum intensity projection (MIP) and volume-rendering (VR) reconstructions

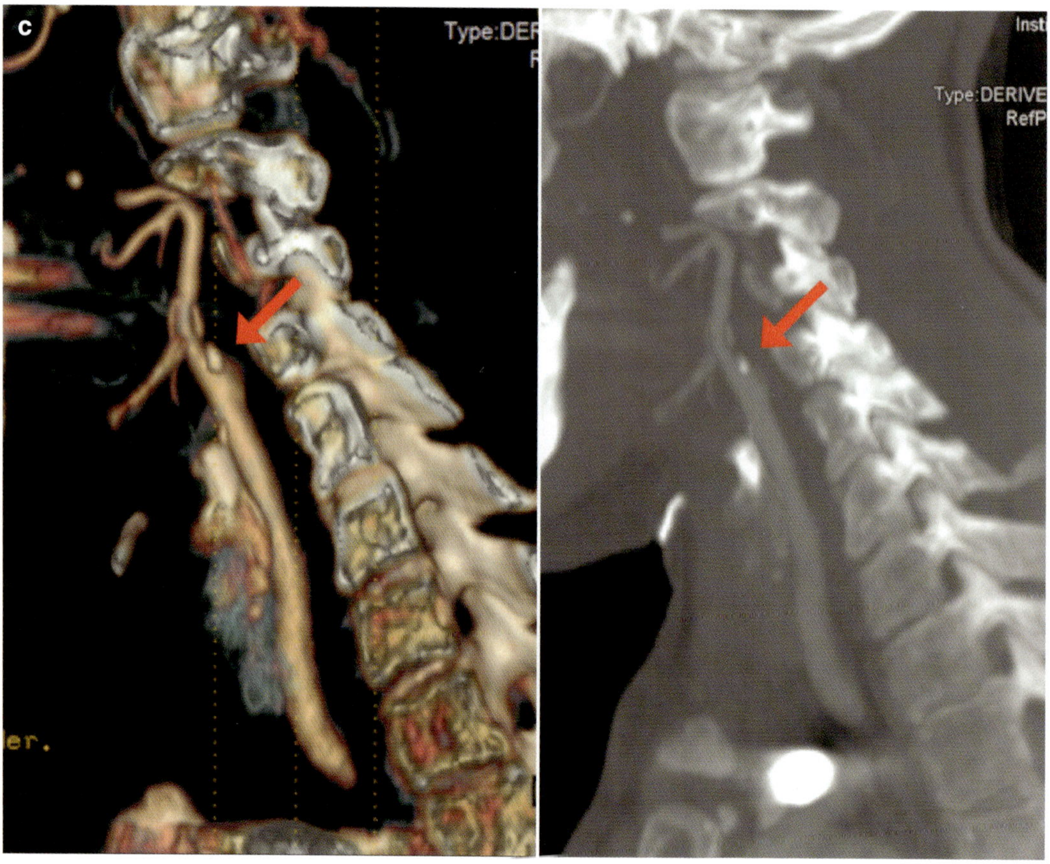

Fig. 6.2 (continued)

The protocol of epi-aortic vessel angiography follows:

- Balanced steady-state gradient echo sequence in axial and coronal planes to evaluate correctly the extension and course of the vessels
- T_1-weighted images with fat saturation in coronal and axial plane
- T_2-weighted images in coronal and axial plane
- Time-of-flight sequence (TOF)
- 3D FAST spoiled gradient echo with elliptical K-space sampling; contrast enhancement angiography sequence
- 0.2 ml gadolinium contrast enhanced 0.5 mol with a flow of 2.0 ml/s
- Bolus tracking is mandatory at the level of the aortic arch

6.5.3.2 MR Signs of Pathology

T_1-weighted imaging with fat saturation allows visualization of a hematoma inside the vessel wall, with different characteristics depending on the paramagnetic effect evolution of signal intensity during the hemoglobin degradation process.

In the very early and chronic stage, the hematoma is usually iso-intense when compared to the other structures. In the subacute phase (between 7 days and 2 months after the accident), the hematoma appears hyperintense in T_1-weighted images.

TOF sequences also allow us to evaluate a subacute hematoma because it does not completely suppress short T_1 tissue values. Contrast enhancement angiography allows the visualization of only the lumen of the arterial vessels.

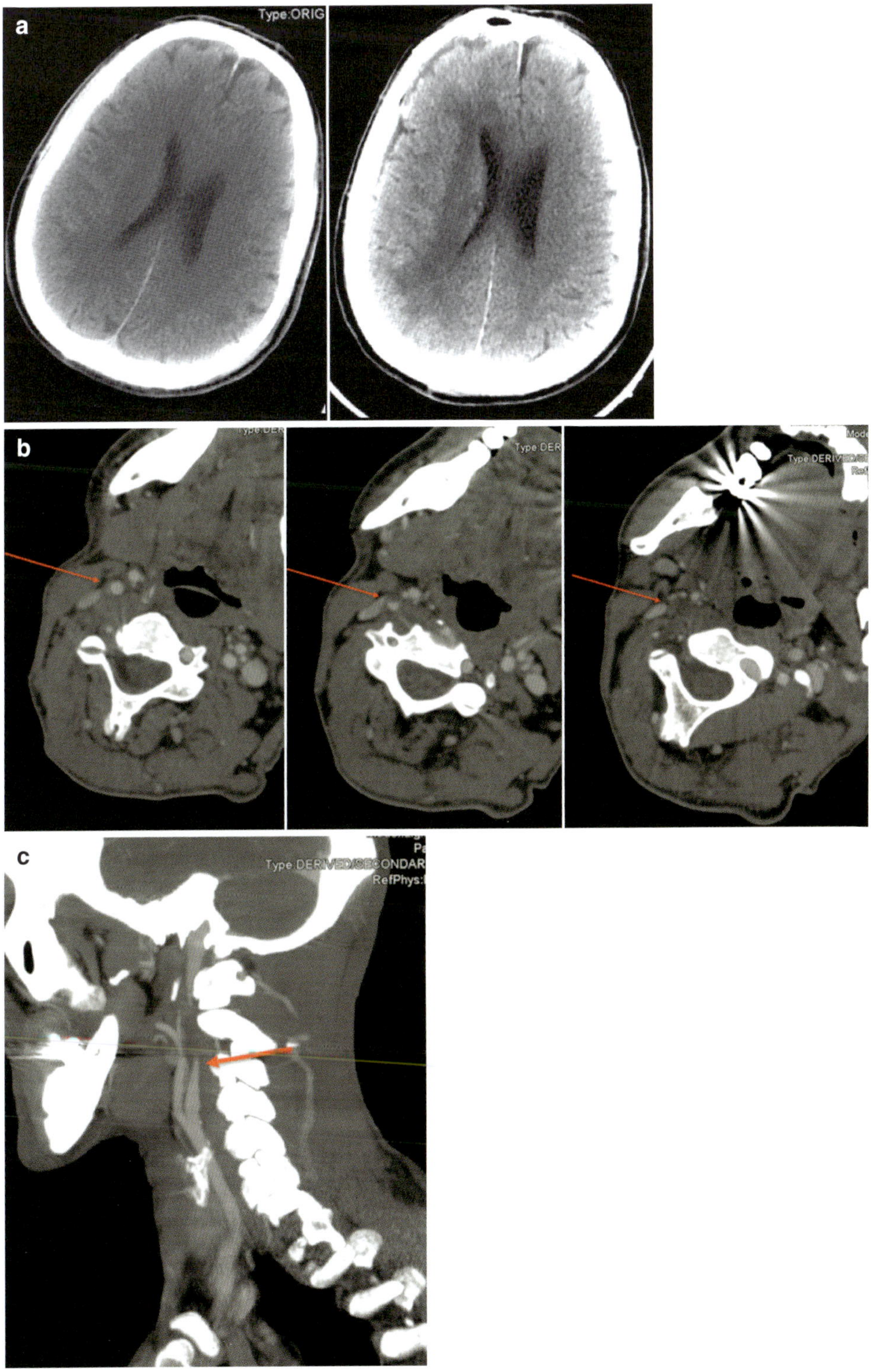

Fig. 6.3 (**a**) Brain parenchyma the day of the trauma (*A*) and 2 days after (*B*). Neck vessels were not included in the first examination. The scan 2 days later included the neck arterial vessels, confirming the right internal carotid dissection and occlusion (**b**, **c**)

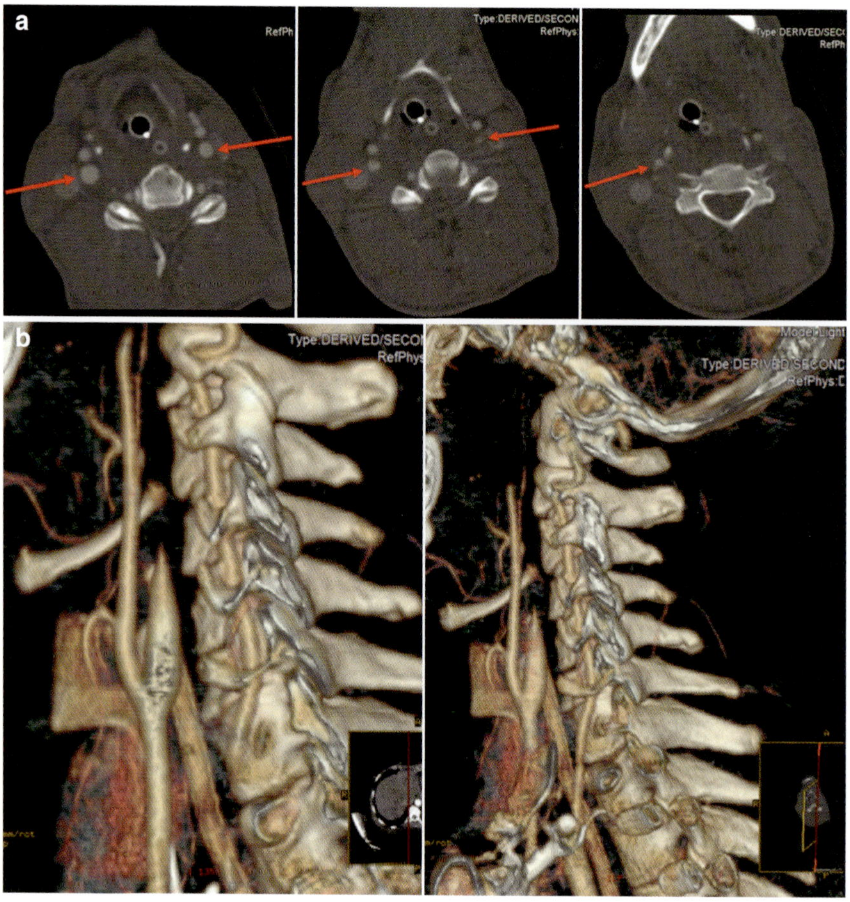

Fig. 6.4 Bilateral dissection of internal carotid arteries. (**a**) Axial images demonstrate the bilateral dissection of internal carotid arteries (*red arrows*). (**b**) Tridimensional volume rendering reconstruction images of the bilateral dissection of internal carotid arteries

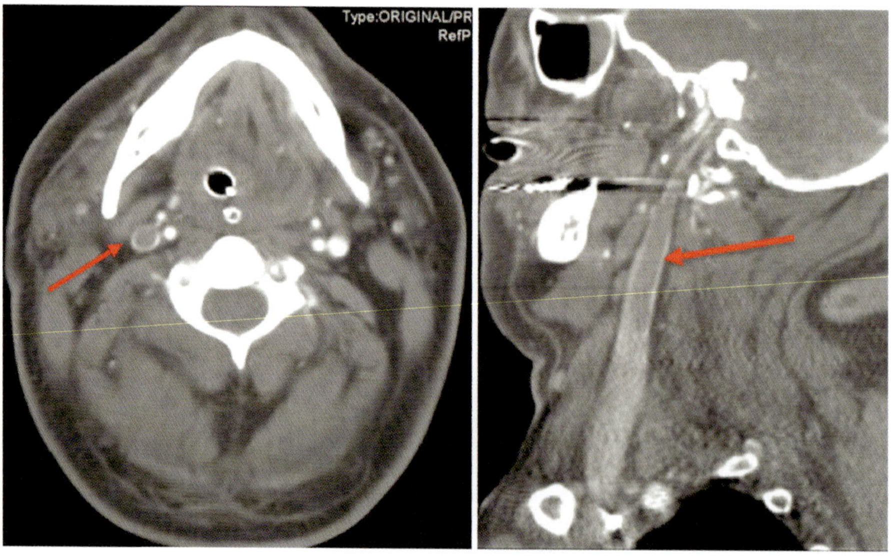

Fig. 6.5 Traumatic thrombosis of the right jugular vein

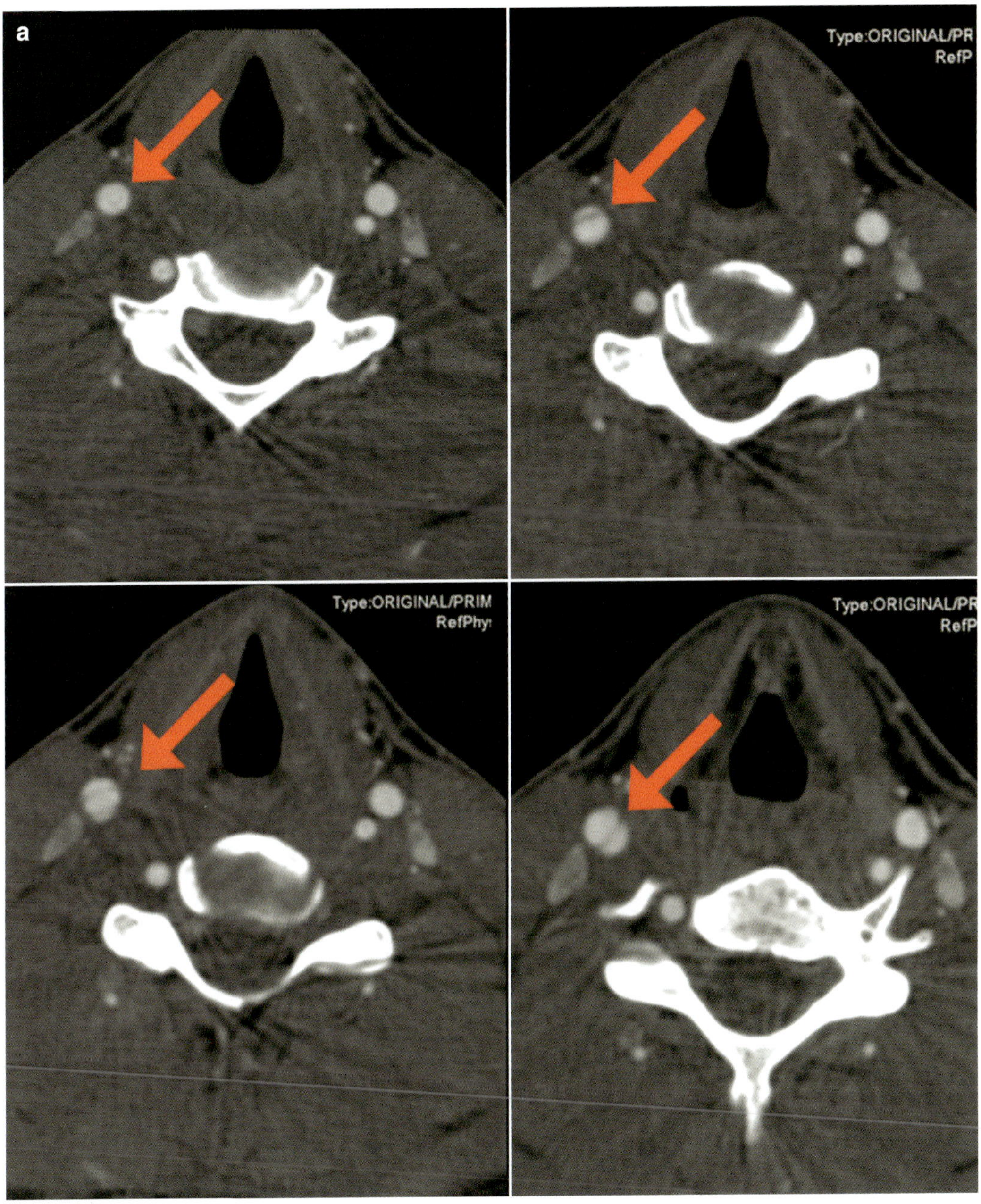

Fig. 6.6 Traumatic partial dissection of the right common carotid artery after a blow with the elbow during a sports activity. Axial CT images (**a**), multiplanar (MPR) curve reconstruction; magnetic resonance (MR) examination control (**b**, **c**)

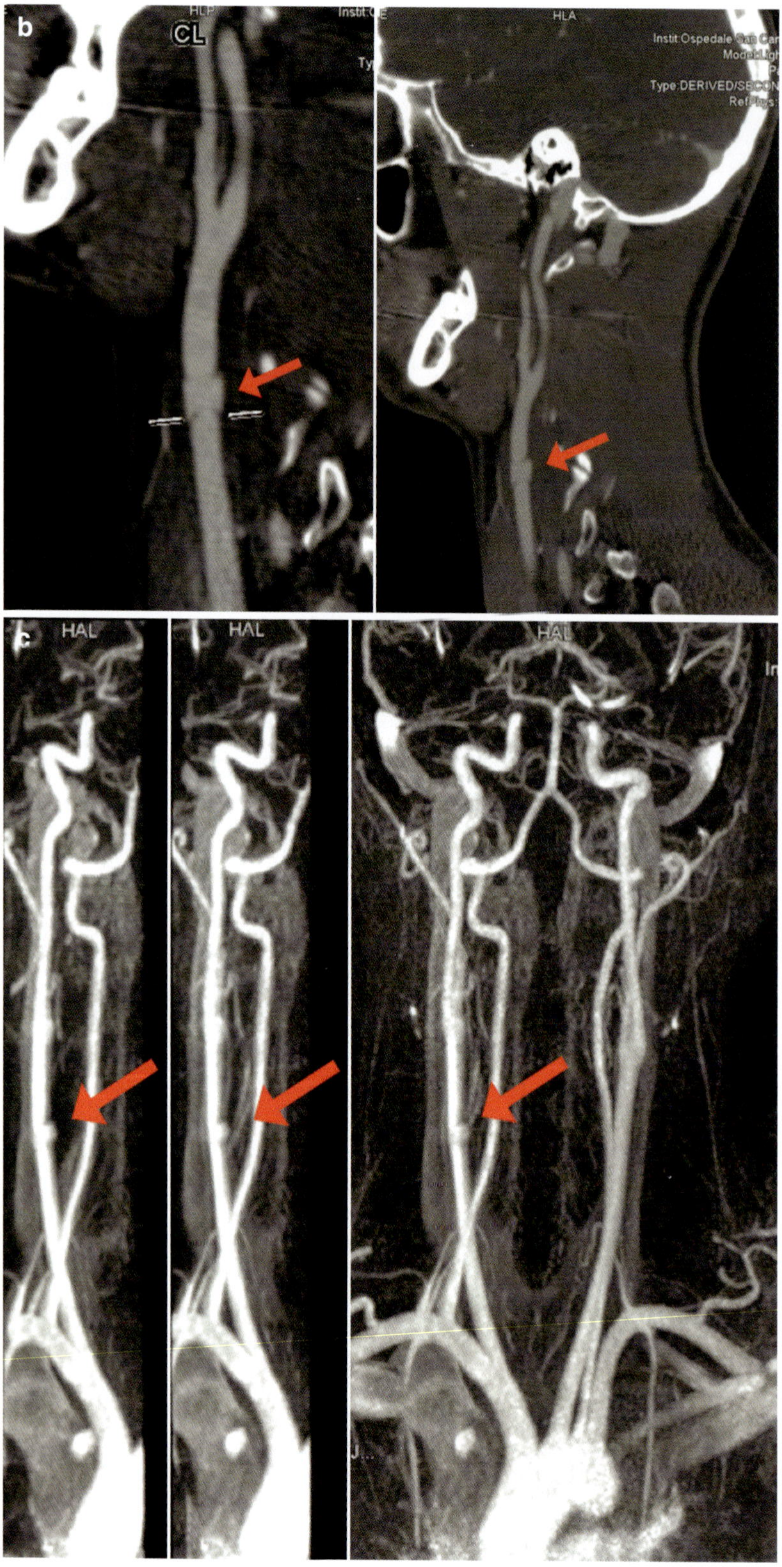

Fig. 6.6 (continued)

There is some experience using phase-contrast sequences to evaluate blood flow.

The signs of carotid artery dissection include increased external diameter and narrowing of the lumen, which therefore are not specific signs. High specificity and sensitivity (84% and 99%, respectively) are reported. The percentages of correct diagnosis decrease when evaluating the vertebral artery (specificity, 60%; sensitivity, 58%). We discuss the presence of artifacts at the level of the foramen magnum. It is therefore difficult to evaluate the first part of the vertebral arteries because of the limitation of the reception coil in the scan volume [25].

6.5.4 Digital Subtraction Angiography

Digital subtraction angiography is never the first diagnostic choice because of the impossibility of evaluating the vessel wall. It is of course the gold standard in diagnostic procedures and in evaluation of the vessel lumen. The string sign is a long eccentric and irregular stenosis beginning distal to the carotid bulb and is the sign of dissection. A dilatation aneurysm is another typical sign [26].

6.6 Differential Diagnosis

Many conditions can mimic or should be differentiated from the epi-aortic dissection stenosis. Many of them are not coherent with the history of trauma of the patient and can be readily dismissed.

6.6.1 Fibromuscular Dysplasia

This noninflammatory vascular disease of the medium–small vessels has a low prevalence in the population (0.6–1.1%). It is more frequent in middle-aged women and affects the renal artery (75%) less frequently than the epi-aortic vessels (25%). The disease spares the proximal part of the vessel and is very often bilateral in the carotid artery. Vertebral arteries are less commonly involved. Tight stenosis and subarachnoid hemorrhage are the main symptoms.

6.6.2 Dysgenesis of the Internal Carotid Artery (ICA)

With a very low prevalence of disease (0.13%), dysgenesis of the carotid artery could be asymptomatic for a long time. The dysgenesis could mimic a long stenosis.

6.6.3 Atherosclerosis

Atherosclerosis disease is a very common syndrome involving the carotid bulb and bifurcation that usually occurs in the elderly. The vertebral arteries are more frequently involved at the ostium. The disease evolves in steps starting from soft lipomatous plaque to calcified plaque. It can be differentiated well from acute trauma disease by the presence of calcification.

6.6.4 Takayasu Arteritis

This chronic inflammatory disease involves the large vessels, primarily the aorta and its main branches, including supraaortic vessels and the pulmonary arteries.

It is a very rare pathology (2.6 per million), occurring more frequently in young women. More common in Asia and Mexico, it is rare in Europe and North America. The disease involves primarily the media and adventitia, causing occlusion and aneurysm.

6.6.5 Behçet Disease

This multi-systemic recurrent inflammatory disease involves the vasa vasorum of arteries and veins, causing occlusion and thrombophlebitis; it more frequently affects people from 30 to 50 years of age in the Mediterranean and Asian areas.

6.6.6 Giant Cell Arteritis

This inflammatory disease more frequently involves patients more than 50 years old and more often affects the temporal artery. It can cause occlusion, especially of the vertebral artery; the carotid artery is less frequently involved.

The most typical manifestation is headache with an increased erythrocyte sedimentation rate. Giant cell arteritis is a rare cause of stroke, most often in the vertebrobasilar territory. The diagnosis is generally made with a temporal biopsy.

References

1. Jones O. http://teachmeanatomy.info/neck/vessels/arterial-supply/
2. Steenburg SD, Sliker CW, Shanmuganathan K, et al. Imaging evaluation of penetrating neck injuries Radiographics. 2010;30:869–86. doi:10.1148/rg.304105022.
3. Biffl WL, Moore EE, Rehse DH, et al. Selective management of penetrating neck trauma based on cervical level of injury. Am J Surg. 1997;174:678–82.
4. Asensio JA, Valenziano CP, Falcone RE, et al. Management of penetrating neck injuries: the controversy surrounding zone II injuries. Surg Clin North Am. 1991;71:267–96.
5. LeBlang SD, Nunez DB Jr, Rivas LA, et al. Helical computed tomographic angiography in penetrating neck trauma. Emerg Radiol. 1997;4:200–6.
6. Núñez DB, Torres-León M, Múnera F. Vascular injuries of the neck and thoracic inlet: helical CT-angiographic correlation. Radiographics. 2004;24:1087–98. doi:10.1148/rg.244035035.
7. Singh RR, Barry MC, Ireland A, et al. Current diagnosis and management of blunt internal carotid artery injury. Eur J Vasc Endovasc Surg. 2004;27:577–84. doi:10.1016/j.ejvs.2004.01.005.
8. Biffl WL, Moore EE, Offner PJ, et al. Optimizing screening for blunt cerebrovascular injuries. Am J Surg. 1999;178:517–22.
9. Bromberg WJ, Collier BC, Diebel LN, et al. Blunt cerebrovascular injury practice management guidelines: the Eastern Association for the Surgery of Trauma. J Trauma. 2010;268:471–7. doi:10.1097/TA.0b013e3181cb43.
10. Fanelli F, Salvatori FM, Ferrari R, et al. Stent repair of bilateral post-traumatic dissections of the internal carotid artery. J Endovasc Ther. 2004;11:517–21. doi:10.1583/04-1207.1.
11. Chen CJ, Tseng YC, Lee TH, et al. Multisection CT angiography compared with catheter angiography in diagnosing vertebral artery dissection. AJNR Am J Neuroradiol. 2004;25:769–74.
12. Miele V, Di Giampietro I. Diagnostic imaging in emergency. Salute Soc 2014;(2EN):127–38. doi:10.3280/SES2014-002010EN.
13. Demetriades D, Salim A, Brown C, et al. Neck injuries. Curr Probl Surg. 2007;44:13–85. doi:10.1067/j.cpsurg.2006.10.004.1.
14. Rodallec MH, Marteau V, Gerber S, et al. Craniocervical arterial dissection: spectrum of imaging findings and differential diagnosis. Radiographics. 2008;28:1711–29.
15. Vanninen RL, Manninen HI, Partanen PL, et al. Carotid artery stenosis: clinical efficacy of MR phase-contrast flow quantification as an adjunct to MR angiography. Radiology. 1995;194:459–67. doi:10.1148/radiology.194.2.7824727.
16. Utter GH, Hollingworth W, Hallam DK, et al. Sixteen-slice CT angiography in patients with suspected blunt carotid and vertebral artery injuries. J Am Coll Surg. 2006;203:838–48. doi:10.1016/j.jamcollsurg.2006.08.003.
17. Kasbekar AV, Combellack EJ, Derbyshire SG, Swift AC. Penetrating neck trauma and the need for surgical exploration: six-year experience within a regional trauma centre. J Laryngol Otol. 2017;131:8–12.
18. Provenzale JM. Dissection of the internal carotid and vertebral arteries: imaging features. AJR Am J Roentgenol. 1995;165:1099–104. doi:10.2214/ajr.165.5.7572483.
19. Munera F, Soto JA, Palacio DM, et al. Penetrating neck injuries: helical CT angiography for initial evaluation. Radiology. 2002;224:366–72. doi:10.1148/radiol.2242010973.
20. Brywczynski JJ, Barrett TW, Lyon JA, et al. Management of penetrating neck injury in the emergency department: a structured literature review. Emerg Med J. 2008;25:711–5.
21. Regine G, Stasolla A, Miele V. Multidetector computed tomography of the renal arteries in vascular emergencies. Eur J Radiol. 2007;64:83–91.
22. Lombardi M, Bartolozzi C. Risonanza Magnetica del Cuore e dei Vasi. Mailand: Springer; 2004.
23. Laghi A, Ferrari R. Protocolli di studio in TC spirale multistrato. Vol. 2: Vascolare. Mailand: Springer; 2008.
24. Montorfano MA, Pla F, Vera L, et al. Point-of-care ultrasound and Doppler ultrasound evaluation of vascular injuries in penetrating and blunt trauma. Crit Ultrasound J. 2017;9:5. doi:10.1186/s13089-017-0060-5.
25. Günther A, Witte OW, Freesmeyer M, et al. Clinical presentation, magnetic resonance angiography, ultrasound findings, and stroke patterns in patients with vertebral artery dissection. Eur Neurol. 2016;76:284–94.
26. Brueck M, Heidt MC, Szente-Varga M, et al. Hybrid treatment for complex aortic problems combining surgery and stenting in the integrated operating theater. J Interv Cardiol. 2006;19:539–43.

Airway Injuries

7

Luigia Romano, Antonio Pinto, Ciro Acampora, Nicola Gagliardi, Sonia Fulciniti, and Massimo Silva

7.1 Introduction

Thoracic trauma causes 25% of the annual traffic deaths in the United States. Among patients suffering chest blunt trauma, tracheo-bronchial injury is rare, occurring in only 0.8–2% of cases [1–3].

The causes of injury include height fall, impact with the car steering wheel, the handlebars of a motorcycle or a steel plate. Furthermore, blunt trauma to the neck can determine laceration, transection or shattering injury of both cervical and mediastinum trachea.

Closed injury to the cervical trachea can also result from a strong impact against the cervical spine, while closed injury to the mediastinal trachea and main bronchus can depend on a knock against the thoracic spine. The consequence could be a fracture of the cartilage rings, frequently associated with lesions of other deep neck structures as larynx, oesophagus, nerves and vessels.

In addition, tracheal or bronchial rupture can be determined by intubation manoeuvre and post-intubation injuries [4].

Depending on the depth of damage, a wide spectrum of lesions may occur and can determine, as consequence, a mucosal-tracheal stenosis, tracheo-malacia and full-thickness stricture.

Pathogenesis of intubation manoeuvre injury is frequently proportional to pressure necrosis determined by the cuff of endotracheal tube. In addition, the tip of the endotracheal tube may predispose to erosions or granulomas within the wall of the trachea (Fig. 7.1).

Post-intubation injuries occur because of tracheal irritation from the endotracheal tube or for tracheostomy stoma. There are different predisposing factors, including too large a stoma, infection in the stoma and excessive pressure from the connecting systems. Granulation tissue can determine a narrowing of the tracheal lumen (Fig. 7.1).

Acquired tracheo-oesophageal fistula (Fig. 7.2) could be the result of prolonged erosion by the endotracheal tube positioned postero-laterally, while the tracheo-innominate artery fistula may result from prolonged cuff erosion inferiorly and anteriorly to the trachea. Inappropriate low stoma may further increase the probability of a direct erosion of the trachea by the innominate artery.

L. Romano (✉) • A. Pinto • C. Acampora
N. Gagliardi • S. Fulciniti • M. Silva
Department of Radiology, A.O.R.N. A. Cardarelli,
Via Cardarelli n.9, 80131 Naples, Italy
e-mail: luigia.romano1@yahoo.com

V. Miele, M. Trinci (eds.), *Diagnostic Imaging in Polytrauma Patients*,
https://doi.org/10.1007/978-3-319-62054-1_7

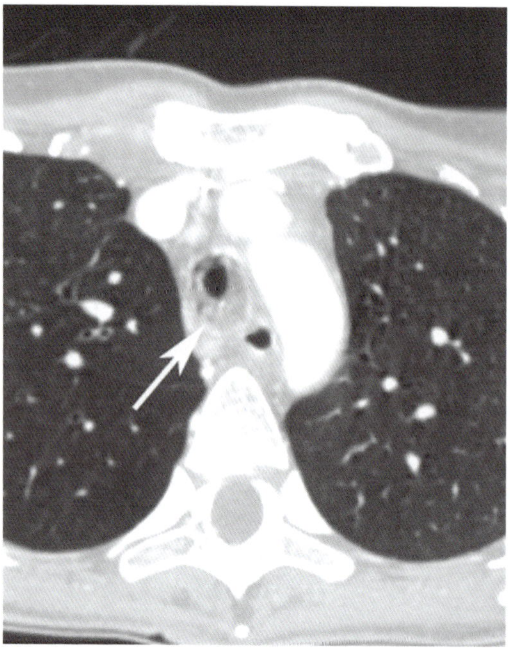

Fig. 7.1 Post-contrast axial CT scan at the level of the upper mediastinum depicts a circumferential granulomas within the wall of the trachea (*white arrow*) with stenosis of the lumen

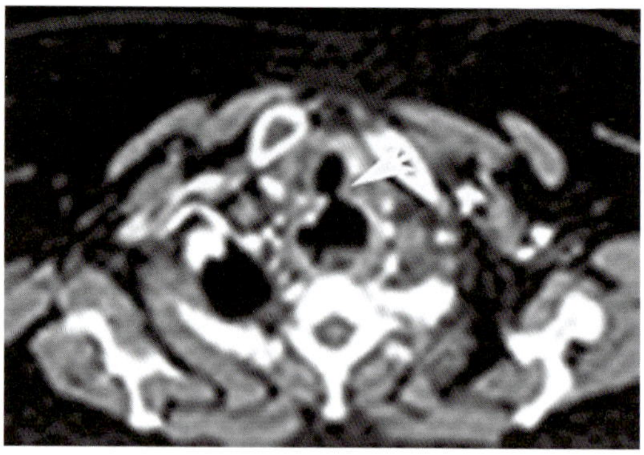

Fig. 7.2 Post-contrast axial CT scan at the level of the upper mediastinum depicts a defect of the posterior wall of the trachea continuing in the lumen of the oesophagus (*white arrow head*), due to a post-traumatic tracheo-oesophageal fistula

Also penetrating injury to the cervical or mediastinum trachea is often the cause of a tracheo-bronchial rupture. However, high speed traffic accidents are the most frequent cause of tracheal and bronchial injuries.

Tracheal rupture is associated with a higher morbidity and mortality [1, 5, 6].

It is supposed that 50% of patients die at the trauma scene from severe respiratory insufficiency or other associated injuries, especially significant traumatic lesions of thoracic cage, lungs and thoracic aorta [7, 8]. In patients that survive, airway injuries have an overall mortality rate of 30% [9].

Generally, airway injuries are mainly located on the initial part of the respiratory tract. In 15–27% of cases, rupture is tracheal (Fig. 7.3) and 76% is exclusively bronchial, either on the right main-stem bronchus (47%) (Fig. 7.4) or on the left main-stem bronchus (32%) [10].

Laceration of the cervical trachea is rare for the elasticity of the cartilagineus rings and the presence of many hard bones as the jaws, the sternum manubrium, the clavicles ant the cervical spine that protect this upper segment of the airways.

Bronchial injuries occur more commonly than tracheal, usually on the right side and between 2.5 cm from the carina [11] (Fig. 7.4), while 80% of tracheal lacerations occur generally 2 cm above the carena.

Most major airway injuries are not recognized initially. Diagnosis of tracheal rupture may be delayed as a result of its rare incidence, subtle and not specific clinical and radiological manifestation and the presence of additional clinical findings of other more common associated injuries of the thorax and other body districts [6, 12].

A significant number of cases are undiagnosed until complications develop either at the site of rupture, such as bronchial stenosis, or in the lung distal to the rupture such as lung infection and atelectasis (Fig. 7.5) [13, 14].

In fact, in two thirds of airway injuries, the diagnosis is delayed with subsequent high morbidity for serious complications, such as recurrent pneumonia, empyema (Fig. 7.6), pulmonary abscesses, mediastinitis (Fig. 7.7), sepsis, airway obstruction and atelectasis [10, 15].

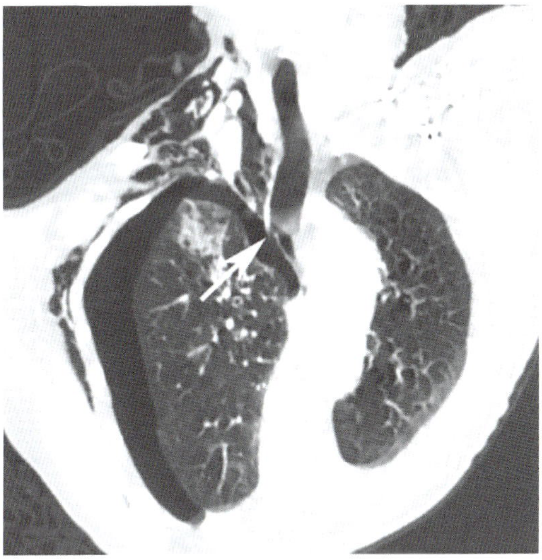

Fig. 7.3 Coronal CT reconstruction demonstrates a focal discontinuity of the right wall of the trachea (*white arrow*) associated with ipsilateral pneumothorax and subcutaneous emphysema

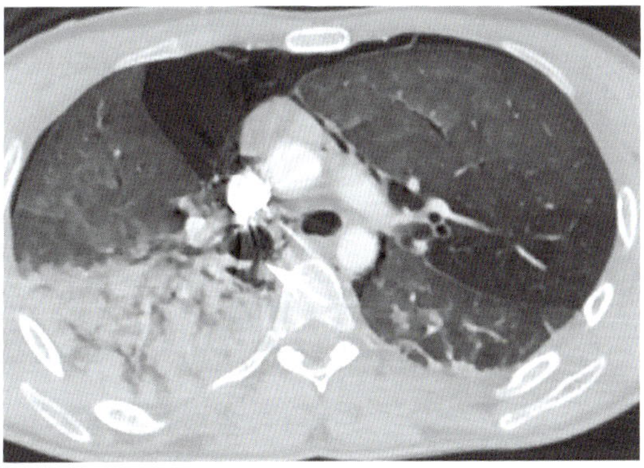

Fig. 7.4 Post-contrast axial CT scan depicts the disruption of the right main-stem bronchus with a visible posterior wall defect (*white arrow*). There is a bilateral pneumothorax associated with lung contusions and parenchymal haemorrhage of the right inferior lobe due to a diffuse laceration

Generally, the most frequent symptoms of all blunt airway injuries are dyspnoea (76–100%), hoarseness (46%), subcutaneous emphysema (35–85%) and haemoptysis (14–25%) [16].

In many cases, the diagnosis is missed in the acute phase and is detected only because of persistent lung or lobar atelectasis. Bronchoscopy should be performed in any cases in which the features described previously provide at least some suspicion of an airway lesion.

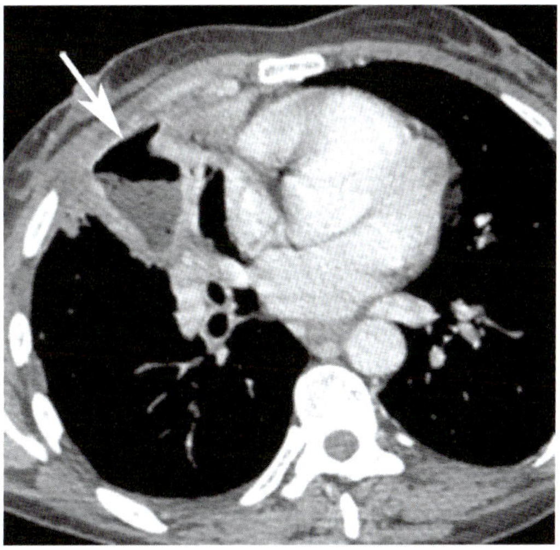

Fig. 7.5 Post-contrast axial CT scan shows a middle lobe atelectasis associated with an abscess (*white arrow*)

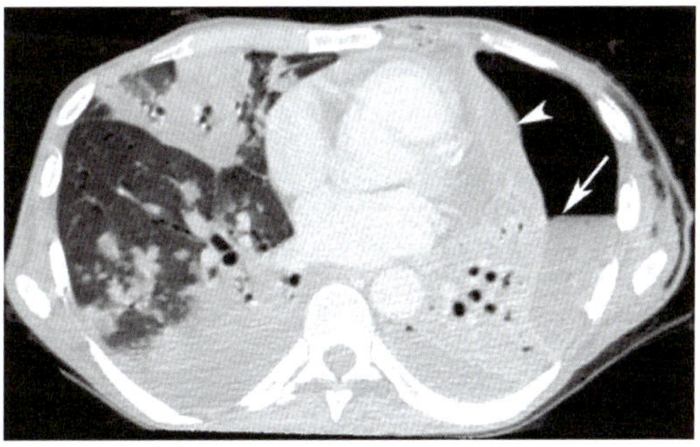

Fig. 7.6 Post-contrast axial CT scan shows a left side empyema with air-fluid level (*white arrow*) correlated to pulmonary atelectasis (*white arrow head*). The right lung shows multiple, lobular, patchy, confluent consolidation areas, due to bronchopneumonia associated with pleuric fluid

7.2 Clinical Features

Clinical findings of airway rupture are sometimes unclear and may be hidden by other traumatic injuries. Alternatively, some obvious airway rupture features may be wrongly assigned to lesions of other structures, especially oesophagus.

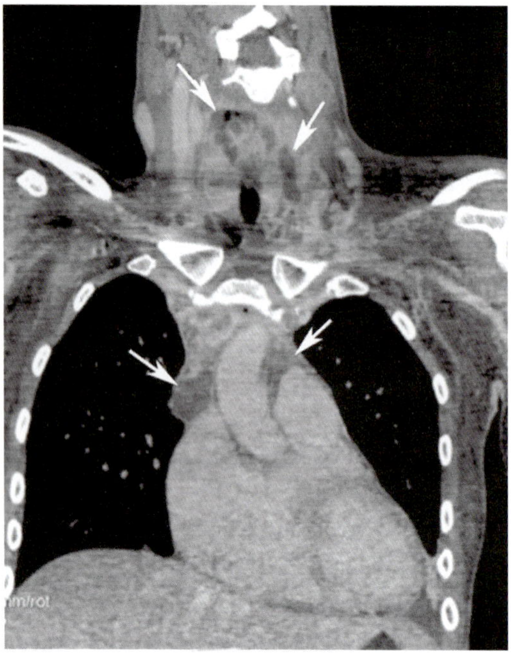

Fig. 7.7 Post-contrast CT coronal reconstruction shows multiple neck and mediastinal fluid collections (*white arrows*) mixed to air bubbles due to a post-traumatic cervical-mediastinitis

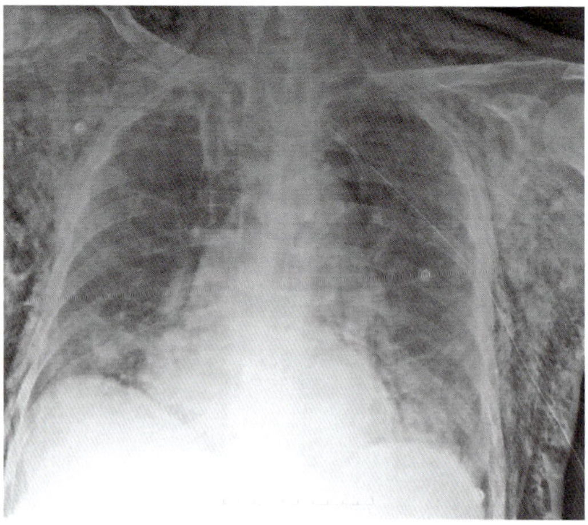

Fig. 7.8 Chest radiograph shows extensive subcutaneous emphysema diffused into shoulders and chest fat planes; it is also present pneumo-mediastinum, with multiple lucencies along mediastinal planes

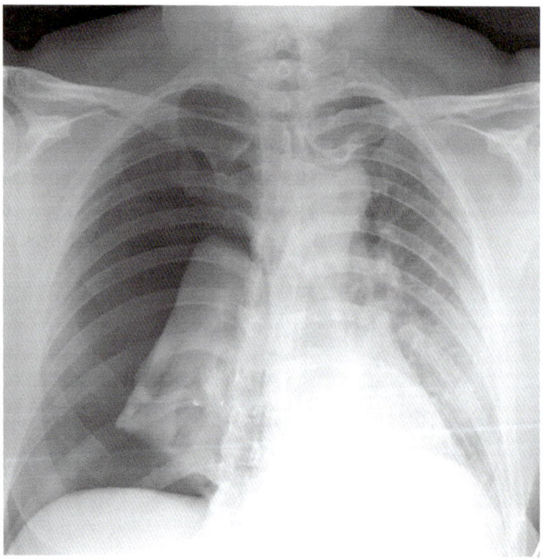

Fig. 7.9 X-ray film performed immediately after the admission, evidences an extensive right pneumothorax with complete collapse of the ipsilateral lung

Pain associated with swallowing and skin contusion, neck emphysema, pneumo-mediastinum and hoarseness are clinical findings that can allow suspecting the diagnosis.

Other symptoms are dyspnoea, cough, bloody saliva, haemoptysis and dysphagia. These symptoms are frequently associated with physical features as cyanosis, pneumothorax, vocal cord paralysis, aphonia and subcutaneous emphysema diffused also into shoulders and chest fat planes (Fig. 7.8).

The pneumothorax is frequently large and under tension (Fig. 7.9). The air leak may be persistent after introduction of pleural drainage. In these circumstances, the lung fails to expand. One unusual but characteristic feature that may be evidenced in cases of bronchial tear and a large pneumothorax is that bronchial rupture may allow the lung to bulge downwards from the hilum giving rise the "fallen lung" sign (Fig. 7.10). Normally, in the presence of a pneumothorax, the lung recoils towards the hilum, the vascular pedicle persists in its normal site and the lung remains perfused although under-ventilated.

If the "fallen lung sign" is present, the consequent ventilation-perfusion discrepancy may result in hypoxia and cyanosis.

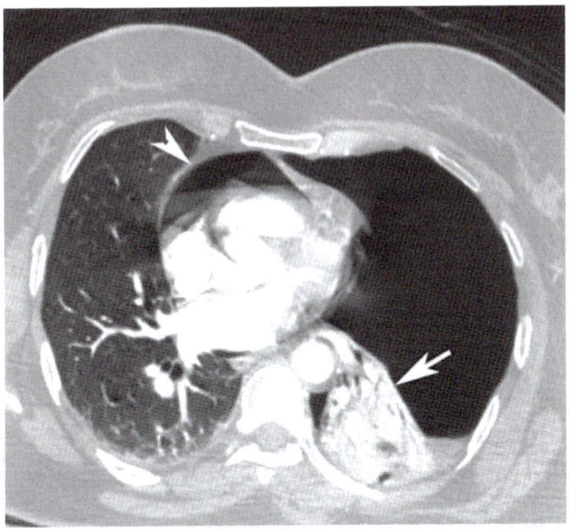

Fig. 7.10 Post-contrast axial CT scan demonstrates a left undertension pneumothorax. The ipsilateral lung bulges downwards from the hilum, giving the "fallen lung" sign (*white arrow*); it is also evidenced the presence of pneumopericardium (*white arrow head*)

It is also necessary to evaluate if tracheal injury is partial or complete.

Clinical signs of partial tracheal rupture include gradually increasing dyspnoea, haemoptysis, hoarseness and subcutaneous emphysema. In complete tracheal rupture, the skin of the anterior neck moves in and out with breathing movement and a gap in the tracheal rings can be felt beneath the moving skin.

Tracheo-bronchial injuries could also be suspected in the presence of subcutaneous cervical emphysema expanding with mechanical ventilation, pneumo-mediastinum and recurrent pneumothorax due to the persisting air leak (Fig. 7.11) [17].

Sometimes, patients have other blunt lesions as laryngeal trauma, cervical spine or mandibular fractures, oesophageal injury, clavicular, scapular or ribs fractures. Oesophageal perforation is present in up to 20% of cases (Fig. 7.12).

Clinical features of tracheal stenosis (Fig. 7.13), as a consequence of a tracheal injury, include dyspnoea on effort, stridor or wheezing and episodes of obstruction even with small amounts of mucus. Other complications could be the development of a tracheo-oesophageal fistula (Fig. 7.14) or a tracheo-innominate fistula.

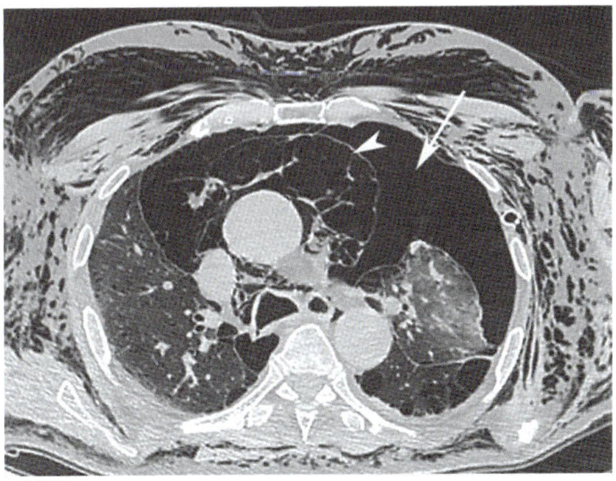

Fig. 7.11 Post-contrast axial CT scan evidences a diffuse subcutaneous chest cage emphysema associated with a large pneumo-mediastinum (*white arrow head*) and left pneumothorax (*white arrow*) due to air leak

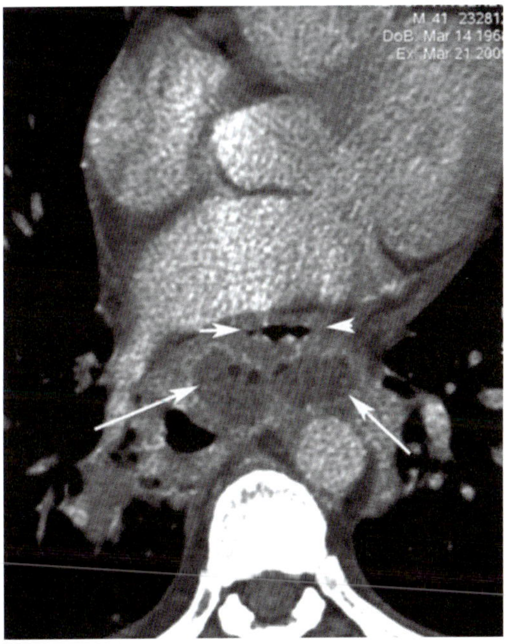

Fig. 7.12 Post-contrast CT axial image at the level of inferior mediastinum shows a mediastinal fluid collection (*white arrows*) mixed to air bubbles, posteriorly to the oesophagus (*white arrow heads*), due to oesophageal injury and perforation

The most common clinical manifestation of a post-traumatic tracheo-oesophageal fistula is represented by considerable secretion associated

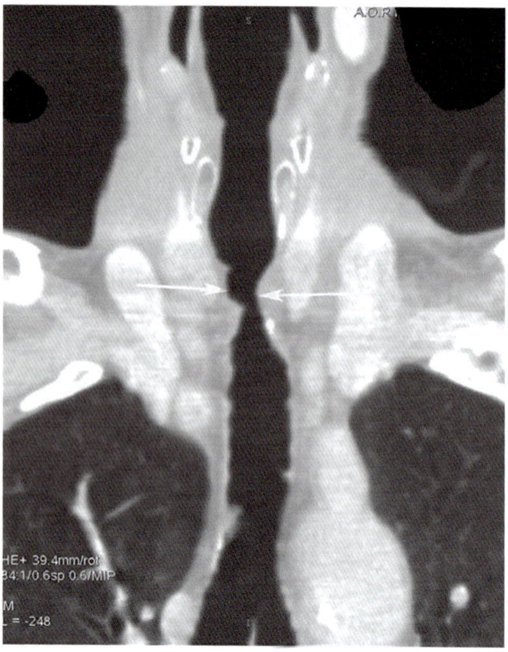

Fig. 7.13 CT coronal reconstruction of the trachea shows a post-traumatic stenosis (*white arrows*)

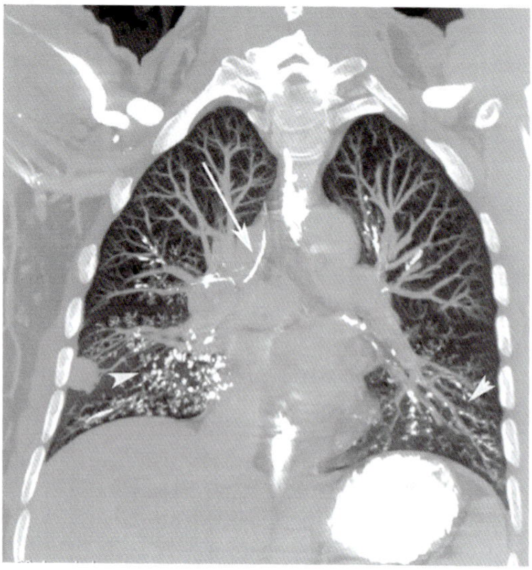

Fig. 7.14 CT coronal reconstruction obtained after administration of oral contrast demonstrates the passage of the c.m. from the lumen of the oesophagus in the lumen of the main right bronchus (*white arrows*) due to a post-traumatic broncho-oesophageal fistula. The oral contrast is also spread in the lumen of bilateral bronchial tree (*white arrow heads*)

with cough and recurrent broncho-pneumonia. Gastric lumen enlargement may also occur.

Tracheo-innominate fistula may be associated with severe haemoptysis.

7.3 CT Technique

CT is considered the more relevant diagnostic tool in patients with blunt chest trauma following the basic and indispensable chest X-ray film [18].

When a closed injury to the airways is suspected, it is important to perform immediate neck and chest CT scan, including three-dimensional image reconstruction of the trachea and the main bronchus.

Traditionally, the gold standard for the diagnosis is bronchoscopy because it enables visualization both the side and extent of the tracheo-bronchial injury. But in patients with severe respiratory insufficiency or in haemodinamically unstable patients, it may be impossible to perform. Bronchoscopy is not only time consuming, but also not always immediately available. Differently from bronchoscopy, CT is non-invasive, quicker and more ready available [5].

CT can clearly demonstrate fascial fat planes, arterial and venous vessels, larynx, trachea, bronchus and oesophagus traumatic lesions (Figs. 7.12 and 7.14), and it is the most important preoperative diagnostic imaging modality for determining the location, extent and type of airway lesions [6, 19].

7.4 MDCT Protocol Design Consideration

The MDCT protocol that is illustrated is designed for 64-row CT scanner; images are acquired at 0.625 collimation, with reconstruction axial slice of 2.5 mm, pitch of 0.984 and gantry rotation time of 0.5 s.

Preliminary unenhanced neck and chest CT is obtained to detect free air bubbles into the superficial and deep fascial fat planes or in fluid collections to depict blood clots inside haemothorax, haemopericardium and haemomediastinum.

Intravenous administration of contrast medium is mandatory for clearly evidencing neck and chest injuries.

Intravenous injection of a volume of 70–90 of iodine c.m. is generally sufficient for evaluating the enhancement of vessel lumen and surrounding other structures.

The contrast medium (c.m.) is injected with an 18–20 gauge needle through the ante-cubital vein by the use of a dual syringe power injector.

The c.m. transit time is determined by using a test-bolus in the ascending aorta lumen.

The optimal delay time corresponds to the peak arrival time of a test-bolus in the aortic lumen. The image acquisition is triggered at an attenuation threshold of 150 UH.

For better viewing, the enhancement alterations of the neck and chest tissues and vessels, contrast agents with higher concentration of iodine (400 mg/mL) and high injection rates (at least 3–4 mL/s) are preferred and are followed by a 30–50 mL saline chaser, also injected at a rate of 3–4 mL/s.

The c.m. arterial phase is mandatory to detect neck and chest arterial injuries.

The portal phase acquisition, obtained with a scan delay of 70 s, gives maximum airway wall, neck and mediastinum tissues and venous lumen enhancement.

In selected cases, orally administration of iodine contrast material could be helpful for demonstrating tracheo-oesophageal fistulization.

Sagittal and coronal MIP reformatted images are useful for localizing the ruptured segment of tracheo-bronchial tree and evaluating the map of the distribution of air bubbles, pneumothorax and blood collections. The post-processing procedure mainly requires a minimum-intensity projection technique for airway imaging. If tracheo-bronchial injury is suspected, three-dimensional (3D) extraction of the airway may be useful by focusing the 3D volume-rendering technique on the tracheo-bronchial tree. This technique is classically utilized for depicting stenosis or distortion of the tracheo-bronchial lumen, but may also allow the diagnosis of tracheo-bronchial injury by demonstrating a wall defect and/or an abnormal position of lobar and segmental bronchi [20].

7.5 Radiological Findings

As the clinical symptoms of acute airway injuries may not be specific and initially hidden by the presence of traumatic lesions of other organs and structures; the chest radiograph and CT scan are both important methods for diagnostic evaluation.

There are two main radiographic manifestations of tracheal and bronchial injuries: evidence of air leakage at the site of rupture and dysfunctional ventilation of the lung distal to the rupture. Evidence of air leakage is the more critical finding, and the absence of air leakage makes the diagnosis of a tear of the tracheo-bronchial tree very difficult (Fig. 7.15) [9].

The predominant radiographic findings could be attributed to air leak evidenced by cervical and thoracic subcutaneous emphysema and various degrees of pneumo-mediastinum and pneumothorax (Fig. 7.8). The coexistence of a pneumothorax and pneumo-mediastinum is the strongest manifestation of a bronchial rupture. On the other hand, if the outer adventitial layer of the bronchus remains intact, no air leak may exist, a situation that occurs in approximately 10% of cases of tracheo-bronchial lesion.

The presence of pneumo-mediastinum is a critical finding in patients with severe chest

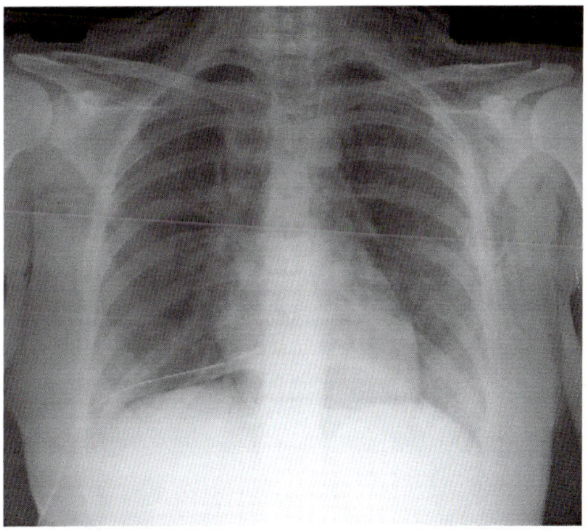

Fig. 7.15 Chest radiograph shows subcutaneous emphysema especially diffused into supraclavicular fat planes; it is also present pneumo-mediastinum, with multiple lucencies along mediastinal planes and pericardium. A pleural tube has been inserted on the right

trauma and may be the only visible sign of an air leak associated with tears of tracheal wall or intra-mediastinal portion of the bronchi. It is a more specific sign of a breaking of airway integrity.

Air in the mediastinum is seen as streaky lucencies in the carinal region extending superiorly as the air dissects in the tissue planes around the trachea, aorta and great vessels. On the margins of the mediastinum, the air dissects and elevates the mediastinal parietal pleura from the aorta, the venous vessels and the heart (Fig. 7.15). On lateral films, a pneumo-mediastinum is best appreciated inside the retrosternal space.

Subcutaneous emphysema is a non-specific sign. It is most likely the result of decompression of pneumo-mediastinum [21] and is more commonly found in the acutely traumatized patients after difficult intubation, penetrating chest wounds or multiple rib fractures [22].

Conventional chest radiography shows pneumo-mediastinum in 60% of cases. Absence of pneumo-mediastinum in the presence of tracheo-bronchial tear has been attributed to preservation of the integrity of the paratracheal or peribronchial connective tissue layer or transitory occlusion of the tear by an endotracheal balloon cuff or by fibrin [23].

However, the most common X-ray film finding is pneumothorax (Fig. 7.16), found in 60% up to 100% of cases. Other radiographic signs include over-distension of endotracheal tube cuff, displacement of endotracheal tube or, in the case of complete transection, the fallen lung sign of Kumpe (Fig. 7.10) [24].

A pneumothorax is also a frequent sign associated with rib fractures and its potential significance may be overlooked.

CT performed with appropriate window settings can frequently demonstrate the exact site of tracheo-bronchial tear, by showing a circumferential absence of the tracheal wall, a parietal defect of the posterior wall of the trachea (Fig. 7.17) or bronchus (Fig. 7.4), a contour deformity (Figs. 7.18, 7.19, and 7.20), a fracture of the cartilage rings of the trachea or a fistulization with other mediastinal structures, especially oesophagus (Fig. 7.14) and innominate artery [25].

Other specific CT findings include over-distension of the tracheal tube balloon (Fig. 7.21a, b), the herniation of the deformed endotracheal tube balloon beyond the trachea (Fig. 7.22) or an extra-luminal position of the endotracheal tube [26].

In addition, CT can evidence other associated findings as cervical and thoracic subcutaneous emphysema, pneumothorax, pneumo-mediastinum

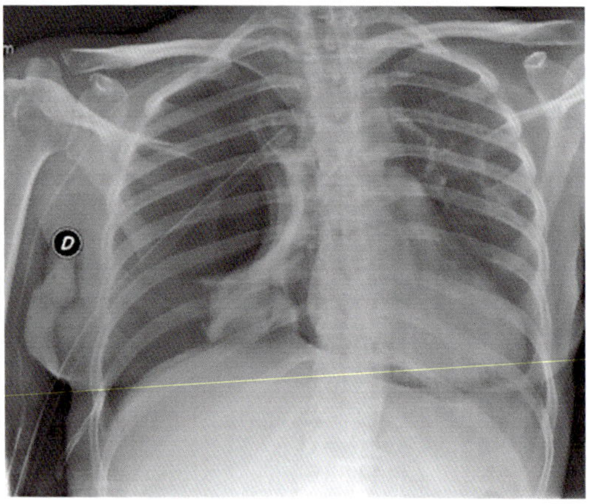

Fig. 7.16 Chest radiograph shows a right undertension pneumothorax. Right lung is seen to be collapsed below the hilus (fallen lung sign). A pleural tube has been inserted on the right

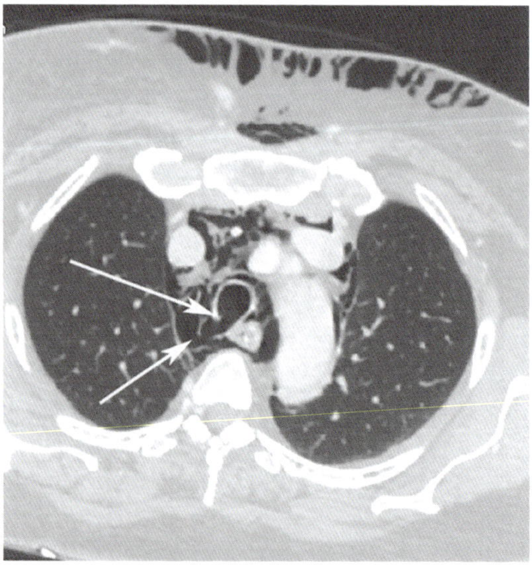

Fig. 7.17 Post-contrast axial CT scan at level of upper mediastinum shows a parietal defect of the posterior wall of the trachea (*white arrows*), associated with pneumo-mediastinum and subcutaneous emphysema

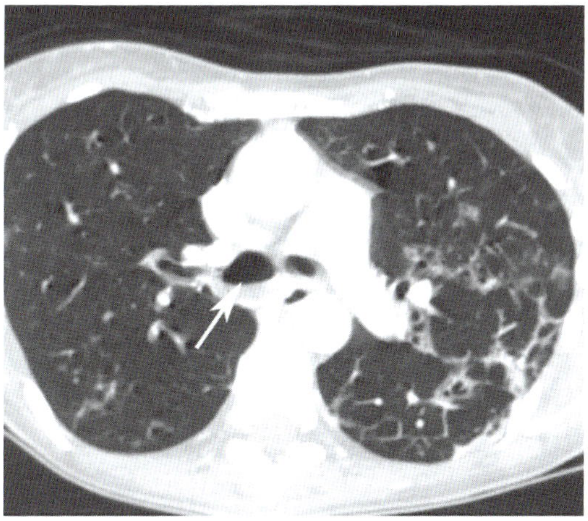

Fig. 7.18 Post-contrast axial CT scan at level of middle mediastinum shows an enlargement of main right bronchus due to a partial tear of the wall

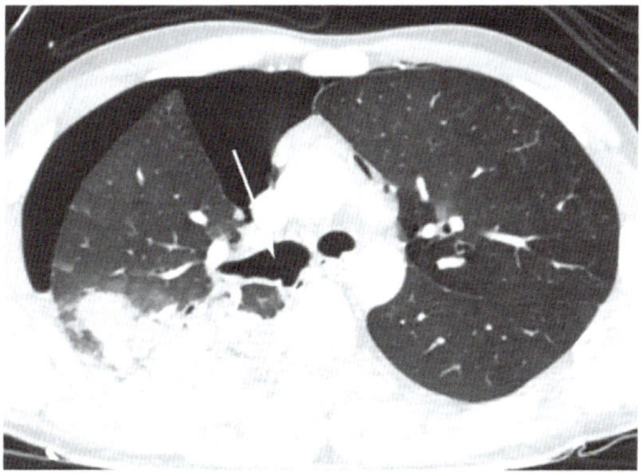

Fig. 7.19 Post-contrast axial CT scan at level of mainstem bronchus depicts an enlargement with contour deformity of the main right bronchus (*white arrow*). There is a right pneumothorax associated with a large lung contusion with alveolar haemorrhage

and air surrounding a bronchus (Fig. 7.23), abnormalities in the appearance of an endotracheal tube, with over-distension of the cuff or extra-luminal position of the tip, the "fallen lung sign" and upper thoracic fractures that involve the clavicles, scapula, sternum and ribs. Among these features, cervical and thoracic subcutaneous emphysema are the most consistent CT findings in tracheal injury caused by blunt trauma [27].

If the source of the subcutaneous air is unknown and it does not increase in amount, it may be considered of little clinical significance.

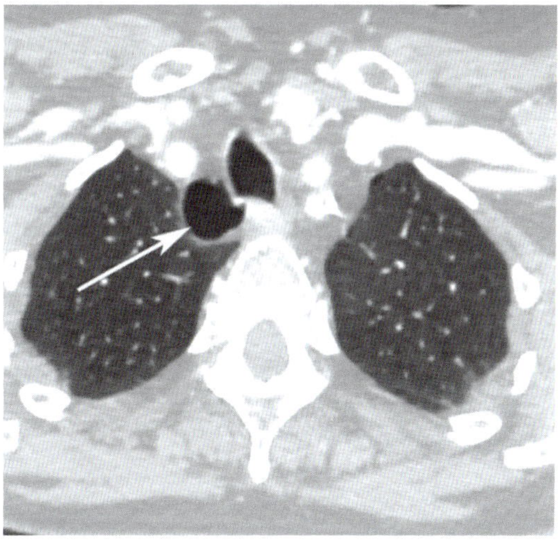

Fig. 7.20 Axial CT scan at level of middle mediastinum shows a pseudo-diverticulum of the right posterior wall of the trachea, as a consequence of a partial tear

In the presence of tracheo-bronchial laceration, when air inside the fascial fat planes is a consequence of continuing air leak, the subcutaneous emphysema would be expected to persist or increase (Fig. 7.23).

Oesophageal injury is sometimes associated with tracheo-bronchial tear. It is associated with a clear tear of the oesophageal wall or with the presence of air bubbles around the oesophagus (Fig. 7.12).

Persistent pneumothorax after pleural drainage tube application is correlated with the "fallen lung" sign and is demonstrated by the collapsed lung, recoiling away from the hilum, towards the dependent portion of the haemithorax (Fig. 7.16) [28]. The term "fallen lung" refers to the peripheral displacement rather than the usual central position of the collapsed lung. This is usually the result of complete rupture of a bronchus wall [28, 29].

The airway tear associated with haemorrhage can occlude the bronchial tree lumen by clots and blood aspiration and interfere with the ventilation of the related pulmonary lobe, with consequential atelectasis. In these cases, there are differential diagnostic difficulties because in severely traumatized patients, atelectasis may develop also for a severe lung contusion with alveolar haemorrhage.

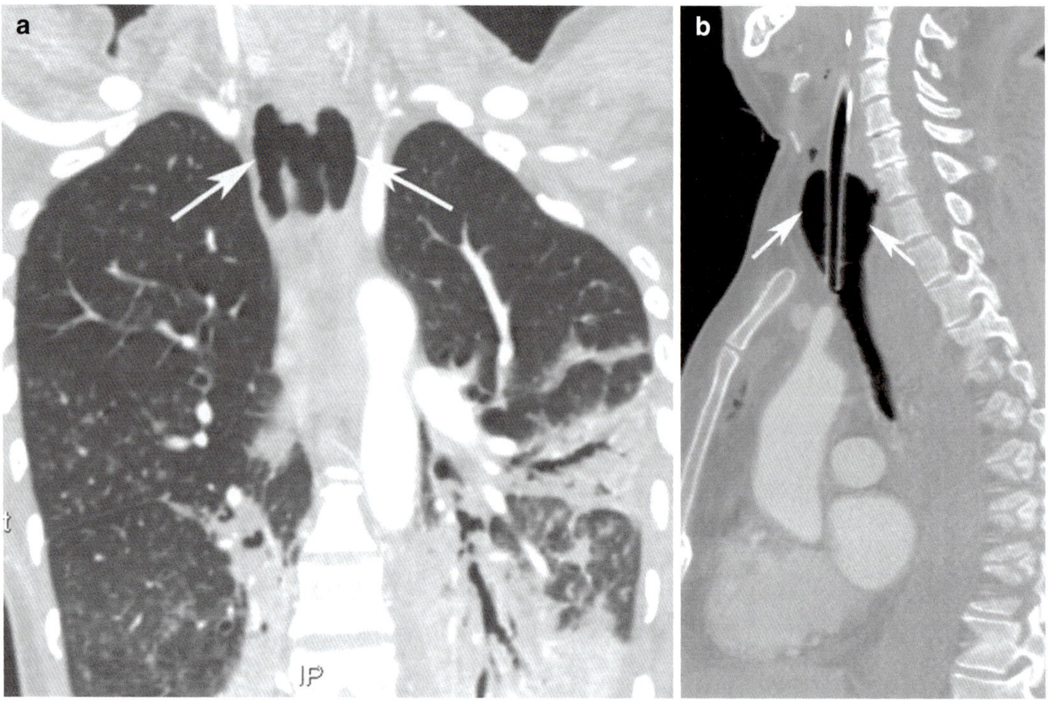

Fig. 7.21 CT coronal (**a**) and sagittal (**b**) reconstruction evidence the over-distension of the tracheal tube balloon, herniating through injury site

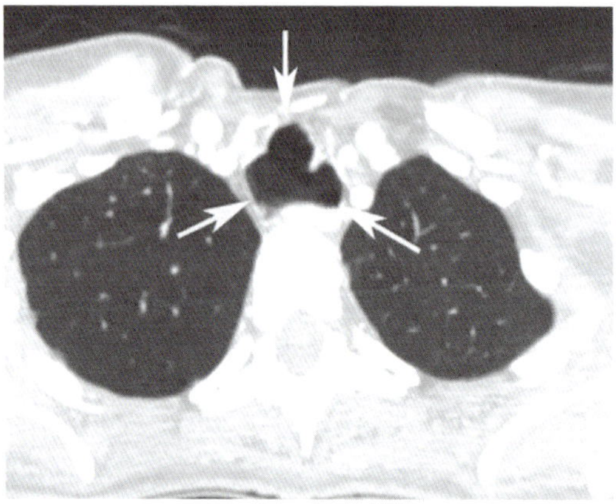

Fig. 7.22 Axial CT scan at level of middle mediastinum shows the "Mickey Mouse head" sign demonstrated by the over-distension of the tracheal tube balloon, herniating besides the tracheal wall

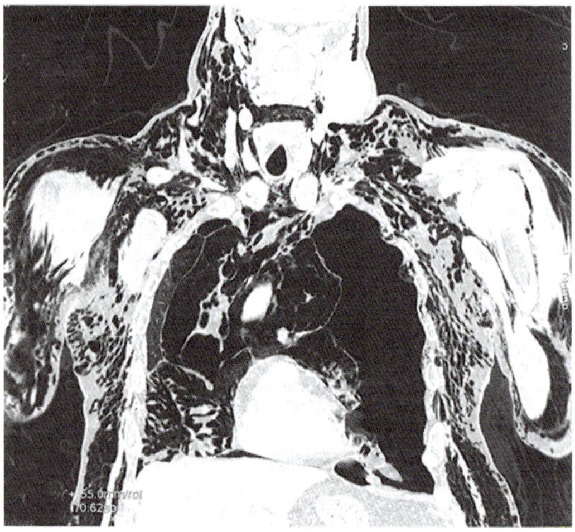

Fig. 7.23 CT coronal reconstruction demonstrates extensive cervical and thoracic subcutaneous emphysema diffused also into shoulders and superior limbs, left pneumothorax and severe pneumo-mediastinum

Atelectasis correlated with bronchial rupture is usually persistent and unresponsive to normal therapeutic procedures. Collapse of the lung is also waited in the presence of pneumothorax, particularly if it is large and under tension.

In a small number of cases, the CT diagnosis of major airway injury has been supposed by observing an unusual configuration of the air-filled cuff of the mechanical ventilation tube or an abnormally positioned endotracheal tube. Normally, the walls of the trachea circumscribe the cuff of the tube. In the presence of a tracheal rupture, the diameter of the over-distended endotracheal balloon cuff can be greater of the normal diameter of the trachea (Figs. 7.21 and 7.22).

In cases in which the tracheo-bronchial tear depends on a traumatic intubation, the tip of the endotracheal tube may be seen to be positioned outside the tracheal lumen [30].

Pneumothorax in patients with tracheobronchial transection is the result of rupture of the mediastinal pleura, or injury to the right mainstem bronchus or distal left bronchus, allowing air to enter the pleural space on the same side.

Tears in the trachea or proximal left main bronchus produce central air dissection with cervical and mediastinal emphysema without pneumothorax [31].

Other associated CT findings could be haemothorax, myocardial contusion, haemopericardium and oesophageal tear.

The presence of any kind of bone fractures involving the upper thorax associated with airway injuries is approximately 40%.

Especially fractures involving one or more of the upper three ribs in addition to an ipsilateral pneumothorax are considered to provide an important diagnostic indication to tracheobronchial transection. Although fracture of an upper rib may suggest the possibility of a contemporary fractured bronchus, rib fractures generally occur more often in the absence of airway injury [6]. Frequently, the rupture of the first three ribs is on the opposite side of the bronchus transection.

These fractures are common in patients over 30 years age, with reports of their frequency varying from 40 to 90%; on the other hand are uncommon in children and young adults with tracheo-bronchial tears because of the greater flexibility of the thoracic cage [12]. The thoracic fractures may also involve the clavicles, scapula and sternum.

Three-dimensional reconstruction of the airway associated with multiple oblique reformations of the lungs is particularly useful for evidencing a complete bronchial rupture, especially if it is located just below the origin of the bronchus and associated with a partial or total collapse of the pulmonary lobes.

7.6 Management of Tracheal Injuries

Early repair of injuries to the airways helps to preserve the function of these structures (b). The main therapeutic aim is to maintain the airway patency.

The management may be difficult and includes endotracheal intubation or eventually emergency tracheostomy [18].

At the admission, all patients suspected for neck and/or thoracic trauma have to receive fluid resuscitation and vital signs should be stabilized.

As soon as possible, the patient should also be assessed and treated for eventual consequent haemorrhagic shock and other important organs and apparatus lesions. If it is necessary, blood transfusion has to be done.

If a III or IV degree of dyspnoea is present, a tracheotomy is needed.

Cervical tracheal injury management has a different approach than mediastinal one.

If a small partial laceration of cervical trachea is identified and there is a good apposition of lacerated tissue and there are no other associated injuries, the tear can be treated conservatively.

In this case, the endotracheal tube is placed distal to the lesion, and the cuff is kept inflated for some days. Cervical tracheal injury may also be treated with primary repair without tracheostomy. This approach is indicated with most knife and gunshot wounds and occasional cases of blunt transection.

For complex shattering injuries, the tracheostomy may be best done through the damaged tract of the cervical trachea.

For injuries to mediastinal trachea, the surgical approach is based on thoracotomy. Tracheostomy is rarely needed. Most patients have selective intubation of the main-stem bronchus, double lumen tube or jet ventilation.

There is debate regarding whether airway patency is best maintained by tracheal intubation or by tracheotomy [31]. Blind oral intubation in patients with tracheal injury can lead to false extra-tracheal intubation and irreversible damage to the airway. If tracheotomy is performed before confirmation of the diagnosis, the distal end of the injured trachea may retract into the thoracic cavity, causing airway obstruction and death.

After validation of diagnosis, the patient with significant tracheal injury should undergo standard tracheostomy to reduce the risk of potential damage of airway.

The diagnosis of tracheo-bronchial rupture should be performed before proceeding with any treatment.

In patients with partial tracheal rupture, oral-tracheal intubation may worsen the damage and lead to massive haemorrhage causing worsening of dyspnoea [32]. The distal end of the trachea may retract into the thoracic cavity and intubation attempts may increase the separation between the ends of the tracheal borders and can cause additional trauma and haemorrhage in the tracheal lumen and inside surrounding tissues.

If the endotracheal tube cannot be successfully placed in the distal end of disrupted trachea, respiratory distress may increase and the patient may die owing to airway obstruction.

Tracheal fracture should be repaired as soon as possible, before the development of surrounding adhesions and scars, for preventing the development of granulation tissue, scarring and tracheal stenosis (Figs. 7.1 and 7.13).

A tracheal stenosis rarely demands a definitive procedure either electively or emergently. However, emergency management of obstruction may include the placement of the tracheostomy through the stricture, then through the old tracheostomy site, then remote from the lesion.

Conservative measures can be added on a chronic basis with a stent, especially if the patient is of poor risk or has a partial thickness lesion with potential for regression.

Conclusions

Closed injury of the airways due to blunt trauma is rare and presents diagnostic and management challenges. Early diagnosis is important and a high suspicion is required, particularly in cases of head, neck or chest trauma and in patients with discordant clinical findings who respond poorly to therapeutic measures. We vigorously advise CT scan before bronchoscopy, as reliable diagnostic modality for closed injury to the cervical trachea. Early recognition and airway management are important [12, 33, 34].

Although always symptomatic, tracheo-bronchial injury is a rare entity, not easy to diagnose. The lack of specificity of subcutaneous emphysema, stridor, pneumo-mediastinum, haemoptysis, pneumothorax and the occult nature of the rupture frequently result in a delayed diagnosis. In addition, associated injuries such as head and abdominal severe trauma can hide the diagnosis in the early period following hospital admission, and the emergency procedure may also interfere with the diagnostic one.

Among all clinical and radiological signs that are frequently observed in tracheo-bronchial rupture, both the presence of pneumo-mediastinum and cervical emphysema appears to be the most frequent association [26, 35]. The pneumo-mediastinum is related to the tracheal or bronchial rupture into the hilum with a retrograde dissection into the mediastinum.

Logically, tracheo-bronchial rupture should not be associated with pulmonary interstitial emphysema, a radiological sign resulting from alveolar rupture at the lung periphery [36].

The interstitial emphysema could not be related to airway injuries, but it is frequently associated, suggesting that alveolar barotrauma and tracheo-bronchial injuries might be associated in many patients with severe blunt chest trauma [37].

Early diagnosis and treatment of airway injuries are mandatory because the severity of the injury is frequently life threatening [1, 38].

The diagnosis of tracheo-bronchial rupture should be confirmed before undertaking surgical repair.

Traditionally, the gold standard for the diagnosis is bronchoscopy because it enables direct visualization of both the side and extent of the tracheo-bronchial tear. But in patients with severe respiratory insufficiency or in haemodinamically unstable patients, it may be impossible to perform.

In fact, bronchoscopy is a procedure that requires specific skills and therefore is not always and easily available under emergency conditions [39].

Furthermore, endotracheal intubation often precludes the use of rigid bronchoscopy, necessary for clearing the airways from blood, clots and secretions. Sometimes, the technical conditions of the bronchoscopy are unreliable, for the presence of large blood quantity inside the airway lumen and a rapid drop of arterial oxygen saturation, all factors that preclude the procedure.

Differently from bronchoscopy, CT is non-invasive, quicker and more ready available.

CT has an overall sensitivity of 85% [26]. It is the most important preoperative diagnostic imaging modality for determining the location, extent and type of airway lesions.

CT is also considered the more relevant diagnostic tool in patients with blunt chest trauma following the basic and essential chest X-ray film [26].

References

1. Conn JH, Hardy JD, Fain WR, et al. Thoracic trauma: analysis of 1022 cases. J Trauma. 1963;3:22–40.
2. Shorr RM, Critten M, Indeck M, et al. Blunt thoracic trauma: analysis of 515 patients. Ann Surg. 1987;206:200–5.
3. Lee RB. Traumatic injury of the cervicothoracic trachea and major bronchi. Chest Surg Clin N Am. 1997;7:285–304.
4. Glinjongol C, Pakdirat B. Management of tracheobronchial injuries: a 10 year experience at Ratchaburi Hospital. J Med Assoc Thail. 2005;88:32–40.
5. Bertelsen S, Howitz P. Injuries of the trachea and bronchi. Thorax. 1972;27:188–94.
6. Wiot JF. Tracheobronchial trauma. Semin Roentgenol. 1983;18:15–22.
7. Kaewlai R, Avery LL, Asrani AV, et al. Multidetector CT of blunt thoracic trauma. Radiographics. 2008; 28:1555–70.
8. Symbas PN, Justics AG, Ricketts RR. Rupture of the airways from blunt trauma: treatment of complex injuries. Ann Thorac Surg. 1992;54:177–83.
9. Karmy-Jones R, Wood DE. Traumatic injury to the trachea and bronchus. Thorac Surg Clin. 2007;17:35–46.
10. Kiser AC, O'Brien SM, Detterbeck FC. Blunt tracheobronchial injuries: treatment and outcomes. Ann Thorac Surg. 2001;71:2059–65.
11. Sangster GP, Gonzales-Beicos A, Carbo AL, et al. Blunt traumatic injuries of the lung parenchyma, pleura, thoracic wall and intratoracic airways; multidetector computer tomography imaging findings. Emerg Radiol. 2007;14:297–310.
12. Burke JF. Early diagnosis of traumatic rupture of the bronchus. JAMA. 1962;181:682–6.
13. Valerio P, Ivan M, Francisco R, et al. Survival after traumatic complete laryngotracheal transection. Am J Emerg Med. 2008;26(837):e3–4.
14. Loh KS, Irish JC. Traumatic complications of intubation and other airway management procedures. Anesthesiol Clin North Am. 2002;20:953–69.
15. Cassada DC, Munyikwa MP, Monitz MP, et al. Acute injuries of the trachea and major bronchi: importance of early diagnosis. Ann Thorac Surg. 2000;69: 1563–7.
16. Rossbach MM, Johnson SB, Gomez MA, et al. Management of major tracheobronchial ruptures: a 28 year experience. Ann Thorac Surg. 1998;65:182–6.
17. Tcherveniak A, Tchalakov P, Tcherveniak P. Traumatic and iatrogenic lesions of the trachea and bronchi. Eur J Cardiothorac Surg. 2001;19:19–24.
18. Trupka A, Waydhas C, Hallfeldt KK, et al. Value of thoracic computed tomography in the first assessment of severely injured patients with blunt chest trauma: results of a prospective study. J Trauma. 1997;43:405–11.
19. Hood RM, Sloan HE. Injuries of the trachea and major bronchi. J Thorac Cardiovasc Surg. 1959;38: 458–80.
20. Silverman PM, Zeiberg AS, Sessions RB, et al. Helical CT of the upper airway: normal and abnorml findings on three-dimensional reonstructed images. AJR. 1995;165:541–6.
21. Macklin MT, Macklin CC. Malignant interstitial emphysema of the lungs and mediastinum. Medicine. 1944;23:281–358.
22. Tocino IM, Miller MH. Mediastinal trauma and other acute mediastinal conditions. J Thorac Imag. 1987;2:79–100.
23. Chesteman JT, Satsangi PH. Rupture of the trachea and bronchi by closed injury. Thorax. 1966;21:21–7.
24. Stark P. Imaging of tracheobronchial injuries. J Thoracic Imaging. 1995;10:206–19.
25. Epelman M, Ofer A, Klein V, et al. CT diagnosis of traumatic rupture in children. Pediatr Radiol. 2002;1(32):888–91.
26. Chen JD, Shanmuganathan K, Mirvis SE, et al. Using CT to diagnose tracheal rupture. AJR. 2001;176:1273–80.
27. Meislin HW, Iserson KV, Kaback KR. Airway trauma. Emerg Med Clin North Am. 1983;1:295–312.
28. Thack D, Defrance P, Delcour C, et al. The CT fallen lung sign. Eur Radiol. 2000;10:719–21.

29. Wintermark M, Schnyder P, Wicky S. Blunt traumatic rupture of a main bronchus: spiral CT demonstration of the fallen lung sign. Eur Radiol. 2001;11:409–11.
30. Almasi M, Andrasovska M, Koval J. Blunt external trauma to the trachea: report of two cases. B-ENT. 2005;1:93–6.
31. Kirsh MM, Orriger MB, Behrendt DM, et al. Management of tracheobronchial disruption secondary to nonpenetrating trauma. Ann Thorac Surg. 1976;22:93–101.
32. Rollins RJ, Tocino I. Early radiographic signs of tracheal rupture. AJR. 1987;148:695–8.
33. Ejigelaar A, Homan van der Heide JN. A reliable early symptom of bronchial or tracheal rupture. Thorax. 1970;25:120–5.
34. Karaaslan T, Meuli R, Androux R, et al. Traumatic chest lesions in patients with severe head trauma: a comparative study with computed tomography and conventional chest roentgenograms. J Trauma. 1995;39:1081–6.
35. Atkins BZ, Abbate S, Fisher SR, et al. Current management of laryngotracheal trauma: case report and literature review. J Trauma. 2004;56:185–90.
36. Nishiumi N, Maitani F, Yamada S, et al. Chest radiography assessment of tracheobronchial disruption associated with blunt chest trauma. J Trauma. 2002;53:372–7.
37. Macklin CC. Transport of air along sheats of pulmonic blood vessels from alveoli to mediastinum: clinical implications. Arch Inter Med. 1939;64:913–26.
38. Balci AE, Eren N, Eren S, et al. Surgical tratment of post traumatic tracheobronchial injuries: 14 year experience. Eur J Cardiothorac Surg. 2002;22:984–9.
39. Mussi A, Ambrogi MC, Ribecchini A, et al. Acute major airway injuries: clinical features and management. Eur J Cardiothorac Surg. 2001;20:46–51.

Lung/Pleural Injuries

8

Chiara Moroni, Alessandra Bindi, Edoardo Cavigli, Diletta Cozzi, Monica Marina Lanzetta, Peiman Nazerian, and Vittorio Miele

8.1 Introduction

Trauma is the most common cause of death during the first three decades of life in occidental countries, followed only by malignancies, and deaths for thoracic trauma account for about 25% of all trauma deaths [1]. As thoracic trauma may produce injuries to endothoracic organs that play a vital role in normal physiology and homeostasis, some injuries to the chest and its contents, if unrecognized or untreated, may produce death within minutes [2]. In the diagnostic algorithm of thoracic trauma, clinical data are of extreme importance and must be well recognized by the emergency physician. But, because of the low specificity of most of them consisting mainly in dyspnea, cough, hemoptysis, chest pain and, in very critical cases, in severe hypoxia or shock, imaging plays an essential role in the diagnostic work-up of these events permitting in most cases a fast and definite diagnosis and, therefore, a prompt adequate treatment.

Thoracic traumas are frequently due to blunt traumas (70–90%), generally consequent to road accidents (85%) and, less frequently, to working or domestic accidents [2]; open traumas from wounds, either ballistic or non-ballistic, are rare [3]. Lung and pleural involvement is very frequent in each of these as they are involved in approximately 65–75% [4] in blunt thoracic traumas and in nearly 95% of open traumas [5].

In blunt thoracic trauma, we find at least three different mechanism of action: direct force, rapid deceleration, and barotrauma. Usually, each modality is responsible for different effects on thoracic structures. Direct trauma generally interests structures near the site of impact and, very often, damages the thoracic cage. In deceleration traumas, intrathoracic mobile organs or regions, such as heart, ascending aorta, or pulmonary parenchyma, are thorn off from adjacent organs or structure that are fixed to the thoracic cage (such as descending aorta, trachea, and main bronchi) or may hit nearby bony structures as ribs or spine [2]. Blunt trauma has got a very peculiar

C. Moroni, M.D. (✉) • A. Bindi • E. Cavigli
D. Cozzi • M.M. Lanzetta • V. Miele
Department of Radiology, Careggi University Hospital, L.go G. A. Brambilla 3, 50134 Florence, Italy
e-mail: chiaramoroni73@gmail.com; bindialessandra@gmail.com; edoardocavigli@yahoo.it; dilettacozzi@gmail.com; monica.lanzetta@virgilio.it; vmiele@sirm.org

P. Nazerian
Department of Emergency Medicine, Careggi Univeristy Hospital, Florence, Italy
e-mail: nazerianp@aou-careggi.toscana.it

V. Miele, M. Trinci (eds.), *Diagnostic Imaging in Polytrauma Patients*,
https://doi.org/10.1007/978-3-319-62054-1_8

mechanism of action due to the drastic increment of intrathoracic pressure. In this case, the principal organs involved are lungs and airways. But, very frequently, the three mechanisms coexist in many traumatic events, and the involvement of thoracic organs consists in different associations of injuries [2].

In open trauma, we can find different mechanisms of damage starting from the direct stab of non-ballistic wounds to the complex mechanism of injury of a bullet wound. The resultant injuries are the same as in blunt trauma but, as in open traumas there are imaging peculiarities that should be acknowledged [5], we will discuss them separately at the end of the chapter.

8.2 Imaging Modalities

In an emergency context, three imaging modalities are helpful in the diagnosis of a thoracic trauma: chest X-ray, ultrasound (US) examination, and multidetector computed tomography (MDCT). Chest plain film and US examination play an important role in the initial emergency work-up of post-traumatic thoracic injuries as they are cheap and bedside available [2, 6] and should be considered the first and last imaging approach in unstable patients as MDCT is the technique of choice in stable ones.

Chest radiography is the first-line examination for assessment of thoracic trauma in the emergency setting [7]. Generally, in the emergency room with patients obliged in a supine position, single-view anteroposterior radiographs have many limitations characterized mainly by the incapacity to distinguish alterations in superimposed opacification from bones or damaged lung parenchyma and the impossibility to see air-fluid levels as the XR beam is perpendicular to the air-fluid level surface. Furthermore, the scarce inspiratory status and the heart magnification effect can produce apparent increases in pulmonary vascularity and pseudo-cardiomegaly [7].

Actually, many studies confirmed its lacking in sensibility and specificity compared to chest MDCT [1, 8, 9]. In particular, in 2007 Brink et al. [8] demonstrated the higher accuracy of routine chest CT in detecting lung injuries in post-traumatic patients compared to elective CT acquired only post-positive chest X-ray. More recently, Corbacioglu et al. confirmed this statement [9]. Both the authors, furthermore, proved that the nonselective CT method had changed the course of patient management in 2–22% of the patients [8, 9].

Nevertheless, chest X-ray is a useful tool for the patient evaluation in the emergency setting of thoracic trauma as it should be considered a completion of the history and physical examination [7]. Furthermore, in unstable patient's chest X-ray can rapidly detect tension pneumothorax and massive hemothorax while the patient is still in the emergency room, thus permitting immediate treatment of these life threatening conditions [2].

Chest US examination is a bedside procedure with rapid availability, absence of ionizing radiation (children and pregnant patients can be safely examined), easy repeatability, and lack of contraindications and can be performed at patient supine in the emergency room. Furthermore, US can guide invasive procedures, e.g., drainage of pleural effusions or of tension pneumothorax [10, 11].

Its limitations consist mainly in its dependence on the patient constitution (obese patients cannot be easily explored) and clinical conditions (chest US is not feasible in the presence of extensive subcutaneous emphysema) and in its dependence on the skills of the examiner, which implies that adequate training in US of the chest is a prerequisite for proper results [10]. Another important disadvantage is that pulmonary lesions can only be detected if they are pleura based [10].

Since 2008, the BLUE protocol included chest US for detection of pleuropulmonary emergencies, including pneumothoraces, pleural effusions, and pulmonary consolidations, in patients with respiratory failure admitted to the emergency department, demonstrating that chest US is a rapid and helpful tool in reducing diagnostic time in critical patients [12]. More recently, Zanobetti et al. demonstrated, in a very large cohort of patients, a higher sensitivity of US, compared to chest X-ray, for pneumothorax, free pleural effusion, and pulmonary consolidations in dyspnoic patients presenting in the emergency department [13].

Regarding post-traumatic patients, Hyacinthe et al. demonstrated that chest US acquired in the emergency room is a better diagnostic test than objective examination plus chest X-ray in comparison with CT scanning, particularly for diagnosing pneumothorax and lung contusion [14].

Actually, US examination of the thorax is strongly suggested in addiction to abdominal examination as part of the extended-FAST (focused assessment with sonography for trauma) [6, 15, 16] which has been developed in order to rule out pleural and pericardial post-traumatic alterations along with the abdominal ones [6].

The US chest examination in post-traumatic patients is generally performed with a linear probe. A range of frequencies (4–12 MHz) can be used to visualize the lungs. High frequencies are useful to look at the periphery of the lung with a high resolution as in looking for signs of pneumothorax. Lower US frequencies help with the imaging of deep lung tissues as in looking at consolidation. The examination consists mainly of longitudinal and oblique scans acquired on anteromedial, anterolateral, and posterolateral thoracic wall areas [6]. In polytraumatized patients, it is targeted to the detection of specific US patterns identified according to the international recommendations on point-of-care lung US for pulmonary contusion, pneumothorax, and pleural effusion (in particular hemothorax) [16, 17]. US signs of normal and injured pleura and lung are based mainly on the high acoustic mismatch between aerated lung tissues and the pleura which casts a total reflection of the sound wave [18]. When air content within the lungs decreases (e.g., in lung contusion), the acoustic mismatch is lowered, and the ultrasound wave can partly demonstrate the deeper pulmonary parenchymal structures. It is important to note that many signs at lung US represent artifacts occurring naturally because of acoustic mismatch of tissues reflecting sound waves [18].

Actually, MDCT has established itself as the preferred imaging method for the evaluation of polytrauma patients [19]. MDCT is widely available, quick, permits a whole-body imaging, offers the possibility of multiplanar and three-dimensional reconstructions, and it has been established as more sensitive and specific than chest radiography [1, 8, 9, 19].

MDCT in a post-traumatic chest should always include a direct acquisition with at least three window levels: one dedicated to the visualization of lung parenchyma; one for soft (mediastinal) structures; and one for the evaluation of bones. These permit us to respectively detect: pulmonary injuries and pneumothoraces, recent hematic extravasations inside (hemothorax) or outside the pleural space (hemopericardium or hematoma), and scheletric disruptions.

Successively, it is mandatory to perform an angio CT of the thoracic aorta in order to rule out large vessels injuries and to depict any contrast media extravasation suggesting arterial active bleeding. A venous and a delayed acquisition are important in order to rule out the non-arterial bleedings [3]. Furthermore, we must not forget that a traumatized patient is often a thoraco-abdominal one. This statement is particularly true in open traumas where stab or bullet trajectories often include supra- and infra-diaphragmatic structures [5].

Isotropic acquisition is necessary in order to obtain high quality multiplanar and tridimensional reconstructions, helpful in detecting irregular or complex wound trajectories and in exactly evaluating the site and the extension of post-traumatic injuries.

In this chapter, we will discuss the principal MDCT aspects of lung and pleural injuries following blunt and open thoracic trauma.

8.3 Pleural Injuries

Pleura is frequently involved in chest trauma [2] due to its ubiquitarian localization along the inner surface of the chest wall. Generally, when a mechanical breach to the pleural surface occurs after a penetrating or blunt injury, the collapsed interpleural space may fill with air, blood, or both, forming, respectively, a pneumothorax, a hemothorax, or a hemopneumothorax [20]. The percentage of their incidence in chest traumas is approximately 28% for hemothorax, 28% for pneumothorax, and 11% for hemopneumothorax [2].

8.3.1 Pneumothorax

Pneumothorax refers to an air collection in the pleural space, and it is found in about 15% to 50% of cases of blunt trauma [2]. The rate of bilateral pneumothorax is reported to be 8–10%. In 52% of these cases, pneumothorax develops in the right hemithorax; in 44%, it develops in the left; and in 4% it developed bilaterally [21].

Following blunt trauma, the main mechanism accountable for a pneumothorax is usually laceration to the visceral pleura from the sharp edges of fractured ribs. It can also be caused, in the absence of rib fractures, by peripheral lung lacerations or by ruptured alveoli and visceral pleura due to the drastic increase of intrapulmonary pressure in barotraumas or even, more rarely, by rupture of the proximal airways [20]. This last rare event is achieved only if the lesion affects the pleura-covered bronchial wall nearby the pulmonary hilum. Otherwise, airways lesions more frequently generate pneumomediastinum [20]. Penetrating injuries are also likely to produce pneumothorax due to direct pleural laceration, with air entering the interpleural space via either the chest wall or the lacerated lung [7].

The diagnosis of pneumothorax with chest X-ray in a supine patient relies on few, scarcely visible, signs. In particular, as in supine patients the free air collects anteriorly, medially, and basally, we should search for one or more of the next signs: hyperlucency at the lung base, a better definition of the mediastinal contour, the "deep sulcus" sign (an apparent deepening of the costophrenic angle) and the "double diaphragm" sign, the latter consisting in the presence of two diaphragm-lung interfaces [7]. Actually, 10–50% of pneumothoraces are not diagnosed on chest radiographs acquired on supine chest X-rays in emergency rooms [19] also if it frequently permits to depict rib fractures (Fig. 8.1).

Due to the lack of sensitivity of chest X-ray in the supine position, US has progressively been taken into account. In 2010, an evidence-based review of chest X-ray and US in post-traumatic pneumothorax, found a US sensitivity ranging from 86 to 98% in the enrolled studies, an US specificity of 97–100%, a supine chest X-ray sensitivity of 28–75%, and a chest X-ray specificity of 100%, suggesting that bedside thoracic US is a more sensitive screening test than supine chest X-ray in detecting pneumothorax in blunt chest trauma [16, 22]. In a recent study, compared to

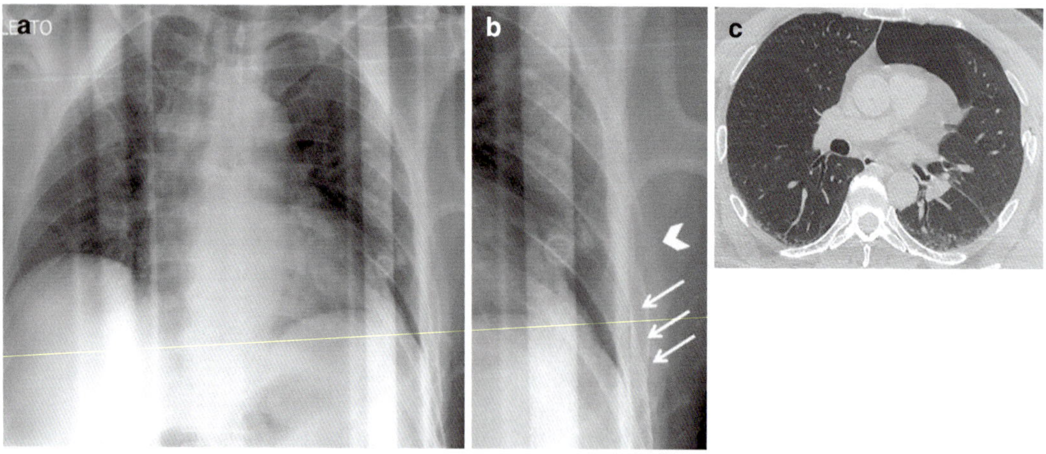

Fig. 8.1 Left pneumothorax. Supine chest X-ray acquired in the emergency room (**a**) (note the opacity of the spinal support over imposed) where is scarcely appreciable a "deep sulcus sign" at the basal left of the radiogram (*arrows*) suggesting a subtle layer of anterobasal left PNX, associated with a rib fracture (*arrowhead*). The signs are better depictable in the magnification (**b**). The chest CT examination in (**c**) confirms the diagnosis

chest CT as gold standard, the sensitivity of bed US to detect pneumothorax was 88% and the specificity 99.5%; these results are very similar to those reported in the previous review [21].

To detect a pneumothorax, the area of interest corresponds to the anterior part of the chest on both sides of the thoracic wall, approximately the third to eighth intercostal space between the parasternal and the midclavicular lines. It is essential that the results obtained have to be compared with the contralateral site. The probe is moved longitudinally in order to study the intercostal tissues on the real-time image. The hyperechogenic pleural line between the shadows of two ribs must be detected. The necessary criteria to diagnose a pneumothorax sonographically have been assessed in the "International evidence-based recommendations for point-of-care lung ultrasound" [17] and consist in absence of respiratory lung movement during dynamic examination (the so-called lung sliding sign), absence of lung pulse at power color Doppler imaging, absence of B-lines (vertical narrow based lines arising from the pleural line to the edge of the ultrasound screen, the so-called comet-tail image), detection of a "lung point" that reflects the border between the movement of the lung during respiration, and the area of absence of the sliding sign due to the pneumothorax [17] (Fig. 8.2).

While the absence of lung sliding can be seen in conditions in which there is no lung movement

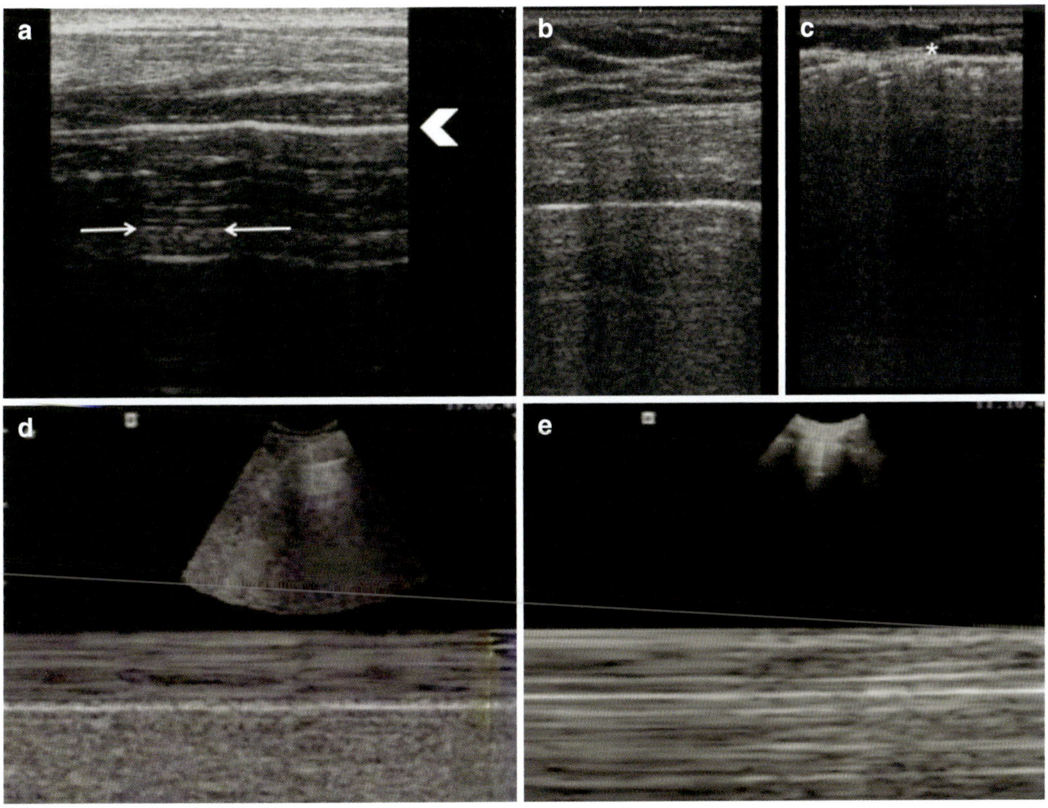

Fig. 8.2 US images to detect a pneumothorax. Despite the fact that diagnosis is purely dynamic, we have to find some basic features: first of all, the hyperechogenic pleural line between the *shadows* of two ribs must be detected (*arrowhead* in **a**). It is crucial to find the "lung point sign" (*arrows* in **a**) that reflects the border between the movement of the lung during respiration and the area of absence of the sliding sign due to the pneumothorax. It is essential that the results obtained have to be compared with the contralateral site: in (**b**) it's possible to detect the hyperechogenic pleural line in the left lung, instead in the right one (**c**) there is subcutaneous emphysema that creates an acoustic barrier (*asterisk*). M-mode on a physiological pleura (**d**), and on a pathological one (**e**). (Courtesy of Dr. G. Volpicelli, Department of Emergency Medicine, San Luigi Gonzaga University Hospital, Turin)

against the thoracic wall, for example, after pneumonectomy, pleuroparenchymal adhesion, or subpleural bullae [23], the "lung point" sign has been shown to be 100% specific for pneumothorax and should routinely be sought in all the patients with loss of lung sliding [24].

In spite of its high sensibility and specificity, we must take into account US limitations. In addition to the above-mentioned referring to the patient constitution, the presence of anterior subcutaneous emphysema and the operator skill, we must not forget that small, apical, and dependent pneumothoraces are poorly detected using thoracic US. A perspective study in 2012 correlated the site of pneumothoraces detected with chest CT with the capability of the previously acquired chest US to detect them. They found that the frequency and the extent of pneumothoraces both increments moving towards the medial and inferior thoracic regions which should always, in the authors opinion, be the first to be scanned [25]. Another limitation of chest US examination is that quantification of the pneumothorax is not easy [10] even if Volpicelli et al. in 2014 demonstrated that in supine patients, the more posterior the lung point is located, the greater the pneumothorax is, as compared to CT volume measurement [26].

MDCT offers confident diagnosis of the pneumothorax itself plus a panoramic view of all thoracic structures allowing the detection of associated injuries and accompanying pathological processes. In particular, it allows to detect the exact number and site of rib fractures, the associated lung injuries and the definition of presence and extent of an eventual subcutaneous emphysema, the latter frequently associated with pneumothorax when rib fractures are involved [11, 19, 27] (Fig. 8.3).

Intrapleural air usually collects in the nondependent regions of the thorax and, in particular, as the patients during CT scan is in a supine position, in the anteromedial basal pleural recesses [27] (Fig. 8.4). Sometimes however, especially in little pneumothorax, air can be detected nearby the rib fracture, wherever the fracture is (also if in a dependent region). This fact may be due to preexisting or trauma-related pleural adhesions which can delimitate small air collections (Fig. 8.5).

A tension pneumothorax is a less common and more dangerous variant of the simple pneumothorax and occurs when air continues to

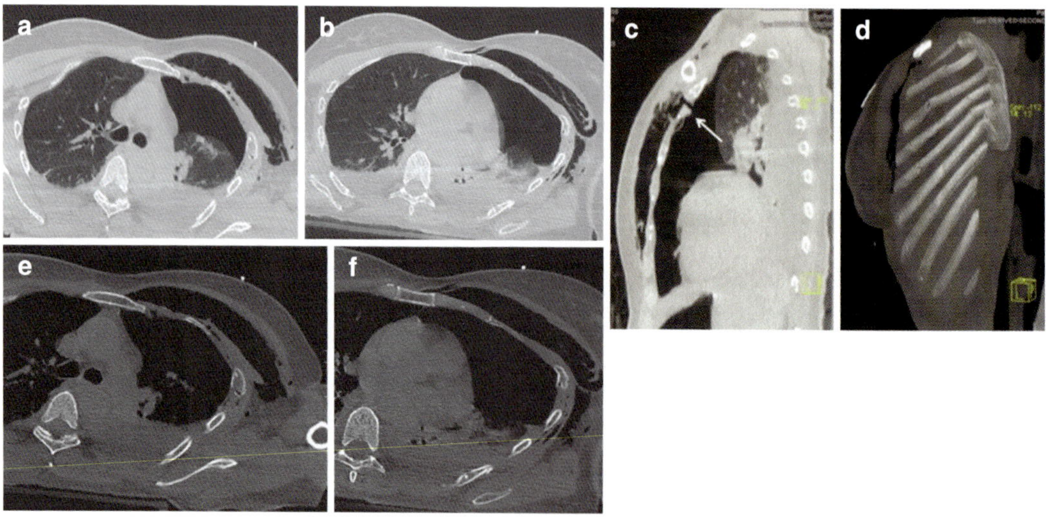

Fig. 8.3 Left pneumothorax. Axial CT-scans in (**a–f**) shows large pneumothorax located in the anteromedial regions with extensive chest wall emphysema. Lung parenchyma window (**a–c**) best helps to detect the intrapleural and intramural air collections while bone-window (**e–f**) permits to determine site and number of rib fractures. Note the panoramic views, often very useful for surgeons or clinicians, offered by sagittal (**c**), and maximum intensity projection (**d**) images. In the sagittal CT-image, you can also depict the mural disruption which permits the passage of the air from the interpleural to the intramural space (*arrow*)

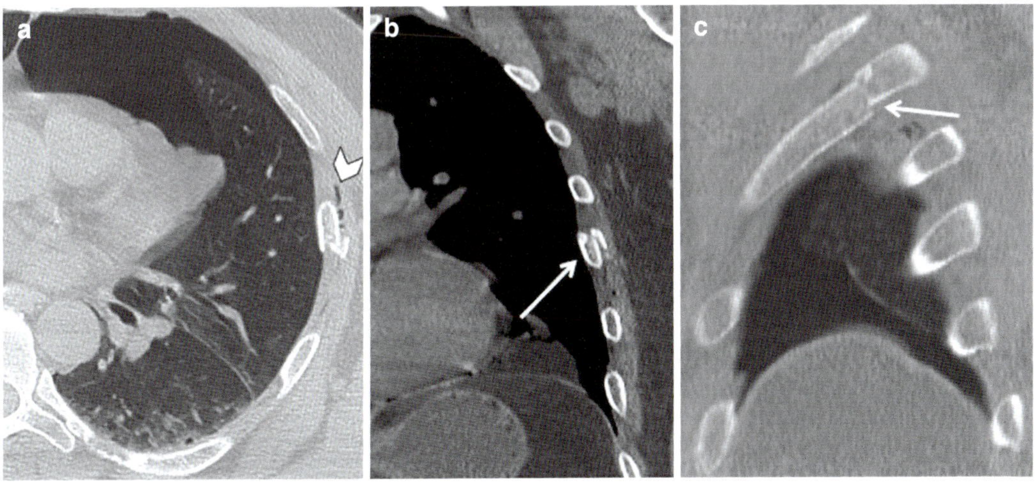

Fig. 8.4 Left pneumothorax. Axial CT-scan (**a**) shows a pneumothorax localized in the anterior-basal site, associated with rib fracture (*arrow*) and subcutaneous emphysema (*arrowhead*), as it is shown in coronal (**b**) and sagittal (**c**) reconstruction

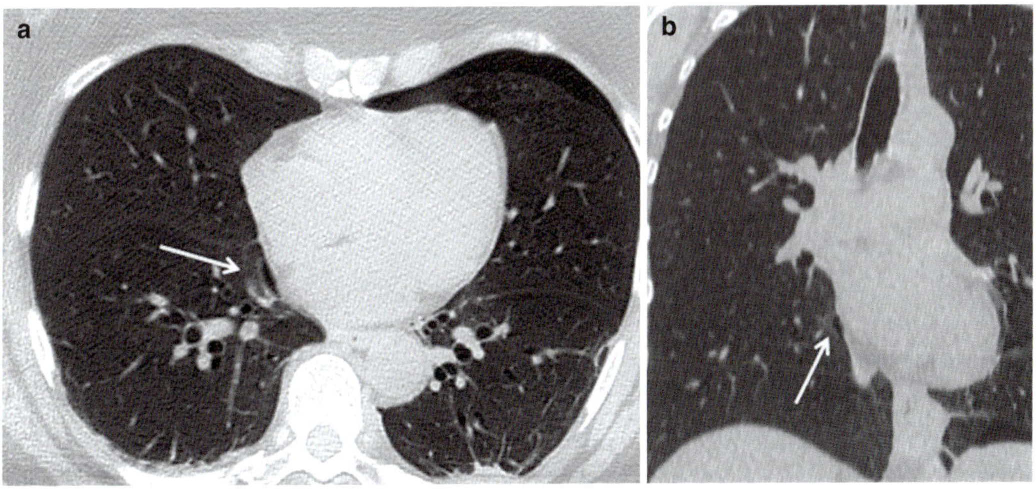

Fig. 8.5 Bilateral pneumothorax. Left pneumothorax located anteromedially and a very small air collection in the right para-mediastinal space (*arrows*): axial (**a**) and coronal (**b**) CT-scan. Note the absence of rib fractures in the right hemithorax: here, the main mechanism involved in the intrapleural air collection may have been parenchymal disruption due to the high increase in intrapulmonary pressure

enter the interpleural space with each breath, either via laceration in the chest wall or via an injured lung, but cannot escape [20]. The resultant progressive increase in volume of trapped air will compress the adjacent lung and diminish its expansion leading initially to respiratory distress and hypoxemia. As the interpleural volume of air continues to increase, the mediastinal structures, including the vena cava, are also displaced and compressed, producing an eventual drop in cardiac preload due to diminished venous cardiac filling pressures. The result is compromised cardiac output which usually rapidly progresses to cardiogenic shock and eventual cardiac arrest [20].

In this life-threatening situation, chest X-ray permits to depict in a few minutes the hyperlucency of a hemithorax plus the opacification of the contralateral (occupied by the mediastinal structures and by the contralateral collapsed lung) thus permitting immediate pleural drainage which is necessary as promptly as possible in order to save the patient's life [7] (Fig. 8.6). We must remember that only a mediastinal shift from its median localization is not a definite sign of a tension pneumothorax as it can also occur in a massive lung athelectasia. So it is important to look for hyperlucency of a hemithorax associated with the ancillary signs of overinflation: flattened or inverted diaphragm profile and enlarged intercostal spaces [7]. Sudden evacuation of a large pneumothorax with tube drainage can be complicated by re-expansion pulmonary edema [28, 29] which is clearly visible in a chest radiogram, being characterized mainly by immediate appearance of subtle opacifications in the ipsilateral lung that can rapidly progress to the total opacification of the entire hemithorax. The complication is more common in younger patients (20–50 years of age), occurs more often than was previously believed, and it has a reported variable mortality rate reaching 20% [29]. So, a control chest X-ray should always be acquired after positioning a drainage tube in a hypertension pneumothorax as it exactly localizes the tube apex and helps us to rapidly diagnose acute complications of the invasive maneuver [7].

MDCT signs are much the same as in conventional radiography, namely contralateral mediastinal shift and collapsed ipsilateral and contralateral lung in a hyperexpanded ipsilateral hemithorax. Also in MDCT imagines, we can find a flattened or inverted ipsilateral diaphragm [19] (Fig. 8.7). Sometimes, with MDCT we are able to find the exact site of the laceration responsible for the intrapleural air accumulation.

8.3.2 Hemothorax

Hemothorax represents blood in the pleural space. It is seen in 50% of blunt thoracic trauma [19] with many possible bleeding sources including pleura, chest wall, lung, mediastinal structures, and diaphragm [20]. The main reported sources of bleeding are intercostal vessels (in rib fractures) and lung parenchyma which, respectively, represent the 50 and 30% of sources [20]. In the left hemothorax, we must also be aware that the 15% of blood is derived from the aortic isthmus [20].

Chest X-ray is scarcely sensible in the depiction of pleural effusion in the supine position, as it has been demonstrated that between 50 and 100 cm^3 of pleural fluid can be detected on upright chest radiograph while about 170–200 cm^3 are usually neces-

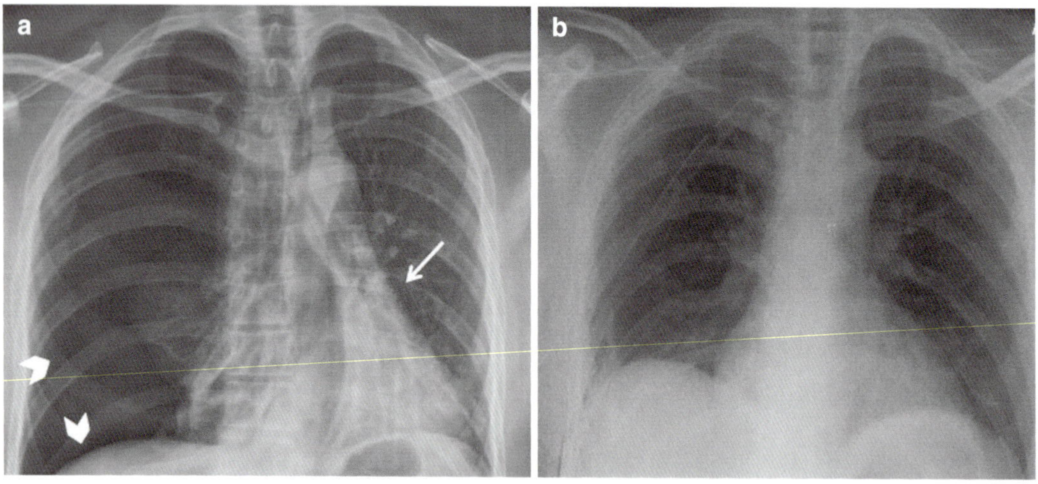

Fig. 8.6 Tension pneumothorax. Chest X-ray (CXR) in (**a**) shows the radiological signs of massive tension pneumothorax: contralateral dislocation of the mediastinum (*arrow*), hyperlucency of the ipsilateral hemithorax associated with flattening of the diaphragm and increment of the intercostal spaces (*arrowheads*). (**b**) CXR control after drainage positioning. Note the complete re-expansion of right lung without any sign of edema

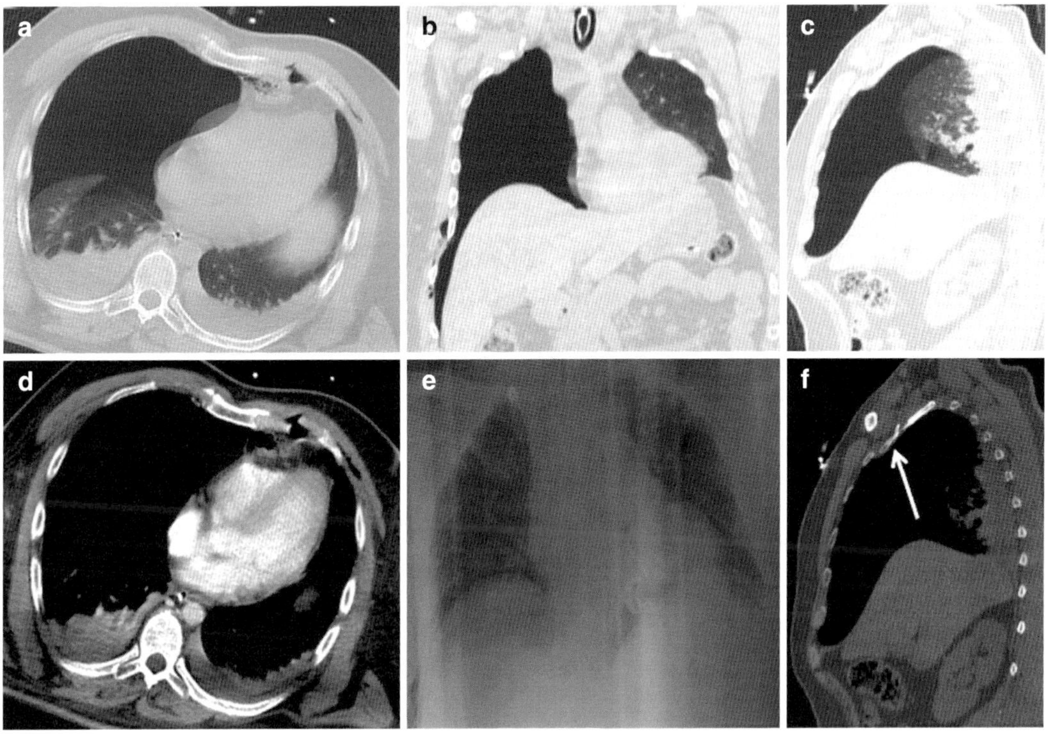

Fig. 8.7 Tension pneumothorax: axial (**a–d**), coronal (**b**), and sagittal (**c**) CT-scans show a massive-right pneumothorax associated with contralateral mediastinal shift collapsed ipsilateral and contralateral lung and hyperexpanded ipsilateral hemithorax. It is also visible a rib fracture in (**f**) (*arrow*), sagittal bone-window. Chest X-ray control after drainage positioning (**e**)

sary for detection when the radiograph is taken with the patient supine [30]. Chest X-ray, however, can diagnose complete opacification of a hemithorax that, in unstable post-traumatic patients, is highly suggestive of massive hemothorax, actually defined as a pleural collection of blood exceeding 1 L with clinical signs of shock [31] and so a life-threatening condition [31] (Fig. 8.8).

Following the actual international evidence-based recommendations for point-of-care lung ultrasound [17], the optimal site to detect a free pleural effusion is at the posterior axillary line above the diaphragm and the main standardized US signs to look for are a space (usually anechoic) between the parietal and visceral pleura and respiratory movements of the lung within the anechoic space. It has been demonstrated that US is an accurate methodic not only to detect even small pleural effusions but also to differentiate its nature [32]. In fact, visualization of internal echoes, mobile particles, or septa is highly suggestive of hemothorax. Unfortunately, if depicting anechoic fluid, US alone can't differentiate between pleural effusion and hemothorax (Fig. 8.9) [33].

Although it has been stated that even very small quantities of fluid can be detected with ultrasound, with one study estimating that as little as 20 cm^3 of pleural fluid can be visualized [30], a recent meta-analysis pursued in 2016 [34] showed that the sensitivity of US in detection of hemothorax is higher than radiography but it is still at a moderate level (67%), while the specificity of both imaging modalities was found to be very high. In this review, the performance of US was influenced, in the different studies, mainly by the operator skill and by the transducer frequency [34].

MDCT readily characterizes pleural fluid in the setting of trauma and can show even subtle fluid collections [8]. As blood may not be the only fluid encountered in the injured pleural space, with serous effusion and chyle being other possibilities, attenuation measurement may be

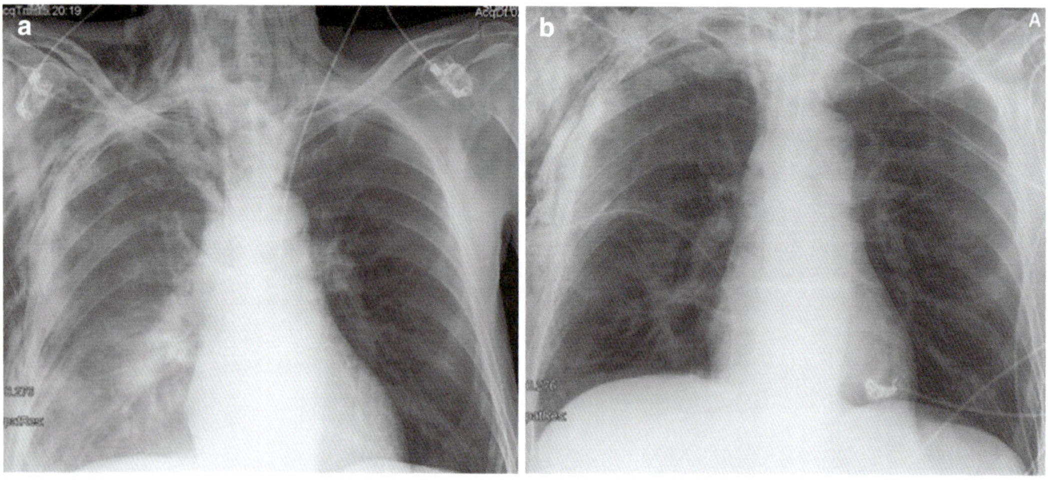

Fig. 8.8 Chest X-ray (CXR) in (**a**) shows an opacification of the right hemithorax caused by a massive hemothorax; subcutaneous emphysema is associated. CXR control after drainage positioning (**b**)

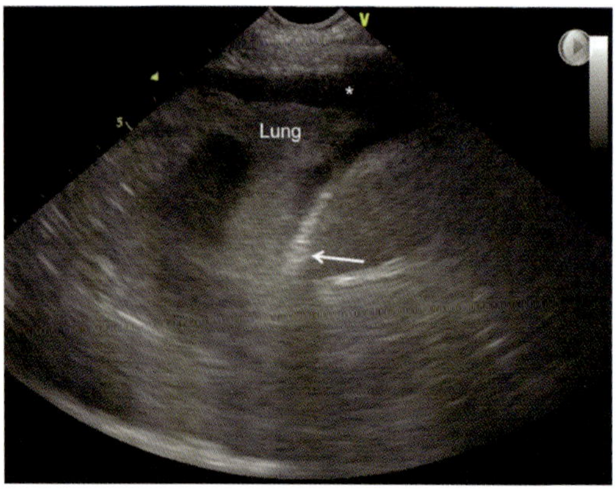

Fig. 8.9 US hemothorax. The optimal site to detect a free pleural effusion is at the posterior axillary line above the diaphragm (*arrow*) and the main standardized US signs to look for are: a space (usually anechoic) between the parietal-visceral pleura and respiratory movements of the lung within the anechoic space (*asterisk*). It has been demonstrated that US is an accurate method not only to detect even small pleural effusions but also to differentiate its nature. In fact, visualization of internal echoes, mobile particles or septa, is highly suggestive of hemothorax. Unfortunately, if depicting anechoic fluid, US alone can't differentiate between pleural effusion and hemothorax

employed to try to differentiate the various entities although this is not a simple effort due to the frequent coexistence of various fluids in the pleural space with different proportion [2]. However, all the authors recommend that measurement of attenuation of pleural space fluid should be routinely performed in the appropriate setting [2]. Usually, a mean density <15 HU is indicative of serous effusion, liquid blood attenuation typically measures 30–45 HU, and clotted blood is 50–90 HU. A mixture of serous and blood fluid can present as a homogeneous fluid with an intermediate density or as a very inhomogeneous one where hyperdense areas or stripes can be seen in the contest of a more hypodense fluid collection, usually the first located in the depending regions of the pleural space [2].

It is mandatory to perform an angio CT of thoracic aorta in order to identify active intrapleural bleeding and to differentiate arterial bleeding from venous one. Arterial hemorrhage is characterized by rapidly increasing hemothorax volume, mainly with hyperdense fluid, with depiction of active arterial bleeding by extravasation of contrast material into the pleural space in the arterial phase, having density similar to that of the contrast-enhanced arterial vessels [3] (Fig. 8.10). In active venous hemorrhage, you can find the presence of contrast media into the pleural space in the venous or delayed phase of the contrast-enhanced examination with the extravasated contrast media showing density values similar or inferior to venous vessels. When an active bleeding is suspected, a delayed acquisition at 5 min is highly recommended, provided that the patient's hemodynamic stability allows for it [3] (Fig. 8.11).

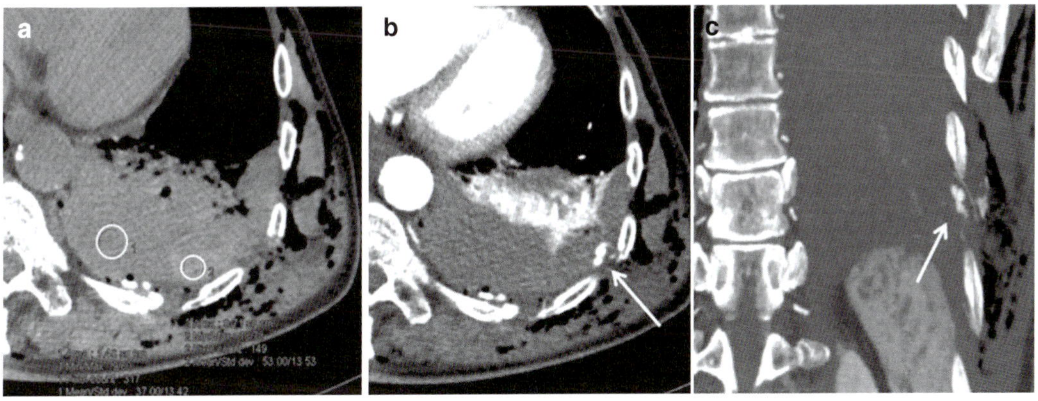

Fig. 8.10 Hemothorax. Axial CT-scan at baseline (**a**) shows a posterior pleural fluid collection. As blood may not be the only fluid encountered in the injured pleural space, measurement of the attenuation of pleural space fluid collection should be performed. In (**a**), the pleural fluid is homogeneous with a marginal hyperdense area: one roi (*red circle*) shows an attenuation of 37 HU (liquid blood attenuation measures 30–45 HU) and another roi (*yellow circle*) has 53 HU (clotted blood is 50–90 HU). Angio-CT is performed (**b**, **c**) and shows an extravasation of contrast material, proving the active arterial bleeding from an intercostal artery (*arrows*)

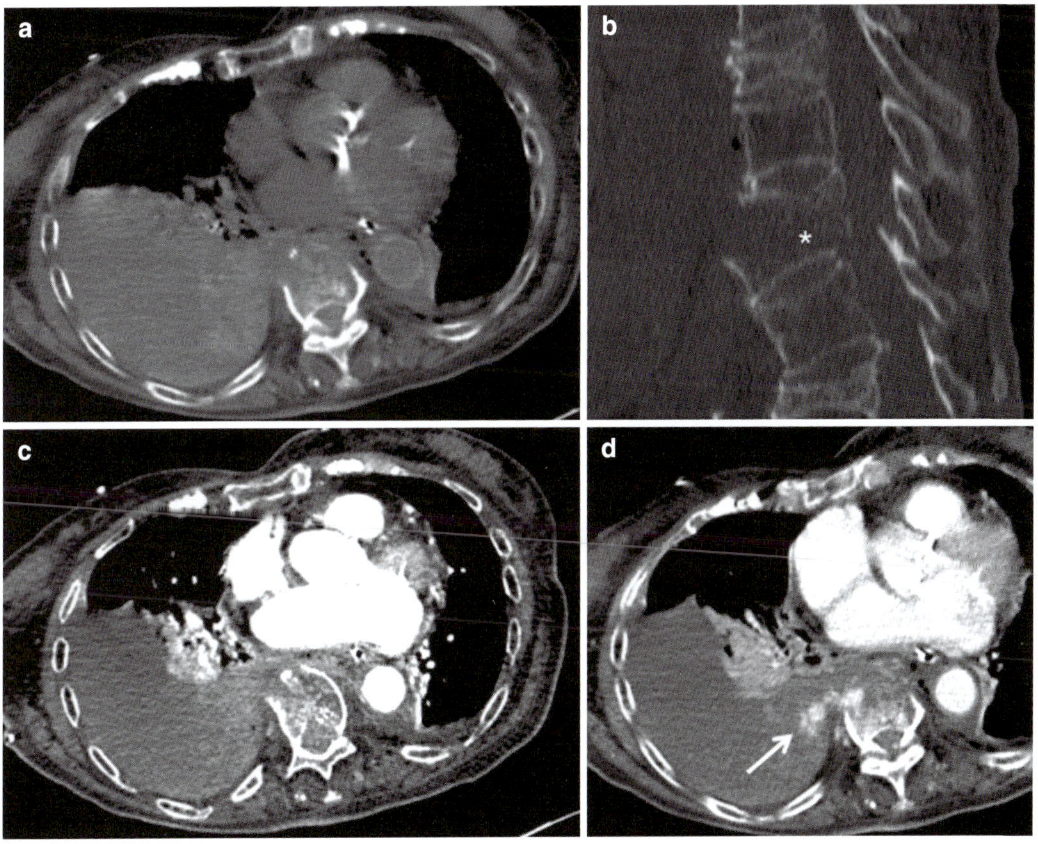

Fig. 8.11 Right hemothorax with active venous bleeding: axial CT-scan at baseline (**a**) shows an inhomogeneous fluid collection with iso- and slightly hyperdense coexisting areas. No extravasation of contrast media can be seen in arterial phase (**c**). The venous phase in (**d**) proves the active blood supply from a lumbar artery (*arrow*), in a vertebral fracture, (**b**) (*asterisk*)

8.4 Lung Injuries

The spectrum of pulmonary injuries consequent to thoracic blunt or open trauma consists in pulmonary contusion, pulmonary laceration, and pulmonary extrathoracic herniation [2].

8.4.1 Lung Contusion

It is the most common type of lung injury in blunt chest trauma with a reported prevalence of 17–70% [35].

Although the pathophysiology of pulmonary contusion is complex and poorly understood, three possible mechanisms have been hypothesized [36, 37]:

1. Inertial effect: the lighter alveolar tissue is sheared from the heavier hilar structures due to different tissue densities and therefore different rates of acceleration or deceleration.
2. Spalling effect: lung tissue bursts or is microsheared where a shock wave meets the lung tissue at interfaces between gas and liquid.
3. Implosion effect: it occurs when a pressure wave passes through a tissue containing bubbles of gas; the overexpansion of gas bubbles stretches and tears alveoli walls [36] with no macroscopic disruption of pulmonary parenchyma.

These injuries damage alveolar capillaries, so blood and other fluids accumulate in the alveolar spaces. Then, the different blood components entering the lung tissue most likely cause the release of multiple inflammatory factors which act as starter for many processes as damage to type II pneumocytes and enrollment of many flogistic cells and molecules into pulmonary parenchyma [36].

Recently, studies on rats demonstrated a rising level in bronchoalveolar lavage (BAL) of inflammatory cellules and molecules. They all decline to baseline in about 1 week [38]. This inflammatory response probably leads to multiple events including endoalveolar and endobronchial mucus production. Aufmkolk et al. in 1999 and Raghavendran et al. in the first 2000s [39, 40] reported some abnormalities in surfactant lipid composition in BAL from trauma patients which reflect type II cell injury or dysfunction. Such surfactant activity deficits were most severe 24 h after contusion and returned to normal state over 48–96 h in parallel with improving lung parameters. Furthermore, tracheal instillations of bovine surfactant in rats with trauma-induced pulmonary contusion improve pulmonary function at 24 h post-injury [40] and surfactant therapy was to be found beneficial in suine with unilateral induced lung contusion [41].

So, contusion has been proved to be sustained by multiple, non-completely known, mechanisms, including alveolar and interstitium filling with hematic and non-hematic fluids, flogistic activation (which can be responsible also for systemic effects as fever or contralateral pulmonary edema), and surfactant abnormalities. All these mechanisms lead to a precocious lung dysfunction which rapidly tends to resolve, usually with complete restitution [36, 37].

The principal complications of lung contusion are ARDS and pneumonia [37]. ARDS develops in 17% of patients with isolated pulmonary contusion, while 78% of contusions with additional injuries develop ARDS [42]. Globally, significant pulmonary contusion leads to ARDS in 50 to 60% of cases while pneumonia develops in about 20% of cases [43].

Systemic activation of neutrophils after trauma is likely to be the leading cause of acute respiratory distress syndrome and multiple organ failure in post-contusion hospitalization [44, 45].

Lung contusion is also a well-known risk factor for development of pneumonia. However, the reason for this increased susceptibility is not clear. It has been supposed that acute lung injuries of lung contusion create in the local pulmonary immune system a sort of vulnerability from a "second" hit bacterial infection [46].

The respiratory impairment of lung contusion includes ventilation/perfusion mismatching, increased intrapulmonary shunting, increased lung water, segmental lung damage, and loss of compliance [36, 37]. Clinically, patients with pulmonary contusion present very unspecific signs as hypoxemia, hypercapnia, and dyspnea [36, 37].

In lung contusion, findings on chest radiography are nonspecific, varying from irregular, patchy areas of opacification to diffuse and extensive homogeneous hypolucency. These changes are usually evident within 6 h after trauma and resolve rapidly, typically within 3–10 days [2, 7, 37]. The scarce specificity of pulmonary post-contusion changes on chest X-ray suggest clinicians to refer as pulmonary contusion every opacification seen on radiograms in post-traumatic patients with the reported time evolution, until proven otherwise [36, 37].

As already stated, lung pulmonary changes in lung contusion consist mainly in three phases characterized, respectively, by: a precocious hematic or serous flooding of alveolar cavities, an intermediate (1–2 h after the traumatic event) edematous infiltration of lung interstitium and a successive flooding of air spaces with inflammatory cells associated with local surfactant deficiency [47]. This last phase, occurring from 6 to 24 h after the trauma and developing in consolidation, is the one visible on chest X-ray [7]. As it has been demonstrated the US accuracy in diagnosing pulmonary interstitial edema [48], we can assume that US is able to depict pulmonary contusion changes in the interstitial phase, earlier than chest X-ray. A study by Soldati et al. [47] confirmed this statement as demonstrated a sensibility of an admission ultrasound examination of 94.6% and a specificity of 100% (in the selected trauma population) compared to CT as gold standard. This specificity cannot be reached in a clinical population, since there are other lung diseases that show the same US patterns, and although US is able to recognize different alterations in lung parenchyma, its specificity in a general population is not so high [47].

As a bedside technique, lung US is performed focusing on the anterior and lateral walls and on the most posterior accessible region beyond the posterior axillary line, not compromising patient immobilization in supine position [18]. The US signs for lung contusion [17] are: the presence of the gliding sign (that is generated by the lung parenchyma movement under the parietal pleural and that indicates the absence of pneumothorax or pleural effusion) associated with the presence of an alveolo-interstitial syndrome defined as the presence of multiple B-lines, in a patient with no clinical suspicion of cardiogenic pulmonary edema, or peripheral parenchymal lesions defined as subpleural echo-poor (or with tissue-like echotexture) regions, allowing ultrasound transmission, from which B-line-like artifacts arise [17, 47]. Lower frequency ultrasound scanning may allow for better evaluation of the extent of a consolidation [17] (Fig. 8.12).

In a recent article [49], the diagnostic accuracy of US was compared to that of combined clinical examination and chest radiography for pneumothorax, lung contusion, and hemothorax, with thoracic CT-scan as reference. It tested also the ability of an US score, measuring the extent of lung contusions, to predict ARDS. It confirmed the major accuracy of US than that of combined clinical examination and chest radiography for all the three injuries, and it demonstrated that the suggested US score can identify patients at risk of developing ARDS after blunt trauma [49].

The more frequent MDCT findings of contusion consist of poorly defined, generally

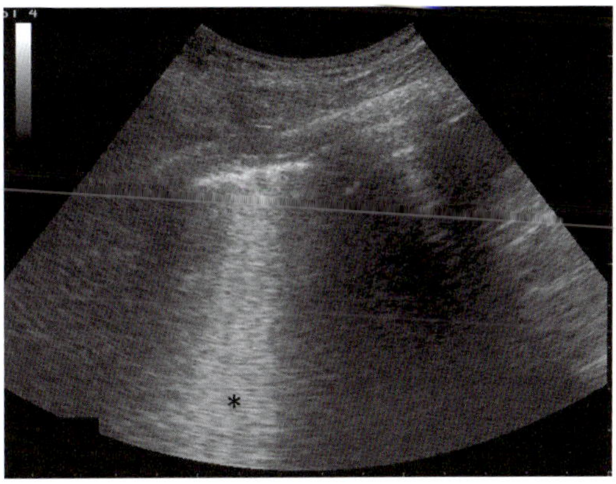

Fig. 8.12 Lung contusion: US image shows an early pulmonary contusion, which was not yet detectable with a standard chest X-ray. The interstitial involvement is shown by the vertical hyperechoic lines, the so-called B-lines (*asterisk*)

non-segmental areas of consolidation and ground glass alterations [2] sometimes (especially in children) sparing 1–2 mm of subpleural lung parenchyma adjacent to the injured chest wall [43]. Contusion areas generally do not show air bronchograms as the bronchioles are often filled with fluid. These signs are well visible with MDCT, unlike chest X-ray, immediately after the traumatic event though it reaches the major increment within the first 6–24 h [19, 37, 50] (Fig. 8.13). As in chest X-ray, clearance of an uncomplicated contusion in MDCT begins at 24–48 h with complete resolution after 3–14 days [2] (Fig. 8.14).

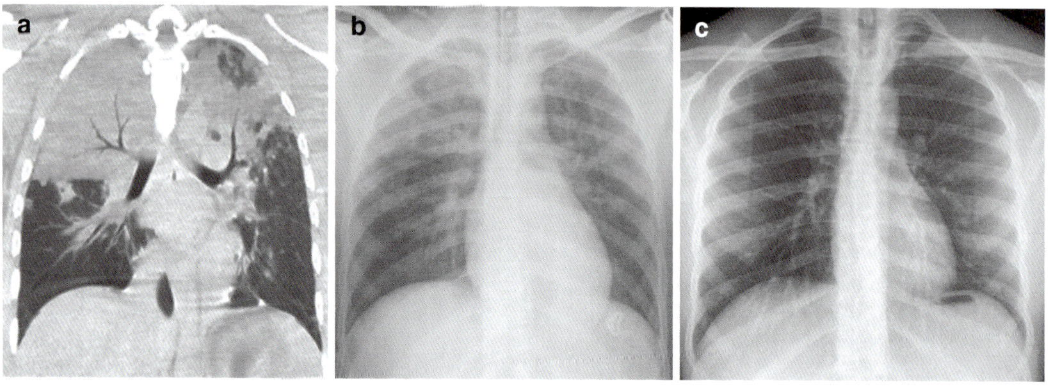

Fig. 8.13 Bilateral parenchymal contusion. Coronal CT-reconstruction immediately after trauma (**a**) shows large parenchymal consolidations. Chest X-ray (CXR) acquired 2 h after the trauma (**b**) shows patchy areas of opacification in the upper lobes. CXR after 14 days shows a complete resolution (**c**)

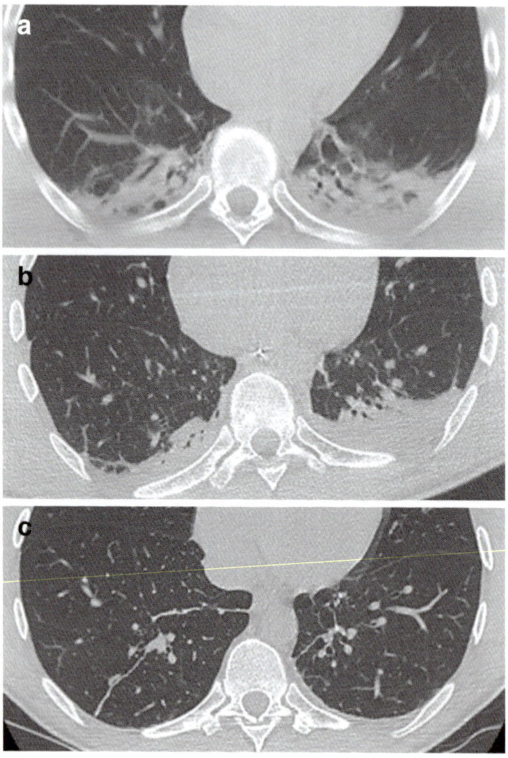

Fig. 8.14 Contusion of the posterior-lower lobes (**a**), that improves in the controls after 5 (**b**), and 10 days (**c**)

Despite the high sensibility, MDCT is poorly specific so in clinical practice, any kind of densitometric increment in lung parenchyma that shows the same temporal pattern is related to contusion damage (Figs. 8.15 and 8.16). At the same time, any kind of parenchymal increase in density arising after 24 h from the traumatic event should be referred to other lung injuries rather than contusion (the more frequents, in a post-traumatic setting, being pneumonia or aspiration) (Fig. 8.17). On the other hand, any kind of lung alterations that do not resolve within a week in a traumatic patient should be regarded as contusion complications, in particular as infection or ARDS [2, 27] (Fig. 8.18).

MDCT is the most useful tool not only in the depiction and in the recognition of contusion injuries but also in its quantification. In fact, it has been proved that, in a large post-traumatic population, the Thoracic Trauma Score (TTS) which considers patients' characteristics as long as CT measurement of contusion extent plus associated thoracic injuries significantly correlates with the occurrence of ARDS.

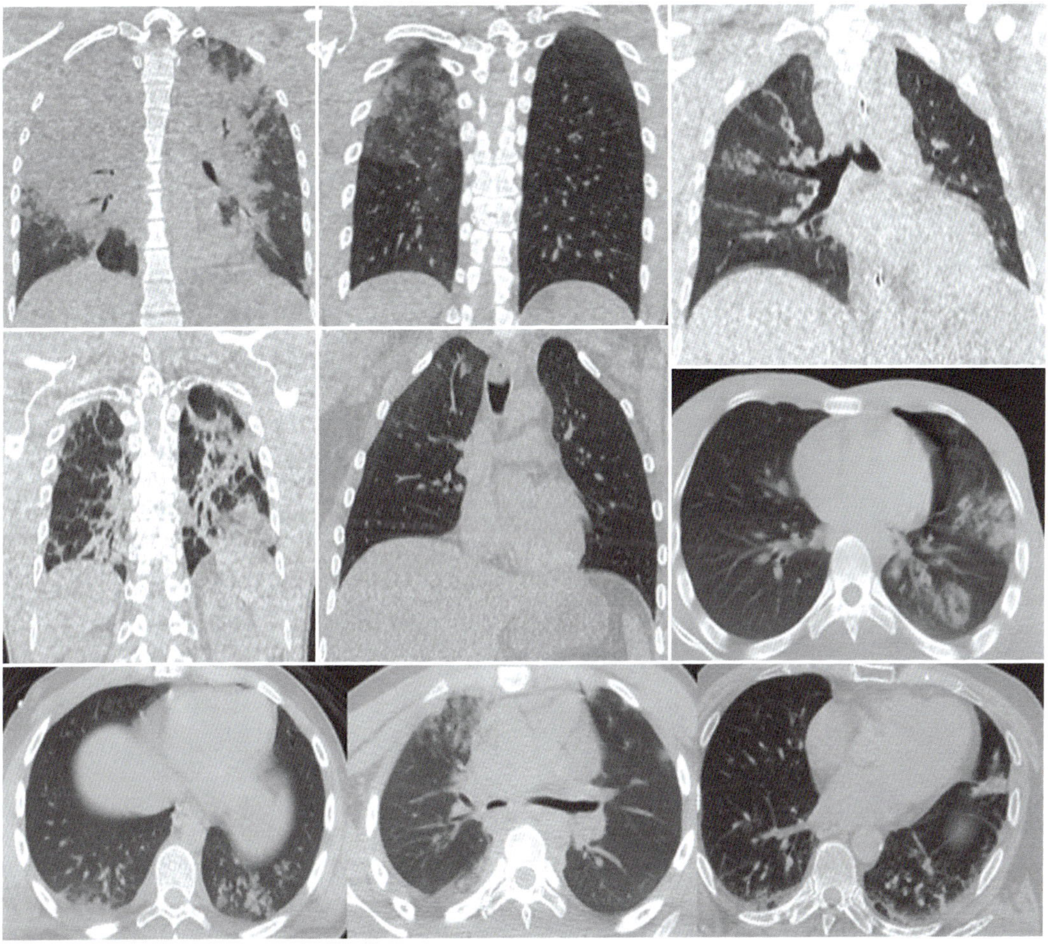

Fig. 8.15 Several examples of pulmonary contusion: it generally consists of poorly defined and non-segmental areas of consolidation and/or ground glass alteration adjacent to the injured chest wall. As we can see, the heterogeneity of lung contusion doesn't permit a differential diagnosis based only upon CT-scan aspect. Thus, every consolidation or ground glass alteration seen on CT-scan after a thoracic trauma should be considered pulmonary contusion until proven otherwise

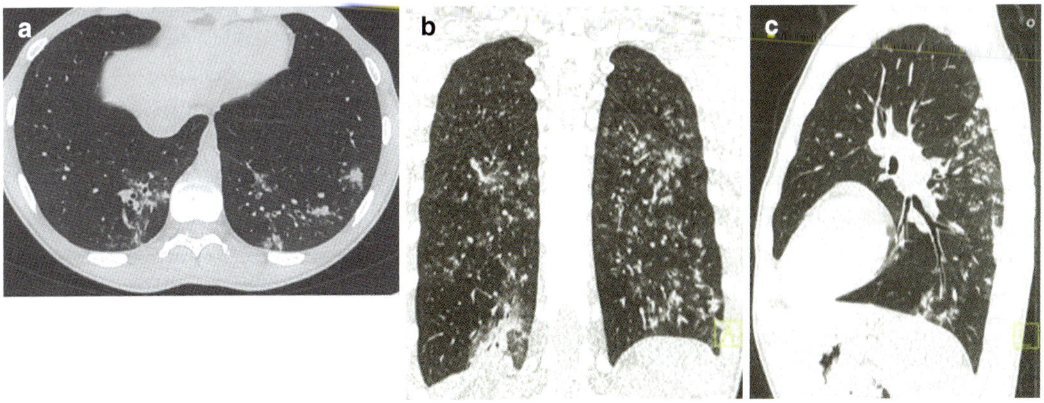

Fig. 8.16 Atypical contusion areas in the posterior segments of the inferior lobes. Post-traumatic CT-scan in axial (**a**), coronal (**b**), and sagittal (**c**) reconstructions. Their clarification in less than 10 days from the traumatic event suggested the hypothesis of pulmonary contusions unless their atypical aspect

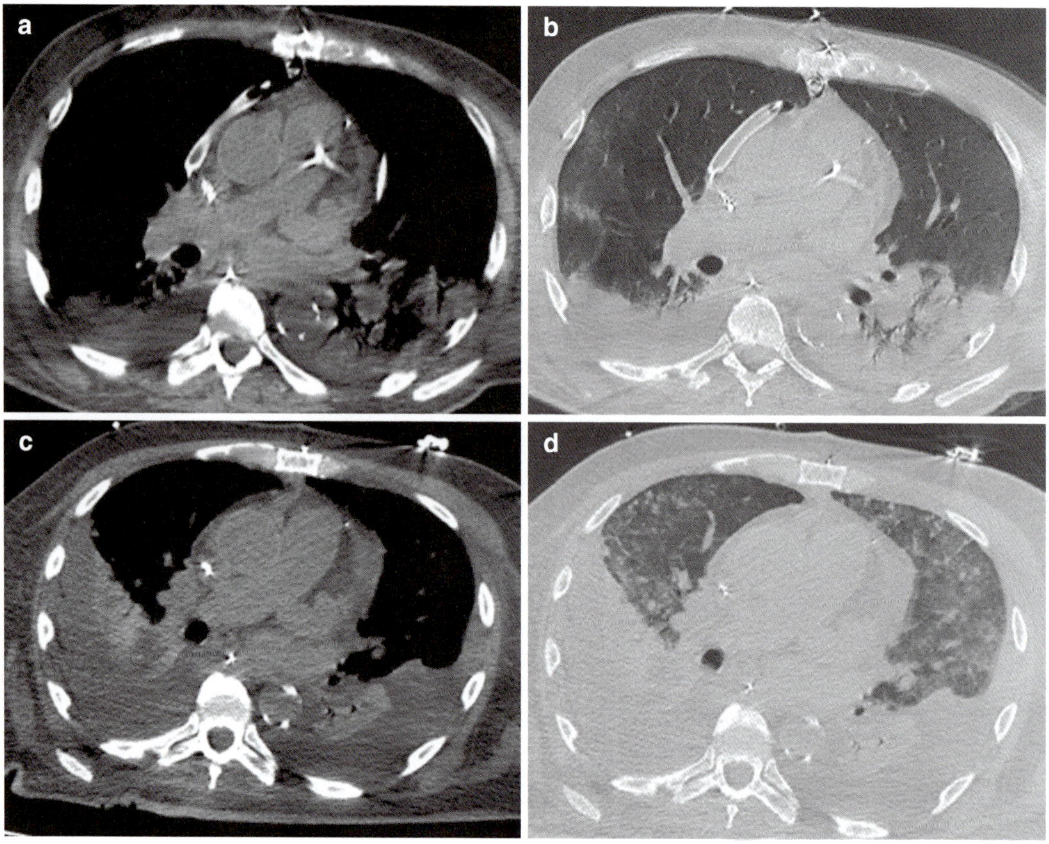

Fig. 8.17 Complication of a pulmonary contusion. (**a**, **b**) Axial CT-scans show the parenchymal areas of consolidation immediately after trauma. Any kind of parenchymal increase in density seen after 24 h should be referred to other causes, such as pneumonia as in this case (**c**, **d**) where pleural effusion and fever appeared

8.4.2 Laceration

Pulmonary laceration occurs when there is a macroscopic disruption of pulmonary parenchyma. Although lung lacerations occur more frequently with penetrating traumas, they may occur also in blunt traumas, caused by much the same mechanisms as pulmonary contusions: the direct effects of pressure on the thorax, the damage of rib fracture, the sudden tears of mobile pulmonary tissue from still structures [19].

The mechanism of laceration consists in lung parenchyma disruption and subsequent filling of intraparenchymal defects with air and/or blood. Due to the elastic recoil properties of lung tissue, normal tissue surrounding pulmonary lacerations recoils to form oval or round defects as opposed to linear or branching defects seen in solid organ tissues [2, 27].

It is difficult to detect lacerations as hyperlucency areas with chest radiography as they usually overlap opacifications due to contusions, hemothorax, or lung collapse [7, 28]. Furthermore, as in their evolution generally fill with fluids and persists for weeks or months, in a later depiction on chest X-ray, they may be misdiagnosed as pulmonary nodules, having the shape of a rounded opacification [28].

CT [35] is significantly superior to chest radiography in detecting even a small laceration and in revealing their overall extent. In the acute setting, it is visualized as a rounded cystic lesion, with air or fluid in its cavity, usually surrounded by ground glass or consolidated area due to surrounding contusion [2, 19, 27]. When filled with fluid and surrounded by consolidation, it is more difficult to detect a laceration even with a CT examination. Lacerations may range from a solitary lesion to multiple confluent small ones; these ones, when surrounded by consolidated parenchyma, are defined as "swiss cheese appearance" [51].

Lacerations have been classified into four types according to the mechanism of injury, the morphological pattern, and their localization [35]:

Type 1: Compression rupture injury is centrally located, can become very large, and is produced by compressing or tearing off the lung parenchyma from the adjacent tracheobronchial tree (Fig. 8.19).

Type 2: Compression shear injury is produced when the lower lobes are suddenly squeezed against the spine. It is located paraspinally and may be tubular in morphology (Fig. 8.20).

Type 3: Rib penetration tear is peripherally located, is small and round, and is very often multiple and associated with pneumothorax and subcutaneous emphysema (Figs. 8.21 and 8.22).

Type 4: The adhesion tear is seen adjacent to a previous pleuropulmonary adhesion and is

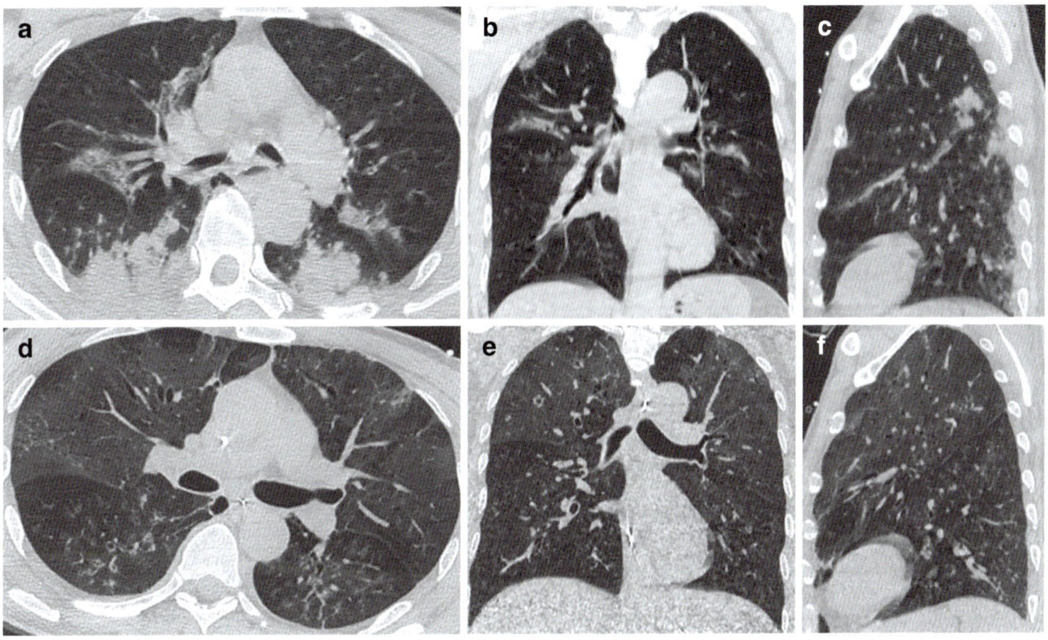

Fig. 8.18 Complication of a pulmonary contusion. (**a**–**c**) Post-traumatic CT-scans show bilateral areas of contusion. Although the relative clarification of contusion areas in the posterior regions, we can appreciate the emerging ground glass alteration of the entire parenchyma at the control CT-scan in (**d**–**f**), acquired 1 week after the hospital admission. The patients experienced a serious ARDS despite the rapid and appropriate respiratory support

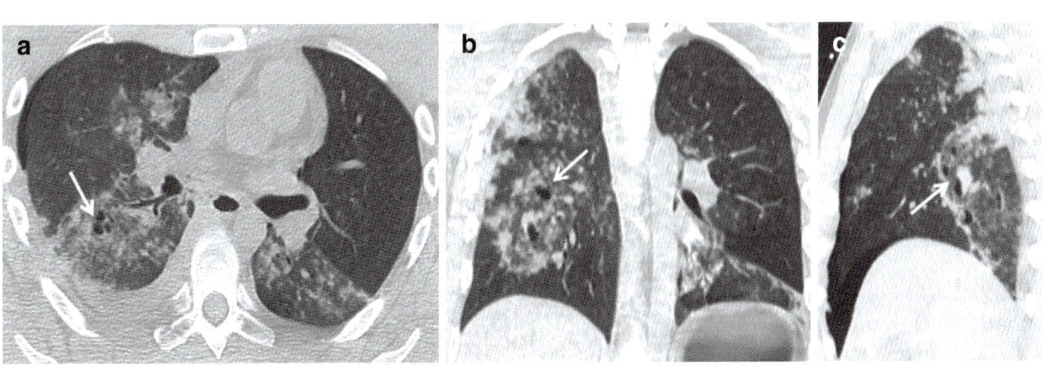

Fig. 8.19 Type 1 lacerations (*arrows*). In (**a**–**c**) are centrally located, surrounded by extensive contusion areas and without any rib fracture visible nearby. Note the ipsilateral hemopneumothorax

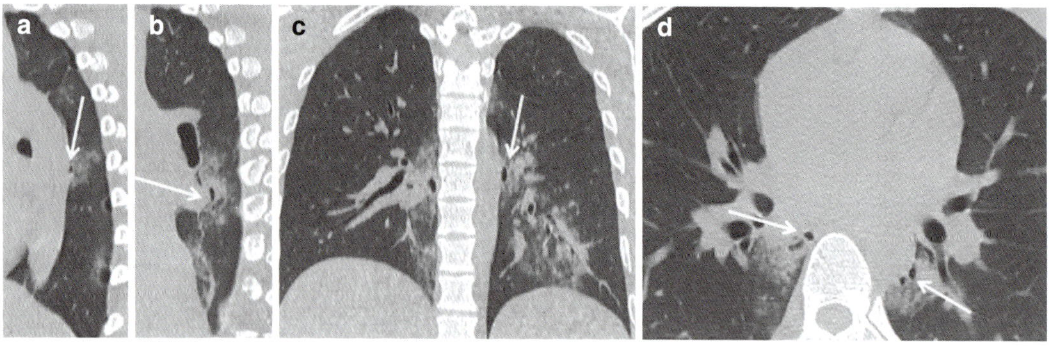

Fig. 8.20 Type 2 lacerations: these injuries (showed in **a**-**b**-**c**-**d**) are produced when the lower lobes are suddenly squeezed against the spine. These lacerations are generally paraspinally located (*arrows*) and bilateral

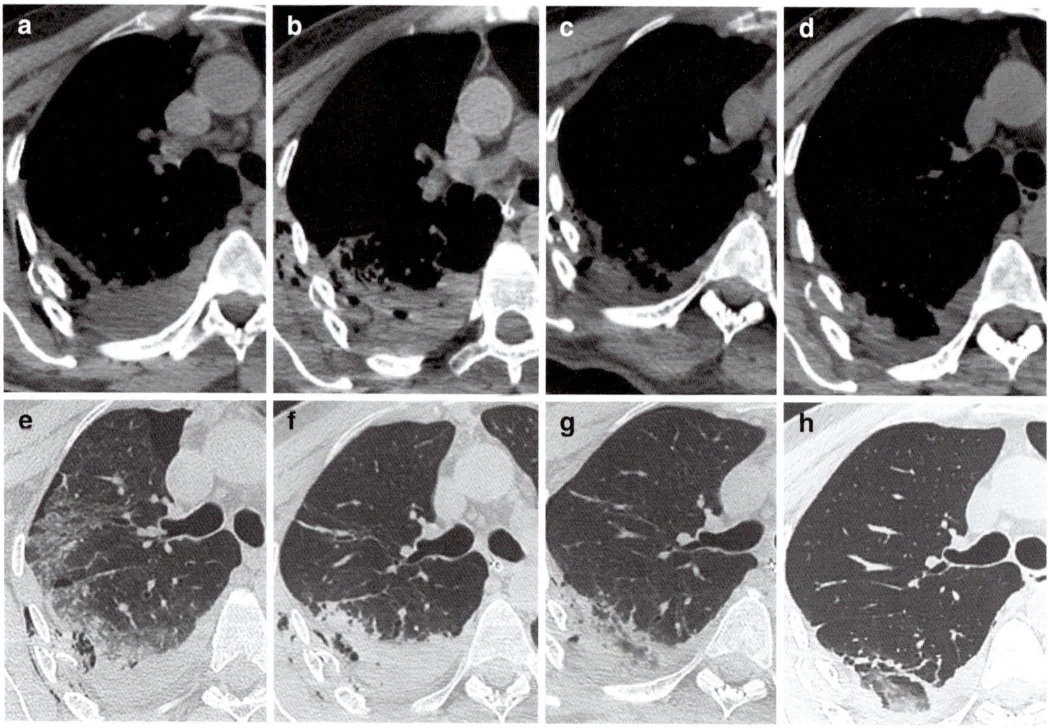

Fig. 8.21 Axial CT-images show contusions and type 3 lacerations (*arrow*). Immediately after trauma (**a**–**e**) the lacerations are small peripheral and associated with local rib fractures, pneumothorax, and chest wall emphysema. In the following controls after 1 (**b**–**f**), 4 (**c**–**g**), and 10 days (**d**–**h**), the lacerations are evolving: become increasingly filled with blood or fluid, so less appreciable (**c**–**g**) and regress slowly, often ending in a residual scar

almost always seen at surgery or at autopsy, not recognizable in MDCT images.

Lacerations resolve more slowly than contusions, and clearance may take months. Over time, they become increasingly filled with blood/fluid and then regress, often ending in residual scarring [52] (Fig. 8.23). Complications of laceration are uncommon and can be: pulmonary abscesses, bronchopleural fistula, or very large pneumatoceles generated by a ball-valve mechanism [19, 28].

Intrapulmonary hematoma is a special kind of laceration consisting in the presence of an organizing hematoma inside the rounded cavity of lacerated parenchyma. It is well depicted with CT that shows a solid rounded consolidation with high density values at the direct examination and no significant increase in Hounsfield Units after administration of contrast media (Fig. 8.24).

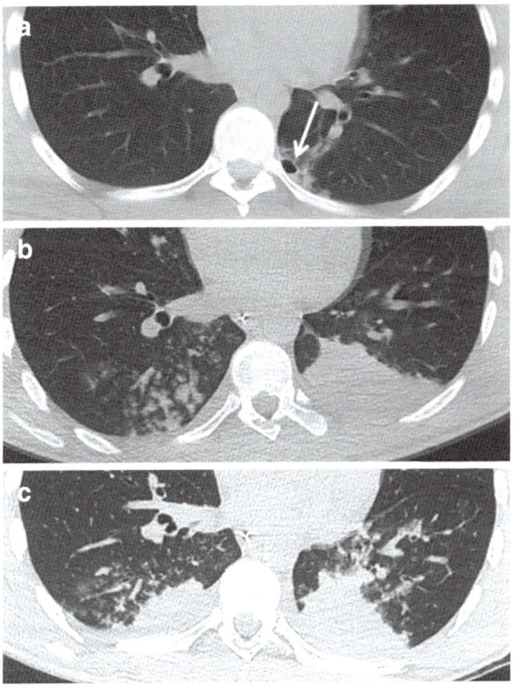

Fig. 8.22 Left lower lobe contusion associated with a small type 3 parenchymal laceration (*arrow*) in a young boy: axial CT-scan immediately after trauma (**a**). Images in (**b**, **c**) show the CT controls after 5 and 10 days: the progressively filling of the small laceration with fluids does not permit its depiction in the successive CT controls

8.4.3 Pulmonary Hernia

Traumatic lung herniation occurs when a pleura-covered part of the lung extrudes through a traumatic defect in the chest wall [2]. It is generally an acquired condition, mainly caused by trauma (52% of cases), which is more often a penetration than a blunt injury [53]. Any chest trauma may cause bones or joint disruption, resulting in acquired chest wall defects and allowing lung herniation; however, lung protrusion is more likely when the trauma causes a sudden marked increase in intrathoracic pressure; many ribs are broken or a focal blunt trauma occurs [53].

Generally, anterolateral chest wall is more susceptible to traumatic lung herniation because of the lesser soft tissue support compared to the posterior wall. The first, in fact, relies only to intercostal muscles while the latter is supported also by the trapezius, latissimus dorsi, rhomboid, and paravertebral muscles [50]. Herniation caused by penetrating trauma occurs, naturally, at the site of the wound [53].

In case of lung hernia, symptoms are aspecific including pain, coughing, hemoptysis, and breathlessness while chest examination may reveal a soft mass that moves paradoxically with respiration and/or is more evident in Valsalva maneuver [53]. Sometimes, lung hernias can remain asymptomatic and uncomplicated and presentation can be delayed. Delays of a few months to 40 years have been reported [54].

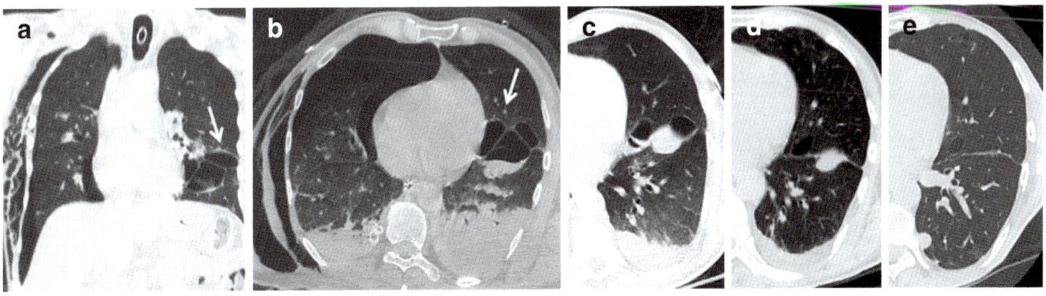

Fig. 8.23 Multiple parenchymal lacerations (*arrows*): coronal (**a**) and Axial (**b**) CT-scans done immediately after trauma; note the large subcutaneous emphysema and ipsilateral pneumothorax. Controls after 10 days (**c**), 3 months (**d**), and 1 year (**e**). Note the progressive filling of the cavities and their slow involution in irregular residual scars

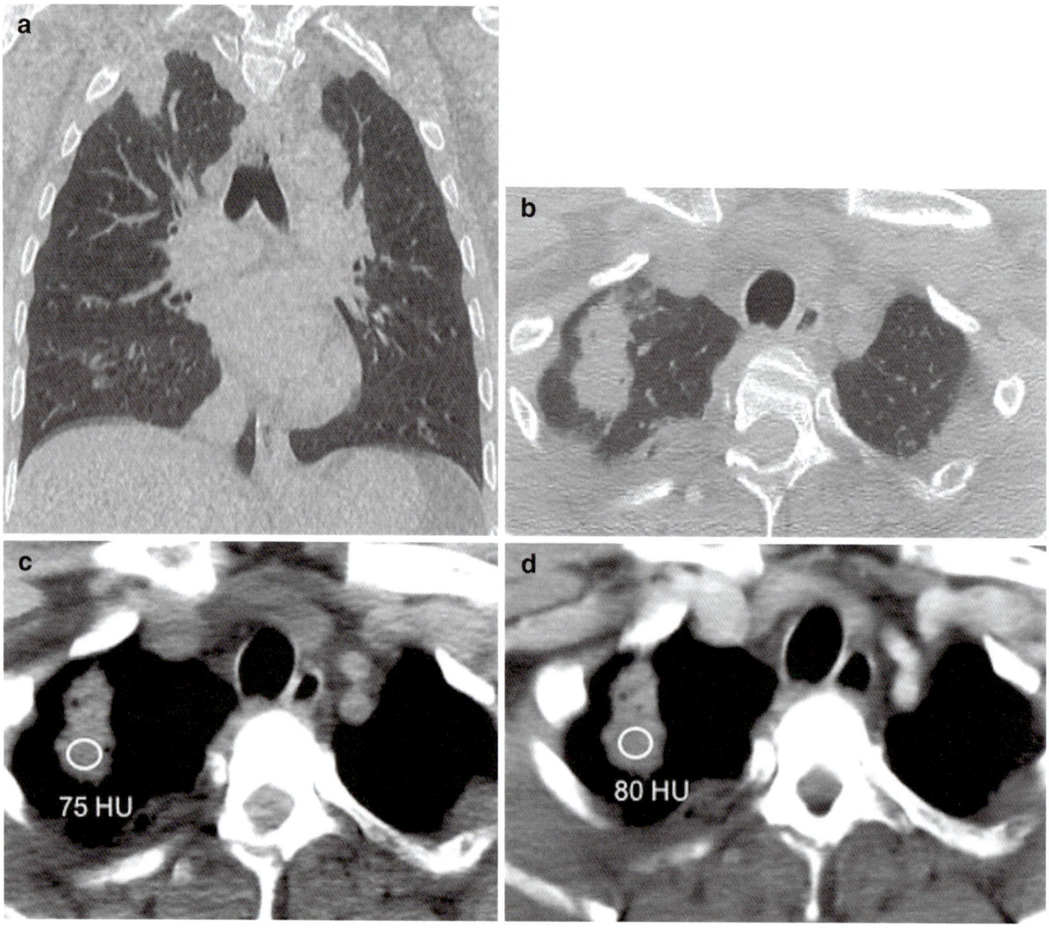

Fig. 8.24 Intrapulmonary hematoma: it is an organizing hematoma inside the rounded cavity of lacerated parenchyma (**a**, **b**). CT-scan shows a solid rounded consolidation with high density at baseline (**c**), and no significant increment after administration of contrast media (**d**)

Lung hernia, when symptomatic, may be a life threatening condition as can be itself complicated with tension pneumothorax or strangulation of the protruding lung and as it is usually associated with other severe injuries of thoracic structures, due to the high energy mechanism that implies this event [50].

Plain chest may see bone or joint rupture [53]. Sometimes, owing to the opacity difference between herniated lung and surrounding soft tissues, the hernia itself may be apparent [7, 53] (Fig. 8.25). Chest X-ray acquired during the Valsalva maneuver have also been demonstrated to be of value for diagnosis because of the increasing hernia volume [54]. Utilization of plain radiographs is not

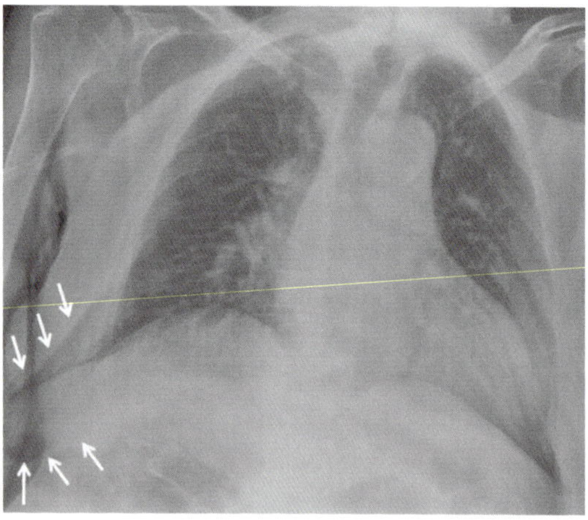

Fig. 8.25 Suspect of right basal lung herniation (*arrows*) in the chest X-ray done immediately after trauma

recommended when a CT-scan can be rapidly performed [53].

MDCT can easily depict the herniated lung portion and evaluate the adjacent altered thoracic wall structures [50] (Fig. 8.26). Furthermore, during the contrast-enhanced phase, MDCT enables to suspect a strangulation of the herniated region when we do not find any opacification of the herniated lung vessels [53] (Fig. 8.27). Owing to the panoramic visualization of all thoracic structures, MDCT can also depict pneumothorax, pneumomediastinum, and hemothorax, which are often associated, and permits to evaluate any other injured thoracic structure. Minimum intensity projection reconstructions may be of value to the cardiothoracic surgeon managing the patient, particularly with regard to their surgical strategy [53] (Fig. 8.28).

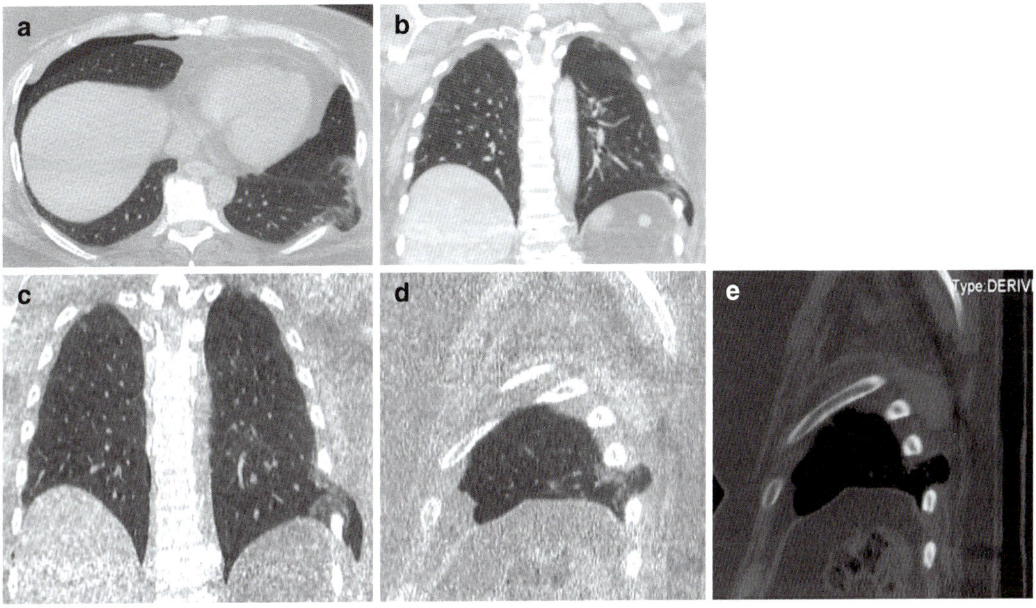

Fig. 8.26 Lung herniation of the posterolateral chest wall. Axial (**a**), coronal (**b**, **c**) and sagittal reconstructions, the latter with both lung (**d**), and bone (**e**) window. While the lung window allows to depict and localize the herniated lung, the bone window provides optimal visualization of the rib cage. As we can see, the hernia wasn't associated to any rib fracture

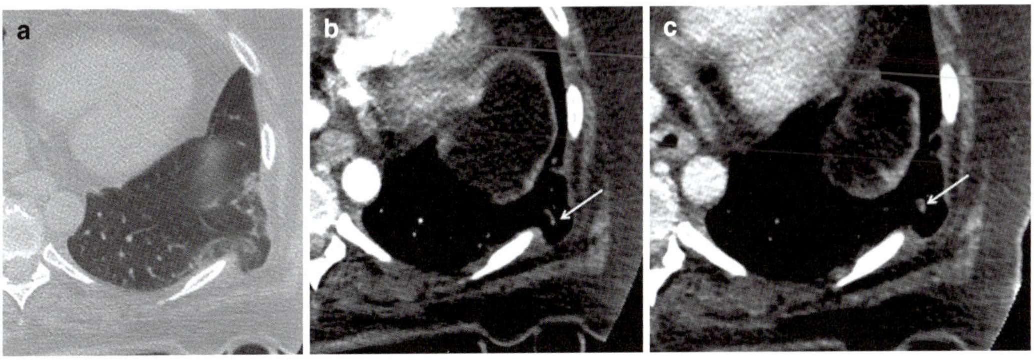

Fig. 8.27 Same patient as Fig. 8.25. Axial CT-scans after administration of contrast media (**a**–**c**). We can appreciate the lack if opacification on arterial (**b**) and venous (**c**) vessels of the herniated portion of the lung, suggesting the possibility of its strangulation (*arrows*). In the lung window image in (**a**), the protruding lung shows subtle increment in density as in aspecific suffering

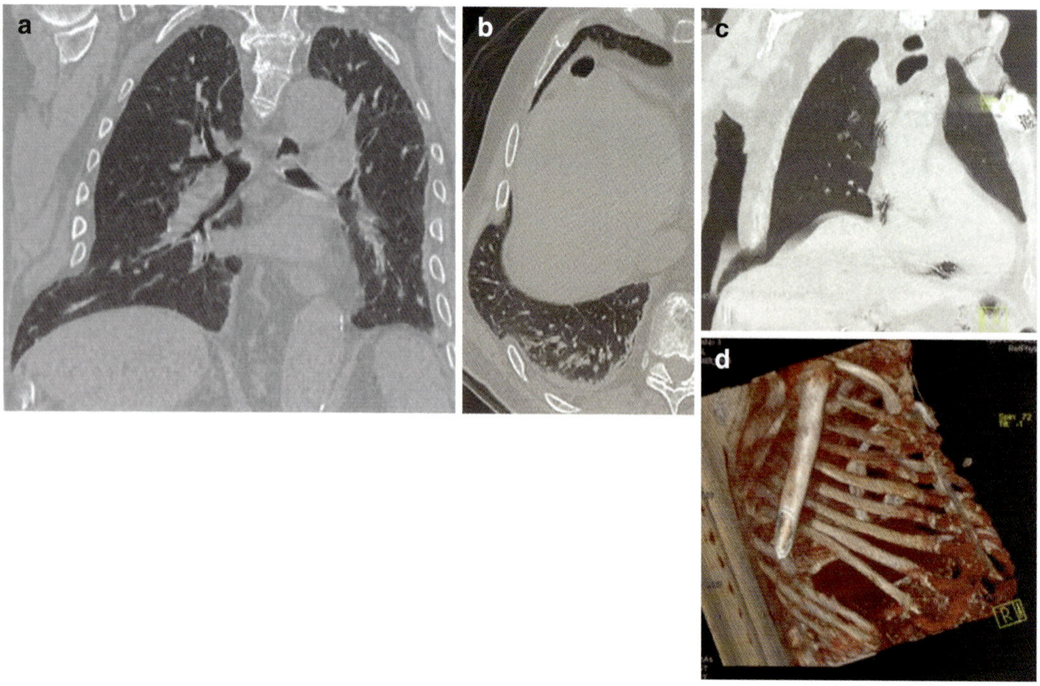

Fig. 8.28 Same patient as in Fig. 8.26: CT confirms the herniation and enables to evaluate the chest wall disruption: coronal (**a**), axial (**b**), minimum intensity projection (**c**), and 3D reconstructions (**d**)

As lung herniation is a rare condition with a wide spectrum of causes, severities, associations, and complications, some of which are life threatening, it is important for the radiologist to recognize the condition as fast as possible [27]. This is particularly true in dyspnoic or hypoxic patients as herniation may increase with positive-pressure ventilation [50, 53].

8.4.4 Open Trauma

Although blunt trauma accounts for approximately 70% of trauma cases, penetrating trauma should not be overlooked as a cause of significant morbidity and mortality. In fact, gunshot wounds are the second leading cause of injury death after motor vehicle crashes in the United States [55]. Overall, the exact incidence of penetrating chest injury varies according to the geographical location with incidence ranging from 1 to 13% of all trauma admissions [56]. These injuries are frequently serious and, particularly in gunshot wounds, any region of the chest may be involved. Also, as many as 20% of open thoracic trauma will have associated abdominal injuries [56]. Generally, less than one-third of knife wounds and approximately one half to two-thirds of gunshot wounds in stable patients will require surgical repair [5] and, in unstable patients (event not rare due to the frequent involvement of vascular structures along the stab trajectory), an acute exploration is required in 5–15% of cases [56].

The lung parenchyma and the pleural sheets are involved in the great majority of open thoracic traumas. From 88 to 97% of penetrating chest injuries involve the chest wall, pleura, or lung [5] and the tissue damage has the same anatomo-pathological characteristics as in blunt trauma. There are, however, peculiarities in imaging of penetrating trauma, especially in gunshot injuries, that are worth considering by the emergency radiologist.

Penetrating trauma can be divided into ballistic and non-ballistic. The first cause tissue disruption and laceration along their trajectory and damage tissue nearby their entrance [55]. In the second, we can identify at least three major mechanism of disruption: the direct tissue laceration occurring along the bullet trajectory, as in non-ballistic wounds (called permanent cavity); the damage caused by the pressure gradients resulting in tissue separation in a radial direction along the bullet trajectory (called "temporary cavity"); and the damage obtained by the ballistic pressure preceding the bullet [55]. While the term "temporary cavity" refers to the effect of bullet shockwaves on gelatin in experimental studies, in vivo it is usually referred to the "concussion zone" located radially with respect to the bullet path [55]. So, the wound is not in a linear shape (as in stab wounds) but involves also tissues around the trajectory. The degree of injury will depend on how the projectile transfers its kinetic energy into the target tissues. In vital organs, the transfer of energy is influenced by the velocity of the projectile, the bullet shape and design, and the intrinsic tissue characteristics. Experimental studies demonstrated that the temporary cavitation size becomes more significant at higher velocities with almost an exponential relationship between the bullet velocity and the cavity size [55]. Regarding tissue characteristics, damage increases with tissue density and decreases with tissue elasticity [5]. As lung has got more elasticity than abdominal organs (as liver, kidney, or spleen), it can better absorb the perforating forces thus experiencing less damage from the same ballistic trauma [55]. So, while renal, hepatic, and splenic parenchyma show greater degrees of tissue destruction and fragmentation, a surrounding contusion around the bullet path in the highly elastic lung is often the most commonly visible injury of the "concussion zone" [5].

The clinical presentation of a patient with penetrating trauma is highly variable depending mainly on two interrelated factors: the hemodynamic stability and the mechanism and location of the wound and can range from a stable to a comatose condition [55].

Although from 88 to 97% of patients who are admitted with penetrating injuries to the chest have involvement of the chest wall, pleura, or lung, it has been demonstrated that up to 62% of patients are asymptomatic and have normal chest radiographs [57]. Furthermore, other studies and case series reported rates of delayed pneumo- or hemothorax of 8–12%, after a negative admission chest X-ray in asymptomatic patients with penetrating thoracic wounds [58]. In order to prevent this, many studies explored the utility of sequential chest X-rays acquired during the first hours after the patient's admission. In particular, a 2013 study based on a population of 88 patients with thoracic penetrating injuries suggested a hospitalized observational period in asymptomatic patients with normal initial chest radiographs, with repeat chest X-ray, at intervals approaching 1 h, for at least 3–6 h [58]. As a matter of fact, already in 2007, Magnotti et al. [59] demonstrated that after an initial chest CT there was no need for repeat chest radiograph after penetrating thoracic trauma. Actually, chest X-ray in penetrating thoracic traumas, as in blunt trauma, should be considered a helpful tool in the prior evaluation of patients and provides, along with bedside US, immediate useful information in the unstable patient as it rapidly recognizes hemothorax and pneumothorax [3].

The evidence for the use of chest US in the evaluation of thoracic penetrating trauma is more limited than that for blunt trauma [60]. Current literature, however, demonstrates that US is a valid screening tool for penetrating thoracic injuries with a high sensitivity for detecting injury requiring acute intervention [60] as hemothorax, pneumothorax, and pericardial effusion.

In particular, since 1997, it has been demonstrated the high sensitivity of US in detecting hemothorax in penetrating thoracic injury compared to CT and tube thoracostomy as gold standard [30]. In this study was found a sensitivity and specificity of US of 100% in detecting hemothorax in 18 patients with thoracic penetrating trauma [30].

Other studies have also evaluated US for the depiction of pneumothorax in penetrating trauma, and recently Ku et al. [61] compared, in 47 patients, thoracic US for pneumothorax with computed tomography, tube thoracostomy, and supine chest radiograph followed by clinical observation. In this case report, US demonstrated a sensitivity of 57% and a specificity of 99% with respect to the CT examination [61]. The lack in sensitivity may be explained by the high "operator dependence" of US as this study was performed with many operators, each of them with different experience [61].

Finally, we must not forget that, in penetrating traumas, US is a valuable instrument to detect also a pericardial effusion. In 2015, in a large cohort of injured patients, US demonstrated a sensitivity of about 86% [62].

MDCT has certainly become the modality of choice in stable patients with penetrating torso trauma [63]. The mayor utility of MDCT in penetrating trauma relies in its capability to detect the trajectory of non-ballistic and ballistic wounds, the so-called CT trajectogram [5]. This is particularly true since the advent of multidetector technology which permits to achieve rapid isotropic acquisitions and, thus, to perform multiplanar and 3D reconstructions,

It has been demonstrated that the depiction of the wound trajectory allows a better management of the patient in the acute setting, reducing the frequency of diagnostic surgery, and has got forensic utility as it provides valuable data regarding the dynamic of the traumatic event and the nature of the injuring object [5].

Non-ballistic wound trajectories are often not entirely evaluable, even with MDCT, as tissues tend to return to the one adjacent to the other after releasing the stab [5] (Fig. 8.29). Ballistic wounds path, on the other hand, are better depicted as

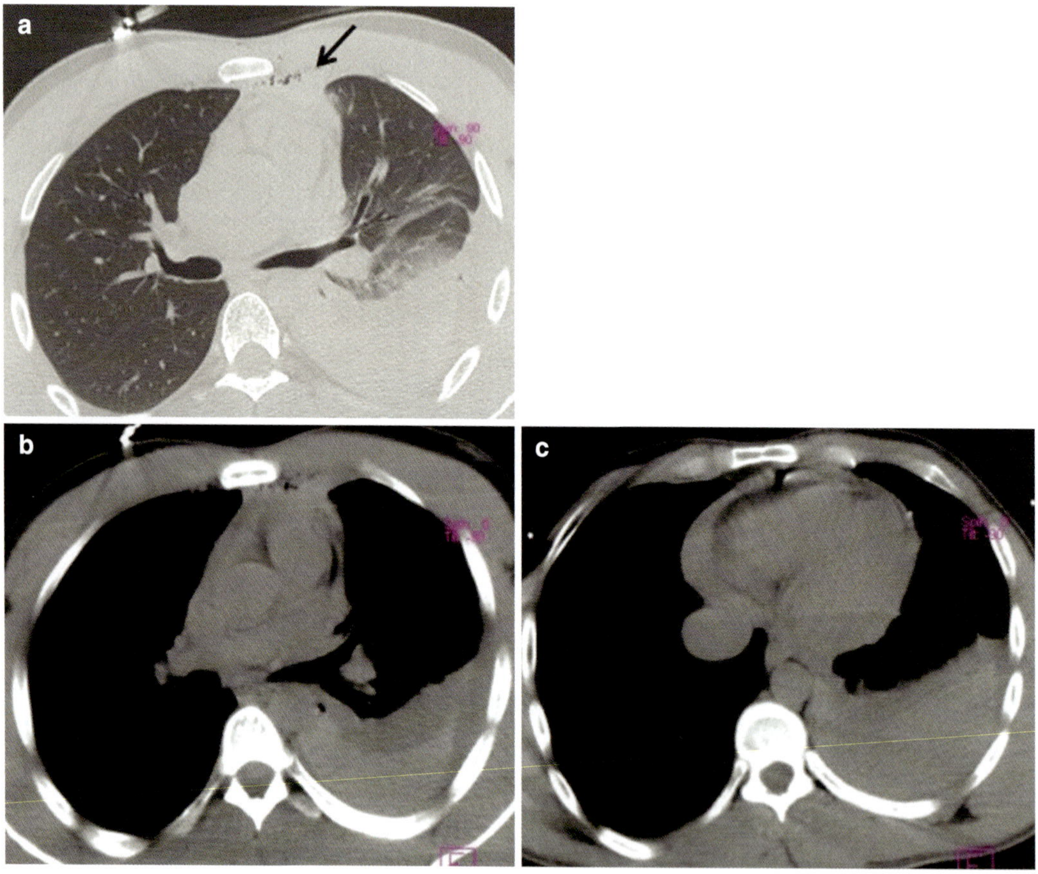

Fig. 8.29 Young man stabbed to the anterior left chest wall. In (**a**) (lung parenchyma window), it is possible to notice the small air bubbles behind the sternum (*arrow*), an indirect knife-penetration sign. We have no more appreciation of the stab trajectory but have indirect signs of pericardial and pleural disruption in the axial CT-scans with smooth tissues window (**b**, **c**) that show left hyperdense pleural and pericardial effusion, signs of left hemothorax and hemopericardium

there is a greater tissue disruption as the damage is not only along the wound tract but also in surrounding tissues. Furthermore, since MDCT has high sensitivity in finding and exactly localizing metallic external fragments, air, hemorrhage, and small bone or bullet fragments (lead dust) along the wound track, it allows better identification of the course of the bullet compared to a stab wound [28] (Fig. 8.30). Unfortunately, pitfalls may occur, especially in cases of multiple penetrating injuries, or when there is not a linear trajectory, for example when projectiles or stab are rebounded off or deviated by bony structures [5]. It is important, in order to reduce pitfalls, to use more than one window setting in order to adequately identify CT trajectograms in the thorax. In fact, it is suggested to use wide CT windows in order to identify the exact wound entry site in the subcutaneous fat, as well as the intrapulmonary path and the bone damage, while we will need a "soft tissues" CT window to identify the relationship of the bullet path with the mediastinal structures [28] (Fig. 8.31).

As just said, since 88–97% of penetrating wounds involve the chest wall, pneumothorax, and hemothorax are the most common complications following these events. In particular, in penetrating traumas, open or communicating pneumothorax occurs, also called "sucking chest wound," which develops when the skin and pleura are both injured [7]. This kind of pneumothorax may more easily develop in tension pneumothorax (up to one-third of patients) [5]. Air location in the pleural space, as in blunt traumas, depends mainly on the patients' position and only rarely on the site of laceration or on previous or newly generated pleural adhesions.

Hemothorax is more frequently seen in open injuries than in blunt traumas [5]. It is usually the result of a laceration or contusion of lung parenchyma (associated to a disruption of the visceral pleura), or of diaphragm, internal mammary, and intercostal vessels, heart or great vessels. Also, more frequently than in blunt trauma, there can be active bleeding that can became rapidly massive and life threatening [5].

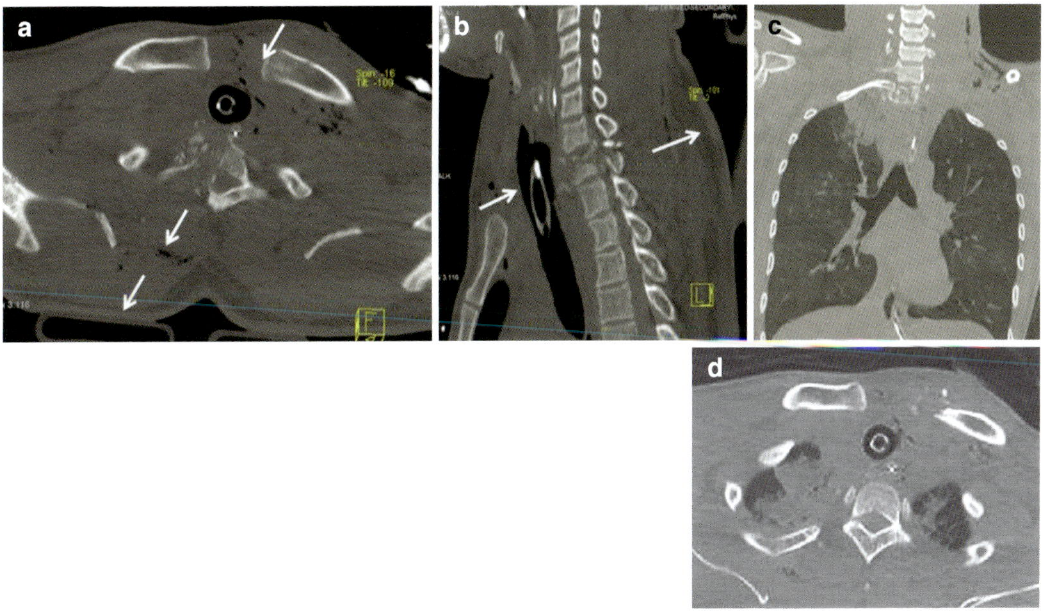

Fig. 8.30 The wide disruption of soft tissues and of bones permits to depict quite exactly the projectile trajectory along the cervicothoracic outlet (*arrows*). In these axial (**a**–**d**), sagittal (**b**), and coronal (**c**), CT-scans we appreciate that the bullet entered from the anterior left jugular region and emerged from the right suprascapular region, crossing the first thoracic vertebral body. Note that, although not directly involved, right lung apex shows a wide contusion area related to the "concussion zone" (**c**, **d**)

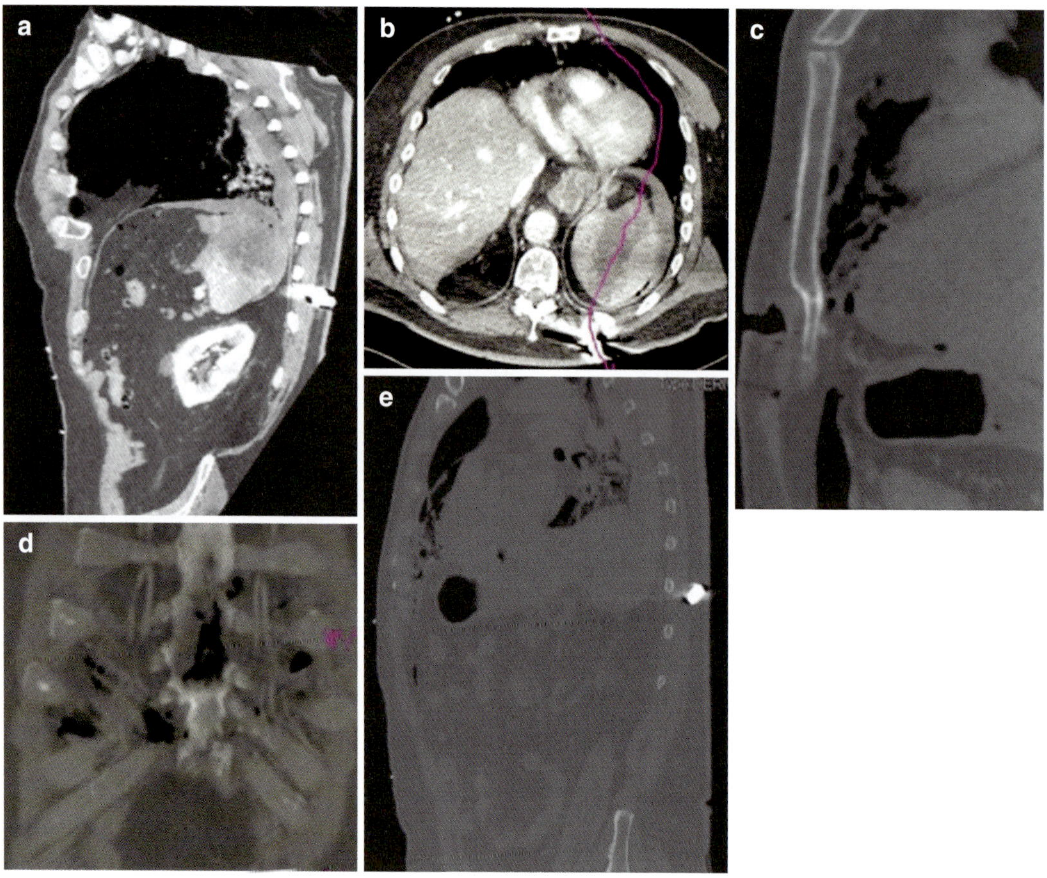

Fig. 8.31 CT trajectogram. CT allows to depict the trajectogram using multiple window levels and multiplanar reconstruction (**a–e**). If the trajectory is not linear, as often occurs due to the different densities of crossed tissues, curved reconstruction along the bullet pathway (**a**, **b**) allows to evaluate correctly all the involved organs in just one image. More wide windows width allows to highlight the bullet entry hole in the subcutaneous fat and in the sternum and the bullet itself, in this case, stopped in the posterior chest wall (**e**)

As already stated, compared to many solid organs, lung is more elastic and is less damaged by bullet wounds and the extent of parenchymal damage depends on the energy of the projectile.

Lung contusion is the main injury after penetrating chest trauma as it occurs along the wound track and in the concussion zone as a result of microscopic disruption of small vessels and alveolar walls which lead to hemorrhage into the parenchyma at the time of trauma, followed in 1–2 h by interstitial edema, which peaks 24 h after injury [28].

Laceration are the most frequent lung injury seen along the wound trajectory and, in penetrating traumas lacerations are much more frequent than in blunt ones [5].

Due to the increase in temperature in lung parenchyma along the bullet path, caused by the high energy released, blood in lacerated parenchymal cavities may tend more frequently to coagulate and pulmonary hematomas are more easily seen.

In all these injuries, MDCT multiplanar images are very useful not only to depict the wound trajectory and to evaluate the site and extent of lung damage [28].

Finally, we must not forget that in thoracic penetrating wound, very often is involved the abdomen and MDCT permits, in a single acquisition, a view of the whole body [5] (Fig. 8.32).

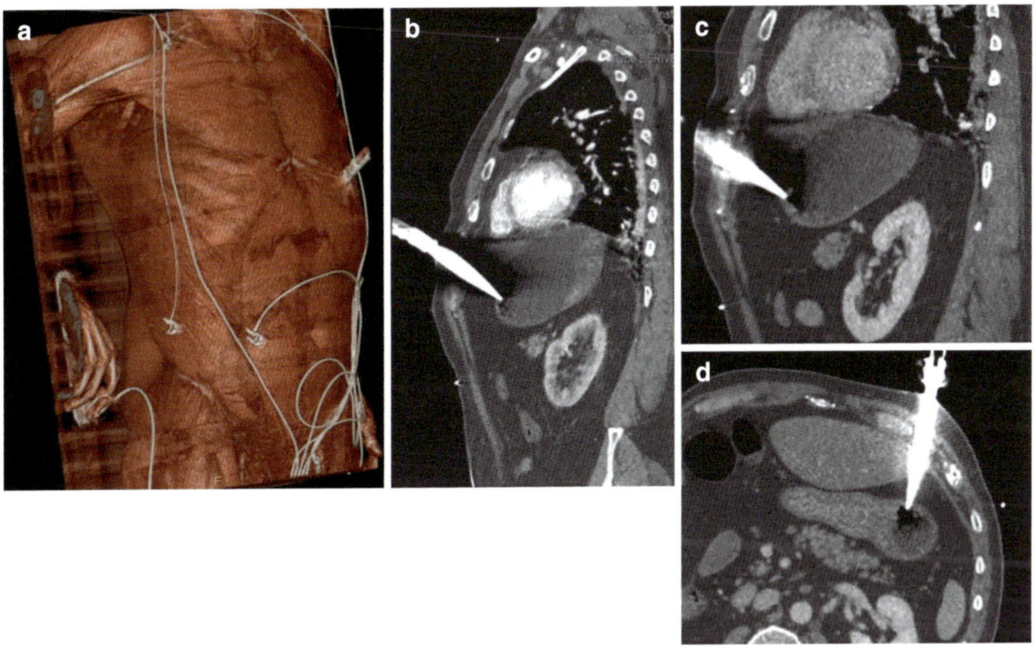

Fig. 8.32 Computed tomography allows to have multiplanar reconstruction to better visualize the penetrating trauma. More than the 3D spectacular reconstruction (**a**), are useful the sagittal (**b**), and the oblique (**c**, **d**) multiplanar imagines that allow to depict the transdiafragmatic trajectory of the stab and the small lesion of the gastric wall and of the left hepatic lobe

References

1. Elmali M, Baydin A, Nural MS, et al. Lung parenchymal injury and its frequency in blunt thoracic trauma: the diagnostic value of chest radiography and thoracic CT. Diagn Interv Radiol. 2007;13:179–82.
2. Kaewlai R, Avery LL, Asrani AV, et al. Multidetector CT of blunt thoracic trauma. Radiographics. 2008; 28:1555–70. doi:10.1148/rg.286085510.
3. Scaglione M, Pinto A, Pedrosa I, et al. Multi-detector row computed tomography and blunt chest trauma. Eur J Radiol. 2008;65:377–88.
4. Demirhan R, Onan B, Oz K, et al. Comprehensive analysis of 4205 patients with chest trauma: a 10-year experience. Interact Cardiovasc Thorac Surg. 2009;9:450–3. doi:10.1510/icvts.2009.206599.
5. Dreizin D, Munera F. Multidetector CT for penetrating torso trauma: state of the art. Radiology. 2015;277:338–55. doi:10.1148/radiol.2015142282.
6. Richards JR, McGahan JP. Focus assessment with sonography in trauma (FAST) in 2017: what radiologist can learn. Radiology. 2017;238:30–48. doi:10.1148/radiol.2017160107.
7. Ho ML, Gutierrez FR. Chest radiography in thoracic polytrauma. AJR Am J Roentgenol. 2009;192:599–612. doi:10.2214/AJR.07.3324.
8. Brink M, Deunk J, Dekker HM, et al. Added value of routine chest MDCT after blunt trauma: evaluation of additional findings and impact on patient management. AJR Am J Roentgenol. 2008;190:1591–8. doi:10.2214/AJR.07.3277.
9. Çorbacioglu SK, Erhan E, Aslan S, et al. The significance of routine thoracic computed tomography in patients with blunt chest trauma. Injury. 2014;46:849–53. doi:10.1016/j.injury.2014.12.022.
10. Kreuter M, Mathis G. Emergency ultrasound of the chest. Respiration. 2014;87:89–97. doi:10.1159/000357685.
11. Ianniello S, Merola MG, Trinci M, et al. Priorità diagnostiche nel management del trauma maggiore: ruolo dell'E-FAST e della TCMD. Il Giornale Italiano di. Radiol Med. 2015;2:715–20. doi:10.17376/girm_2-4-07082015-19.
12. Lichtenstein DA, Mezière GA. Relevance of lung ultrasound in the diagnosis of acute respiratory failure: the BLUE protocol. Chest. 2008;134:117–25. doi:10.1378/chest.07-2800.
13. Zanobetti M, Scorpiniti M, Gigli C, et al. Point-of-care ultrasonography for evaluation of acute dyspnea in the emergency department. Chest. 2017;151(6):1295–301. doi:10.1016/j.chest.2017.02.003.
14. Hyacinthe AC, Broux C, Francony G, et al. Diagnostic accuracy of ultrasonography in the acute assessment of common thoracic lesions after trauma. Chest. 2012;141:1177–83. doi:10.1378/chest.11-0208.
15. Kirkpatrick AW, Sirois M, Laupland KB, et al. Handheld thoracic sonography for detecting post-traumatic

pneumothoraces: the extended focused assessment with sonography for trauma (EFAST). J Trauma. 2004;57:288–95.
16. Ianniello S, Di Giacomo V, Sessa B, et al. First-line sonographic diagnosis of pneumothorax in unstable major trauma: accuracy of e-FAST and comparison with multidetector computed tomography. Radiol Med. 2014;2014(119):674–80. doi:10.1007/s11547-014-0384-1. Epub 2014 Jan 28.
17. Volpicelli G, Elbarbary M, Blaivas M, et al. International evidence-based recommendation for point-of-care lung ultrasound. Intensive Care Med. 2012;38:577–91. doi:10.1007/s00134-012-2513-4.
18. Wongwaisayawan S, Suwannanon R, et al. Emergency thoracic US: the essentials. Radiographics. 2016;36:640–59. doi:10.1148/rg.2016150064.
19. Peters S, Nivolas V, Heyer CM. Multidetector computed tomography-spectrum of blunt chest wall and lung injuries in polytraumatized patients. Clin Radiol. 2010;65:333–8. doi:10.1016/j.crad.2009.12.008.
20. Ursic C, Curtis K. Thoracic and neck trauma. Part two. Int Emerg Neurs. 2010;18:99–108. doi:10.1016/j.ienj.2008.11.011.
21. Kaya S, Cevik AA, Acar N, et al. A study on the evaluation of pneumothorax by imaging methods in patients presenting to the emergency department for blunt thoracic trauma. Ulus Trauma Acil Cerrahi Derg. 2015;21:366–72. doi:10.5505/tjtes.2015.91650.
22. Wilkerson RG, Stone MB. Sensitivity of bedside ultrasound and supine anteroposterior chest radiographs for the identification of pneumothorax after blunt trauma. Acad Emerg Med. 2010;17:11–7. doi:10.1111/j.1553-2712.2009.00628.x.
23. Rowan KR, Kirkpatrick AW, Liu D, et al. Traumatic pneumothorax detection with thoracic US: correlation with chest radiography and CT-initial experience. Radiology. 2002;225:210–4.
24. Gillman LM, Kirkpatrick AW. Portable bedside ultrasound: the visual stethoscope of the 21st century. Scand J Trauma Resusc Emerg Med. 2012;9:20–18. doi:10.1186/1757-7241-20-18.
25. Mennicke M, Gulati K, Oliva I, et al. Anatomical distribution of traumatic pneumothoraces on chest computed tomography: implications for ultrasound screening in ED. Am J Emerg Med. 2012;30:1025–31. doi:10.1016/j.ajem.2011.06.020.
26. Volpicelli G, Boero E, Sverzellati N, et al. Semi-quantification of pneumothorax volume by lung ultrasound. Intensive Care Med. 2014;40:1460–7. doi:10.1007/s00134-014-3402-9.
27. Oikonomou A, Prassopulos P. CT imaging of blunt chest trauma. Insights Imaging. 2011;2:281–95.
28. Miller LA. Chest wall, lung, and pleural space trauma. Radiol Clin N Am. 2006;44:213–24.
29. Kim YK, Kim H, Lee CC. New classification and clinical characteristics of reexpansion pulmonary edema after treatment of spontaneous pneumothorax. Am J Emerg Med. 2009;27:961–7. doi:10.1016/j.ajem.2008.07.036.
30. Ma OJ, Mateer JR. Trauma ultrasound examination versus chest radiography in the detection of hemothorax. Ann Emerg Med. 1997;29:312–5.
31. Chen SW, Huang YK, Liao CH, Wang SY. Right massive haemothorax as the presentation of blunt cardiac rupture: the pitfall of coexisting pericardial laceration. Interact Cardiovasc Thorac Surg. 2014;18:245–6. doi:10.1093/icvts/ivt483.
32. Sajadieh H, Afzali F, Sajadieh V, et al. Ultrasound as an alternative to aspiration for determining the nature of pleural effusion, especially in older people. Ann N Y Acad Sci. 2004;1019:585–92.
33. Brooks A, Davies B, Smethhurrst M, et al. Emergency ultrasound in the acute assessment of haemothorax. Emerg Med J. 2004;21:44–6.
34. Movaghar V, Yousefifard M, Ghelichkhani P, et al. Application of ultrasound and radiography in detection of hemothorax; a systematic review and meta-analysis. Emerg (Tehran). 2016;4:116–26.
35. Wagner RB, Crawford WO, Schimpf PP. Classification of parenchymal injuries of the lung. Radiology. 1988;167:77–82.
36. Ganie FA, Lone H, Lone GN, et al. Lung contusion: a clinico-pathological entity with unpredictable clinical course. Bull Emerg Trauma. 2013;1:7–16.
37. Cohn SM, Dubose JJ. Pulmonary contusion: an update on recent advances in clinical management. World J Surg. 2010;34:1959–70. doi:10.1007/s00268-010-0599-9.
38. Raghavendran K, Davidson BA, Woyatsh JA, et al. The evolution of isolated bilateral lung contusion from blunt chest trauma in rats: cellular and cytokine responses. Shock. 2005;24:132–8.
39. Aufmkolk M, Fischer R, Voggenreiter G, et al. Local effect of lung contusion on lung surfactant composition in multiple trauma patients. Crit Care Med. 1999;27:1441–6.
40. Raghavendran K, Davidson BA, Knight PR, et al. Surfactant dysfunction in lung contusion with and without superimposed gastric aspiration rat model. Shock. 2008;30:508–17. doi:10.1097/SHK.0b013e3181673fc5.
41. Strohmaier W, Trupka A, Pfeiler C, et al. Bilateral lavage with diluted surfactant improves lung function after unilateral lung contusion in pigs. Crit Care Med. 2005;33:2286–93.
42. Miller DL, Mansour KA. Blunt traumatic lung injuries. Thorac Surg Clin. 2007;17:57–61.
43. Tovar JA. The lung and paediatric trauma. Semin Pediatr Surg. 2008;17:53–9.
44. Miller PR, Croce MA, Kilgo PD, et al. Acute respiratory distress syndrome in blunt trauma: identification of independent risk factors. Am Surg. 2002;68:845–50.
45. Moore EE, Moore FA, Harken AH, et al. The two-event construct of postinjury multiple organ failure. Shock. 2005;1:71–4.
46. Dolgachev VA, Yu B, Reinke JM, et al. Host susceptibility to gram-negative pneumonia after lung con-

tusion. J Trauma Acute Care Surg. 2012;72:614–22. doi:10.1097/TA.0b013e318243d9b1.
47. Soldati G, Testa A, Silva FR, et al. Chest ultrasonography in lung contusion. Chest. 2006;130:533–8.
48. Lichtenstein DA, Mezière GA, Biderman P, et al. The comet-tail artifact. An ultrasound sign of alveolar-interstitial syndrome. Am J Respir Crit Care Med. 1997;156:1640–6.
49. Leblanc D, Bouvet C, Degiovanni F, et al. Early lung ultrasonography predicts the occurrence of acute respiratory distress syndrome in blunt trauma patients. Intensive Care Med. 2014;40:1468–74. doi:10.1007/s00134-014-3382-9.
50. Sangster GP, Gonzales-Beicos A, Carbo AI. Blunt traumatic injuries of the lung parenchyma, pleura, thoracic wall, and intrathoracic airways: multidetector computer tomography imaging findings. Emerg Radiol. 2007;14:297–310.
51. Mirvis SE. Imaging of acute thoracic injury: the advent of MDCT screening. Semin Ultrasound CT MR. 2005;26:305–31.
52. Novelline RA. Imaging chest trauma. In: Diseases of the heart, chest & breast. Part 1. Milan: Springer; 2007.
53. Clark AJ, Huges N, Chisti F. Traumatic extrathoracic lung herniation. Br J Radiol. 2009;82:e82–4. doi:10.1259/bjr/24198593.
54. Forty J, Wells FC. Traumatic intercostal pulmonary hernia. Ann Thorac Surg. 1990;49:670–1.
55. Durso AM, Caban K, Munera F. Penetrating thoracic injury. Radiol Clin N Am. 2015;53:675–93. doi:10.1016/j.rcl.2015.02.010.
56. Karmy-Jones R, Namias N, Coimbra R, et al. Western Trauma Association critical decisions in trauma: penetrating chest trauma. J Trauma Acute Care Surg. 2014;77:994–1002. doi:10.1097/TA.0000000000000426.
57. Ball CG, Dente CJ, Kirkpatrick AW, et al. Occult pneumothoraces in patients with penetrating trauma: does mechanism matter? Can J Surg. 2010;53:251–5.
58. Berg RJ, Inaba K, Recinos G, et al. Prospective evaluation of early follow-up chest radiography after penetrating thoracic injury. World J Surg. 2013;37:1286–90. doi:10.1007/s00268-013-2002-0.
59. Magnotti LJ, Weinberg JA, Schroeppel TJ, et al. Initial chest CT obviates the need for repeat chest radiograph after penetrating thoracic trauma. Am Surg. 2007;73:569–72.
60. Governatori NJ, Saul T, Siadecki SD, et al. Ultrasound in the evaluation of penetrating thoraco-abdominal trauma: a review of the literature. Med Ultrason. 2015;17:528–34. doi:10.11152/mu.2013.2066.174.evp.
61. Ku BS, Fields JM, Carr B, et al. Clinician-performed bedside ultrasound for the diagnosis of traumatic pneumothorax. West J Emerg Med. 2013;14:103–8. doi:10.5811/westjem.2012.12.12663.
62. Aj N, Navsaria PH, Beningfield S, et al. Screening for occult penetrating cardiac injuries. Ann Surg. 2015;261:573–8.doi:10.1097/SLA.0000000000000713.
63. Chiu WC, Shanmuganathan K, Mirvis SE, Scalea TM. Determining the need for laparotomy in penetrating torso trauma: prospective study using triple-contrast enhanced abdominopelvic computed tomography. J Trauma. 2001;51:860–8.

9 Aortic Injury

Mario Moroni, Giulia Grazzini,
Monica Marina Lanzetta, Silvia Pradella,
Manlio Acquafresca, and Vittorio Miele

9.1 Introduction

Injury to the aorta and the arch vessels can occur following blunt and penetrating trauma. Penetrating trauma commonly occurs secondary to gunshot and stab wounds, is uncommon, and is a highly lethal injury (90%), with most patients dying rapidly in the field. Blunt trauma is almost invariably resulting from high-impact trauma (collision >50 km/h), usually with rapid deceleration forces. Patients sustaining blunt traumatic aortic injury (BTAI) usually have many concomitant injuries that will distract from studying the aorta.

BTAI is relatively rare. Incidence of BTAI in polytrauma victims transported to hospitals is of 0.3%, and it occurs in about 2% of cases with massive chest trauma [1].

M. Moroni, M.D. (✉) • G. Grazzini • M.M. Lanzetta
S. Pradella • M. Acquafresca • V. Miele
Department of Radiology, Careggi University Hospital, Florence, Italy
e-mail: elleci77@libero.it

Despite its relative rarity, BTAI has a high mortality and remains the second leading cause of death, after head injury, in polytrauma patients [2–4]. Approximately 80% of patents with TAI die before even reaching the hospital, 4% die during transportation, and 19% die during triage in the hospital [5, 6].

These potentially life-threatening conditions need urgent detection and treatment.

Significant advancements have been made in the diagnosis and treatment of aortic injuries over the past two decades. These include the widespread use of computed tomography angiography (CTA) for diagnosis, medical management of minimal aortic injuries (MAI), delayed repair (>24 h) for stable patients, and broad implementation of endovascular repair. Previously, around 50% patients that reached the hospital with TAI died within 24 h, but now with better imaging, improving surgical techniques, and percutaneous interventions, the mortality among these patients has decreased up to approximately 5% [7].

Especially, following treatment, the mortality rate varies from 5 to 28% depending on the technique used and the extent of the associated lesions. However, with modern therapeutic techniques, particularly endovascular repair, it is close to 9% according to more recent studies [8].

Patients with BTAI are mainly males (72%) and the mean age is 41 (±20) [6].

V. Miele, M. Trinci (eds.), *Diagnostic Imaging in Polytrauma Patients*,
https://doi.org/10.1007/978-3-319-62054-1_9

Hospitalized BTAI patients have frequently concurrent chest wall injuries (as bone fractures) and severe injuries elsewhere in about 40% of cases, as head injury, pulmonary contusion, hepatic and splenic injury, pelvic trauma, upper extremity trauma, and spine injury [9].

9.2 Anatomy

The thoracic aorta can be divided into four segments (Fig. 9.1).

The first two segments, which are intrapericardial, are the Valsalva sinus (segment 0), where the coronary arteries originate, and the ascending aorta (segment 1), which originates 1–2 cm above the coronary ostia. From the aortic arch (segment 2) arise the brachiocephalic, left common carotid and left subclavian arteries (LSAs), which are the three major branches of the arch in most patients. The brachiocephalic artery bifurcates to form the right common carotid and right subclavian arteries. The ligamentum arteriosus is the remnant of the patent ductus arteriosus, which shunts blood from the pulmonary artery to the aorta during development. Finally, the descending aorta (segment 3) is situated beyond the subclavian artery and extending to the diaphragmatic orifice, where it becomes the abdominal aorta [10]. The isthmus is the portion of the proximal descending thoracic aorta located between the origin of the left subclavian artery and the site of attachment of the ligamentum arteriosus [11].

A variety of congenital alterations to the aortic arch exist, such as the true bovine arch and the so-called bovine arch. The true bovine arch (Fig. 9.2a) is a rare variant in which a single, large common brachiocephalic trunk comes off the arch and separates into the right and LSAs and the bicarotid trunk. This bicarotid trunk then bifurcates to form the right and left common carotid arteries. A more common variant is the so-called bovine arch, present in as many as 20% of patients. The so-called bovine arch (Fig. 9.2b) includes a brachiocephalic trunk that splits into the right subclavian, right common carotid, and left common carotid arteries. The LSA comes off separately from the arch of the aorta. Other variants include the left vertebral artery coming off directly from the arch in 2.5% of patients (Fig. 9.3) and the existence of a right-sided aortic arch in patients with dextrocardia or situs inver-

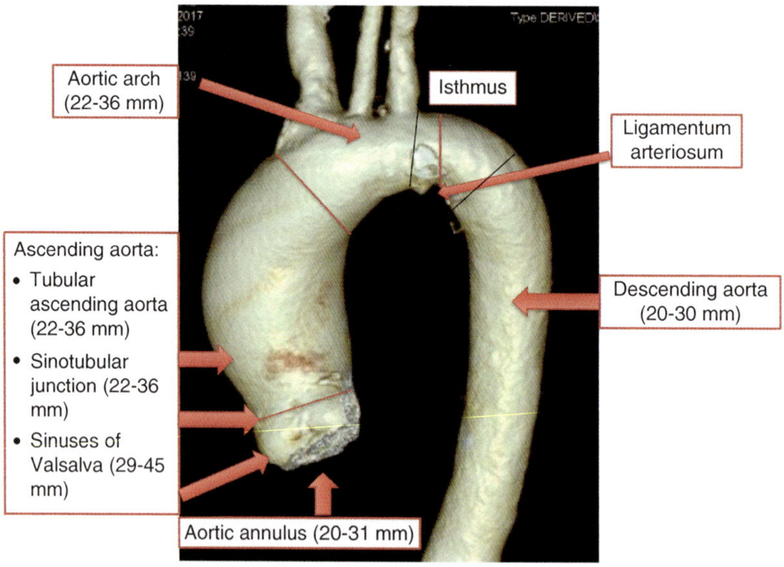

Fig. 9.1 Three-dimensional volume-rendered (3D-VR) image shows the segments of the thoracic aorta

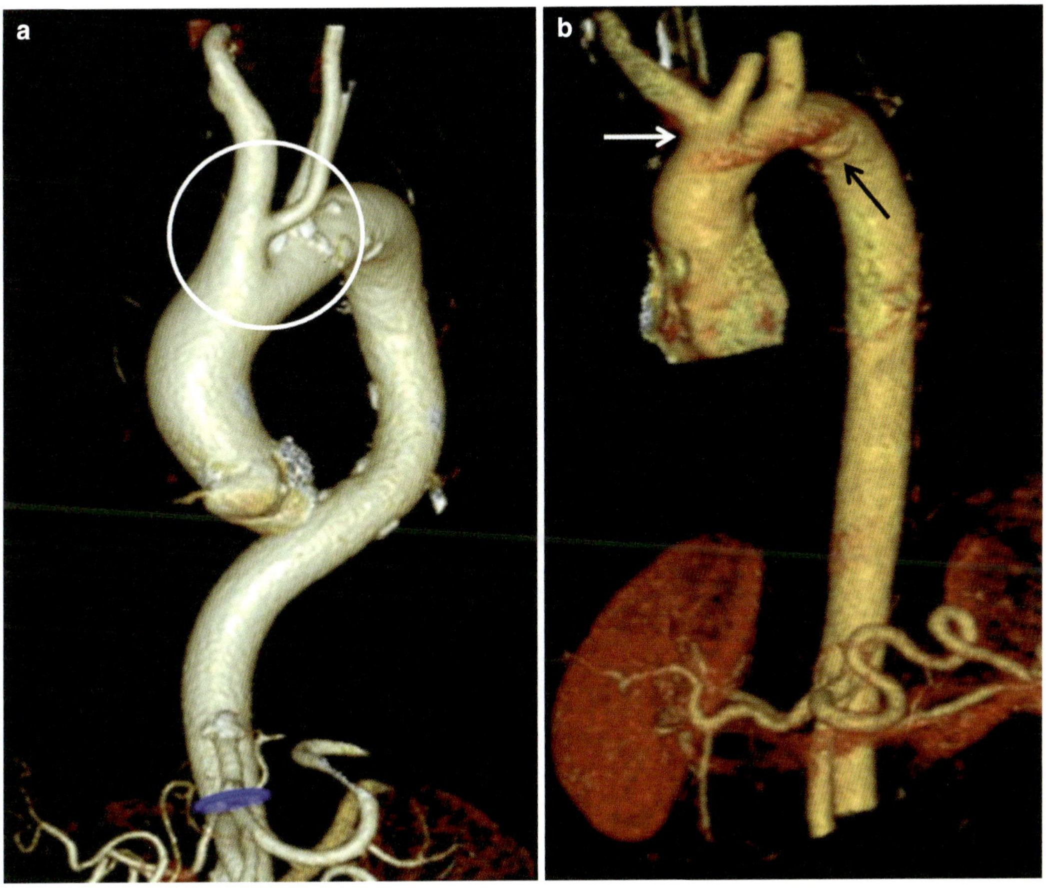

Fig. 9.2 Three-dimensional volume-rendered (3D-VR) images show in (**a**), bovine arch (*white circle*); in (**b**), the so-called bovine arch (*white arrow*); see also small pseudoaneurysm isthmus (*black arrow*)

sus. Anatomic variants of the aorta can mask as traumatic injury. For example, a ductus diverticulum may be present along the anterior surface near the ligamentum arteriosus, which may be confused with pseudoaneurysm formation. An aortic spindle may present as circumferential dilatation between the LSA and ligamentum arteriosus [12].

9.3 Pathophysiology and Location

There are several causes of traumatic aortic injury, but the common factor is the violence of the shock. Motor vehicle accidents make up 75–80% of the cases, while motorcycle, aircraft, pedestrian accidents, fall from height, and crush injury to chest account for the remainder [5].

Injury to the aortic wall is likely a result of any or a combination of several potential mechanisms include torsion and shearing forces, rapid deceleration, stretching, increased intravascular pressure (water-hammer effect), and compression of the aorta (osseous pinch) [13, 14] (Fig. 9.4). Osseous pinch results from direct compression of the aorta between the vertebral column and the anterior chest wall (sternum, clavicles, and ribs). Torsion indicates rotational forces of the aorta along its longitudinal axis. Shearing forces are caused by differential relative motion at different points of fixation; at the

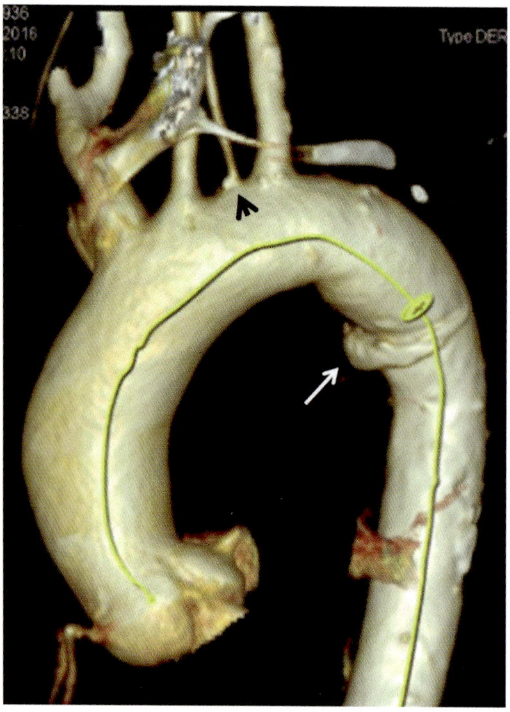

Fig. 9.3 Three-dimensional volume-rendered (3D-VR) image shows normal anatomic aortic arch variant. *Black arrowhead* shows left vertebral artery coming off directly from the aortic arch; *white arrow* shows pseudoaneurysm isthmus

aortic root, the ligamentum arteriosus attachment, and the diaphragmatic crus, the aorta is connected to other tissues, so it's submitted to increasing regional strain by different deceleration characteristics of the joined tissues. Stretching of the aorta from displacement of vertebrae is the so-called stretch injury. The water-hammer effect, proposed by Lundevall, results when the flow of a non-compressible fluid is occluded dramatically; this condition leads to high-pressure waves being reflected back along the vessel wall, and it could happen after a compression on the abdomen or lower chest. Sudden deceleration is the most common cause of traumatic aortic injury, and it concerns particularly the front seat passenger of a vehicle going at speeds 100 km/h, (sudden deceleration >32 km/h) subjected to frontal or lateral or rear shock [15]. This mechanism causes displacement of the heart, with torsion and shearing forces against the aorta at levels of relative immobility, mainly the ligamentum arteriosus, aortic root, diaphragm, and intercostal arteries.

Direct penetration from fractured ribs, sternum, vertebrae or from gunshot and stab wounds may

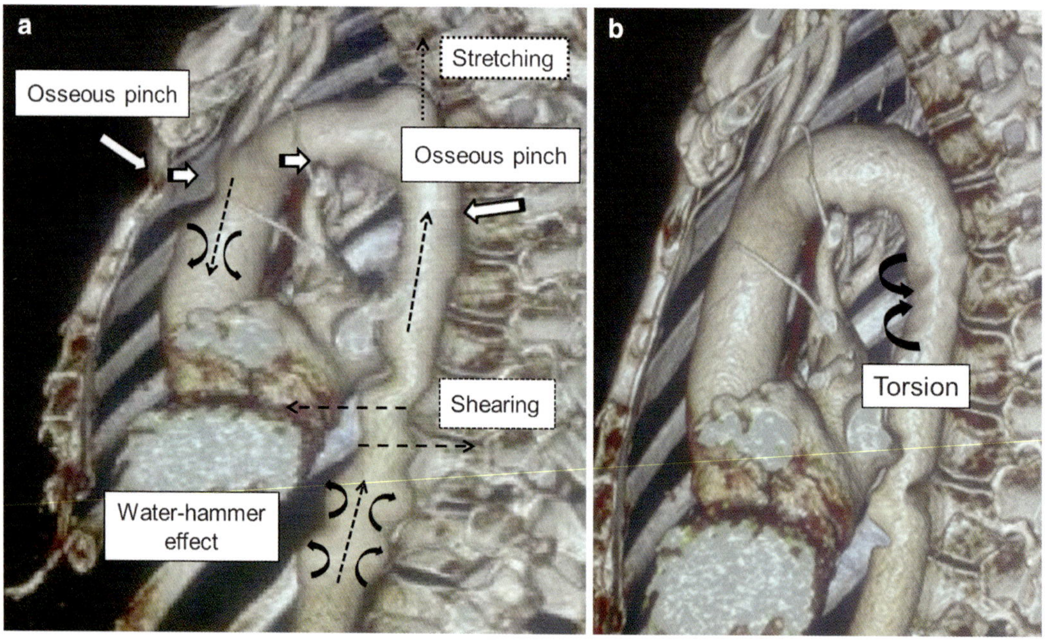

Fig. 9.4 Three-dimensional volume-rendered (3D-VR) image shows various mechanisms of injury: in (**a**), osseous pinch, shearing, stretching, and water-hammer effect; in (**b**), torsion

also occur. Penetrating injuries to the thoracic aorta are uncommon. When present, they are likely to lead to rapid exsanguination, and many of these patients do not survive transport to the hospital.

Depending on the forces in play, the aorta injury site can be the root, ascending aorta, arch, isthmus, descending aorta, or even abdominal aorta (less common). A considerable number of patients have aortic injury at multiple sites.

The isthmus is the commonest location for lesions (approximately 90% of all cases of patients who have been subjected to thoracic trauma) [16]. Its relatively immobile position in the thorax due to its attachment by the ligamentum arteriosus explains the reason for this site being involved in many injuries (Fig. 9.5).

Lesions of the root of the aorta are sometimes associated with damage to the aortic valve. Lesions of the ascending aorta are rare (between 5 and 8% of the cases) [17] and mainly occur close by the brachiocephalic origin. In contrast, injuries infrequently occur at the proximal portion of the ascending aorta [18]. These two types of lesions are sometimes associated with hemopericardium.

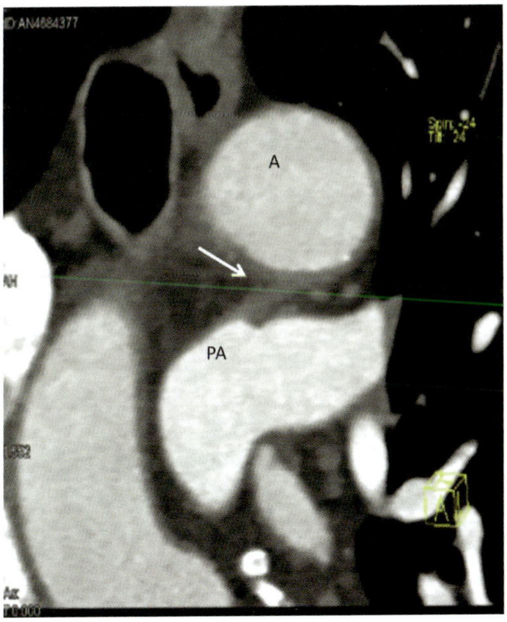

Fig. 9.5 Oblique multiplanar reformation (MPR). *White arrow* shows site of attachment for ligamentum arteriosus (*A* aorta, *PA* pulmonary artery)

Involvement of the aortic arch and its branches is not so common. While involvement of the aortic arch itself is rare (about 2% of the cases) [18], the incidence of aortic arch branch involvement varies considerably in the literature (about 3% have a combined aortic and aortic branch vessel injury, whereas the great vessels alone are injured in about 16%) [19].

At multidetector CT, a careful search for a branch vessel injury should be performed in the presence of mediastinal hematoma when there is no direct sign of aortic injury. The innominate artery accounts for 50% of these injuries and is the second most common injured vessel after the thoracic aorta [20]. The left common carotid and left subclavian artery account for the remaining injuries. Innominate artery and left carotid injuries almost always occur proximally at the vessel origin; anatomically, this is where the vessel is tightly fixed onto the aortic arch, whereas the distal part is more mobile and flexible (Fig. 9.6).

In contrast, blunt subclavian injuries tend to be more distal; these can be explained by adding the direct force of posterior dislocated clavicles [21].

In 1–12% of the cases, there is trauma to the descending thoracic aorta [17]. The distal descending aorta is attached to the adjacent vertebral column by the diaphragm. When there is a shock to the thorax, the resulting shear forces are responsible for lesions at this site. Injuries to this segment of the thoracic aorta can be associated with diaphragm injury in 10% of cases and with adjacent compression fractures of the thoracic spine [22].

In the abdomen, the most common site of injury is the infrarenal abdominal aorta. These injuries are typically related to lap belt compression. There are a number of additional abdominal injuries that are associated with traumatic abdominal aortic injury, including lumbar spine fracture, splenic injury, pelvic fractures, bowel injury, and solid organ injury. Lumbar spine fracture has the highest association with traumatic abdominal aortic injury [23] and if seen should prompt a careful evaluation of the aorta and vice versa.

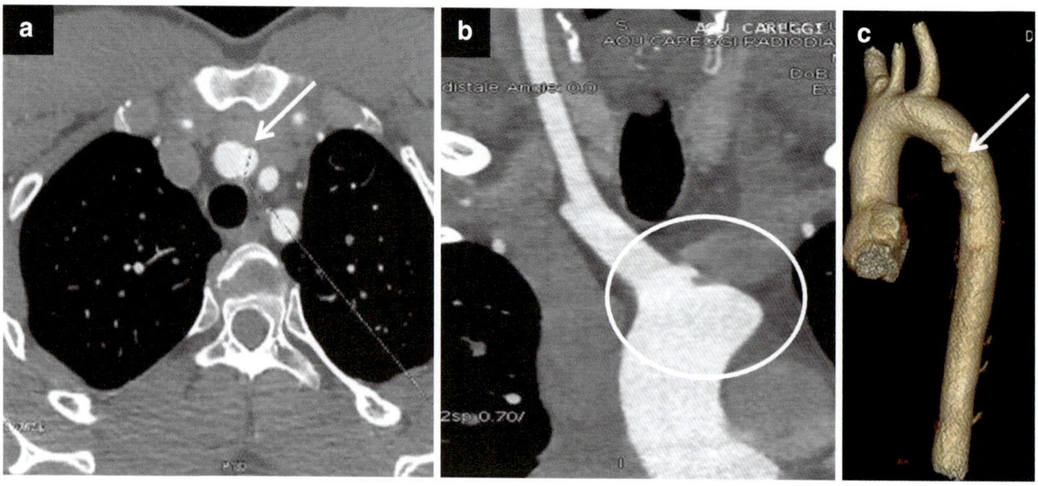

Fig. 9.6 Combined thoracic aorta and aortic branch vessel injury. (**a**) Axial CT scan and (**b**) multiplanar reformation (MPR) show small pseudoaneurysm artery innominate proximally at the vessel origin (*white arrow* in **a** and *white circle* in **b**); (**c**) three-dimensional volume-rendered (3D-VR) image shows combined pseudoaneurysm isthmus (*white arrow*) in the same patient

9.4 Clinical Presentation

Clinical signs and symptoms (Table 9.1) are nonspecific and insensitive for the diagnosis and exclusion of BTAI. A majority of patients with BTAI have no clinical signs of aortic injury until the sudden onset of hemodynamic instability [24].

Symptoms of BTAI are thought to be due to stretching of the mediastinal connective tissues by mediastinal blood and include retrosternal pain, referred interscapular pain, dyspnea, and cough [25].

Clinical signs of BTAI are absent in up to one-third of patients but when present include upper limb hypertension and lower limb hypotension with diminished femoral pulses due to "pseudo-coarctation syndrome," systemic hypotension, systolic murmur, external chest wall injuries, fractures (sternal, rib, or vertebral column), and paraplegia [26].

Factors negatively influencing prognosis are a systolic blood pressure < 90 mmHg and hypothermia with $T < 35$ °C.

Therefore, the clinical picture of patients with BTAI varies from asymptomatic to profound shock.

Table 9.1 BTAI signs and symptoms

Symptoms	Signs
Chest pain	Unexplained systemic hypotension
Dyspnea	"Pseudocoarctation syndrome" (upper limb hypertension and lower limb hypotension with diminished femoral pulses)
Cough	Systolic murmur
Dysphagia	Chest wall ecchymosis
Hemoptysis	Sternal, rib, or thoracic spine fractures

9.5 Diagnosis

The most important factor in preventing a delay in diagnosis is the arousal of clinical suspicion based on mechanism of injury. Patients sustaining massive chest trauma associated with rapid deceleration (motor vehicle accidents or falls) should carry suspicion of thoracic aortic injury.

9.5.1 Chest X-Ray

A chest X-ray (CXR) has long been a part of the initial imaging assessment of suspected BTAI with a long list of signs described (Table 9.2), including a widened mediastinum (>8 cm at the

Table 9.2 Thoracic aortic injuries: radiographic signs

Widened mediastinum >8 cm
Loss or abnormal aortic contour
Left apical cap
Loss of the aortopulmonary window
Depression of the left main stem bronchus
Fractures (sternal, vertebral, 1–2 rib, clavicular)
Nasogastric tube and/or trachea displacement to the right midline
Pneumothorax
Pulmonary contusion
Left-sided hemothorax

arch), irregular aortic knob, loss of aortic-pulmonary window, an apical cap, tracheal deviation to the right, nasogastric shifting to right, widening of the left paraspinal line, and the presence of a basilar hemothorax, with sensitivities ranging from 80 to 92% [27, 28].

Furthermore, scapular, sternal, thoracic spine, or multiple rib fractures should heighten suspicion of thoracic aortic injury. Patel et al. combined positive chest radiograph findings with clinical suspicion and elevated the sensitivity of plain radiographs to 98% [29].

The most common radiographic abnormality is widened mediastinum (>8 cm) although only 20–43% of patients with a widened mediastinum have a thoracic aortic injury. The finding of a widened mediastinum may be an indirect determinant of thoracic aortic injury being a result more from bleeding small vessels contained within the mediastinum hemorrhage than from aortic bleeding or an aortic pseudoaneurysm, therefore giving low positive predictive values [27] (Fig. 9.7).

The utility of chest radiographs in the diagnosis of blunt aortic injury was questioned because radiographic signs on plain chest films carry low specificity and no improvement in overall accuracy [30].

An important factor to bear in mind is that these RX findings are based on upright chest radiographs, thus decreasing projection and magnification artifact appreciated on supine studies. This is complicated by the difficulty in obtaining upright plain films during initial trauma resuscitations secondary to a patient's injury status. Furthermore, there are several reports documenting thoracic aortic rupture with normal initial chest radiographs [31], so a normal CXR does not exclude an aortic injury. Therefore, plain chest radiographs should not be used as sole criteria for either excluding or confirming thoracic aortic injury and the utility of CXR in the setting of suspected BTAI is low. However, in the acute trauma setting, the supine chest radiograph is still frequently obtained mainly to detect immediate life-threatening lesions requiring immediate treatment (massive hemothorax or tension pneumothorax).

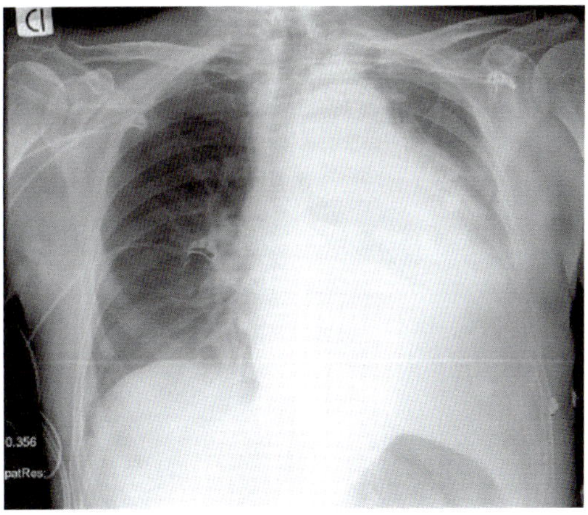

Fig. 9.7 Chest X-ray (CXR) in blunt thoracic trauma shows widened mediastinum, abnormal aortic contour, loss of the aortopulmonary window, left-sided pleural effusion, and pulmonary contusion

CRX could be used in the long-term follow-up of young BTAI patients after endovascular treatment to reduce radiation exposure as compared with CT; it enables to detect stent-graft migration or collapse [32].

9.5.2 Angiography

Conventional angiography was considered the gold standard for the diagnosis of BTAI for decades with sensitivity and specificity nearing 100%. The publication of the Eastern Association for the Surgery of Trauma (EAST) practice management guideline for the diagnosis and management of blunt aortic injury in 2000 still defined angiography as the "gold standard" for the diagnosis of BTAI [33, 34].

Even though aortography is safe, it is a resource intensive, invasive, expensive and, most importantly, time consuming. It does not demonstrate intramural hematoma and may miss less severe injuries, such as intimal flaps. A false-positive interpretation can occur due to focal atheroma, particularly if ulcerated, an overlapping vessel, and a ductus diverticulum. A rapid development of computed tomography (CT) techniques has rendered CT more sensitive than conventional angiography, mostly due to the detection of extra-luminal abnormalities, either confined to the aortic wall or beyond.

Catheter angiography is now most commonly used to plan endovascular intervention.

9.5.3 Transesophageal Echocardiography (TOE)

Currently, the use of transoesophageal echocardiography (TOE) is very restricted: about 1% of BTAI patients receive TOE [35].

This technique is reported to identify intimal tears, intramural hematoma, pseudoaneurysms, pseudocoarctation, and active bleeding with a sensitivity of 91–100% and a specificity of 98% [36, 37].

TOE is an operator-dependent technique, and even in experienced hands there is incomplete visualization of the entire aortic circumference in a third of patients. Another disadvantage is the relatively poor visualization of the distal ascending aorta and proximal arch.

Patients with facial injuries, unstable cervical spine injuries, or where cervical spine injuries have not been excluded are unsuitable. TOE does not demonstrate the full spectrum of injuries that cross-sectional imaging can.

The primary use currently is to evaluate cardiac dysfunction and injury or hemodynamic state and response to treatment. In hemodynamically unstable patients, transoesophageal echocardiography can be performed quickly at the bedside or in the operating room, which is seen as its main advantages. Thus, unlike the other imaging techniques, TEA can be used intraoperatively to immediately affect surgical and anesthesia decisions.

9.5.4 Intravascular US

Endoluminal or intravascular US is another useful adjunctive imaging modality that can be used to provide high-resolution cross-sectional images of the vessel wall and the surrounding tissues. The findings of aortic injury at intravascular US include vessel wall disruption, intimal flap, focal pseudoaneurysm, intramural and periaortic hematoma, and complete transection. Although these findings are considered to be specific for BTAI, false-positive results have been described [38].

Patel et al. demonstrated better sensitivity compared to angiography especially for picking up MAI, before the era of CT angiography (CTA) as a gold standard [39, 40]. It can be performed concurrently with conventional aortography and has been shown to be a useful complementary modality. Intravascular US is an operator- and experience-dependent invasive procedure, requiring arterial puncture, and complete evaluation of the aorta can be time consuming and may not allow complete visualization of the brachiocephalic artery [24].

9.5.5 Magnetic Resonance Imaging (MRI)

MRI combines safety with an acceptable diagnostic performance [41]. Nonetheless, this technique is not at present used in emergency situations. The duration of acquisitions and the immobility required of the patient prohibit the use of this modality. Furthermore, It may be contraindicated by the support or immobilization equipment required in polytrauma. MRI, however, may have a role in the follow-up when delayed surgery is contemplated, particularly as a strategy for radiation dose reduction in young trauma victims [42].

MRI is useful in the follow-up of patients who have been treated with MR-compatible stent grafts decreasing radiation dose in a usually young patient population although its poorer spatial resolution could lead to a lowered sensitivity for subtle complications and will not detect stent-graft migration.

9.5.6 Computed Tomography Angiography (CTA)

The diagnostic value of chest CT became of increasing interest throughout the 1990s. Previously, chest and abdominal CT have been used as a screening tool detecting periaortic hematomas or posterior mediastinal blood, both of which are highly specific for thoracic aortic rupture, but CT had decreased sensitivity if compared to aortography [43]. During the past 20 years, the wider use of newer, helical CT angiograms (CTA) have increased sensitivity and specificity to as high as 98–100% and a 100% negative predictive value [44], so that CTA is able to exclude aortic injuries without doing any other diagnostic test (Table 9.3) [45–48].

Two studies sponsored by the American Association for the Surgery of Trauma in 1997 and 2007 showed how in this decade the diagnosis of BTAI shifted from angiography and TEE to CT scanning [49]. BTAI patients underwent angiography and TEE in 87% and 12% of cases, respectively, in 1997 and only in 8% and 1% in 2007; in contrast, use of CT scan for the diagnosis of thoracic aortic injuries was increased from 34.8 to 93.3% (1997 to 2007).

Dyer et al. also noted significant cost savings of CTA when compared to traditional aortography for diagnosis [50].

With the arrival of multidetector CT (MDCT), the acquisition time was intensely reduced and the scan of whole body, from the base of the skull through the symphysis pubis, can be achieved in few second depending on the scanning parameters (Fig. 9.8).

In addition to faster image acquisition, other MDCT benefits are the panoramicity and an elevated spatial resolution due to axial thin slice (<1 mm) acquisition that can be utilized for "real" multiplanar reformations (MPRs) and 3D reformations.

These features of new CT scanners permit improved diagnosis of BTAI. The advent of dual-source CT scanners and scanners with 64 or more slices has revolutionized the cardiovascular applications of CT [51]. These scanners have the spatial resolution ranging from 0.25 to 0.47 mm, with most newer scanners offering 0.33 mm. These scanners also have a very high temporal resolution due to faster gantry rotation. Newer dual-energy and 256/320 slice CT machines have

Table 9.3 Angiography versus computed tomography angiography (CTA)

Angiography (%)		CTA (%)
94–100	Sensitivity	96–100
93	Specificity	100
99	Diagnostic accuracy	99.9
92.3	Negative predictive value	99.9
99	Positive predictive value	92.3

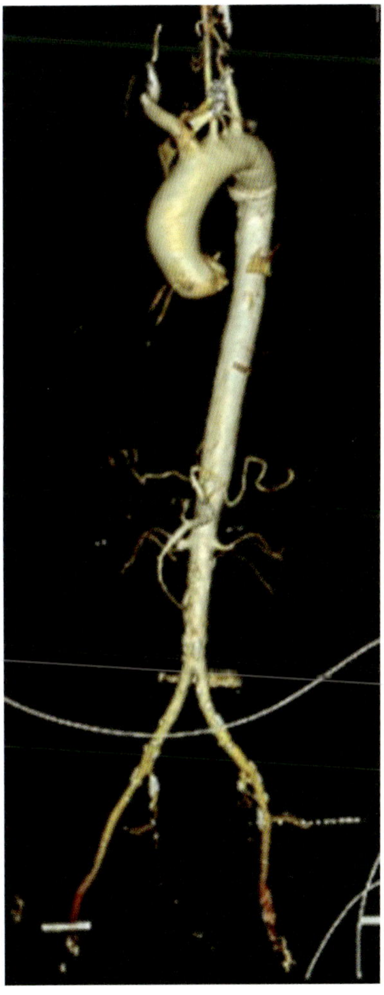

Fig. 9.8 Multidetector CT (MDCT) angiography three-dimensional volume-rendered (3D-VR) image allows scan of whole body

allowed coverage of the entire aorta in <3 s [52]. Due to the faster image acquisition, still or motion-free images of even the ascending aorta can be obtained without any ECG gating. Also, motion artifacts from patient breathing are minimal. Dual-energy CT scanners can also produce diagnostic images at a lower kV for most patients allowing a reduced contrast administration and a lowering of the radiation dose.

Computed tomography angiography (CTA) is currently the modality of choice for the acute diagnosis of BTAI replacing conventional angiography.

The practice management guideline from the Eastern Association for the Surgery of Trauma published in 2015 "strongly recommend CT with intravenous contrast for the diagnosis of BTAI" [5].

CT of the chest with intravenous contrast has the advantage of being readily available, less invasive, being less time consuming, and allowing for identification of other intrathoracic injuries and for assessment of subtle intimal abnormalities and indirect signs of aortic injury such as periaortic hematoma.

Imaging protocols for MDCT evaluation of the thoracic aorta vary considerably, depending on the technical specifications of the CT scanner (e.g., number of detector rows, the availability of electrocardiographic (ECG) gating). Opinions on the use of multiple phases differ between institutions and a variety of imaging protocols is recommended in the literature.

The protocol that is classically followed is that of the multiple trauma patient. This consists of a pre-contrast acquisition of the head, chest, and abdomen (most useful for diagnosis of intramural hematoma), followed by an arterial phase acquisition covering the neck, chest, and abdomen.

This is usually followed by a portal phase acquisition of the abdomen, so that any injuries to wholly intra-abdominal organs can be better studied [10].

A low-dose delayed phase scan of abdomen and pelvis is performed if the injury is confirmed on portal venous phase or if kidney or bladder injury is suspected.

ECG-gated CT can only be considered when the patient is hemodynamically stable. This technique, which overcomes the issue of artifacts related to movements caused by the patient's heartbeat, can prove to be very useful in some cases by removing doubts over diagnosis.

Different protocols exist to administer iodinated intravenous contrast material, with either single-bolus, split-bolus, or triple-bolus administration being used.

It should be injected high concentration contrast media (370/400 mg/mL) at a high rate (5 mL/s), followed by another injection saline at the same rate. To avoid streak artifacts from high concentrations of iodine in the left brachiocephalic vein, contrast material should preferably be administered via the right arm whenever possible. Contrast medium should be administered via an 18 G or 20 G cannula. Depending on scanner manufacturer and type, an empirically fixed delay or a bolus-triggering mode can be used. In our institute, we generally use bolus tracking with the region of interest (ROI) placed over the descending thoracic aorta and trigger set at 100–120 HU.

At our institution, all examinations are performed by a 128-slice MDCT with slice thickness of 5–3 or 1 mm (reconstruction 1 mm), collimation of 128 × 0.6 mm, and rotation time of 0.33/0.5 s; intravenous contrast material consists 90–100 mL iodinated contrast agent at 400 mg/mL, concentration injected at 4–5 mL/s, followed by 40 mL of saline at the same flow rate. An automated bolus tracking, with region of interest placed in the descending aortic at an attenuation threshold of 120 HU, is used to time the beginning of the arterial phase. The venous phase is performed at 50–60-s delay from the end of the injection [53].

Our CT trauma protocol is summarized in Table 9.4.

To detect and evaluate vascular injuries, it is mandatory to use thin slices (0.6 mm) so that it is possible to make post-processing works, as multiplanar reformations (MPRs), three-dimensional volume-rendered (VR) images, and maximum intensity projection (MIP) (Figs. 9.9, 9.10, and 9.11).

Multiplanar reconstructions are sensitive for the detection of small grade I or II lesions, which are sometimes difficult to see on standard axial images. They also allow the lesions and their extent to be better understood.

Table 9.4 CT trauma protocol

High concentration contrast agent	400 mg/mL
Mdc ev.	80–100 mL
Saline	40–50 mL
Injection	Bolus tracking
Injection rate	5 mL/s through 18 G cannula (right arm)
Pre-contrast acquisition	Head, chest, and abdomen
Arterial phase acquisition	Neck, chest, and abdomen
Portal phase acquisition (70 s after the injection)	Abdomen
Equilibrium phase acquisition (180 s after the injection)	If it is necessary
Collimation	128 × 0.6
Rotation rate	0.5/0.3
Pitch	>1.2 (to reduce cardiac pulsation artifacts)
Slice thickness	0.6 mm (arterial phase)–5/3 mm (other phases)
Voltage	100–120 Kv
Current (mA)	Optimized relative to body attenuation

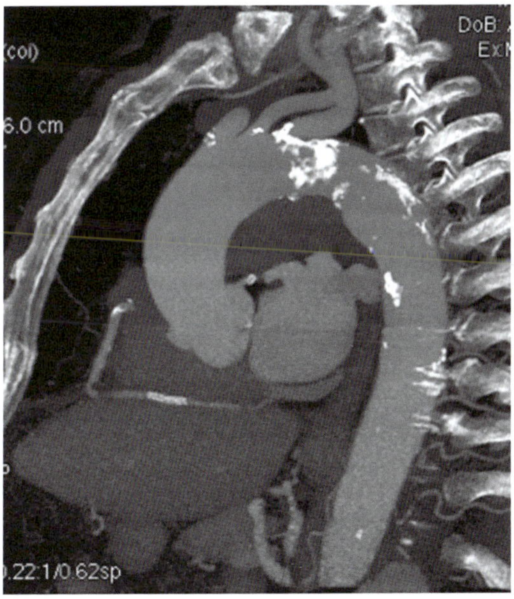

Fig. 9.9 Thoracic aorta. Reformat—maximum intensity projection (MIP) shows the map of the parietal calcifications

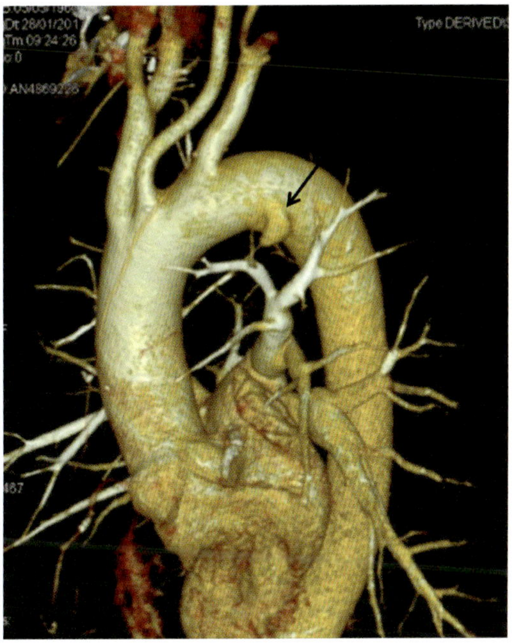

Fig. 9.10 Thoracic aorta vessel-rendering 3D shows pseudoaneurysm isthmus (*black arrow*)

A sagittal-oblique reconstruction is especially useful since it shows the entire length of the thoracic (and possibly abdominal) aorta and is most helpful to evaluate the relationship of the injury with the left subclavian artery because they give a longitudinal view of the aorta comparable to standard angiographic projections (Fig. 9.12).

To obtain a more accurate vascular analysis, a dedicated software should be used; it should able to provide accurate and reproducible measurements through reformat linear/curved images and axial analysis for choosing the appropriate management.

Finally, they are an essential tool for assessing the required dimensions of an endoprothesis when endovascular treatment is planned (Fig. 9.13).

CTA reports should include the information on location, length, severity and type of aortic injury, aortic diameter above and below the injury, and proximity to the origin of left subclavian artery (in case of isthmic injuries). CTA reports should specify aortic arch anatomy and anatomical variants, any significant preexistent atherosclerotic disease or stenosis, prior

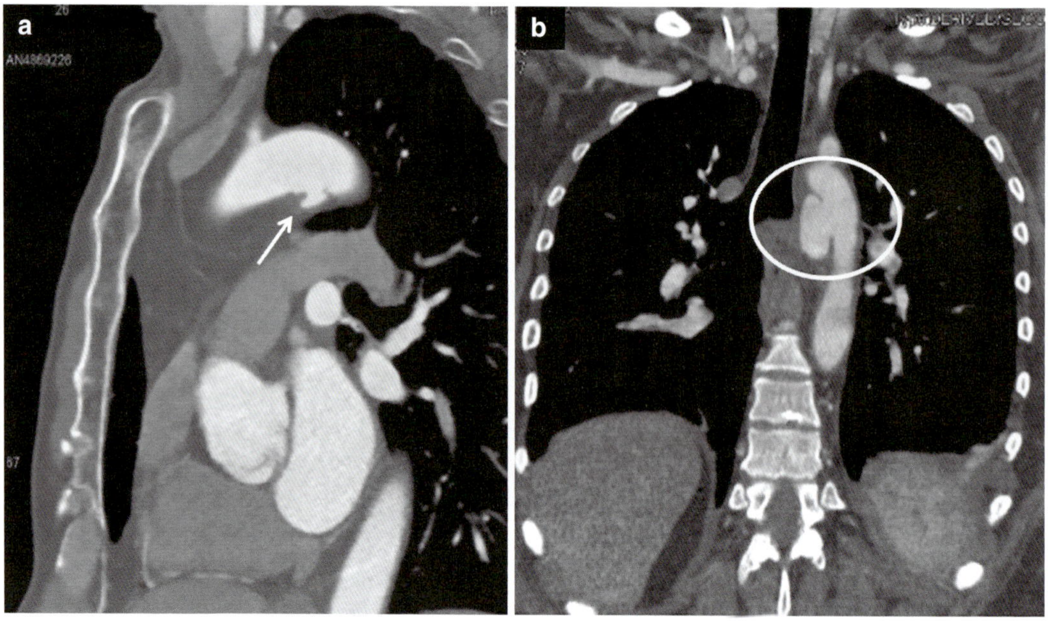

Fig. 9.11 Thoracic aorta multiplanar reformations (MPRs) show in (**a**) (sagittal reformat aortic arch) small pseudoaneurysm isthmus (*white arrow*); in (**b**), (coronal reformat), large pseudoaneurysm aortic descendens (*white circle*)

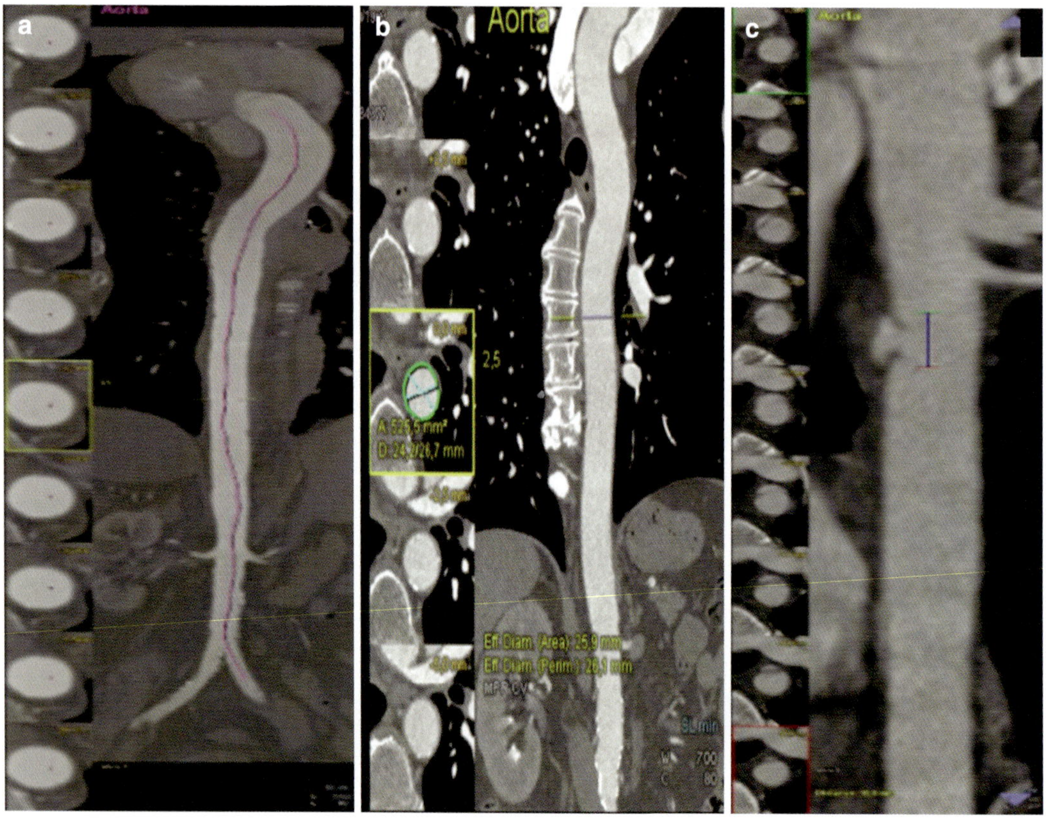

Fig. 9.12 Aorta. (**a**) Reformat linear image with axial analysis; (**b**) reformat curved image with axial analysis; (**c**) reformat linear image with axial analysis shows small pseudoaneurysm isthmus

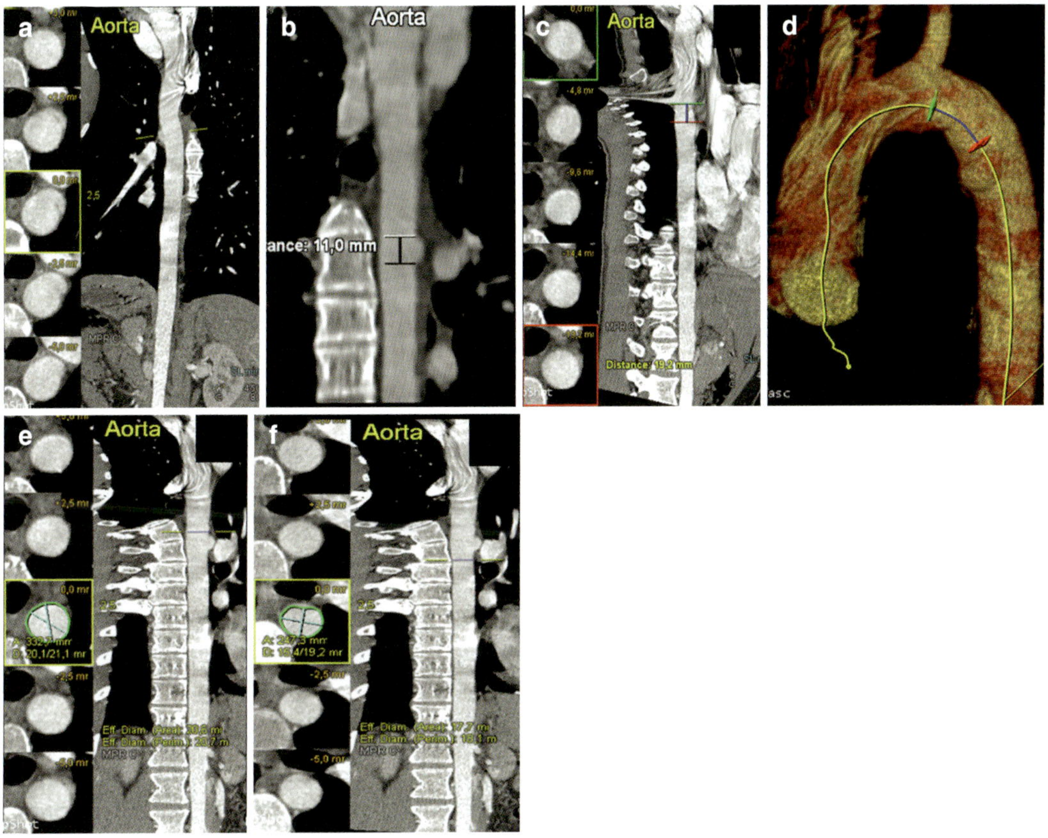

Fig 9.13 Blunt trauma thoracic aortic injury. (**a**) Reformat and vessel analysis and (**b**) reformat linear image show small pseudoaneurysm isthmus; (**c**) reformat and vessel analysis show the distance measurement from left subclavian artery; (**d**) shows representation of volume-rendered 3D image; (**e**, **f**) reformat and vessel analysis show diameter aorta pre-/post-lesion

postoperative changes (like CABG—coronary artery bypass graft surgery) and comment on anatomic variation or anomalous origin of the great vessels. The radiologist should look for possible coexisting branch vessel injuries and assess femoral or brachial access. Vertebral artery dominance should be determined, if present, on the basis of a measurable larger difference in caliber of one vertebral artery. This information helps the clinician to decide between the treatment options and also guides the intervention.

9.5.6.1 CT Imaging Findings

Based on the layer of the aortic wall involved, BTAI are called aortic dissection (when only intima and deep media are involved), intramural hematoma (when media is involved), pseudoaneurysm (injury contained by adventitia), or rupture (when also adventitia lost its integrity). Based on anatomo-pathological analysis, post-traumatic aortic injuries are generally transverse, segmented, and circumferential, rarely spiral.

Table 9.5 CT imaging findings

Direct signs	Indirect signs
Intimal flap	Hemomediastinum
Luminal thrombus	Hemothorax
Aortic dissection	Hemopericardium
Intramural hematoma	Obliteration of the retrocrural periaortic fat
Pseudoaneurysm	Unexplained acute renal infarcts
Pseudocoarctation	
Rupture	

The spectrum of findings (Table 9.5) in thoracic aortic injury includes the following direct signs [13, 45, 54, 55]:

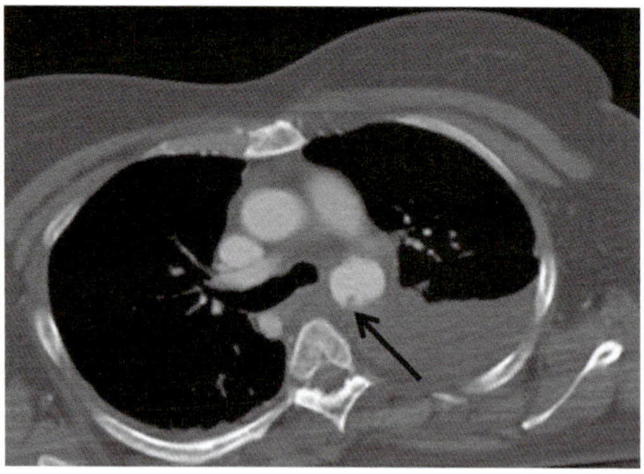

Fig. 9.14 Axial CT scan shows (*black arrow*) intraluminal aortic thrombus (minimal aortic injury)

- Intimal tears/flaps (Figs. 9.14 and 9.15): luminal thrombus abutting the intima often demonstrated as a small, round contrast-filling defect (10 mm in length or width) on the axial images, without external contour abnormality. An intimal flap is a more linear hypodense structure projecting into the lumen of the aorta, connected to the wall.
- Intramural hematoma alone (Fig. 9.16): can be seen as thickening of the aortic wall, separating the intima and adventitia by hematoma in the media. It can be focal or rather long and usually are not circumferential. If a non-

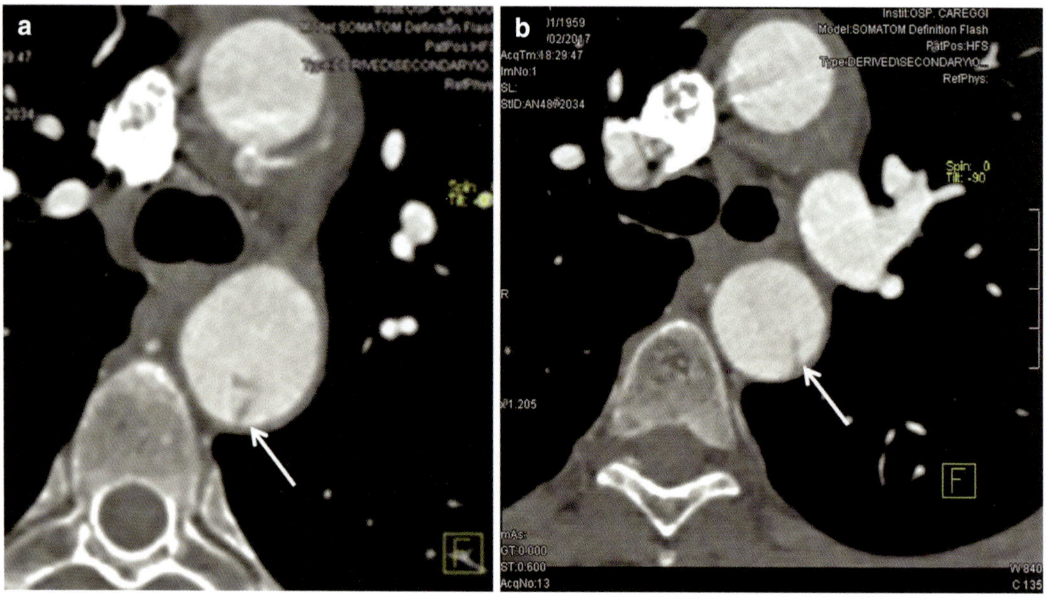

Fig 9.15 Axial CT scan shows in (**a**, **b**) (*white arrows*) intimal tear (intimal flap isthmus)

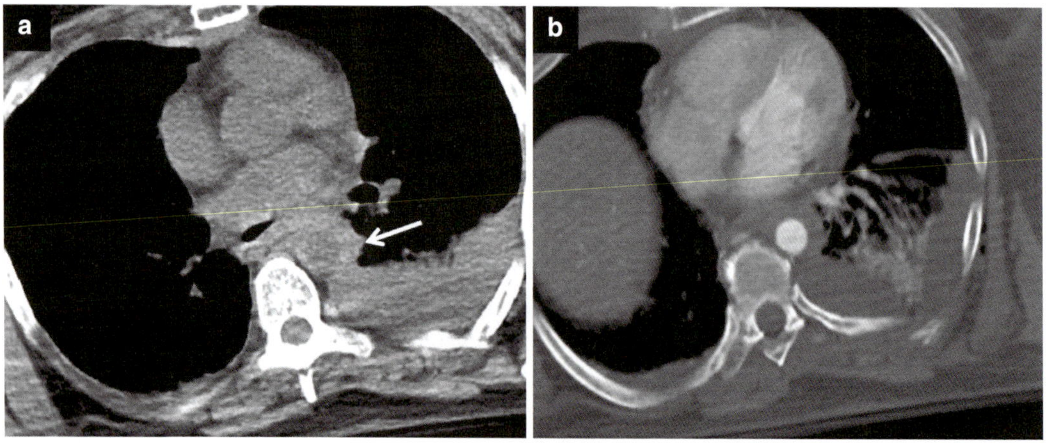

Fig. 9.16 Post-traumatic intramural aortic hematoma (see also rib fracture and pleural effusion). (**a**) CT axial non-contrast image show (*white arrow*) high attenuation material into aortic wall; (**b**) postcontrast image

contrast-enhanced CT is performed, this portion of the aortic wall will demonstrate increased attenuation (around 40–60 HU), a feature that is less obvious if contrast was given. Intramural hematoma plus is characterized by contour changes and/or intimal flaps (Fig. 9.17).

- Pseudoaneurysm: focal abrupt change in the aortic contour with a regular (Fig. 9.18) or irregular outpouching, most commonly just distal to the left subclavian artery (Fig. 9.19). Pseudoaneurysm has one or both acute angles with the aortic wall (Fig. 9.20). Especially if there are irregular outlines and surrounding hematoma, there is a high chance of rupture (Fig. 9.21). It has been proposed that a circumferential abrupt change in the aortic contour with an irregular outpouching is at higher risk of rupture.
- True aortic dissection (long flap indistinguishable from spontaneous dissection and managed in the same way as spontaneous dissections). This is an uncommon injury (Fig. 9.22).
- Pseudocoarctation (obstructive flap reducing the caliber of the descending aorta) (Fig. 9.23).
- Active extravasation (rare and often an immediately antemortem finding) (Fig. 9.24).

Indirect signs of aortic injury are hemomediastinum and hemothorax. The location of hemomediastinum is an important data because the

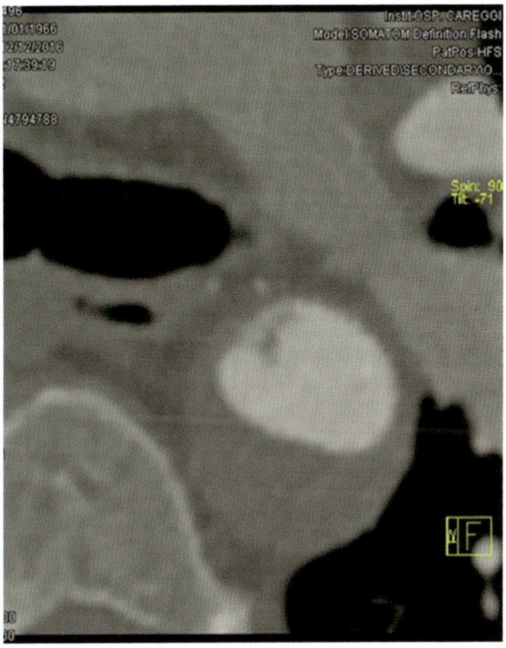

Fig. 9.17 Contrast-enhanced thoracic multidetector CT (MDCT) scan of a patient with blunt trauma shows hematoma post-isthmic aortic with intimal flap (intramural hematoma plus)

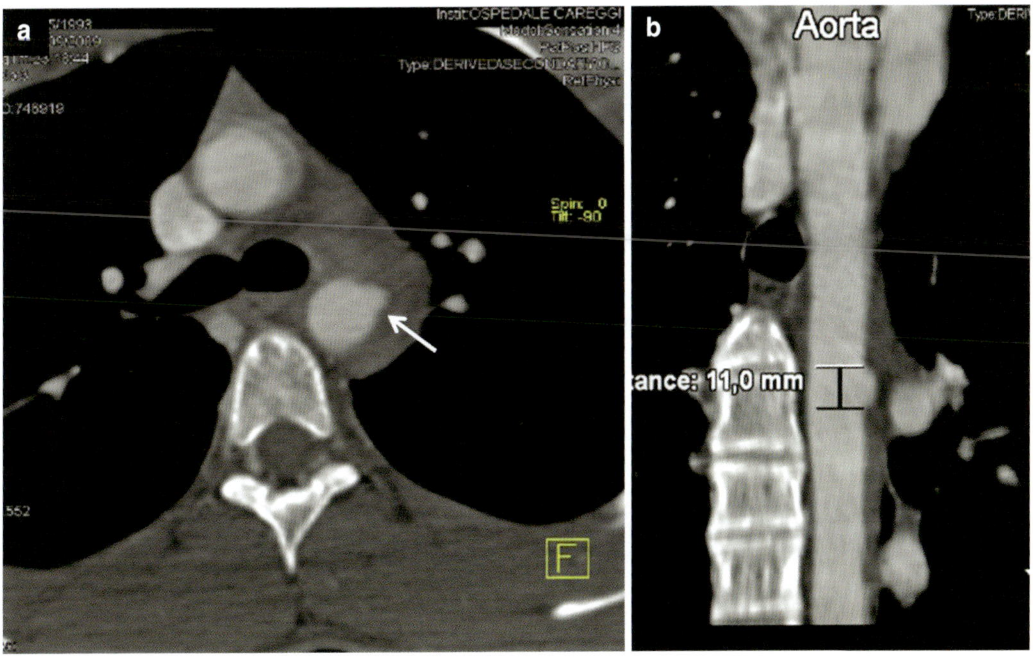

Fig. 9.18 Isthmus, small pseudoaneurysm with periaortic hematoma. (**a**) Axial CT scan (*white arrow*); (**b**) reformat linear 2D image (size 11 mm)

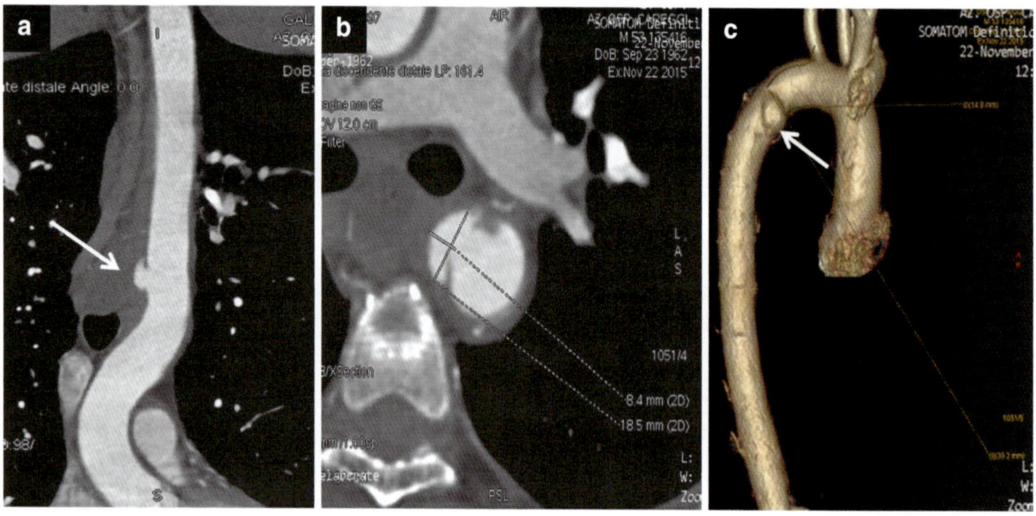

Fig. 9.19 Aortic isthmus, same large post-traumatic pseudoaneurysm (white arrows). (**a**) Reformat linear image; (**b**) axial CT scan; (**c**) reformat 3D image

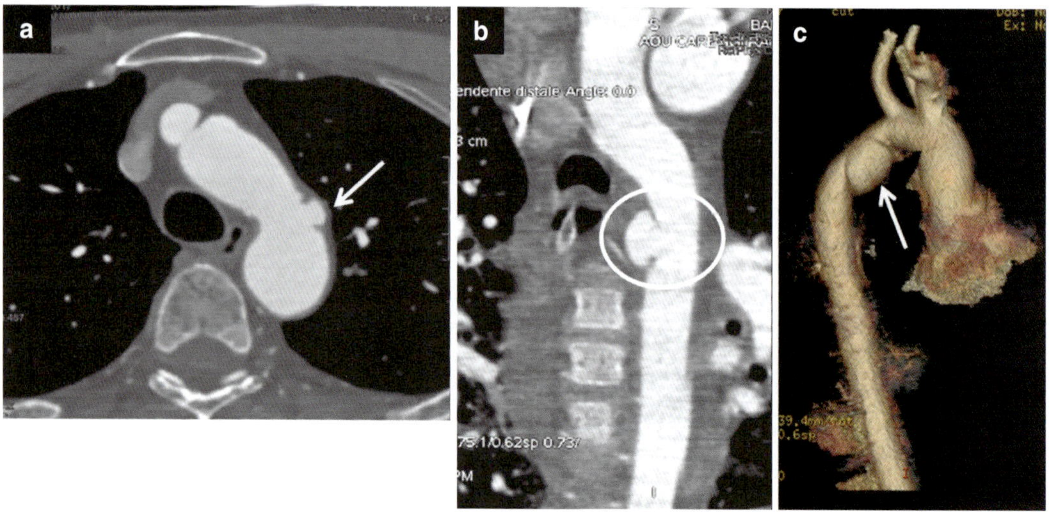

Fig. 9.20 Pseudoaneurysm (acute angles with the aortic wall). (**a**) Axial CT scan shows small pseudoaneurysm isthmus (*white arrow*); (**b**) reformat oblique image and (**c**) reformat 3D image show large pseudoaneurysm isthmus (*white circle* in **b** and *white arrow* in **c**)

immediate periaortic region or beyond is mostly related to the bleeding from the aortic injury. Periaortic hematoma is used to describe hematoma directly bordering the aortic adventitia and obliterating the periaortic fat plane (Fig. 9.25). If periaortic hematoma is present, the aorta should be scrutinized for the presence of injury. However, lesser grade injury is possible if periaortic hematoma is absent, around 21–22% of such cases occurring without surrounding hematoma [56, 57]. In the presence of periaortic hematoma without direct signs of major vessel injury seen on a technically adequate study, debate exists about whether or not to perform follow-up scans in 48–72 h. Mediastinal hematomas not immediately adjacent to the aorta

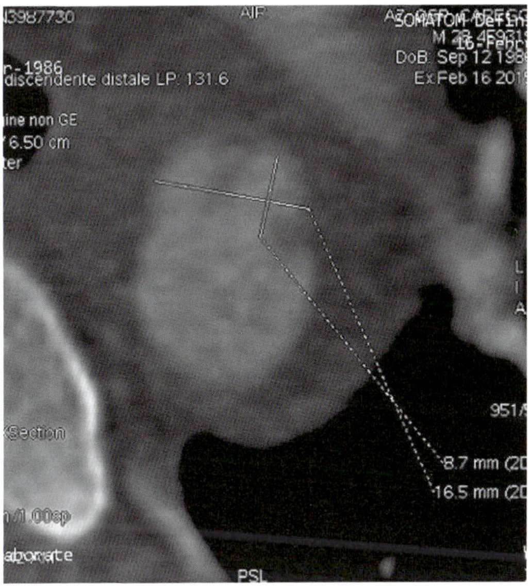

Fig. 9.21 Axial CT scan shows pseudoaneurysm: irregular outlines and surrounding hematoma

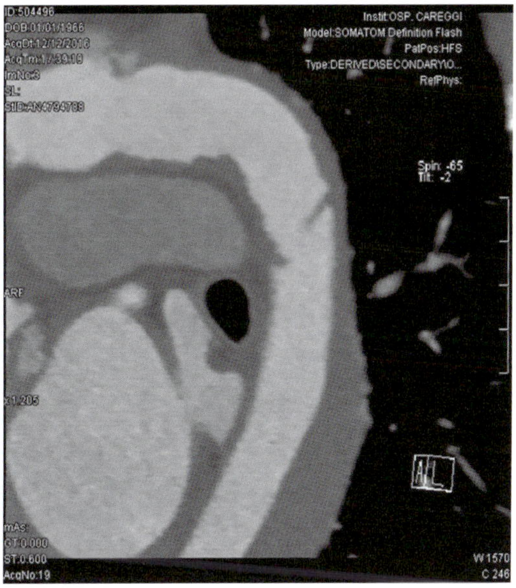

Fig. 9.22 Multiplanar reformation (MPR) shows post-traumatic aortic dissection

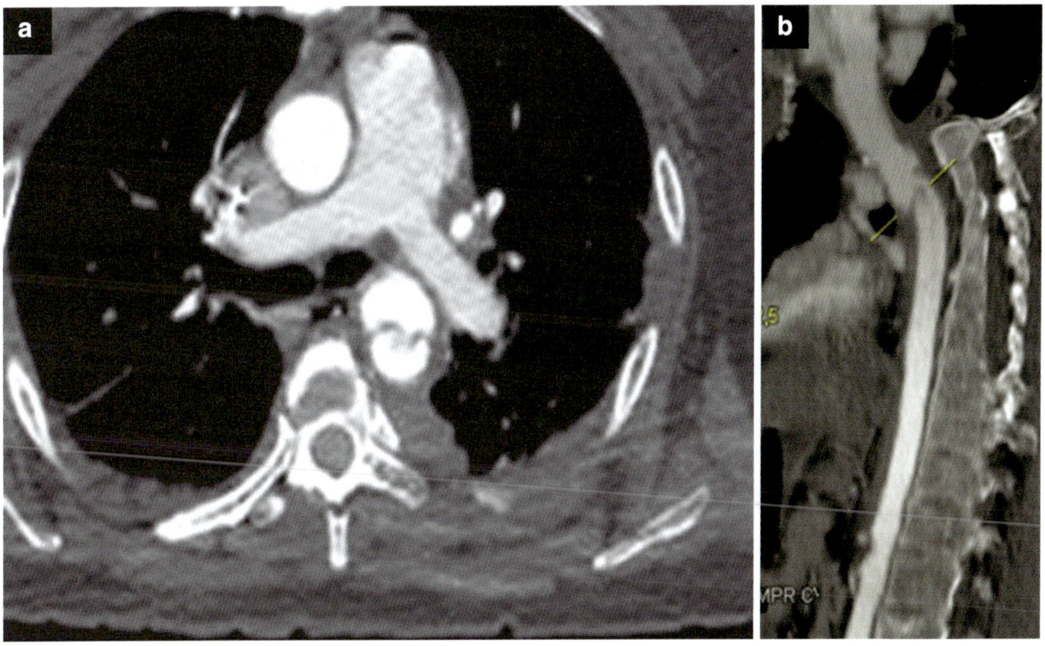

Fig. 9.23 Traumatic pseudoaneurysm with pseudocoarctation (obstructive flap reducing the caliber of the descending aorta). (**a**) Axial CT scan; (**b**) reformat linear image

(with a obliterating the periaortic fat plane) are likely to be secondary to venous bleeding (Fig. 9.26). Isolated anterior mediastinal hematoma is unlikely to be due to BTAI; injuries to the internal mammary artery (which may be life threatening), bronchial arteries, superior intercostals veins and ribs, clavicles, and sternal fractures are all more likely culprits.

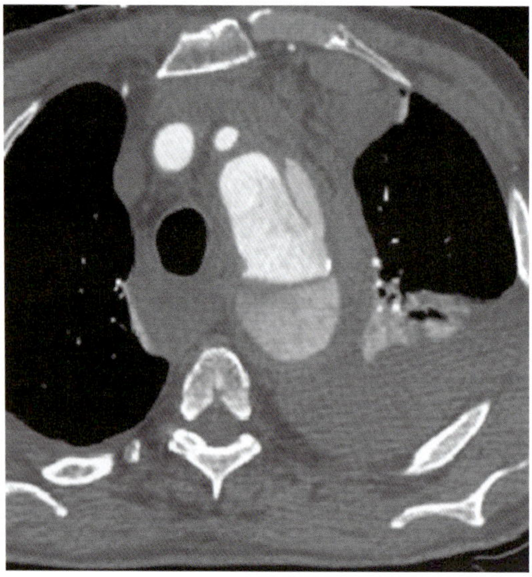

Fig. 9.24 Axial CT scan shows aortic dissection with active extravasation (hematoma periaortic, hemothorax)

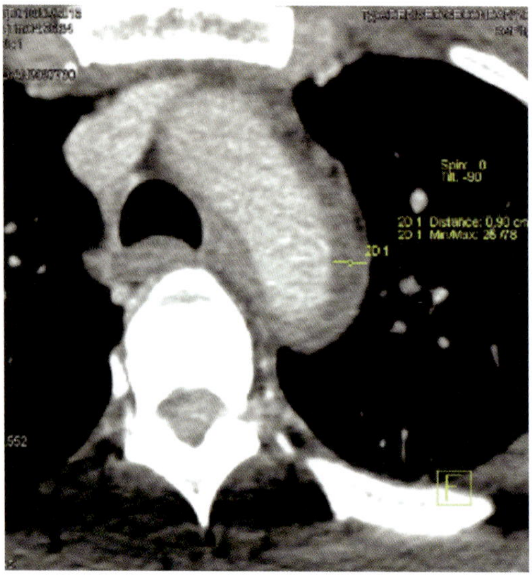

Fig. 9.25 Axial CT scan shows periaortic hematoma (obliterating the periaortic fat plane)

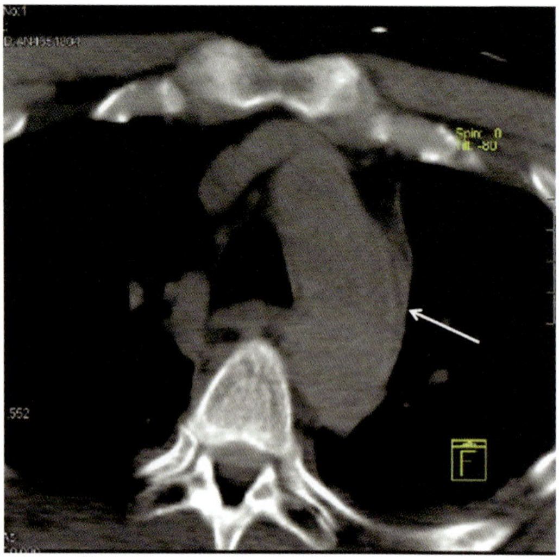

Fig. 9.26 Axial CT scan shows mediastinal hematoma (*white arrow* shows preserved periaortic fat plane)

Bleeding from the aortic injury can extend into the pleural space (Fig. 9.27) or pericardium, depending on the location of the injury, giving rise to hemopericardium or hemothorax. Usually, hemopericardium is homogenously hyperdense, whereas hemothorax can have mixed densities with more hyperdense areas indicating cloth. However, if pleural effusion has densities similar to fluid (0–20/30 HU), differentiating hyperacute hematoma from reactive effusion can be difficult.

Other two indirect signs can be seen on abdominal CT and should mandate further investigation of the thoracic aorta. These are obliteration of the retrocrural periaortic fat (possibly indicating caudal extension of more cranially located periaortic hematoma) and otherwise unexplained acute renal infarcts, especially when bilateral, that can originate from luminal thrombus of more cranially located BTAI.

Secondary signs of injury (SSI) were recently defined as pseudocoarctation, extensive mediastinal hematoma (with mass effect), and large left hemothorax [58, 59]. The SSI seem to be associated with a higher risk of rupture.

Chronic pseudoaneurysms can develop at the sites of undiagnosed and/or untreated aortic injury. These often have extensive peripheral calcification and may also contain thrombus. The peripheral calcification is thought to be protective against aneurysm rupture.

Concurrent injuries in patients with blunt TAI include major abdominal injury (57%), closed head injury (50%), major peripheral vascular injury (46%), multiple rib fractures (46%), pulmonary contusion (38%), pelvic trauma (31%), upper extremity trauma (20%), flail chest (12%), and spine injury (12%) [9].

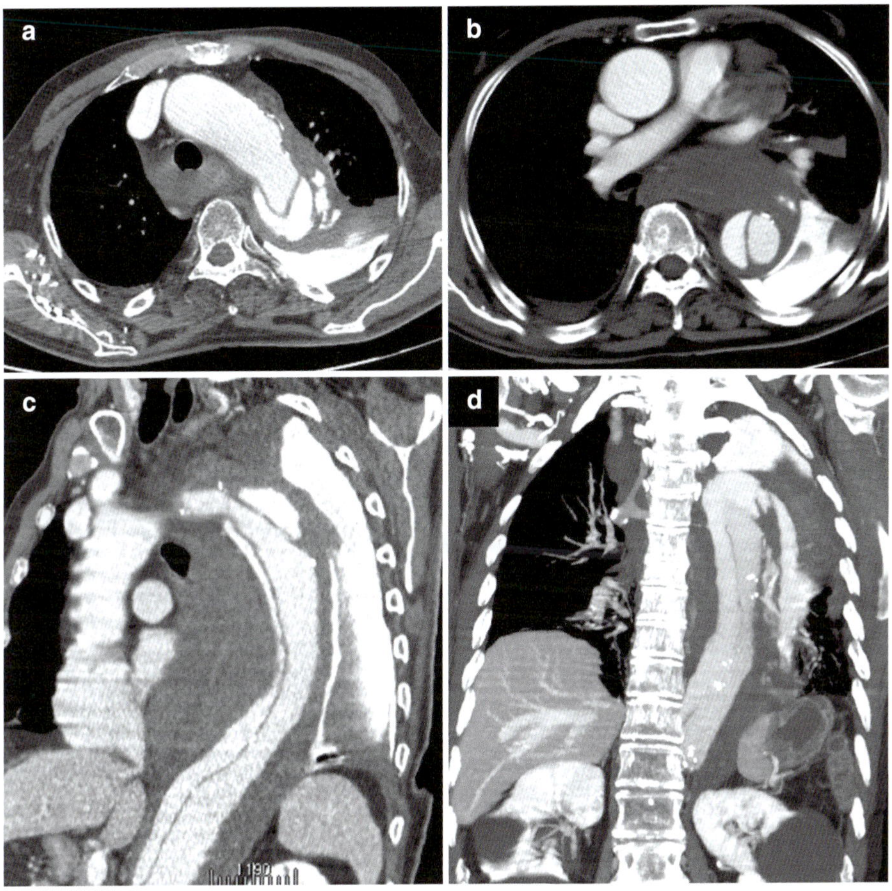

Fig. 9.27 Aortic rupture with active extravasation. (**a**, **b**) Axial CT scan show traumatic aortic injury (isthmus-descending aorta) with hemothorax and hemomediastinum. (**c**) Multiplanar reformation (MPR) oblique reformat image; (**d**) elaborate maximum intensity projection (MIP) image

9.6 Differential Diagnosis and Pitfalls

A number of artifacts can mimic a traumatic injury of the thoracic aorta.

Diagnostic pitfalls (Table 9.6) can be divided into two categories: anatomic and technical [13, 60].

The classic example of technical pitfall is that of the cardiac pulsation artifact, which is particularly present at the root of the aorta and in the ascending aorta that simulates an intimal pseudo-flap (Fig. 9.28). This image continues in the mediastinal fat giving a blurred interface with the hyperdense lumen of the aorta, which can help with diagnosis. Otherwise, these artifacts can be removed by ECG-gated CT in stable patients if there is any doubt. Breathing and patient movement artifacts can also be found. They are revealed by visualizing the thorax in the lung parenchymal window.

Table 9.6 The most common diagnostic pitfalls

Cardiac pulsation artifacts
Ductus diverticulum
Branch vessel infundibula
Anatomic variants
Superior intercostal artery/vein
Ulcerative plaques
Pulmonary atelectasis adjacent
Kammerell's diverticulum

Anatomic pitfalls that can be mistaken for BTAI mainly reside around the level of the isthmus, namely a ductus diverticulum, patent ductus

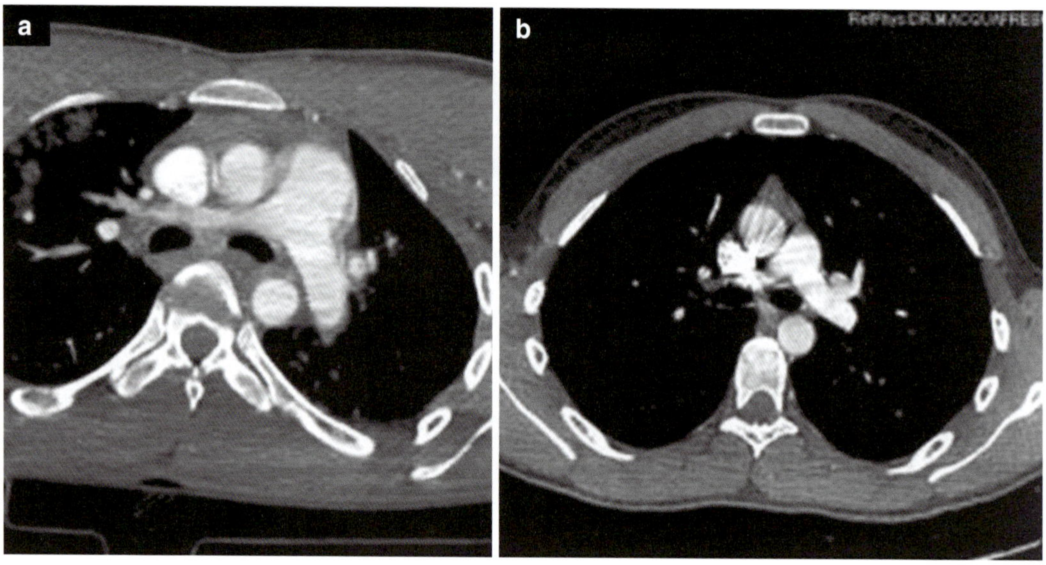

Fig. 9.28 Artifact. (**a**) Axial CT image shows motion artifact at the aortic ascendant. (**b**) Axial CT image shows dense contrast media in the superior vena cava

arteriosus, and aortic spindle. The ductus diverticulum, found in 9% of the arteriograms in the adult, is a remnant of the closed or partially closed ductus arteriosus which connects the pulmonary artery to the aorta in fetal circulation. Ductal remnants are located at the inferior surface of the aortic arch near the aortic isthmus which leads to confusing them with BTAIs. Ductus diverticulum has typically smooth, obtuse angles with the aortic wall and are often calcified, whereas BTAI usually is more irregular and steeply angled (Fig. 9.29).

A patent ductus arteriosus is a rarity in itself, and it can be recognized as a tubular structure with regular contours, where the differential of active contrast extravasation in BTAI is usually irregular and situated within hematoma.

Aortic spindles are located just distal to the isthmus and are smooth, regular fusiform mild dilatations of the aorta, without periaortic hematoma (Fig. 9.30).

Branch vessel infundibula can also be confused with a small pseudoaneurysm. They can have a similar appearance to a ductal remnant, but are found at the origin of bronchial or intercostal arteries. They are typically cone shaped and smooth walled with a small artery extending from the apex (Fig. 9.31).

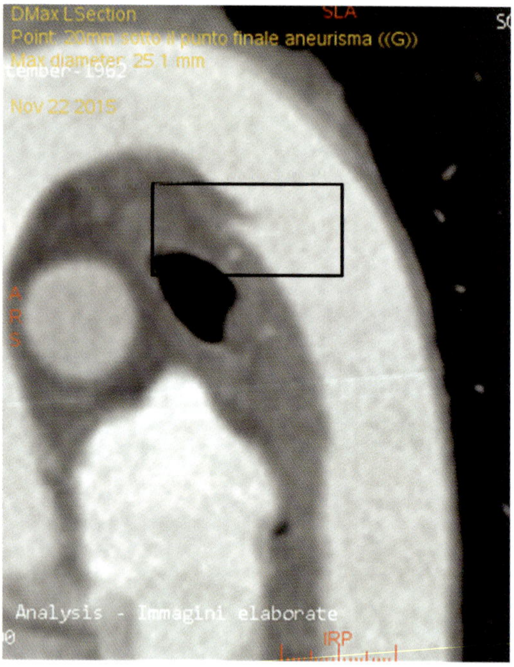

Fig 9.29 Ductus diverticulum. Multiplanar reformation (MPR), sagittal-oblique reconstruction, shows smooth, obtuse angles with the aortic wall (*white rectangle*)

Penetrating ulcerated atherosclerotic plaques (Fig. 9.32) is a focal contrast-medium filled outpouching within the media wall. Focal outpouching can present a substantial diagnostic problem

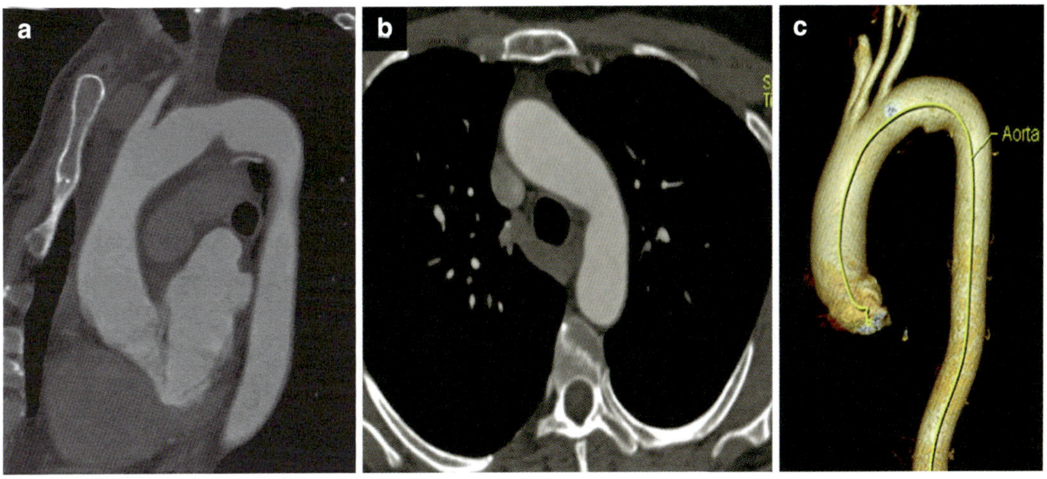

Fig 9.30 (**a**) Multiplanar reformation (MPR), oblique reconstruction, (**b**) axial CT scan, and (**c**) three-dimensional volume-rendered (3D-VR) image show aortic spindle, regular fusiform mild dilatation of the aortic isthmus

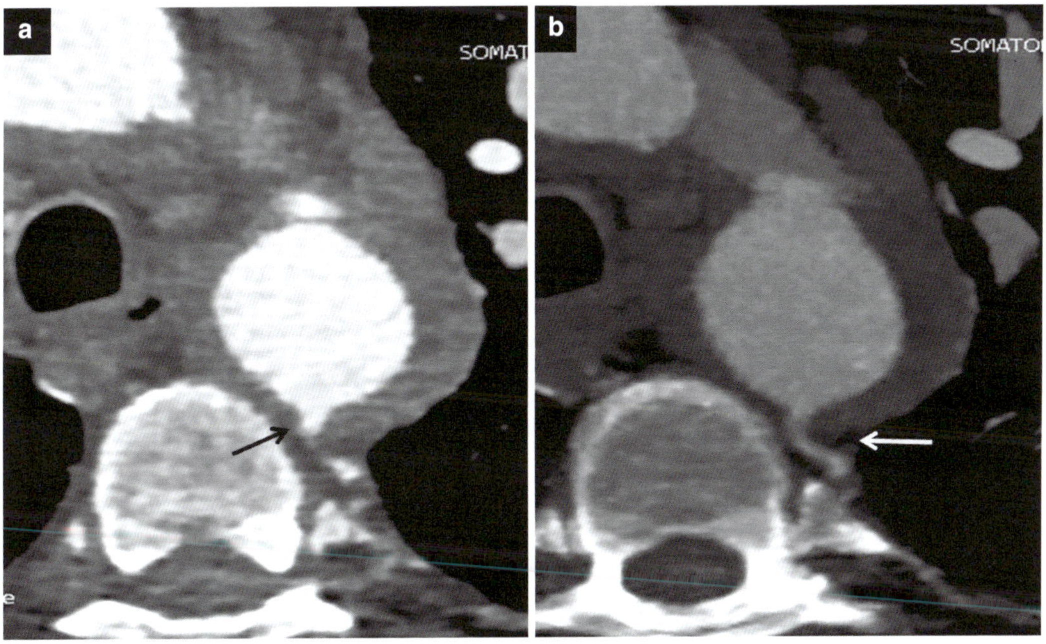

Fig. 9.31 Post-traumatic periaortic hematoma isthmus. (**a**) Axial CT scan shows ostium intercostal artery mimics small pseudoaneurism posterior wall (*black arrow*); (**b**) elaborate maximum intensity projection (MIP) image shows small artery extending from the apex (*white arrow*)

due to post-traumatic pseudoaneurysm. The presence of atherosclerotic plaques associated with intramural hematoma, thickening of aortic wall, displaced calcifications, and irregular and multiple outpouching can be helpful in distinguishing; as an alternative to exclude the evolution, CT follow-up would be helpful.

Finally, enhancement of the collapsed lung adjacent to the aorta may also simulate an intimal flap.

Furthermore, not all mediastinal bleeding corresponds to aortic injury. Mediastinal hematomas can be due to injury to other structures including the pulmonary artery, great vessels

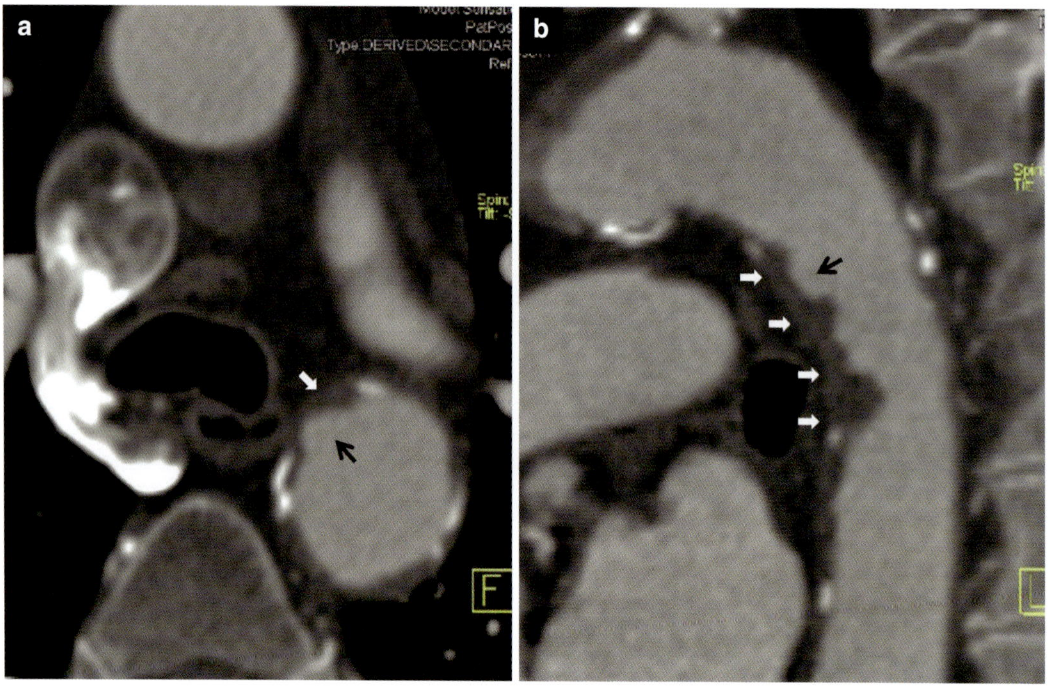

Fig. 9.32 (**a**) Axial CT scan and (**b**) oblique MPR show ulcerative (*black arrows*) plaques (*white arrows*)

or mediastinal veins, or even fractures of vertebral bodies. It is important to pay specific attention to detect abnormalities of the supra-aortic vessels, possibly using 3D reconstructions. These dangerous lesions are a therapeutic challenge. They are often associated with aortic injuries although they can sometimes be isolated. The literature describes trauma injuries to the great veins like the superior vena cava; these injuries are rare, but they can be life threatening.

9.7 Minimal Aortic Injury (MAI)

The term "minimal aortic injury" (MAI) was used for the first time in 1999 in "Presley Trauma Center CT Grading System of Aortic Injury" by Gavant [61] to describe injuries that are minor in nature.

Recent studies estimated that this injury is present in 25–35% of patients with BTAI [56], whereas it was initially estimated to be present in approximately 10% [40].

The increased detection of MAI may be related to a combination of factors including increased availability of CTA, improvement in CTA technology, and better vehicle safety [62].

The most common site for MAI are descending aorta and the aortic isthmus [63].

MAI is an evolving concept and there currently is no unanimity definition of this aortic injury (Table 9.7).

The definition ranges from injuries in which outer aortic wall contour is preserved (luminal thrombus; intimal flap or hematoma smaller than 10 mm) (Figs. 9.33 and 9.34) to those including pseudoaneurysm of up to 50% of the normal aorta diameter (Fig. 9.35).

As with the definition of MAI, there is also no consensus on management and follow-up of these injuries. Relatively to low risk of rupture of MAI, most studies in the literature have suggested that it can be safely managed with medical treatment, by controlling blood pressure and heart rate [63, 64]. However, the selection of appropriate treatment for patients with MAI should be done on individual basis, keeping in

Table 9.7 Definition of MAI in various studies

Gavant ML	Minimal aortic injury = Grade II; IIa. Intimal flap or pseudoaneurysm <1 cm. No mediastinal hematoma IIb. Intimal flap or pseudoaneurysm <1 cm. Mediastinal hematoma present
Malhotra et al.	Intimal flap <1 cm in size with no or minimal periaortic hematoma
Azizzadeh et al.	Grade 1 = Intimal tears
Paul et al.	Presley CT Grade I and II (normal aorta with/without mediastinal hematoma, intimal flap or pseudoaneurysm <1 cm with/without mediastinal hematoma)
Mosquera et al.	Intramural hematoma without intimal tear Intimal flap <10 mm
Kidane et al.	Intimal flap with minimal or no periaortic hematoma
Riesenman et al.	Intimal tears (Grade 1 classification system proposed by Azizzadeh et al.)
Starnes et al.	Absence of aortic external contour abnormality and intimal defect and/or thrombus of <10 mm in length or width
Estrera et al.	Intimal tears (Grade 1 classification system proposed by Azizzadeh et al.)
Forman et al.	Aortic contour abnormality Intimal flap with or without attached thrombus Intramural hematoma Pseudoaneurysm <10% of the normal aortic diameter as measured at the level of the pseudoaneurysm
Gunn et al.	Abnormality of the internal contour of the vessel wall projecting into the lumen, not thought to represent an atheromatous plaque Intimal flap Intraluminal filling defect Intramural hematoma No evidence of an abnormality to the external contour of the aorta (i.e., no pseudoaneurysm)
Rabin et al.	Intimal tears, intramural hematoma, or small pseudoaneurysm (< 50% circumference)
Osgood et al.	Intimal tear or intramural hematoma without external contour deformation (Grades 1 and 2 classification system proposed by Azizzadeh et al.)
Heneghan et al.	No external contour abnormality Intimal tear and/or thrombus <10 mm

Reproduced with permission from Nagpal P et al. Advances in Imaging and Management Trends of Traumatic Aortic Injuries. Cardiovasc Intervent Radiol (2017) 40: 643–654. Doi:10.1007/s00270-017-1572-x

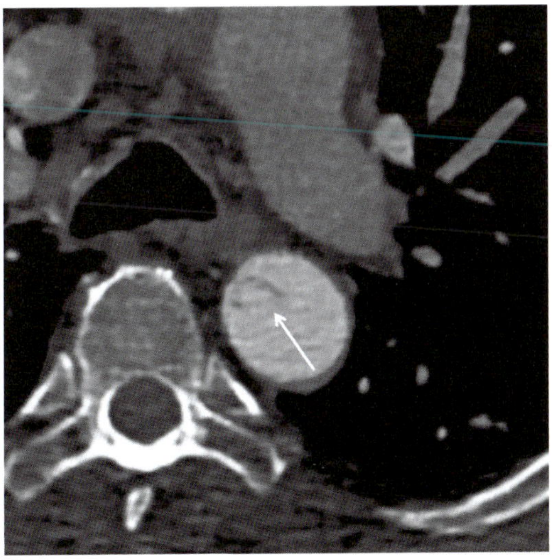

Fig. 9.33 MAI. Axial CT scan shows intraluminal filling defect (intimal flap) (*white arrow*)

mind other comorbidities. Nonoperative management is based on the use of negative inotropes (most commonly β-blockers) with a goal of systolic blood pressure (BP) of 100–120 mmHg and heart rate goal of 60–80 beats per min to decrease vascular shear stress [65].

Even clinical practice guidelines published by the Society for Vascular Surgery in 2011 suggested expectant management for minimal aortic injuries with serial imaging follow-up for intimal injuries (type I by Azizzadeh's classification) [8].

There is a lack of specific recommendation on "expectant" management and follow-up protocol, so that the imaging surveillance of MAI is usually variable and based on each particular institution's experience and their observations. Although there is no consensus on the timeline, the surveillance should end when the aorta

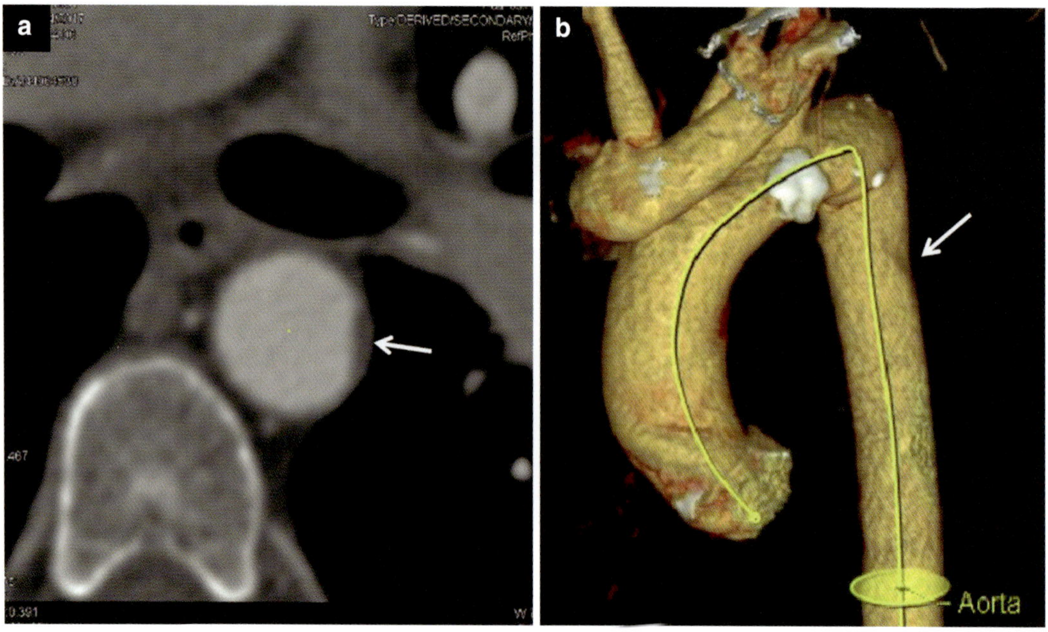

Fig. 9.34 MAI. (**a**) Axial CT scan and (**b**) three-dimensional volume-rendered (3D-VR) image show small hematoma in the wall of the aorta (*white arrows*)

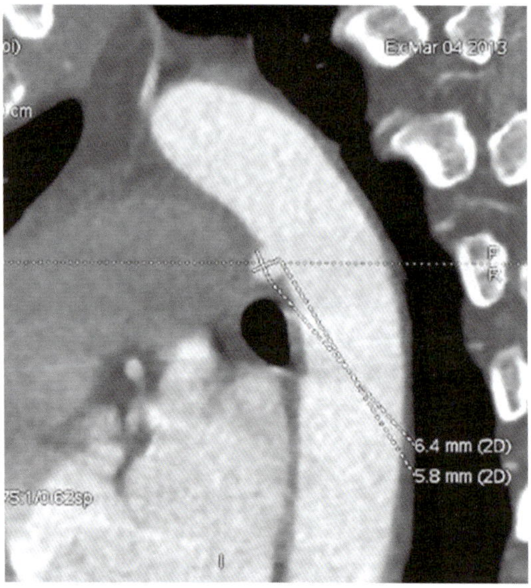

Fig. 9.35 MAI. Sagittal oblique Multiplanar Reformation (MPR) image of the aortic isthmus shows small pseudoaneurysm (< 50% of the normal aortic diameter)

returns to normal appearance, as many studies suggest [47, 64].

The nonoperative management of MAI has been proposed according to the evidence of no progression of disease in the majority of patients, and if it occurs, it happens in the first month of injury [63, 64]. To resume, in the presence of a small intimal flap or pseudoaneurysm without periaortic hematoma, the literature suggests that it can be safely followed with serial CTA (at 24 h, every 48–72 h for 7 days and after 4 weeks). However, if the injury is associated with significant thrombus or periaortic hematoma, it could be recommended to proceed with endograft coverage.

9.8 Classification

Currently, there is neither common classification nor grading of BTAI, and several different classification systems have been proposed (Table 9.8).

The first classification system has been published by Parmley et al. in 1958 on the basis of a large autopsy study; it was an accurate description of the relationship between injury and layer of the aortic wall involved. Parmley classified the lesions into six groups: (1) intimal hemorrhage; (2) intimal hemorrhage with laceration; (3) medial laceration; (4) complete transection; (5) pseudoaneurysmal formation; (6) periaortic hemorrhage [16].

Table 9.8 BTAI classification systems

Gavant	I. Normal aorta
	Ia. Normal thoracic aorta on CT
	Ib. Normal thoracic aorta on CT. Mediastinal hematoma present
	II. Minimal aortic injury
	IIa. Intimal flap or pseudoaneurysm <1 cm. No mediastinal hematoma
	IIb. Intimal flap or pseudoaneurysm <1 cm. Mediastinal hematoma present
	III. Confined thoracic aorta injury
	IIIa. >1 cm, regular, well-defined pseudoaneurysm with intimal flap or thrombus. No involvement of ascending aorta, arch, or great vessels. Mediastinal hematoma present
	IIIb. >1 cm, easily identified, regular, well-defined pseudoaneurysm with intimal flap or thrombus. Ascending aorta, arch, or great vessels present. Mediastinal hematoma present
	IV. Total aortic disruption
	Easily identified, irregular, poorly defined pseudoaneurysm with intimal flap or thrombus. Mediastinal hematoma present
Azizzadeh et al. (endorsed by SVS)	1. Intimal tear
	2. Intramural hematoma
	3. Aortic pseudoaneurysm
	4. Free rupture
Vancouver	1. Intimal flap, thrombus, or intramural hematoma <1 cm
	2. Intimal flap, thrombus, or intramural hematoma >1 cm
	3. Pseudoaneurysm (simple or complex, no extravasation)
	4. Contrast extravasation (±pseudoaneurysm)
Harborview	Minimal
	No external contour abnormality
	Intimal tear and/or thrombus is <10 mm
	Moderate
	External contour abnormality or intimal tear >10 mm
	Severe
	Active extravasation
	Left subclavian artery hematoma >15 mm
Starnes	I. Intimal tear = No aortic external contour abnormality: tear and/or associated thrombus is <10 mm
	II. Large intimal flap = No aortic external contour abnormality: tear and/or associated thrombus is >10 mm
	III. Pseudoaneurysm = Aortic external contour abnormality: contained
	IV. Rupture = Aortic external contour abnormality: not contained, free rupture
Rabin	Grade I: Intimal tear or localized hematoma
	Grade II: Pseudoaneurysm involving less than 50% of the total aortic circumference
	Grade III: Pseudoaneurysm involving more than 50% of the total aortic circumference
	Grade IV: Rupture or complete section

Reproduced (modified) with permission from Nagpal P et al. Advances in Imaging and Management Trends of Traumatic Aortic Injuries. Cardiovasc Intervent Radiol (2017) 40: 643–654. Doi: 10.1007/s00270-017-1572-x

With the arrival of the new generation of CT scanners, able to detect the architecture of aortic injuries, a CT-based grading system became necessary to evaluate the severity of traumatic aortic injury and identify what patients needed urgent or emergency therapy and what patients needed only medical management. Many classification systems were proposed to stratify injury severity.

Gavant et al. published the first classification system based on CT images in 1999, very comprehensive but somewhat difficult to use [61], because the first three grades were split into two subgroups and not correlating with clinical outcome. The injury classification was based on the progressive involvement of the aortic wall. Gavant identified four grades: (I) normal aorta; (II) minimal aortic injury; (III) confined thoracic aorta injury; (IV) total aortic disruption. The cut-off between grades I and II was 10 mm.

In 2011, the Society for Vascular Surgery (SVS) published clinical practice guidelines for endovascular repair of BTAI [8], using the classification system by Azizzadeh et al. [66] that divides injuries into four grades: (Grade 1) intimal tear; (Grade 2) intramural hematoma or large intimal flap; (Grade 3) pseudoaneurysm; (Grade 4) free rupture (Fig. 9.36).

Lamarche et al. [67] proposed Vancouver classification. This grading system was reproducible among radiologists, and they showed that the grade correlated well with patient outcome, but it does not provide direct grade-based management recommendations. The Vancouver classification, like most other classifications, has four grades. Grade 1 and grade 2 essentially have preserved outer aortic contours and consist of luminal thrombus, intimal flap, and/or intramural hematoma, these lesions in grade 1 being smaller than 1 cm and in grade 2 larger than

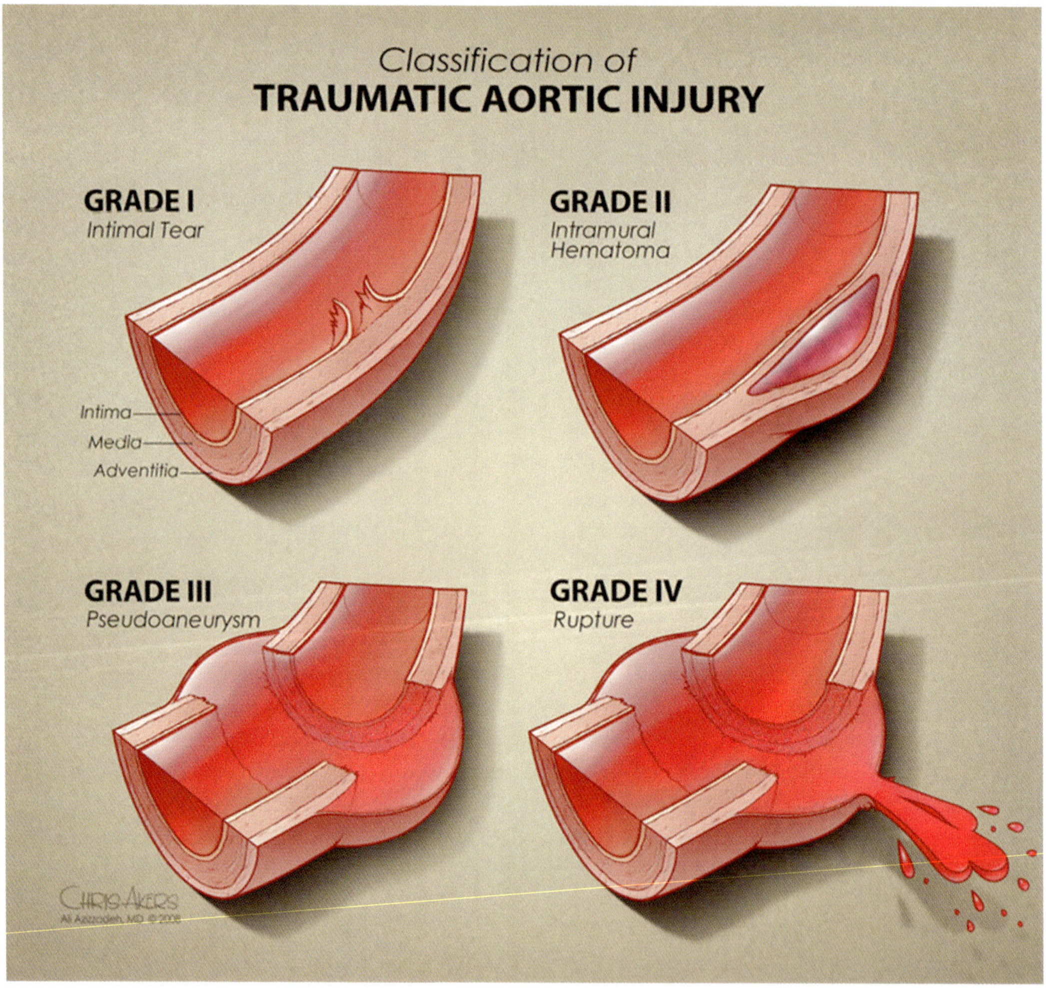

Fig. 9.36 Classification of BTAIs (With permission: Anthony L. Estrera, Charles C. Miller III, Gustavo Guajardo-Salinas, Sheila Coogan, Kristofer Charlton-Ouw, Hazim J. Safi, and Ali Azizzadeh; Update on blunt thoracic aortic injury: Fifteen-year single-institution Experience. The Journal of Thoracic and Cardiovascular Surgery c March 2013, Doi: 10.1016/j.jtcvs.2012.11.074 Copyright 2013 by The American Association for Thoracic Surgery)

1 cm. Grade 3 and grade 4 lesions demonstrate abnormality of the outer wall of the aorta, with grade 3 lesions being pseudoaneurysms of any size and grade 4 lesions showing frank contrast extravasation. Correlating the severity of aortic trauma to clinical outcome, grades 1 and 2 show a survival rate of 100%, grade 3 has a survival rate of 29%, and grade 4 of 33%. A recent study proved these data showing similar survival rate (grades I/II 100%, grades III 88%) among BTAI patients who mainly underwent to surgical approach [68].

Starnes et al. [69] have proposed a classification based on the CT angiography images, allowing a distinction to be made from the outset between two clear groups: patients with no abnormality to the external contours of the aorta (grades I and II); patients with an external contour abnormality to the thoracic aorta (grades III and VI). Concurrent periaortic hematoma >15 mm at the aortic arch is a severe sign associated with a higher risk of death. Grades I and II show a survival rate of 100% (except for not aortic-correlated death).

Rabin et al. utilized the dimension of the pseudoaneurysm to distinguish grade II (including psuedoaneurysm <50% of the normal aorta diameter) from grade III (including pseudoaneurysm >50%). They suggested to incorporate the following criteria for serious injury into the classification: significant mediastinal hematoma, extent of left hemothorax, and the presence of pseudocoarctation [58]. The presence of these criteria worsens the grade of injury. According to this classification, survival rate is of 13% for grade I, 20% for grade II, 21% for grade III, and 17% for grade IV.

Recently, Heneghan et al. [7] proposed the “Harborview Classification” of BTAI, which also helps to guide management based on the grade of injury. Harborview classification divides BTAI into minimal, moderate, and severe injury and suggests that patients should be managed, respectively, by follow-up imaging, initial stabilization of concomitant injuries, and urgent repair of aortic injury.

In the future, more accurate indications for treatment modality could be made possible by the use of a common, simple classification system for the description of traumatic aortic injury.

9.9 Management and Treatment

There is an ongoing debate among the best management option for BTAI patients.

The initial treatment requires strict adherence to advanced trauma life support (ATLS) principles. Once the stability and assessment of a patient have been achieved and the presence of a thoracic aortic injury has been established, the subsequent management can vary considerably.

The rationale for treating BTAI is to prevent early rupture from the acute injury and prevent late aneurysm formation and rupture.

In BTAI patients, the treatment of choice may be interventional (immediate or delayed, surgical or endovascular repair) or conservative (medical management) depending on clinical judgement on an individual basis related to the degree of aortic disruption, the safety of controlling blood pressure, the clinical assessment, and other associated injuries [21].

9.9.1 Medical Management

Nonoperative management is a therapeutic option with acceptable survival in carefully selected patients with aortic injuries that could benefit from delayed repair or with multiple severe associated injuries or high-risk comorbidities.

Medical management is based on blood pressure control by the use of antihypertensive medication (100–120 mmHg) and β-blockers (60–80 bpm) since this circumstance, by decreasing aortic shear forces, proved to be able to avoid progression of aortic injuries.

Conservative management became the treatment of choice for low-grade lesions, in particular for MAI, because these aortic injuries, even when not repaired, either have a spontaneous resolution or no progression, with a survival rate of 100%.

A retrospective study on BTAI patients undergone medical treatment, showed how 78% of grade I-III (based on Rabin’s classification) remained stationary, 18% had spontaneous resolution, and only 4% evolved. The conclusion of this study was that "deliberate nonoperative management of selected patients with traumatic aortic injuries may be a reasonable alternative in the polytrauma patient" [70].

Another recent retrospective study showed similar conclusion: among 44 grades I and II (based on Azizzadeh's grading) patients undergone conservative treatment (86 days of follow-up), 55% had spontaneous resolution, 40% had stable lesions, and only 5% evolved to grade III (pseudoaneurysm) [63].

The aortic injuries undergone medical treatment are closely followed with serial CTA at 48–72 h from the trauma and, in case of stationary lesions, at 30 days, 6 and 12 months and annually thereafter. For the follow-up, currently, magnetic resonance scans have been proposed as alternative to CTA in order to decrease the radiation dose in a usually young patient population [71].

9.9.2 Operative Repair

The first acute repair of aortic rupture was reported in the 1950s by DeBakey et al. For decades, open repair of aortic injuries was considered the standard of care.

During the years, the operative repair for blunt aortic injury has undergone a number of modifications that have reduced the morbidity associated with the procedure. Until the mid-1970s, most of these procedures were completed with an expeditious clamp-and-sew technique that usually included an interposition graft of woven or knitted Dacron to bridge the defect. Although there are isolated reports of reasonable outcomes [72], a meta-analysis of this technique reported an associated mortality of 16% and a striking 19% incidence of paraplegia.

Various methods of distal aortic perfusion have evolved for use during the period of aortic clamping in order to protect the spinal cord. The use of a blood pump (active perfusion) further reduced the rate of paralysis to 2.3% [73].

Most centers with extensive experience in such procedures now use active bypass. Active perfusion can be performed by two main techniques: bypass from the left atrium to the femoral artery (or descending aorta) or venoarterial bypass that involves cannulation of the pulmonary artery (or the right atrium) and the femoral artery (or descending aorta). The downside of these techniques is that they all require systemic heparinization. Typically, the thoracic aorta is not injured in isolation; closed head injuries, solid organ, and pulmonary contusions, as well as pelvic and long bone fractures, are all adversely affected by systemic anticoagulation.

Despite technical advances, a prospective series of 274 cases of blunt aortic injury collected from 50 trauma centers during a 2.5-year period involving a variety of operative techniques showed an overall rate of death of 31% and rate of paraplegia of 8.7% [2].

The best management strategies for ascending aortic injury is a topic of an ongoing debate, but open surgical repair remains the treatment of choice for traumatic ascending aortic injuries.

9.9.3 Endovascular Repair

The most significant advance for the treatment of blunt aortic injury in the past 50 years has been endovascular grafting, first described by Parodi et al. in 1991 for the treatment of abdominal aortic aneurysms [74].

Endografts are placed through a femoral artery. A guide wire is advanced under fluoroscopic guidance to the site of injury. The position is identified on angiography and the stent graft deployed across the injured aorta, excluding it from the circulation. Endovascular grafting has numerous advantages. It is a minimally invasive procedure. Single-lung ventilation is not required. The procedure can be accomplished with minimal or no heparin, and there is no need for a bypass of any kind.

Thin slice CTA with multiplanar and three-dimensional reconstruction allows for appropriate visualization of the vascular injuries as well as the planning for thoracic endovascular repair (TEVAR).

The various multiplanar reconstructions allow to assess the caliber of the aorta, which assists in the choice of aortic endoprothesis, keeping in mind how the diameter of the aorta is influenced by the hemodynamic status of the patient [75, 76]. Hemodynamically unstable patients have smaller diameters and require more oversizing than hemodynamically stable patients. Abdominal and pelvic images allow to assess the various femoral or brachial accesses and if they are of sufficient diameter to deliver the stent graft. The existence of any anatomical variant must be noted in the pre-treatment CT angiogram report. For example, an arteria lusoria may need to be occluded before an endoprothesis can be placed in the descending thoracic aorta.

Table 9.9 lists what information should be present in CTA reports to aid in planning TEVAR.

Currently, endovascular repair has replaced open surgery as the primary treatment of blunt aortic injuries in several institutions. The American Association for the Surgery of Trauma (AAST) confirmed endovascular repair is currently performed more commonly than open repair in patients with BTAI, demonstrating that 64.8% of the patients were treated with endovascular stent grafts in 2007 in contrast to 0% in 1997 (open repair 100% in 1997 versus 35.2% in 2007) [49].

Clinical practice guidelines published by the Society for Vascular Surgery in 2011 recommended TEVAR as the first policy for the treatment of BTAI, supporting the progressive shift in management from open to endovascular repair. From a review of many studies (1990–2009), they detected a lower mortality for patients managed with endovascular repair versus open repair (9% vs. 19%). Comparing TEVAR with open surgical repair, also the rate of paraplegia as iatrogenic complication was lower for endovascular repair (3% vs. 9%) [8], whereas the incidence of stroke was slightly higher for endovascular when compared to open repair (2.5% vs. 1%) [5].

Table 9.9 What CTA reports should include to aid in planning TEVAR

Anatomy of aortic injury (location, length, severity, and type)
Distance from the origin of left subclavian artery (at least 15–20 mm; if <15 mm covering LSA and possible bypass from the left common carotid artery to the LSA)
Suitable femoral or brachial access (femoral access >6–9 mm; optional iliac access)
Aortic diameter (value aortic stent 16–20 mm/36–44 mm)
Curving angle between aortic arch and descending aorta (>90°)
Winding of aorta
Atherosclerotic disease of aorta (vascular calcification)
Vascular stenosis

TEVAR shows a technical success rate which often reaches 100%, with cause-specific mortality at 30 days hovering around 2.1%, and a 2-year survival rate of 93.7% [77, 78]. The practice management guideline from the Eastern Association for the Surgery of Trauma published in 2015 "strongly recommend the use of endovascular repair in patients who do not have contraindications to endovascular repair" [5] (Fig. 9.37).

Table 9.10 shows the benefits of TEVAR as compared with open repair.

Nevertheless, as with any endovascular procedure, placement of an aortic endoprothesis is not devoid of risk, with mortality during the intervention of around 4% and periprocedural mortality of around 16%. This mortality rate is of course more often attributable to the traumatic injury itself rather than to endovascular procedure. Among iatrogenic complication, spinal cord ischemia remains a very rare complication in this condition, estimated to arise in fewer than 1% of cases [79].

There are currently some technical limitations to endografting. Injuries that occur adjacent to a sharp bend in the aorta may result in poor apposition of the covered stent to the aortic wall. This leads not only to failure in covering the injury, but also to device collapse [80]. Another technical issue relates to the management of the left subclavian artery. Lesions adjacent to the left subclavian artery may require covering this vessel in order to achieve adequate repair. Although usually well tolerated, coverage of the left subclavian artery (LSA) can result in ischemia of the upper extremity or territory perfused by the left vertebral artery. In such cases, bypass from the left common carotid artery to the left subclavian artery may be required. Patients with

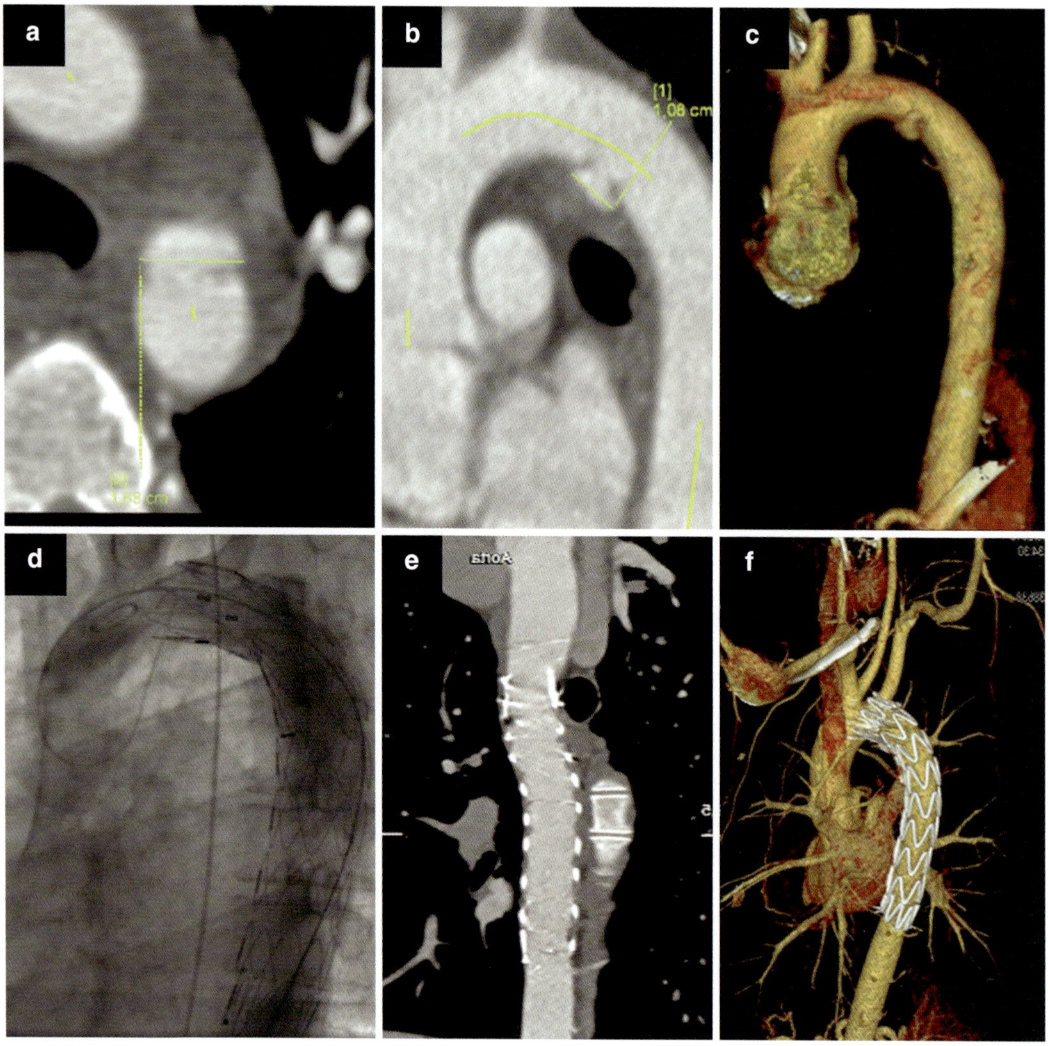

Fig. 9.37 Treatment BTAI of isthmus (grade 3). (**a**) Axial CT scan, (**b**) Multiplanar reformation (MPR), and (**c**) three-dimensional volume-rendered (3D-VR) image show traumatic pseudoaneurysm isthmus grade 3 with periaortic hematoma. (**d**) Angiography image after placement of the endovascular stent; (**e**) reformat linear image; and (**f**) three-dimensional volume-rendered (3D-VR) image show that the stent has expanded correctly and there is no leakage

Table 9.10 Benefits of TEVAR as compared with open repair

No thoracotomy
No single-lung ventilation
No aortic clamping
No cardiopulmonary bypass
Reduced systemic heparinization (and decreased hemorrhagic risk)
Reduced blood loss
Lesser postoperative pain
Lower mortality and incidence of paraplegia

a dominant left vertebral artery (relative to the right) should be considered for left subclavian artery revascularization before coverage.

Finally, the durability of endografts is unknown. There are questions about long-term device integrity as well as the natural history of the aorta itself after this type of injury and repair. These issues are particularly important when considering the relatively young age of trauma patients, in comparison to patients with aneurysmal disease. Therefore, several trauma centers still perform open repair awaiting long-term outcomes. However, the short-term complication rate for endovascular repair is substantially lower when compared to open repair.

In 2008, Demetriades et al. detected device-related complications in 20% (endoleaks in 14%) [49]. In the years thereafter, many studies demonstrated a significant decrease of the rate of device-related complications.

In 2014, Azizzadeh et al. [81] published the follow-up results of 82 consecutive patients who underwent endovascular repair for BTAI. Average time to follow-up was 2.3 years, and the incidence of device-related complications was 2.4%.

Follow-up imaging after TEVAR aims to diagnose potential adverse events such as device migration, disconnection, or endoleak, which might need additional treatment. However, there are no guidelines regarding follow-up imaging after TEVAR for BTAI. The RESCUE trial, published in 2013, defined its follow-up protocol as follows: "a CTA or magnetic resonance angiogram at 1, 6, and 12 months and annually thereafter for 5 years. Multiple view chest x-rays will also be acquired at 1, 3, and 5 years to assess for device integrity." [82].

Evaluation at the time of immediate or delayed follow-up imaging should assess any residual contrast material flow within the pseudoaneurysm, compare pseudoaneurysm size and configuration with those at prior examination or initial repair, and compare stent position with that at prior examination. Other anatomic features that should be reviewed are the diameter and appearance of the aorta proximal and distal to the injury, completeness of injury exclusion by the stent, apposition or seal of the stent along the length of the aortic wall (particularly at the endograft ends), stent patency and luminal configuration, adjacent branch vessels, and surrounding soft tissues and organs.

Complications after endograft repair (Table 9.11) can manifest immediately or in a delayed fashion. The reported complications (many of which are rare) include endoleak (Fig. 9.38), graft collapse, branch vessel complications including both stroke and left upper

Table 9.11 Endograft-related complications

Stent migration
Endoleak
Endograft collapse
Stroke
Upper extremity ischemia
Graft infection
Access site complications (infection, dissection, thrombus, pseudoaneurysm)
Paraplegia
Endograft structural failure
Retrograde dissection

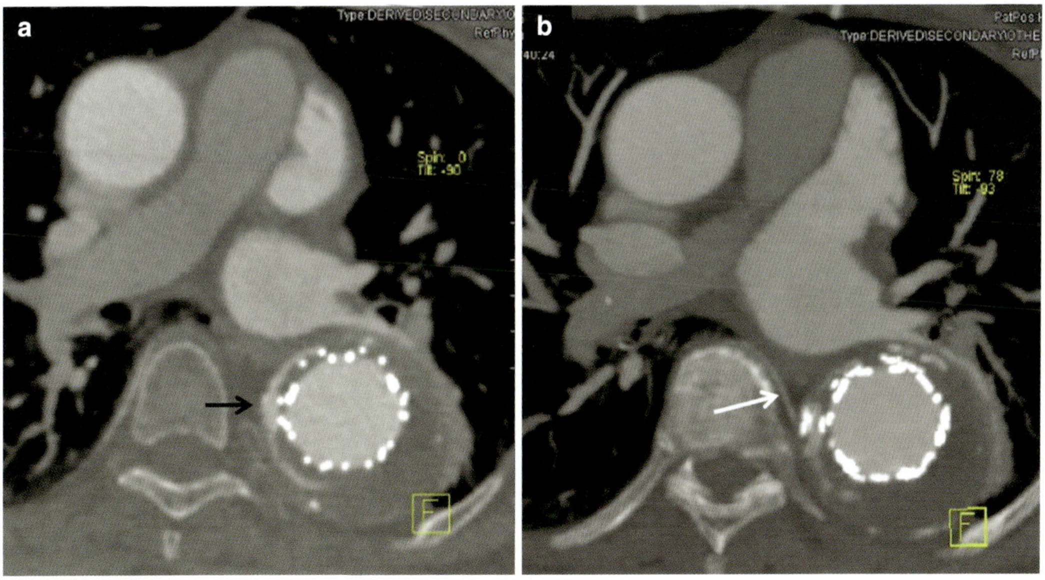

Fig. 9.38 Endoleak tipe II. (**a**) Axial CT scan (*black arrow*); (**b**) elaborate maximum intensity projection (MIP) shows intercostal artery (*white arrow*)

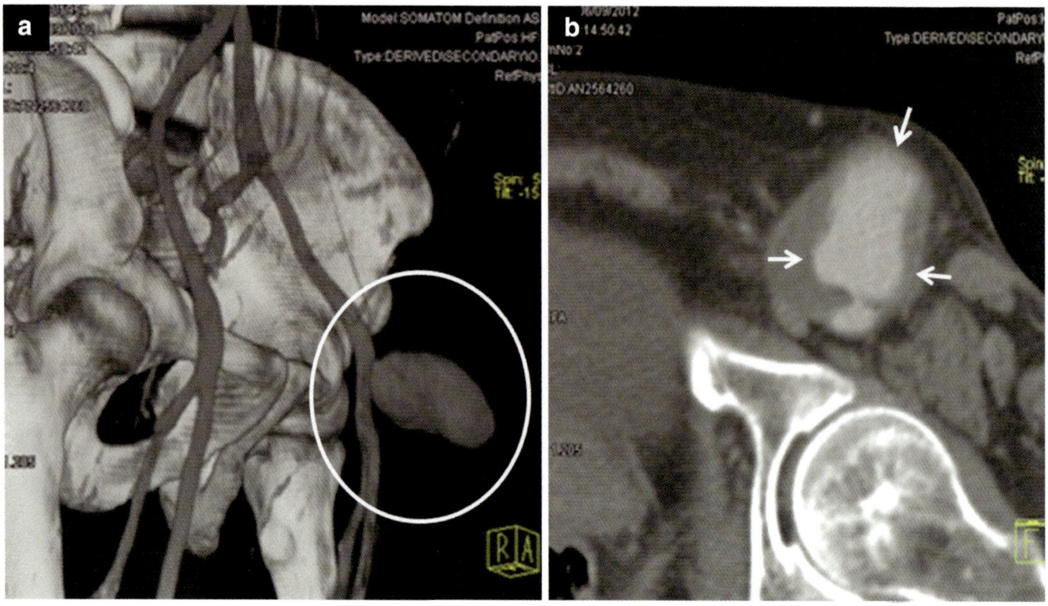

Fig. 9.39 TEVAR, access site complications. (**a**) Volume-rendered (3D-VR) image and (**b**) axial CT scan show large pseudoaneurysm of left common femoral artery (*white circle* in **a** and *white arrows* in **b**)

extremity ischemia (from covering LSA as yet explained), endograft infection, graft material failure, missed injury or stent migration, and complications related to the access site (Fig. 9.39).

Endoleak is the most common complication after endovascular repair with a prevalence ranging from 3.2 to 14.4% [49, 80].

Small endoleaks are sometimes managed conservatively with imaging follow-up, but most require rapid intervention with either additional overlapping stent placement or conversion to open surgical repair. Three designated types of endoleaks (Table 9.12) have been described and are adapted from endoleak types originally described after stent repair of non-traumatic abdominal aortic aneurysms. Type I is the most frequently reported [83] and is defined as blood flow into the aneurysm sac secondary to incomplete or inadequate sealing of the graft end. Type Ia endoleaks occur at the proximal end of the graft and are more common. Type Ib endoleaks occur at the distal end. A shorter proximal neck length between the LSA and the injury has been shown to correlate with an increase in the prevalence of type Ia endoleaks.

Table 9.12 Types of endoleaks

I.	Incomplete or inadequate seal at either side of the stent graft
II.	Blood accumulation in the excluded segment as a result of opposing retrograde flow from a collateral vessel
III.	Blood leakage between overlapping stent grafts due to breakdown of graft material or fracture of the metallic skeleton.

A type II endoleak is defined as blood flow into the aneurysm sac as a result of opposing retrograde flow from a collateral vessel. Type II endoleak has been associated with stent coverage of the LSA [84].

A type III endoleak is defined as blood flow within the aneurysm sac from inadequate sealing at the junction of two stent grafts, from breakdown of graft material, or from fracture of the metallic skeleton.

Endograft collapse is a serious potential complication of endograft repair that can result in high morbidity and mortality. A short neck above the level of injury and sharp angulation or bend of the aortic arch can cause poor apposition of the endograft to the aortic intima. Device collapse can also occur when the endograft is oversized in comparison to the thoracic aorta [85].

A focal collapse may appear as a focal concavity in the endograft. Partial or complete collapse will appear as narrowing and irregularity of the endograft lumen or even apposition of the endograft walls, with blood flow diverted between the aortic wall and endograft.

Endograft infections are rare but are associated with significant morbidity and mortality [86].

Patients with graft infection can present with nonspecific clinical findings such as leucocytosis, fever, and chest pain. CT findings suggestive of endograft infection after BTAI repair include perigraft soft-tissue or fluid collection, pseudoaneurysm, perigraft air, adjacent soft-tissue stranding or abscess formation, and graft thrombosis or expansion [87].

The long-term integrity of endografts used for repair of acute thoracic injury has not been well established because of a lack of long-term data. Endograft material failure is a lifelong complication risk. Close inspection of the integrity of the graft should be performed during every follow-up CT study. The configuration of the stent should be compared with the ones in previous examinations. Sharp angulation of the metallic framework or irregularity in contour of the stent-graft material should raise suspicion of an endograft disruption.

Stent migration can also occur and lead to reexposure of the aortic injury. Patients with endografts that lack complete exclusion of the aortic injury may have the same risk of aortic rupture and mortality as nontreated aortic injury patients [88], and urgent reintervention is always required. Both the position of the endograft in comparison with the ones at previous examinations and its relation to the entire aortic injury should be assessed at every follow-up CT angiography examination.

Access site complications are among the most common problems after endograft repair. In a meta-analysis by Tang et al. [79], the access site complication rate was 2.8%. Complications include arterial rupture, dissection, pseudoaneurysm, mycotic aneurysm, thrombosis, and subcutaneous infection.

9.9.4 Delayed Vs. Immediate Repair

The timing of repair is based both on the extent of the patient's coexisting injuries as well as the extent of injury to the thoracic aorta [21].

The risk of rupture of contained BTAI is highest within the first 24 h of injury. For this reason, immediate repair of BTAI was advocated and considered the standard of care for decades.

Although the traditional approach to BTAI has been emergency (<24 h) repair, currently there is a trend toward delayed repair (open or endovascular). During the last years, several studies have suggested that not all traumatic injuries of the thoracic aorta require emergency treatment and that some patients can be safely managed with medical treatment, adequately controlling blood pressure and contractility [58].

Demetriades et al. compared the findings of two studies conducted by of the American Association for the Surgery of Trauma in 1997 and in 2007. They found that the mean time from traumatic event to surgical repair increased from 16.5 h in 1997 to 67.6 h in 2007 and the mean time from injury to endovascular repair was 48.1 h [49].

From a literature review of seven comparative studies (1998–2013), Fox et al. found that mortality decreased from 21 to 9%, paraplegia from 5.5 to 0.6%, and stroke from 9 to 7% when delayed repair was adopted when compared with emergency repair. The only exception was renal insufficiency that increased from 8.6 to 9.3% when delayed repair was chosen. Based on results, they suggested that in hemodynamically stable patients the definitive management of TAI should be delayed until other acute life-threatening injuries are adequately managed and appropriately resuscitated, enphasizing that in these cases an effective blood pressure control with antihypertensive medication must be used. If instead the patient is hemodynamically unstable and there are direct signs of the aortic injury on CT, definitive emergent management of the aortic injury is suggested [5, 89] (Table 9.13).

Table 9.13 The management algorithm of BTAI (Reproduced with permission from Nagpal P et al., Advances in Imaging and Management Trends of Traumatic Aortic Injuries. Cardiovasc Intervent Radiol 40: 643–654. Doi:10.1007/s00270-017-1572-x)

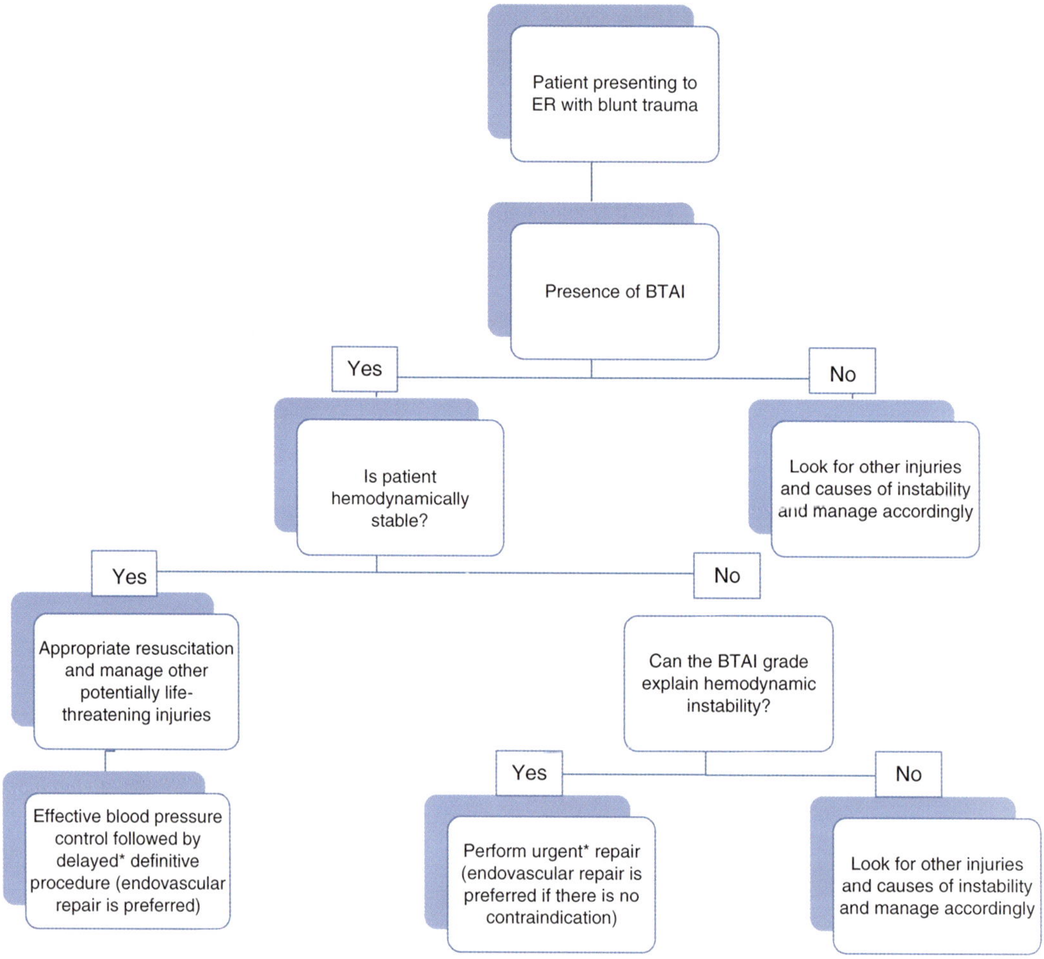

* Decision for urgent or delayed repair should be based on combination of patient-specific risk of aortic rupture, clinical suspicion, imaging characteristics, and/or grade of injury.

Aside from patients presenting signs of complications (significant left hemothorax, pseudocoarctation, or extensive mediastinal hematoma), trauma injuries can be traditionally classified into two distinct groups according to their course:

- injuries in which the external wall of the aorta is spared: these are grade I and II injuries and they can be treated medically, combined with close monitoring. Over half of grade I and II injuries will resolve spontaneously with medical treatment only. Just 5% of grade I and II injuries deteriorate [59].
- injuries with abnormality of the outer wall of the aorta; they must be treated as an emergency. Traditionally, these included traumatic aortic pseudoaneurysms (grade III) and contrast extravasation on CTA (grade IV) although the management of BTAI varies per operator and among trauma centers.

Recent research shows that an expectant approach is also justified for patients with traumatic pseudoaneurysms [58, 70], especially if these grade III injuries don't show signs of serious damage and other trauma injuries. Akins et al. reported a 24–14% decrease in the mortality of patients when operative intervention was delayed at least 48 h [90]. Several studies since then have demonstrated both the safety and reduction in mortality in delayed traumatic aortic repair (>24 h) [91].

Delaying immediate operative intervention allows time to assess for further injuries, assess prognosis (especially in severe head injury), and maximize resuscitation. Delay does not equate observation; rather, it means pharmacologic intervention and rigorous intensive care unit (ICU) monitoring. The cornerstone for delayed therapy involves precise control of blood pressure in an effort to reduce aortic wall tension. Initial nonoperative management is predicated on the concept that maintaining a mean arterial pressure of less than or equal to 80 mmHg is possible since late rupture is uncommon under these circumstances [92] β-blockers are the preferred antihypertensive agents.

When applied more broadly, medical management has enabled more patients with advanced aortic lesions to undergo delayed aortic repair [93, 94].

9.9.5 Practice Management Guideline

About the treatment of BTAI, clinical practice guidelines published by the Society for Vascular Surgery in 2011 recommended TEVAR as treatment of BTAI preferentially over open surgical repair or nonoperative management. They suggested urgent repair (<24 h) except for minimal aortic injuries for which they advocated an expectant management with serial imaging for type I injuries. TEVAR is the treatment of choice, regardless of age; only if anatomical criteria aren't permissive they suggested to consider conventional open repair [8].

However, appropriate patient selection remains challenging and must balance poorer outcomes associated with emergency repair against the risk of aortic rupture. Multiple radiographic grading systems exist to stratify the severity of aortic injuries although none of the current systems quantify a lesion's risk of rupture. A recent study developed an aortic injury risk score that predicts early rupture based on patient physiology, lesion characteristics, and secondary signs of aortic injury [91]. The objective was to help to appropriately select patients for early vs delayed intervention and to reduce the number of unnecessary emergency procedures in patients with high-grade (Society for Vascular Surgery grade III and IV) aortic lesions but otherwise low-risk lesions for aortic rupture. From their study, they conclude that a patient is at high risk of early rupture if any two of the following three factors are present: admission lactate >4 mM, posterior periaortic hematoma >10 mm, or lesion/normal aortic diameter ratio > 1.4 (meaning an aortic diameter increased more than 40% when compared to the nearest normal aortic diameter).

Another recent study sought parameters for successful nonoperative management of BTAI. They concluded that grade 3 aortic injuries (pseudoaneurysms involving more than 50% the circumference of the aorta in their study) with secondary signs of injury (SSI) (pseudocoarctation, extensive mediastinal hematoma, and large left hemothorax) needed urgent repair, whereas those without SSI could undergo delayed repair [58].

Starnes et al. proposed a well-structured management for patients with BTAI. They recommended a nonoperative management with follow-up CTA, respectively, within 1 week for intimal tear (< 10 mm) and within 1 month for large intimal tear (>10 mm), suggesting for the last one an endovascular repair in case of progression. All patients with an aortic external contour abnormality should be considered for semielective (≤1 week) endovascular repair in case of a high likelihood of survival from other associated injuries. An earlier repair is considered in the presence of an aortic arch hematoma >15 mm on CT scan or in patients with hypotension on presentation (Table 9.14) [69].

Table 9.14 University of Washington clinical treatment guidelines for blunt aortic injury

1.	All patients with radiographic evidence of blunt aortic injury (BAI) should undergo anti-impulse therapy with β-blockade, if tolerated, coupled with antiplatelet therapy (81 mg aspirin).
2.	Observation alone with interval follow-up computed tomography angiography (CTA) within 30 days is appropriate for all intimal tears <10 mm.
3.	Selective management of large intimal flaps (>10 mm) is appropriate with repeat imaging within 7 days to assess for progression. Evidence of progression should be managed, when possible, with endovascular repair.
4.	All patients with an aortic external contour abnormality should be considered for semielective (≤1 week) endovascular repair if there is a high likelihood of survival from other associated injuries. These patients should be monitored with CT imaging as follows: 1 month, 6 months, 1 year, and every other year thereafter. Patients with hypotension on presentation and aortic arch hematoma >15 mm should be repaired with endovascular methods on a more *urgent* basis.
5.	Intentional left subclavian artery coverage *without* revascularization is well tolerated in a majority of patients with BAI.
6.	Patients with traumatic brain injury and an aortic external contour abnormality should be considered for earlier repair if a deliberate increase in mean arterial pressure is deemed beneficial for the patient.

Reproduced with permission from: Starnes BW et al., A new classification scheme for treating blunt aortic injury. J Vasc Surg 55:47–54. Doi: 10.1016/j.jvs.2011.07.073

References

1. Ungar TC, Wolf SJ, Haukoos JS, et al. Derivation of a clinical decision rule to exclude thoracic aortic imaging in patients with blunt chest trauma after motor vehicle collisions. J Trauma. 2006;61:1150–5. doi:10.1097/01.ta.0000239357.68782.30.
2. Neschis DG, Scalea TM, Flinn WR, Griffith BP. Blunt aortic injury. N Engl J Med. 2008;359:1708–16. doi:10.1056/NEJMra0706159.
3. Arajärvi E, Santavirta S, Tolonen J. Aortic ruptures in seat belt wearers. J Thorac Cardiovasc Surg. 1989;98:355–61.
4. Teixeira PG, Inaba K, Barmparas G, et al. Blunt thoracic aortic injuries: an autopsy study. J Trauma. 2011;70:197–202. doi:10.1097/TA.0b013e3181df68b3.
5. Fox N, Schwartz D, Salazar JH, et al. Evaluation and management of blunt traumatic aortic injury: a practice management guideline from the Eastern Association for the Surgery of Trauma. J Trauma Acute Care Surg. 2015;78:136–46. doi:10.1097/TA.0000000000000470.
6. Arthurs ZM, Starnes BW, Sohn VY, et al. Functional and survival outcomes in traumatic blunt thoracic aortic injuries: an analysis of the National Trauma Databank. J Vasc Surg. 2009;49:988–94. doi:10.1016/j.jvs.2008.11.052.
7. Heneghan RE, Aarabi S, Quiroga E, et al. Call for a new classification system and treatment strategy in blunt aortic injury. J Vasc Surg. 2016;64:171–6. doi:10.1016/j.jvs.2016.02.047; Epub 2016 Apr 27.
8. Lee WA, Matsumura JS, Mitchell RS, et al. Endovascular repair of traumatic thoracic aortic injury: clinical practice guidelines of the Society for Vascular Surgery. J Vasc Surg. 2011;53:187–92. doi:10.1016/j.jvs.2010.08.027; Epub 2010 Oct 25.
9. Fabian TC, Richardson JD, Croce MA, et al. Prospective study of blunt aortic injury: multicenter trial of the American Association for the Surgery of Trauma. J Trauma. 1997;42:374–80; discussion 380–383.
10. Ait Ali Yahia D, Bouvier A, Nedelcu C, et al. Imaging of thoracic aortic injury. Diagn Interv Imaging. 2015;96:79–88. doi:10.1016/j.diii.2014.02.003; Epub 2014 Dec 22.
11. Costa DN, Rubin GD, Rofsky NM, Hallett RL. Thoracic aorta. In: Rubin GD, Rofsky NM, editors. CT and MR angiography: comprehensive vascular assessment. Philadelphia: Lippincott Williams & Wilkins (LWW); 2009.
12. Desai SS, Lidsky M, Pascarella L, Shortell CK. Principles of vascular surgery in clinical review of vascular surgery. In: Desai SS, Shortell CK, editors. Clinical review of vascular surgery. Durham: Surgisphere Corporation; 2010.
13. Steenburg SD, Ravenel JG, Ikonomidis JS, et al. Acute traumatic aortic injury: imaging evaluation and management. Radiology. 2008;248:748–62. doi:10.1148/radiol.2483071416.
14. Riesenman PJ, Brooks JD, Farber MA. Acute blunt traumatic injury to the descending thoracic aorta. J Vasc Surg. 2012;56:1274–80. doi:10.1016/j.jvs.2012.04.035; Epub 2012 Jun 23.
15. Horton TG, Cohn SM, Heid MP, et al. Identification of trauma patients at risk of thoracic aortic tear by mechanism of injury. J Trauma. 2000;48:1008–13; discussion 1013–1014.
16. Parmley LF, Mattingly TW, Manion WC, Jahnke EJ Jr. Nonpenetrating traumatic injury of the aorta. Circulation. 1958;17:1086–101.
17. Kodali S, Jamieson WR, Leia-Stephens M, et al. Traumatic rupture of the thoracic aorta. A 20-year review: 1969–1989. Circulation. 1991;84(5 Suppl):III40–6.
18. Carter Y, Meissner M, Bulger E, et al. Anatomical considerations in the surgical management of blunt thoracic aortic injury. J Vasc Surg. 2001;34:628–33. doi:10.1067/mva.2001.117143.
19. Macura KJ, Corl FM, Fishman EK, Bluemke DA. Pathogenesis in acute aortic syndromes: aortic aneurysm leak and rupture and traumatic aortic transection. AJR Am J Roentgenol. 2003;181:303–7. doi:10.2214/ajr.181.2.1810303.

20. Prêtre R, Chilcott M, Mürith N, Panos A. Blunt injury to the supra-aortic arteries. Br J Surg. 1997;84:603–9.
21. O'Connor JV, Byrne C, Scalea TM, et al. Vascular injuries after blunt chest trauma: diagnosis and management. Scand J Trauma Resusc Emerg Med. 2009;17:42. doi:10.1186/1757-7241-17-42.
22. Murakami R, Tajima H, Ichikawa K, et al. Acute traumatic injury of the distal descending aorta associated with thoracic spine injury. Eur Radiol. 1998;8:60–2. doi:10.1007/s003300050339.
23. de Mestral C, Dueck AD, Gomez D, et al. Associated injuries, management, and outcomes of blunt abdominal aortic injury. J Vasc Surg. 2012;56:656–60. doi:10.1016/j.jvs.2012.02.027; Epub 2012 Jul 12.
24. Williams DM, Simon HJ, Marx MV, Starkey TD. Acute traumatic aortic rupture: intravascular US findings. Radiology. 1992;182:247–9. doi:10.1148/radiology.182.1.1727291.
25. Merrill WH, Lee RB, Hammon JW Jr, et al. Surgical treatment of acute traumatic tear of the thoracic aorta. Ann Surg. 1988;207:699–706.
26. Kram HB, Wohlmuth DA, Appel PL, Shoemaker WC. Clinical and radiographic indications for aortography in blunt chest trauma. J Vasc Surg. 1987;6:168–76. doi:10.1067/mva.1987.avs0060168.
27. Fishman JE. Imaging of blunt aortic and great vessel trauma. J Thorac Imaging. 2000;15:97–103.
28. Mirvis SE, Bidwell JK, Buddemeyer EU, et al. Value of chest radiography in excluding traumatic aortic rupture. Radiology. 1987;163:487–93. doi:10.1148/radiology.163.2.3562831.
29. Patel NH, Stephens KE Jr, Mirvis SE, et al. Imaging of acute thoracic aortic injury due to blunt trauma: a review. Radiology. 1998;209:335–48. doi:10.1148/radiology.209.2.9807557.
30. Cook AD, Klein JS, Rogers FB, et al. Chest radiographs of limited utility in the diagnosis of blunt traumatic aortic laceration. J Trauma. 2001;50:843–7.
31. Symbas PJ, Horsley WS, Symbas PN. Rupture of the ascending aorta caused by blunt trauma. Ann Thorac Surg. 1998;66:113–7.
32. O'Conor CE. Diagnosing traumatic rupture of the thoracic aorta in the emergency department. Emerg Med J. 2004;21:414–9.
33. Sturm JT, Hankins DG, Young G. Thoracic aortography following blunt chest trauma. Am J Emerg Med. 1990;8:92–6.
34. Pozzato C, Fedriga E, Donatelli F, Gattoni F. Acute posttraumatic rupture of the thoracic aorta: the role of angiography in a 7-year review. Cardiovasc Intervent Radiol. 1991;14:338–41.
35. Demetriades D, Velmahos GC, Scalea TM, et al. Diagnosis and treatment of blunt thoracic aortic injuries: changing perspectives. J Trauma. 2008;64:1415–8. doi:10.1097/TA.0b013e3181715e32; discussion 1418–1419.
36. Wintermark M, Wicky S, Schnyder P. Imaging of acute traumatic injuries of the thoracic aorta. Eur Radiol. 2002;12:431–42. doi:10.1007/s003300100971; Epub 2001 Jun 30.
37. Smith MD, Cassidy JM, Souther S, et al. Transesophageal echocardiography in the diagnosis of traumatic rupture of the aorta. N Engl J Med. 1995;332:356–62. doi:10.1056/NEJM199502093320603.
38. Uflacker R, Horn J, Phillips G, Selby JB. Intravascular sonography in the assessment of traumatic injury of the thoracic aorta. AJR Am J Roentgenol. 1999;173:665–70. doi:10.2214/ajr.173.3.10470899.
39. Patel NH, Hahn D, Comess KA. Blunt chest trauma victims: role of intravascular ultrasound and transesophageal echocardiography in cases of abnormal thoracic aortogram. J Trauma. 2003;55:330–7. doi:10.1097/01.TA.0000078696.27012.5C.
40. Malhotra AK, Fabian TC, Croce MA, et al. Minimal aortic injury: a lesion associated with advancing diagnostic techniques. J Trauma. 2001;51:1042–8.
41. Patterson BO, Holt PJ, Cleanthis M, et al. Imaging vascular trauma. Br J Surg. 2012;99:494–505. doi:10.1002/bjs.7763; Epub 2011 Dec 22.
42. Fattori R, Celletti F, Descovich B, et al. Evolution of post-traumatic aortic aneurysm in the subacute phase: magnetic resonance imaging follow-up as a support of the surgical timing. Eur J Cardiothorac Surg. 1998;13:582–6; discussion 586–587.
43. Wong H, Gotway MB, Sasson AD, Jeffrey RB. Periaortic hematoma at diaphragmatic crura at helical CT: sign of blunt aortic injury in patients with mediastinal hematoma. Radiology. 2004;231:185–9. doi:10.1148/radiol.2311021776.
44. Mirvis SE, Shanmuganathan K, Buell J, Rodriguez A. Use of spiral computed tomography for the assessment of blunt trauma patients with potential aortic injury. J Trauma. 1998;45:922–30.
45. Steenburg SD, Ravenel JG. Acute traumatic thoracic aortic injuries: experience with 64-MDCT. AJR Am J Roentgenol. 2008;191:1564–9. doi:10.2214/AJR.07.3349.
46. Ting J. Blunt traumatic aortic injury. Eur J Trauma. 2003;29:129–38. doi:10.1007/s00068-003-1291-7.
47. Kirsh MM, Behrendt DM, Orringer MB, et al. The treatment of acute traumatic rupture of the aorta: a 10-year experience. Ann Surg. 1976;184:308–16.
48. Fabian TC, Davis KA, Gavant ML, et al. Prospective study of blunt aortic injury: helical CT is diagnostic and antihypertensive therapy reduces rupture. Ann Surg. 1998;227:666–76; discussion 676–677.
49. Demetriades D, Velmahos GC, Scalea TM, et al. Operative repair or endovascular stent graft in blunt traumatic thoracic aortic injuries: results of an American Association for the Surgery of Trauma multicenter study. J Trauma. 2008;64:561–70. doi:10.1097/TA.0b013e3181641bb3; discussion 570–571.
50. Dyer DS, Moore EE, Mestek MF, et al. Can chest CT be used to exclude aortic injury? Radiology. 1999;213:195–202. doi:10.1148/radiology.213.1.r99oc49195.
51. Rogalla P, Kloeters C, Hein PA. CT technology overview: 64-slice and beyond. Radiol Clin N Am. 2009;47:1–11. doi:10.1016/j.rcl.2008.10.004.

52. Voitle E, Hofmann W, Cejna M. Aortic emergencies-diagnosis and treatment: a pictorial review. Insights Imaging. 2015;6:17–32. doi:10.1007/s13244-014-0380-y; Epub 2015 Feb 1.
53. Iacobellis F, Ierardi AM, Mazzei MA, et al. Dual-phase CT for the assessment of acute vascular injuries in high-energy blunt trauma: the imaging findings and management implications. Br J Radiol. 2016;89:20150952. doi:10.1259/bjr.20150952; Epub 2016 Feb 17.
54. Scaglione M, Pinto A, Pinto F, et al. Role of contrast-enhanced helical CT in the evaluation of acute thoracic aortic injuries after blunt chest trauma. Eur Radiol. 2001;11:2444–8. doi:10.1007/s003300100836; Epub 2001 Feb 23.
55. Berger FH, van Lienden KP, Smithuis R, et al. Acute aortic syndrome and blunt traumatic aortic injury: pictorial review of MDCT imaging. Eur J Radiol. 2010;74:24–39. doi:10.1016/j.ejrad.2009.06.023; Epub 2009 Aug 8.
56. Forman MJ, Mirvis SE, Hollander DS. Blunt thoracic aortic injuries: CT characterisation and treatment outcomes of minor injury. Eur Radiol. 2013;23:2988–95. doi:10.1007/s00330-013-2904-0; Epub 2013 May 31.
57. Aladham F, Sundaram B, Williams DM, Quint LE. Traumatic aortic injury: computerized tomographic findings at presentation and after conservative therapy. J Comput Assist Tomogr. 2010;34:388–94. doi:10.1097/RCT.0b013e3181d0728f.
58. Rabin J, DuBose J, Sliker CW, et al. Parameters for successful nonoperative management of traumatic aortic injury. J Thorac Cardiovasc Surg. 2014;147:143–9. doi:10.1016/j.jtcvs.2013.08.053.
59. Harris DG, Rabin J, Kufera JA, et al. A new aortic injury score predicts early rupture more accurately than clinical assessment. J Vasc Surg. 2015;61:332–8. doi:10.1016/j.jvs.2014.08.007; Epub 2014 Sep 5.
60. Mokrane FZ, Revel-Mouroz P, Saint Lebes B, Rousseau H. Traumatic injuries of the thoracic aorta: the role of imaging in diagnosis and treatment. Diagn Interv Imaging. 2015;96:693–706. doi:10.1016/j.diii.2015.06.005; Epub 2015 Jun 27.
61. Gavant ML. Helical CT grading of traumatic aortic injuries. Impact on clinical guidelines for medical and surgical management. Radiol Clin N Am. 1999;37:553–74,vi.
62. de Mestral C, Dueck A, Sharma SS, et al. Evolution of the incidence, management, and mortality of blunt thoracic aortic injury: a population-based analysis. J Am Coll Surg. 2013;216:1110–5. doi:10.1016/j.jamcollsurg.2013.01.005; Epub 2013 Mar 13.
63. Osgood MJ, Heck JM, Rellinger EJ, et al. Natural history of grade I–II blunt traumatic aortic injury. J Vasc Surg. 2014;59:334–41. doi:10.1016/j.jvs.2013.09.007; Epub 2013 Dec 15.
64. Kidane B, Abramowitz D, Harris JR, et al. Natural history of minimal aortic injury following blunt thoracic aortic trauma. Can J Surg. 2012;55:377–81. doi:10.1503/cjs.007311.
65. Erbel R, Aboyans V, Boileau C, et al. 2014 ESC guidelines on the diagnosis and treatment of aortic diseases: document covering acute and chronic aortic diseases of the thoracic and abdominal aorta of the adult. The Task Force for the Diagnosis and Treatment of Aortic Diseases of the European Society of Cardiology (ESC). Eur Heart J. 2014;35:2873–926. doi:10.1093/eurheartj/ehu281; Epub 2014 Aug 29.
66. Azizzadeh A, Keyhani K, Miller CC 3rd, et al. Blunt traumatic aortic injury: initial experience with endovascular repair. J Vasc Surg. 2009;49:1403–8. doi:10.1016/j.jvs.2009.02.234.
67. Lamarche Y, Berger FH, Nicolaou S, et al. Vancouver simplified grading system with computed tomographic angiography for blunt aortic injury. J Thorac Cardiovasc Surg. 2012;144:347–54, 354.e1. Doi: 10.1016/j.jtcvs.2011.10.011; Epub 2011 Nov 8.
68. Forcillo J, Philie M, Ojanguren A, et al. Outcomes of traumatic aortic injury in a primary open surgical approach paradigm. Trauma Mon. 2015;20:e18198. doi:10.5812/traumamon.18198; Epub 2015 May 25.
69. Starnes BW, Lundgren RS, Gunn M, et al. A new classification scheme for treating blunt aortic injury. J Vasc Surg. 2012;55:47–54. doi:10.1016/j.jvs.2011.07.073; Epub 2011 Nov 29.
70. Caffarelli AD, Mallidi HR, Maggio PM, et al. Early outcomes of deliberate nonoperative management for blunt thoracic aortic injury in trauma. J Thorac Cardiovasc Surg. 2010;140:598–605. doi:10.1016/j.jtcvs.2010.02.056; Epub 2010 Jun 25.
71. DuBose JJ, Leake SS, Brenner M, et al. Contemporary management and outcomes of blunt thoracic aortic injury: a multicenter retrospective study. J Trauma Acute Care Surg. 2015;78:360–9. doi:10.1097/TA.0000000000000521.
72. Razzouk AJ, Gundry SR, Wang N, et al. Repair of traumatic aortic rupture: a 25-year experience. Arch Surg. 2000;135:913–8; discussion 919.
73. von Oppell UO, Dunne TT, De Groot MK, Zilla P. Traumatic aortic rupture: twenty-year metaanalysis of mortality and risk of paraplegia. Ann Thorac Surg. 1994;58:585–93.
74. Parodi JC, Palmaz JC, Barone HD. Transfemoral intraluminal graft implantation for abdominal aortic aneurysms. Ann Vasc Surg. 1991;5:491–9. doi:10.1007/BF02015271.
75. Chandra V, Greenberg JI, Maggio P, et al. Aortic diameter varies in trauma patients: a function of hemodynamic status. J Vasc Surg. 2012;56:586–7. doi:10.1016/j.jvs.2012.05.042.
76. Jonker FH, Verhagen HJ, Mojibian H, et al. Aortic endograft sizing in trauma patients with hemodynamic instability. J Vasc Surg. 2010;52:39–44. doi:10.1016/j.jvs.2010.02.256; Epub 2010 May 23.
77. Oberhuber A, Erhard L, Orend KH, Sunder-Plassmann L. Ten years of endovascular treatment of traumatic aortic transection—a single center experience. Thorac Cardiovasc Surg. 2010;58:143–7. doi:10.1055/s-0029-1240779; Epub 2010 Apr 7.

78. Zipfel B, Chiesa R, Kahlberg A, et al. Endovascular repair of traumatic thoracic aortic injury: final results from the relay endovascular registry for thoracic disease. Ann Thorac Surg. 2014;97:774–80. doi:10.1016/j.athoracsur.2013.09.034; Epub 2013 Nov 22.
79. Tang GL, Tehrani HY, Usman A, et al. Reduced mortality, paraplegia, and stroke with stent graft repair of blunt aortic transections: a modern meta-analysis. J Vasc Surg. 2008;47:671–5. doi:10.1016/j.jvs.2007.08.031; Epub 2007 Nov 5.
80. Neschis DG, Moaine S, Gutta R, et al. Twenty consecutive cases of endograft repair of traumatic aortic disruption: lessons learned. J Vasc Surg. 2007;45:487–92. doi:10.1016/j.jvs.2006.11.038; Epub 2007 Jan 24.
81. Azizzadeh A, Ray HM, Dubose JJ, et al. Outcomes of endovascular repair for patients with blunt traumatic aortic injury. J Trauma Acute Care Surg. 2014;76:510–6. doi:10.1097/TA.0b013e3182aafe8c.
82. Khoynezhad A, Azizzadeh A, Donayre CE, et al. Results of a multicenter, prospective trial of thoracic endovascular aortic repair for blunt thoracic aortic injury (RESCUE trial). J Vasc Surg. 2013;57:899–905.e1. doi:10.1016/j.jvs.2012.10.099; Epub 2013 Feb 4.
83. Moainie SL, Neschis DG, Gammie JS, et al. Endovascular stenting for traumatic aortic injury: an emerging new standard of care. Ann Thorac Surg. 2008;85:1625–1629.; ; discussion 1629–1630. doi:10.1016/j.athoracsur.2008.01.094.
84. Geisbüsch P, Leszczynsky M, Kotelis D, et al. Open versus endovascular repair of acute aortic transections—a non-randomized single-center analysis. Langenbeck's Arch Surg. 2009;394:1101–7. doi:10.1007/s00423-009-0468-x; Epub 2009 Mar 3.
85. Idu MM, Reekers JA, Balm R, et al. Collapse of a stent-graft following treatment of a traumatic thoracic aortic rupture. J Endovasc Ther. 2005;12:503–7. doi:10.1583/04-1515R.1.
86. Brown KE, Eskandari MK, Matsumura JS, et al. Short and midterm results with minimally invasive endovascular repair of acute and chronic thoracic aortic pathology. J Vasc Surg. 2008;47:714–722. ; discussion 722–723. doi:10.1016/j.jvs.2007.12.003.
87. Orton DF, LeVeen RF, Saigh JA, et al. Aortic prosthetic graft infections: radiologic manifestations and implications for management. Radiographics. 2000;20:977–93. doi:10.1148/radiographics.20.4.g00jl12977.
88. White GH, Yu W, May J, et al. Endoleak as a complication of endoluminal grafting of abdominal aortic aneurysms: classification, incidence, diagnosis, and management. J Endovasc Surg. 1997;4:152–68. doi:10.1583/1074-6218(1997)004<0152:EAACOE>2.0.CO;2.
89. Nagpal P, Mullan BF, Sen I, et al. Advances in imaging and management trends of traumatic aortic injuries. Cardiovasc Intervent Radiol. 2017;40:643–54. doi:10.1007/s00270-017-1572-x; Epub 2017 Jan 11.
90. Akins CW, Buckley MJ, Daggett W, et al. Acute traumatic disruption of the thoracic aorta: a ten-year experience. Ann Thorac Surg. 1981;31:305–9.
91. Maggisano R, Nathens A, Alexandrova NA, et al. Traumatic rupture of the thoracic aorta: should one always operate immediately? Ann Vasc Surg. 1995;9:44–52. doi:10.1007/BF02015316.
92. Carter YM, Karmy-Jones R, Aldea GS. Delayed surgical management of a traumatic aortic arch injury. Ann Thorac Surg. 2002;73:294–6.
93. Holmes JH 4th, Bloch RD, Hall RA, et al. Natural history of traumatic rupture of the thoracic aorta managed nonoperatively: a longitudinal analysis. Ann Thorac Surg. 2002;73:1149–54.
94. Rabin J, Harris DG, Crews GA, et al. Early aortic repair worsens concurrent traumatic brain injury. Ann Thorac Surg. 2014;98:46–51. doi:10.1016/j.athoracsur.2014.04.025; discussion 51–52. Epub 2014 May 21.

Cardiac Trauma

10

Silvia Pradella, Marta Brandani, Giulia Grazzini, Mario Moroni, Manlio Acquafresca, and Vittorio Miele

10.1 Background

Patients victim of trauma with blunt cardiac injury (BCI) aren't uncommon even if the exact incidence is unknown. Subtler cases of BCI are often misdiagnosed, frequently overshadowed by concomitant consequences of the trauma, while severe injuries can cause the patient's death. Indeed, cardiac injury includes a spectrum of pathology ranging from clinically silent, transient arrhythmias to deadly cardiac wall rupture [1]. The cardiac contusion is the most frequent possibility and the management of that is still debated [2, 3]. Actually, in patients with traumatic injuries cardiac contusions might remain hidden.

However, laboratory data as troponin release have been observed far from the occurrence of the chest trauma [4]. After cardiac injury, arrhythmias, cardiac wall motion abnormalities, cardiac failure, cardiogenic shock, septum, papillary muscles or valves rupture can occur and great attention to these clinical signs should be paid to these patients [5, 6]. Due to their anterior position, right ventricle (RV) and right atrium (RA) are most frequently involved, whereas left-sided lesions are less frequent. On the contrary, lesion of septum, coronary arteries, and valve injuries rarely occur [7].

Pericardium or myocardium laceration and/or coronary artery or vein lesions frequently result in life-threatening hemopericardium and cardiac tamponade. The prompt diagnosis and treatment (pericardiocentesis and/or surgical repair of the lesion) are crucial.

Evaluation of trauma patients with suspected cardiac injury can be complex and include electrocardiography (ECG), measurement of cardiac biomarkers, and imaging examinations. ECG and cardiac biomarkers are useful screening tools for injury, while echocardiography is allowing to evaluate function and anatomic abnormalities.

The patient may not notice or be capable of reporting chest trauma. If the injury occurs in the hospital (e.g., perforation of a cardiac chamber by catheters) in a conscious patient, the individual often complains of severe chest discomfort.

The occurrence of hemopericardium, with or without clinical signs of hemodynamic impairment,

S. Pradella (✉) • M. Brandani • G. Grazzini
M. Moroni • M. Acquafresca • V. Miele
Department of Radiology, Careggi University Hospital, Florence, Italy
e-mail: pradella3@yahoo.it; marta86brandani@gmail.com; grazzini.giulia@gmail.com; elleci77@libero.it; manlioacquafresca@gmail.com; vmiele@sirm.org

V. Miele, M. Trinci (eds.), *Diagnostic Imaging in Polytrauma Patients*,
https://doi.org/10.1007/978-3-319-62054-1_10

could be the main sign of cardiac injury. The multislice spiral computed tomography (MSCT), with administration of intravenous iodinated contrast material, can detect a spectrum of complications related to the trauma [8]. The careful assessment of patients with cardiac trauma, with or without penetrating injuries, is a challenging and time-critical issue. Clinical data and imaging findings provide complementary information necessary for an accurate diagnosis, therapeutic planning, and prognosis also in hemodynamically stable patients. In addition to transthoracic and transesophageal echocardiography, chest radiography and computed tomography (CT), other available modalities such as nuclear medicine, and magnetic resonance imaging (MRI) may play a role in selected cases [9].

10.2 Definitions, Diagnosis, and Treatments

BCI historically refers to a broadly defined group of injuries typically occurring after a rapid deceleration or a direct blow to the chest. BCI has been associated with valvular or myocardial dysfunction leading to heart failure, dysrhythmias, free wall rupture causing pericardial effusion and tamponade, and, rarely, coronary artery damage leading to acute myocardial infarction (AMI).

Myocardial rupture, contusion, and laceration account for almost 90% of deaths secondary to non-penetrating cardiac trauma [1]. Penetrating cardiac trauma is characterized by high mortality rate and those who survive to hospital discharge still have an overall mortality approaching 80% [10]. Evaluation for cardiac trauma should be mandatory for patients with anterior chest wall injury.

10.2.1 Definition

BCIs, based on specific injuries, will be addressed:

Myocardial contusion, extremely variable in severity, is usually caused by blunt chest trauma (car or motorcycle accidents) or chest compression during cardiopulmonary resuscitation (CPR) maneuvers. Palpitations, arrhythmias, or unexplained tachycardia or hypotension may occur. Some patients develop conduction abnormalities. Normal troponin I or T assay in combination with an ECG are exclusion criteria for cardiac injury/damage and the patient can be safely discharged [11].

Cardiac camera ruptures are usually associated with quick death. Sometimes, in case of limited wall damage, such as in case of trauma involving the atrium, the junction with vena cava, or the right ventricle, the clinical presentation can be characterized by hemopericardium (Fig. 10.1). In these cases, a timely diagnosis is crucial. Both ultrasound and CT examination can provide useful information leading to emergent surgery.

Similar to the previous conditions, *valve injuries*, such as leaflet rupture, rapidly lead to a clinical

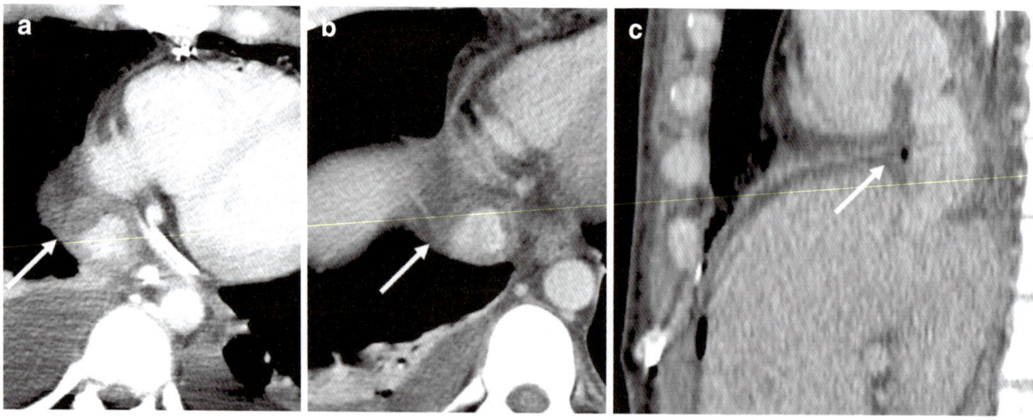

Fig. 10.1 Traumatic inferior cava disconnection. Contrast enhanced MSCT—post-surgical control after 1 day (**a**) and after 1 week (**b**, **c**). In (**a**) (*arrow*) is still present a hematoma; in (**b**, **c**) the hematoma decreased (*arrow*)

scenario of heart failure (rapidly evolving respiratory insufficiency due to pulmonary edema, pulmonary crackles, and hemodynamic instability) [12].

Septal rupture can cause delayed heart failure. It is important to understand if septal defect (SD) is a preexisting situation or it is caused by trauma. Acquired ventricular SD could be associated with a third heart sound, a loud systolic murmur, and signs of left or right ventricular failure. Finally, *commotio cordis* is characterized by sudden death following a blunt chest impact in patients without preexisting or traumatic structural heart diseases. Common situations of commotio cordis are those that occur during sport activities [13]. Although the pathophysiology is unclear, the temporal correlation between the trauma and the death keeps the ventricular fibrillation the most likelihood etiopathogenesis [13].

10.2.2 Diagnosis

In multiple trauma, the chest trauma is considered to cause up to 25% of the causes of death. Therefore, chest trauma should always be taken into serious consideration even in the absence of external signs or specific symptoms. The dynamics of the event is also important in the stratification of the risk of damage (impact on steering, airbags, etc.) [14]. Cardiac involvement should be suspected in patients with significant chest injury or polytrauma referring palpitations, ore suffering of arrhythmias, presenting new cardiac murmur, or unexplained tachycardia or hypotension. ECG ST segment might change by mimicking myocardial ischemia after cardiac trauma. The most common conduction abnormalities include atrial fibrillation, bundle branch block (mostly right), unexplained sinus tachycardia, and single or multiple ventricular ectopic beats. Cardiac biomarkers (i.e., troponin, CPK-MB) are useful tools for the screening of blunt cardiac injury. If cardiac biomarkers and ECG are within normal limits and there are no arrhythmias, blunt cardiac injury can be excluded. Rarely, chest trauma can cause a coronary artery damage causing myocardial infarction (Fig. 10.2). In addition, in approximately 20% of patients with penetrating lesions of the heart, and in patients with non-penetrating trauma, a delayed form of pericarditis, similar in character and natural history to those occurring after AMI, can occur [15]. In these cases, the medical history before chest trauma is of major importance in diagnosing the cardiac disease.

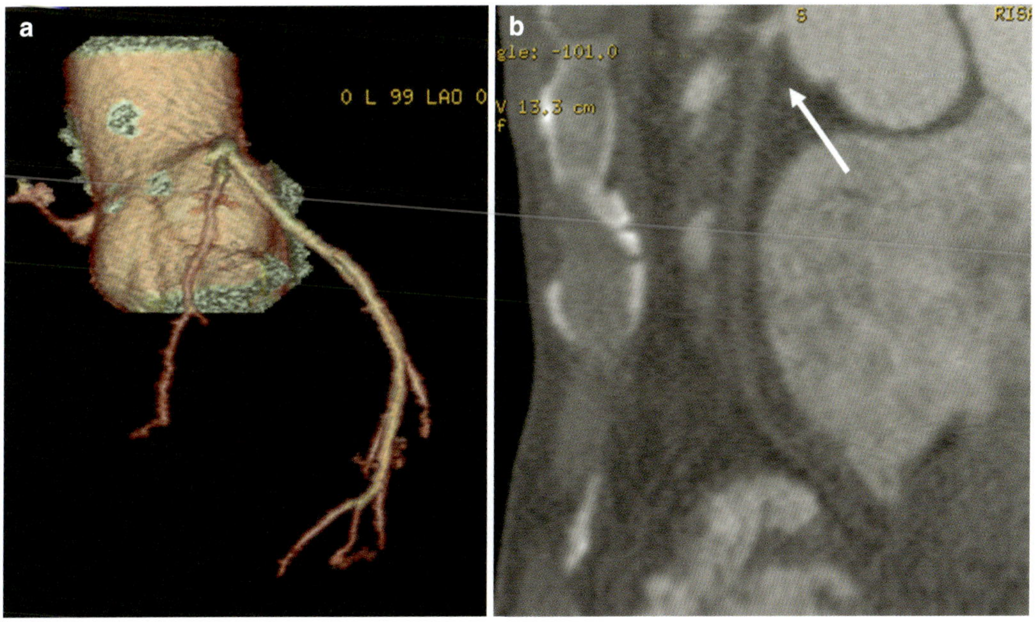

Fig. 10.2 Post-traumatic right coronary occlusion. (**a**) VRT reconstruction and (**b**) MIP reconstruction

Nuclear medicine. Until now, the role of nuclear medicine (including PET using 18F-2-fluoro-2-deoxy-D-glucose) has not well established in the setting of blunt thoracic trauma [16]. In selected cases, the same nuclear medicine techniques that are successfully used to diagnose myocardial ischemia have been attempted in evaluating trauma patients.

Angiography. Angiography, although not specifically indicated, can visualize or suspect some of the mechanical consequences of a chest trauma such as pericardial effusion, ventricular septal defects (VSDs), fistulae, and ventricular or aortic aneurysms [17].

Echocardiography. Ultrasound techniques, in the setting of trauma, has gained wide acceptance in the form of the Focused Assessment with Sonography for Trauma (FAST), in which echography is used to detect free fluid in the pericardium [16].

Echocardiography usually performed during the early phases of resuscitation can show wall motion abnormalities, pericardial fluid, or chamber or valvular rupture.

In addition, regurgitant valvular lesions, aortic-atrial or ventricular fistulae, and VSDs can produce left ventricular dilatation or hypercontractility at the echocardiographic examination. Valvular regurgitation and shunt flow can be detected and quantified by means of the Doppler evaluation. Myocardial contusion and MI result in regional hypokinesis or akinesis [2].

Chest X-ray (CXR): CXR continues to be an appropriate primary screening modality in thoracic trauma assessment, as noted in "ACR Appropriateness Criteria Blunt Chest Trauma" [16]. Antero-Posterior (AP) chest radiography is essential to quickly exclude rough displacement of lines and tubes that could be difficult to detect in the setting of polytrauma. Although AP chest radiographs are often of pore quality in case of polytrauma, they still are considered essentials. Signs include cardiomegaly secondary to hemopericardium or pericardial effusion; signs of left ventricular failure (vascular redistribution, interstitial or alveolar edema, pleural effusion) secondary to myocardial contusion, ventricular aneurysm, valvular disruption, intracardiac fistula, or VSD; and mediastinal widening secondary to aortic disruption and tracheal deviation. In addition, chest X-ray can easily investigate the occurrence of further findings, such as fractured ribs, hemo/pneumothorax, or pulmonary infiltrates in patients with trauma. However, it is widely known that AP chest radiography has lower accuracy for blunt traumatic injuries than CT and the use of this as the only diagnosis tool in trauma does not seem appropriate [16].

CT how and when. CT represents a gold standard modality in polytrauma. Contrast enhanced chest CT is known as a reliable modality for the investigation of thoracic trauma [16]. A cardiac injury can be present in patients with high kinetic energy trauma associated with sternum or rib fractures, lung contusions, pneumothorax, and vascular lesions. Although CT clearly allows detailed evaluations of trauma patients, the use of ionizing radiation have raised some safety concerns related to the extensive use of CT. In fact, ionizing radiation derived from medical use has increased, and the use of CT should be limited to the necessity [18]. There are conflicting data on whether routine chest CT is necessary in the setting of blunt trauma so far.

Depending on CT available apparatus, a collimation of 0.6 mm is recommended. The radiation dose should be kept as lower as possible, especially by applying dose reduction software wherever available. Nevertheless, the use of 120 KV and 300 mA is currently considered appropriate. Intravenous administration of contrast medium is imperative for imaging polytrauma patients. Usually, pre- and post-contrast imaging is performed in arterial phase (as not to miss any injury of the major vessels) and in venous phase. In case of suspected bleeding, a delayed acquisition at 5 min is highly recommended, taking into account patient's hemodynamic stability. Optimal opacification may be obtained with injection of 100–140 mL of iodinated contrast medium (preferable high concentration) at a flow rate of 3–4 mL/s followed by a saline flush injection. Importantly, pericardial effusion must be considered a red flag sign (Fig. 10.3). ECG gating for thoracic trauma is quite controversial as it provides a high diagnostic

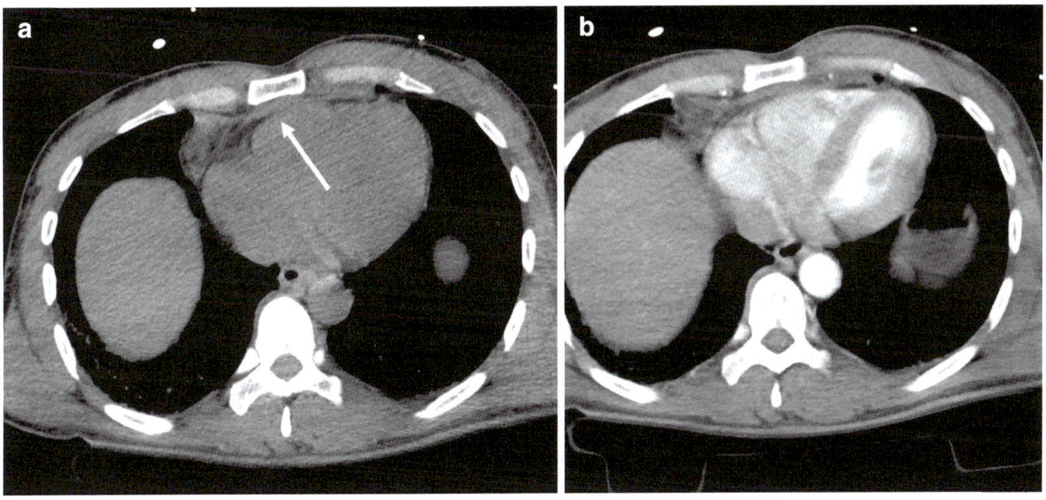

Fig. 10.3 (**a**) Non-contrast enhanced CT shows a hyperdense pericardial effusion; this must be a warning sign (*arrow*). The CT study may require the completion of a gated exam. (**b**) Contrast enhanced MSCT doesn't show any change in the pericardial effusion

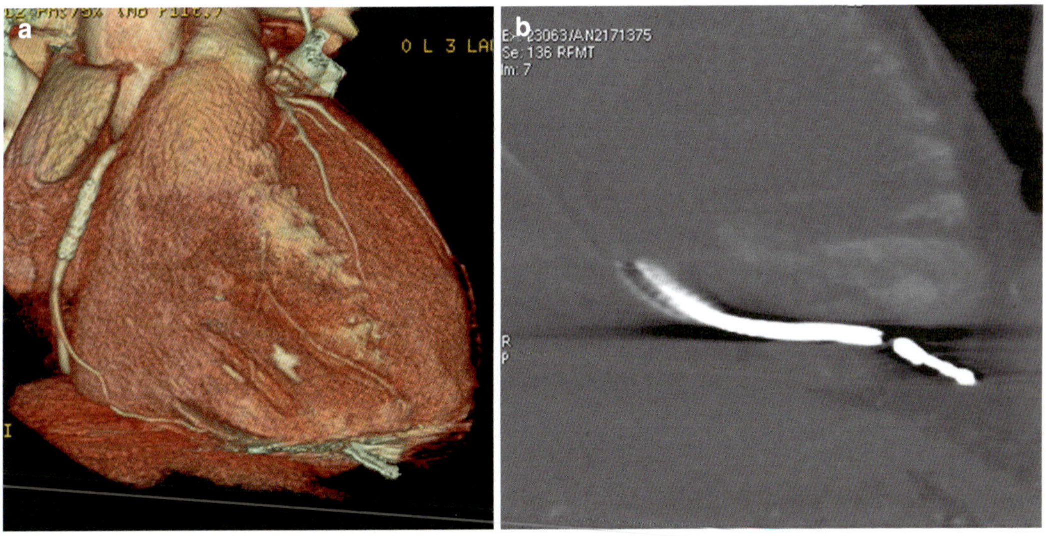

Fig. 10.4 Myocardial laceration caused by cardiac catheter. Gated cardiac CT acquisition. (**a**) VRT reconstruction shows the catheter end that goes beyond the myocardial wall. (**b**) MIP reconstruction

quality for vascular structures (aortic, coronary, or cardiac injury) but may reduce the quality of bone and lung injury. Given the fact that retrospective ECG gating compared with prospective ECG gating increases the radiation dose significantly, and that polytrauma patients may have an unstable heart rate higher than 80 beats/min, one should weigh the use of ECG gating carefully so as not to lose valuable time [14]. When a cardiac trauma or great vessels heart connection injury are suspected in stable patients, a gated CT examination could be useful after the initial CT as extending. A gated cardiac CT can be useful also in a suspect of iatrogenic cardiac trauma as post-surgery or vascular procedures (Fig. 10.4).

Post-mortem computed tomography is now an emerging method which is employed in forensic medicine before autopsy for "violent" death [19].

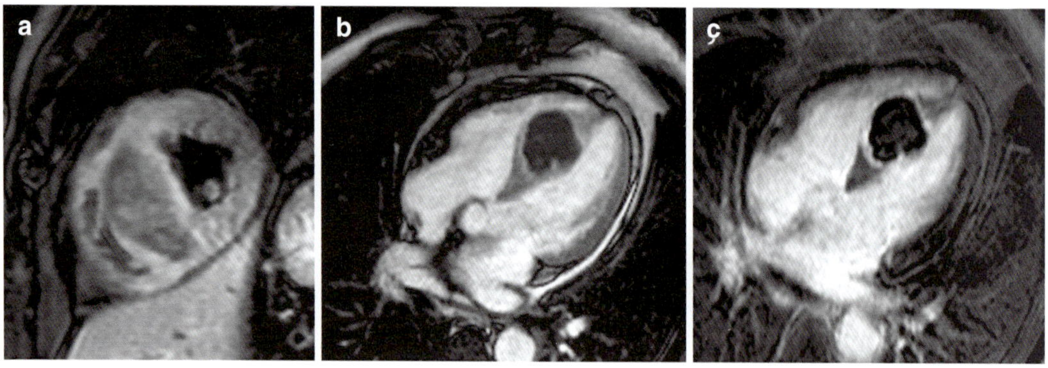

Fig. 10.5 Septal post-traumatic hematoma after cardiac catheterization. (**a**) T2w SPAIR short axis acquisition shows a septal thickening with the presence of focal well-circumscribed hypointense lesion. (**b**, **c**) Post-contrast cine bTFE and PSIR images show septal non-enhanced core

MRI: how and when. MRI is not widely used in the trauma setting since, differently to radiography, ultrasound, and CT, a rapid image acquisition is not possible with MRI. In addition, cardiac assessment is usually performed with breath-hold sequences which imply a cooperation frequently impossible in trauma patients.

Moreover, in emergency, the patient's past medical history, often unknown, could hide a dangerous contraindication to MRI examination. But, in conditions of clinical stability, MRI can be used to solve any residual doubt. The cine images can highlight areas of hypokinesia and also to assess the possible presence of myocardial or pericardial tearing. T1 w and T2 w sequences could underline the presence of pericardial effusion (and eventually blood content) as well as the presence of myocardial edema [16].

The assessment of perfusion and late gadolinium enhancement (LGE) may reveal ischemic injury or the presence of complications such as post-traumatic pericarditis.

Also, MRI in special cases helps to characterize possible injury as the presence of intramyocardial or pericardial hematoma (Fig. 10.5) [9].

10.2.3 Treatment

Patients with myocardial contusion causing conduction abnormalities require cardiac monitoring for 24 h due to the risk for sudden major arrhythmias. Treatment is mainly supportive (e.g., treatment of symptomatic arrhythmias or heart failure) and a further therapy is seldom needed. In severe injury, medical therapy (as volume loading) could be necessary awaiting surgical treatment. But, medical therapy could be enough, as in case of cardiac contusion, resembling that of non-Q wave myocardial infarction. Heart failure usually can be managed with conventional treatments, including vasodilators, diuretics, and inotropes.

In case of myocardial or valvular damages, surgical repair could be indicated, and in such cases, valve reconstruction is commonly successful. Fistulae and significant septal defects usually must be surgically repaired since spontaneous recover does not usually occur. Patients with commotio cordis are treated for their arrhythmias (e.g., resuscitation with CPR and defibrillation followed by in-hospital observation). Post-traumatic pericarditis treatments are similar to those that follow an infarction. Transient or permanent conduction disturbances may require temporary or permanent transvenous pacing. Laceration or rupture of a coronary vessel, a cardiac chamber, or the aorta requires urgent surgical repair. A coronary artery bypass could be necessary.

Key Points

- In case of chest trauma, the occurrence of palpitations, arrhythmias, new cardiac murmur, or unexplained tachycardia and/or hypotension could suggest blunt cardiac injury.

- ECG and cardiac biomarkers are useful tools for screening. Echocardiography is a simple and promptly available method to evaluate cardiac function and anatomic abnormalities.
- Chest radiography and chest CT or computed tomography angiography (CTA) are complementary first-line imaging modalities in the evaluation of patients with blunt trauma. Whether the combination of clinical conditions and mechanism of injury suggest a low probability of damage, a chest radiograph could be enough as first line of investigation.
- Transthoracic echocardiography is always indicated when cardiac injury is suspected.
- Cardiac CTA, cardiac MRI, and transesophageal echocardiography may be useful additional tools in selected cases

References

1. Saar S, Lomp A, Laos J, et al. Population-based autopsy study of traumatic fatalities. World J Surg. 2017;41(7):1790–5. doi:10.1007/s00268-017-3929-3.
2. Clancy K, Velopulos C, Bilaniuk JW, et al. Screening for blunt cardiac injury. J Trauma Acute Care Surg. 2012;73:S301–6. doi:10.1097/TA.0b013e318270193a.
3. Duke JC. Blunt Cardiac Trauma. Sci York. 2001:3–5.
4. Babuin L, Jaffe AS. Troponin: the biomarker of choice for the detection of cardiac injury. CMAJ. 2005;173:1191–202. doi:10.1503/cmaj/051291.
5. Smedira NG, Zikri M, Thomas JD, et al. Blunt traumatic rupture of a mitral papillary muscle head. Ann Thorac Surg. 1996;61:1526–8. doi:10.1016/0003-4975(95)01180-3.
6. Stahl RD, Liu JC, Walsh JF. Blunt cardiac trauma: Atrioventricular valve disruption and ventricular septal defect. Ann Thorac Surg. 1997;64:1466–8. doi:10.1016/S0003-4975(97)00843-6.
7. Ghoneim A, Bouhout I, El-Hamamsy I, et al. Traumatic transection of the posterior descending coronary artery. J Trauma Acute Care Surg. 2017;1:1. doi:10.1097/TA.0000000000001392.
8. Baxi AJ, Restrepo C, Mumbower A, et al. Cardiac injuries: a review of multidetector computed tomography findings. Trauma Mon. 2015;20(4):e19086. doi:10.5812/traumamon.19086.
9. Burrell AJ, Kaye DM, Fitzgerald MC, et al. Cardiac magnetic resonance imaging in suspected blunt cardiac injury: a prospective, pilot, cohort study. Injury. 2017;48(5):1013–9. doi:10.1016/j.injury.2017.02.025.
10. Connor JO, Ditillo M. Scalea T trauma reviews penetrating cardiac injury. J R Army Med Corps. 2009;155(3):185–90.
11. Sybrandy KC, Cramer MJM, Burgersdijk C. Diagnosing cardiac contusion: old wisdom and new insights. Heart. 2003;89:485–9. doi:10.1136/heart.89.5.485.
12. Singh H, Ali S, Luni FK, et al. Isolated rupture of bicuspid aortic valve following blunt chest trauma: a case report and systematic review of literature. Cardiovasc Diagn Ther. 2017;7:89–91. doi:10.21037/cdt.2016.05.03.
13. Rodríguez-González F, Martínez-Quintana E. Cardiogenic shock following blunt chest trauma. J Emerg Trauma Shock. 2010;3:398–400. doi:10.4103/0974-2700.70772.
14. Oikonomou A, Prassopoulos P. CT imaging of blunt chest trauma. Insights Imaging. 2011;2:281–95. doi:10.1007/s13244-011-0072-9.
15. Anderson EM, Jaroszewski DE, Arabia FA. Blunt trauma as a suspected cause of delayed constrictive pericarditis: a case report. J Med Case Rep. 2011;5:76. doi:10.1186/1752-1947-5-76.
16. Chung JH, Cox CW, Mohammed T-LH, et al. ACR appropriateness criteria blunt chest trauma. J Am Coll Radiol. 2014;11:345–51. doi:10.1016/j.jacr.2013.12.019.
17. Co SJ, Yong-Hing CJ, Galea-Soler S, et al. Role of imaging in penetrating and blunt traumatic injury to the heart. Radiographics. 2011;31:E101–15. doi:10.1148/rg.314095177.
18. Lin EC. Radiation risk from medical imaging. Mayo Clin Proc. 2010;85:1142–6. doi:10.4065/mcp.2010.0260.
19. Sifaoui I, Nedelcu C, Beltran G, et al. Evaluation of unenhanced post-mortem computed tomography to detect chest injuries in violent death. Diagn Interv Imaging. 2017. Doi:10.1016/j.diii.2016.08.019.

Traumatic Chest Wall Injuries

11

Michele Tonerini, Francesca Pancrazi, Silvia Lorenzi, Giulia Angelini, Giacomo Aringhieri, Piercarlo Rossi, and Giuseppe Zocco

11.1 Introduction

A chest wall injury can occur as the result of an accidental or a deliberate penetration of foreign objects into the chest. This type of injury can also result from blunt trauma causing rib bruises, fractures, lung or heart contusions.

Blunt chest wall injuries account for over 15% of all trauma admissions to emergency departments (ED) worldwide [1], with a mortality that ranges between 4 and 60%, depending on the grade of the trauma suffered [2].

The patients may present minor chest wall injuries, with rib fractures being the most common findings, (about 50% of cases); the overall incidence is probably higher because not all rib fractures are detected, in the acute phase, on chest X-ray (CXR). Other minor chest wall injuries include soft-tissue contusions and hematoma that might result from arterial or venous bleeding. A hematoma from a high-pressure arterial injury may enlarge rapidly requiring an intra-arterial embolization, whereas a bleeding from a low-pressure venous injury is usually self-limiting. Patients treated with anticoagulants are at higher risk for developing hemorrhagic complications even from minor trauma.

The pain is normally the only symptom referred to the clinician in the ED, and few risk factors have to be taken into account in the management of chest wall trauma patients: age, pre-existing disease, number of fractured ribs, and the onset of respiratory and vascular complications, 24–72 h after the trauma [2].

Major chest wall traumatic injuries include deep organs laceration and flail chest syndrome (seen in 6% of patients with rib fractures), an immediate life-threatening injury that require evaluation and treatment during the primary survey.

The AAST (American Association of the Surgery of Trauma) developed a scale, where site, extent of fractures, and concomitant soft-tissue injuries define the grade [3].

M. Tonerini (✉) • G. Zocco
Department of Emergency Surgery,
Cisanello University Hospital, Pisa, Italy
e-mail: m.tonerini@tiscali.it; g.zocco@med.unipi.it

F. Pancrazi • S. Lorenzi • G. Angelini • G. Aringhieri
P. Rossi
Department of Diagnostic and Interventional
Radiology, University of Pisa, Pisa, Italy
e-mail: pancrazi.francesca@gmail.com;
lorenzisilvia1@gmail.com; giu.angelini@gmail.com;
g.aringhieri@gmail.com; rossi-piercarlo@live.it

V. Miele, M. Trinci (eds.), *Diagnostic Imaging in Polytrauma Patients*,
https://doi.org/10.1007/978-3-319-62054-1_11

Trauma scoring might be considered evaluating the following:

Grade I	Contusion	Any size
	Laceration	Skin and subcutaneous tissue
	Fracture	<3 adjacent ribs
		Nondisplaced clavicle
Grade II	Laceration	Skin, subcutaneous, and muscle
	Fracture	>3 adjacent ribs
		Open or displaced clavicle
		Nondisplaced sternum
		Scapular body
Grade III	Laceration	Full thickness including pleura
	Fracture	Displaced or flail sternum
		Unilateral flail segment <3 ribs
Grade IV	Laceration	Avulsion of chest wall tissues with underlying rib fractures
	Fracture	Unilateral flail chest >3 ribs
Grade V	Fracture	Bilateral flail chest

More than two-thirds of cases of chest wall trauma are the result of a motor vehicle collision (MVC). Other causes include falls from height, sport injuries, motorcycle/bike accident, or of blows from blunt objects.

Imaging plays an important role in the diagnosis. CXR is typically used as the first and, in most cases, as the only diagnostic technique. Multidetector computed tomography (MDCT) must be performed in stable polytrauma patients or in doubtful cases at initial plain film study and has a very high sensibility and specificity; it can demonstrate significant disease in patients with negative initial CXR images, thus changing their clinical management [4].

11.2 Anatomy of the Chest Wall

11.2.1 Bones

The rib cage surrounds the thoracic cavity and supports the pectoral girdle (shoulder girdle, scapulae, and clavicles), enclosing the thoracic organs and with its muscle being a component of the human respiratory system.

In its normal shape, the human thoracic cage consists of 12 pair of ribs, the sternum, and the 12 thoracic vertebrae.

11.2.1.1 Ribs

About 1 in 200–500 people have an additional cervical rib, with female predominance. Bifid ribs (with the sternal end cleaved in two) occur in about 1.2% of the population. An extra cervical rib, from the seventh vertebra is also a common variant, which may mechanically interfere with the nerves (brachial plexus) going to the arm.

Ribs that articulate directly with the sternum are called true ribs (the first seven), whereas those that connect indirectly via cartilage are termed false ribs.

The last two pair of ribs are called floating rib, attached only to the vertebrae, not to the sternum.

Between the ribs there are the intercostal spaces, containing the intercostal muscles, nerves, arteries, and veins.

Each rib consists of a posterior head and neck, attached posteriorly to the thoracic vertebrae (the insertion point of the longissimus dorsi muscle), a body and a cartilaginous anterior part articulating with the sternum.

Ribs body has a flattened shape with a lateral convex face and a concave medial face, two margins: a smooth superior one and an inferior one, where there is a rut due to the passage of the intercostal nerves and vessels.

11.2.1.2 Thoracic Spine

Dorsal vertebrae, in number of 12, compose the middle segment of the vertebral column, between cervical and lumbar spine.

They are distinguished from the other ones by the presence on either side of the bodies of two semi-facets articulating with the ribs heads and the presence of complete facets on the transverse processes, except for the 11th and 12th one, joining them with the ribs tubercula.

Pedicles and laminae are broad, thick, and directed backward and slightly upward.

Spinous processes are long and triangular shaped, directed obliquely downward, arising from the lamina with a pointed end.

Superior and inferior articular processes arise at the junction between pedicles and laminae, articulating the vertebrae with the one below and above.

Posterior to the latter ones the transverse processes arise, directed obliquely backward and laterally.

11.2.1.3 Sternum

The sternum is a flat bone, forming the middle portion of the front of the thorax. It consists of three parts, from the top: manubrium, body, and xiphoid process.

The manubrium is the upper part of the sternum. It has a quadrangular shape, with a superior jugular notch, located in the middle part of the manubrium; its lateral surface presents two clavicle notches, articulating with the medial parts of the clavicles and the costal notches, articulating with the first pair of ribs.

The manubrium, in his lower part, articulates with the body of the sternum, with a synarthrosis, (the angle between the manubrium and the body is named angle of Louis) laterally at this point there is the attachment of the second pairs.

The sterno-pericardial ligament attaches the pericardium to the posterior side of the manubrium.

The body of the sternum, the longest part, is flat with a front and back surface. Laterally, there are the costal notches, articulating with the ribs.

The xiphoid process is located at the inferior end of the body of the sternum and might remain cartilaginous also in the elderly people.

11.2.1.4 Clavicle

Clavicle or collarbone is a long bone between the scapula and the sternum, with a body, a medial and a lateral end. Clavicle body is flat, forming a superior and posterior face with two margins; the superior and posterior face gives attachment to many muscles: deltoid, trapezius, subclavius, pectoralis major, sternocleidomastoid, and sterno-hyoid muscles.

11.2.1.5 Scapula

The scapula is a flat bone with a lower apex and a triangular shape, attached to the rear face of the rib cage, forming the shoulder skeleton, articulating with humerus at its lateral margin with the glenoid cavity.

It has an anterior and a posterior face, with three margins: a medial, a lateral, and an upper one. The anterior face is concave, with the attachment of the subscapular muscles.

The posterior one is divided into two parts due to a bone process, named spine, dividing it into a small supraspinous fossa and in the larger infraspinous fossa.

The spine becomes more prominent assuming a triangular shape, constituting the so-called acromion, articulated with the clavicle.

The superior margin has a bone process called coracoid process, giving attachment to ligaments and muscles (biceps and pectoralis minor muscle) [5].

11.2.2 Muscles

Chest muscles may be divided into intrinsic and extrinsic according to their origin and insertion entirely in the thorax. Intercostal, levatores costarum and transversus thoracis muscles are the only intrinsic chest muscles.

11.2.2.1 Intrinsic Muscles

Intercostal muscles are a group of three muscles, located between the ribs in order to reduce or increase the size of the rib cage during respiration. They are the external intercostal, internal intercostal, and the innermost intercostal muscles.

External intercostal muscles are obliquely oriented, from the lower edge of a rib to the upper part of the lower one and functioning to elevate the ribs as an inspiratory muscle. The internal intercostal muscles are oriented postero-inferiorly and functions to depress the ribs, as an expiratory muscle. The innermost intercostal muscles are a thin layer of fibers oriented similarly to those of the internal intercostal, separated from them by the intercostal neurovascular bundles.

The intercostal blood supply is derived from the posterior intercostal branches of the aorta and the anterior intercostal branches of the internal thoracic artery.

Other intrinsic muscles are the levatores costarum muscles: they are 12 in number on either side, with a triangular shape, lateral to the spine, originating from the transverse processes of the vertebrae ending on the upper edge of the rib below, with the role of helping in inspiration.

Another intrinsic muscle is the transversus thoracic muscle that is a flat muscle, originating from the body and the xiphoid process of the sternum, ending on the cartilaginous part of the ribs from the second to the sixth, helping in expiration.

11.2.2.2 Extrinsic Muscles

Extrinsic muscles include thoracoappendicular, spinoappendicular, spinocostal muscles, and the diaphragm.

The pectoralis major is a fan-shaped muscle, originating from the medial clavicle, the anterolateral surface of the sternum, the costal cartilages (from second to sixth ribs) and inferiorly from rectus muscle fibers and the aponeurosis of the external oblique muscle; inserting on the lateral lip of the bicipital groove of the humerus. Its actions are to flex, adduct, and rotate the arm medially.

The pectoralis minor muscle is located deep to the pectoralis major and mainly acts as an inspiratory muscle, also stabilizing the scapula. It originates from the outer face and the posterior margin of the third, fourth, and fifth ribs, near the costal cartilages. Its fibers are obliquely oriented superiorly and converge at the apex of the coracoid process of the scapula.

The serratus anterior is located on the side of the chest wall; this muscle is embedded in the vertebral border of the scapula and originates from the first ten ribs. It is usually divided, given its size, in three parts depending on where the fibers originates from the ribs and where they fit exactly in the shoulder bone. This muscle mainly acts abducting and externally rotating the scapula as well as make it adhere to the chest (the latter action coupled to the rhomboids and trapezius muscles). It lowers the shoulder blades with his lower beams, raises them with the upper beams. If taken as a fixed point elevates the coasts participating in the forced inspiration (inspiratory accessory muscle) [6].

11.3 Mechanisms of Injury

Four main mechanisms of injury are responsible for chest wall injury: direct chest impact, thoracic compression, rapid acceleration/deceleration, and blast injury.

Direct impact injuries are normally less risky, affecting mainly only the soft tissues and muscles of the chest wall (hematomas, bruises, cuts, and scratches). On occasion, a localized injury to the osseous part may occur, mainly rib fractures, but also sternal fracture and sternoclavicular dislocation. Rarely direct impact forces may be transmitted through the chest wall to the deeper organs, causing serious injury to the heart, lung, or large mediastinal vessels.

In the thoracic compression injuries, the chest wall is put against a fixed anatomical bone structure, anteriorly the ribs or sternum and posteriorly the vertebrae causing deep organs laceration, contusion, or rupture. Thoracic compression may cause contusion or laceration of lung parenchyma, pneumothorax or hemothorax, tracheobronchial fractures as well as rupture of the diaphragm.

In acceleration/deceleration injuries, the production of shearing forces causes direct compression against fixed points. This type is the most common and potentially lethal injury, may causing major tracheobronchial disruption, cardiac contusions, aortic, and diaphragmatic rupture [7].

Blast injuries are increasing recently, resulting from the sudden conversion of a solid or liquid material into gas after activation of explosive material. A primary blast injury results from the creation of a blast pressure wave, applying pressure differentials, mostly at air-tissue interfaces within the chest wall, affecting mainly the pulmonary and gastrointestinal systems.

Secondary blast injuries result from objects driven by the explosion impacting the individual and creating a chest wall injury. Tertiary blast injuries might also be indirect, due to the blown out of the individual subject to the explosion [8, 9].

11.4 Anterior Rib Fractures, First Rib and Lateral Rib Fractures

11.4.1 Pattern of Injury

Rib fractures are the most common injury after blunt chest trauma which occurs in approximately 50% of patients. It is important to consider the specific location of rib fractures because this is an important indicator of related injury. Rib fractures can be studied as three distinct patterns according to their location: (1) fractures of the first rib and those of the second to fourth ribs, (2) fractures of the fifth to ninth ribs, and (3) fractures of the 10th to 12th ribs. These three distinct patterns of rib fractures represent different pathophysiology and associated morbidity. A rib score has been proposed to predict adverse pulmonary outcomes [10].

A high-energy trauma is necessary to result in fracture of the first, second, or third ribs because these ribs are well protected by the scapulae, clavicles, and musculature. The presence of this fracture should prompt the evaluation of vascular thoracic injuries, brachial plexus injury, or subclavian vascular injuries [11].

Isolated first rib fractures are seen in association with cranial and maxillofacial injuries and are probably secondary to avulsion of the first rib by its muscular attachment rather than direct trauma to the rib, which is relatively protected.

Fractures of the fourth up to the eighth ribs are the most common [12].

The compression of the rib cage with associated fracture of the 10th, 11th, or 12th rib might cause internal abdominal organs injuries, of course fractures of the right lower ribs are more often associated with hepatic injury, fractures of the left lower ribs with splenic injury, and fractures of the posterior portion of the lower ribs with renal injury.

Injury to the liver might result in tearing, intraparenchymal or subcapsular hematoma, active bleeding, or there might be injury of major liver vessels. Injury of the spleen or kidney might result in subcapsular hematoma or abdominal rupture in greater force impact. Even hemorrhage around and within the adrenal glands represents a risk that is associated with fractures of the lower ribs.

Fracture of any rib can be associated with pneumothorax, hemothorax, or extrapleural hematomas. Although lung trauma is generally seen immediately, the occurrence of a pneumothorax and hemothorax may be delayed for hours after the injury. Hemothorax of a significant degree secondary to rib fractures is usually the result of laceration of an intercostal artery rather than bleeding from the lung. It is important in the evaluation of rib fractures to check in particular the lower sulcus of the ribs where the intercostal arteries are located; fractures that involve the sulcus are more prone to hematomas and the hemothorax resulting from a laceration of an intercostal artery can be life threatening.

The risk of intra-abdominal or intrathoracic injury increases if two or more rib fractures are present at the same level [13–15]. These injuries should always be ruled out by MDCT [16].

Elderly individuals are prone to rib fractures because of decreased rib cage compliance; limited respiratory movement may cause an increased prevalence of atelectasis and subsequent pneumonia which lead to pulmonary insufficiency, even from single rib fractures, that may increase morbidity and mortality [11, 17].

A study showed that in elderly people more than three rib fractures may indicate the need to transfer to a trauma center, and the more ribs broken, the greater the death rate [18].

In contrast, children's bones are immature and more compliant, due to the greater pliability of children's ribs, greater force is required to produce a fracture and rib fractures in this group of patients are indicative of high-energy transfer trauma [4, 9].

Anyway in elderly and not elderly people, knowing the number of ribs fractured might influence treatment decisions and might change morbidity and mortality.

A single blow may cause rib fractures in multiple places. At the level of the rib cage, the typical pattern of fractures varies depending on the site of compression: if the compression comes

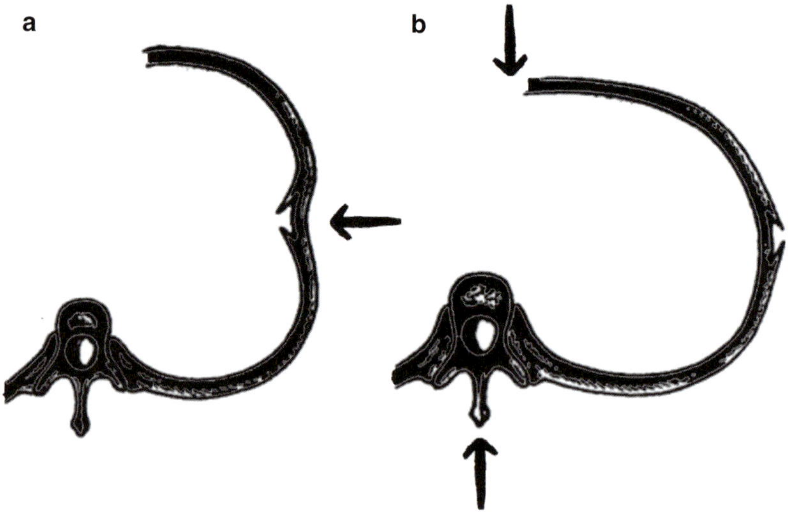

Fig. 11.1 Chest trauma: different mechanisms of injury secondary to different axial load force (*arrows*). (**a**) Lateral impact. (**b**) Anterior-posterior impact

from the front we usually observe sternal compression fractures and antero-lateral rib fractures; if the compression comes from the back we usually observe posterior rib fractures; if a lateral force occurs, we usually observe posterior fractures and detachment from the costochondral cartilage or anterior fractures.

If the compression is anterior and posterior, lateral rib fractures occur on the lateral cortical margins; if the force is laterally direct to the ribs, internal cortical rib fracture might occur (Fig. 11.1).

Traumatic fractures most often occur at the site of impact or the posterolateral bend, where the rib is the weakest. Both displaced and nondisplaced fractures can be seen in adults and children.

Fractures might be anterior; there might be lateral fracture with rib cage deformation and posterior fractures occasionally involving the costovertebral joint; it is important to note that buckle fractures are easy to overlook even at CT and additional coronal image scan be helpful in the diagnosis of rib fractures that are not seen on axial images [19, 20].

11.4.2 Imaging Evaluation and Findings

11.4.2.1 Plain Radiography

A standard CXR is almost always the initial study for the evaluation of non-traumatic chest pain and for traumatic injuries. If rib fractures are suspected clinically, a rib plain film series might be performed; this radiograph consists of oblique views and optimization of the X-ray parameters by the technologist to highlight bony detail. The decision to image a rib fracture in the absence of other underlying abnormalities or associated injuries depends on the clinical scenario.

Even in the absence of associated injuries, radiographic confirmation of a rib fracture can help prevent complications such as atelectasis and is particularly important in patients with comorbidities such as chronic obstructive pulmonary disease, cardiac disease, hepatic disease, renal disease, dementia, and coagulopathy.

Despite its routinary use, CXR, even with dedicated oblique rib series, has limited sensitivity, showing only 40–50% of rib fractures [21, 22].

11.4.2.2 MDCT

MDCT is the study of choice to fully evaluate trauma-associated injuries and bony details; it is the most sensitive technique for imaging rib fractures since it can help determine the site and number of fractures. It is however relatively costly, time-consuming, not always 24 h available, and exposes the patient to a significant amount of radiation [21].

With the help of reconstructed maximum intensity projections (MIP) and volume-rendered (VR) images, MDCT depicts with great detail the number and sites of rib fractures [12].

MDCT angiography plays a crucial role in the evaluation of the vascular injuries associated with chest trauma and should be considered in stable patients with first rib fractures if there are absent or decreased upper extremity pulses, if regional hemorrhage, and/or brachial plexus injury are present. Additional criteria for angiographic MDCT include displacement of bone fragments and multiple thoracic injuries.

11.4.2.3 US

Ultrasonography (US) can be used to look for broken ribs and costal cartilage fractures, in cases in which they occur in an accessible thoracic point, especially in pediatric population and in young women. Unfortunately, US is unable to adequately assess certain portions of the thorax such as the first rib under the clavicle, and the upper ribs under the scapula.

Other limitations include subcutaneous emphysema and the pain at the site of the transducer compression, making it difficult in traumatized patients; and its results depend greatly on the skill of the performer [23]. Even if with these limitations, US might demonstrate cortical discontinuity, linear edge shadow (Fig. 11.2), and acoustic reverberation artifacts in accessible points and associated injuries such as pneumothorax and hemothorax; abdominal organ injuries might be evaluated too.

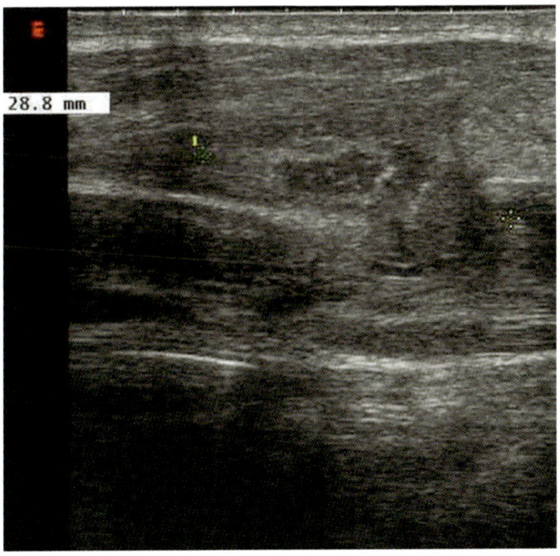

Fig. 11.2 US imaging showing interruption of cortical margins and a 2.9 cm hematoma after chest wall trauma (calipers)

Studies have found it to be much more sensitive than plain radiography in detecting rib fractures, whereas other studies have suggested that it is only equally sensitive or slightly better, but it should be underlined that US is not as panoramic as plain radiography and MDCT.

11.4.2.4 MRI

Magnetic resonance imaging (MRI) has not yet a role in rib fracture evaluation and is not considered appropriate for evaluating rib fractures, due to the fact that it is time-consuming and not easily available in trauma centers. However, it may be useful if there is concern about soft-tissue or vascular abnormalities [21].

11.4.3 Natural History and Mortality

Pain from rib fractures can be severe for several days following the injury and even if most of them heal within 6 weeks, many patients are able to resume daily activities much sooner. Follow-up CXR after the injury are not routinely recommended and should be performed only if indicated by clinical findings or if in complicated cases [24]. Clinical signs of worrisome might be unilateral decreased breath sounds suggesting pneumothorax or persistent pain suggesting difficult consolidation or nonunion. A follow-up examination 6–8 weeks after the injury is reasonable to assess the patients, if they are unable to return to sports or work by that time.

The number of displaced rib fractures and fracture location could be a significant predictor for developing pulmonary and other organs complications. For patients with fewer than three rib fractures without rib displacement and initial lung or other organ injuries, conservative management could be safe and efficient [25].

As the number of rib fractures increases, morbidity and mortality grows substantially in all age groups owing to major risk of complications such as pneumothorax, pneumonia, and acute respiratory distress syndrome (ARDS).

Other associated injuries such as concomitant great vessel injury might happen in 3% of traumatic injuries to the first rib that affect prognostic outcome. Pneumothorax occurs in about 14–35% of rib fractures, hemopneumothorax in 20–25%, pulmonary contusions in 17%, and a flail chest in 5.8%.

Chest wall injuries in older people should not be dismissed. Older patients have twice the morbidity and mortality compared with younger people; for every increase in the number of ribs fractured, mortality increases by 19% while the risk of pneumonia increases by 27%.

11.4.4 Treatment

Simple rib fractures themselves are usually not significant in isolation and are treated symptomatically. They have a good prognostic outcome and are rarely life threatening [12].

Virtually, all non-pathologic rib fractures heal well with conservative management. Some patients are able to return to work within a few days, depending on their occupation. One small case series suggests that some patients experience prolonged pain and disability [26]. It found that patients with an isolated rib fracture regain pain-free function at a mean of 51 days.

11.5 Costochondral Injuries

Costochondral injuries refer to the fracture at the joints between each rib and its costal cartilage. They are primary cartilaginous joints and represent the demarcation of the unossified and ossified part of the rib. There is no movement at these joints. Costal cartilages form part of the thoracic cage and anterior chest wall. There are ten costal cartilages, one for rib 1–10, each of which forms a costochondral joint. Costal cartilages 1–7 articulate with the sternum at sternocostal joints, and costal cartilages 8–10 are attached to each other via small interchondral synovial joints forming the costal margin.

11.5.1 Patterns of Injury

Costal cartilage fractures are rare lesions, which may be located at the chondrocostal or chondrosternal junction.

While in adult patient pain is the primary complaint, in young children, a costal cartilage fracture may present as a thoracic wall mass associated with pain.

Costochondral injuries might occur in three locations: costochondral, midchondral, and sternochondral. Disruptions or fractures of costal cartilage might result in an unstable rib cage and may expose thoracic contents, such as the heart, to injury.

While the more fixed first and second rib seems to be easily subjected to costochondral separation, the lower ribs can suffer costal cartilage fracturing more frequently.

11.5.2 Imaging Evaluation and Findings

11.5.2.1 Plain Radiography

Fractures of the costal cartilages are challenging to establish on physical examination and on plain radiographs, where they are easily overlooked. However, when there is severe calcification of the cartilage, a traumatic interruption might be displayed at this level [27, 28].

CXR is indicated to show associated findings such as pneumothorax, hemothorax, pulmonary contusion, and subcutaneous emphysema.

11.5.2.2 MDCT

MDCT is the gold standard technique to represent costal cartilage fractures and eventually associated injuries such as thoracic wall hematoma, pneumothorax, subcutaneous emphysema, hemothorax, and pulmonary contusions [21, 29].

11.5.2.3 US

US is a reliable method to diagnose costal cartilage fractures and can increase the sensitivity of their detection when used together with MDCT scanning. US is preferable in a pediatric population, in young or pregnant women and for follow-up examinations [30].

In pediatric population, US examination might be useful when costal cartilage fracture presents as a chest wall mass associated with pain to exclude neoplasm or post-traumatic hematoma.

Furthermore, it is suggested an US examination when there is a high clinical suspicion and other modalities have not demonstrated an injury.

Sonographic signs of a cartilage damage include a fracture line, disruption of the anterior echogenic margin, a step-off deformity or gas located at the costochondral junction [27, 31].

Pitfalls in US examination include false fractures that might be produced when the probe overlies the rib and partly the intercostal space. Also costal cartilage calcifications, running parallel to the rib margin, at the costochondral junction, may give rise to the false identification of a fracture due to normal sharp indentation (less likely in pediatric population) [32].

11.5.2.4 MRI

MRI can easily demonstrate costal cartilage fractures and, like US, doesn't result in radiation exposure.

Costal cartilage injuries are detected on MRI due to the high T2 signal from the surrounding edema, and they are often more easily detectable than on MDCT. Even in cases of remote injury, persistent high T2 signal at the site of fracture might be seen, presumably due to nonunion in persistent clinical symptoms.

When costochondral injury is suspected, a fat-saturated T2-weighted or STIR sequence in the coronal view are recommended [33].

11.5.3 Natural History and Mortality

Costochondral fractures slightly increases mortality rate as they may determine rib cage instability and flail chest, impairing respiratory function [34].

11.5.4 Treatment

These injuries are usually treated like the osseous rib fractures, typically with nonsurgical management involving ice, nonsteroidal anti-inflammatory medications and taping of the ipsilateral chest wall or use of a rib belt; in addition, athletes are restricted from sport for 3 weeks or longer [33, 35, 36].

However when returning to sports, especially contact sports at risk for direct trauma (e.g., hockey, rugby), a protective padding may be used to allow for further healing while reducing the risk of any repeated injury.

11.6 Flail Chest

A flail chest deformity may be a severe consequence of multiple rib fractures. It occurs when three or more contiguous ribs are fractured in two site, or five or more contiguous ribs are fractured in one site with or without associated sternal fractures [37].

With regard to injury mechanism, such trauma may be caused by MVC, falls, and assaults in younger, healthy patients.

The initial diagnosis of flail chest is performed with physical examination, when paradoxical or reverse motion of a chest wall segment is detected while spontaneously breathing. This pattern of injury gives the rib cage an unstable dynamic of motion because a segment can act as a flail segment. The movements of this segment are opposite to the expected in the dynamic of the rib cage motion: in inspiration the unstable segment of the rib cage is attracted towards the pleura and in expiration it goes away from it. In this pattern of fracture in a non-ventilated patient, this segment of the rib cage movement is contrary to the expected and is called paradoxical. The segment of the chest wall that is flail is unable to contribute to lung expansion. This abnormal movement hinders the creation of negative intrathoracic pressure during inspiration and positive airway pressure during expiration.

The force that is needed to produce a flail chest varies on the structure on which it impacts, if the structural components (i.e., the ribs) are weakened for any reason (i.e., osteoporosis, total sternotomy, and multiple myeloma, as well as individuals with congenital absence of the sternum), then much lower force may be required. Mechanically, however flail chest generally requires a significant traumatic energy diffused over a large area (i.e., the thorax) to create multiple anterior and posterior rib fractures.

The motion of the flail segment is usually limited by the surrounding structural components, the intercostalis, and the surrounding musculature. This mechanical limitation of motion affects the actual size of the changes in thoracic volume and patient-generated tidal volume. Underlying pulmonary or cardiac disease determines the physiologic perturbations to respiration caused by the flail segment.

Although the diagnosis of flail chest is initially clinical, it always requires radiological studies including CXR and MDCT.

11.6.1 Patterns of Injury

The chest wall is inherently stable, with 12 ribs attaching posteriorly to the spinal column and anteriorly to the sternum. Intercostal muscles with fascial attachments, coupled with other muscle groups, including the trapezius and the serratus groups, add further strength to the bony cage around the thoracic organs.

Borrelly and Aazami [38] reported that contraction of the serratus anterior muscle digitations pulls the flail segment posteriorly and superiorly. Canine flail chest experiments have also shown that the degree of inward inspiratory displacement is related to force differences between intrapleural pressure and parasternal muscle activity [39].

Frontal and lateral impact may result in multiple anterior and posterior rib fracture points. Severe anterior compressive forces may cause sternochondral disruption and a subsequent sternal flail.

Flail chest can be subdivided into anterior and posterior flail chest depending on the presence of fractures along the anterior or posterior rib angles, respectively [40]. Flail segment might include the sternum with ribs on both sides of the thoracic cage fractured.

The rib cage is a flexible ring-like structure; the arch design of the ribs allows some flexing in trauma. The rib cage is less compliant in adults rather than in children and in the latter can absorb small amounts of blunt kinetic energy. Consequently, flail chest in children is observed with lower frequency, rather than injury to the underlying structures. Contrary in an adult, a transfer of significant kinetic energy in blunt trauma to the rib cage or a crushing rollover injury is the most frequent cause of flail chest.

11.6.2 Imaging Evaluation and Findings

Patients with flail chest, resulting from a high-energy trauma, need to be considered at risk for severe associated injuries such as massive pulmonary contusion or laceration, pneumothorax with subcutaneous emphysema, hemothorax (which are the major contributors to respiratory insufficiency) and vertebral fractures.

11.6.2.1 Plain Radiography

CXR is the first examination performed in case of acute chest trauma and the strict definition of three ribs broken in two or more places, or more than five contiguous ribs injured can be confirmed eventually by means of specific ribs plain films too. The inherent structural stability of the chest wall due to the ribs and intercostal muscles usually does not show abnormal or paradoxical motion without three or more ribs involved.

11.6.2.2 MDCT

CXR is less sensitive than MDCT for the diagnosis of flail segments, and thoracic MDCT is routinary performed in case of severe trauma with paradoxical chest movements to exclude associated complications, such as pulmonary contusions, usually subjacent to the point of impact or on the counterpoint; lung laceration frequently masked by the surrounding pulmonary contusion; pneumothorax that is very common, but might be not clearly evident on supine CXR; hemothorax; pneumomediastinum; subcutaneous emphysema; mediastinal hemorrhage; and major vascular injuries (Figs. 11.3, 11.4, 11.5, 11.6, 11.7, and 11.8).

11.6.3 Natural History and Mortality

The incidence of flail segments is 10–15% in major thoracic trauma and might be associated with cranial, thoracic, and abdominal injuries.

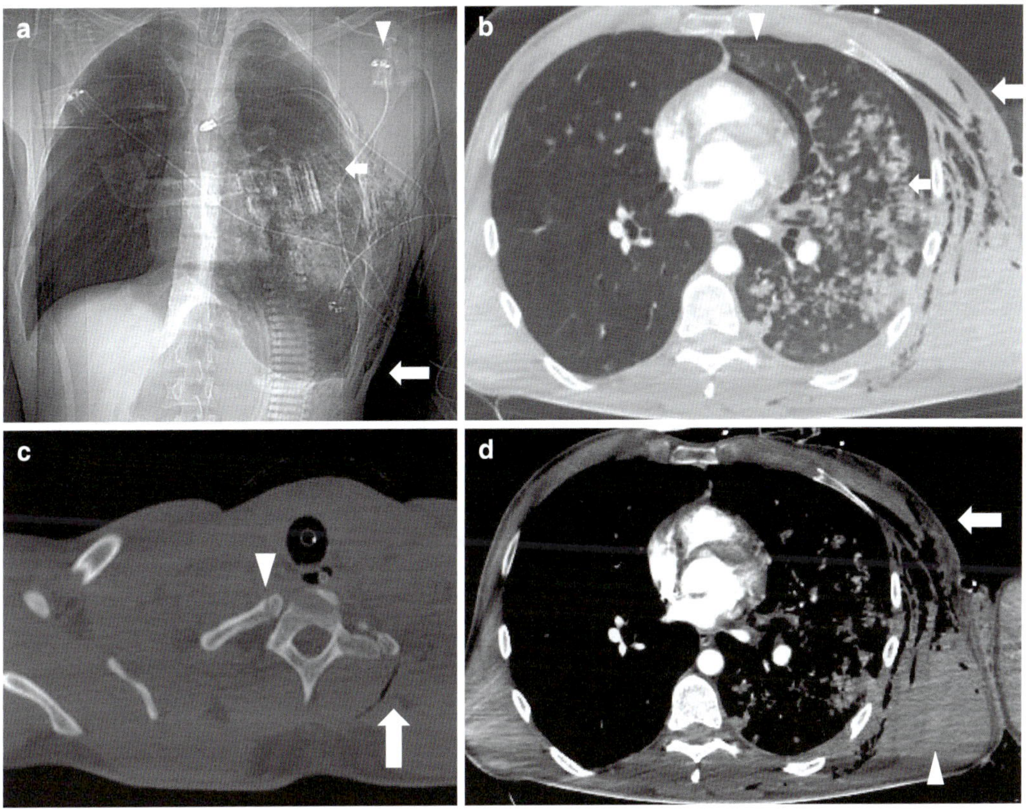

Fig. 11.3 CT scout of a patient underwent to a severe chest trauma after MVA, showing subcutaneous emphysema (*long arrow* in **a**, arrow in **b**) of the left thoracic wall, lung contusions (*short arrow* in **a** and in **b**). Left scapular fracture (*arrowhead* in **a**). Not dislocated fracture of the proximal part of the first right rib of the same patient (*arrowhead* in **c**). Subcutaneous emphysema in the left neck (*arrow* in **c**). Chest wall hematoma without active bleeding (*arrowhead* in **d**)

Early mechanical ventilatory assistance is provided to patients with severe concomitant injuries. The paradoxical movements of the flail segment disappears after intubation with positive pressure ventilation.

Patients may demonstrate only the paradoxical chest wall motion, with minimal respiratory insufficiency, although they usually show some tachypnea with a notable decrease in resting tidal volume due to painful fractures. The impairment of respiratory function is typically related to the underlying lung injury and loss of negative intrathoracic pressure, rather than the chest wall abnormality. It can cause the development of atelectasis and adult respiratory distress syndrome secondary to impaired pulmonary drainage, with progressive hypoxemia, elevated airway pressures, and a progressive infiltrate in the affected lung [41].

Flail chest can lead to severe respiratory failure and requires prompt intensive respiratory ventilation, sometimes also for prolonged periods in more than 50% of cases [12, 37].

Flail chest has a reported mortality rate between 10 and 15% that is primarily caused by associated injuries.

The mortality rate of patients with severe associated injuries may be decreased from 50% to 6% if mechanical ventilation is instituted within 24 h of injury; on the opposite, the mortality rate can exceed 90%, however, when there is hypotension and hypoxia for a period of more than 24 h [40].

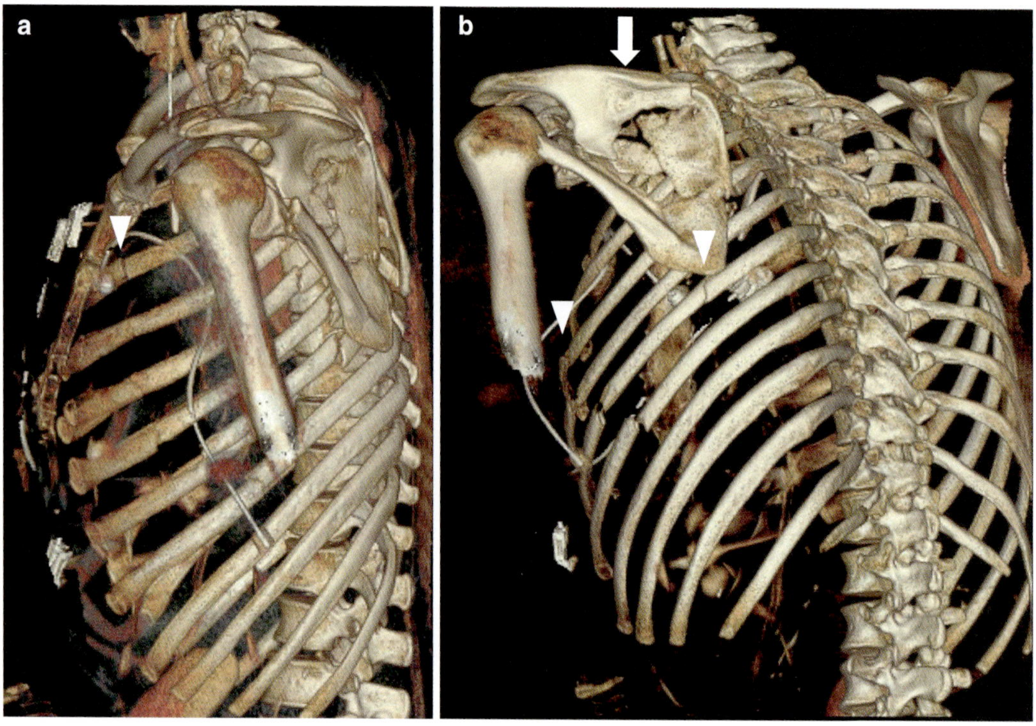

Fig. 11.4 3D reconstruction (**a**. Left lateral view; **b**. Left posterolateral view) of a patient underwent to a severe chest trauma, after a MVA, showing flail chest with fractures, in two points, from the second to seventh rib (*arrowheads*). Left scapular fracture (*arrow*). Chest, endotracheal, and nasogastric tube placement

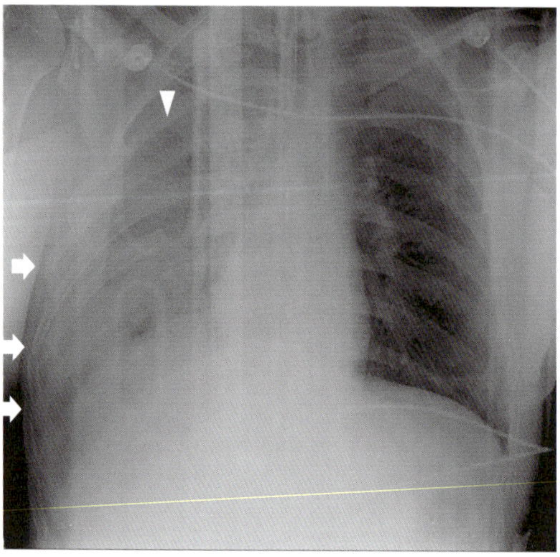

Fig. 11.5 Chest X-ray performed in shock room in supine position on the spinal board, in a patient who underwent a severe chest trauma after a MVA, showing subcutaneous emphysema of the right chest wall, multiple rib fractures (*arrows*), lung contusions (*arrowhead*). Endotracheal tube placement

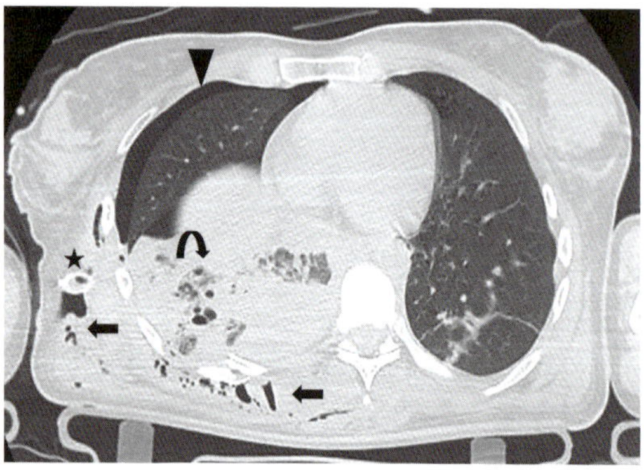

Fig. 11.6 CT axial imaging of the same patient showing subcutaneous emphysema (*arrow*) of the right chest wall, lung contusions (*curved arrow*). Right pneumothorax (*black arrowhead*). Chest tube placement (*star*)

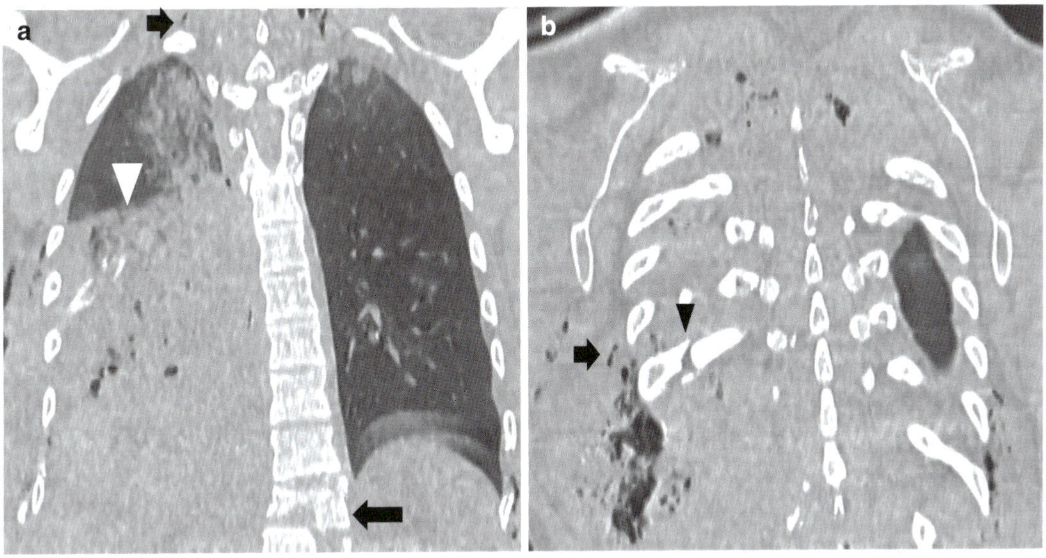

Fig. 11.7 MPR images (**a**, **b**) of the same patient showing lung contusions and subcutaneous emphysema (*black arrow* in **b**) of the right chest wall and lower portion of the neck (*short black arrow* in **a**). Multiple rib fractures (*arrowhead* in **b**) and T12 vertebral fracture (*long black arrow* in **a**)

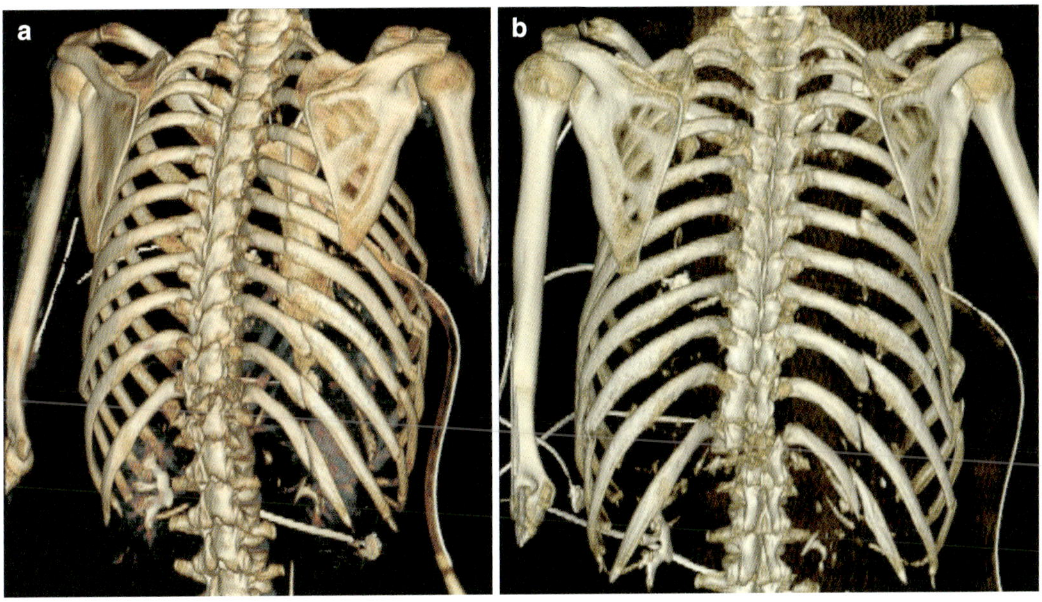

Fig. 11.8 3D reconstruction (**a**. Right posterolateral view; **b**. Posterior view) of the same patient showing flail chest with fractures from the seventh to twelfth rib. Chest drainage, endotracheal tube, venous catheter placement

Prolonged mechanical ventilation and pulmonary contusion are associated with the development of pneumonia and a poor outcome.

11.6.4 Treatment

Flail chest is usually managed supportively, with adequate analgesia and chest physiotherapy to assist volume expansion and secretion management, and to prevent secondary complications of atelectasis and pneumonia. Adequate analgesia is of paramount importance and may contribute to the return of normal respiratory mechanics.

Chest tube insertion might be necessary in case of complications such as hemo- or pneumothorax.

Posterior flail segments are easier to manage clinically because of the presence of strong muscular and scapular support and because of a patient's natural tendency to lie with his or her back against the mattress.

The surgical management has traditionally been reserved for the following indications: flail chest who require thoracotomy for other intrathoracic injuries, severe chest wall instability, persistent pain secondary to fracture malunion, and persistent or progressive loss of pulmonary function [40]. Surgical stabilization can effectively reduce the duration of mechanical ventilatory support and facilitating a shorter intensive care unit (ICU) stay and quicker recovery. The long-term benefits include restoration of normal chest wall geometry and improved pulmonary function testing.

Open fixation is also indicated for flail chest when thoracotomy is performed for other concomitant injuries. Rarely, severe rib injuries (e.g., flail chest) may be treated with open reduction internal fixation (ORIF), often in the setting of other severe traumatic injuries and in the hope that respiratory function will improve [12].

11.7 Sternal Fractures, Sterno-chondral Injuries, and Sternoclavicular Dislocation

11.7.1 Sternal Fractures

Sternal fractures usually occur in patients who involved in high-speed motor vehicle collision, with an incidence of 8–10%. Their importance lies in the high frequency of associated injuries such as fractured ribs, pulmonary and cardiac trauma, cranio-cerebral injuries, thoracic and lumbar spinal fractures, whiplash, and lower-extremity injuries [42].

Sternal fractures have associated mediastinal injuries in more than 50% of cases and a mortality of 22% due to cardiac and great vessel lesions.

11.7.1.1 Patterns of Injury

Fractures may occur in any segment of the sternum but most commonly affect the upper third of the sternal body and the manubrium. In 18% of cases, fractures occur at the manubriosternal joint. The fractures of the manubrium, rather than the ones at the sternal body, require higher force [43, 44].

The degree of displacement is proportional to the energy of the impact and, thus, to the likelihood of concomitant injuries.

The most common mechanism of sternal injuries is a direct impact between the sternum and the steering wheel or seat belt or air bag as a result of sudden deceleration. These injuries are more common in front-seat and/or restrained passengers and in frontal collisions.

Fractures may be displaced or undisplaced: an isolated undisplaced sternal fracture is considered a benign entity not associated with appreciable morbidity [45].

On the contrary, a sternal fracture with displacement or multisystemic trauma may alert the clinician to search for possible associated serious injury. In these cases, displaced fragments are often associated with soft-tissue and cardiothoracic damage due to the posterior shift of the lower fragment. The manubrial fractures may be associated with aortic and brachiocephalic vessel injuries, while the depressed sternal body fractures may determine myocardial injuries in 1.5–6% of patients. A general rule is: the more displaced the fracture, the higher the association with additional chest injuries.

Clinically, sternal fractures can be detected by inspection and palpation of the chest wall, but usually the diagnosis relies on imaging.

11.7.1.2 Imaging Evaluation and Findings

Plain Radiography

Frontal CXR detects only sternal fractures with lateral displacement and may be useful in detecting concomitant injuries (rib fractures, pulmonary contusions, hemothorax/pneumothorax). The presence of widened mediastinum, usually reflects a mediastinal hematoma; however, a hematoma due to a sternal fracture may be indistinguishable from one that is secondary to an acute aortic injury [46].

The essential radiographic projection required to establish the diagnosis of sternal injury is the lateral projection. Although lateral CXR is the best view to depict sternal fractures with sensitivity of 70%, it is hard to be obtained in the acute trauma setting and furthermore, it cannot show the associated thoracic injuries [22, 47].

US

Chest US may demonstrate sternal fractures as a focal discontinuity, or stepping of the anterior cortex, sometimes associated with a localized presternal hematoma, pericardial effusion, cardiac wall motion abnormalities, or hemopneumothorax [48]. US pitfalls are determined by its inaccuracy for the evaluation of the degree of fracture displacement and misdiagnosis in case of incomplete sternal fusion in children and in case of subcutaneous emphysema [49].

MDCT

In multitrauma patients, chest US and X-rays are replaced by MDCT examination because it identifies not only all sternal fractures and dislocations but also internal thoracic injuries and retrosternal hematomas. Moreover, multiplanar reconstructions (MPR) allow to visualize horizontal fracture lines [37], which may be missed on the axial scans (Fig. 11.9).

Electrocardiography (ECG), echocardiography, serial enzyme analysis, and telemetry monitoring are useful to show pericardial effusion or other signs of myocardial injury in case of depressed, displaced sternal fractures. In 40% of

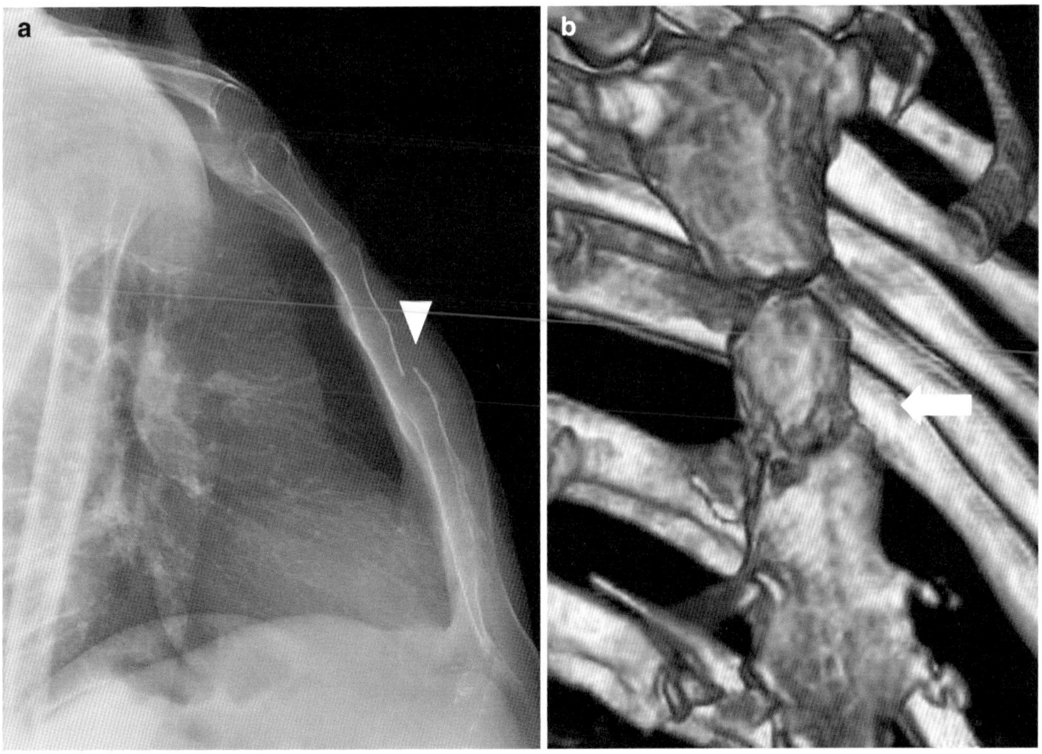

Fig. 11.9 Lateral X-ray projection of the sternum (**a**) showing a fracture in the upper third of its body (*arrowhead*) confirmed in 3D reconstruction of MDCT (**b**) (*arrow*)

cases, there are also compression fractures of the upper thoracic spine and more rarely of the cervical and lumbar spine. Clinically, there is violent chest pain, tenderness, bruising, and a stair-step sometimes palpable at the fracture line [44].

11.7.1.3 Natural History and Mortality

The isolated sternal fractures have a very good outcome in patients without abnormality in the ECG and no underlying chest pathology, with conservative management; most healing in a few months with a very low mortality rate (<1%).

The sternal fractures associated with other injuries have a higher mortality rate, ranging from 25–45%. Two-thirds of displaced or unstable sternal fractures have concomitant injuries which can be subdivided into three categories:

- soft-tissue injuries
- injuries to the chest wall
- injuries to the spine, extremities, and skull

Chest wall injuries include rib fractures, flail chest, and sternoclavicular dislocation. Pneumothorax, hemothorax, cardiac tamponade, and pulmonary contusions, as well as injuries to the abdomen and diaphragm are common soft-tissue injuries. Thoracic spine compression fractures, as well as trauma to the head, neck, and extremities are also common [50, 51].

The complications following sternal fractures may include short-term sequelae, such as chest pain post-injury and long-term problems such as nonunion and painful pseudarthrosis that may require surgical correction.

11.7.1.4 Treatment

Satisfactory pain control is usually achieved with oral analgesics as well as codeine and non-steroidal anti-inflammatory drugs (NSAIDs), in case of noncomplicated sternal fractures. Otherwise, the treatment of the underlying complication is necessary.

11.7.2 Sternochondral Injuries

There are few published papers on sternochondral injuries as they are often misdiagnosed.

11.7.2.1 Patterns of Injury

Most reported cases are in young males as the result of blunt trauma or a fall in sports, and they are represented by fractures and dislocations. The sternochondral dislocations are encountered especially in children and, when multiple, they produce an anterior flail chest. The most frequently reported site of injury is the sternochondral junction of first or second rib; in particular, Subhas et al. reported a characteristic pattern of injury at the sternochondral junction of the first rib, in which a small triangular chondral fragment remains attached to the sternum [29, 33].

11.7.2.2 Imaging Evaluation and Findings

Plain Radiography

The clinical presentation of sternochondral injuries may be identical to that of rib fractures, but cartilage injuries are not detectable with CXR, unless considerable costal calcification is present, so these injuries are usually overlooked on plain films.

US

US have been reported as effective in revealing sternochondral fractures [29].

On sonographic examination, the cartilages appear hypoechoic than the adjacent muscle and are delineated by a thin echogenic anterior margin. US has the advantage of an easy multiplanar scanning, the lack of ionizing radiations, and the opportunity of a bedside examination.

MDCT

Axial and MPR images from thin MDCT slices demonstrate focal interruption in the relatively high sternochondral density. Moreover, MDCT shows displacement of the adjacent segments and adjacent soft-tissue swelling [44], allowing to detect a hematoma with or without an active bleeding (Fig. 11.10).

MRI

MRI, with its intrinsic soft-tissue contrast and the ability to evaluate cartilage elsewhere in the musculoskeletal system, is very suitable for the evaluation of sternochondral junction; however, this approach has received low attention in literature, with only a single published series by Subhas et al. [33].

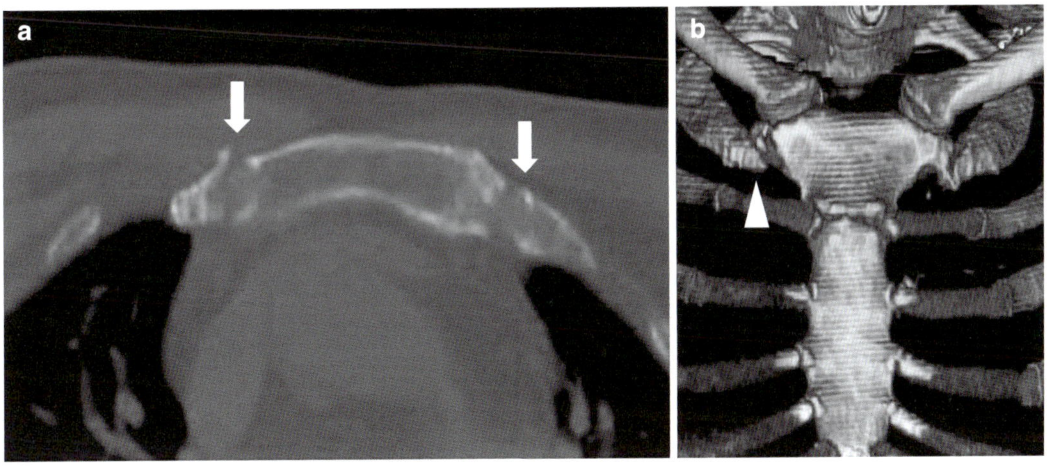

Fig. 11.10 Axial CT image (**a**) and 3D reconstruction (**b**) of a fracture of the first sternochondral joint (*arrows* in **a**) with right dislocation (*white arrowheads* in **b**)

11.7.2.3 Natural History and Mortality

Fracture or subluxation of the sternochondral joints is very common in wrestlers and mixed martial arts artists as a result of leverage and twisting again resistance. Symptoms are dyspnea, chest pain, worsening with deep breaths or arm movements, and tenderness (touching the joint area makes the pain worse). The outcome of these injuries is very good if they are isolated, while the presence of associated lesions (such as myocardial contusion, aortic rupture, pneumothorax, and hemothorax) worsens prognosis.

11.7.2.4 Treatment

Pain relief is the most common treatment. Oxygen terapy is used in response to possible hypoxemia and to decrease workload on the myocardium; cardiac monitoring is employed to treat eventual cardiac arrhythmias due to trauma. Pain management is used during the initial setting; the later rehabilitation allows healing and deep breathing, in order to prevent atelectasis, pneumonia, and other lung expansion complications.

In conclusion, these injuries are managed nonsurgically like osseous rib fractures.

11.7.3 Sternoclavicular Dislocation

The sternoclavicular dislocation are rare; they represent only 2–3% of shoulder dislocations, usually result from blunt or sport trauma and are distinguished in anterior or posterior.

11.7.3.1 Patterns of Injury

The anterior dislocations usually result from an anterior blow to the shoulder. They are more common than posterior ones and typically less dangerous because there is no significant risk of great vessel injury.

The posterior (or retrosternal) displacement results from a posterior blow to the shoulder or a blow to the medial clavicle; in particular, the most common mechanism is a massive direct trauma to the anterior chest wall, driving the medial end of the clavicle posteriorly or posterolaterally. It is frequently associated with life-threatening complications caused by the compression of vital structures such as the trachea, great vessels, and nerves [52].

Posterior dislocations at the left sternoclavicular joint are particularly dangerous considering the contiguity with the left subclavian vessels [53].

11.7.3.2 Imaging Evaluation and Findings

Even if all these fractures/dislocation can be detected by inspection and palpation of the chest wall, usually the diagnosis relies on imaging studies.

Plain Radiography

Standard view of a CXR may not provide a definitive diagnosis, but an abnormal position of the clavicle may arouse suspicion about the presence of sternoclavicular joint dislocation. Alternative views such as "*serendipity view*" (40° cephalic tilt) may provide more information.

MDCT

MDCT gives a detailed depiction of the sternoclavicular joint [46] and helps distinguish dislocation as either anterior or posterior and to assess an eventual vascular compromise (Figs. 11.11 and 11.12).

11.7.3.3 Natural History and Mortality

Clinically, they may present with pain, tenderness, a large hematoma and ecchymosis of the upper anterior chest wall, and a palpable or visible abnormality of the injured joint.

The main symptom of anterior dislocation is the deformity with palpable bump while in posterior dislocations there are dyspnea, dysphagia, tachypnea, and stridor, worsening in supine position. At physical examination, there is a prominence that increases with arm abduction and paresthesias increasing in elevation of the affected upper extremity; also venous congestion or diminished pulse when compared with contralateral side might be present [54, 55].

Many complications have been reported in the literature related to retrosternal dislocation of the medial end of the clavicle including subclavian compression and laceration, mediastinal com-

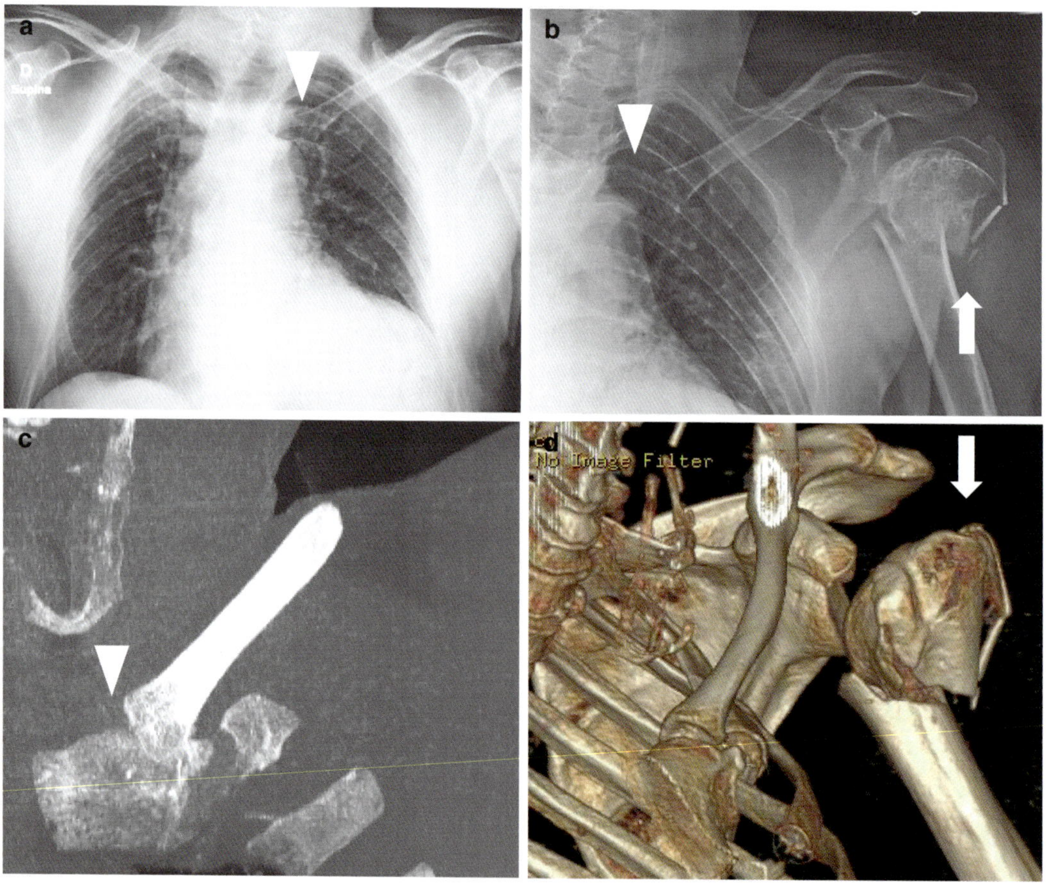

Fig. 11.11 Chest X-rays showing posterior dislocation of the left clavicle (*arrowhead* in **a**). Shoulder X-plain film of the same patient demonstrating subluxation of the left sternoclavicular joint (*arrowhead* in **b**) and left humeral head comminuted fracture (*arrow* in **b**). MIP (**c**) and 3D reconstruction of left shoulder at MDCT (**d**) confirms the left sternoclavicular subluxation (*arrowhead* in **c**) and the comminuted fracture of the left humeral head (*arrow* in **d**)

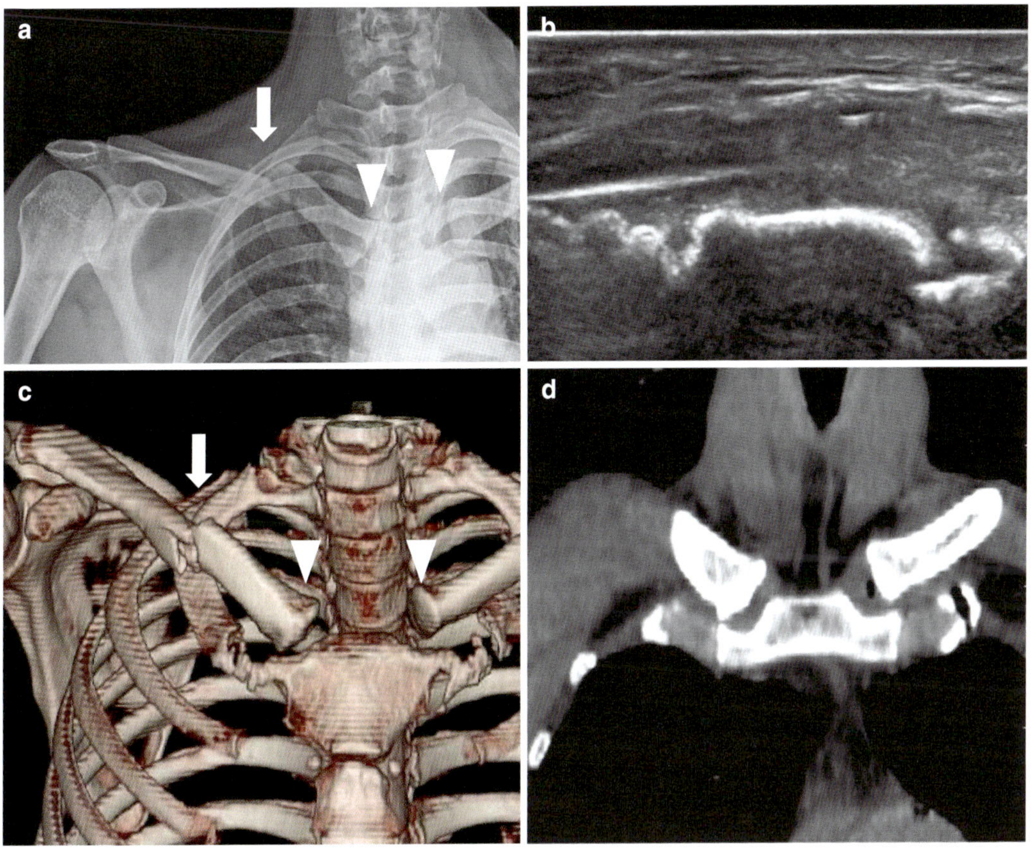

Fig. 11.12 (**a**) Chest X-rays showing a fracture of the medial third of the right clavicle (*arrow*) with a sternoclavicular subluxation (*arrowheads*) in a polytrauma patient; (**b**) US of the same patient demonstrates subluxation of the sternoclavicular joint; (**c**) 3D reconstruction confirming the right sternoclavicular subluxation (*arrowhead*) and clavicular fracture (*arrow*); (**d**) coronal MPR image of the bilateral sternoclavicular dislocations

pression, pneumothorax, esophageal rupture, and tracheal tear [56].

Anterior dislocations typically have a more benign course and conservative treatments are usually justified. However, they may result in chronic pain, ankylosis, and deformity.

11.7.3.4 Treatment

It consists of conservative therapy with ice, analgesia, and shoulder sling for immobility leading usually to complete recovery in about 1 week. Subluxation of the sternoclavicular joint will require the application of a clavicular splint or sling for 3–6 weeks.

Different therapies will be requested if the dislocation is associated to other chest wall or internal thoracic structures injuries.

11.8 Costovertebral Dislocation

The costovertebral articulations permit the respiratory movements of the ribs and consist of two gliding type of synovial joints, the costocentral joint (between the head of the rib and the lateral portion of the vertebral body) and the costotransverse articulation (between the tubercle of the rib and the tip of the transverse process).

In costovertebral joints, the head of a rib has two facets separated by a ridge which articulate with two vertebra, in particular the lower rib facet articulates with the upper costal facet of its own vertebra and the upper facet articulates with the lower facet of the vertebral body above.

The first rib articulates with the T1 vertebra only and the lowest three ribs articulate only with their own vertebral body [57].

The costovertebral joints are stabilized by articular capsules, the radiate ligaments, and the intra-articular ligaments (where they exist), the latest binding the medial ends of the ribs to the intervertebral disks.

The first, tenth, eleventh, and twelfth costocentral joints have no intra-articular ligament, so they have only one synovial compartment.

The costotransverse joints consist the tubercle of a rib articulating with the transverse process. The tubercle has two facets, the medial and the lateral articulating, respectively, with the tip of the transverse process (forming a plane synovial joint, reinforced by a capsule) and with the transverse process through three ligaments—lateral costotransverse, costotranverse, and superior costotransverse. Superior costotransverse ligament attaches the superior border of the neck of the rib to the transverse process, immediately above. The first rib has no superior costotransverse ligament [58]. All ribs have a feeble posterior costotransverse ligament which attaches the neck of the rib to the base of the transverse process and lateral border of the inferior articular process of the vertebra immediately above [59].

The lower two floating ribs are only attached by ligaments and do not form costotransverse joints.

11.8.1 Pattern of Injury

When subjected to severe trauma, these joints may be subluxated or dislocated. The costotransverse joint is the more likely of the two to be injured. The first costotransverse joint is especially vulnerable because of its unique position at the top of the rib cage [59].

The predominant mechanism of injury is a blunt trauma such as motor vehicle collision, sports, fall, and gunshot. Significant associated injuries include fracture dislocation of the spine and of the sternum. Symptoms include pain, swelling, deformity, altered motility, anesthesia, or paresthesia up to paraplegia (especially with a fracture of the spine associated).

11.8.2 Imaging Evaluation and Findings

11.8.2.1 Plain Radiography

CXR is the first radiological examination performed in case of suspected costovertebral dislocation but it is not the best because these displacements can be subtle, especially when CXR is performed with portable devices on the spinal board, as in multitrauma patients. On AP view, the more significant finding is an asymmetric rib interspace narrowing above and widening below the level of injury.

11.8.2.2 MDCT

The effect on ligamentous disruption and/or fracture may be assessed with axial MDCT images.

An important anatomic reference on MDCT axial images is the position of the head of the rib that is located at the level of the intervertebral disk enabling to evaluate this structure and the number the vertebral level as well. MDCT findings include the displacement of the costal head from the pedicle and the transverse process with its associated rib displaced out of view usually anteriorly (naked transverse process) [57].

11.8.3 Natural History and Mortality

Because these costovertebral articulations provide the contact points of the rib cage, disruption could impede the thoracic spine's ability to resist normal physiologic loads; particularly when it is involved the first costovertebral joint, associated with massive trauma to other part of the body, including the thorax, head, and abdomen [59]. The most common associated injuries are pneumothorax, hemothorax, pulmonary contusion, and flail chest. Local injuries more directly related to the first costovertebral fracture/dislocation include trauma of the brachial plexus, Horner's syndrome, and tear of the subclavian artery.

The outcome of these injuries depends on associated fractures and on the presence of neurologic impairment.

11.8.4 Treatment

Treatment ranges from strapping or bandaging of the chest and immobilization in uncomplicated cases up to surgical reduction in severe cases [60].

11.9 Scapulo-Thoracic Dissociation

The scapulo-thoracic dissociation (STD) is defined as the lateral displacement of the scapula from the thoracic cage after severe scapular girdle trauma [61], which leads to the disruption of the attachments of the shoulder girdle to the trunk, either by acromioclavicular or sternoclavicular dislocation or a fracture of the clavicle [62].

Closed rupture of the subclavian or axillary vessels, paralysis of the brachial plexus, and complete or partial avulsion of the shoulder muscles might be associated [63]. First described by Oreck et al. in 1984, STD is a rare situation and only a few other similar cases have been reported. It has different variants, from the absence of neurovascular injury [64] to bilateral involvement [65].

11.9.1 Patterns of Injury

STD is related to high-energy trauma, and it is usually caused by a lateral traction injury to the shoulder girdle. Approximately half of the cases is related to motorcycle accidents. Less frequently, other injury mechanisms are reported: motor vehicle crashes, rollover accidents, pedestrian accidents, and falls from heights [66]. The traction force disrupts the muscular tissues and the acromioclavicular ligaments/sternoclavicular ligaments making the neurovascular tissues vulnerable to injury [67].

Significant cardiac, chest wall and pulmonary injuries might be associated, while the skin is usually intact.

The concomitant lesions might be:

- arterial (88% [68]), such as subclavian or, less frequently, axillary artery ruptures
- osteo-articular, such as scapula or clavicle fractures, acromioclavicular dislocation/separation, sternoclavicular dislocation, or flail extremity (complete loss of motor and sensory function)
- neurologic, such as complete or, less frequently, partial brachial plexus paralysis with root avulsion or trunk rupture, or phrenic nerve injury with diaphragmatic paralysis

11.9.2 Imaging Evaluation and Findings

In STD, the first imaging procedure required is CXR in anterior-posterior projection; lateral view of the chest and shoulder plain film is recommended. STD diagnosis should be considered in patients with major trauma, with neurovascular upper limb deficit and if on CXR the ratio of distances between affected and the non-affected sides is 1.5 centimeters or greater (measured between the spine and the medial border of scapula) [66]. Widely displaced clavicle fracture, acromioclavicular separation, and sternoclavicular dislocation are usually related findings. If the diagnosis is uncertain, additional trans-scapular or oblique views of the affected scapula as well as MDCT scan are recommended [67].

MDCT angiography is indicated to detect injury of subclavian and axillary artery and is recommended in hemodynamically stable patient before surgery.

Bone and joints injuries must be reported on X-ray examinations, but the diagnosis is frequently missed [69], because of the presence of other severe associated injuries and the limited quality of radiographs performed in shock room (Figs. 11.12, 11.13, 11.14, and 11.15).

In the case of brachial paralysis, an MRI must be used to assess the nervous damage. This is essentially a preoperative assessment for the possibility of repair by nerve graft from an intact root [70].

11.9.3 Natural History and Mortality

The typical clinical presentation of STD is a swollen shoulder containing a large hematoma and extending to the thoracic wall; absent distal

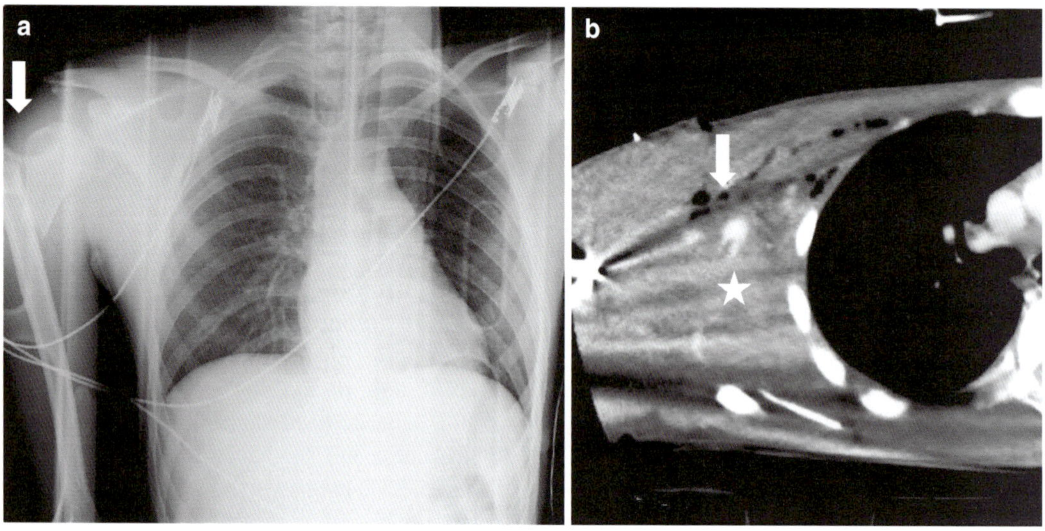

Fig. 11.13 Chest X-rays after MVA in a 14-year-old patient showing humeral shaft fracture with medial dislocation of the humeral head (*arrow* in **a**). Intraluminal axillary artery thrombosis (*star* in **b**) and subcutaneous emphysema (*arrow* in **b**)

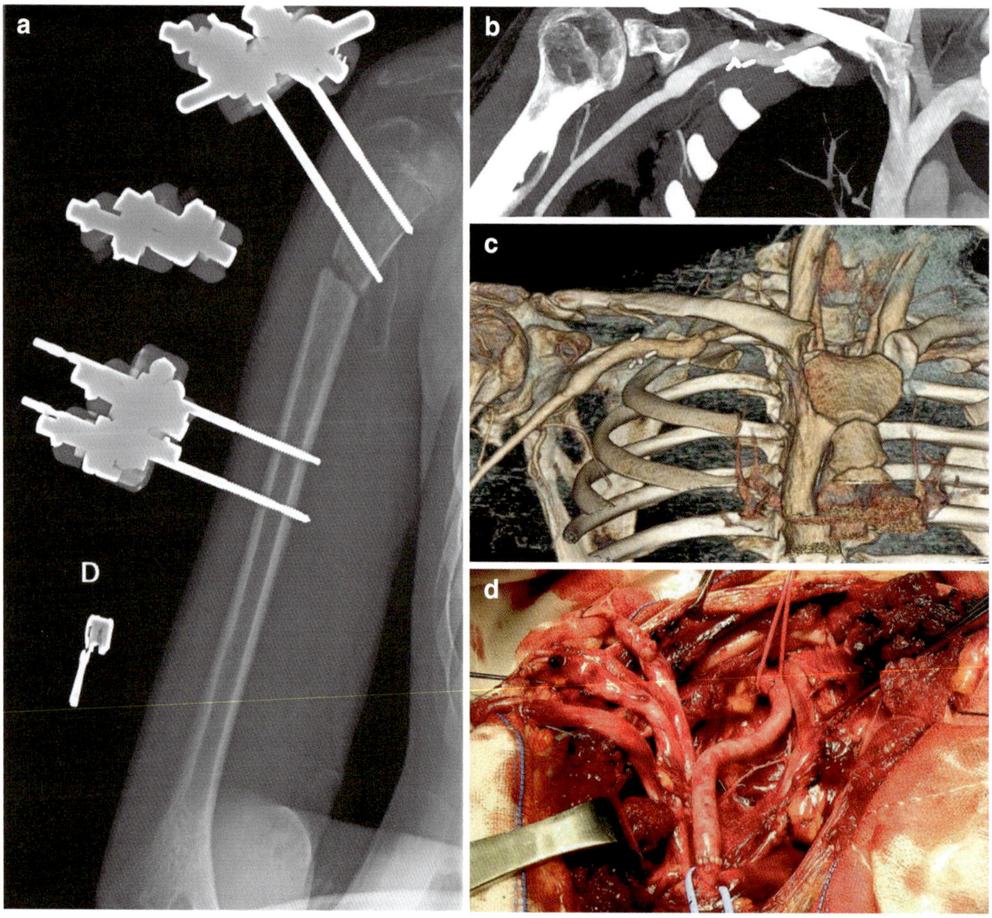

Fig. 11.14 Humeral X-ray after external fixation in the same patient (**a**). MIP (**b**) and VR reconstruction (**c**) of the subclavian and axillary artery after surgical repair. Surgical imaging of vascular reconstruction with saphenous vein stent graft of the axillary artery (**d**). Courtesy of Professor Seccia

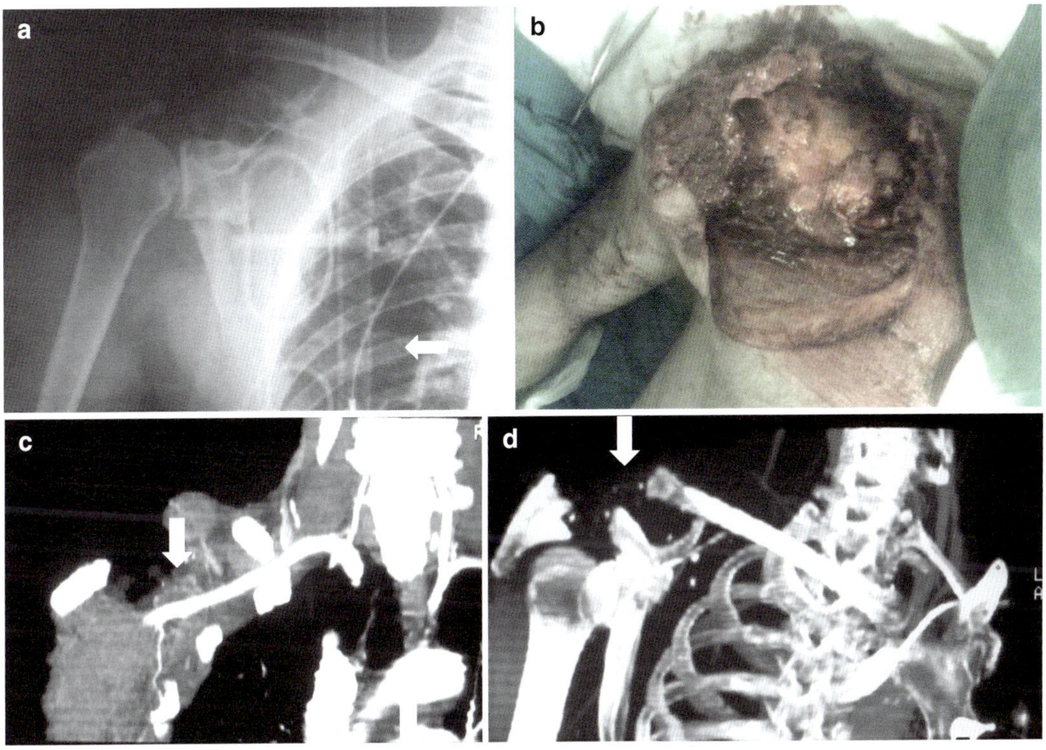

Fig. 11.15 (**a**) Shoulder X-ray of a 51-year-old patient after a MVA with clavicular fracture and scapulo-thoracic dissociation; (**b**) macroscopic appearance of the right shoulder's injury at the arrival in the emergency room. (**c**) MIP imaging with intravenous contrast medium of the shoulder showing clavicular fracture (*arrow*) with integrity of the subclavian and axillary artery; (**d**) 3D volume rendering reconstruction of the shoulder showing scapulo-thoracic dissociation

pulses with pallor of the distal end of the upper limb; a brachial plexus palsy and a sternoclavicular dislocation; a displaced fracture of the clavicle or a dislocation of the acromioclavicular articulation [62, 63, 71]. Common symptoms are pain and numbness or tingling in involved upper extremity. STD is often a missed or delayed diagnosis because in polytrauma patients the presence of concomitant severe injuries represents a sort of "distraction" for the emergency physician.

The arterial injury may be lethal in case of ongoing bleeding, and there is a 10% death rate in those who reach hospital, due to failure to treat hypovolemic shock or associated injuries [62]. Despite of arterial injuries are frequent, upper limb ischemia is a quite rare situation (12.5%), probably due to the good collateral arterial network around the shoulder [62]. It is important to notice that diagnosis of upper limb ischemia in this clinical situation is not so obvious because radial pulse might be absent due to the hypovolemic shock.

Nerve injuries occur in 94% of the patients [66]. Brachial plexus paralysis is usually complete, and it is associated with supraclavicular root avulsions or even rupture of the trunks in the interscalene space [61]. Partial damage is more frequently observed in retro- and infraclavicular injuries, and spontaneous recovery occurs in some cases but this is never complete [72].

It is important to emphasize that double lesions might occur in this type of traumatic injury: root lesions upper in the neck region and trunk ruptures lower down the arm [63]. Damage of the plexus determines the functional prognosis of STD.

There is a classification system for the injury severity of the STD [73]:

Type 1: Musculoskeletal injury alone
Type 2A: Musculoskeletal injury with vascular disruption
Type 2B: Musculoskeletal injury with incomplete neurological impairment of the upper extremity
Type 3: Musculoskeletal injury with incomplete neurological impairment of the upper extremity and vascular injury
Type 4: Musculoskeletal injury with complete brachial plexus avulsion

11.9.4 Treatment

The STD is usually associated with other life-threatening injuries, which lead the further management. In hemodynamically stable patients, MDCT angiography is widely recommended prior to surgery or interventional radiology. In hemodynamically unstable cases, however, urgent surgical intervention is required to control the arterial bleeding [66]. In arterial injuries, emergency revascularization is recommended only in patients with signs of severe ischemia, such as cold, temperature, and blue mottled color of the limb (compared with the opposite side) [62].

When the patient is stable, the shoulder is investigated in depth and then a decision regarding the final treatment could be taken. Shoulder stability in such cases can be obtained later by an arthrodesis. In many cases, scapulohumeral arthrodesis as a primary or secondary procedure has proven to be satisfactory [66, 71, 74]. In summary, the nerve reconstructions must try to restore elbow flexion. If it is weak and/or the shoulder is unstable and painful, a shoulder arthrodesis may be indicated [62].

Management of the nerve lesions is not in itself an emergency, but their severity means that there should be early assessment to plan the most appropriate time for surgical intervention. Nerve reconstruction by neurotization and/or nerve graft, preferably within a period of 2–6 months of the accident, is performed with the sole objective of recovering elbow flexion [62]. In case of complete brachial plexus avulsion, the functional recovery is usually poor and results mostly in a flail, anesthetic upper extremity [66].

Upper arm amputation remains a radical procedure which is only indicated when upper extremity function is not restorable. In these cases, the recommended treatment is an early above-elbow amputation with immediate prosthetic fitting in order to obtain a better functional outcome [66, 75].

The analysis of the previous literature about STD shows that approximately 11% of the reported patients died. However, probably the mortality of STD is overestimated because many of these patients die from the concomitant injuries during the preclinical course [66].

11.10 Scapular Fractures

Scapular fractures are about the 3–5% of all fracture of the shoulder girdle, where the most frequent fractures occur in the clavicle and proximal humerus [76].

This low fracture rate might be explained by its high mobility, helping in dissipating energy during trauma, together with the anatomical protection of the rib cage and the surrounding muscles [77].

The new evidences recently acquired show that the scapula plays an important role as dynamic stabilizer of the shoulder joint complex [78].

This is supported by several studies in the last two decades which have reported poor results following nonoperative management of both intra- and extra-articular fractures [79–81].

11.10.1 Pattern of Injury

Usually, scapular fractures are caused by high-energy injury (motor vehicle accidents account for 50%) through direct trauma to the shoulder region or indirect trauma by falling on outstretched hand. Non-accidental causes might be found in children injuries [82, 83].

Scapular fractures might be initially underestimated because attention is centered on the other frequent associated chest lesions such as a pneumothorax, hemothorax, pulmonary contusion, and spinal injuries [77]. In a retrospective review of data in the national trauma database, Baldwin et al. assessed that in association with scapular fractures rib fractures were present in 52.9% spine fractures, in 29.1%, lung injury in 47.1%, head injury in 39.1%, and clavicle fractures in 25.2% [84].

Also neurovascular lesions might be associated, especially regarding the brachial plexus, which is present in 13% of scapular fractures [85].

They are divided into three main groups:

- fractures of the body (50%); due to direct impact to the scapula or sudden muscular contraction (seizures or electric shocks) and respond well to conservative management.
- fractures of the scapular neck and glenoid fossa; among which, the fractures of the anatomic neck are rare, unstable, and necessitate surgical treatment. The variant, called "floating shoulder," is a scapular-neck fracture associated with an ipsilateral clavicular fracture.
- fractures of the acromion and the coracoid process [77].

11.10.2 Imaging Evaluation and Findings

A standard CXR should be initially performed in order to evaluate associated injuries, such as pneumothorax. Eventually, MDCT scan should be indicated to evaluate associated parenchymal lesions and exclude spinal fractures [76]. A correct radiographic study for scapular fractures should include an upright anterior-posterior scapula (called Grashey view), axillary, and scapula Y views.

In the Grashey view, we evaluate the glenopolar angle (GPA) and the lateral border offset (LBO). First measure is created by the intersection of a line drawn from the inferior glenoid fossa to the superior apex of the glenoid fossa and a line drawn from the superior apex of the glenoid fossa to the inferior angle of the scapula. The second measure concerns the medial displacement of the proximal fragment, relative to the distal fragment at the lateral border. In the Y view, we should draw a line parallel to the proximal fragment and a line parallel to the distal fragment and then measured the resulting angle in order to evaluate the angulation of the scapular fracture. The indications for surgery are based on these X-ray parameters. The axillary view is helpful to show fracture of the acromion and coracoid [76], subluxation or dislocation and intra-articular step-off (Figs. 11.16, 11.17, 11.18, and 11.19).

As scapular fractures are often encountered in polytrauma patients, MDCT scan is almost always performed with higher accuracy in defining the scapular deformity, especially thanks to the presence of MPR and three-dimensional imaging [86].

11.10.3 Natural History and Mortality

The physical examination, as well as prognosis, may depend on the commonly associated injuries, especially those that are life threatening, usually located to the spine, skull, and thorax. When possible, the suspected shoulder should be assessed preferably while patient is sitting or standing and the clinical findings are medial and caudal displacement of the shoulder with marked asymmetry [85].

11.10.4 Treatment

Treatment approaches are decided on the basis of imaging evaluation and measurements, in particular on angular deformity and displacement. However, it is recommended to take into account other ipsilateral injuries, patient activity level, hand dominance, and any comorbidities. In the review article of P. A. Cole et al. about scapular fractures nonoperative management of extra-articular scapula fractures is recommended for displacement smaller than 15–20 mm and angle lower than 30°–45° (minimal displacement) in order to obtain a better clinical outcome. When a clear deformity of scapula is depicted on X-ray, a MDCT scan with

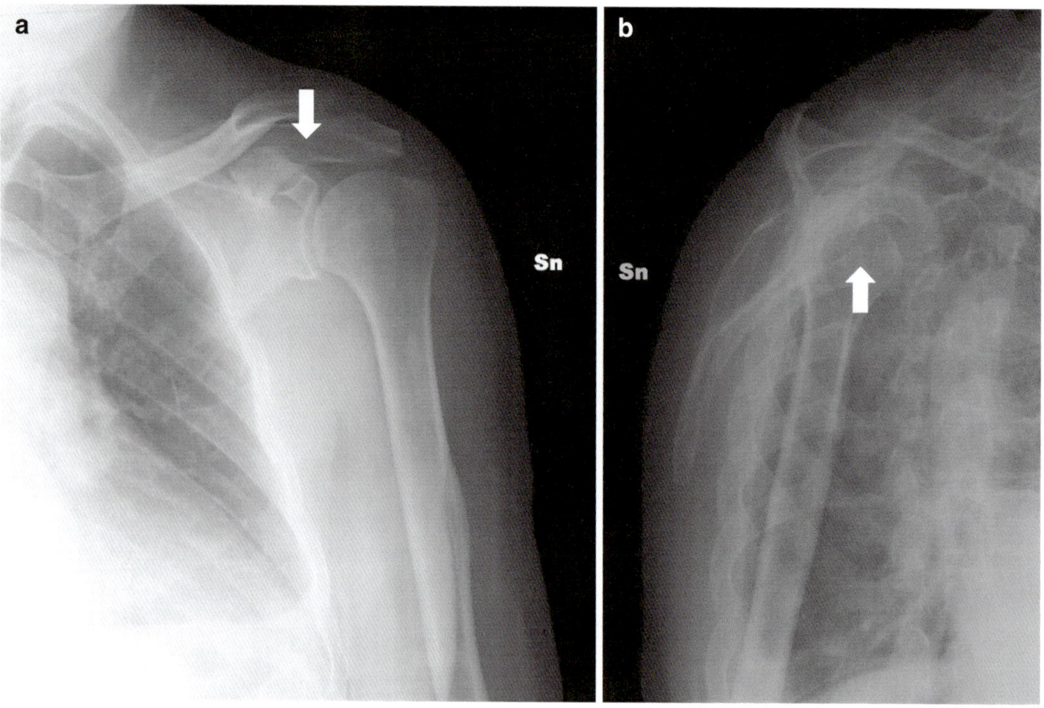

Fig. 11.16 Anterior-posterior (**a**) and Y (**b**) X-ray shoulder projections of a 64-year-old man after thoracic blunt trauma showing multiple fractures of the left scapula with fragments displacement (*arrows*)

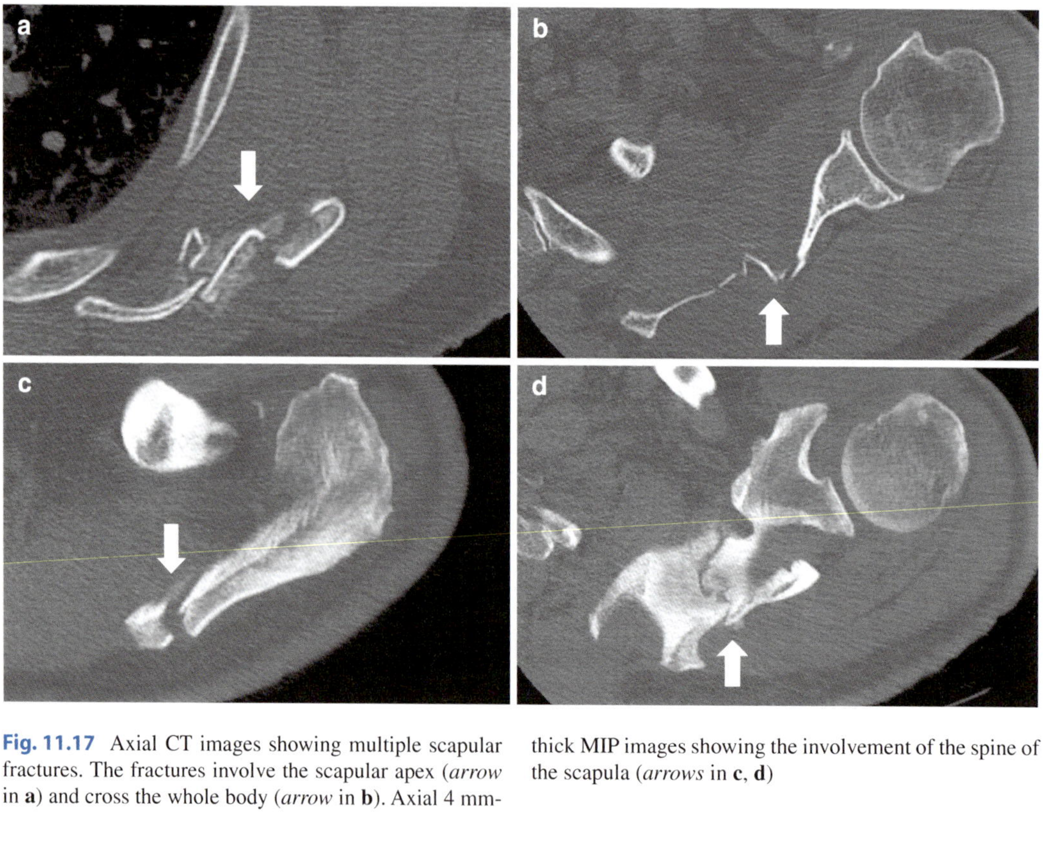

Fig. 11.17 Axial CT images showing multiple scapular fractures. The fractures involve the scapular apex (*arrow* in **a**) and cross the whole body (*arrow* in **b**). Axial 4 mm-thick MIP images showing the involvement of the spine of the scapula (*arrows* in **c**, **d**)

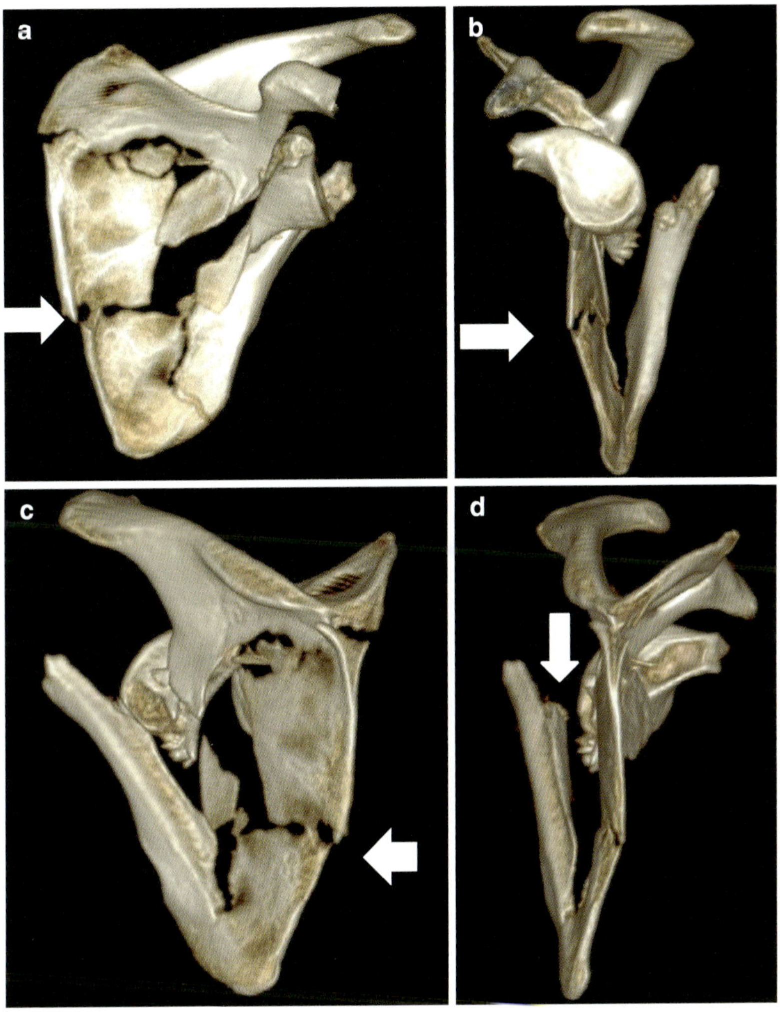

Fig. 11.18 Selective 3D reconstruction images of a 26-year-old man showing multiple fractures of the scapular bone involving the whole body. Anterior (**a**), lateral (**b**), posterior-medial (**c**), and medial view (**d**). Displacement and angulation of the multiple fragments of the body are here depicted (*arrows*). These images demonstrate that the acromial process and the glenoid cavity are not involved

3D reconstruction should be performed prior to surgical intervention to confirm the entity of displacement. Surgical intervention is indicated if GPA $\leq$ 22°, LBO $\geq$ 2 cm, angulation $\geq$ 45°, and articular gap/step-off $\geq$ 4 mm. In case of multiple shoulder elements, fractures involving the superior shoulder suspensory complex (SSSC, which consists in the shoulder's osseo-ligamentous connection of the acromion, coracoid, and glenoid processes of the scapula and their respective capsule–ligamentous connections) causing instability of the displaced floating shoulder the threshold for open reduction internal fixation is lower: LBO $\geq$ 15 mm and angulation $\geq$ 30° [87].

It is important to note that skin integrity should be assessed for appropriate timing of surgery. It is preferable to wait on surgery until the skin has re-epithelialized [76].

11.11 Chest Wall Hematoma

Chest wall hematoma often is caused by traumatic event or iatrogenic procedures and it is usually treated conservatively due to his self-limiting course [88].

Post-traumatic expanding chest wall hematomas, with underlying active arterial bleeding, are a rare eventuality and they require urgent surgical

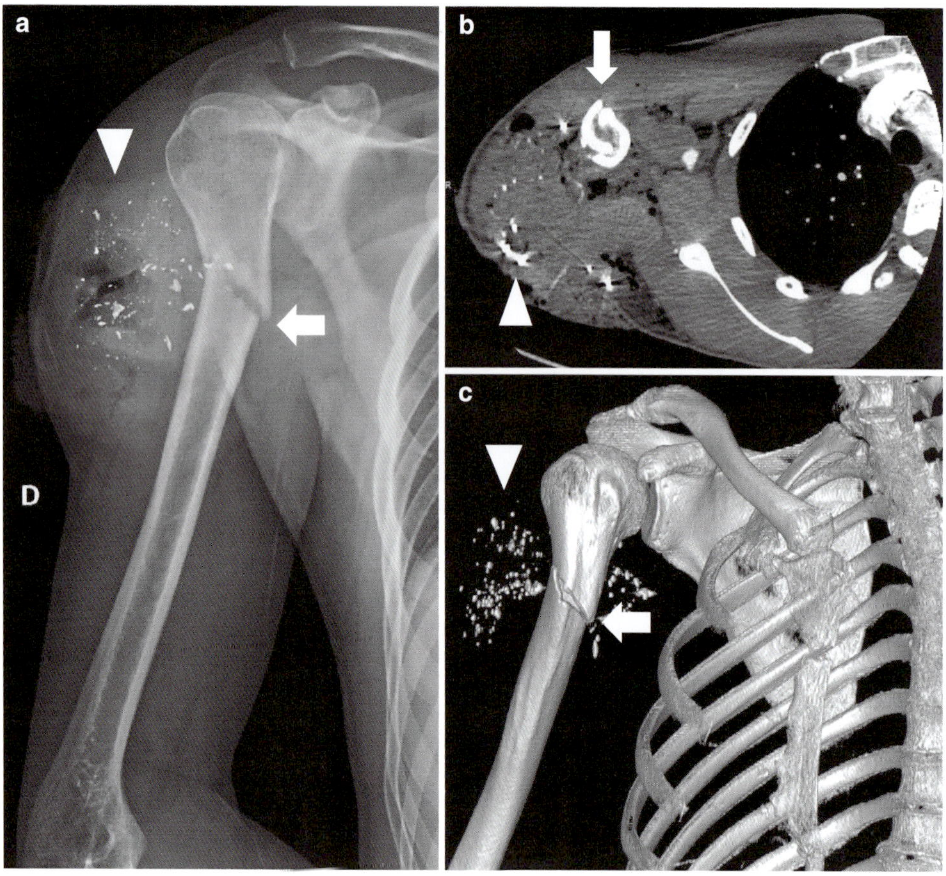

Fig. 11.19 Shoulder X-rays (**a**) in a 39-year-old patient after a gunshot. Axial CT imaging (**a**) and VR reconstruction (**b**) showing humeral shaft fracture (*arrows* in **a–c**) and multiple metallic fragments (*arrowheads* in **a–c**)

exploration with hemostasis and/or angiographic embolization [89].

11.11.1 Pattern of Injury

Chest wall hematoma are usually associated with blunt and penetrating trauma, in particular when rib fractures occur. Frequently in traumatic rib fractures, the intercostal, internal mammary, or subclavian arteries might be injured, creating a blood collection between parietal pleura and endothoracic fascia, defined as extrapleural hematomas [37].

The mandatory use of seat belts resulted in the last decades in a significant decrease of injuries and deaths from car accidents [90].

At the same time, hollow viscus and soft-tissue injuries number increased because of the seatbelt itself, especially in women [91].

In female population, the seat belt during motor vehicle accident might represent a potential cause of injuries of the breast due to the shear and compressive forces from the chest strap over the breast and bony thorax [92, 93].

Soft-tissue injuries are most of the time represented by nonexpanding hematomas or ecchymosis or avulsion.

11.11.2 Imaging Evaluation and Findings

Radiographically, extrapleural hematoma might be depicted as bulging convex chest wall mass that may project into the thoracic cavity.

11.11.2.1 MDCT-US

Usually, a MDCT scan is performed in polytrauma patients. Imaging studies like US or MDCT might help to confirm the diagnosis by differentiating the belonging chest wall compartment. The typical imaging features are the same as bleeding in the other areas. US scan shows inhomogeneous hypoecoic fluid collection in the chest wall thickness. Non-contrast-enhanced MDCT scan might confirm the hyperdense fluid collection within the wall. Contrast-enhanced MDCT is able to differentiate arterial or venous origin of the hematoma. In arterial bleeding, we can find hyperdense spot in the arterial phase within the collection and we might identify the source of bleeding. In subsequent phases, the density of the fluid should increase due to the contrast medium accumulating within the collection. The typical clinical low-pressure and self-limiting features together with the absence of hyperdense spot in arterial phase of enhanced MDCT allows to diagnose the venous origin of hematoma (Figs. 11.20 and 11.21).

Angiography is usually performed in order to treat active arterial bleeding, when indicated (Fig. 11.22).

11.11.3 Natural History and Mortality

Chest wall hematoma could be induced by arterial or venous injuries. Arterial bleeding usually leads to rapidly enlarging hematomas with mass effect and displacement of adjacent structures. Venous blood collection are commonly low-pressure and self-limited. Diagnosis might be made clinically by swelling/bruising or might be nonspecific findings like chronic anemia, fever, and plural effusion. Usually, the clinical presentation is characterized by a painful, pulsating mass was on the chest wall. Physical examination might show distended discoloration of the involved chest wall area. The active

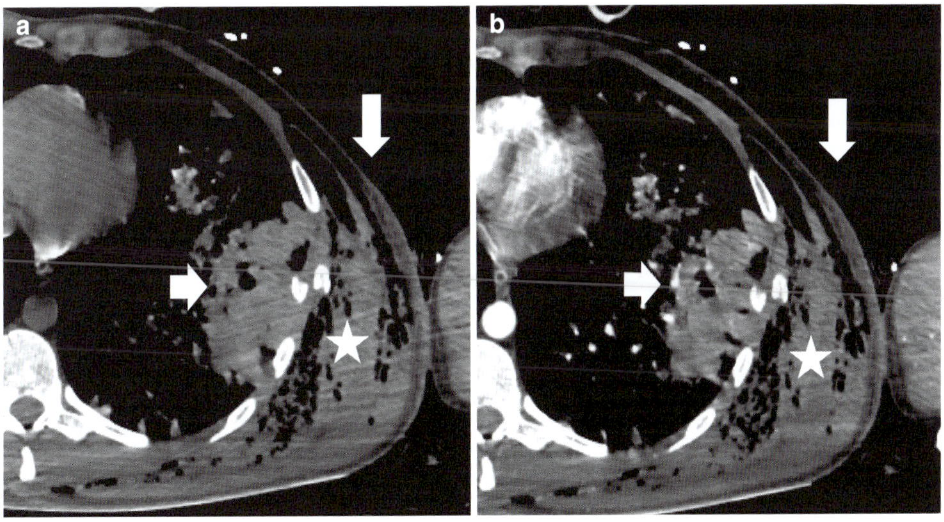

Fig. 11.20 Axial CT images of a 26-year-old man after thoracic blunt trauma showing a hematoma of the posterior-lateral thoracic wall (*stars* in **a**–**d**) associated with subcutaneous emphysema (*long arrows* in **a**–**d**) and with left lateral rib fracture and lung contusions (*short arrows* in **a**–**d**). Different phases acquired: unenhanced CT scan (**a**), arterial (**b**), venous (**c**), and delayed (**d**) scan show there is no active bleeding

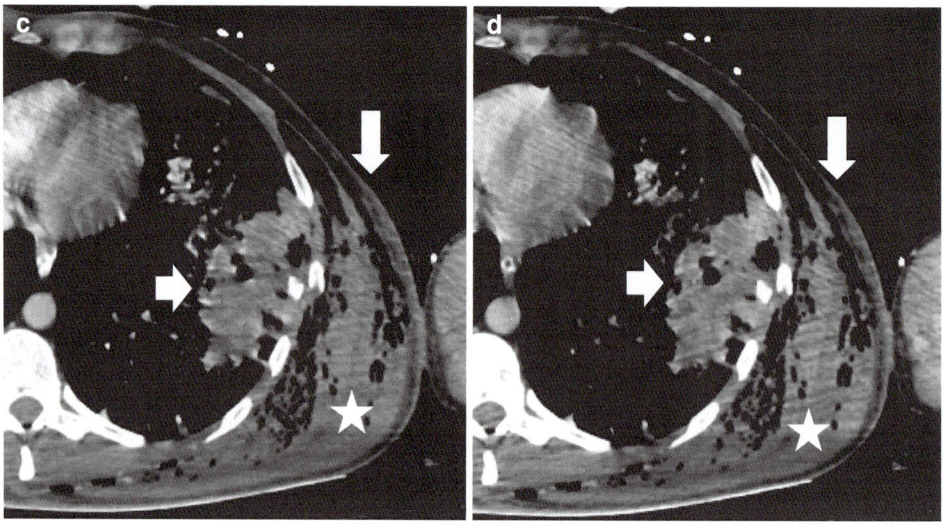

Fig. 11.20 (continued)

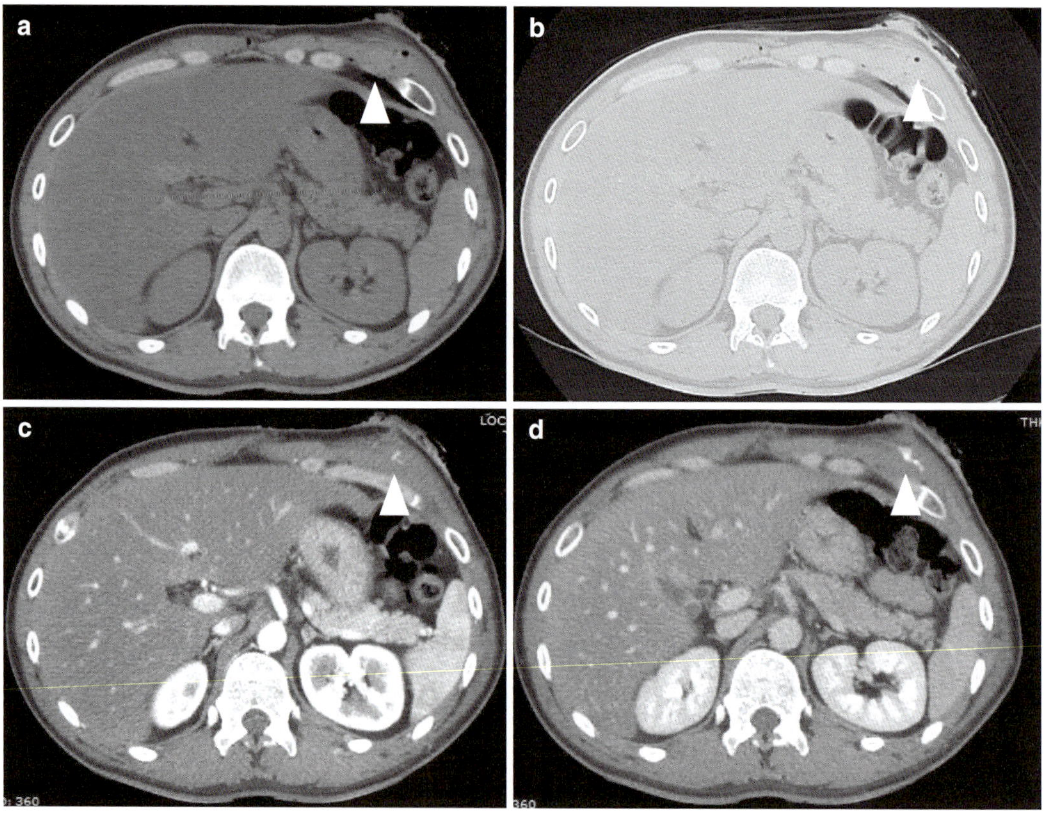

Fig. 11.21 Anterior left chest wall trauma after stab wound injury, in a 26-year-old patient, showing chest wall hematoma with subcutaneous emphysema (*arrowheads* in **a**, **b**) and signs of active bleeding in arterial (**c**) and venous (**d**) phase (*arrowheads*)

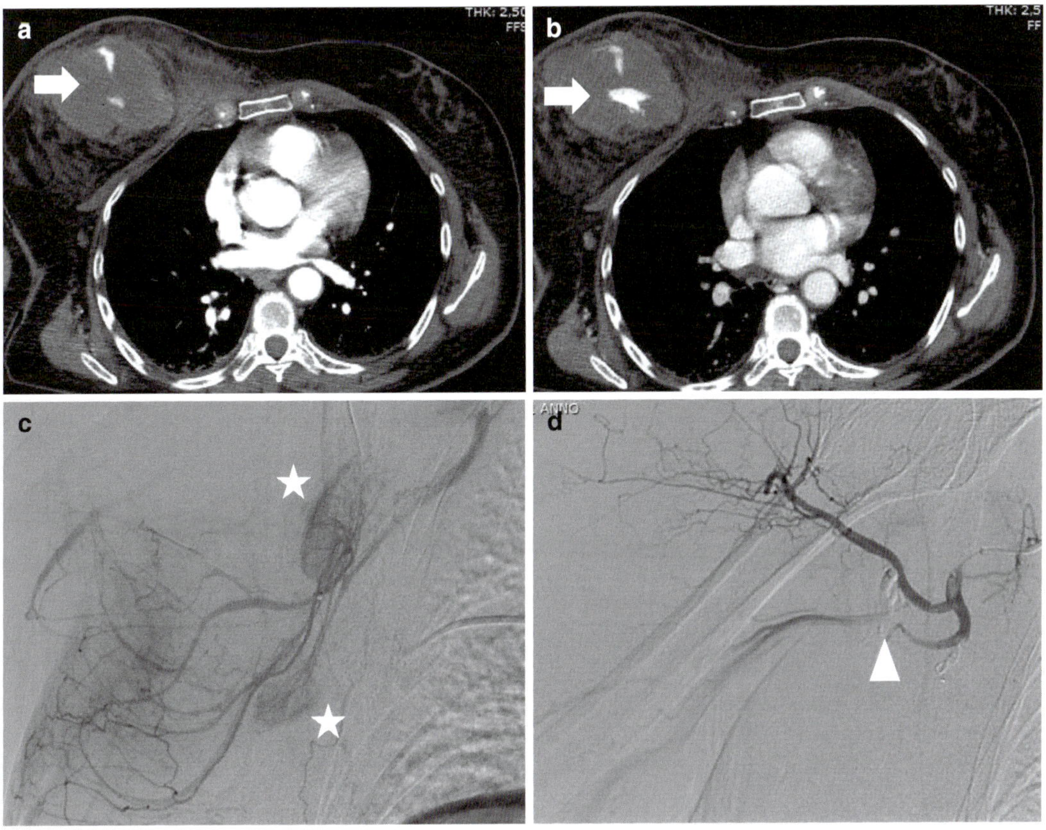

Fig. 11.22 Blunt traumatic hematoma of right breast showing signs of active bleeding in arterial (**a**) and venous (**b**) phase (*arrows*); Diagnostic angiographic procedure (**c**) showing arterial blush (*stars* in **c**). Angiographic endovascular embolization imaging post coils placement showing resolution of bleeding (*arrowheads* in **d**)

range of motion over the ipsilateral shoulder might also be limited because of this expanding anterior chest wall hematoma. Large chest wall hematomas with important active arterial bleeding might be life-threatening due to their systemic and hemodynamic consequences [88].

11.11.4 Treatment

Venous hematomas are usually self-limiting and treated conservatively. In case of arterial bleeding, there are several ways to manage the hemorrhage: selective angiographic embolization, US-guided hemostatic injection, and conservative management, such as compression [94].

When there's no injury of the great vessels, MDCT angiography often allows to detect bleeding from branches of the internal mammary artery, which can be embolized successfully with low complication rates [95].

If blunt injury to the subclavian artery is described, surgical intervention is needed in order to guarantee the blood supply to the upper limb [96].

References

1. Demirhan R, Onan B, Oz K, Halezeroglu S. Comprehensive analysis of 4205 patients with chest trauma: a 10-year experience. Interact Cardiovasc Thorac Surg. 2009;9:450–3.
2. Battle CE, Hutchings H, Evans PA. Risk factors that predict mortality in patients with blunt chest wall trauma: a systematic review and meta-analysis. Injury. 2012;43:8–17.
3. Moore E, et al. Organ injury scaling III: chest wall, abdominal vascular, ureter, bladder and urethra. J Trauma. 1992;33(3):337–9.
4. Mayberry JC. Imaging in thoracic trauma: the trauma surgeon's perspective. J Thorac Imaging. 2000;15: 76–86.

5. Cattaneo L. Compendio di anatomia umana. 1986.
6. Anastasi G. Trattato di anatomia umana, vol. 1; 2010.
7. Scaglione M, et al. Multi-detector row computed tomography and blunt chest trauma. Eur J Radiol. 2008;65:377–88.
8. Wolf SJ, et al. Blast injuries. Lancet. 2009;374:405–15.
9. Wanek S, Mayberry JC. Blunt thoracic trauma: flail chest, pulmonary contusion, and blast injury. Crit Care Clin. 2004;20:71–81.
10. Chapman BC, et al. A novel radiographic score based on fracture pattern that predicts pneumonia, respiratory failure and tracheostomy. J Trauma Acute Care Surg. 2016;80(1):95–101.
11. Rathachai Kaewlai MD, et al. Multidetector CT of blunt thoracic trauma. Radiographics. 2008;28:1555–70. doi:10.1148/rg.286085510.
12. Oikonomou A, Prassopoulos P. CT imaging of blunt chest trauma. Insights Imaging. 2011;2:281–95. doi:10.1007/s13244-011-0072-9.
13. Easter A. Management of patients with multiple rib fractures. Am J Crit Care. 2001;10(5):320.
14. Sirmali M, et al. A comprehensive analysis of traumatic rib fractures: morbidity, mortality and management. Eur J Cardiothorac Surg. 2003;24(1):133.
15. Al-Koudmani I, et al. Chest trauma experience over eleven-year period at al-mouassat university teaching hospital-Damascus: a retrospective review of 888 cases. J Cardiothorac Surg. 2012;7:35; Epub 2012 Apr 19.
16. Collins J. Chest wall trauma. J Thorac Imaging. 2000;15:112–9.
17. Barnea Y, Kashtan H, Skornick Y, Werbin N. Isolated rib fractures in elderly patients: mortality and morbidity. Can J Surg. 2002;45:43–6.
18. Stawicki SP, Grossman MD, Hoey BA, Miller DL, Reed JF. Rib fractures in the elderly: a marker of injury severity. J Am Geriatr Soc. 2004;52:805–8.
19. Cho SH, Sung YM, Kim MS. Missed rib fractures on evaluation of initial chest CT for trauma patients: pattern analysis and diagnostic value of coronal multiplanar reconstruction images with multidetector row CT. Br J Radiol. 2012;85(1018):e845–50.
20. Love JC, Symes SA. Understanding rib fracture patterns: incomplete and buckle fractures. J Forensic Sci. 2004;49(6):1153–8.
21. Bhavnagri SJ, Mohammed TL. When and how to image a suspected broken rib. Cleve Clin J Med. 2009;76(5):309–14. doi:10.3949/ccjm.76a.08026.
22. Primack SL, Collins J. Blunt nonaortic chest trauma: radiographic and CT findings. Emerg Radiol. 2002;9:5–12.
23. Hurley ME, Keye GD, Hamilton S. Is ultrasound really helpful in the detection of rib fractures? Injury. 2004;35(6):562–6. doi:10.1016/S0020-1383(03)00263-8.
24. Bansidhar BJ, et al. Clinical rib fractures: are follow-up chest X-rays a waste of resources? Am Surg. 2002;68(5):449–53.
25. Chien CY, et al. The number of displaced rib fractures is more predictive for complications in chest trauma patients. Scand J Trauma Resusc Emerg Med. 2017;25:19. doi:10.1186/s13049-017-0368-y.
26. Kerr-Valentic MA, et al. Rib fracture pain and disability: can we do better? J Trauma. 2003;54(6):1058.
27. Orth RC, Laor T. Isolated costal cartilage fracture: an unusual cause of an anterior chest mass in a toddler. Pediatr Radiol. 2009;39(9):985–7. doi:10.1007/s00247-009-1276-8.
28. Ontell FK, Moore EH, Shepard JA, et al. The costal cartilages in health and disease. Radiographics. 1997;17(3):571–7. doi:10.1148/radiographics.17.3.9153697.
29. Malghem J, Vande Berg B, et al. Costal cartilage fractures as revealed on CT and sonography. Am J Roentgenol. 2001;176:429–32.
30. Lopez V, et al. Costal cartilage fractures and disruptions in a rugby football player. Clin J Sport Med. 2013;23(3):232–4. doi:10.1097/JSM.0b013e31825b55ed.
31. Turk F, Kurt AB, Saglam S. Evaluation by ultrasound of traumatic rib fractures missed by radiography. Emerg Radiol. 2010;17(6):473–7. doi:10.1007/s10140-010-0892-9.
32. Griffith JF, Rainer TH, Ching AS, et al. Sonography compared with radiography in revealing acute rib fracture. AJR Am J Roentgenol. 1999;173(6):1603–9. doi:10.2214/ajr.173.6.10584808.
33. Subhas N, Kline MJ, et al. MRI evaluation of costal cartilage injuries. Am J Roentgenol. 2008;191:129–32.
34. Nummela M. et al. The incidence and effect on mortality of costochondral fractures in blunt polytrauma patients—a review of 1461 consecutive whole body CT studies for trauma. Radiological Society of North America 2016.
35. Piao Z, et al. The response of costal cartilage to mechanical injury in mice. Plast Reconstr Surg. 2007;119(3):830–6. doi:10.1097/01.prs.0000240817.11002.3e.
36. Gregory PL, Biswas AC, Batt ME. Musculoskeletal problems of the chest wall in athletes. Sports Med. 2002;32(4):235–50.
37. Sangster GP, González-Beicos A, et al. Blunt traumatic injuries of the lung parenchyma, pleura, thoracic wall, and intrathoracic airways: multidetector computer tomography imaging findings. Emerg Radiol. 2007;14:297–310. doi:10.1007/s10140-007-0651-8.
38. Borrelly J, Aazami M. New insights into the pathophysiology of flail segment: the implication of anterior serratus muscle in parietal failure. Eur J Cardiothorac Surg. 2005;28:742–9.
39. Cappello M, Legrand A, De Troyer A. Determinants of rib motion in flail chest. Am J Respir Crit Care Med. 1999;159:886–91.
40. Pettiford BL, et al. The management of flail chest. Thorac Surg Clin. 2007;17:25–33.
41. Athanassiadi K, et al. Management of 150 flail chest injuries: analysis of risk factors affecting outcome. Eur J Cardiothorac Surg. 2004;26:373–6.
42. Oyetunji TA, Jackson HT, et al. Associated injuries in traumatic sternal fractures: a review of the National Trauma Data Bank. Am Surg. 2013;79(7):702–5.

43. Crestanello JA, Samuels LE, et al. Sternal fracture with mediastinal hematoma: delayed cardiopulmonary sequelae. J Trauma. 1999;47:161–4.
44. Jurik AG, editor. Imaging of the sternocostoclavicular region. Heidelberg: Springer. isbn:103-540-33147-6.
45. Khoriati A-A, Rajakulasingam R, et al. Sternal fractures and their management. J Emerg Trauma Shock. 2013;6(2):113–6.
46. Restrepo CS, Santiago Martinez MD, et al. Imaging appearances of the sternum and sternoclavicular joints. Radiographics. 2009;29:839–59.
47. Soto J, Lucey B. Emergency radiology: the requisites. 2nd ed. Philadelphia, PA: Elsevier. isbn:978-0-323-37640-2.
48. Fisher DA. Imaging in sternal fractures. Medscape, Jan 11, 2016.
49. Wongwaisayawan S, Suwannanon R, et al. Emergency thoracic US: the essentials. Radiographics. 2016;36(3):640–59. doi:10.1148/rg.2016150064.
50. Grosse A, Grosse C, et al. MRI findings of prolonged post-traumatic sternal pain. Skelet Radiol. 2007;36(5):423–9.
51. Roy Shapira A, Levi I, et al. Sternal fractures: a red flag or a red herring? J Trauma. 1994;37(1):59–61.
52. Laffosse JM, Reina N, et al. Variations du syndrome d'impaction de l'épaule: la luxation sternoclaviculaire postérieure. Revue de Chirurgie Orthopédique et Traumatologique. 2010;96(7):869–73.
53. Peters S, Nicolas V, et al. Multidetector computed tomography-spectrum of blunt chest wall and lung injuries in polytraumatized patients. Clin Radiol. 2010;65(4):333–8.
54. Morell DJ. Thyagarajan. Sternoclavicular joint dislocation and its management: a review of the literature. World J Orthop. 2016;7(4):244–50.
55. Kirby JC, Edwards E, et al. Management and functional outcomes following sternoclavicular joint dislocation. Injury. 2015;46(10):1906–13.
56. Cruz MF, Erdeljac J, et al. Posterior sternoclavicular joint dislocation in a division football player: a case report. Int J Sports Phys Ther. 2015;10(5):700–11.
57. O'Brien SD, Bui-Mansfield LT. Costovertebral fracture dislocations: important radiographically difficult diagnosis. J Comput Assist Tomogr. 2009;33:748Y751.
58. Saker E, Graham RA. Ligaments of the costovertebral joints including biomechanics, innervations, and clinical applications: a comprehensive review with application to approaches to the thoracic spine. Cureus. 2016;8(11):e874.
59. Christensen EE, Dietz GW. Injuries of the first costovertebral articulation. Radiology. 1980;134:41–3.
60. Brooksher WR, Smith F. Costovertebral dislocation of the twelfth rib. JAMA. 1933;100(11):816.
61. Leffert RD. Brachial plexus. In: Green DP, Hotchkiss RN, Pederson WC, editors. Green's operative hand surgery. 4th ed. New York: Churchill Livingstone; 1999. p. 1557–87.
62. Masmejean EH, et al. Brachial plexus injuries in scapulothoracic dissociation. J Hand Surg Br. 2000;25(4):336–40.
63. Oreck SL, Burgess A, Levine AM. Traumatic lateral displacement of the scapula: a radiographic sign of neurovascular disruption. J Bone Joint Surg. 1984;66-A:758–63.
64. An HS, Vonderbrink JP, et al. Open scapulothoracic dissociation with intact neuro-vascular status in a child. J Orthop Trauma. 1988;2:36–8.
65. Lange RH, Noel SH. Traumatic lateral scapular displacement: an expanded spectrum of associated neurovascular injury. J Orthop Trauma. 1993; 7:361–6.
66. Brucker PU. Scapulothoracic dissociation: evaluation and management. Injury. 2005;36:1147–55.
67. Jangir R, et al. Scapulothoracic dissociation: a rare variant: a case report. Malays Orthop J. 2014;8(2):46–8.
68. Damschen DD, et al. Scapulothoracic dissociation caused by blunt trauma. J Truama. 1997;42:537–40.
69. Tüzüner S, et al. Scapulothoracic dissociation: a case report. Isr J Med Sci. 1996;32:70–4.
70. Alnot JY, Narakas A. Traumatic brachial plexus injuries, Monographie de la SocieÂ teÂ FrancË aise de Chirurgie de la Main. Vol. 22. Paris: Expansion Scientifique Francaise; 1996. p. 275.
71. Sampson LN, et al. The neurovascular outcome of scapulothoracic dissociation. J Vasc Surg. 1993;17:1083–9.
72. Ebraheim NA, et al. Scapulothoracic dissociation (closed avulsion of the scapula, subclavian artery, and brachial plexus). A new recognized variant, a new classification, and a review of the literature and treatment options. J Orthop Trauma. 1987;1:18–23.
73. Zelle BA, et al. Functional outcome following scapulothoracic dissociation. J Bone Joint Surg Am. 2004;86:2–7.
74. Rubenstein JD, et al. Traumatic scapulothoracic dissociation. Radiology. 1985;157:297–8.
75. Clements RH, Reisser JR. Scapulothoracic dissociation: a devastating injury. J Trauma. 1996;40:146–9.
76. Cole PA, et al. Scapula fractures. Curr Rev Musculoskelet Med. 2013;6:79–87.
77. Mazaheri P, et al. Advanced imaging of the scapula: what every radiologist needs to know. J Comput Assist Tomogr. 2016;40(4):567–75.
78. McClure PW, et al. Shoulder function and 3-dimensional scapular kinematics in people with and without shoulder impingement syndrome. Phys Ther. 2006;86:1075–90.
79. Van Noort A, et al. The floating shoulder. A multicentre study. J Bone Joint Surg Br. 2001;83:795–8.
80. Cole PA, et al. Extra-articular malunions of the scapula: a comparison of functional outcome before and after reconstruction. J Orthop Trauma. 2011;25:649–56.
81. Bozkurt M, et al. Conservative treatment of scapular neck fracture: the effect of stability and glenopolar angle on clinical outcome. Injury. 2005;36:1176–81.
82. Egol K, et al. Handbook of fractures. Philadelphia, PA: Lippincott Williams & Wilkins; 2010.

83. Rockwood CA, et al. Rockwood and green's fractures in adults. Philadelphia, PA: Lippincott Williams & Wilkins; 2010.
84. Baldwin KD, et al. Scapula fractures: a marker for concomitant injury? A retrospective review of data in the national trauma database. J Trauma. 2008;65: 430–5.
85. Mayo KA, et al. Displaced fractures of the glenoid fossa. Results of open reduction and internal fixation. Clin Orthop Relat Res. 1998;347:122–30.
86. Armitage BM, et al. Mapping of scapular fractures with three-dimensional computed tomography. J Bone Joint Surg Am. 2009;91:2222–8.
87. Goss TP. Double disruptions of the superior shoulder suspensory complex. J Orthop Trauma. 1993;7:99–106.
88. Antevil JL, Holmes JF, Lewis D, Battistella F. Successful angiographic embolization of bleeding into the chest wall after blunt thoracic trauma. J Trauma. 2006;60(5):1117–8.
89. Yu P-C, et al. Angiographic embolization in chest wall hematoma due to handlebar injury—a rare case report. Am J Emerg Med. 2015;33:1328.e3–5.
90. McDermott FT, Hough DE. Reduction in road fatalities and injuries after legislation for compulsory wearing of seatbelts: experience in Victoria and the rest of Australia. Br J Surg. 1979;66:518–21.
91. Newman RJ. Chest wall injuries and seatbelt syndrome. Injury. 1984;16:110–3.
92. Murday AJ. Seatbelt injury of the breast—a case report. Injury. 1982;14:276–7.
93. Dawes RFH, et al. Seatbelt injury to the female breast. Br J Surg. 1986;73:106–7.
94. Yoo DH. Transcatheter arterial embolization of intramuscular active hemorrhage with N-butyl cyanoacrylate. Cardiovasc Intervent Radiol. 2012;35:292–8.
95. Jonsson K, Karlsson S. Angiography of the internal mammary artery. Acta Radiol. 1985;26:113–20.
96. Costa M, Robbs J. Non-penetrating subclavian artery trauma. J Vasc Surg. 1988;8:71–5.

12 Traumatic Diaphragmatic Injuries

Michele Tonerini, Silvia Lorenzi,
Francesca Pancrazi, Barbara Mugellini,
Alessandra Scionti, and Veronica Iodice

12.1 Introduction

A traumatic diaphragmatic injury (TDI) is a severe lesion that often produces an interruption in the continuity of muscular and tendinous fibers of the diaphragm, resulting in a communication between thorax and abdomen. It may be due to both a severe blunt trauma, from motor vehicle accidents, and penetrating trauma, from knife or gunshot wounds. The frequency, with which either of these mechanisms leads to a diaphragmatic lesion , mainly depends on the geographic location and socioeconomic status of traumatic patients [1, 2]. TDIs are estimated to occur in 0.8–8% of patients with blunt abdominal trauma and in 10% of patients with penetrating trauma, representing a diagnostic challenge for both emergency radiologists and surgeons; indeed, especially blunt TDIs are missed at initial presentation in 7–66% of cases [1, 3]. There are several reasons why these injuries often remain early undiagnosed. Firstly, the specific clinical and radiologic signs may be absent or very subtle, and, considering the high frequency of concurrent visceral lesions, especially in polytrauma patients, a TDI may be overshadowed by life-threatening multiple organ involvement. The diagnosis results easier when clinical manifestations is related to a complication: the latter is mostly caused by a massive visceral herniation through the diaphragm (that is responsible for respiratory compromise due to lung compression) and by the organ strangulation, secondary to visceral incarceration. Such kind of complication may occur long after the trauma and, if symptoms are not conspicuous, the TDI is missed. The radiologic interpretation is difficult too; each imaging technique has advantages and pitfalls related to the type of injury. The chest X-ray (CXR) is still the first imaging evaluation performed in trauma patients at the Emergency Department, but, in the hemodynamically stable multitrauma patients, it is fundamental a total body examination with multi-detector computed tomography (MDCT) that is consid-

M. Tonerini (✉)
Department of Emergency Radiology, Cisanello University Hospital, Pisa, Italy
e-mail: m.tonerini@tiscali.it

S. Lorenzi • F. Pancrazi • B. Mugellini • A. Scionti
V. Iodice
Department of Diagnostic and Interventional Radiology, University of Pisa, Pisa, Italy
e-mail: lorenzisilvia1@gmail.com; pancrazi.francesca@gmail.com; barbara.mugellini87@gmail.com; alessandra86sc@gmail.com; veronica.iodice@hotmail.it

V. Miele, M. Trinci (eds.), *Diagnostic Imaging in Polytrauma Patients*,
https://doi.org/10.1007/978-3-319-62054-1_12

ered the modality of choice, with a high sensitivity rate for both blunt and penetrating TDIs [3–6].

Another reason that emphasizes the importance of detecting diaphragmatic injuries with imaging techniques concerns the fact that emergency surgeons increasingly tend to perform a nonoperative management (NOM) both for blunt and penetrating abdominal trauma; indeed, these patients are treated conservatively, without immediate surgical intervention, that could lead to a prompt diagnosis and a treatment of the smallest and insidious diaphragmatic tears. Finally, there is a general lack of awareness about this serious traumatic entity on the part of both clinicians and radiologists and a lack of familiarity with all the imaging signs of TDI [1, 4, 6–9].

Considering that diaphragmatic tears do not heal spontaneously and that delayed life-threatening complications, such as visceral herniation and strangulation, may occur, an early diagnosis and a prompt surgical repair are crucial. The better way to improve TDI detection is to maintain a high degree of suspicion in every case of severe thoracoabdominal trauma to have a good knowledge of the mechanism of injury and familiarity with specific and nonspecific radiological signs.

12.1.1 Anatomy

The diaphragm is a dome-shaped musculotendinous structure with upper convexity that separates the thoracic from the abdominal cavity. It is composed by a peripheral striated muscular component that originates from the circumference of the thoracic outlet and converges to a central tendinous component; these two parts, respectively, arise from the pleuroperitoneal membrane and from the septum transversum. The muscular fibers belong to three different groups according to the anatomic structure on which they insert: sternal, with attachment to the posterior margins of the lower sternum and xiphoid process; costal, with insertion on the inner margins of the sixth through twelfth rib; lumbar, with attachment to the medial and lateral arcuate ligaments and to right and left crura. There are three normal orifices through the diaphragm: the aortic hiatus, the inferior vena cava foramen, and the esophageal hiatus [2, 10–13].

The diaphragmatic anatomy is not well appreciated in all its components on conventional CT axial images because the dome is tangential to transverse plane; therefore, thinner sections and multiplanar reformations (MPR) are needed to improve the diagnosis. MDCT allows the detection of the diaphragmatic lumbar aspect made of the crura and the arcuate ligaments that may appear thickened or nodular; the sternal and costal sections are much more difficult to depict on axial images (Figs. 12.1 and 12.2). Besides, only the portions of the diaphragm outlined by fat will be clearly represented; instead, the parts bordering structures of similar attenuation, such as liver or spleen, are not well recognizable, a fact that partially explains some of the limitations in the diagnosis of diaphragmatic tears at MDCT [4, 14].

The pattern and site of TDIs may be influenced by some typical regions of muscular weakness that predisposes to injury and are directly related to embryological development. These points of weakness are located where groups of muscle fibers from different embryological origins meet: the right and left sternocostal triangles and the lumbocostal triangles. Indeed, the majority of injuries occur in the posterolateral areas of the left diaphragm between lumbar and costal muscular attachment, where the pleuroperitoneal membrane finally join with the septum trasversum during embryogenesis [1, 15, 16]. On the right side, the diaphragm is more protected by liver parenchyma from blunt traumatic injuries.

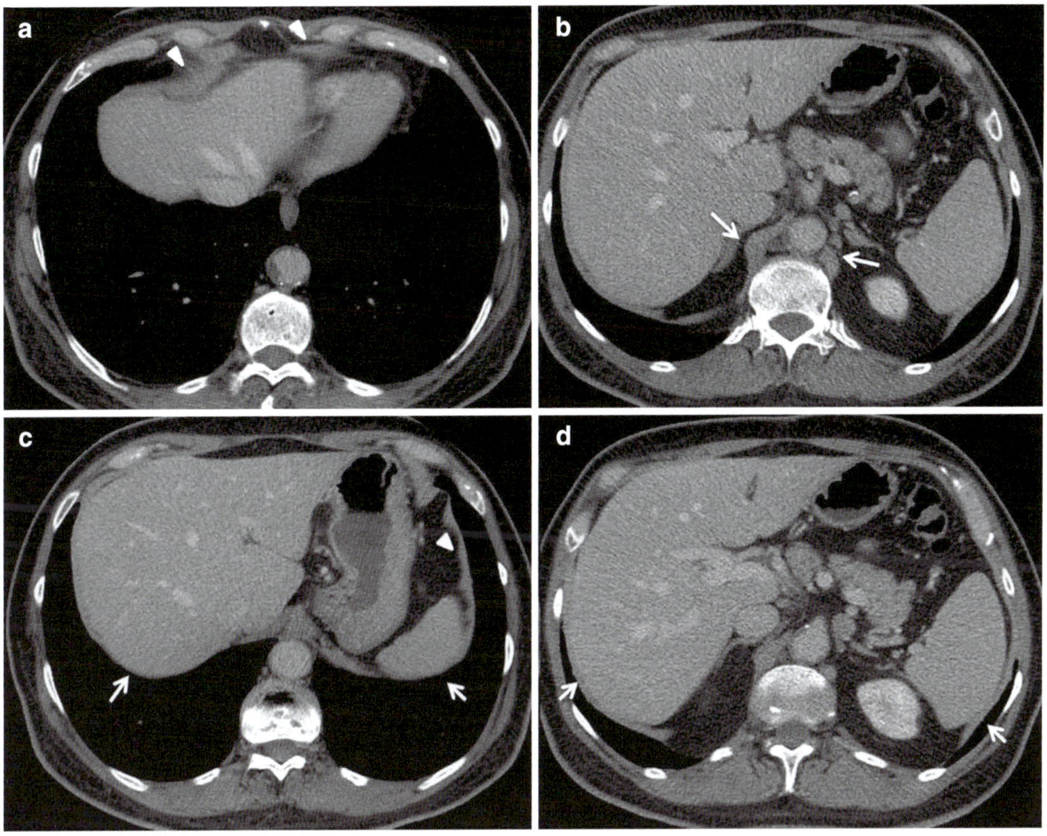

Fig. 12.1 Normal CT anatomy of the anterior, posterior, and lateral/costal part of the diaphragm. (**a**, **b**) Axial MDCT images show the anterior diaphragmatic component (*arrowheads*) and the crura (*arrows*). (**c**, **d**) Axial MDCT scans of the lateral/costal part of the diaphragm show incomplete detection of the muscle where it abuts structures of similar attenuation, such as liver and spleen (*arrows* in **c**, **d**). The diaphragm is well appreciated when it is defined by peritoneal, retroperitoneal, or extraperitoneal fat (*arrowheads* in **c**)

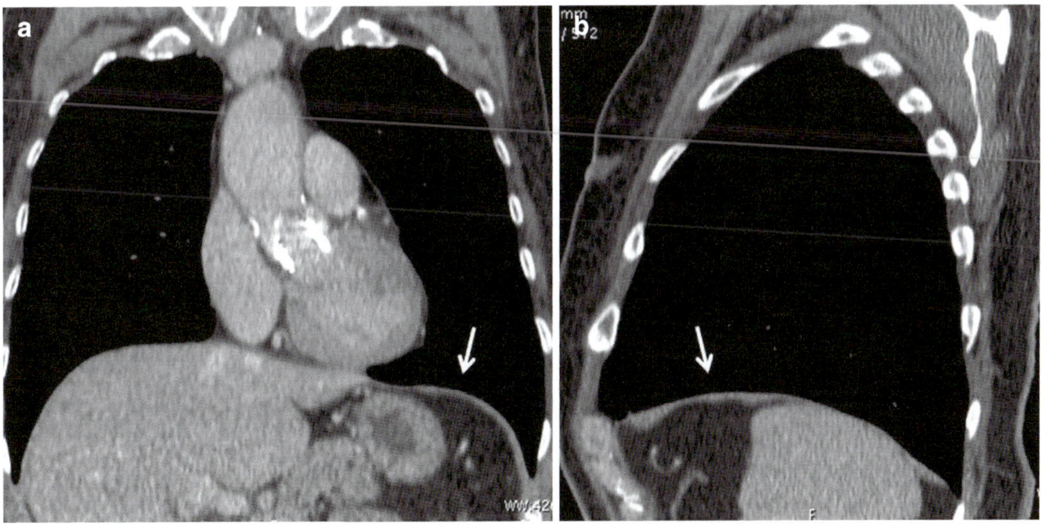

Fig. 12.2 Normal CT anatomy. Coronal (**a**) and sagittal (**b**) MPR images contribute to the evaluation of the diaphragmatic profile (*arrows*). Note the poor visualization of the muscle in the portions next to the liver and the spleen

12.1.2 Mechanism of Injury

The most common mechanisms of TDI include blunt and penetrating diaphragmatic trauma: the former results from considerable force and most often occur in high-energy vehicular impact, a fall from a height or a crushing blow; the latter is variable and largely dependent on the nature, velocity, and path of the weapon or projectile [1, 4].

The pattern of a blunt TDI is partially determined by the direction of impact. A lateral impact distorts and elongates anterior-posteriorly the chest wall, shears the stretched dome of the diaphragm, and results in avulsion of its peripheral attachment. A frontal impact leads to a sudden and abrupt increase of the abdominal pressure, with rise of the diaphragmatic gradient and transmission of force to the diaphragm through the abdominal viscera, resulting in a large rupture. In the context of a blunt thoracoabdominal trauma, the diaphragm may also be injured by fractured or fragmented ribs that penetrate the muscle [4, 8, 17, 18].

The penetrating thoracoabdominal wounds, at risk for a diaphragmatic involvement, generally occur anteriorly beneath the fourth intercostal space, laterally beneath the sixth intercostal space and posteriorly beneath the eighth intercostal space [19].

Once the diaphragmatic tear has occurred, the positive pressure gradient, that exists between the peritoneal and pleural spaces, induces abdominal viscera herniation into the thoracic cavity [20].

The mechanism of injury is also influenced by other important factors like the respiratory phase and the position of the patient at the time of the impact, preexistent and congenital alterations of the diaphragm, volume and fullness of abdominal viscera [19].

The knowledge of the mechanism of injury and of the circumstances of trauma, as well as imaging signs, represents an important contribution to the detection of TDIs and helps to avoid a misdiagnosis.

12.1.3 Patterns and Site of Injury

A blunt TDI is generally large, measuring 5–15 cm, and most often occurs in the posterolateral aspect of the muscle, with spread in a radial direction toward the central tendon, following the structurally weak area, corresponding to the embryologic origin of the pleuroperitoneal membrane. Other blunt ruptures of the diaphragm can occur in its central portion and at the costal attachment spreading in a transverse direction. The peripheral diaphragmatic detachment is the least frequent type of rupture observed at surgery (Fig. 12.3) [1, 3, 4, 17].

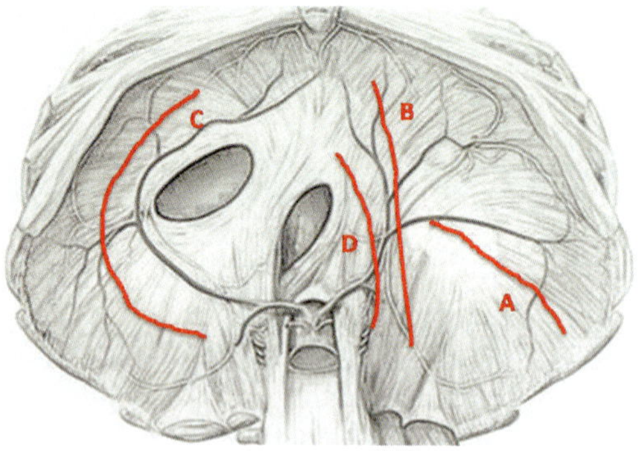

Fig. 12.3 A drawing showing sites and patterns of diaphragmatic injuries: radial (*A*), transverse (*B*), central (*C*) ruptures, and peripheral detachment (*D*)

A penetrating trauma, due to stab or gunshot wounds, causes a diaphragmatic injury along the trajectory of the weapon, so it is more variable in location and are usually shorter, measuring 1–4 cm, unless associated with blast injuries. These small defects may be easily missed on the initial MDCT (and even intraoperatively) unless deliberately sought for, especially when accompanied by other more threatening injuries [3, 4, 21]. A left-sided blunt diaphragmatic injury occurs three times more frequently than right-sided one, and this is due to multiple factors. First of all, the liver protects the right diaphragm preventing transmission of increased intra-abdominal pressure generated by the trauma and acting as a sort of buffer. Furthermore, the area between the lumbar and intercostal tendinous attachment represents a congenital structural weakness of the left diaphragm to which contributes the presence of the esophageal hiatus. The relative minority of right-sided injuries may also be associated with the missed diagnosis: indeed, a correct detection of right diaphragmatic lesions results more difficult because the radiologic signs may be subtle, the breach may be obscured by the liver and the herniation may be delayed or absent [1, 8, 20, 22, 23]. Even if an equal incidence of left- and right-sided TDIs is expected from penetrating trauma, the left injuries result to be predominant because most people are right handed [8].

12.1.4 Associated Injuries

The anatomic site of the diaphragm, its adjacency to thoracic and abdominal organs, and the severity of the trauma represent the reason why a blunt diaphragmatic trauma rarely occurs as an isolated lesion and results in a high percentage of associated life-threatening injuries (44–100% of patients) [1, 4, 8, 20]. The most common injuries, associated with a left-sided blunt TDI, involve the spleen, while liver lesions are more frequent with right-sided blunt diaphragmatic injuries. Rib fractures, pneumothorax, and pleural effusion are present in 90% of cases. Associated renal and aortic lesions and pelvic or spine fractures are less frequently encountered [1, 4, 8, 18, 24].

Emergency radiologists have to keep in mind the importance of suspecting a diaphragmatic rupture, especially in cases of high-energy trauma with multiple severe thoracoabdominal injuries.

Concerning penetrating trauma, the occurrence of associated injuries is variable and mainly dependent on the kind of weapon or projectile, on its velocity and trajectory [4, 18]. Anyway, it is fundamental to exclude a TDI before a chest tube placement (in example to drain a pneumothorax) in order to avoid iatrogenic perforations of the herniated viscera, especially in case of a left diaphragmatic rupture.

12.2 Imaging Evaluation and Findings

As previously mentioned, the role of imaging is to identify the abnormality as soon as possible to avoid acute or delayed severe complications that can result from a missed diagnosis. However, the radiologic interpretation is often difficult. The CXR is performed as initial screening study to evaluate the patient in the emergency room, but most radiographic features, concerning a TDI, are often subtle and nonspecific. The MDCT examination represents the second-level imaging necessary to stage a traumatized hemodynamically stable patient; particularly, it allows an accurate evaluation of the injuries, because of the higher quality of axial and MPR images compared to conventional single-slice CT, that showed a lower diagnostic accuracy for the TDI [7, 25–27].

12.2.1 X-Ray Signs

Despite its technical limitations, which include the supine positioning, the use of portable radiography, and the limited patient's cooperation, a CXR remains valuable as first radiological examination in the acute phase for the detection of a TDI [4]. It is generally performed only in the supine position and frequently it is acquired on the long spine board (LSB) in the shock room. For these reasons, the CXR has a relatively poor sensitivity and specificity, resulting normal or nonspecific in 20–50% of cases of a traumatic TDI, due to the high range of initially unrecognized injuries. Generally, the diagnosis or the suspicion of a left-sided injuries is easier (with detection sensitivity up to 60% of patients) than for right-sided injuries (18–33%) [8, 26, 28]. Indeed, a right TDI is more difficult to detect on CXR, as the liver blocks herniation of abdominal contents into the lower right side of the chest. Moreover, herniation of the liver is often overlooked and differentiation of a herniated liver through a TDI, from other causes of elevated diaphragm, such as atelectasis, pleural effusion, or pulmonary contusion or laceration, remains difficult [4].

The following two are the main radiographic findings that are specific of TDI:

- the presence of intrathoracic gastrointestinal air due to the herniation of abdominal viscera into the lower thorax (stomach, small bowel, or colon), with or without an associated focal

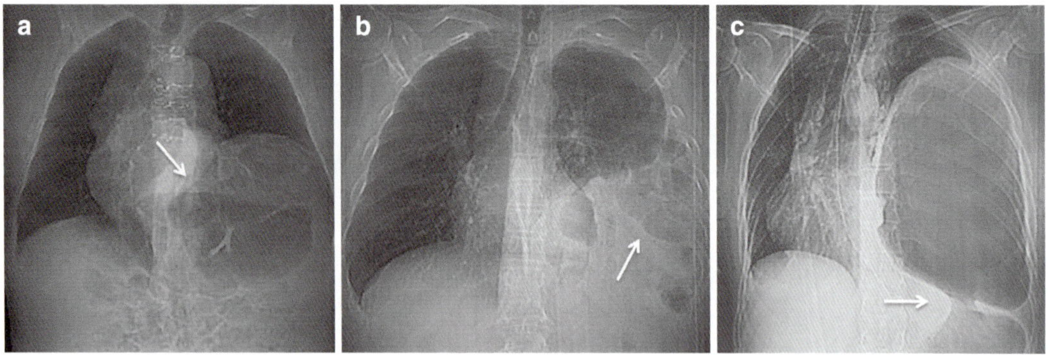

Fig. 12.4 Diaphragmatic rupture: specific CXR signs. Left diaphragmatic elevation associated to abdominal viscera above the diaphragm (*arrow* in **a**) and to the presence of intrathoracic gastrointestinal air (*arrow* in **b**). Left hemithorax mostly occupied by a gas-filled herniated stomach, associated with a focal constriction at the site of the diaphragmatic tear, indicative of collar sign (*arrow* in **c**)

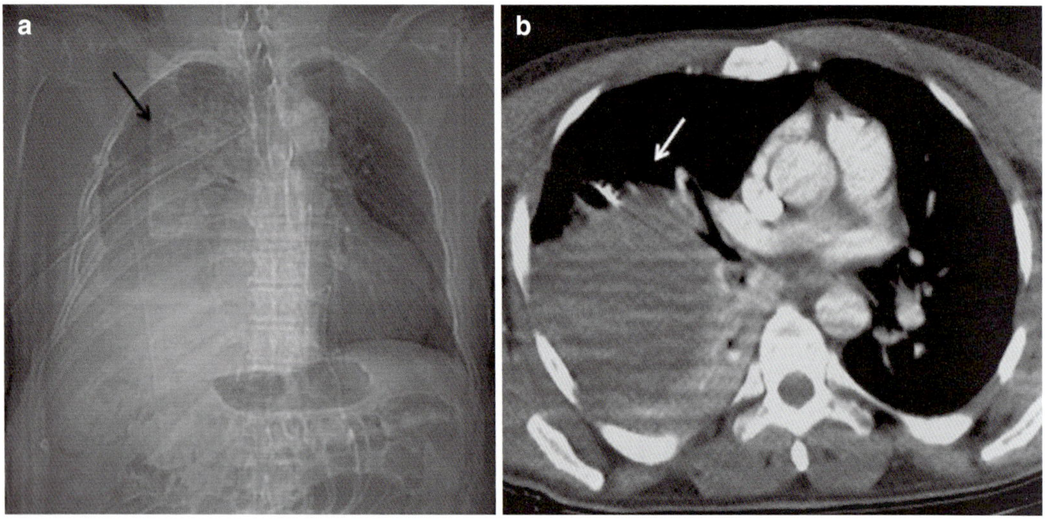

Fig. 12.5 Right diaphragmatic elevation with undefined diaphragmatic contour (*black arrow* in **a**), pulmonary atelectasis, and left mediastinal shift, consistent with right TDI and liver herniation, then confirmed by MDCT (*white arrow* in **b**). In this case, a right chest tube was improperly positioned, in shock room, to drain a pneumothorax, before having excluded a diaphragmatic rupture

constriction of the herniated mass at the site of the diaphragm tear, the so-called collar sign (Fig. 12.4)

- the visualization of the nasogastric tube above the left diaphragm, when stomach has herniated, with an abnormal U-shaped course [29]

Other common and suggestive, but nonspecific findings of TDI on CXR are:

- a diaphragmatic elevation (4–6 cm, or more, above the level of the contralateral diaphragm), especially when the right one is involved (Fig. 12.5)
- a contralateral mediastinal shift, toward the not affected side (Figs. 12.4 and 12.5)
- an obliteration or distortion of the diaphragmatic contour (Fig. 12.6)
- a pleural effusion (when the TDI develops a pleural effusion, the underlying diaphragmatic injury may be masked, particularly with small tears not associated with the herniation of abdominal content) [30]

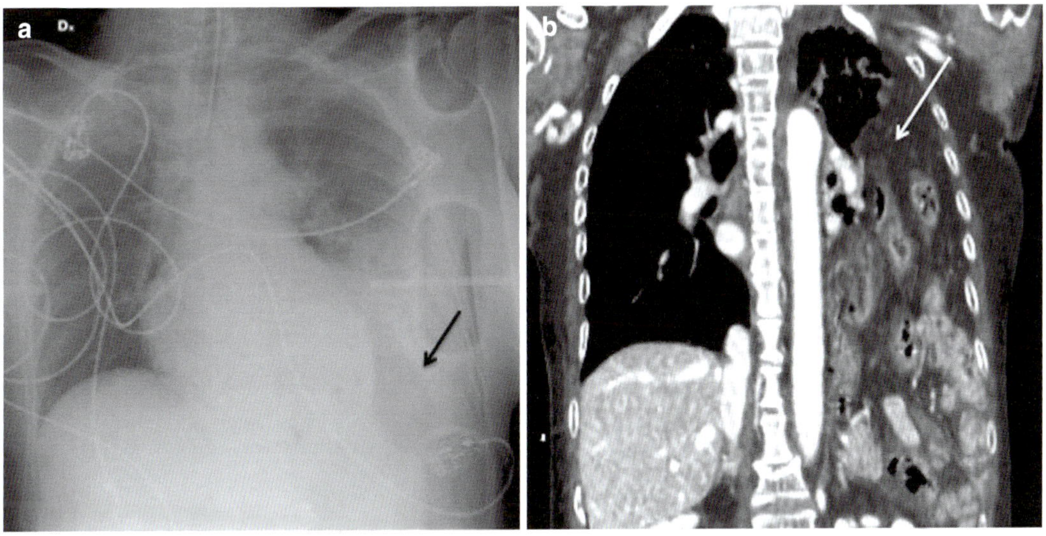

Fig. 12.6 Left diaphragmatic rupture. (**a**) Supine CXR on spinal board shows nonspecific signs: opacification of the left hemithorax base with lack of visualization of the left diaphragm (*black arrow*). (**b**) MDCT: a coronal MPR image clearly demonstrates the left diaphragmatic rupture with hollow abdominal viscera and mesenteric fat herniation (*white arrow*)

– an association with other traumatic thoracic injuries such as pneumothorax, pulmonary contusion, and multiple fractures of the ribs, spine, or both [11, 31]

It is important to underline how concurrent pulmonary abnormalities, related to the trauma, such as hemothorax, pulmonary contusion or laceration, atelectasis, and phrenic nerve palsy may mimic or mask a TDI on CXR. In addition, the positive pressure of ventilatory support may delay herniation of abdominal contents through a torn diaphragm. Therefore, the rate of a missed TDI on CXR ranges from 12 to 66%, with the potential risk of a late visceral herniation through the diaphragmatic defect. Anyway, in the presence of both specific and nonspecific CXR findings a MDCT examination is warranted in hemodynamically stable patients to confirm a TDI to assess potential associated injuries and to guide clinical management [1, 4].

12.2.2 CT Signs

The MDCT is nowadays considered the gold standard imaging study for the assessment of a TDI, with a specificity of 76–99% and a sensitivity of 61–100%, considerably higher if compared with the single-layer CT era [8, 10, 20, 32]. Indeed, the improvement of the MDCT technology, such as the use of multilayer scanners, with higher spatial resolution and speed, reduces artifacts and produces high quality MPR images, which are fundamental for diagnosis [33]. If a TDI is suspected, on a clinical and/or a radiographic basis, the hemodynamically stable patients should undergo a whole-body MDCT examination, whereas hemodynamically unstable patients (or patients with signs of acute peritonitis) must be directed to a surgical exploration as soon as possible [6, 20, 34]. The MDCT protocols vary depending upon the type of scanner available, the institution, and the patient's clinical conditions. Usually, a whole-body MDCT, with intravenous (IV) contrast is performed. In our emergency department, the MDCT examination is composed by three phases: a first non-enhanced phase, from the thoracic inlet through the symphysis pubis to appreciate hyperdense features (such as calcification or blood), an arterial phase (for which it is advisable to use high-flow IV contrast, by means of a power injector) to detect arterial lesion and a venous phase for visualization of parenchymal injuries. The arterial and portal venous scan can be acquired using, respectively, delays of 30 and 70 s, but, for the arterial phase, a bolus tracking or a smart prep technique is preferred. The images should have a thin collimation (2.5–3 mm) and they might afterwards be reconstructed at 0.625–1 mm for the interpretation and post-processing.

Several MDCT findings have been described over the years, which have been classified into three groups [10]: direct and indirect evidence of rupture; uncertain-controversial signs; and associated signs, according to Table 12.1. These signs are highly specific but the sensibility is lower because, in the setting of penetrating trauma, the herniation might be of small size and it might be overshadowed by more critical and severe traumatic injuries. The fundamental role of MDCT is to establish the best therapeutic management for patients with TDI giving clear indications to the emergency clinician and surgeon. As summarized in Table 12.2, the findings specific for a diaphragmatic rupture directly refer the patient to the operating room, while nonspecific findings need a radiological follow-up [8].

Table 12.1 Summary of the TDI findings, classified in three groups, according to their radiological meaning: direct evidence of diaphragmatic rupture, indirect signs hiding the presence of a diaphragmatic lesion, and uncertain/associated findings suspected for a diaphragmatic involvement

Direct signs
Discontinuity of diaphragmatic profile
Segmental non-visualization of diaphragm
Dangling sign
Indirect signs
Intrathoracic visceral herniation
Collar sign
Hump sign and band sign
Dependent viscera sign
Contiguous injury on either side of the diaphragm
Elevated abdominal organs
Signs of uncertain-controversial origin or associated signs
Thickening of the diaphragm
Hypoattenuated diaphragm
Fractured rib
Diaphragmatic/peridiaphragmatic contrast extravasation

Table 12.2 Management of the TDI

Specific findings		
Fat/abdominal viscera thoracic herniation	⇨	Surgery
Collar sign		
Dependent viscera sign		
Nonspecific findings		
Diaphragm thickening	⇨	X-ray/CT follow-up
Discontinuity of the diaphragmatic profile		
Segmental non-visualization of diaphragm		

When specific radiological findings are detectable, a surgical approach is warranted, as a TDI do not heal spontaneously. On the other side, when only nonspecific signs are present a radiological follow-up is indicated

Discontinuity of the diaphragmatic profile. It is the most frequent and important sign of a TDI since it represents the direct evidence of the tear of the musculotendinous component, which can be located both centrally and peripherally (Fig. 12.7). This sign is observed in almost 96% of all traumatic diaphragmatic hernia, and it is considered to be very significant since its sensitivity has been reported to be 58–82.7% and its specificity 88–95%. The free edges of the ruptured diaphragm are usually thickened by post-traumatic edema, hemorrhage, or muscle retraction [10, 20].

Segmental non-visualization of diaphragm. It is an isolated absence of a part of the diaphragm in the site of the injury. This sign has a sensitivity of 86% and a specificity of 68% since it may be falsely positive in elderly patients, in whom the non-visualization of a section of diaphragm might be a normal variant, or when the outline of the diaphragm is blurred due to retroperitoneal hematoma, hemothorax, pulmonary contusion, or atelectasis of pulmonary bases [20].

Dangling sign. This sign has been recently described for a large TDI. The free edges of the torn diaphragm are retracted and they curl inward toward the abdominal cavity, assuming the appearance of a comma-shaped fragment (Figs. 12.7 and 12.8). The dangling sign has a sensitivity of 54% and a specificity of 98% [35].

Intrathoracic visceral herniation. At the time of the TDI, the sharp increase of intra-abdominal

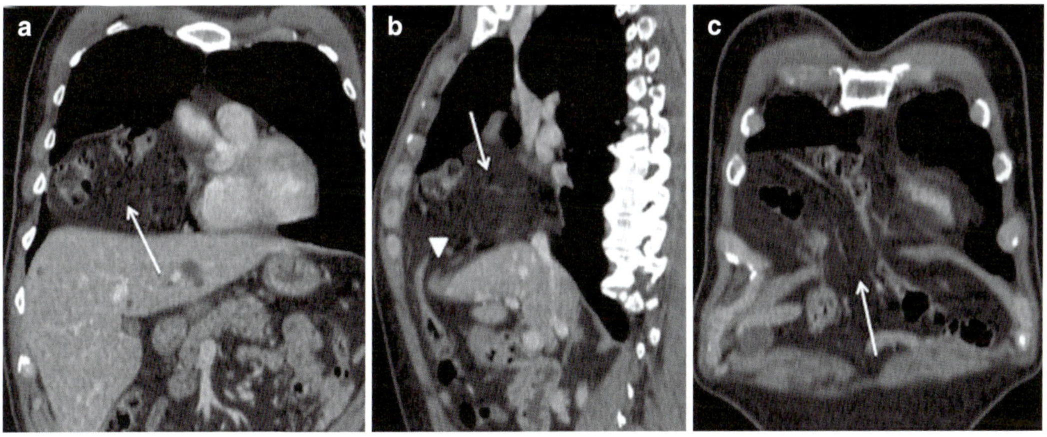

Fig. 12.7 Coronal (**a**, **c**) and sagittal (**b**) MPR images show right diaphragmatic rupture characterized by a large interruption of the muscle profile with concomitant intrathoracic herniation of fat, part of the colon, and small bowel (*arrows*). Sagittal MPR view shows also the dangling sign: the free edge of the diaphragm at the level of the traumatic tear bends outwards the abdominal cavity (*arrowhead*)

pressure and the negative intrathoracic pressure causes the abdominal viscera to herniate into the thoracic cavity. The thoracoabdominal pressure gradient, that develops after the acute phase, may also induce an enlargement of the diaphragmatic tear, facilitating the herniation of viscera. In case of a left diaphragmatic rupture, the most likely organs to herniate are the stomach, the colon, the omentum, and the retroperitoneal fatty tissue; rarely small bowel, spleen, and/or kidney migrate into the chest. On the other hand, in the right side, the most likely organs to herniate are the right colic flexure, the liver, the gallbladder, or even the small bowel (Figs. 12.7, 12.8, 12.9, and 12.10). This sign has a specificity of 94–100%, whereas its sensitivity is of 90.9%, if the TDI is on the left side (because hollow viscera are very well visible in the thoracic cavity), but it lowers to 8–81%, if the injury is on the right side. A visceral herniation might be absent in case of high intrathoracic pressure due to a hemothorax or a positive pressure ventilation. A very rare case of abdominal visceral migration into the chest is the intrapericardial herniation, which is caused by the tear of the central tendon of the diaphragm into the pericardium. It can be an acute or subacute complication following the trauma, or it can also occur after several years. It might cause cardiac luxation into the peritoneal cavity, acute/chronic cardiac tamponade, or symptoms related to the obstruction/strangulation of the herniated viscera [8, 10, 20, 36].

Collar sign. It is a waist-like area of constriction of the herniated viscera or omental fat at the level of the diaphragmatic defect. It usually concerns the stomach (Fig. 12.9) on the left side and the liver on the right side. It may be associated with a vascular compromise of the herniated abdominal organ. This sign has a high specificity (80–100%) but once again sensitivity is lower, especially for right-sided injuries (25–85%).

Hump sign and band sign. They are considered to be two variants of the collar sign in the right-sided injuries of the diaphragm, specifically in the herniation of the liver. The hump sign refers to a rounded portion of liver bulging through the diaphragm and forming a hump-shaped mass; it has a sensibility of 83% [8, 20]. The band sign, which has a lower sensitivity of 33%, is a linear lucency of low attenuation across the liver, especially on the liver dome, at the site of the diaphragmatic breech. It is thought to be due to hypo-perfusion of the liver parenchyma at the level of the narrow herniation caused by the compressive edge of the torn diaphragm [6, 7, 20].

Dependent viscera sign. This sign is caused by the herniated viscera that, in the supine position, are not more supported by the torn diaphragm and

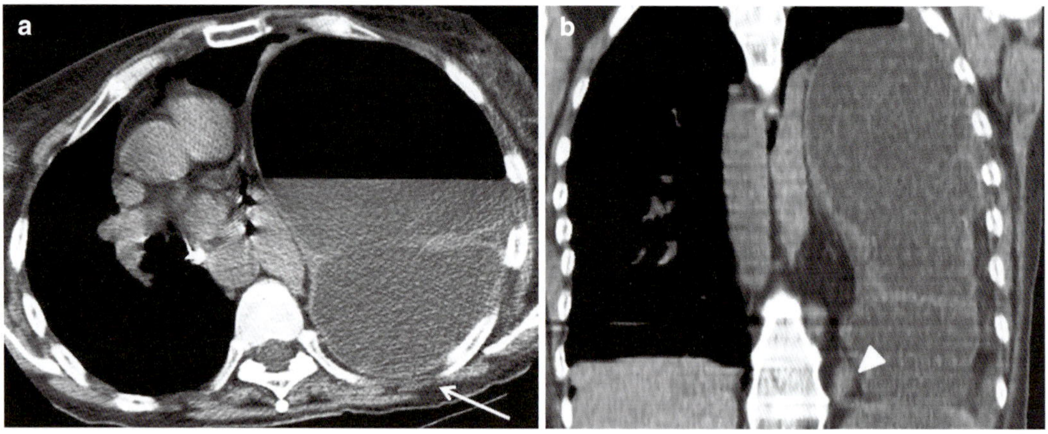

Fig. 12.8 The axial MDCT scan (**a**) and the coronal MPR image (**b**) show a left diaphragmatic rupture with herniated stomach that occupies most part of the thorax and lies on the posterior chest wall, in a declivous position, the so-called dependent viscera sign (*arrow* in **a**). In the coronal MPR image, it is appreciable also the dangling sign (*arrowhead*)

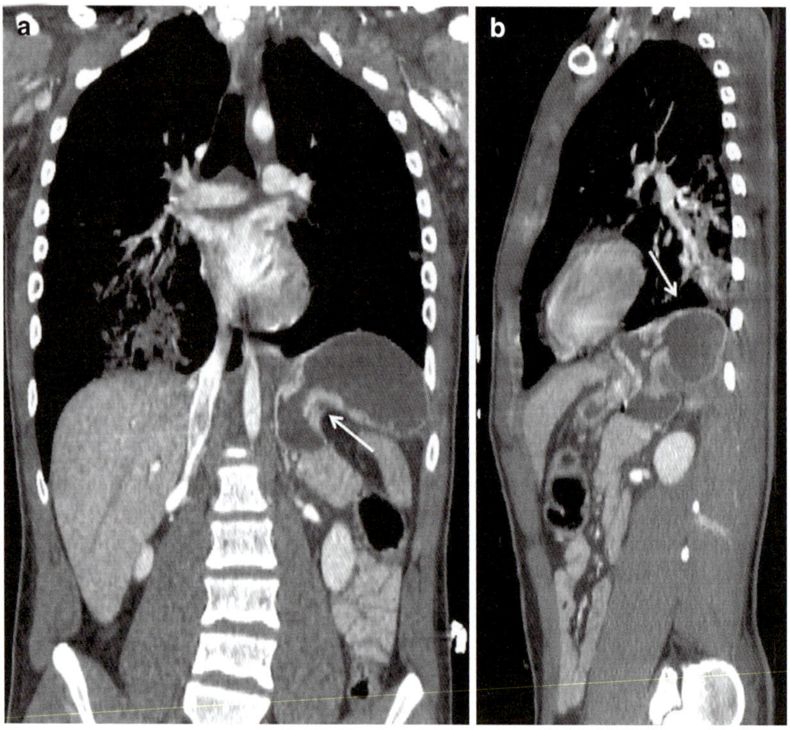

Fig. 12.9 Left diaphragmatic rupture. The coronal MPR image shows an area of constriction of the herniated stomach, the so-called collar sign (*arrow* in **a**); the sagittal MPR image also depicts the dependent viscera sign, represented by the stomach lying on the posterior chest wall (*arrow* in **b**)

they shift posteriorly, to lie in a "dependent" position, against the chest wall (Figs. 12.8, 12.9, and 12.10). This sign is usually associated with a wide diaphragmatic tear and has a sensitivity and a specificity, respectively, of 52–90% and 71–96% [20]. It involves the upper one-third of the liver, if the rupture is on the right side, whereas, if the tear is on the left, it interests the stomach, the spleen, or the bowel abutting the posterior ribs. It can also be bilateral in case of major trauma [8, 10, 37].

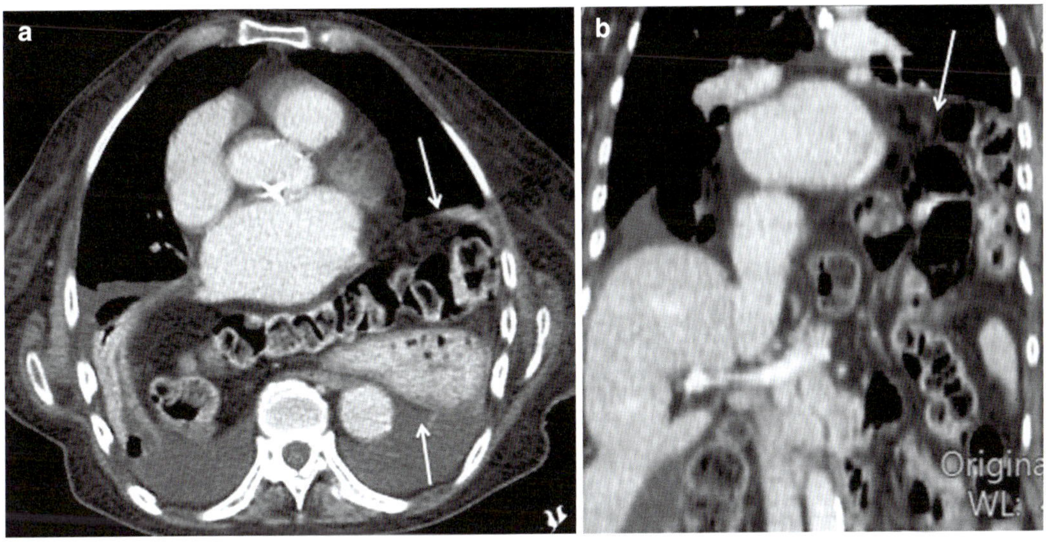

Fig. 12.10 Blunt left diaphragmatic rupture. Axial MDCT scan (**a**) and coronal MPR image (**b**): herniated colon, stomach, small bowel, and fat (*arrows*) are shifted posteriorly when the patient assumes the supine position in the scan, in a "dependent" position

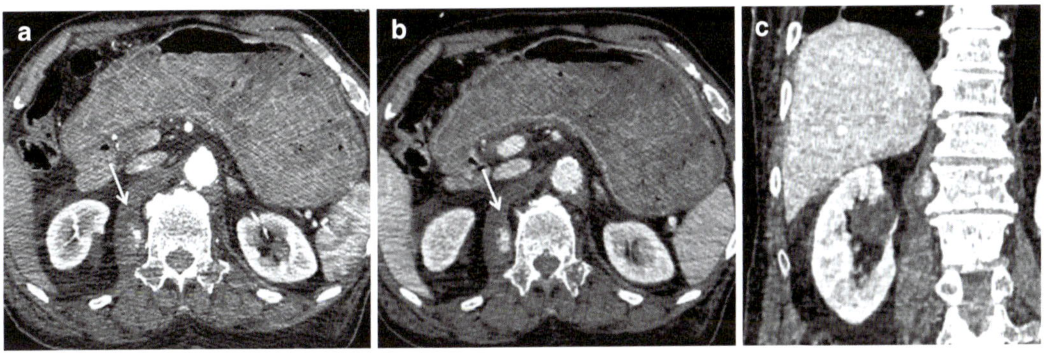

Fig. 12.11 Axial MDCT scan (**a**, **b**) and coronal MPR image (**c**) show a TDI characterized by a lacerocontusion of the right lumbar vertebral insertion: the right crura is thickened with active bleeding demonstrated by contrast medium extravasation in the arterial phase (*arrow* in **a**) that increases in the venous phase (*arrow* in **b**). The patient was treated with angiographic embolization

Elevated abdominal organs. They are considered to be abnormally elevated if the left-sided organs are 4 cm or more above the dome of the right diaphragm and if the right-sided viscera are 5 cm or more above the dome of the left diaphragm [10]. This sign is yet clear at the preliminary MDCT scout of view, and it is a good first predictor of a TDI, with a sensitivity and specificity of 78.1% and 92.8%, respectively.

Thickening of the diaphragm. It may be caused by the retraction of the tendinous insertions or by the edema and hemorrhagic infarction of the diaphragm, especially in its peripheral portion (Figs. 12.11, 12.12, 12.13, 12.14, and 12.15). Sensitivity and specificity have been showed to be, respectively, 36–60% and 58.4–77%, even if false-positive cases might be due to the presence of intra- or retroperitoneal hematoma. For a better evaluation of the thickening of the injured diaphragm, a comparison with the controlateral one should be done and the measurement should be taken at the same level on both side, 10 mm from the midline. However, this sign may be confusing since thickening of the diaphragmatic crus

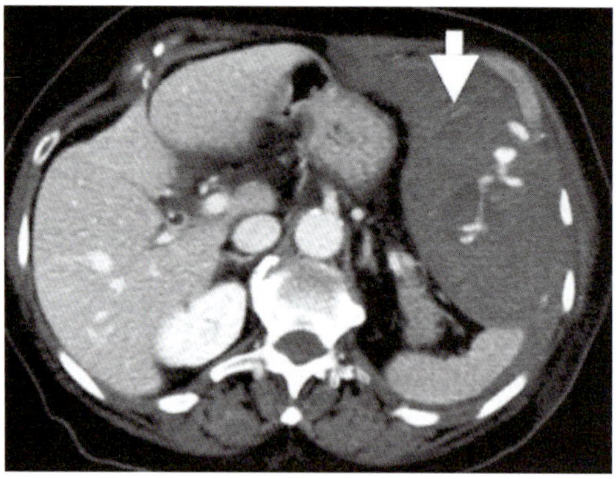

Fig. 12.12 Axial MDCT image shows a voluminous hematoma of the anterior-lateral costal part of the left diaphragm with contrast medium extravasation due to active arterial bleeding (*arrow*). Angiographic embolization was the treatment of choice

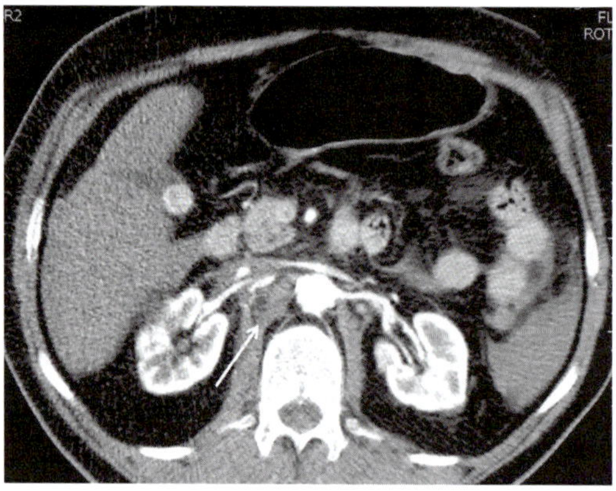

Fig. 12.13 Axial MDCT scan shows inhomogeneous thickening and hemorrhagic infiltration of the right crus and of perirenal fat tissue (surrounding right renal artery and vein) without arterial bleeding, consistent with a diaphragmatic contusion (*arrow*)

may vary in non-traumatic healthy patients accordingly to the age [10].

Hypoattenuated diaphragm. It is due to the hypo-perfusion of the diaphragmatic muscle, and it is considered to be associated to a TDI especially if there are others signs, such as rib fractures or thickening of the diaphragm; otherwise, on its own it has a poor sensitivity [10].

Contiguous injury on either side of the diaphragm. Tracing the pathway of a penetrating wound, the presence of contiguous injury on either side of the diaphragm is considered an indirect but highly specific sign of a penetrating TDI. Patients suffering from penetrating trauma should be carefully evaluated looking for organ laceration, blood, and gas along the trajectory of the injury (Figs. 12.16 and 12.17).

12.2.3 Diagnostic Pitfalls

False-negative findings. Hemothorax, pulmonary contusion, and atelectasis are common findings in polytrauma patients and can mask a TDI, especially on CXR. It is frequently difficult to identify the margins of the diaphragm, following thoracic trauma, because of pleural effusion, particularly in small tears and in the absence of herniation of abdominal viscera. In addition, the types of diaphragmatic tears due to blunt trauma are not correlated with the sensitivity of CT for detection of diaphragmatic rupture.

False-positive findings. Some conditions can simulate TDI at MDCT evaluation, like congenital

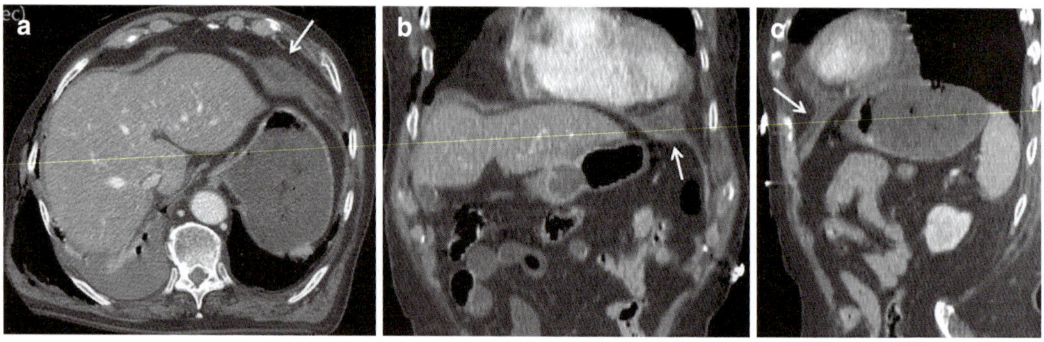

Fig. 12.14 Axial MDCT image (**a**), coronal (**b**), and sagittal MPR images (**c**): thickening of the left anterior part of the costal diaphragm caused by contusion and edema (*arrows*)

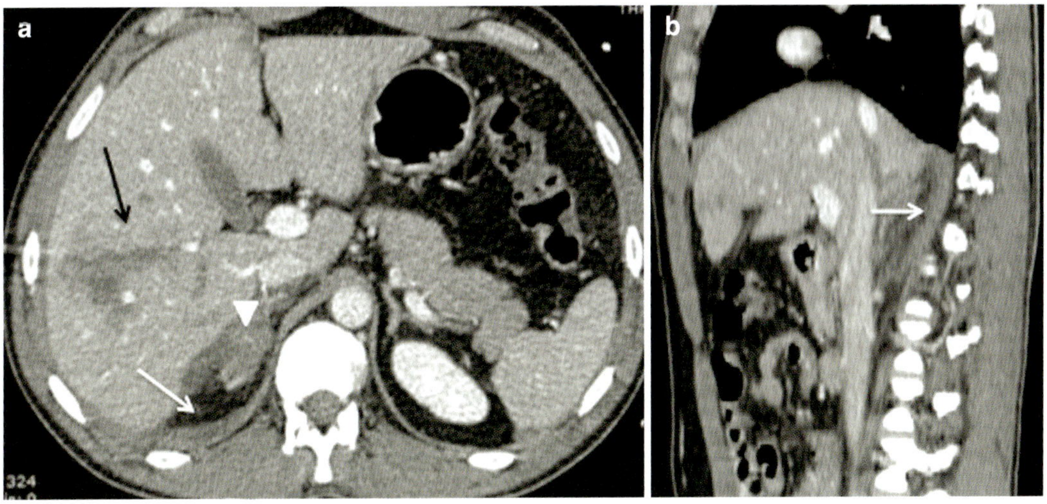

Fig. 12.15 Axial MDCT scan (**a**) and sagittal MPR image (**b**): hepatic laceration (*black arrow*) associated to right adrenal contusion (*arrowhead*) and right posterior costal diaphragmatic thickening, caused by contusion (*white arrows*)

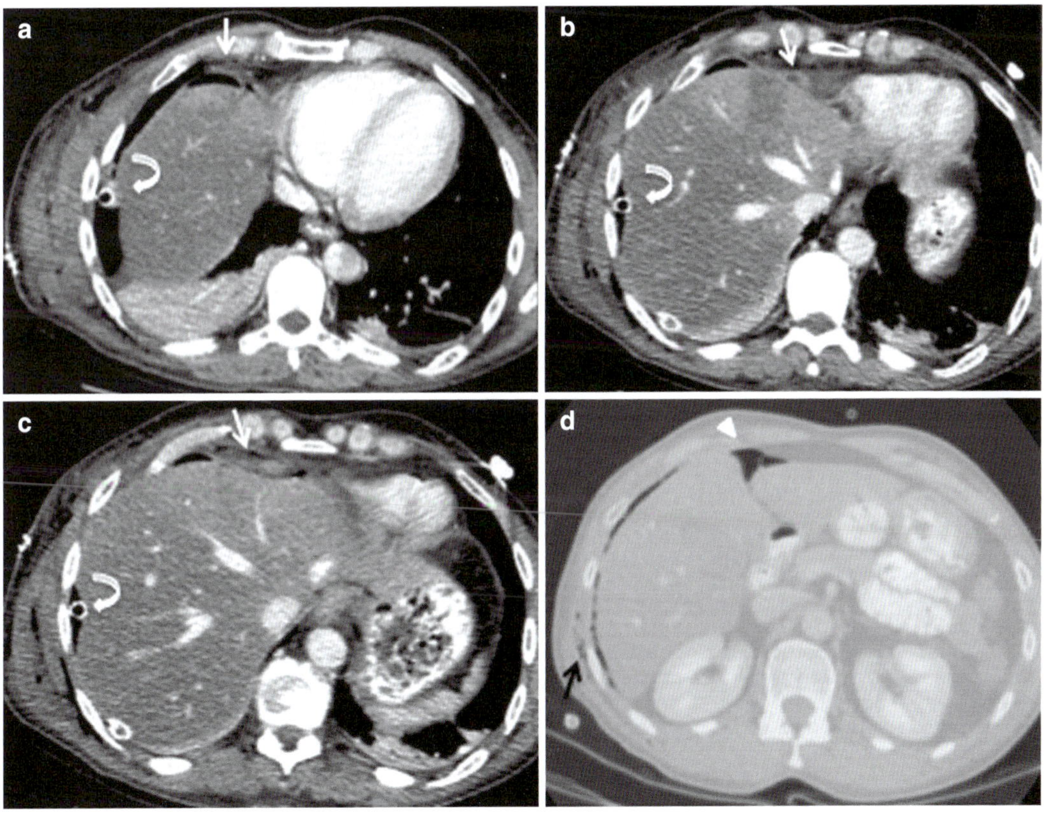

Fig. 12.16 (**a–c**) Axial MDCT scans show a right anterior diaphragmatic injury (*white arrows*) due to a penetrating wound, caused by a knife, associated with a right thoracic wall subcutaneous emphysema (*black arrow*) and pneumothorax drained by a chest tube (*curved arrows*). (**d**) The lung window of the axial scan displays free abdominal gas adjacent to the liver and just beneath the diaphragm, confirming the presence of a diaphragmatic laceration (*arrowhead*)

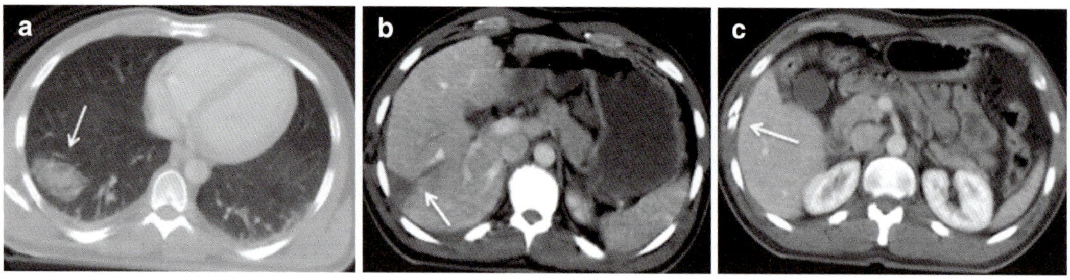

Fig. 12.17 Axial MDCT scans of a patient injured by a knife shows contiguous lesions on both side of the diaphragm: pulmonary laceration (*arrow* in **a**), hepatic contusion (*arrow* in **b**), and rib fracture (*arrow* in **c**). These are indirect but specific signs of a right diaphragmatic penetrating injury

or acquired diaphragmatic abnormalities including congenital hernias, acquired diaphragmatic defect and diaphragmatic eventration. The most common type of congenital diaphragmatic hernia is the Bochdalek hernia, which occurs more commonly on the left side, in correspondence of posterolateral diaphragmatic defects, where the pleuroperitoneal membranes fuse. This kind of hernia is detected on MDCT in approximately 6% of asymptomatic adults, it is generally small and contains fat. Sometimes, they can be larger containing also abdominal organs. Another common type of congenital hernia is the Morgagni hernia, which results from a congenital defect of the anteromedial part of the diaphragm, the sternocostal triangle [38]. An acquired diaphragmatic defect is a discontinuity that can be found in any region of the diaphragm, but results to be most often located in its posterior aspect or at the crura. It is seen more commonly in elderly women with emphysema [15, 39]. Finally, the term diaphragmatic eventration refers to an abnormal area of diaphragmatic relaxation and elevation, generally affecting the left side, that consists of a thinned but intact portion of the diaphragm (Fig. 12.18). It's generally a congenital condition, but sometimes injuries to the phrenic nerve, with subsequent paresis or paralysis of the left or right diaphragm, can cause a diaphragmatic eventration. Coronal and sagittal MPR images are helpful to avoid false-positive diagnosis of TDI and to identify the site of injury. Motion artifacts due to respiratory movement decrease the quality of MPR images and can mimic a diaphragmatic rupture, especially on the right side with pseudoherniation of the liver.

12.2.4 Role of MRI

It is not the imaging study normally performed for the evaluation of a TDI in the acute trauma setting, but it can be helpful in selected cases, such as uncertain CT diagnosis or delayed signs of TDI. In addition to its intrinsic high contrast resolution, it can be useful to optimally visualize the entire profile of the diaphragm also thanks to respiratory and cardiac gating and to the coronal and sagittal planes of acquisition [40].

T1-weighted and gradient-echo sequences display the normal diaphragm as a continuous hypointense band. Injuries are so seen as defects in the low signal intensity diaphragm, as interruption of the diaphragmatic signal, associated with visualization of abdominal viscera or omentum through the diaphragm tear (characterized by relative hyperintensity); so T1-weighted sequences are considered by some authors the most important, eventually associated with gadolinium injection and fat-sat sequences [41].

Nevertheless, the high quality of current MDCT scanners has significantly reduced the necessity of using MRI in clinical practice.

12.3 Natural History, Complications, and Mortality

According to the classification originally proposed by Carter et al., the natural history of a TDI can be divided into three main stages [20, 42].

The "*acute phase*" (within 14 days) is the period immediately following the traumatic event, and the diagnosis of TDI is frequently missed, especially if shock, respiratory insufficiency, mechanical ventilation, severe visceral injuries, and coma are present [43]. Acute mortality in patients with TDI is entirely dependent on associated injuries and rarely on the diaphragmatic involvement itself. This is the reason why more severe lesions may overshadow a TDI and why it is important to have a high index of suspicion. The need for a radiographic follow-up is emphasized to detect a TDI at an earlier stage [44].

In case of undiagnosed injury or not repairing lesions, begin the so-called *latent phase*, which ranges from a few days to tens of years; it is characterized by nonspecific and heterogeneous symptoms such as dyspnea, orthopnea, abdominal cramps, and decreased breathing sounds [43]. Usually, the "*latent phase*" is diagnosed through clinical and instrumental examinations performed for other purposes, often after several years of injury [20]. Sometimes, a TDI is diagnosed on CXR at the end of the mechanical ventilation in the intensive care unit.

With time, a missed diaphragmatic defect may enlarge and coupled with the gradient between the negative intrathoracic pressure and positive intra-abdominal pressure and may result in a subsequent herniation of intra-abdominal contents into the chest. The stomach is the organ with the highest rate of involvement (48%), followed by the spleen (26%), and the small bowel, large bowel, and omentum (13%). Although less frequent, there are right diaphragmatic ruptures with the herniation of the liver [45].

The "*obstructive phase*" is represented by the dramatic evolution of the "*latent phase.*" It is generally characterized by a massive herniation of the abdominal organs into the thoracic cavity with mediastinal "shift" and cardiorespiratory impairment. This event may be associated with ischemia and/or perforation of the herniated organs. The clinical evolution is associated to significant increase in morbidity (30–80% of cases) [20]. High mortality has been reported if patients have strangulated viscera in chronic traumatic TDI (30%) [46].

12.4 Treatment

Timely diagnosis and correct identification of a TDI and any associated lesions are essential for proper clinical management and surgical treatment [47].

Surgical repair is the standard management of TDI and should be applied as soon as the diagnosis is confirmed in order to limit expansion of the traumatic tear to prevent or reduce herniation of intrathoracic abdominal viscera and to avoid late complications.

Two principles must be observed when repairing acute traumatic diaphragmatic hernias: complete reduction of the herniated organs back into the abdomen and watertight closure of the diaphragm to avoid recurrence [45].

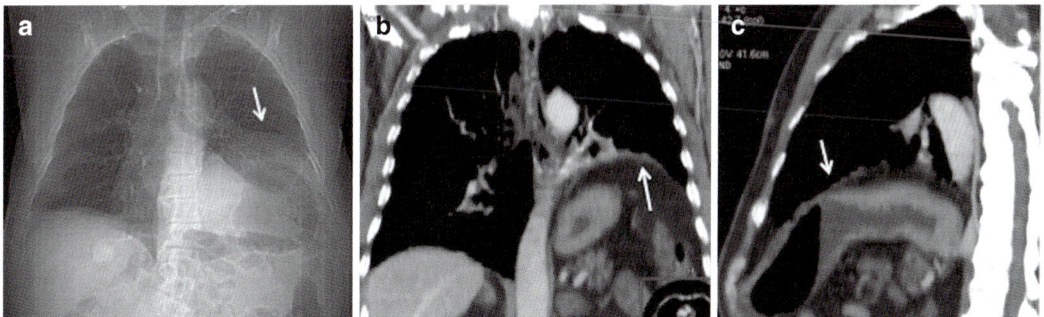

Fig. 12.18 (**a**) Chest X-ray, (**b**) coronal, and (**c**) sagittal MPR images show: elevation of the left diaphragm that is thinned but intact (*arrows*); no dependent viscera sign or collar sign is depicted. These radiological findings are consistent with a diaphragmatic eventration

The choice for surgical approach is controversial, being possible both an abdominal and a thoracic approach. It is closely related to patient's hemodynamic status, associated injuries. and surgeon's experience [48].

According to Lesquen e al., three patterns can be described for surgical indications in the first 48 h:

- Traumatic TDI in unstable patients with abdominal associated injury: laparatomy is mandatory, offering the opportunity to repair diaphragmatic tears and associated lesions at the same time.
- Traumatic TDI in stable patients without abdominal associated injuries: thoracotomy should be performed. As alternative, mini invasive approach like video-assisted thoracoscopic surgery (VATS) could be proposed.
- Traumatic TDI suspected in stable patients without thoracic or abdominal injury: VATS or laparoscopy is required for diagnosis and treatment [48]. Indeed, there are reports of the use of laparoscopy for the diagnosis of TDI in the setting of acute trauma, when intra-abdominal injuries are suspected but not found with noninvasive imaging modalities [41, 48].

However, chronic traumatic diaphragmatic herniation is somewhat different from the acute injury. It induces intense fibrosis and severe adhesion, which leads to difficulty in the reduction of the herniated viscera and repair of the diaphragmatic defect [49].

In the majority of cases, repair is successfully accomplished using either interrupted or continuous non-adsorbable sutures with or without mesh reinforcement; in fact, large defect can be bridged by synthetic mesh and recurrence after repair is uncommon [50].

References

1. Desir A, Ghaye B. CT of blunt diaphragmatic rupture. Radiographics. 2012;32:477–98.
2. Nchimi A, Szapiro D, et al. Injuries of the diaphragm. In: Dondelinger RF, editor. Imaging and intervention in abdominal trauma. Berlin: Springer; 2004. p. 205–36.
3. Panda A, Kumar A, et al. Traumatic diaphragmatic injury: a review of CT signs and the difference between blunt and penetrating injury. Diagn Interv Radiol. 2014;20:121–8.
4. Iochum S, Ludig T, et al. Imaging of diaphragmatic injury: a diagnostic challenge? Radiographics. 2002;22:S103–18.
5. Nchimi A, Szapiro D, et al. Helical CT of blunt diaphragmatic rupture. AJR Am J Roentgenol. 2005;184(1):24–30.
6. Dreizin D, Bergquist PJ, et al. Evolving concepts in MDCT diagnosis of penetrating diaphragmatic injury. Emerg Radiol. 2015;22:149–56.
7. Rees O, Mirvis SE, et al. Multidetector-row CT of right hemidiaphragmatic rupture caused by blunt trauma: a review of 12 cases. Clin Radiol. 2005;60(12):1280–9.
8. Mirvis SE, Shanmuganathan K. Imaging hemidiaphragmatic injury. Eur Radiol. 2007;17:1411–21.
9. Como JJ, Bokhari F, et al. Practice management guidelines for selective non operative management of penetrating abdominal trauma. J Trauma. 2010;68:721–33.
10. Kaur R, Prabhakar A, et al. Blunt traumatic diaphragmatic hernia: pictorial review of CT signs. Indian J Radiol Imaging. 2015;25:226–32.
11. Shackleton KL, Stewart ET, et al. Traumatic diaphragmatic injuries: spectrum of radiographic findings. Radiographics. 1998;18:49–59.
12. Nason LK, Walker CM, et al. Imaging of the diaphragm: anatomy and function. Radiographics. 2012;32:E51–70.
13. Chavhan GB, Babyn PS, et al. Multimodalityimaging of the pediatric diaphragm: anatomy and pathologic conditions. Radiographics. 2010;30:1797–817.
14. Scaglione M, Grassi R, et al. Delayed presentation of traumatic left-sided diaphragmatic avulsion. A case report. Acta Radiol. 2000;41:165–6.
15. Restrepo CS, Eraso A, et al. The diaphragmatic crura and retrocrural space: normal imaging appearance, variants, and pathologic conditions. Radiographics. 2008;28(5):1289–305.
16. Schumpelick V, Steinau G, et al. Surgical embryology and anatomy of the diaphragm with surgical applications. Surg Clin North Am. 2000;80(1):213–39, xi.
17. Sangster G, Ventura Pietro V, et al. Diaphragmatic rupture: a frequently missed injury in blunt thoracoabdominal trauma patients. Emerg Radiol. 2007;13:225–30.
18. Shanmuganathan K, Killeen K, et al. Imaging of diaphragmatic injuries. J Thorac Imaging. 2000;15(2):104–11.
19. Volterrani L, Mazzei MA, et al. Parete toracica e diaframma. In: Miele V, Scaglione M, et al., editors. Diagnostica per immagini nel trauma maggiore. Milan, Italy: Elsevier Masson; 2010. p. 121–8.
20. Bocchini G, Guida F, et al. Diaphragmatic injuries after blunt trauma: are they still a challenge? Emerg Radiol. 2012;19:225–35.

21. Bodanapally UK, Shanmuganathan K, et al. MDCT diagnosis of penetrating diaphragm injury. Eur Radiol. 2009;19:1875–81.
22. Sliker CW. Imaging of diaphragm injuries. Radiol Clin N Am. 2006;44:199–211, vii.
23. Chen HW, Wong YC, et al. Computed tomography in left-sided and right-sided blunt diaphragmatic rupture: experience with 43 patients. Clin Radiol. 2010;65(3):206–12.
24. Reiff DA, McGwin G Jr, et al. Identifying injuries and motor vehicle collision characteristics that together are suggestive of diaphragmatic rupture. J Trauma. 2002;53(6):1139–45.
25. Tresallet C, Menegaux F, et al. Usefulness of CT reconstructed pictures for diaphragmatic rupture after blunt trauma. J Am Coll Surg. 2004;198:666–7.
26. Gelman R, Mirvis SE, et al. Diaphragmatic rupture due to blunt trauma: sensitivity of plain chest radiographs. AJR Am J Roentgenol. 1991;156:51–7.
27. Demos TC, Solomon C, et al. Computed tomography in traumatic defects of the diaphragm. Clin Imaging. 1989;13:62–7.
28. Shanmuganathan K, Mirvis SE. Imaging diagnosis of nonaortic thoracic injury. Radiol Clin N Am. 1999;37:533–51.
29. Perlman SJ, Rogers LF, et al. Abnormal course of nasogastric tube in traumatic rupture of left hemidiaphragm. AJR Am J Roentgenol. 1984;142(1):85–8.
30. Gavelli G, Canini R, et al. Traumatic injuries: imaging of thoracic injuries. Eur Radiol. 2002;12(6):1273–94.
31. Pikoulis E, Delis S, et al. Reliability of initial chest radiographs in the diagnosis of blunt diaphragmatic rupture. Ann Chir Gynaecol. 2000;89(1):10–3.
32. Scaglione M, Pinto F, et al. CT assessment of blunt diaphragmatic injury. A retrospective study on 35 cases. Radiol Med. 2000;99:46–50.
33. Larici AR, Gotway MB, et al. Helical CT with sagittal and coronal reconstructions: accuracy for detection of diaphragmatic injury. AJR. 2002;179:451–7.
34. Hammer MM, Flagg E, et al. Computed tomography of blunt and penetrating diaphragmatic injury: sensitivity and inter-observer agreement of CT signs. Emerg Radiol. 2014;21:143–9.
35. Desser TS, Edwards B, et al. The dangling diaphragm sign: sensitivity and comparison with existing CT signs of blunt traumatic diaphragmatic rupture. Emerg Radiol. 2010;17:37–44.
36. Tonerini M. Urgenze dell'esofago e del diaframma. Radiol Med. 2010;115(Suppl):75–80.
37. Bergin D, Ennis R, et al. The "dependent viscera" sign in CT diagnosis of blunt traumatic diaphragmatic rupture. AJR. 2001;177:1137–40.
38. Panicek DM, Benson CB, et al. The diaphragm: anatomic, pathologic, and radiologic considerations. Radiographics. 1988;8(3):385–425.
39. Caskey CI, Zerhouni EA, et al. Aging of the diaphragm: a CT study. Radiology. 1989;171(2):385–9.
40. Barbiera F, Nicastro N, et al. The role of MRI in traumatic rupture of the diaphragm. Our experience in three cases and review of the literature. Radiol Med (Torino). 2003;105:188–94.
41. Eren S, Kantarci M, et al. Imaging of diaphragmatic rupture after trauma. Clin Radiol. 2006;61:467–77.
42. Lu J, et al. Delayed traumatic diaphragmatic hernia. A case-series report and literature review. Medicine. 2016;95(32):e4362.
43. Shah R, et al. Traumatic rupture of diaphragm. Ann Thorac Surg. 1995;60(5):1444–9.
44. Crandall M, et al. Post traumatic hernias: historical overview and review of the literature. Am Surg. 2007;73(9):845–50.
45. Hanna WC, et al. Acute traumatic diaphragmatic injury. Thorac Surg Clin. 2009;19(4):485–9.
46. Liao CH, Chu CH, et al. The feasibility and efficacy of laparoscopic repair for chronic traumatic diaphragmatic herniation: introduction of a novel technique with literature review. Hernia. 2015;20(2):303–9.
47. Thiam O, Konate I, et al. Traumatic diaphragmatic injuries: epidemiological, diagnostic and therapeutic aspects. SpringerPlus. 2016;5:1614.
48. De Lesquen H, Avaro JP, et al. Surgical management for the first 48 h following blunt chest trauma state of the art (excluding vascular injuries). Interact Cardiovasc Thorac Surg. 2014;20(3):399–408.
49. Yildar M, Yaman I, et al. Laparoscopic repair in simultaneous occurrence of recurrent chronic traumatic diaphragmatic hernia and transdiaphragmatic intercostal hernia. Arq Bras Cir Dig. 2015;28(1):90–2.
50. Safdar G, Slater R et al. Laparoscopically assisted repair of an acute traumatic diaphragmatic hernia. BMJ Case Rep. 2013. pii: bcr2013009415.

Thoracic Trauma: Interventional Radiology

13

Gianpaolo Carrafiello, Chiara Floridi,
Francesca Patella, Francesco Morelli,
Filippo Pesapane, and Matteo Crippa

13.1 Introduction

Polytrauma is a leading cause of death and disability worldwide; the major cause is road traffic collisions but other causes exist such as workplace and battlefield injuries [1, 2].

Thoracic injuries both blunt and penetrating mechanisms account for approximately one quarter of deaths due to trauma and contribute to 25–50% of the remaining deaths [3, 4]. Trauma to the thorax is responsible for 20–25% of all motor collision-related deaths, and the thorax is the third most common site of traumatic injury after the head and extremities [5]. Trauma patients are at risk for shock, coagulopathy, acidosis, and multi-organ system failure: their treatment is a race against time and most patients with thoracic trauma die at the crash scene [6]. Among those who survive the traumatic event, aortic injury is usually lethal if left untreated although 70% of patients survive with intervention [7]. In the absence of aortic injury, thoracic trauma may usually be managed with appropriate life support and monitoring [8].

The increased prevalence of penetrating chest injury and improved prehospital and perioperative care have resulted in an increasing number of critically injured but potentially salvageable patients presenting to trauma centers [9]. Moreover, a rapid recovery and mobility will allow patients to resume work and other activities thus resulting in a reduced overall cost to the social and healthcare systems.

In the last decades, there has been an acknowledged improvement in trauma care, and there are constant ongoing developments, especially there has been a growing role for both diagnostic and interventional radiology (IR) in all types of trauma affecting different areas of the body, thorax included, with imaging becoming an integral part of the multidisciplinary approach to modern trauma care [10].

Computed tomography (CT) has sensitivity as high as 98% for depiction of aortic injury [11]. Injuries range from subtle intimal damage to active extravasation, with the latter rarely seen

G. Carrafiello (✉)
Diagnostic and Interventional Radiology Department, San Paolo Hospital, Università degli Studi di Milano, Milan, Italy
e-mail: gcarraf@gmail.com

C. Floridi
Diagnostic and Interventional Radiology Department, Fatebenefratelli Hospital, Milan, Italy

F. Patella • F. Morelli • F. Pesapane
Postgraduation School in Radiodiagnostics, Diagnostic and Interventional Radiology Department, San Paolo Hospital, Università degli Studi di Milano, Milan, Italy

M. Crippa
Vascular Surgery Department, San Paolo Hospital, Università degli Studi di Milano, Milan, Italy

V. Miele, M. Trinci (eds.), *Diagnostic Imaging in Polytrauma Patients*,
https://doi.org/10.1007/978-3-319-62054-1_13

because of its high lethality [6]. Dissection, seen as intimal flaps, is often present in conjunction with pseudoaneurysm, whose appearance varies from an eccentric irregular outpouching of contrast material to a sudden change in caliber that is sometimes referred to as pseudocoarctation [12]. Endovascular intervention (EVI) has emerged as the preferred treatment in patients with such injuries. The multisciplinar team (MT) decision to perform EVI rather than conventional surgical repair is typically made on the basis of CT angiographic findings [12].

Among the MT, interventional radiologists are ideally qualified to play an important role in the management of thoracic trauma patients [13]. Aside from their specialized training in the delivery of transcatheter therapies, IRs receive broad-based multimodality imaging training, which renders them highly capable of correlating findings from preprocedural imaging studies to speed diagnosis and treatment of trauma patients in the emergency setting [14].

Aortic injury may be safely excluded if no luminal or mural abnormality is seen, irrespective of the presence of mediastinal hematoma [15]. When it abuts the aorta, hematoma may result from injury to the vasa vasorum, and when it is isolated to the anterior or posterior mediastinum, it likely is related to sternal or spinal injuries [16]. No treatment or further imaging is needed in either case; however, attention should be paid to the great vessels because periarterial hematoma in the superior mediastinum may be a sign of a great vessel injury [16].

Rupture of the hilar pulmonary arteries may result in brisk extravasation with massive hemothorax, respiratory compromise, and exsanguination [17]. The pulmonary trunk and the anterior aspect of the intrathoracic IVC are intrapericardial structures, and injury to these regions will likely lead to hemopericardium. The ensuing rapid increases in intrapericardial pressure that result from bleeding into an intact pericardium cause cardiac tamponade and hemodynamic compromise.

Although the primary role of whole-body CT angiography in patients with chest trauma is to identify or exclude the presence of aortic or other types of major vascular injury, important nonvascular injuries may also be identified. In elderly patients, even a solitary rib fracture may lead to pulmonary insufficiency requiring prolonged periods of mechanical ventilation [18]. CT is able to depict large pneumothoraces that require immediate chest tube insertion [18]. However, detection of small pneumothoraces is also important because their size may increase in patients who are intubated [19]. Although parenchymal lung injuries such as contusion and laceration are typically treated conservatively, early diagnosis is important because these injuries may contribute to respiratory failure [18]. Diaphragmatic injuries are uncommon in patients with chest trauma but also in this case an early diagnosis is essential to prevent herniation and strangulation of abdominal contents [18, 19].

In conclusion, thoracic trauma patients need to be rapidly and accurately assessed to determine the nature of their injuries with treatments prioritized by injury severity [11].

13.2 Blunt Traumatic Aortic Injuries

13.2.1 Introduction

Blunt traumatic aortic injury (BTAI) is the second most common cause of death after blunt trauma among patients with major traumatic injuries although it accounts for 1% of adult admissions to level I trauma centers [20].

Indeed, an estimated 80–90% of all victims die at the scene of the accident [20]. The prognosis for patients who survive the initial injury remains poor: nearly 30% will die within the first 6 h, and 50% of these patients will not live beyond the first 24 h after the injury [20].

The affected population is generally young with an average age of 40 years [21].

The classic injury mechanism of blunt thoracic aorta is related to the combination of sudden deceleration and traction on the inner curvature of the arch at the ligamentum arteriosum, which represents the junction between the relatively mobile aortic arch and the fixed descending aorta. Thus, the isthmus is the most common location for rupture (50–70%), followed by the ascending aorta or aortic arch (18%) and the distal thoracic aorta (14%) [22].

Given the location of injury, conventional surgical repair typically involves a high posterolateral thoracotomy with or without cardiopulmonary bypass, aortic cross clamping, and significant blood loss, which can negatively impact the status of the patient. Historically, open repair of traumatic aortic injuries has been associated with a 28% mortality rate [23] and a 16% paraplegia rate [24]. There has been a risk of delayed rupture in the unrepaired thoracic transection that has been estimated to be 2–5% [25].

Thoracic endovascular aortic repair (TEVAR) is a rapidly evolving alternative therapy in the treatment of a variety of thoracic aortic pathologies, consisting in placing an endovascular stent graft into the thoracic aorta from a remote peripheral location under imaging guidance.

To date, no randomized controlled trials have sought to determine whether use of TEVAR for treatment of BTAI is associated with reduced mortality and morbidity when compared with conventional open surgery [26]. However, clinicians are moving forward with EI of BTAI on the basis of a number of meta-analyses and large clinical series, which assessed that TEVAR is a safe and effective procedure for patients with traumatic aortic injuries and involves lower mortality and spinal ischemia rates, as well as reduced risk of graft infection and systemic infection when it is compared with open repair [26].

13.2.2 Technique

TEVAR procedures can be performed under local or general anesthesia in an IR operating room. The abdomen and bilateral groins are prepared in standard way. Single femoral access may be achieved using an open or percutaneous technique. Then, the location of the injury is identified during an arch aortography. The cerebrovascular anatomy should also be evaluated based, especially if left subclavian artery coverage is planned. If angiography is equivocal, IVUS can be used. The patient is then anticoagulated with heparin with a smaller dose than the standard weight-based protocol especially in patients with intracranial hemorrhage. The thoracic device(s) is selected on the basis on contrast enhanced CT images according to the manufacturer's sizing recommendations. The device(s) is delivered over a stiff wire and then deployed using the standard technique without any pharmacological adjunct. The subclavian artery can be covered in order to obtain a proximal landing zone or gain better apposition with the lesser curvature of the aortic arch, and if necessary the vessel can be selectively revascularized. Post-deployment balloon angioplasty is generally not performed given the high risk of rupture [27, 28]. The procedure is supposed to end with a diagnostic angiography to check the position of the graft and the resolution of the injury (Fig. 13.1).

13.2.3 Indications and Guidelines

According to the most recent consensus of the Society for Vascular Surgery (SVS) the use of TEVAR is supposed to follow some guidelines that the committee suggested on the basis of a systematic review and meta-analysis of the literature including 7768 patients from 139 studies [29]. As it was said before, only observational studies, case series and unsystematic observations or expert opinion are available to date; thus, using the GRADE system, all of the following indications should be regarded as Grade 2, Level C statements:

1. *Timing of TEVAR in a stable patient*

   The committee suggests urgent (24 h) repair in the absence of other serious concomitant non-aortic injuries, or repair immediately

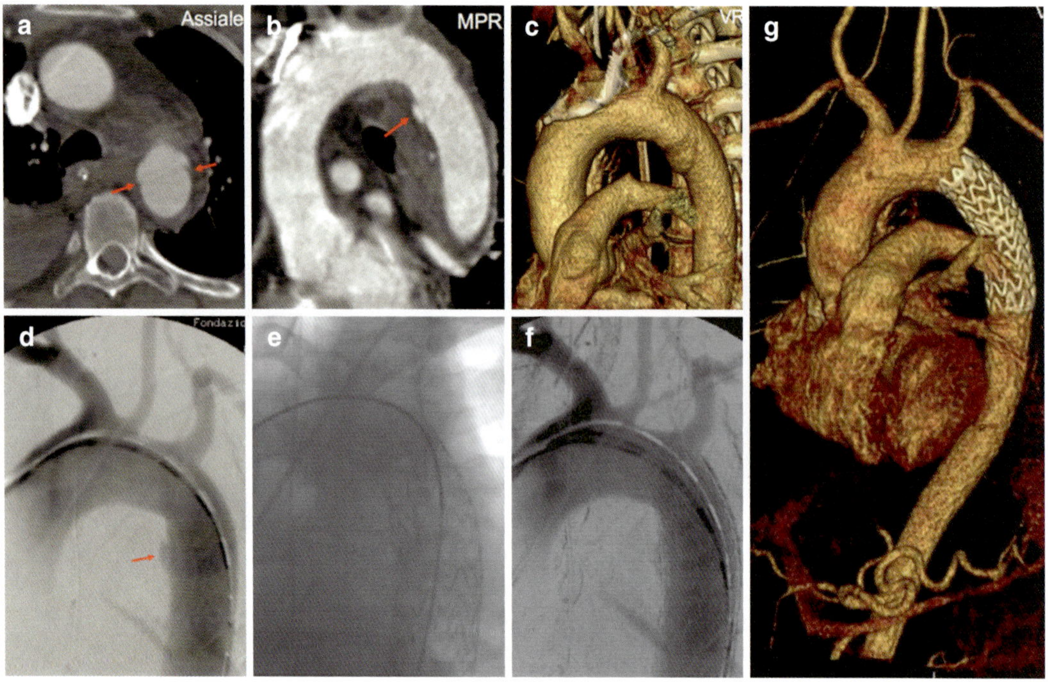

Fig. 13.1 (**a–c**) CT-angiography showing intimal tear at the aortic istmus (*arrows*); (**d**) DSA confirms the presence of an intimal tear (*arrow*); (**e**, **f**) placement of the stent graft; (**g**) follow-up CTA showing the correct placement of the stent graft with disappearance of intimal tear

after other injuries have been treated, but at the latest prior to hospital discharge [30, 31]. This is consistent with the available evidence in which mortality was 46% in those managed nonoperatively [32].

2. *Management of "minimal aortic injury"*

   Based on imaging, BTAI can be classified in four grades of severity:

   - type I: intimal tear
   - type II: intramural hematoma
   - type III: pseudoaneurysm (presence of a thin layer of adventitia that covers a transverse tear in the intima and media preventing complete rupture)
   - type IV: rupture

     The committee suggests expectant management with serial imaging for type I injuries, while types II to IV should be repaired. This is consistent with the evidence that most type I injuries can be managed with medical therapy (anti-impulse control). Decision to intervene and its timing should be guided by progression of the initial radiographic abnormality and/or symptoms [33].

3. *Choice of repair in the young: TEVAR vs. open*

   Age should not be a factor influencing the choice of the type of repair. The risks of death and spinal cord ischemia are significantly lower in all age groups after endovascular repair compared with open surgery, and these advantages overcome the concerns of potential late complications [34].

4. *Management of left subclavian artery*

   LSA is generally covered in 30% [32]. The committee suggests selective revascularization (either before or after TEVAR) depending on the status of the vertebral anatomy, especially whether the right vertebral artery is atretic or hypoplastic with or without an intact Circle of Willis.

5. *Systemic heparinization*

   The committee suggested routine heparinization, but at a lower dose than in elective TEVAR.

6. *Spinal drainage*

   Given the low risk of spinal cord ischemia during TEVAR for BTAI treatment (3%) [32], the proximal location of the injury involving limited coverage of the thoracic aorta, and the risk of epidural hematoma in a coagulopathic patient, the committee suggests that spinal drainage is not routinely indicated, and it should only be placed for symptoms of spinal cord ischemia.

7. *Choice of anesthesia: general vs. regional vs. local*

   The committee endorses general anesthesia because of unreliable cooperation of an agitated trauma patient and the presence of concomitant injuries that may require additional surgery.

8. *Femoral access technique*

   The committee suggests open femoral exposure

9. *Optimal follow-up strategy*

   In the absence of any abnormalities on imaging (i.e., stable endograft position, no endoleak) in the first 12–36 months, some have suggested decreasing the frequency to 2–5 years, while others have expressed that, lacking any evidence to the contrary, follow-up for traumatic thoracic aortic injuries should be no different than those treated with TEVAR for other pathologies. There was, however, some consensus suggesting that a combination of a multi-view chest X-ray and a magnetic resonance angiography (MRA) may be preferable over conventional contrast computed tomographic angiography (CTA) for long-term imaging, with due consideration of the metallic composition of the endograft.

13.2.4 Challenges and Limits

Despite TEVAR is associated with a lower risk of complications compared to open repair, there remains a number of controversial issues:

1. *Young age of affected population*:

   As mentioned before, BTAI tends to affect younger populations, in contrast to the aneurysm population. It is not uncommon that adolescent or pediatric patients may present with this injury [29].

   This carries some challenges:

   - Poor conformability of grafts to the aortic arch:
   - Young patients present not only a smaller aortic diameter, but also a shorter radius of aortic curvature compared to elderly patients. As individuals age, not only does the aorta enlarge, but the radius of curvature also increases [29]. This is potentially problematic for devices that are designed to mimic the stiffness of older patients with thoracic aneurysms. As such, their conformability is not ideal along the lesser curvature of the arch, potentially resulting in proximal endoleaks.

     Furthermore, when coupled with the increased aortic impulse in young patients, a lack of proximal conformability can also cause an aortic pseudocoarctation from compression of the device.

     Both device collapse and endoleaks are not always predictable and avoidable occurrences. They can, however, be treated when they occur.
   - Uncertain natural history of the repair:

     Given the morphologic changes of the aorta that come with age, the possibility of stent-graft migration as the aorta enlarges must be considered [29].

2. *Stent sizing*:

   Severe hypovolemia can lead to aortic contraction with underestimation of the aortic diameter ranging from 5 to 40% [35]. This can result in potential problems because undersized devices are associated with type I endoleak, persistent lesion perfusion, and bleeding. Oversizing the device would help minimize this risk but excessive oversizing can also lead to major complications as the aforementioned device compression [20].

3. *Manipulation of an endograft in the vicinity of the ascending aorta*:

   It is not only technically difficult but also carries a risk of stroke complications [29].

13.3 Interventional Radiology of Thoracic Wall Arteries

13.3.1 Introduction

Chest wall trauma shows a significant morbidity and mortality rate, with reported mortality ranging from 5 to 25% [3, 4].

Pape et al. [36] developed a scoring system for guiding initial clinical decision-making in the blunt chest trauma patient with multiple associated injuries. However, there are no evidence-based guidelines for management in the blunt chest wall trauma patients without associated injuries.

13.3.2 Clinical Considerations

The chest wall is a typical site of injury in patients with thoracic trauma. Rib fractures, sternum fractures, and flail chest are quite common findings, especially in case of blunt chest trauma. Dislocated fractures can induce damages to the pleuro-pulmonary structures and vessels, with formation of hemothorax, pneumothorax, pulmonary hematoma, pulmonary contusion, and hemomediastinum.

Penetrating injuries of the chest wall are lesser associated with bone fractures, but have similar risk to damage the pleuro-pulmonary structures and vessels.

Bone fractures generally undergo to nonoperative management. An exception is flail chest, for which recent studies suggest major benefits from surgical stabilization [37].

Vascular injury is a quite rare finding in chest wall trauma but its prompt recognition and management is fundamental for patient's life. Both blunt and penetrating traumas are recognized to be causes of vascular damages of the chest wall arteries.

Thoracotomy was the only useful treatment in these patients until 1977, when Barbaric et al. first reported the effectiveness of TAE for post-traumatic intercostal arterial hemorrhage [38].

13.3.3 Anatomy

The chest wall is the boundary of the thoracic cavity. Arterial supply originates from the intercostal arteries and the internal thoracic arteries [39]. Knowledge of the anatomy is fundamental in case of EVTs because of the high number of collateral vessels that may cause reperfusion and delayed failure of TAE.

The intercostal arteries (11 for each side) are divided into two branches, anterior and posterior. They lie in the intercostal space near the lower margin of the rib, between the intercostal vein (above) and the intercostal nerve (below).

Posterior branches originate directly from thoracic aorta (except for the first and second branch, which arises from the supreme intercostal artery-collateral of the costo-cervical trunk). They give a dorsal branch which feeds the spinal cord (radicular and spinal arteries).

From the first to the sixth, the anterior branches originate from the two internal thoracic arteries, which give rise to the subclavian arteries; from the sixth space the internal thoracic artery divides into the superior epigastric artery and musculophrenic artery. The latter goes downward and laterally and gives out the remaining anterior intercostal branches.

13.3.4 Management

Arterial injuries of the thoracic wall should be suspected in every case of trauma patient with:

- Abundant hemothorax/hemomediastinum
- Markedly displaced rib fractures

Even if a wide consensus is missing, many authors [40, 41] suggest the following management for these patients.

Patients with chest trauma and evidence of a pneumothorax or hemothorax have to undergo tube thoracostomy. Hemodynamically unstable patients and patients with >200 mL/h of blood loss from the thoracostomy tube should require emergent thoracotomy. When emergent thoracotomy is not indicated, CECT need to be performed. CECT may help to distinguish blood loss from an arterial source versus blood loss from a pulmonary lesion (bleeding from low-pressure pulmonary circulation), which is usually self-limited and in any case cannot be resolved with EVI. If CECT reveals arterial extravasation of contrast medium, angiography with TAE is indicated.

Prompt recognition is important because of the high blood flow in these arteries (150 mL/min for thoracic internal artery), which can be potentially life-threatening in few minutes [42]. Although a lesion of these arteries can achieve temporary hemostasis due to arterial spasm and hypotension, rebleeding may occur after the patient is resuscitated [43].

Active extravasation of contrast medium can be easily detected with CECT, which accurately shows the anatomic location of the bleeding and indicates the probable vascular origin. CECT, therefore, can be used as a guide for angiographic or surgical procedures [44].

CECT can show two types of alterations:

1. Active bleeding: extravasation of contrast medium increasing in the time
2. Pseudoaneurysm: disruption of one or more layers of the arterial wall forming a perfused sac with contrast medium that washes away with bloodstream

Both these lesions require an invasive treatment because pseudoaneurysms are by definition instable lesions and may develop in a real arterial rupture in the time.

In these cases, the patient should be carried in an angiographic suite to have an arterial angiography with TAE. The advent of superselective microcatheters has made the detection of bleeding sources easier and TAE safer [45].

The most common embolic materials used are pushable microcoils and polyvinyl alcohol (PVA) particles. Different embolization strategies can be used depending on the location of the bleeding source:

- If the bleeding source is in the main artery, microcoils can be first placed distal to the bleeding source (to prevent retrograde bleeding and to protect the thoracic wall from embolization). This is followed by placement of further microcoils proximal to the bleeding source. Eventually, final injection of PVA particles can accelerate thrombosis.
- If the source is in a distal part of the artery and could not be reached by the microcatheter, embolization need to be performed by first injecting PVA particles of a medium size (250–500 μm) which can occlude distally to the bleeding source; then, by placing coils proximal to the bleeding afterwards.

These approaches reduce the risk of delayed failure of TAE due to perfusion from other feeding vessels that may be too small to detect during the first angiography [46].

Spinal cord ischemia is the only serious potential complication related to TAE and has been reported by several authors [47].

Nowadays, this adverse event is very rare because microcatheters can go beyond, with their tip, to the origin of medullary branches (Fig. 13.2).

13.3.5 Conclusions

Lesions of thoracic wall arteries are rare but potentially life threatening. Their management includes TEA or thoracotomy, but actually there aren't standardized inclusion and exclusion criteria.

Some authors suggest that the endovascular treatment could be the most effective strategy to control hemorrhage, minimizing potential complications, so that TAE should always be considered before surgery in stable patients [48].

Whigham et al. [43] demonstrated a higher success of TAE with respect to surgery (91.6%

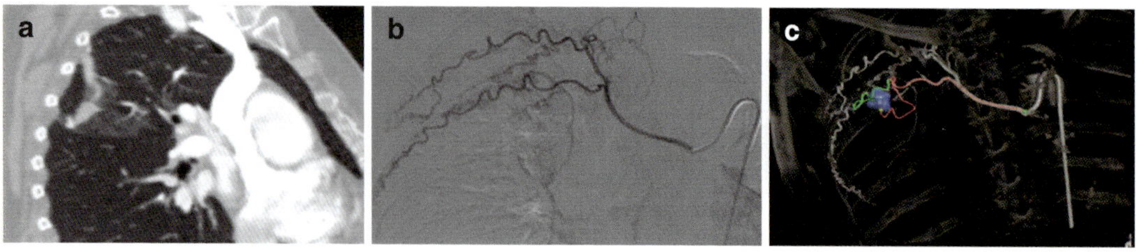

Fig. 13.2 (**a**) CTA shows a small bleeding from a right intercostal artery. (**b**) DSA confirms the presence of a little contrast medium extravasation from the same vessel. (**c**) Embolization planning by the C-arm Cone Beam CT embolization software

vs. 66.0%) to stop the bleeding. Nonetheless, in most centers these traumas are still treated more frequently via thoracotomy.

According to the literature and the state of the art [49–52], stable patient with isolated or not isolated chest wall trauma should always be submitted to CECT. In case of active arterial bleeding, TAE should always be considered before surgery and performed as soon as possible.

13.4 Pleural and Airways Injuries in Trauma Patient

Airways trauma is a life-threatening condition which may be a result of blunt and penetrating injuries to the neck and chest [53]. Therefore, prompt diagnosis is mandatory for the survival of these patients, also because the presence of concomitant severe injuries and unspecific symptoms may delay the diagnosis and lead to early fatal outcome or late sequela such as airway stenosis and recurrent pulmonary infections [54]. The treatment of these patients provides an adequate ventilation and then the repair of the airways injury with a smaller impact on the respiratory function and the quality of life of the patients [55].

Blunt chest trauma causes an abrupt increase in intrathoracic airways pressure. If this happens against a closed glottis, the trachea and major bronchi can be injured secondary to the increased pressure.

The incidence of tracheobronchial injuries (TBI) among trauma patients with thoracic injuries, including those that died immediately, is estimated at 0.5–2% [56, 57]. The mortality from traumatic TBIs has decreased from 36% before 1950 to 9% in 2001 [53]. Laceration of the mediastinal pleura and/or bronchial injuries may allow air to enter in the pleural cavity; pneumothorax occurs in 17–70% of the patients with TBIs [58] and in 30–40% of all patients with a blunt chest trauma [59]. The most common cause is a rib fracture that lacerates the lung, but it also may be caused by rupture of a preexisting bleb at the time of impact [59]. Finally, hemothorax is seen in approximately 50% of patients who sustain blunt chest trauma [60]. Bleeding into the pleural space can originate from injury to the pleura, chest wall, lung, diaphragm, or mediastinum.

Concerning the approach to the patient with thoracic trauma, the airway in a neurologically intact patient is easily assessable: the injured patient who is alert and able to speak normally is maintaining a patent airway. However, especially in polytrauma patient, this must be carefully monitored as facial fractures with associated bleeding or edema, emesis, or foreign bodies can eventually compromise airway patency. The symptoms and signs of TBI depend on the site and the severity of the injury and most of them are not specific for this kind of injury.

Subcutaneous emphysema is the most common finding in TBI occurring in up to 87% of the patients [61]. Dyspnea, tachypnea, and respiratory distress are found in 59–100% of the patients [62], while hemoptysis can be seen in up to 74% of the cases [63].

Clinical signs of pneumothorax can be subtle and difficult to elicit in a patient who has multi-system trauma [60]. Detection of even a small, asymptomatic pneumothorax is important because up to one third can develop into a tension pneumothorax with potential cardiopulmonary decompensation [64].

The most common findings in chest X-rays are subcutaneous emphysema, pneumomediastinum, and pneumothorax.

Subcutaneous emphysema signs include: tracheal deformity, a defect in the tracheal contour, an endotracheal tube out of place, and the tube's cuff over-inflated and protruding beyond the edge of the tracheal wall [65].

Radiographic signs of a pneumothorax can be subtle, and the appearance differs based on the patient position at the time that the radiograph was performed. In the supine position, air collects within the anterior costophrenic sulcus, which extends from the seventh costal cartilage to the 11th rib at the midaxillary line [64]. This appears radiographically as abnormal lucency in the lower chest or upper abdomen, an abnormally wide and deep costophrenic sulcus (the "deep sulcus" sign), a sharply outlined cardiac or diaphragmatic border, depression of the hemidiaphragm, or as a "double diaphragm" sign that is seen when air outlines the dome and anterior insertion of the diaphragm [66].

The appearance of hemothorax on a chest radiograph depends on the amount of blood that has collected in the pleural space and patient position. Plain radiography of the upright chest may be adequate to establish diagnosis by showing blunting at the costophrenic angle or an air–fluid interface if a hemopneumothorax is present. If the patient cannot be positioned upright, a supine chest radiograph may reveal apical capping of fluid surrounding the superior pole of the lung. In the acute trauma setting, the portable supine chest radiograph may be the first and only view available from which to make definitive decisions regarding therapy [60, 67]. When the size of a hemothorax reaches approximately 200 mL, an upright chest radiograph demonstrates blunting of the costophrenic angle. With progressive increase in size, a meniscus-sign will be seen: a concave upward sloping of fluid in the costophrenic angle. In contrast, a straight air–fluid level on the upright chest radiograph indicates a hemopneumothorax. A large hemothorax can opacify the hemithorax completely and cause contralateral shift of the mediastinum as the result of mass effect [68].

It is believed that up to 10–20% of the patients with TBI may have no signs of TBI on chest X-rays [57]; therefore, CT imaging helps the detection of the airways and pleural injury [15], especially the multi-slice detector CT (MDCT) with MPR/3D reconstruction of the images that can significantly increase the diagnostic accuracy of the procedure up to 94–100% [1, 69]. Discontinuity of the tracheal or bronchial wall can be seen, with air leaking around the airway. Among the indirect, more specific signs of tracheobronchial tear, there are the collapsed lung resting on the most dependent area away from the hilum (fallen lung sign), persistent pneumothorax after tube thoracostomy and herniation or overdistention of an endotracheal cuff in an intubated patient [57, 70]. All of these findings can be readily detected with MPR and 3D reconstructions using MDCT, particularly when looking for discontinuity of the airway wall. The MDCT improved significantly the spatial resolution, bringing us isotropic multiplanar and volume-rendering reconstructions and the MDCT's increasingly faster acquisition times have made it more appealing as a screening tool in the trauma setting [18]. Moreover, CT is highly sensitivity in detecting a small hemothorax and the Hounsfield unit (HU) measurement of fluid in the pleural space can be used to identify the origin of the fluid. Hemothorax measures 35–70 HU, depending on the amount of clot present [60]. In contrast, a sympathetic serous pleural effusion, which can be seen in patients who have splenic, hepatic, or pancreatic injuries, typically measures less than 15 HU. Other less common causes of pleural effusion in the patient who has experienced trauma include chylothorax from injury to the thoracic duct [71] and bilious effusion, which is caused by formation of a biliopleural fistula in the patient who has injury to the liver and the right hemidiaphragm [72]. Clues to the source of the bleeding into the pleural space can be gleaned from the appearance on imaging studies. A hemothorax that is due to bleeding from venous origin typically is self-limiting because of the tamponade effect from the lung parenchyma and usually does not increase in size. Arterial bleeding, such as from an intercostal artery, can be inferred by progression of size on radiography or CT [60]. CT also may demonstrate active bleeding within the hemothorax showing a focus of high density of the nearest large artery and multiplanar CT reformatted images can be especially useful to demonstrate the site of active bleeding [60].

It should be recalled that up to 80% of the TBI can be missed during the first 24–48 h after the trauma because of the nonspecific nature of the presenting symptoms and the fact that an airway injury may sometimes allow near normal ventilation [62, 73, 74]. With time the bronchus will be filled with fibro-granulation tissue and organizing hematoma. In the former, recurrent pulmonary infections may lead to bronchiectasis and destruction of the lung parenchyma, while in the later the lung distally to a completely obstructed bronchus is filled with mucus and protected from infections [73].

As a general rule, for patients with severe neck and thoracic trauma, tracheal intubation is required in the presence of the following conditions: severe brain injury, documented or highly suspected thermal inhalation injury, severe pulmonary contusion with hypoxemia or ventilatory insufficiency, high cervical spine injuries, or any injury resulting in pulmonary failure. However, the tracheal intubation in this patients with airway injury may result disastrous [53] because the pressure over a fractured cricoid may dislocate it enough to completely distort the upper airway or even lead to complete airway transection and obstruction [75]. Attempts to blindly overpass an upper airway injury may worsen the laceration and/or create false passage of the tube [76]. Therefore, spontaneous breathing of the patient should be preferred until safe airway has been achieved [53].

The final goals of airways injuries treatment are the following:

1. closing of the airway defect to improve ventilation
2. preventing mediastinal spillage and infection
3. avoiding spontaneous healing complications which can lead to airway stenosis and recurrent pulmonary infections.

The definitive management is essentially with surgery although in the 2001 was published a large revision of patients with blunt tracheobronchial injuries published in the literature [73] showing that conservative management is associated with higher rates of death; since then, several studies have commented on the possibility for nonoperative management in patients with airways injuries [56, 77] and the recent data shows a rating of conservative treatment in patients with TBI that ranges from 33.3 to 94.4% [53, 61].

Concerning the treatment of pneumothorax, patients who are symptomatic or who demonstrate a greater than 20% pneumothorax are generally considered for chest tube [78]. Prophylactic insertion of a chest tube also may be considered in a patient who has a small, asymptomatic pneumothorax who will be placed on a mechanical ventilator or who will be undergoing a lengthy operative procedure.

A tension pneumothorax is a life-threatening condition in which air progressively accumulates in the pleural space as the result of a one-way valve mechanism and causes high ipsilateral intrathoracic pressures. This can cause compression of the vena cava, which impairs venous return and decreases cardiac output. Radiographic signs of a tension pneumothorax include shift of the mediastinum to the contralateral side, abnormal lucency of the hemithorax with a collapsed lung in the hilar region, depression of the ipsilateral hemidiaphragm, and widening of the intercostal spaces. Prompt evacuation with needle aspiration or placement of a chest tube can be life saving.

TBI, bronchopleural fistula, or malpositioning of the chest tube should be considered if a pneumothorax does not respond completely to treatment [60].

References

1. Scaglione M, Pinto A, Pedrosa I, Sparano A, Romano L. Multi-detector row computed tomography and blunt chest trauma. Eur J Radiol. 2008;65(3):377–88.
2. Niska R, Bhuiya F, Xu J. National Hospital Ambulatory Medical Care Survey: 2007 emergency department summary. Natl Health Stat Rep. 2010;(26):1–31.
3. Khandhar SJ, Johnson SB, Calhoon JH. Overview of thoracic trauma in the United States. Thorac Surg Clin. 2007;17(1):1–9.
4. LoCicero J 3rd, Mattox KL. Epidemiology of chest trauma. Surg Clin North Am. 1989;69(1):15–9.
5. Schurink GW, Bode PJ, van Luijt PA, van Vugt AB. The value of physical examination in the diagnosis of patients with blunt abdominal trauma: a retrospective study. Injury. 1997;28(4):261–5.
6. Dreizin D, Munera F. Blunt polytrauma: evaluation with 64-section whole-body CT angiography. Radiographics. 2012;32(3):609–31.
7. Killeen KL, Shanmuganathan K, Poletti PA, Cooper C, Mirvis SE. Helical computed tomography of bowel and mesenteric injuries. J Trauma. 2001;51(1):26–36.
8. Brasel KJ, DeLisle CM, Olson CJ, Borgstrom DC. Splenic injury: trends in evaluation and management. J Trauma. 1998;44(2):283–6.
9. Davis JS, Satahoo SS, Butler FK, et al. An analysis of prehospital deaths: who can we save? J Trauma Acute Care Surg. 2014;77(2):213–8.
10. Glorsky SL, Wonderlich DA, Goei AD. Evaluation and management of the trauma patient for the interventional radiologist. Semin Interv Radiol. 2010;27(1):29–37.
11. Poletti PA, Wintermark M, Schnyder P, Becker CD. Traumatic injuries: role of imaging in the management of the polytrauma victim (conservative expectation). Eur Radiol. 2002;12(5):969–78.
12. Morgan TA, Steenburg SD, Siegel EL, Mirvis SE. Acute traumatic aortic injuries: posttherapy multidetector CT findings. Radiographics. 2010;30(4):851–67.
13. Gould JE, Vedantham S. The role of interventional radiology in trauma. Semin Interv Radiol. 2006;23(3):270–8.
14. Nicholson AA. Vascular radiology in trauma. Cardiovasc Intervent Radiol. 2004;27(2):105–20.
15. Kaewlai R, Avery LL, Asrani AV, Novelline RA. Multidetector CT of blunt thoracic trauma. Radiographics. 2008;28(6):1555–70.
16. Mirvis SE, Shanmuganathan K. Diagnosis of blunt traumatic aortic injury 2007: still a nemesis. Eur J Radiol. 2007;64(1):27–40.
17. Ambrose G, Barrett LO, Angus GL, Absi T, Shaftan GW. Main pulmonary artery laceration after blunt trauma: accurate preoperative diagnosis. Ann Thorac Surg. 2000;70(3):955–7.
18. Sangster GP, Gonzalez-Beicos A, Carbo AI, et al. Blunt traumatic injuries of the lung parenchyma, pleura, thoracic wall, and intrathoracic airways: multidetector computer tomography imaging findings. Emerg Radiol. 2007;14(5):297–310.
19. Stanescu L, Talner LB, Mann FA. Diagnostic errors in polytrauma: a structured review of the recent literature. Emerg Radiol. 2006;12(3):119–23.
20. Clancy TV, Gary Maxwell J, Covington DL, Brinker CC, Blackman D. A statewide analysis of level I and II trauma centers for patients with major injuries. J Trauma. 2001;51(2):346–51.
21. Lin PH, Bush RL, Zhou W, Peden EK, Lumsden AB. Endovascular treatment of traumatic thoracic aortic injury--should this be the new standard of treatment? J Vasc Surg. 2006;43(Suppl A):22A–9A.
22. Jamieson WR, Janusz MT, Gudas VM, et al. Traumatic rupture of the thoracic aorta: third decade of experience. Am J Surg. 2002;183(5):571–5.
23. Cowley RA, Turney SZ, Hankins JR, et al. Rupture of thoracic aorta caused by blunt trauma. A fifteen-year experience. J Thorac Cardiovasc Surg. 1990;100(5):652–60; discussion 660–651.
24. Ott MC, Stewart TC, Lawlor DK, Gray DK, Forbes TL. Management of blunt thoracic aortic injuries: endovascular stents versus open repair. J Trauma. 2004;56(3):565–70.
25. Tehrani HY, Peterson BG, Katariya K, et al. Endovascular repair of thoracic aortic tears. Ann Thorac Surg. 2006;82(3):873–7; discussion 877–878.
26. Pang D, Hildebrand D, Bachoo P. Thoracic endovascular repair (TEVAR) versus open surgery for blunt traumatic thoracic aortic injury. Cochrane Database Syst Rev. 2015;9:CD006642.
27. Piffaretti G, Benedetto F, Menegolo M, et al. Outcomes of endovascular repair for blunt thoracic aortic injury. J Vasc Surg. 2013;58(6):1483–9.
28. Piffaretti G, Carrafiello G, Ierardi AM, et al. Thoracic endovascular aortic repair for blunt thoracic aortic injuries in complex aortic arch vessels anatomies. Ann Vasc Surg. 2015;29(6):1320.e11–5.
29. Lee WA, Matsumura JS, Mitchell RS, et al. Endovascular repair of traumatic thoracic aortic injury: clinical practice guidelines of the Society for Vascular Surgery. J Vasc Surg. 2011;53(1):187–92.
30. Pate JW, Gavant ML, Weiman DS, Fabian TC. Traumatic rupture of the aortic isthmus: program of selective management. World J Surg. 1999;23(1):59–63.
31. Demetriades D, Velmahos GC, Scalea TM, et al. Diagnosis and treatment of blunt thoracic aortic injuries: changing perspectives. J Trauma. 2008;64(6):1415–8; discussion 1418–1419.
32. Murad MH, Rizvi AZ, Malgor R, et al. Comparative effectiveness of the treatments for thoracic aortic transection [corrected]. J Vasc Surg. 2011;53(1):193–9. e191-121.
33. Azizzadeh A, Keyhani K, Miller CC 3rd, et al. Blunt traumatic aortic injury: initial experience with endovascular repair. J Vasc Surg. 2009;49(6):1403–8.

34. Xenos ES, Abedi NN, Davenport DL, et al. Meta-analysis of endovascular vs. open repair for traumatic descending thoracic aortic rupture. J Vasc Surg. 2008;48(5):1343–51.
35. Jonker FH, Verhagen HJ, Mojibian H, et al. Aortic endograft sizing in trauma patients with hemodynamic instability. J Vasc Surg. 2010;52(1):39–44.
36. Pape HC, Remmers D, Rice J, et al. Appraisal of early evaluation of blunt chest trauma: development of a standardized scoring system for initial clinical decision making. J Trauma. 2000;49(3):496–504.
37. Coughlin TA, Ng JW, Rollins KE, Forward DP, Ollivere BJ. Management of rib fractures in traumatic flail chest: a meta-analysis of randomised controlled trials. Bone Joint J. 2016;98-B(8):1119–25.
38. Barbaric ZL, Luka NL. Angiographic demonstration and transcatheter embolic control of post-traumatic intercostal arterial hemorrhage. Surgery. 1977;81(4):409–12.
39. Choi S, Trieu J, Ridley L. Radiological review of intercostal artery: anatomical considerations when performing procedures via intercostal space. J Med Imaging Radiat Oncol. 2010;54(4):302–6.
40. Hagiwara A, Yanagawa Y, Kaneko N, et al. Indications for transcatheter arterial embolization in persistent hemothorax caused by blunt trauma. J Trauma. 2008;65(3):589–94.
41. Kessel B, Alfici R, Ashkenazi I, et al. Massive hemothorax caused by intercostal artery bleeding: selective embolization may be an alternative to thoracotomy in selected patients. Thorac Cardiovasc Surg. 2004;52(4):234–6.
42. Ritter DC, Chang FC. Delayed hemothorax resulting from stab wounds to the internal mammary artery. J Trauma. 1995;39(3):586–9.
43. Whigham CJ Jr, Fisher RG, Goodman CJ, Dodds CA, Trinh CC. Traumatic injury of the internal mammary artery: embolization versus surgical and nonoperative management. Emerg Radiol. 2002;9(4):201–7.
44. Shanmuganathan K, Mirvis SE, Sover ER. Value of contrast-enhanced CT in detecting active hemorrhage in patients with blunt abdominal or pelvic trauma. AJR Am J Roentgenol. 1993;161(1):65–9.
45. Chemelli AP, Thauerer M, Wiedermann F, et al. Transcatheter arterial embolization for the management of iatrogenic and blunt traumatic intercostal artery injuries. J Vasc Surg. 2009;49(6):1505–13.
46. Sekino S, Takagi H, Kubota H, et al. Intercostal artery pseudoaneurysm due to stab wound. J Vasc Surg. 2005;42(2):352–6.
47. Vujic I, Pyle R, Parker E, Mithoefer J. Control of massive hemoptysis by embolization of intercostal arteries. Radiology. 1980;137(3):617–20.
48. Walker TG, Salazar GM, Waltman AC. Angiographic evaluation and management of acute gastrointestinal hemorrhage. World J Gastroenterol. 2012;18(11):1191–201.
49. Aoki M, Shibuya K, Kaneko M, et al. Massive hemothorax due to inferior phrenic artery injury after blunt trauma. World J Emerg Surg. 2015;10:58.
50. Grande AM, Cattadori B, D'Armini AM, Vigano M. Post-traumatic pseudoaneurysm of internal mammary artery: a case report. G Chir. 2006;27(10):377–9.
51. Gutierrez Romero DF, Barrufet M, Lopez-Rueda A, Burrel M. Ruptured intercostal artery pseudoaneurysm in a patient with blunt thoracic trauma: diagnosis and management. BMJ Case Rep. 2014;2014.
52. Carrillo EH, Heniford BT, Senler SO, et al. Embolization therapy as an alternative to thoracotomy in vascular injuries of the chest wall. Am Surg. 1998;64(12):1142–8.
53. Prokakis C, Koletsis EN, Dedeilias P, et al. Airway trauma: a review on epidemiology, mechanisms of injury, diagnosis and treatment. J Cardiothorac Surg. 2014;9:117.
54. Rollins RJ, Tocino I. Early radiographic signs of tracheal rupture. AJR Am J Roentgenol. 1987;148(4):695–8.
55. Amauchi W, Birolini D, Branco PD, de Oliveira MR. Injuries to the tracheobronchial tree in closed trauma. Thorax. 1983;38(12):923–8.
56. Lampl L. Tracheobronchial injuries. Conservative treatment. Interact Cardiovasc Thorac Surg. 2004;3(2):401–5.
57. Chu CP, Chen PP. Tracheobronchial injury secondary to blunt chest trauma: diagnosis and management. Anaesth Intensive Care. 2002;30(2):145–52.
58. Kelly JP, Webb WR, Moulder PV, et al. Management of airway trauma. I: tracheobronchial injuries. Ann Thorac Surg. 1985;40(6):551–5.
59. Tocino IM, Miller MH, Fairfax WR. Distribution of pneumothorax in the supine and semirecumbent critically ill adult. AJR Am J Roentgenol. 1985;144(5):901–5.
60. Miller LA. Chest wall, lung, and pleural space trauma. Radiol Clin N Am. 2006;44(2):213–24. viii
61. Koletsis E, Prokakis C, Baltayiannis N, et al. Surgical decision making in tracheobronchial injuries on the basis of clinical evidences and the injury's anatomical setting: a retrospective analysis. Injury. 2012;43(9):1437–41.
62. Barmada H, Gibbons JR. Tracheobronchial injury in blunt and penetrating chest trauma. Chest. 1994;106(1):74–8.
63. Gabor S, Renner H, Pinter H, et al. Indications for surgery in tracheobronchial ruptures. Eur J Cardiothorac Surg. 2001;20(2):399–404.
64. Rhea JT, van Sonnenberg E, McLoud TC. Basilar pneumothorax in the supine adult. Radiology. 1979;133(3 Pt 1):593–5.
65. Euathrongchit J, Thoongsuwan N, Stern EJ. Nonvascular mediastinal trauma. Radiol Clin N Am. 2006;44(2):251–8, viii.
66. Gordon R. The deep sulcus sign. Radiology. 1980;136(1):25–7.
67. Khan AN, Al-Jahdali H, Al-Ghanem S, Gouda A. Reading chest radiographs in the critically ill (part II): radiography of lung pathologies common in the ICU patient. Ann Thorac Med. 2009;4(3):149–57.

68. Khan AN, Al-Jahdali H, Al-Ghanem S, Gouda A. Reading chest radiographs in the critically ill (part I): normal chest radiographic appearance, instrumentation and complications from instrumentation. Ann Thorac Med. 2009;4(2):75–87.
69. Faure A, Floccard B, Pilleul F, et al. Multiplanar reconstruction: a new method for the diagnosis of tracheobronchial rupture? Intensive Care Med. 2007;33(12):2173–8.
70. Zinck SE, Primack SL. Radiographic and CT findings in blunt chest trauma. J Thorac Imaging. 2000;15(2):87–96.
71. Ikonomidis JS, Boulanger BR, Brenneman FD. Chylothorax after blunt chest trauma: a report of 2 cases. Can J Surg. 1997;40(2):135–8.
72. Franklin DC, Mathai J. Biliary pleural fistula: a complication of hepatic trauma. J Trauma. 1980;20(3):256–8.
73. Kiser AC, O'Brien SM, Detterbeck FC. Blunt tracheobronchial injuries: treatment and outcomes. Ann Thorac Surg. 2001;71(6):2059 65.
74. Richardson JD. Outcome of tracheobronchial injuries: a long-term perspective. J Trauma. 2004;56(1):30–6.
75. O'Callaghan J, Keh SM, D'Souza A. Management of closed tracheal perforation following blunt trauma. Otolaryngol Head Neck Surg. 2009;141(5):661–2.
76. Baumgartner FJ, Ayres B, Theuer C. Danger of false intubation after traumatic tracheal transection. Ann Thorac Surg. 1997;63(1):227–8.
77. Carretta A, Melloni G, Bandiera A, et al. Conservative and surgical treatment of acute post-traumatic tracheobronchial injuries. World J Surg. 2011;35(11):2568–74.
78. Weissberg D, Refaely Y. Pneumothorax: experience with 1,199 patients. Chest. 2000;117(5):1279–85.

Hepatic Injuries

14

Lina Bartolini, Ginevra Danti, Claudio Raspanti, Gloria Addeo, Diletta Cozzi, Margherita Trinci, and Vittorio Miele

14.1 Epidemiology and Mechanism of Action

Trauma is the leading cause of death in the population under 40 years old. In blunt trauma, the liver constitutes, after the spleen, the most common organ involved. On the contrary, in open trauma, the liver is the most commonly injured solid organ [1]. The prevalence of liver injury in patients with blunt multiple trauma, in fact, is about 20%. However, isolated liver lesions are rare and in 77–90% of cases are associated with involvement of other internal organs.

Liver damage in abdominal trauma is generally caused by an accelerative/decelerative force, such as that occurs in road accidents. The right liver lobe, being the most voluminous portion of the hepatic parenchyma, is more often the site of damage. The posterior-superior liver segments are located in close proximity to fixed anatomical structures such as ribs and spine, which play an important role in the genesis of the lesion. Furthermore also the insertion of the coronary ligament in this region contributes to the acceleration–deceleration mechanism. The right hepatic lesions may be associated with lacerations or contusions of the right lower lung lobe, hemothorax, pneumothorax, rib fractures, renal or adrenal lesions. Traumatic lesions of the left hepatic lobe are less frequent and usually occur as a consequence of a compressive direct trauma in the epigastric region, e.g., in case of fractures of the sternum, besides damages of pancreas, duodenum, transverse colon, and myocardium may be associated.

The lesions of the caudate lobe, however, are extremely rare and usually not isolated but associated with other major injuries.

The development of Trauma Centers specialized in the management of critical patients, the diffusion and advancements of imaging techniques, have determined a significant reduction in mortality from trauma; in particular, there was an important decrease of the cases of death for hepatic trauma in the last decades. The most frequent clinical findings in patients with hepatic trauma are represented by pain localized in the right upper quadrant, extending in some cases to the ipsilateral shoulder, hypotension and hemorrhagic shock, biliary peritonitis, and diffused abdominal pain in the absence of intestinal paresis [2].

L. Bartolini (✉) • G. Danti • G. Addeo • D. Cozzi
V. Miele
Department of Radiology, Careggi University Hospital, L.go G. A. Brambilla 3, 50134 Florence, Italy
e-mail: linas4@yahoo.it; ginevra.danti@gmail.com; gloria.addeo@gmail.com; dilettacozzi@gmail.com; vmiele@sirm.org

C. Raspanti
Department of Interventional Radiology, Careggi University Hospital, L.go G. A. Brambilla 3, 50134 Florence, Italy
e-mail: claudio.raspanti@gmail.com

M. Trinci
Department of Emergency Radiology, S. Camillo Hospital, Rome, Italy
e-mail: margherita.trinci@libero.it

V. Miele, M. Trinci (eds.), *Diagnostic Imaging in Polytrauma Patients*,
https://doi.org/10.1007/978-3-319-62054-1_14

14.2 Radiological Diagnosis

In the past years, clinicians and surgeons based their assessments of traumatic lesions on clinical findings because radiological techniques (X-ray) were only able to provide information about bone structures lesions and the presence of free air in the peritoneum.

Patients who were in critical conditions were referred to the surgeons.

Before the introduction of the modern technique of imaging, the diagnostic peritoneal lavage allowed to detect the presence of hemoperitoneum with great sensitivity [3]. However, this instrument was not able to establish both the origin of bleeding and the degree of extension of trauma and did not exclude the possibility of false positives (peritoneal iatrogenic bleeding post-introduction of peritoneal drainage) or false negatives (traumatic injury in the absence of peritoneal bleeding or lesions of the retroperitoneum) [4–6].

The introduction of modern imaging techniques such as US and MDCT has been of great importance in the complete evaluation of the trauma patient [7, 8].

As a multidisciplinary approach is mandatory for the management of traumatic lesions, during the last years the radiologist gained a central role in the identification and staging of traumatic injury, thus providing indications about both clinical and therapeutic priorities.

In fact, the diagnostic evaluation of a polytraumatized patient presents a wide range of variability depending on clinical conditions, first of all hemodynamic stability or instability:

- *Hemodynamically unstable polytrauma patient* (BP <90 mmHg and HPM >120):
  In this case, the imaging tests to be performed are: chest X-ray on AP view, cervical spine X-ray on LL view, pelvis X-ray on AP view, and E-FAST scan. While these radiological investigations are carried out, the patient is lying in a supine position and the resuscitators try to monitor and stabilize the patient's vital signs.
  As soon as the vital functions are stabilized, the patient will be subjected to a whole body MDCT exam for a complete diagnosis.
- *Hemodynamically stable polytrauma patient* (BP >90 mmHg and HPM <120 bpm):
  In this case, the first imaging technique that can be used is MDCT scan. Only in case of low-energy localized trauma it's preferable to use US and CEUS [9].
  Not only diagnosis but also the types of therapeutic approaches have radically changed in the last years.
  Currently, about 80–89% of liver injuries are treated conservatively, with a success rate which ranges from 85 to 94%.
  Moreover, the presence of an interventional radiologist in the Trauma Center group might allow the possibility to treat multiple organ injuries by mini-invasive techniques (embolization and drainage), thus resulting in a significant reduction of postoperative complications as well as in hospital days [10].

14.3 Ultrasonography

When the patient is in emergency room, the purpose of the ultrasound exam is to reveal the presence of hemoperitoneum, which is an indicator of traumatic lesion. In this case, the exam is named Focused Assessment by Sonography for Trauma (FAST) and it doesn't evaluate parenchymal lesion but only the presence of free fluid in abdominal recesses. This examination is widely accepted as an effective initial triage to evaluate trauma victims with suspected blunt abdominal injuries because it can be performed rapidly in the admission area; it's repeatable, noninvasive, non-irradiating, and inexpensive [11]. The sensitivity of US for the detection of free intraperitoneal fluid is generally considered to be excellent.

There is a general consensus that in a polytrauma patient who is hemodynamically unstable at admission, the presence of a large amount of free intraperitoneal fluid on FAST requires surgery [12].

The FAST protocol includes real-time scanning of four regions:

1. Sub-xiphoid region: aimed at seeking a possible pericardial fluid stratum
2. Right upper quadrant: to highlight fluid in the hepatorenal fossa (Morison's pouch)
3. Left upper quadrant: sub-phrenic space and splenorenal recess
4. Pelvis: hemoperitoneum in the recto-vesical space or pouch of Douglas

About the presence of free fluid, there is a semiquantitative model proposed by Federle in 1983 that divided the amount of intraperitoneal fluid into four degrees:

Grade 0, refers to the absence of hemoperitoneum

Grade I, when there is a mild hemoperitoneum (fluid in perihepatic fossa, about 250 cm^3)

Grade II, in the presence of medium hemoperitoneum (fluid in perihepatic and perisplenic recesses, about 500 cm^3)

Grade III, in the case of severe hemoperitoneum (fluid in perihepatic, perisplenic, in parietocolic recesses and/or in the pelvic space, >500 cm^3) [13]

The presence of hemoperitoneum in association with hepatic traumatic injury is an important prognostic factor that can change the management of the patient.

Abdominal US is very useful in emergency setting and may be considered essential as the initial screening method in hemodynamically unstable patients, selecting those with significant hemoperitoneum and so candidates for surgery [14].

Nevertheless, the literature tells us that about 34% of abdominal parenchymal lesions, even severe, which may be managed by interventional endovascular or surgical treatment, cannot be associated with hemoperitoneum or with an amount of fluid collection not proportionate to the severity of damage.

By ultrasound it may be difficult to distinguish if the presence of intra-abdominal fluids is due to non-traumatic conditions, as patients with ascites, patients on peritoneal dialysis treatment or in the post-ovulatory period. Nevertheless, in some cases it is possible to depict the presence of a fluid corpuscular level suggestive for the presence of fresh blood in the abdomen.

As we know, the ultrasound examination has low sensitivity in detection of retroperitoneal fluid, which can also be conspicuous in case of liver damage at the level of the nude hepatic area (posterior-superior region of the segment VII) [15].

By US it is possible to demonstrate a parenchymal liver injury but this technique is severely limited by the operator dependence and also it is conditioned by the body habitus and the clinical condition of the patient, often in such situations uncooperative.

Ultrasonography has low sensitivity in recognizing the small parenchymal lacerations and contusions, especially if they are in the sub-diaphragmatic region (literature tells us that only 12% of post-traumatic hepatic lesions are really identified with this examination) and not associated with free fluid in the peritoneal cavity [16].

The ultrasound characteristics of traumatic lesions of the liver are:

1. In the early phase, during the first 24–48 h: US shows an hyperechoic area, for the presence of recent blood, with irregular morphology and unclear margins.
2. In the latter phase: there will be a changing of echogenicity over the time, the lesion will be hypoechoic, its size reduces, and in case of a favorable prognosis the liver parenchyma will return normal.

In the last years, US limits have been exceeded by the use of CEUS in the study of hepatic injuries.

First of all, it's important to stress that CEUS is indicated in localized low-energy trauma, as well as in the follow-up of abdominal injuries.

Nevertheless, CEUS improves the accuracy of standard ultrasonography, being more sensitive than this in the detection of parenchymal liver injury.

The performing of CEUS does not take much time; the consensus of the patient is needed.

As for the other contrast exam, we have different phases according with the timing of intravenous contrast bolus. The arterial phase is realized in 20–30 s after injection of contrast media and is quickly followed (about 10 s) by the venous phase, lasting about 2 min.

The late phase persists until the complete disappearance of the constituent agents of contrast media (microbubbles) from hepatic parenchyma (4–6 min); there is no correspondence to the equilibrium phase of CT or MRI.

CEUS shows traumatic injuries of liver as low—or not—perfused parenchymal areas, better detectable during the late contrast enhancement phase; the border of the lesion is clear, the distance with the capsule and its integrity is well demonstrated (Fig. 14.1). It is often possible to detect the extracapsular or intralesional active bleeding as an extracapsular or intralesional hyperechoic image.

Regarding traumatic liver injury, there is a good correspondence between CEUS and MDCT; false negatives with CEUS may be represented by minor injuries, without significant consequences for management and prognosis of patient [17].

Many studies have shown that it is possible to monitor the functionality of hepatic microcirculation, in those who suffered an ischemic damage with subsequent reperfusion of parenchyma, through the use of CEUS [18]. Thanks to this method, the dysfunction of liver microcirculation

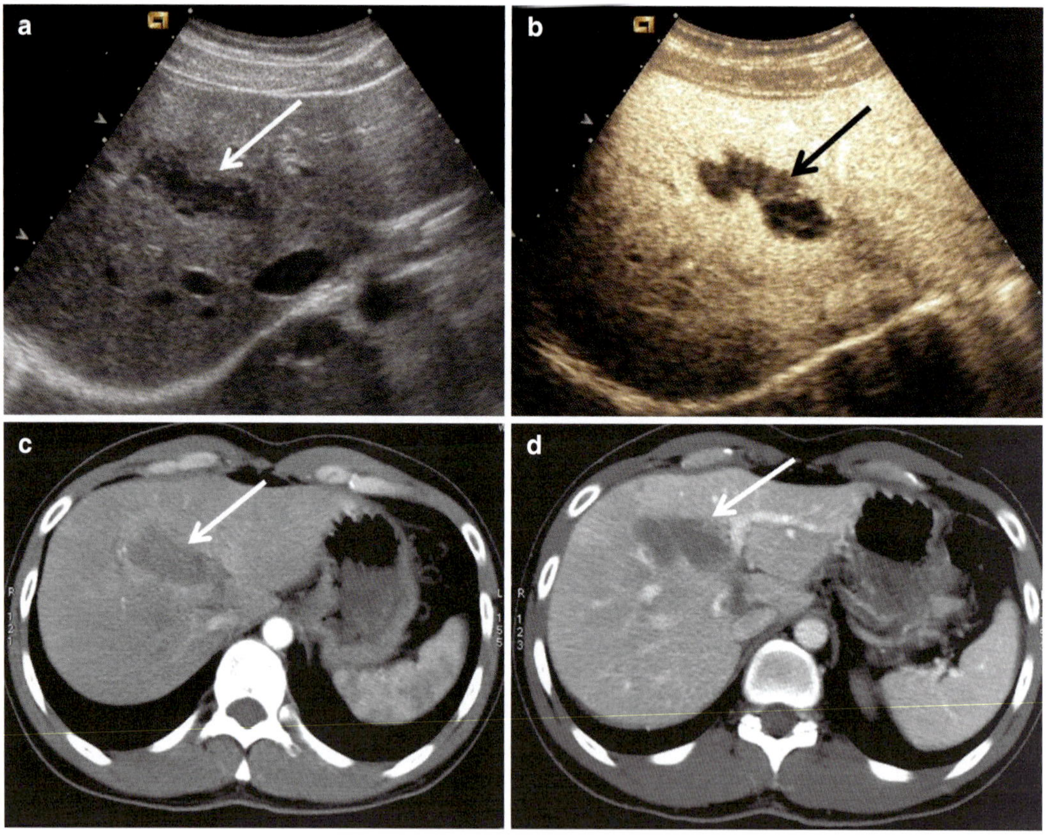

Fig. 14.1 Hepatic laceration. (**a**) Ultrasound shows a hypoechoic area within the right liver lobe (*arrow*); (**b**) CEUS: the laceration appears a nonvascular area (*black arrow*). The CE-MDCT, in arterial phase (**c**) and portal phase (**d**), confirms the presence of a liver laceration (*arrows*) involving segment IV; no active bleeding is appreciable in both CEUS and CE-MDCT imaging techniques.

was evaluated and it was determined how the perfusion of contrast with microbubbles is negatively correlated with the severity of the injury [19].

Some authors suggest the use of CEUS following the execution of a standard ultrasound scan or ultrasound FAST, for those patients who have suffered a low-energy trauma and are hemodynamically stable. Therefore, CT scan would be reserved to high-energy trauma with suspected multiple organ injuries or in cases in which CEUS was not conclusive. CEUS showed a diagnostic accuracy almost comparable to the contrast-enhanced CT scan in the detection of abdominal parenchymal lesions associated with low-energy trauma, with a sensitivity and specificity close to 95% [20]. Another recognized role of CEUS is to be able to highlight blood extravasation and then the possibility of a subsequent therapeutic treatment in a short time.

Other applications are its use for pediatric patients and pregnant women, thanks to the absence of ionizing radiation and of harmful effects on fetus by ultrasound contrast agents. However, CEUS presents some limitations: operator-related method, high costs of contrast media, lack of panoramic view and difficulty to explore deep abdominal regions. Even if, as mentioned, CEUS proved to be more sensitive than baseline ultrasound in the detection of solid organ injury in blunt abdominal trauma, it cannot be deemed to replace CT scan in high-energy trauma. Also in case of isolated trauma, if CEUS detects a liver parenchyma injury, it must be followed by a MDCT examination.

CEUS represents a diagnostic supplement to CT and a radiation protective option in the follow-up of liver lesions, especially in young patients and children [21, 22].

14.4 Computed Tomography

Computed tomography (CT) is the diagnostic examination of choice for polytrauma hemodynamic stable patients. In fact, it represents a time-saving diagnostic technique avoiding the use of other imaging methods and so enabling the Trauma Team to start treatment ahead of time.

MDCT scan allows the panoramic study of the abdomen also in critical patients that may be partially or not collaborating because of their clinical conditions and their need of resuscitation procedures, and this rapid panoramic assessment might be essential to enable treatment onset in a short time [23]. The CT examination has high sensitivity (approximately 99%), specificity (about 96.8%), and diagnostic accuracy (about 97.6%) in the diagnosis of traumatic damage of the liver. It also allows the clinicians to monitor the lesions and highlight the possible occurrence of early and late complications over the time (seromas, bilomas, abscesses, necrosis, pseudoaneurysm), either after conservative therapy or surgical/interventional treatment [24, 25]. MDCT can detect small amounts of free fluid, with sensitivity similar to that of US, but it is superior to US in pointing out injuries of the visceral organs. Moreover CT, compared with US, is less dependent on the operator, less limited by technical factors and is also reproducible [26].

Contrast-enhanced CT scan for polytrauma patients encloses the study of the head, neck, thorax, abdomen, and pelvis, sometimes even the lower and upper limbs are evaluated. It usually is a multiphase examination, with a basal phase followed by an arterial and portal venous phase. Arterial phase is fundamental for the study of vascular injuries, while venous phase is more useful to identify parenchymal liver injuries. It's important to use an appropriate personalized contrast dose based on patient's weight; the exam needs a high-flow intravenous injection (3–4 mL/s). In fact, the amount of contrast greatly improves the visibility of parenchymal lesions and thus the final quality of the examination. In addition to the axial scan, the post-processing with coronal and sagittal multiplanar reconstructions (MPRs) are routinely performed for the evaluation of abdominal structures while maximum-intensity projections (MIPs) and volume rendering (VR) reconstructions are required in case of vascular injuries.

In 1989, Mirvis et al. proposed a classification system of liver lesions based on the size of lesions and the number of involved segments visualized on CT [27]. This classification divides traumatic liver lesions in five degrees.

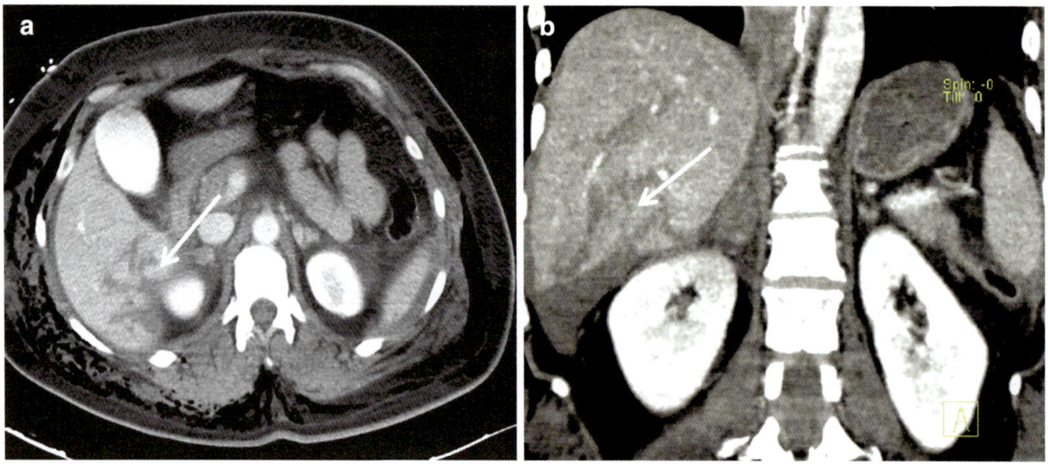

Fig. 14.2 Hepatic trauma, grade III: (**a**) Axial CT scan and (**b**) coronal reconstruction show multiple lacerations with thickness >3 cm

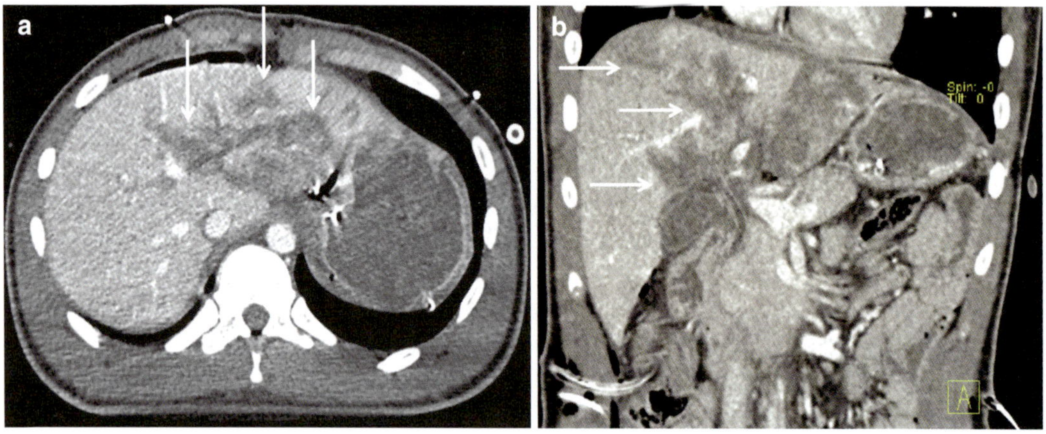

Fig. 14.3 (**a**) Axial CT scan and (**b**) coronal reconstruction show a grade IV parenchymal injury involving from 25 to 75% of a liver lobe (*arrows*)

Grade I includes capsular avulsion, superficial laceration (<1 cm of thickness), sub-capsular hematoma (<1 cm of thickness), and periportal tracking.

Grade II includes laceration with thickness of 1–3 cm and central sub-capsular hematoma with a diameter of 1–3 cm.

Grade III includes lacerations with thickness >3 cm and central sub-capsular hematoma with a diameter >3 cm (Fig. 14.2).

Grade IV includes sub-capsular hematoma with a diameter >10 cm and lobar parenchymal breaking or devascularization (Fig. 14.3, Fig. 14.4).

Grade V includes bi-lobar parenchymal breaking or devascularization [27].

Despite the usefulness of this classification for clinical research purposes, as it allows the description of the severity of injuries, it doesn't seem to be helpful in clinical management because no correlation was reported between lesions grading and required treatment, as it was observed that even in high-grade lesions involv-

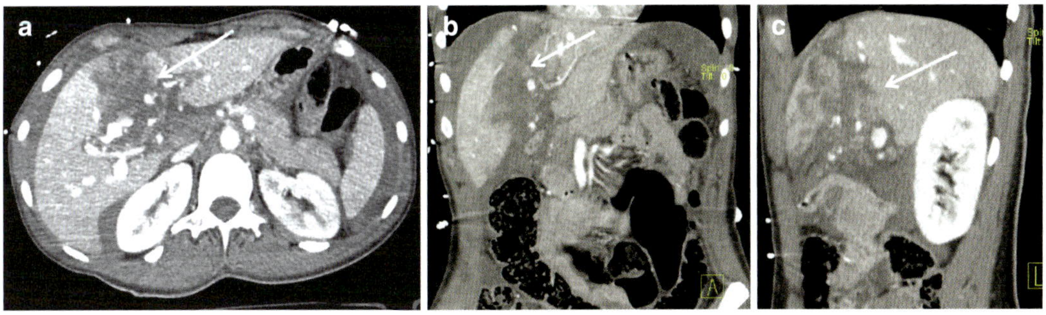

Fig. 14.4 (**a**) Axial CT scan, (**b**) coronal, and (**c**) sagittal reconstruction show a IV grade parenchymal lesion, involving segment IV completely

Table 14.1 The American Association for the Surgery of Trauma (AAST) hepatic injury scale

Degree of injury	Description
I	Hematoma: sub-capsular with liver surface's involvement <10%
	Laceration: capsular lesion with depth <1 cm
II	Hematoma: sub-capsular, interest 10–50% of the surface
	Hematoma: intraparenchymal <10 cm in diameter
	Laceration: capsular injury, depth 1–3 cm and length <10 cm
III	Hematoma: sub-capsular, surfaces's involvement >50% or sub-capsular hematoma with signs of breaking and with active bleeding
	Hematoma: intraparenchymal >10 cm in diameter or with sings of breakage
	Laceration: capsular lesion, depth >3 cm
IV	Hematoma: peritoneal rupture and hemorrhage in progress
	Laceration: parenchymal injury involving from 25 to 75% of a liver lobe or up to three segments of the same lobe
V	Laceration: parenchymal lesions involving over 75% of a liver lobe or more than three segments of the same lobe
	Venous injury: juxta-hepatic (intrahepatic lesion of inferior vena cava) or supra-hepatic veins
VI	Avulsion: of the vascular pedicle
	Laceration: parenchymal extended to both liver lobes

From Moore EE, Shackford SR, Patcher HL et al. (1989) Organ Injury Scaling: Spleen, Liver and Kidney. J Trauma 29:1664–6. Obtained permission from Wolters Kluwer

ing three or more segments, good clinical results can be achieved by conservative treatment [28]..

This CT-based classification system comes from the surgical grading drawn up by the American Association for the Surgery of Trauma (AAST) that divides hepatic trauma in six grades. (Table 14.1) [29] (Fig. 14.5).

The surgical organ-injury scale of the AAST comprises some criteria that cannot be evaluated with CT and wide discrepancies have been seen between the CT injury grade and intraoperative findings, with CT usually underestimating injury gravity [30]. So several studies say that the CT-based injury-grading systems facilitate clinical research as they enable comparison of different series of patients, but their value for predicting the outcome of conservative treatment remains, however, unproven.

The traumatic hepatic injuries detected on CT may be summarized as follows:

Contusion: hypodense area with irregular margins resulting in interstitial blood suffusion. Rarely, contusion is an isolated post-traumatic liver injury, and it is usually associated with tearing or hematoma.

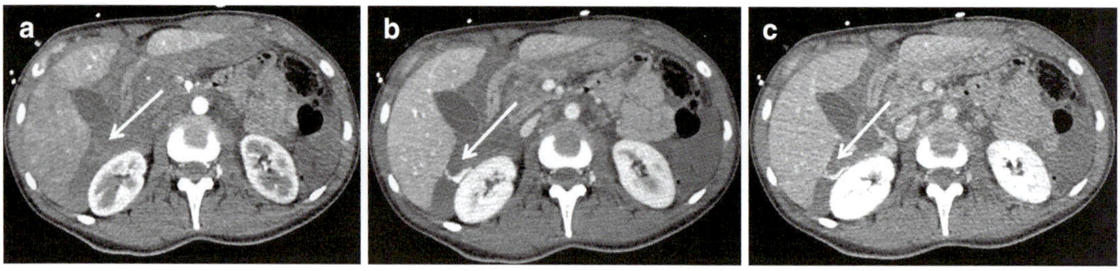

Fig. 14.5 (**a**) Arterial phase axial CT scan shows a perihepatic fluid collection; there is no evidence of arterial bleeding. (**b**) Venous and (**c**) equilibrium phases well depict the active intraperitoneal bleeding

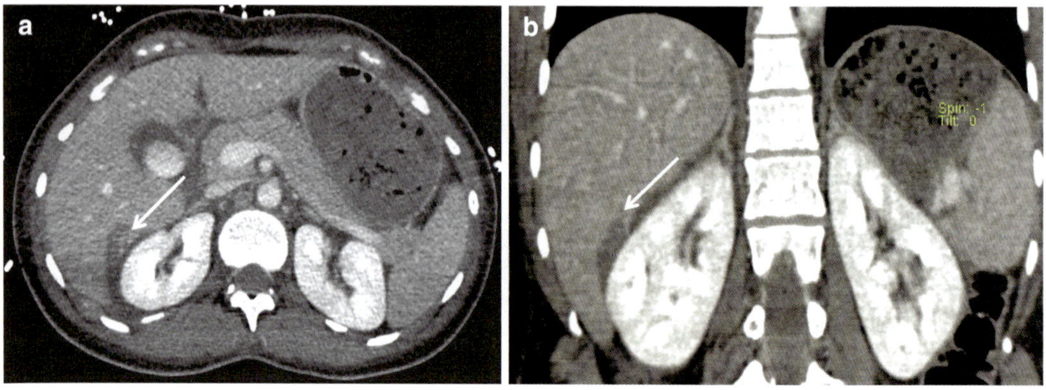

Fig. 14.6 (**a**) Axial CT scan and (**b**) coronal reconstruction show the superficial hepatic laceration (*arrows*): extension is <1 cm deep

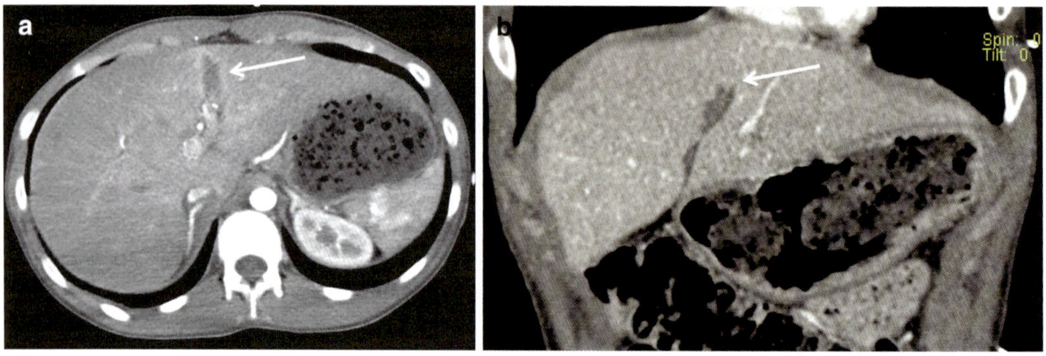

Fig. 14.7 (**a**) Axial CT scan and (**b**) coronal reconstruction show a laceration of hepatic parenchyma between 1 and 3 cm deep (*arrows*)

Laceration: it is the most common traumatic injury of the liver. It appears as a linear or branched image slightly hyperdense on direct examination, caused by the presence of blood and clots of recent deposition, and hypodense in contrast-enhanced scans [31].

Lacerations are often located in the proximity of an intrahepatic portal branch or a supra-hepatic vein; the most frequent lacerations are located parallel to the supra-hepatic veins or to the posterior division of the portal vein's right branch.

They are classified according with their size into: superficial (extension <1 cm deep) (Fig. 14.6), medium (between 1 and 3 cm deep) (Fig. 14.7), and deep (extension >3 cm deep) (Fig. 14.8).

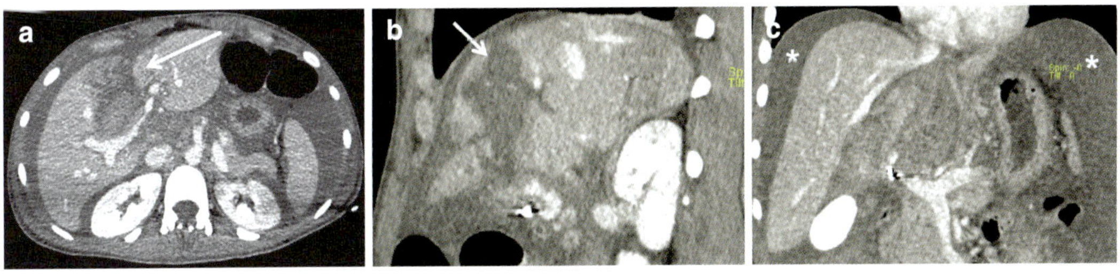

Fig. 14.8 (**a**) Axial CT scan, (**b**) coronal, and (**c**) sagittal reconstruction show a deep hepatic laceration >3 cm deep (*arrows* in **a**) and (**b**). In (**c**), a huge hemoperitoneum is appreciable (*asterisks*)

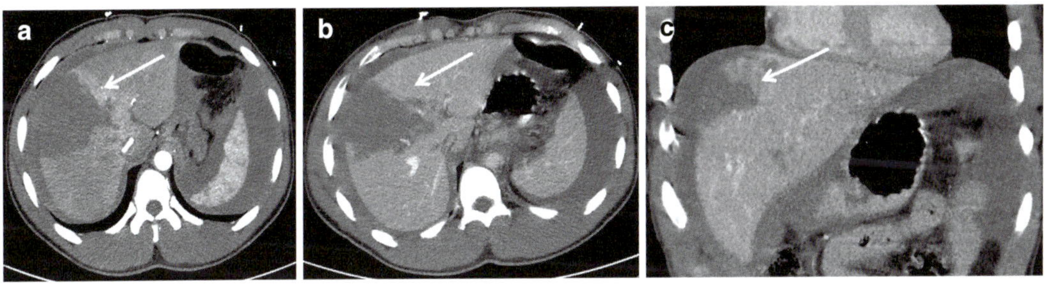

Fig. 14.9 (**a**, **b**) Axial CT scan in arterial (**a**), venous phase (**b**) and (**c**) coronal reconstruction show the hepatic infarction as a hypodense triangular-shaped area (*arrows*). Hepatic infarction is an ischemic area with irregular margins, which doesn't show enhancement during contrast-enhanced phase

Liver lacerations are categorized as deep when affecting the liver parenchyma adjacent to intrahepatic portal branches of first and second order, independently of the involvement of the peripheral parenchyma [29].

If laceration involves the whole surface of the liver, the outcome could be in liver fracture with avulsion of a fragment devoid of vascularization. Depending on the location of the lacerations, they may be associated with other post-traumatic alterations: hemoperitoneum in capsular tears of anterior liver surface, retroperitoneal hematomas adjacent to the inferior vena cava and to the right adrenal gland ("halo sign") in tearing interesting liver's nude area, damage of the biliary tract (hemobilia or bilomas) in tears near the hepatic hilum.

Liver lacerations are particularly serious when affecting the confluence between the suprahepatic veins or intrahepatic vena cava, in this case resulting in massive venous bleeding.

Hepatic infarction: in this case, we see an ischemic area in the liver with irregular margins. It is hypodense in basal phase and doesn't show enhancement during the contrast phase (Fig. 14.9). It's generally caused by thrombotic obstruction or post-traumatic avulsion of one of the main hepatic vessels; the greater is the caliber of the vessel involved, the greater will be the ischemic area.

Hepatic infarction may extend to involve the whole liver in the event of avulsion of vascular pedicle. Disruption of the main vessel can also be associated with massive intraparenchymal or peritoneal hemorrhage, which requires immediate surgical treatment. The rupture of the inferior vena cava or supra-hepatic veins, which cause intraparenchymal and/or extraperitoneal massive bleeding, is a rare and potentially lethal complication [28].

Periportal tracking: this sign is not specific for trauma lesion; it is represented as a hypo-density of periportal fat tissue (Fig. 14.10). It can be determined by:

1. Post-traumatic blood suffusion of periportal interstitium
2. Distension of the periportals lymphatic vessels and lymphedema, which can happen after a

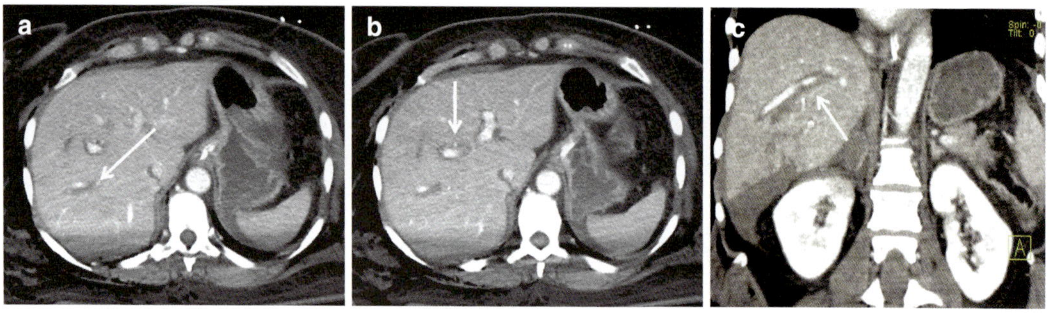

Fig. 14.10 (**a**, **b**) Axial CT scans and (**c**) coronal reconstruction show the periportal tracking characterized by hypodensities of periportal fat tissue (*arrows*)

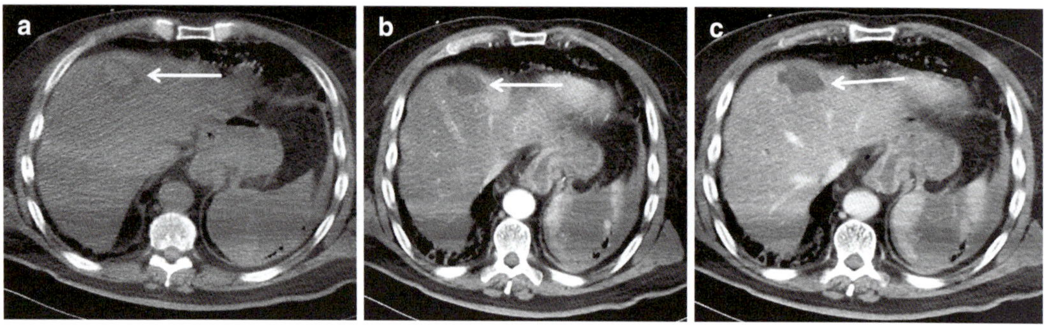

Fig. 14.11 (**a**) CT scan without contrast media administration, (**b**, **c**) CE-MDCT scan in arterial (**b**) and in venous phase (**c**) depict a parenchymal hematoma. The hematoma appears as a round hyperdense area in (**a**) (*arrow*), and hypodense in the post-contrast phases (**b**, **c**) (*arrows*)

rapid increase in central venous pressure (rapid fluid infusion to stabilize the patient, hypertensive pneumothorax, cardiac tamponade, hematoma compressing supra-hepatic veins)

Right liver lobe is the more frequently affected by periportal tracking (63%) [32, 33].

Sub-capsular hematoma: it is a blood collection with biconvex margins between the capsule and liver parenchyma. It appears as hyperdense at direct CT scan and hypodense during contrast-enhanced phase. It is almost always associated with liver lacerations on the surface and generally it is localized along the antero-lateral surface of the right lobe. In contrast to the free fluid in peritoneal cavity, the sub-capsular hematoma determines compression on the adjacent liver parenchyma. This type of hematoma is rare in blunt abdominal trauma, but represents a frequent complication of invasive procedures such as percutaneous liver biopsy.

Intraparenchymal hematoma: is a collection of blood which is developed in the context of a liver laceration. It appears as a round hyperdense area on direct CT scan (45–70 U.H, typical density of coagulated blood) with no enhancement after contrast media administration (Fig. 14.11). If air bubbles appear in the context of collecting blood, you could think of a bacterial superinfection by anaerobic bacteria or necrotic events. These elements are a negative prognostic factor, furthermore yet allowing a conservative treatment [34].

14.4.1 Vascular Contained Lesions: Arterial Pseudo-Aneurysm and Arteriovenous Fistula

Arterial pseudo-aneurysm: it is also known as a false aneurysm, and it is represented by a collection of blood between the two outer layers of an artery, muscularis and adventitia (Fig. 14.12). It's

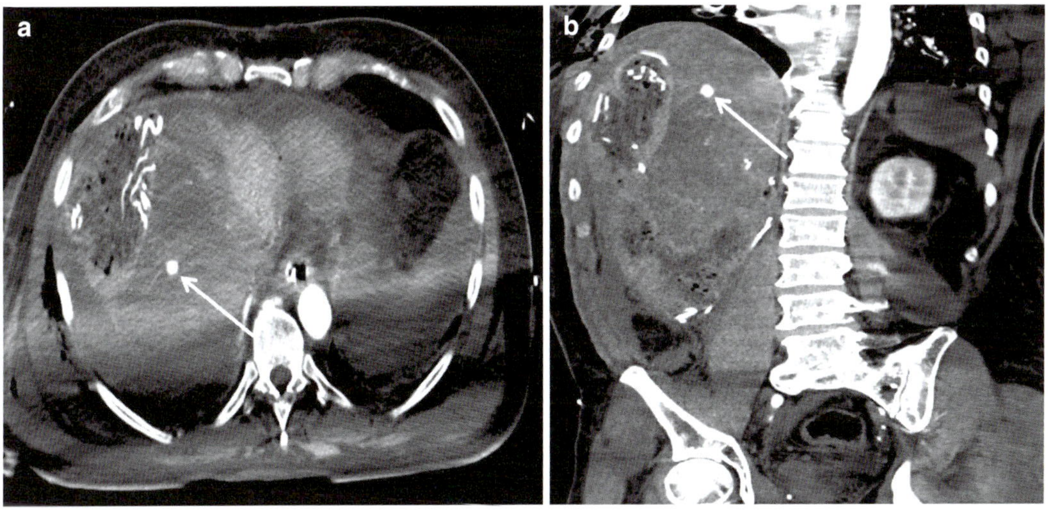

Fig. 14.12 Hepatic trauma treated by surgical packing. (**a**) Axial CT scan and (**b**) coronal reconstruction show a pseudo-aneurysm: it appears as a focal lesion with high attenuation values in the arterial phase (*arrows*)

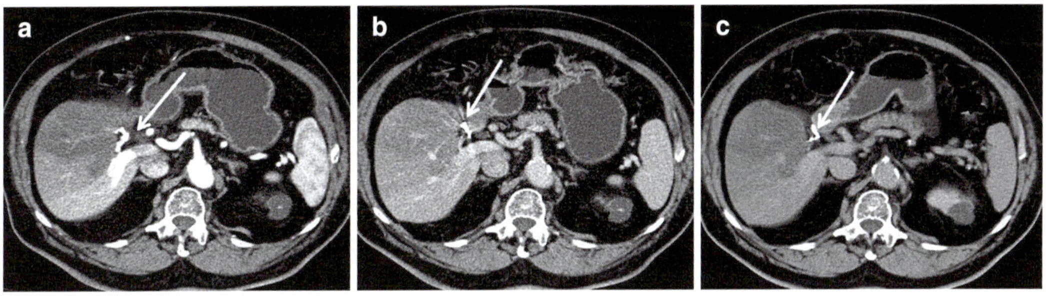

Fig. 14.13 Arteriovenous fistula in the arterial (**a**), venous (**b**), and equilibrium (**c**) phases; it is a communication between the main hepatic artery and a portal vein (*arrows*)

more frequent in open abdominal trauma. In blunt abdominal trauma, it can occur as a result of a bile extravasation. Usually, it can be found in proximity of a hepatic laceration that determines intimal lesion of the vessel.

On CT, it appears as a focal lesion with high attenuation values and featuring similar to normal arteries on contrast-enhanced scans. The morphology of the pseudo-aneurysm does not change during the phases of the exam, and this is important for differentiate it from a pooling. It may not be present at the first examination but it can appear in the following exams. In case of rupture, it can cause massive bleeding, fistula with biliary tract, intra-duodenal rupture, and consequent bleeding of the upper gastro-intestinal tract.

The demonstration of its presence is associated with the need for timely selective embolization of the affected vessel using angiography.

Arteriovenous fistula is a rare event, usually generated by a penetrating hepatic trauma that causes a communication between a main hepatic artery and portal vein or between the hepatic artery and a supra-hepatic vein [35] (Fig. 14.13). In contrast-enhanced CT scans, fistula remains enhanced in both phases, arterial and venous.

The differentiation between arteriovenous fistula and pseudo-aneurysm is easy to perform with angiography that is also useful in therapeutic approach.

Active bleeding: Pooling of contrast material on CT indicates free extravasation of blood as a result of

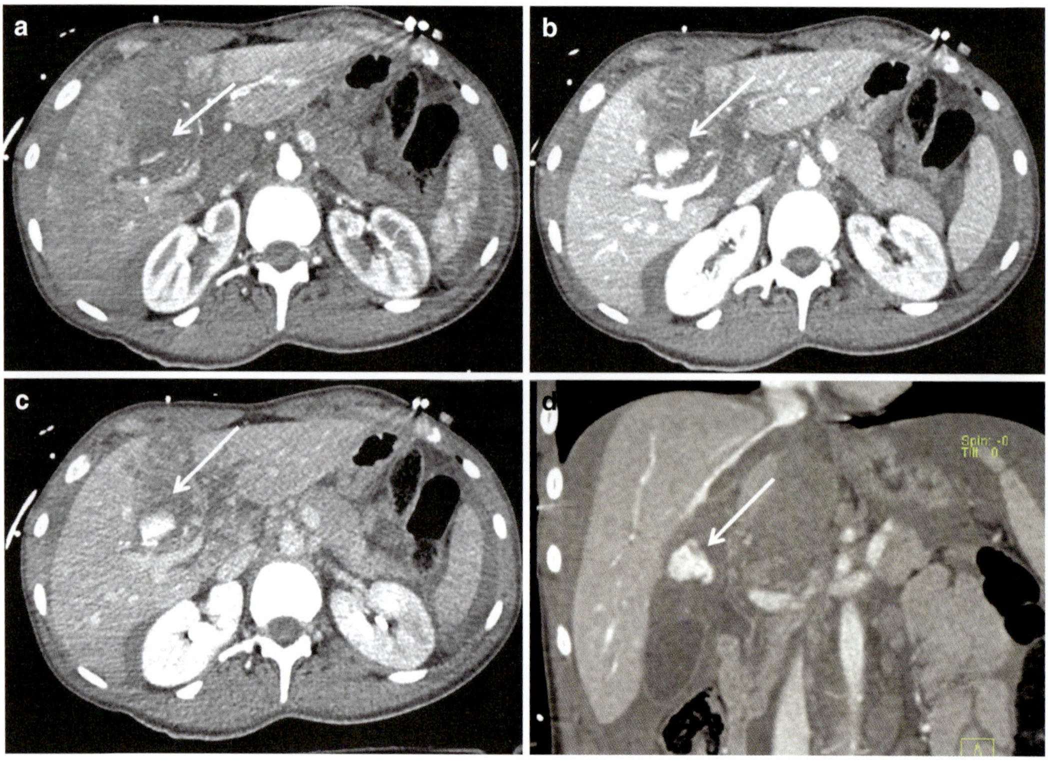

Fig. 14.14 Active bleeding: the extravasation of contrast in the arterial phase (**a**) becomes stronger in the venous (**b**), and the equilibrium (**c**), phases. (**d**) Coronal CT reconstruction confirms the active bleeding (*arrow*)

active bleeding (Fig. 14.14). The presence of active bleeding is an important risk factor for the patient since it can be the cause of hemodynamic instability and determine the need for a timely surgical intervention. The contrast-enhanced CT scan can detect the presence, location, and extent of an active bleeding [36].

Active arterial bleeding has become evident due to the extravasation of contrast medium in the arterial phase in the context of a hematoma, liver laceration, or peritoneal collection. During venous and late phases, the area of active bleeding spreads out. The attenuation values of an active bleeding are >90 U.H; therefore, higher than those of the coagulated blood and the liver parenchyma. To date, the recognition of an active arterial bleeding is an absolute indication to the embolic treatment through angiography.

Both the active bleeding and vascular contained lesions (pseudo-aneurysm and arteriovenous fistula) appear hyperdense in arterial phase. Therefore, it's necessary to differentiate them referring to venous and late phases. In fact, in these subsequent phases, the active bleeding appears more extended and mildly hyperdense, while the vascular contained lesions typically don't change their shape and extension.

In general, the active bleeding in liver trauma is most frequently linked to arterial injury, but may also be due to lesion of the portal vein and supra-hepatic veins. Consequently, the identification of extravasation of contrast in the arterial phase is useful to confirm the origin of the active arterial bleeding.

Venous lesions: lesions of the venous intraparenchymal structures happen in high-grade trauma and in approximately 90% of patients in which there is the failure of conservative therapy [37, 38]. Such injuries should be suspected in the presence of large intraparenchymal hematoma generally located in the sub-diaphragmatic region. Massive retroperitoneal hemorrhage can, however, indicate a lesion of the inferior vena cava, in this case the vein will be thinner than the normal. The lack of enhancement is the hallmark of avulsion of the liver vascular pedicle. Such a post-traumatic vascular lesion turns out to be absolutely the most serious.

14.5 Treatment and Complications

As already mentioned, the use of diagnostic imaging is essential to the therapeutic classification of patients with liver lesions, in order to refer the patient to a nonoperative management—NOM, which is a clinical monitoring—embolization by angiography or operative management by surgery.

To date, the standard therapeutic strategy (50–96%), in hemodynamically stable patients, even with high grading traumatic injuries, is nonsurgical (NOM) [25]. This is possible since it has been seen that the liver has high reparative capacity with restitutio ad integrum, which takes up to 3–6 months. Such conservative treatment has contributed to a clear reduction in mortality for blunt abdominal trauma [39].

If the CT scan shows an active bleeding from an artery, in a hemodynamically stable patient who has undergone a liver trauma, a trans-arterial embolization treatment of the damaged vascular branch is indicated. The interventional treatment should be as selective as possible, in order to minimize the risk of incurring parenchymal ischemia of the liver or the gallbladder, and possibly it should be made using reabsorbable materials [40]. The diagnostic role of angiography in polytrauma patients appears obsolete, after the development of multislice CT technology. On the contrary, it's increasing its application as interventional endovascular procedure. Thanks to the angiographic technique, in fact, it's possible to treat post-traumatic blood spills through active embolization procedures that use specialized instrumentation (metal coils and particles). Interventional endovascular procedures allow to avoid invasive surgery, resulting in reduced hospital stay and postoperative complications [41, 42].

Some studies reported an efficacy of 90–100% of trans-arterial embolization for active bleeding in hemodynamically stable patients (Figs. 14.15 and 14.16).

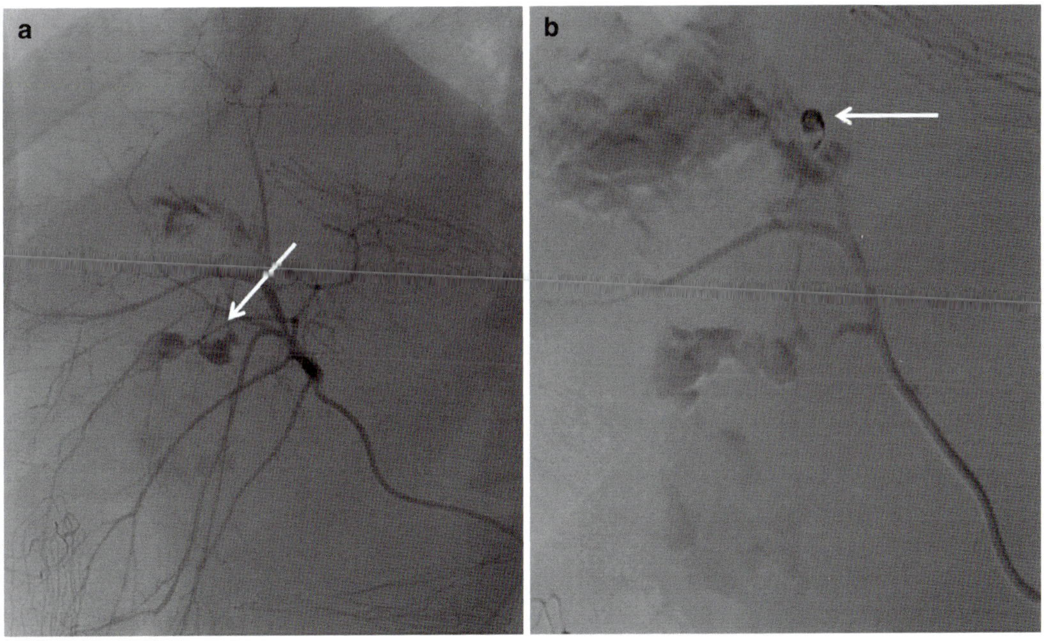

Fig. 14.15 In the same patient of Fig. 14.14, hepatic artery angiography (**a**) confirms active bleeding, previously identified on CE-CT scans. (**b**) Trans-arterial embolization achieved with coils (*arrow*)

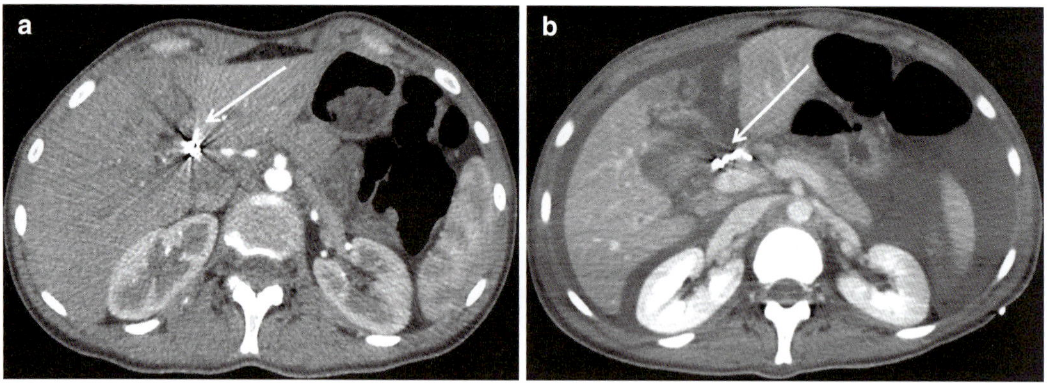

Fig. 14.16 Follow-up CE-MDCT scan (**a**, **b**) after trans-arterial embolization for the treatment of bleeding arteries with coils (*arrows*)

Some authors have also proposed to use the embolization technique for hepatic artery in all patients with traumatic liver lesions of grade III-IV, following the demonstration of a significant clinical improvement in patients treated with conservative method compare to those of the control group [43].

The liver's post-traumatic lesions, on the basis of angiographic findings, are classified according to "Hagiwara et al." in four grades [44].

Grade A includes avascular lesion or irregular accumulation of contrast medium in liver parenchyma or dislocation of the hepatic artery's branches.

Grade B refers to arteriovenous fistula or rupture of the hepatic artery's branches.

Grade C and Grade D indicate, respectively, extravasation of contrast in liver parenchyma and extravasation of contrast over liver parenchyma. The angiographic treatment is indicated for grades C and D if the patient is hemodynamically stable or if it is possible to pharmacologically maintain hemodynamic stability [44].

The new management for polytrauma patients has meant that the intervention of laparoscopic surgery in urgency runs in a small proportion of cases (about 20%). In fact, this is reserved for multiple trauma patients in shock and that present the "lethal triad":

1. pH <7.3
2. Body temperature <35°
3. Need to transfuse more than five units of blood

Liver damage of IV and V degree is often associated with active arterial and venous bleeding; endovascular arterial treatment is not indicated for the latter.

The CT, at times, may not be always able to distinguish the two types of blood extravasation, especially if these are mutually associated and if very extended. Some studies show that CT evidence of IV and V degree injury combined with the need to administer at least 2000 mL/h of fluids to maintain hemodynamic stability of the patient are correlated with a greater likelihood of finding venous blood extravasation.

Anyway if the CT scan highlights an active venous bleeding, an attempt through laparotomy surgery and compression by perihepatic packing is indicated. After intervention of perihepatic packing or trans-arterial embolization of injury, it will be the need to perform a close monitoring of clinical, hemodynamic, and laboratory parameters, in order to prevent the onset of complications which may require a subsequent surgery [45] (Fig. 14.17).

Complications that occur most frequently in trauma patients treated by surgery consist of bile leaks, abscesses, and lung infections.

In 12–28% of cases, a post-surgery trans-arterial embolization may be required if bleeding persists after perihepatic packing or in case of bleeding following the breaking of an arterial pseudo-aneurysm [46].

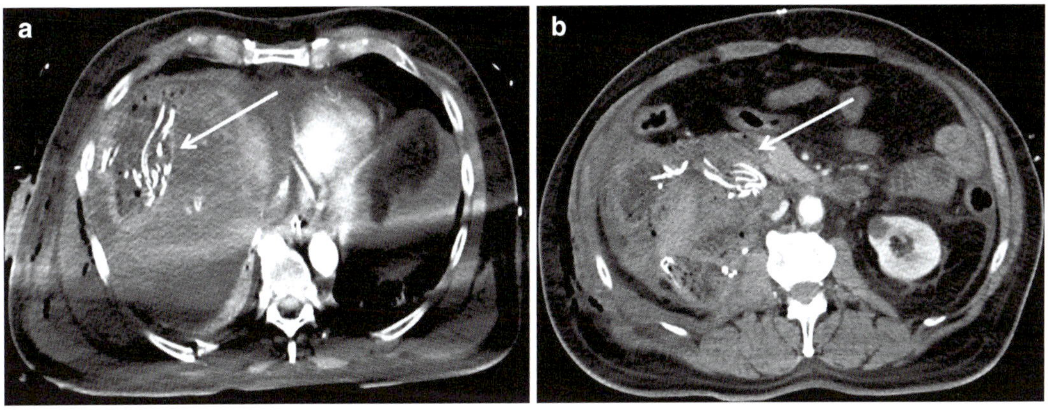

Fig. 14.17 (**a**, **b**) Perihepatic surgical packing: dressings are visible, thanks to the presence of radio-opaque markers (*arrows*)

The probability of complications is greater as the degree of liver damage is greater; particularly for degrees higher than the III and in case it has been necessary to perform trans-arterial embolization of an active bleeding.

The mortality in patients with hepatic trauma of grade IV and V is higher. Many studies, however, tell us how a multidisciplinary approach and the combined use of endovascular embolization treatment, perihepatic packing, and liver's resection lead to a reduction in mortality [47].

In conclusion, the general contraindications for nonoperative management of liver injuries include the hemodynamic instability, extravasations of intravenous contrast on abdominal imaging, expanding hematoma and usually grade IV and V of liver trauma [48, 49].

The prevalence of complications in traumatic liver lesions is about 5–23%, and these are more common in injuries higher than III degree. They consist of late hemorrhage and complications related to injuries involving the bile ducts. Generally, post-traumatic lesions of the bile ducts cause extravasation of bile that is resolved quickly and spontaneously. In 3–5% of cases, however, this doesn't occur, resulting in the appearance of bilomas, hemobilia, coleperitoneum that, instead, require treatment [50].

The liver's main post-traumatic complications are represented by:

1. *Late hemorrhage*: is suspected in the presence of a progressive decrease in hemoglobin. When it happens, contrast-enhanced CT scan must be repeated and, if active bleeding is present, it should be treated with blood transfusion and trans-arterial embolization if the bleeding is arterial, surgical treatment if the bleeding is venous.
2. *Biloma*: is a collection of bile with water density caused by lacerations affecting the bile ducts (Fig. 14.18). Usually small in size, sometimes of greater diameter whether a bile duct of large caliber is involved. Biloma can be intrahepatic, can develop beyond the hepatic parenchyma, or be entirely intraperitoneal. The dividing line for the treatment is the size: if less than 3 cm in diameter biloma can be treated conservatively; if greater than 3 cm in diameter biloma is subjected to guided US or CT drainage.
3. *Hemobilia*: appears with biliary tract hyperdensity at direct examination. It is determined by post-traumatic communication between a vascular branch (usually arterial) and bile duct (arterio-biliary fistula) or, less frequently, by the rupture of a pseudo-aneurysm in a bile duct. Hemobilia can be treated by endovascular arterial embolization. The main complication in this type of treatment, however, includes in the possibility of causing the

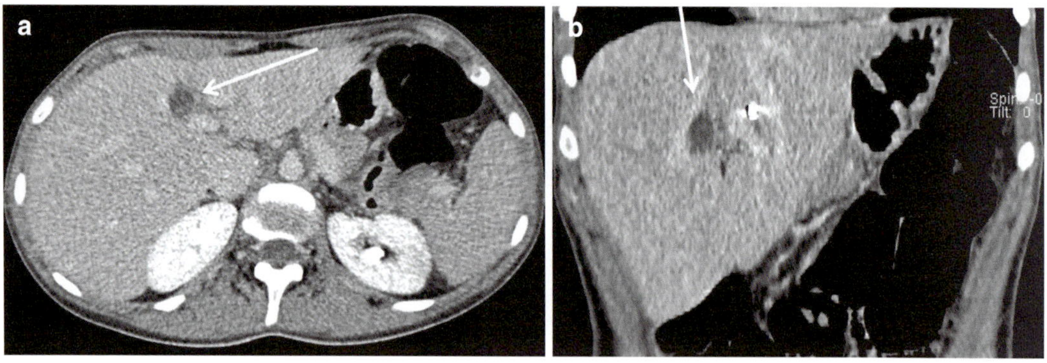

Fig. 14.18 (**a**) Axial CT scan and (**b**) coronal reconstruction show a small biloma (less than 3 cm) caused by lacerations affecting bile ducts (*arrows*)

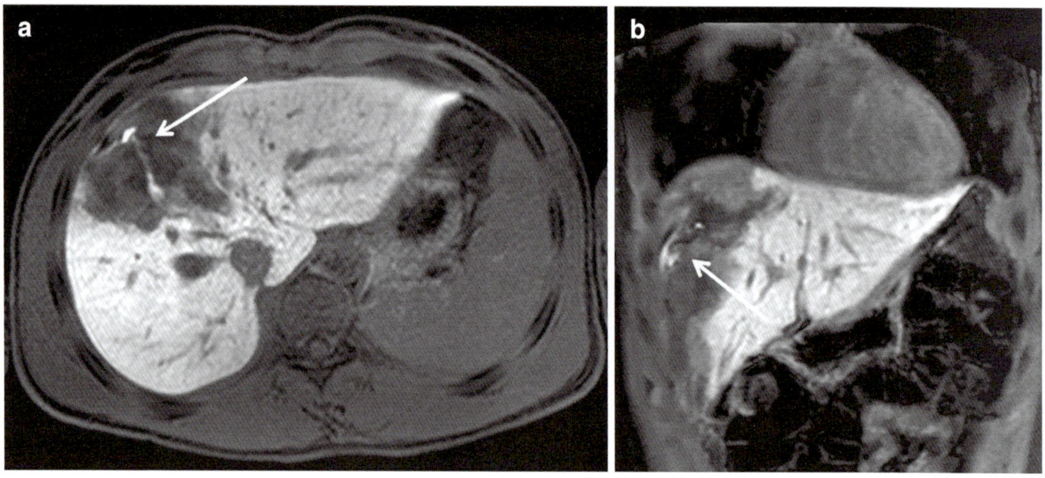

Fig. 14.19 Coleperitoneum is a bile effusion into the peritoneal cavity, diagnosed by MRI with specific liver contrast media in the hepatobiliary phase (T1 W-fat sat). Axial scan (**a**) and coronal scan (**b**)

passage of embolic material in the biliary tract with subsequent stenosis of the same.

4. *Coleperitoneum*: bile effusion into peritoneal cavity. The biliary nature of fluid and the presence of an active bile leakage can be diagnosed by ERCP (with contrast media administered through the retrograde bile duct) or MRI with liver-specific contrast media in hepatobiliary phase (Fig. 14.19).
5. *Abscess*: is a rare complication of high-grade liver injuries. It's achieved, more frequently, as a result of embolization procedure for occlusion of portal vein or a lobar branch. The abscess is identified as a focal area with water density often with air bubbles or air-fluid level in the context (Fig. 14.20). It can be treated by percutaneous drainage with US or CT guidance.

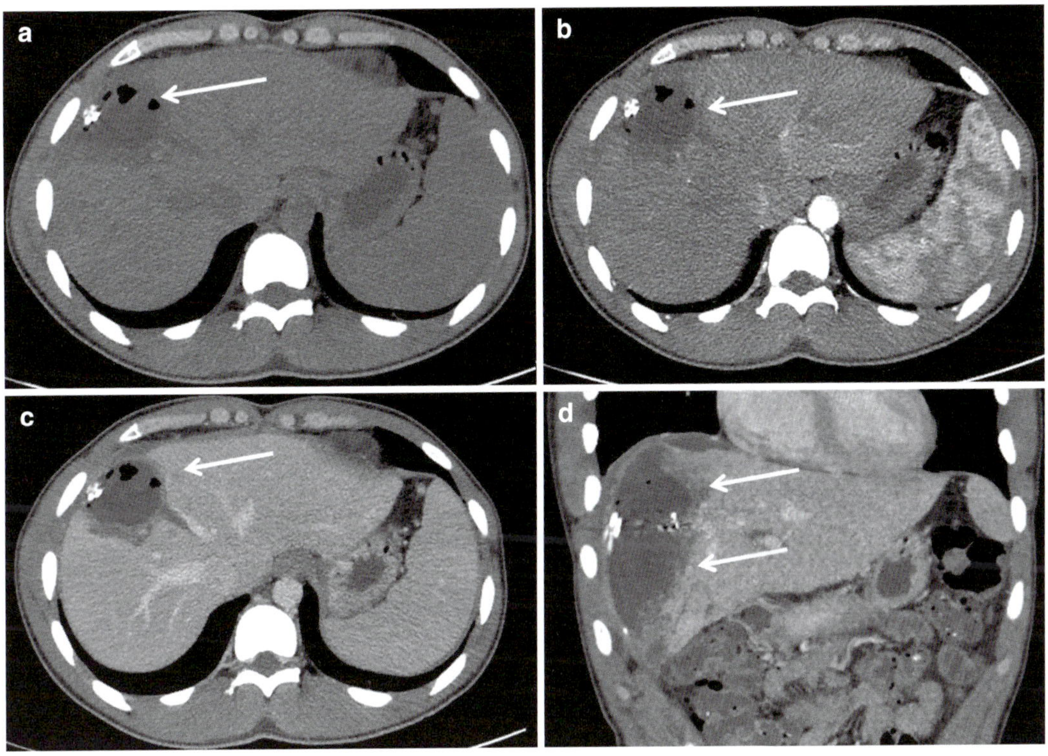

Fig. 14.20 Liver abscess 20 days after trauma. (**a**) Unenhanced CT scan, (**b**, **c**) CE-MDCT in the arterial (**b**) and venous (**c**) phases. (**d**) Coronal reconstruction. CT shows the liver abscess as a hypodense area with some gas bubbles into the lesion (*arrows*)

14.6 Follow-up

As already mentioned, in the last two decades there has been a change in the management of traumatic liver injuries that has led to an increasing number of cases treated by nonoperative methods.

Some studies have shown that the CEUS is almost as sensitive as MDCT in the detection of traumatic lesions in patients with low-energy isolated trauma, with levels of sensitivity and specificity approximately up to 95% [51, 52]. Considering the high number of young people involved in blunt abdominal trauma and the potential risks associated with the use of ionizing radiation and the possible adverse reactions to iodinated contrast media, there is a trend toward the use of CEUS for follow-up of the liver lesions [53–56].

CEUS, however, has some limitations. In fact, it is an operator-dependent technique, with low panoramic views and in case it shows some complications such as abscesses, biloma, vascular complications, a MDCT is needed [57–60].

Nowadays, the use of MRI (magnetic resonance imaging) was considered as a possible diagnostic tool to CEUS in the follow-up of liver injury. This method in fact turns out to be panoramic, devoid of ionizing radiation, and not operator dependent.

In addition, MRI allows a temporal staging of lesions, thanks to the dating of the bleeding through the variation of signal intensity. This is possible in relation with two parameters: the state of hemoglobin oxygenation (which influences the relaxation properties and magnetic susceptibility) and the state of red blood cell membranes (intact or lysed) [61].

In any case, MRI also has some limitations. In fact, it is possible to use it only on compliant patients, it's characterized by long exam duration, and by the inability to use in case of patients who are carriers of non-compatible MRI devices or if they are claustrophobic.

Until now, there isn't a standardized protocol for the follow-up of blunt abdominal trauma conservatively treated, but some studies have shown that it can be effectively done through CEUS at 24 and 72 h after trauma, CEUS and MRI at 1 month and only MRI until the complete resolution of liver injury or the highlighting of a stable residual scar [62].

This point can therefore be made for low-grade lesions (I–III) treated conservatively, while follow-up should be performed differently for high-grade lesions (IV–V).

So for the latter (grades IV and V, with high risk of complications), the timing of follow-up provides at first a CT scan, aimed at demonstrating the hemoperitoneum resolution, 7–10 days after trauma. Subsequent controls that show the resolution of liver lacerations, 40–60 days after trauma [63]. Any precautionary intermediate checks can be performed through ultrasonography.

In general, hemoperitoneum reabsorbs in a variable time, which depends, however, on the amount of fluid collection, lacerations are reduced in size gradually over time becoming more hypodense, fluid collections (biloma, hematoma, seroma) may persist for longer without requiring a percutaneous drainage, unless there is suspicion of superinfection.

Many studies have confirmed that the only reliable prognostic factor for follow-up of traumatized patients, conservatively treated, is hemodynamic stability. It has been proved that other factors, such as the amount of hemoperitoneum or the extension of parenchymal lesions, are not directly related to the need to resort to surgery [64].

References

1. Taurel P, Vernhet H, Suau A, et al. Vascular emergency in liver trauma. Eur J Radiol. 2007;64:73–82.
2. Romano L, Giovine S, Guidi G, et al. Hepatic trauma: CT findings and considerations based on our experience in emergency diagnostic imaging. Eur J Radiol. 2004;50:59–66.
3. Catre MG. Diagnostic peritoneal lavage versus abdominal computed tomography in blunt abdominal trauma: a review of prospective studies. Can J Surg. 1995;38:117–22.
4. Mele TS, Stewart K, Marokus B, et al. Evaluation of a diagnostic protocol using screening diagnostic peritoneal lavage with selective use of abdominal computed tomography in blunt abdominal trauma. J Trauma. 1999;46:847–52.
5. Gonzales RP, Ickler J, Gachassin P. Complementary roles of diagnostic peritoneal lavage and computed tomography in the evaluation of blunt abdominal trauma. J Trauma. 2001;51:1128–34.
6. Fabian TC, Mangiante EC, White TJ, et al. A prospective study of 91 patients undergoing both computed tomography and peritoneal lavage following blunt abdominal trauma. J Trauma. 1986;26:602–8.
7. Brown MA, Casola G, Sirlin CB. Blunt abdominal trauma: screening us in 2,693 patients. Radiology. 2001;218:352–8.
8. Jacobs DG, Sarafin JL, Marxs JA. Abdominal CT scanning for trauma: how low can we go? Injury. 2000;31:337–43.
9. Miele V, Di Giampietro I, Ianniello S, et al. Diagnostic imaging in pediatric polytrauma management. Radiol Med. 2015;120:33–49.
10. Croce MA, Fabian TC, Menke PG, et al. Nonoperative management of blunt hepatic trauma is the treatment of choice for hemodynamically stable patients. Results of a prospective trial. Ann Surg. 1995;221:744–53.
11. Lingawi SS, Buckley AR. Focused abdominal US in patients with trauma. Radiology. 2000;217:426–9.
12. Behboodi F, Mohtasham-Amiri Z, Masjedi N, et al. Outcome of blunt abdominal trauma with stable hemodynamic and positive FAST findings. Emerg (Teheran). 2016;4:136–9.
13. Federle MP, Jeffrey RB. Hemoperitoneum studied by computed tomography. Radiology. 1983;148:187–92.
14. Poletti PA, Wintermark M, Schnyder P, et al. Traumatic injuries: role of imaging in the management of the polytrauma victim (conservative expectation). Eur Radiol. 2002;12:969–78.
15. Shanmuganathan K, Mirvis SE, Sherbourne CD, et al. Hemoperitoneum as the sole indicator of abdominal visceral injuries: a potential limitation of screening abdominal US for trauma. Radiology. 1999;212:423–30.
16. McGahan JP, Wang L, Richards JR. From the RSNA refresher courses: focused abdominal US for trauma. Radiographics. 2001;21:S191–9.
17. Cagini L, Gravante S, Malaspina CM, et al. Contrast enhanced ultrasound (CEUS) in blunt abdominal trauma. Crit Ultrasound J. 2013;5(Suppl 1):S9.
18. Zhang YF, Li H, Zhang BH, et al. Effects of contrast-enhanced ultrasonography in monitoring hepatic microcirculation after rat liver ischemia-reperfusion injury. Exp Clin Transplant. 2016;14:323–8.
19. Zhao DW, Tian M, Yang JZ, et al. Hemostatic mechanism underlying microbubble-enhanced

non-focused ultrasound in the treatment of a rabbit liver trauma model. Exp Biol Med (Maywood). 2017;242:231–40.
20. Catalano O, Aiani L, Barozzi L, et al. CEUS in abdominal trauma: Multi-center study. Abdom Imaging. 2009;34:225–34.
21. Miele V, Piccolo CL, Galluzzo M, et al. Contrast enhanced ultrasound (CEUS) in blunt abdominal trauma. Br J Radiol. 2016;89(1061):20150823.
22. Miele V, Piccolo CL, Trinci M, et al. Diagnostic imaging of blunt abdominal trauma in pediatric patients. Radiol Med. 2016;121:409–30.
23. Soto JA, Anderson SW. Multidetector CT of blunt abdominal trauma. Radiology. 2012;265:678–93.
24. Davis KA, Brody JM, Cioffi WG. Computed tomography in blunt hepatic trauma. Arch Surg. 1996;131:255–60.
25. Kutcher ME, Weis JJ, Siada SS, et al. The role of computed tomographic scan in ongoing triage of operative hepatic trauma: a Western Trauma Association multicenter retrospective study. J Trauma Acute Care Surg. 2015;79:951–6.
26. Wintermark M, Poletti PA, Becker CD, et al. Traumatic injuries: organization and ergonomics of imaging in the emergency environment. Eur Radiol. 2002;12:959–68.
27. Mirvis SE, Whitley NO, Vainwright JR, et al. Blunt hepatic trauma in adults: CT-based classification and correlation with prognosis and treatment. Radiology. 1989;171:27–32.
28. Becker CD, Mentha G, Terrier F. Blunt abdominal trauma in adults: role of CT in the diagnosis and management of visceral injuries. Part 1: liver and spleen. Eur Radiol. 1998;8:553–62.
29. Moore EE, Shackford SR, Patcher HL, et al. Organ injury scaling: spleen, liver and kidney. J Trauma. 1989;29:1664–6.
30. Croce MA, Fabian TC, Kudsk KA, et al. AAST organ injury scale: correlation of CT graded liver injuries and operative findings. J Trauma. 1991;31:806–12.
31. Abramson SJ, Berdon WE, Kaufman RA, et al. Hepatic parenchymal and subcapsular gas after hepatic laceration caused by blunt abdominal trauma. Am J Roentgenol. 1989;153:1031–2.
32. Macrander SJ, Lawson TL, Foley WD, et al. Periportal tracking in hepatic trauma: CT features. J Comput Assist Tomogr. 1989;13:952–7.
33. Yokota J, Sugjmoto T. Clinical significance of periportal tracking on computed tomographic scan in patients with blunt liver trauma. Am J Surg. 1994;168:247–50.
34. Patten RM, Spear RP, Vincent LM. Traumatic laceration of the liver limited to the bare area: CT findings in 25 patients. Am J Roentgenol. 1993;160:1019–22.
35. Tanaka H, Iwai A, Sugimoto H, Yoshioka T, Sugimoto T. Intrahepatic arterio-portal fistula after blunt hepatic trauma: case reports. J Trauma. 1991;31:143–6.
36. Fang JF, Chen RJ, Wong YC, et al. Classification and treatment of pooling of contrast material on computed tomographic scan of blunt hepatic trauma. J Trauma. 2000;49:1083–8.
37. Sher R, Frydman GM, Russel TJ. Computed tomography detection of active mesenteric hemorrhage following blunt abdominal trauma. J Trauma. 1996;40:469–71.
38. Poletti PA, Mirvis SE, Shanmuganathan K, et al. CT criteria for management of blunt liver trauma: correlation with angiographic and surgical findings. Radiology. 2000;216:418–27.
39. Carrillo EH, Spain DA, Wohltmann CD, et al. Interventional techniques are useful adjuncts in nonoperative management of hepatic injuries. J Trauma. 1999;46:619–22.
40. Gaarder C, Naess PA, Eken T, et al. Liver injuries—improved results with a formal protocol including angiography. Injury. 2007;38:1075–83.
41. Am M, Lavery RF, Barone A, et al. Angiographic embolization for liver injuries: low mortality, high morbidity. J Trauma. 2003;55:1077–81.
42. Lai YC, Wu P, Huang CC, et al. Hepatobiliary and pancreatic: intra-hepatic arterio-biliary fistula caused by blunt abdomen trauma. J Gastroenterol Hepatol. 2016;31:1672.
43. Millàn D, Deballon PO. Computed tomography, angiography, and endoscopic retrograde cholangiopancreatography in the nonoperative management of hepatic and splenic trauma. World J Surg. 2001;25:1397–402.
44. Hagiwara A, Murata A, Matsuda T, et al. The efficacy and limitations of transarterial embolization for severe hepatic injury. J Trauma. 2002;52:1091–6.
45. Doklestić K, Stefanović B, Gregorić P, et al. Surgical management of AAST grades III-V hepatic trauma by damage control surgery with perihepatic packing and definitive hepatic repair single centre experience. World J Emerg Surg. 2015;10:34.
46. Ingram MC, Siddharthan RV, Morris AD, et al. Hepatic and splenic blush on CT in children following blunt abdominal trauma: is intervention necessary? J Trauma Acute Care Surg. 2016;81:266–70.
47. Melloul E, Denys A, Demartines N, et al. Management of severe blunt hepatic injury in the era of computed tomography and transarterial embolization: a systematic review and critical appraisal of the literature. J Trauma Acute Care Surg. 2015;79:468–74.
48. Asensio JA, Petrone P, Garcia-Nunez L, et al. Multidisciplinary approach for the management of complex hepatic injuries AAST-OIS grades IV–V: a prospective study. Scand J Surg. 2007;96:214–20.
49. Petrowsky H, Raeder S, Zuercher L, et al. A quarter century experience in liver trauma: a plea for early computed tomography and conservative management for all hemodynamically stable patients. World J Surg. 2012;36:247–54.
50. Gander R, Molino JA, Santiago S, et al. Conservative management of liver trauma and its complications: current gold-standard. Cir Pediatr. 2016;29:19–24.
51. Valentino M, Ansaloni L, Catena F, et al. Contrast enhanced ultrasonography in blunt abdominal trauma:

considerations after 5 years of experience. Radiol Med. 2009;114:1080–93.
52. Clevert DA, Wechbach S, Minaifar N, et al. Contrast enhanced ultrasound versus MS-CT in blunt abdominal trauma. Clin Hemorheol Microcirc. 2008;39:155–69.
53. Mizzi A, Shabani A, Watt A. The role of follow-up imaging in paediatric blunt abdominal trauma. Clin Radiol. 2002;57:908–12.
54. Manetta R, Pistoia ML, Bultrini C, et al. Ultrasound enhanced with sulphur-hex- afluoride-filled microbubbles agent (SonoVue) in the follow-up of mild liver and spleen trauma. Radiol Med. 2009;114:771–9.
55. Menichini G, Sessa B, Trinci M, et al. Accuracy of contrast-enhanced ultrasound (CEUS) in the identification and characterization of traumatic solid organ lesions in children: a retrospective comparison with baseline US and CE-MDCT. Radiol Med. 2015;120:989–1001.
56. Sidhu PS, Cantisani V, Deganello A, et al. Role of contrast-enhanced ultrasound (CEUS) in paediatric practice: an EFSUMB position statement. Ultraschall Med. 2017;38:33–43.
57. Pinto F, Miele V, Scaglione M, et al. The use of contrast-enhanced ultrasound in blunt abdominal trauma: advantages and limitations. Acta Radiol. 2014;55:776–84.
58. Pinto F, Valentino M, Romanini L, et al. The role of CEUS in the assessment of haemodinamically stable patients with blunt abdominal trauma. Radiol Med. 2015;120:3–11.
59. Sessa B, Trinci M, Ianniello S, et al. Blunt abdominal trauma: role of Contrast-Enhanced Ultrasound (CEUS) in the detection and staging of abdominal traumatic lesions compared with US and CE-MDCT. Radiol Med. 2015;120:180–9.
60. Miele V, Piccolo CL, Pallottino AA, et al. Ruolo dell'ecografia e della CEUS nelle urgenze traumatiche dell'addome. Il Giornale Italiano di Radiologia Medica. 2016;3:632–40.
61. Duhem R, Vinchon M, Tonnelle V, Soto-Ares G, et al. Main temporal aspects of MRI signal of subdural hematomas and practical contribution to dating head injury. Neurochirurgie. 2006;52:93–104.
62. Miele V, Piccolo CL, Sessa B, et al. Comparison between MRI and CEUS in the follow-up of patients with blunt abdominal trauma managed conservatively. Radiol Med. 2016;121:27–37.
63. Becker D, Gal I, Baer HU. Blunt hepatic trauma in adults: correlation with CT injury grading with Outcome. Radiology. 1996;201:215–20.
64. Roberts JL, Dalen K, Bosanko CM, et al. CT in abdominal and pelvic trauma. Radiographics. 1993;13:735–52.

15 Pancreatic Injuries

Margherita Trinci, Eva Berardi,
Giovanna Calabrese, Giovanni Maria Garbarino,
Matteo Pignatelli, and Vittorio Miele

15.1 Anatomy

The pancreas is an exocrine and endocrine retroperitoneal gland located transversely across the posterior abdominal wall at level of lumbar (L1–2) spine [1]. It's possible to identify three parts: head that is divided in head proper and uncinated process, body, and tail (Drawing 15.1a).

M. Trinci (✉) • G. Calabrese • M. Pignatelli
Department of Emergency Radiology,
S. Camillo Hospital, Rome, Italy
e-mail: margherita.trinci@libero.it

E. Berardi
Department of Radiology, S. Andrea Hospital,
Sapienza University, Rome, Italy

G.M. Garbarino
Department of Surgery, S. Andrea Hospital, Sapienza
University, Rome, Italy

V. Miele
Department of Radiology, Careggi University
Hospital, Florence, Italy

In adults, the pancreas weighs approximately 100 g and is about 17–20 cm long, it has a soft texture and friable.

The main pancreatic duct of Wirsung (3–4 mm) traverses the entire length of the gland and pours the pancreatic secretion into the duodenum. The caliber of the duct decreases homogeneously from head to tail. The duct receives 25–35 side branches; at the level of the papilla it merges with the choledocus into the Vater ampulla (Drawing 15.1b). There is a secondary duct named Santorini; it is the embryonic vestige of the primitive pancreas and as such may not be working. If it is anatomically functional, it drains the back of the pancreas head. It opens in the duodenum about 2–3 cm above the main duct, in the papilla called "minor" that does not have sphincter, and for this reason, if the ostium is stenotic, it is related to pancreatitis.

Pancreatic vascular supply is owing to the superior pancreaticoduodenal artery from the gastroduodenal artery and the inferior pancreaticoduodenal artery from the superior mesenteric artery which supplies the head of the pancreas.

V. Miele, M. Trinci (eds.), *Diagnostic Imaging in Polytrauma Patients*,
https://doi.org/10.1007/978-3-319-62054-1_15

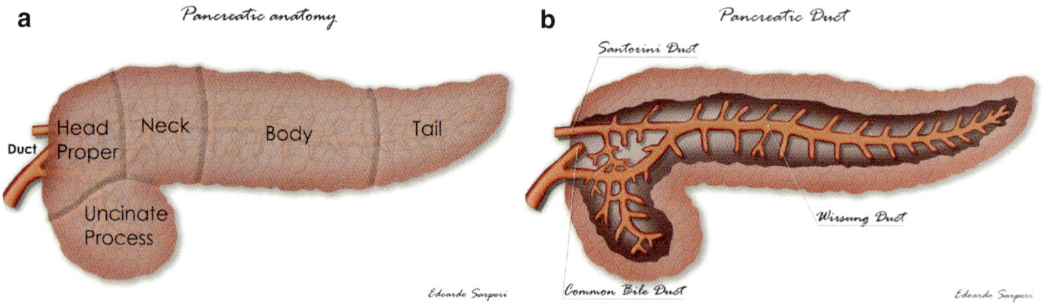

Drawing 15.1 (**a**) Anatomy of the pancreatic gland, (**b**) anatomy of the pancreatic duct

The pancreatic branches of the splenic artery (the largest is called the greater pancreatic artery) supply the neck, body, and tail of the pancreas.

The head of the pancreas drains into the superior mesenteric and portal veins; the neck and the body drains into the splenic vein [2].

15.2 Etiopathogenesis

Pancreatic trauma, due to its retroperitoneal position, is relatively rare especially as an isolated lesion; it is still more frequent in children [3].

Pancreatic traumatic injuries have a mortality rate that can reach 39%, occur in 0.4% of total blunt abdominal trauma with an incidence of 7% (range 2–13%) in major trauma, such as in motor vehicle accidents, pedestrian accidents, or bicycle accidents especially in children "handlebar" trauma [4]. We must not forget that the pancreas for its "central position" is an organ particularly affected in child abuse cases; the injuries of this organ are responsible for about 1/3 of post-traumatic pancreatitis in pediatric age [5].

Nowadays we must take into consideration not only the blunt trauma but also the penetrating trauma as gunshot wounds and blade injuries that is rising in incidence and accounts for 70% of all traumatic pancreas injuries.

With regard to the zone of lesion, body and isthmus are affected in 2/3 of the cases generally for front force vectors (e.g., trauma caused by the steering wheel of the car in the absence of seat belt). The head and tail of the pancreas are involved in 1/3 of the cases generally for lateral force vectors.

Pancreatic lesions are often (in over 90% of cases) associated with other abdominal organ injuries, especially associated with the viscera situated in the upper abdomen [6]. Bone injuries are also often associated.

The absence of specific clinical symptoms and the frequent presence of multiple organ injuries make it difficult to develop a diagnosis. This injury is associated with considerably high morbidity and mortality in cases of delayed diagnosis, incorrect classification of the injury, or delays in treatment.

It's important to notice that in children you may have pancreatic damage even in small claims traumas, due to the lower strength of the abdominal wall [7].

15.3 Clinical Presentation

Ecchymosis in either the upper abdomen or along the flank may be present in cases of pancreatic injury. In the child, in the bicycle handlebars trauma often there is a round bruise in mesogastric region.

The rise in the serum of amylase and lipase is present respectively in 73% and 82% of cases.

The classical clinical triad of pancreatic trauma is upper abdominal pain, leukocytosis, and elevated serum amylase level, that may, however, be absent in the first 24 h (in up to 40% of patients) or even after several days although it does not always indicate the severity of the injury [8].

Amylase may be elevated even in injuries of duodenum, salivary gland, hepatic trauma, and injuries of head and face [1].

The lack of clinical manifestations makes it difficult to diagnose, and delay in diagnosis is the main cause of complications, therefore it is necessary to have a second level radiological diagnosis.

15.4 Classification

Traumatic lesion could interest any site of the pancreas; those that are localized to the head and body (90%) are most frequent and are connected to the compression of the pancreas against lumbar spine.

The most recent grading system for pancreatic injuries was outlined by the American Association for Surgery in Trauma (AAST) [9].

It takes into account both the *type of parenchymal damage* and the *site* of the parenchymal gland in which the damage has occurred, the involvement of the duct of Wirsung, that usually occurs in 15% of cases, or of the ampulla.

The classification is divided into five degrees in relation to the severity of the damage.

In the grade I: there is a minor contusion/hematoma or superficial laceration without ductal injury (Drawing 15.2a, b); sometimes the minor contusion of the gland may be difficult to see especially in a patient with multiple organ lesions. The gland can be enlarged with ill-defined profiles also due to the surrounding fluid often present (see Fig. 15.6).

In the grade II: there is a major contusion/laceration; the lesion is largest than in the first degree but the duct is always intact (Drawing 15.3a, b).

In the grade III: there is a laceration or parenchymal injury with duct injury in *distal* pancreas (Drawing 15.4a, b).

In the grade IV: there is a *proximal* (right of *superior mesenteric vein*) laceration or parenchymal injury with associated injury to *bile duct/ampulla* (Drawing 15.5a, b).

In the grade V: there is a *massive destruction* of pancreatic head (Drawing 15.6).

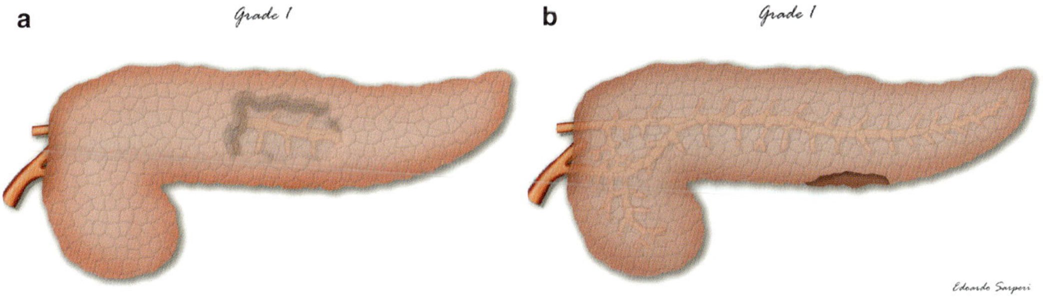

Drawing 15.2 I grade pancreatic lesion (**a**) minor contusion, (**b**) superficial laceration. Note in both cases the integrity of the pancreatic duct

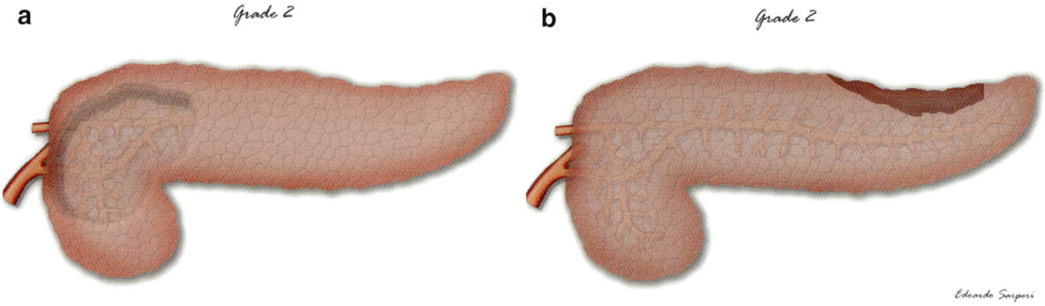

Drawing 15.3 II grade pancreatic lesion. (**a**) Major contusion, (**b**) major laceration. Note in both cases the integrity of the pancreatic duct

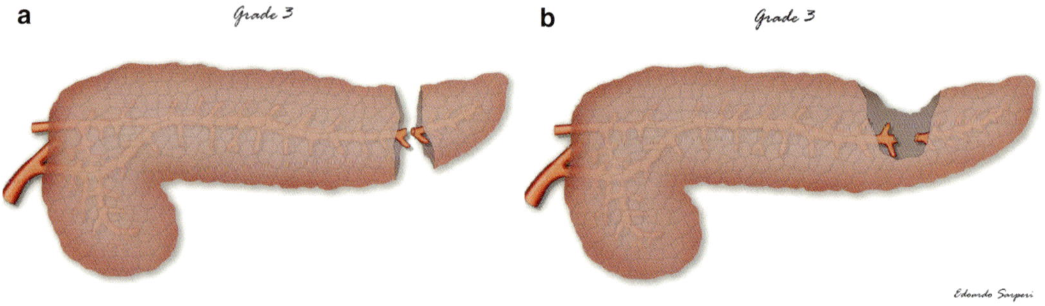

Drawing 15.4 III grade pancreatic lesion. (**a**) Distal laceration (**b**) distal parenchymal injury. In both cases there is a distal duct injury

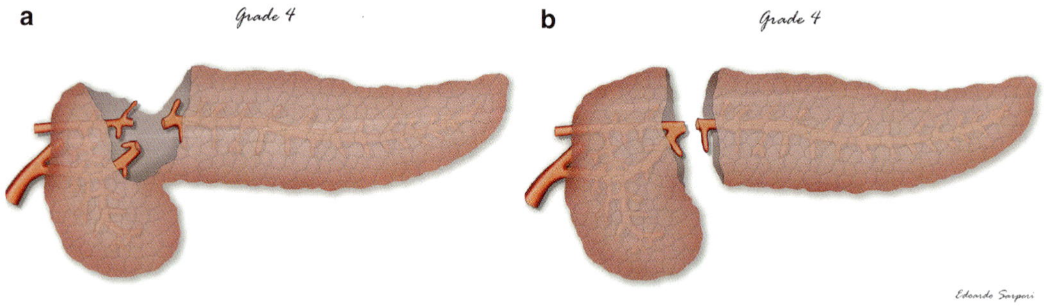

Drawing 15.5 IV grade pancreatic lesion. (**a**) Proximal laceration, (**b**) proximal parenchymal injury. In both cases there is a proximal duct injury

Based on the severity and extent of the lesions that we can find at CT exam:

- Pancreatic contusion: interstitial edema with focal or diffuse enlargement of the gland (Figs. 15.1 and 15.2).
- Pancreatic hematoma: blood collection often intraglandular (Fig. 15.3).
- Pancreatic laceration: partial thickness tear of the pancreas, frequently with vertical axis [10] (Fig. 15.4).
- Pancreatic transection: full thickness tear of the pancreas (Fig. 15.5).

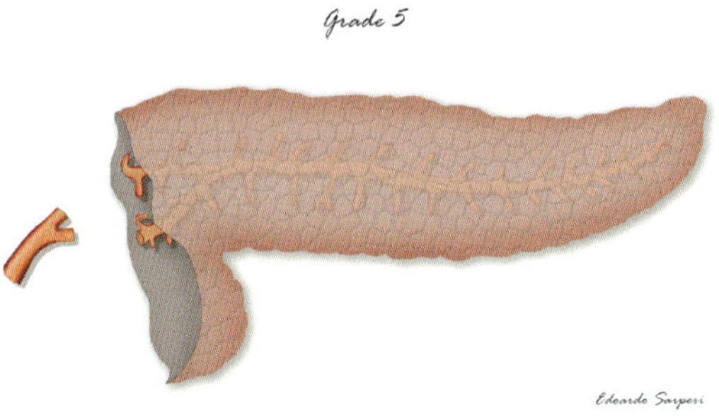

Drawing 15.6 V grade pancreatic lesion. There is a massive destruction of pancreatic head

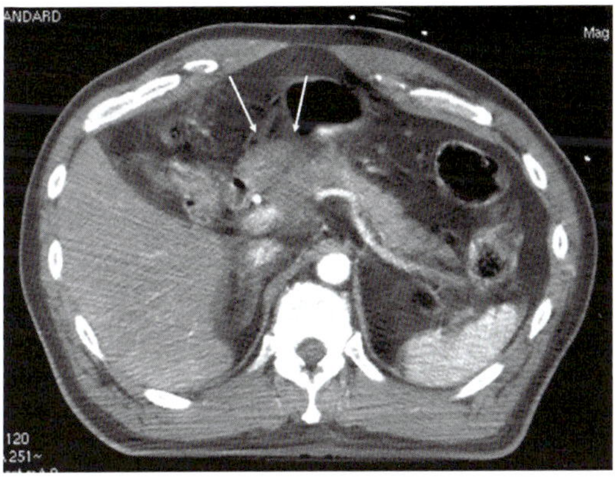

Fig. 15.1 Enhanced CT scan shows pancreatic head contusion as a focal enlarged area with hypodense aspect due to interstitial edema (*white arrows*)

- Intra- or extraglandular active bleeding (Fig. 15.6).

Pancreas head injuries are more severe than those in the body and tail. Pancreatic injury is uncommonly (<10%) an isolated lesion; other organs are frequently involved like: duodenum (involved in 60%), liver (46%), stomach (42%), spleen, kidney, mayor vascular: aorta, inferior cava vein, splenic artery and vein (41%), spine fractures (28–30%), stomach, and other tract of the bowel [11]. The involvement of mayor vessels is responsible for premature mortality for massive bleeding; the bowel involvement increases long-term mortality and late complications for septic state due to perforation and peritonitis. In case of pancreatic lesion, the dehiscence of intestinal anastomosis increases.

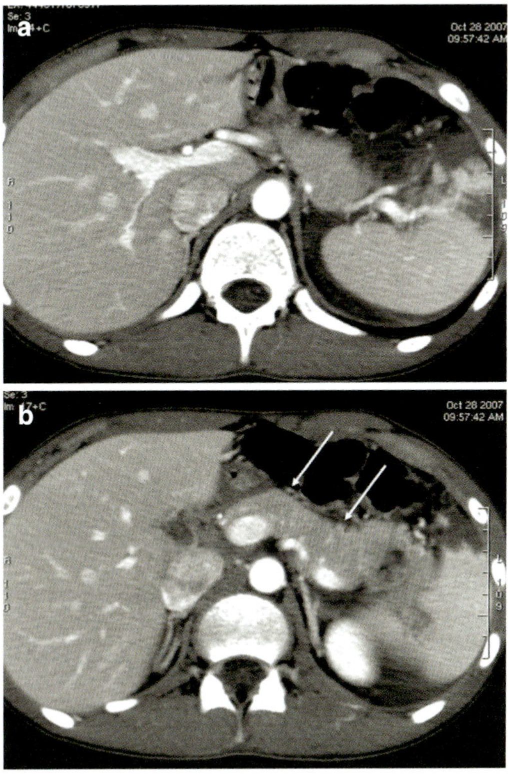

Fig. 15.2 CE-MDCT scans (**a**, **b**) show a fracture of the upper pole of the spleen associated with pancreatic body and tail contusion (*arrows*)

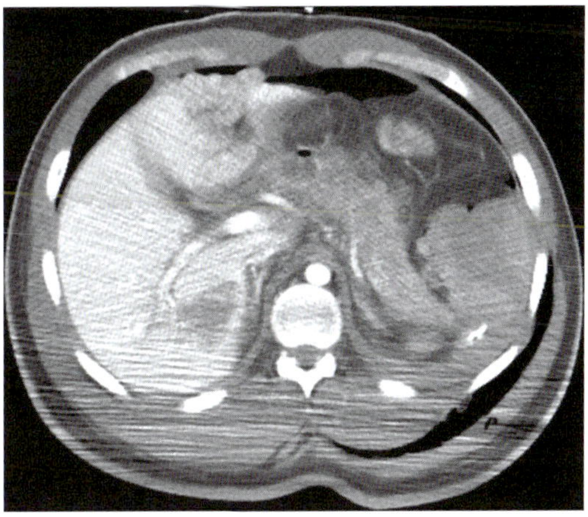

Fig. 15.3 Enhanced CT scan shows pancreatic hematoma: diffuse enlargement inhomogeneous hypodense aspect and irregular borders, in the head there is a focal rounded hypodense area with thin border. Hepatic lesion and free fluid are associated

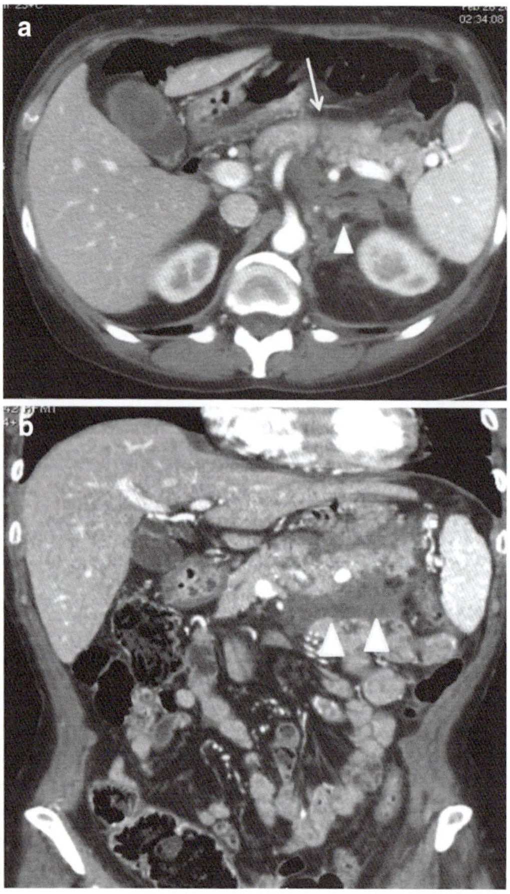

Fig. 15.4 Pancreatic laceration: (**a**) axial CT scan and (**b**) coronal reconstruction show partial thickness tear of the body (*arrow*); there is a fluid collection behind and below the pancreatic body (*arrowheads*)

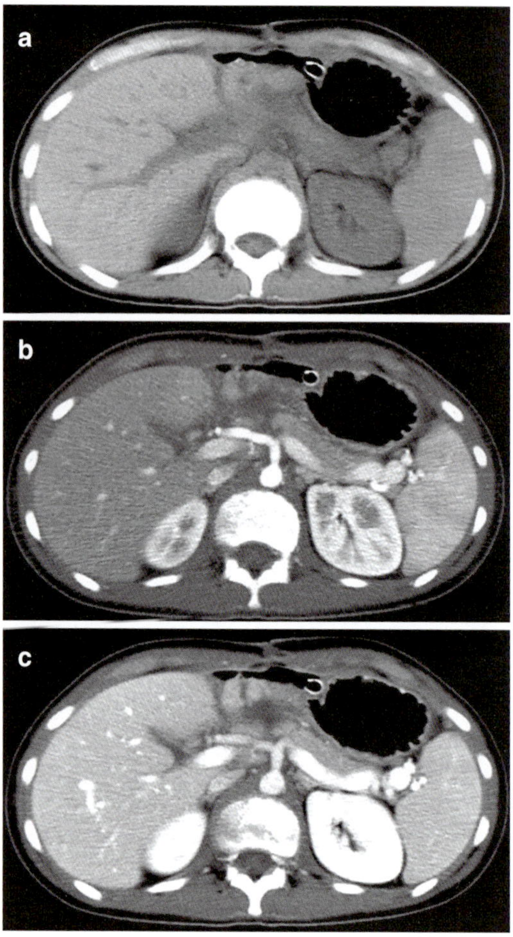

Fig. 15.5 Unenhanced CT (**a**) and enhanced CT scan in arterial (**b**) and portal (**c**) phases show a case of pancreatic body transection. In unenhanced CT (**a**) there is an inhomogeneous aspect of the pancreas body; CE-CT scans (**b**, **c**) well detect the complete transection of the body as a hypodense linear image

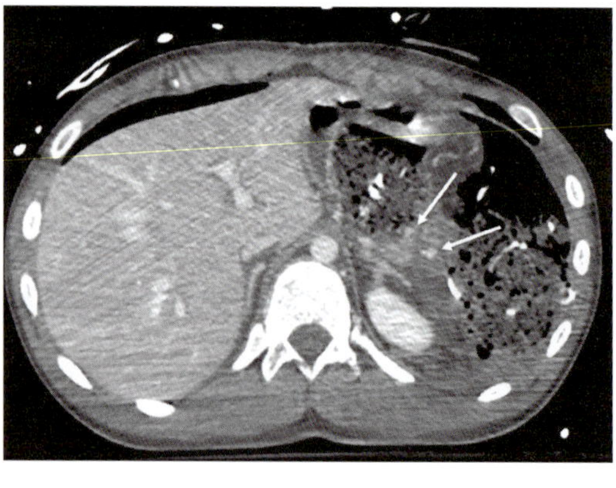

Fig. 15.6 Enhanced CT exam shows a case of pancreatic active bleeding (*white arrows*) complex trauma treated with splenectomy and packing

15.5 CT Imaging

Computed tomography (CT) is the imaging modality of choice in the study of hemodynamically stable polytrauma patient, detecting all grades of pancreatic lesions in 80% [8, 12]. The CT is also able to evaluate most of the prognostic indicators that can change the management of the patient and it is fundamental to follow complications which occur very often.

The pancreas can appear normal in 20–40% of patients in the first 12 h after trauma because pancreatic injuries may produce nuanced hyperdensity which may not be detectable [13].

The CT is not always able to view the pancreatic duct injury but its tear can be suspected in cases of parenchymal injury larger than 50% of the diameter of the pancreas and MPR reconstruction is fundamental in detecting injury. However, it often happens that the ductal lesions are discovered in the operating room. If ductal injury is suspected and the clinical condition of the patient allows further studies, the evaluation of pancreatic duct should be carried out with magnetic resonance (MRI) or endoscopic retrograde cholangio-pancreaticography (ERCP) [14].

15.5.1 CT Protocol

The CT scan is performed with MDCT scanner. The exams are obtained in cranio-caudal direction, in cases of polytrauma patients from "head to toe," and in cases of localized minor trauma the evaluation can be limited to the abdomen.

CT examination includes unenhanced scans, followed by enhanced CT scans, in arterial and portal phases. Arterial phase is performed with bolus tracking (with a ROI located in abdominal aorta below the diaphragm) or with a delay of 30–40 s from the beginning of contrast administration; portal phase is usually performed with a delay of 70–80 s.

The quantity of a nonionic low-osmolar iodinated contrast depends on the patient's weight and on the acquisition speed time of the machine; generally, the quantity is around 120–140 mL injected at a rate of 3–4 mL/s.

A thin collimation is necessary, MPR reconstruction on coronal plane is fundamental to assess the lesion of the duct, even 3D reconstructions can be of help.

The CT findings of acute pancreatic trauma may be separated into specific (direct) features and nonspecific (indirect) features [15].

Direct CT signs of pancreatic trauma include evidence of parenchymal *contusion, hematoma, laceration, and transection* [4, 16].

15.5.1.1 Pancreatic Contusion

Unenhanced CT scan: Contusion cannot be detectable; however, it is possible to find focal or diffuse pancreatic enlargement in case of intraparenchymal edema.

Enhanced CT scan: Small contusion can be difficult to detect; in some cases, it appears as focal or diffuse low attenuation area inside the parenchymal gland without discontinuity at the surface of the gland; the margins of the gland appear irregular, and fluid collection may surround the gland (Fig. 15.7).

15.5.1.2 Pancreatic Hematoma

Unenhanced CT scan: Blood content determines focal hyperdensity that tends to become isodense in later hours.

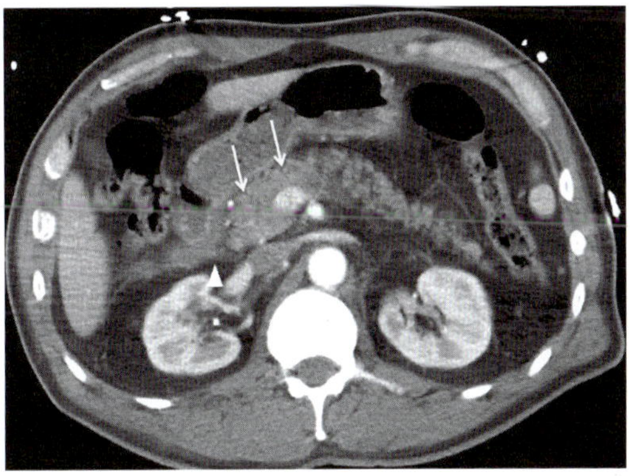

Fig. 15.7 CE-MDCT in a case of pancreatic head and body contusion; note the difference between the hazy irregular contours of the head and part of the body (*arrows*) compared with the rest of the gland. There is also a small fluid collection surrounding pancreatic head and located along the right anterior renal fascia in the retroperitoneal space (*arrowhead*)

Enhanced CT scans: Hematoma can be a very specific sign of pancreatic injury and manifests as an area of focal attenuation within the pancreatic parenchyma. It is often peripherally located and distorts the gland profile (Fig. 15.8).

15.5.1.3 Laceration

Unenhanced CT scan: Lacerations manifest as linear, irregular, low attenuation areas within the pancreatic parenchyma. The laceration is often perpendicular to the long axis of the pancreas. It is often difficult to see in basal conditions and can manifest only as an area of glandular inhomogeneity.

Enhanced CT scans: Lacerations are hypodense but more defined with a linear or irregular aspect. The line, ideally, represents the separation of fragments with fluid or blood within the fragments. This can be classified into superficial laceration (involving <50% of the parenchyma) and deep laceration (>50% pancreatic parenchyma) [4]. It's possible to collect fluid effusion in retroperitoneal space.

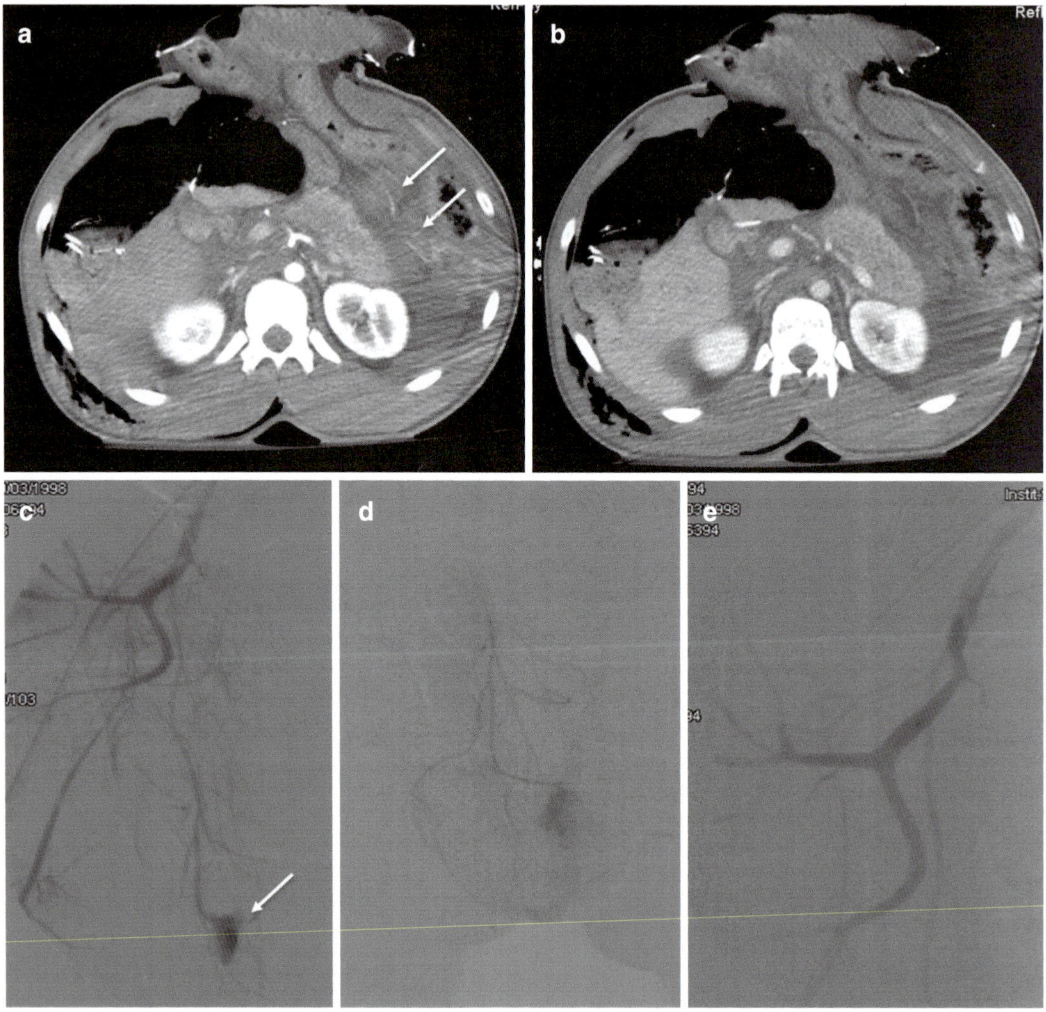

Fig. 15.8 Contrast-enhanced MDCT (**a**, **b**) shows hematoma of the pancreatic body in a polytrauma patient, already undergoing splenectomy. It is possible to detect focal attenuation within the pancreatic tail parenchyma; the tail is enlarged. In arterial phase (**a**) note active bleeding coming from a branch of the left hypogastric artery (*white arrows*). (**c**) Selective arteriography shows the active bleeding (*arrow*), treated by selective embolization with microcoils and spongostan (**d**, **e**)

In case of laceration, the pancreatic duct may be intact or damaged, depending on the extension of the laceration; sometimes the presence of a deep laceration leads to the suspicion of ductal lesion. In doubtful cases, it is recommended to complete the study as soon as possible with magnetic resonance cholangiopancreatography (MRCP) (Fig. 15.9).

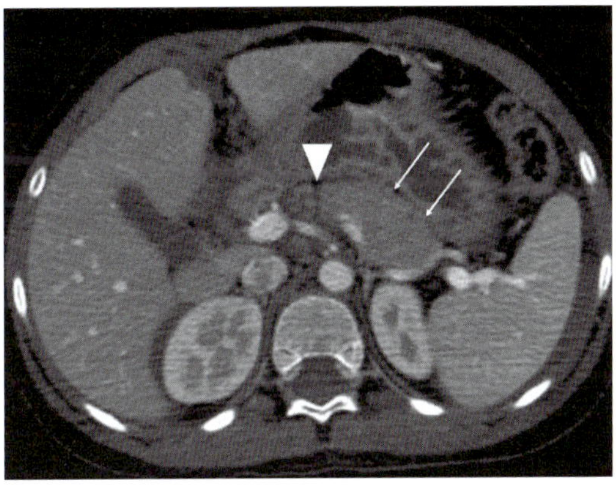

Fig. 15.9 CE-MDCT. Pancreatic body laceration appears as linear, irregular line within pancreatic body (*arrowhead*); note also the enlargement of pancreatic tail expression of contusion (*arrows*)

15.5.1.4 Transection/Fracture

Unenhanced CT scan: Pancreatic transection/fracture was defined as a low-attenuating band extending throughout the thickness of the gland with fluid collection between the two separated fragments. Usually occurs vertical transection of the pancreatic body or head.

Enhanced CT scans: The CT aspects of transection previously described have better evidence in CE-MDCT; furthermore active hemorrhage from the pancreatic parenchyma can be seen as contrast extravasation with hyperdense spots.

In case of transection or fracture of the pancreatic gland, the main duct is always involved; this eventuality determines a change in the management of the patient (Fig. 15.10).

Indirect signs of pancreas trauma are nonspecific and may also be caused by injuries of other organs. However, they are important to know, recognize, and evaluate because they may also be a sign of pancreatic lesion and combined with alteration of specific laboratory analysis may suggest a pancreatic involvement.

- Peripancreatic fluid or hematoma: frequently found between the splenic vein and the pancreas this is the most CT finding suggesting

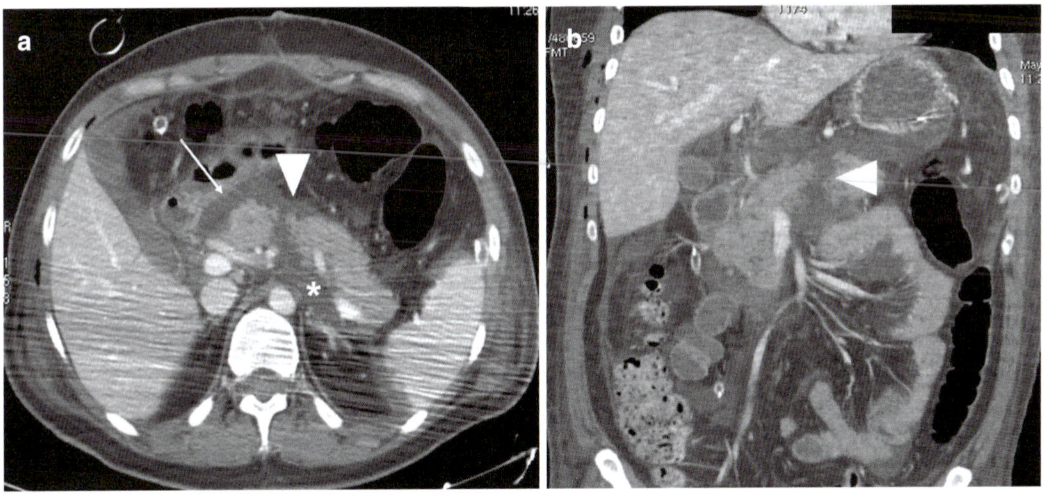

Fig. 15.10 Axial CT scan (**a**) and coronal reconstruction (**b**) show the fracture of the pancreatic body (*arrowheads*) associated at mayor duct injury; fluid collection located in the lesser sac (*arrow*), between the two separated fragments and in peripancreatic space. Note the fluid between splenic vein and the pancreas (*asterisk*)

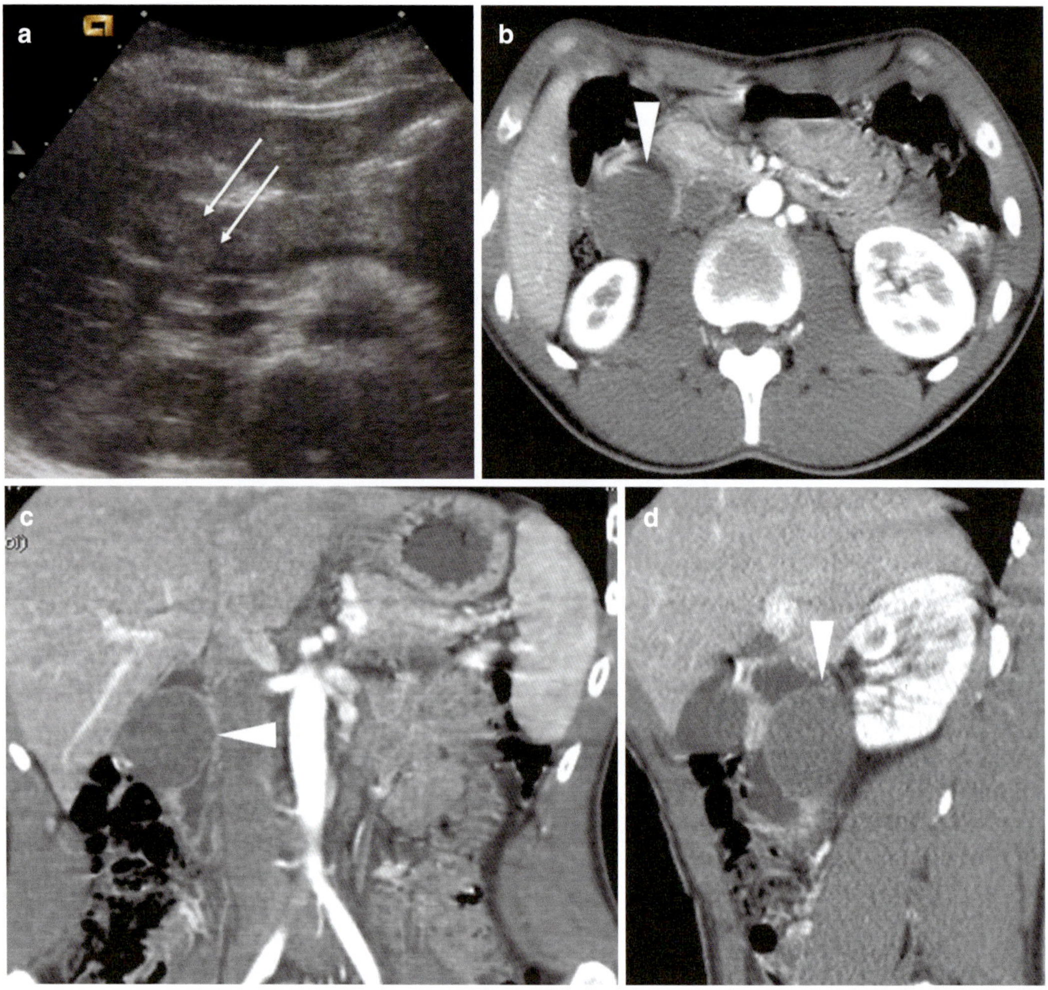

Fig. 15.11 Duodenal injury. Ultrasound (**a**) shows the thickening of the duodenal wall (*arrows*). Contrast-enhanced CT, axial scan (**b**), coronal (**c**) and sagittal (**d**) reconstructions show a duodenal wall rounded hematoma (*arrowheads*)

pancreatic trauma [8], detected in 90% (see Fig. 15.9a).

- Peripancreatic fat stranding.
- Mesenteric fluid.
- Thickening of Gerota's fascia and retroperitoneal free fluid (see Fig. 15.3a).
- Pancreatic ductal dilatation.
- Fluid in the pararenal spaces.
- Fluid in transverse mesocolon and lesser sac (Fig. 15.9a).
- Peritoneal free fluid.

It's very important to evaluate the integrity of duodenum, which is frequently involved. Duodenal contusion should be suspected when it is possible to detect edema or hematoma of the duodenal wall, intramural gas collection, and focal duodenal wall thickening (>4 mm) as in small bowel injury (Fig. 15.11). In the case of duodenum wall rupture, the amount of free air around it may be small, there may be enteric juice, but it does not differ from other free fluid.

15.6 MRI Technique and Manifestation

If the suspicion of pancreatic injury persists after CT and CT findings are negative, endoscopic retrograde cholangio-pancreatography (ERCP) or MRCP can prove useful as important second-line imaging [12, 17].

The outcome of pancreatic trauma in patients depends upon the integrity of the pancreatic duct, and the evaluation of the duct is fundamental. MRI has emerged as an alternative noninvasive diagnostic tool for direct imaging of the pancreatic duct with an accuracy of 100% [12] (Fig. 15.12). The MRI also provides a complete evaluation of the glandular parenchyma and abdominal organs. Compared to the ERCP, the MRI is a faster method and, without being invasive, it does not expose the risk of pancreatitis.

MRI of the pancreas should be performed with height field strength scanners (1.5 T or 3 T); the normal protocol for the study of the pancreas includes coronal and axial T2-weighted single-shot echo train spin echo (SS-ETSE), axial T2-weighted fat suppressed fat spin echo, axial in-phase and out-phase T1-weighted spoiled gradient echo (GRE), and axial T1-weighted fat suppressed 3D GRE images, before and after intravenous administration of gadolinium contrast material. It is important, if possible, the administration of negative oral contrast agent to remove high signal intensity from the fluid inside the stomach and duodenum; if the commercial product is not available, pineapple juice and blueberry juice can be used as alternative negative MR contrast material.

Cholangiopancreatography (MRC) should be performed with coronal and axial T2 sequences (SS-ETSE) for the anatomical display of the common bile duct and 3D images in an oblique coronal projection following the plane of the main pancreatic duct [18].

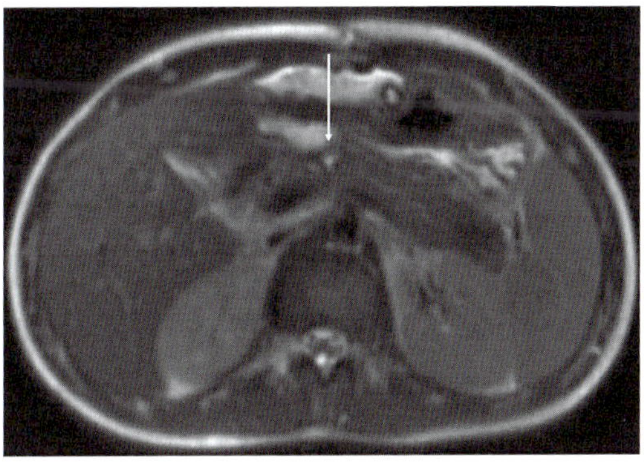

Fig. 15.12 Pancreatic isthmus injury (same patient of Fig. 15.4). MR depicts a subtle dilation of the pancreatic duct in the body and tail. In the site of transection is well appreciated a minimal fluid collection (*arrow*)

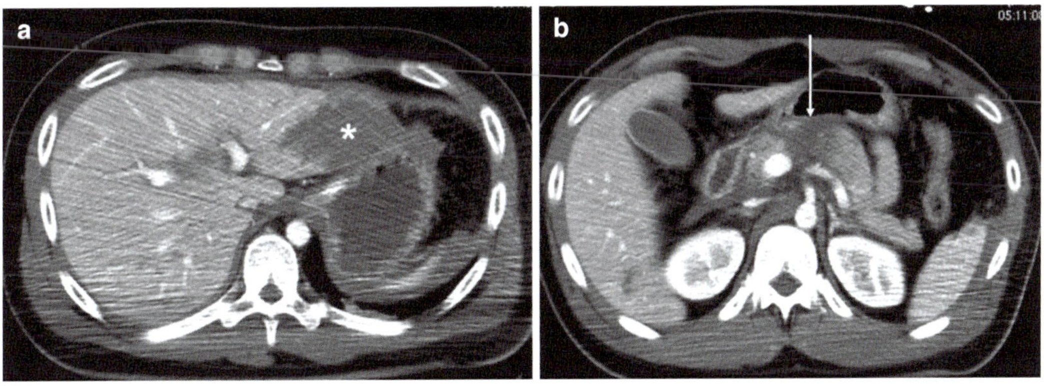

Fig. 15.13 Pancreatic body transection. Axial CT scan (**a**, **b**) and coronal reconstruction (**c**) show the transection as a thick hypodense linear image through the pancreatic body (*arrow*). A traumatic injury of the hepatic left lobe is also depicted (*asterisks*). (**d**) The ERCP highlights a biliary leakage from the injured ducts of the left liver lobe (*arrowhead*)

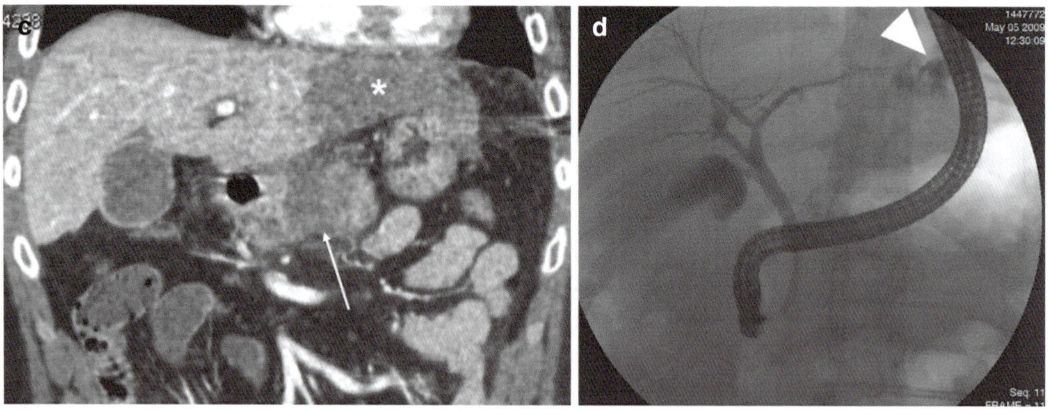

Fig. 15.13 (continued)

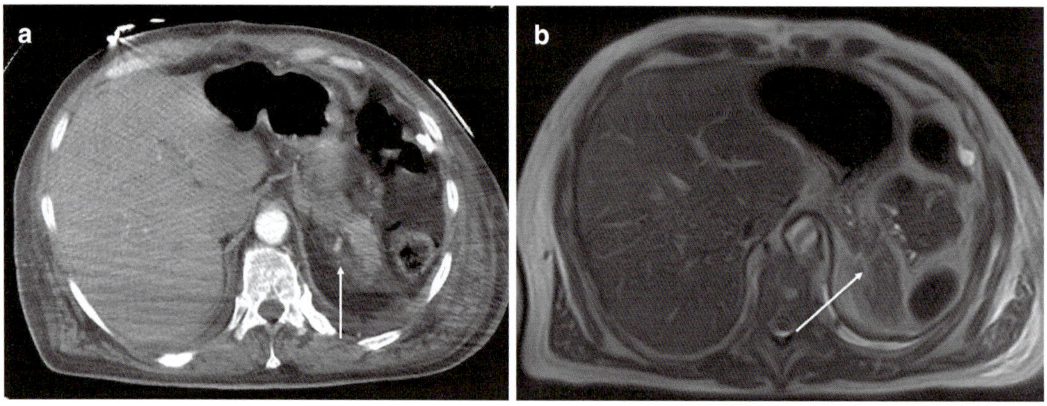

Fig. 15.14 Pancreatic tail injury. The enhanced CT scan (**a**) shows the pancreatic tail enlargement, with inhomogeneous enhancement and a subtle peripancreatic fluid collection (*arrow*). (**b**) One week later, the follow-up T2-weighted MRI scan confirms the well-defined enlargement of the pancreatic tail; there is no fluid collection neither involvement of the peripancreatic fat tissue (*arrow*)

Secretin-enhanced MRCP, obtained after intravenous injection of secretin (0.2 μg/kg), may be helpful to characterize pancreatic ductal anomaly. In fact, secretin increases the signal of pancreatic secretion and can be used to highlight leaks from the destruction of pancreatic duct [19].

ERCP is an invasive method that allows direct imaging guided treatments and in effect ERCP can guide surgical repair or can be used for stent placement (with a rate of complication of 5–15%, such as pancreatitis, cholangitis, and duodenal perforation); it should be used in the suspect of small ductal biliary or pancreatic lesions (Fig. 15.13) that can be treated within 72 h by stent placement, beyond this time increases the incidence of complications [8, 17].

The advantages of MRI is that MRI is a noninvasive study, faster than ERCP, and can illustrate the entire pancreatic parenchymal and ductal anatomy, as well as a pathological fluid collection and ductal destruction [20].

Pancreatic contusion and laceration are seen as focal T2 hyperintense areas within the gland. Pancreatic hematoma is seen as intrapancreatic T1 hyperintense area which has variable signal intensity in T2 [21].

It is important to remember that MRI is also crucial in the follow-up of conservative managed cases or to diagnose sequelae of pancreatic trauma such as pseudocysts, fistulae, etc. (Fig. 15.14) [22].

15.7 Ultrasonography

Pancreatic injuries are difficult to diagnose despite the use of technically adequate sonogram. However, it is a good technique in the follow-up of complications, for example, pseudocysts. The ability to identify a pancreatic lesion and its follow-up is influenced by the patient's constitution and for obvious reasons it's often easier in children and adolescents [23–27].

However, US may show localized traumatic enlargement of pancreas or diffuse pancreatic edema.

Pancreatic laceration can be depicted as a hypoechoic linear image through the glandular parenchyma (Fig. 15.15). An indirect sign of trauma due to the pancreatic head edema is the dilation of the bile ducts. Peripancreatic effusion may also be an indirect sign of pancreatic contusion detectable with US.

With the coming of contrast-enhanced ultrasound (CEUS) the ability to highlight even a small lesion is undoubtedly increased.

At CEUS exam, pancreatic laceration is well depicted as a hypoechoic linear image within the enhanced hyperechoic glandular parenchyma.

It is also easier in the viewing of indirect signs of trauma, for example fluid collection around the gland will appear as a hypoechoic rhyme surrounding the gland, easy to detect even in small amounts (Fig. 15.16).

CEUS exam is not usually performed, as first study, in polytrauma patients but it can be the first choice in minor localized trauma as integration of an ultrasound exam. If a pancreatic lesion shows up at CEUS, it is essential to continue the study with contrast-enhanced CT to evaluate all the other abdomen viscera, the bones, and prognostic factors.

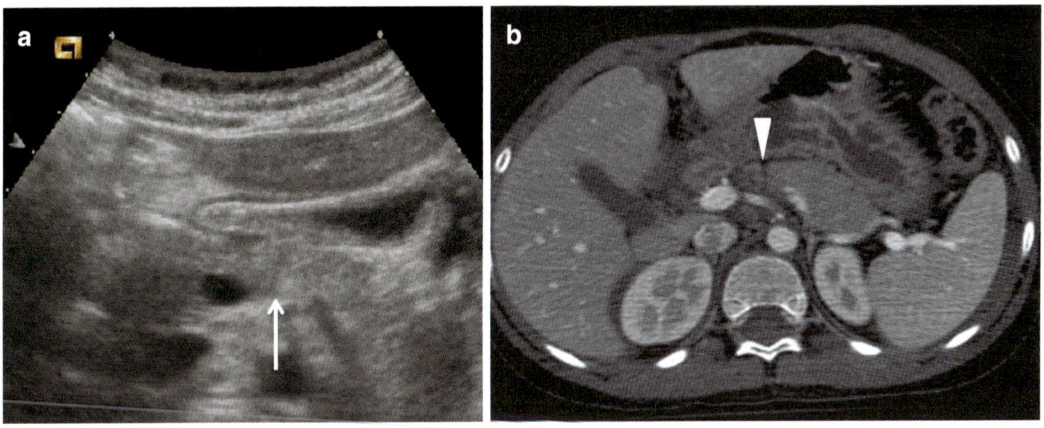

Fig. 15.15 Ultrasonography (**a**) shows pancreatic body transection, which appears as a thin hypodense linear image through the pancreatic body (*arrow*). Contrast-enhanced CT (**b**) confirms the pancreatic lesion (*arrowhead*)

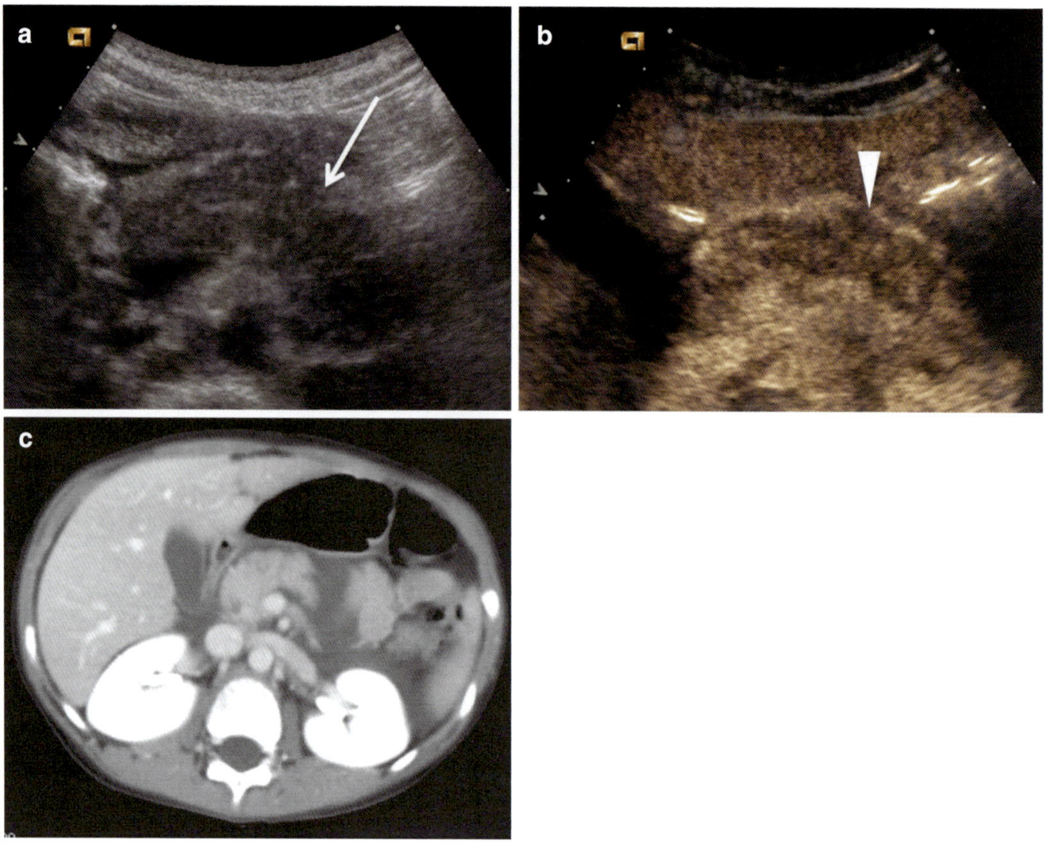

Fig. 15.16 Ultrasonography (**a**) shows a mild inhomogeneity of the pancreatic tail (*arrow*); CEUS (**b**) highlights the parenchymal inhomogeneity of the pancreatic tail, with subtle peripancreatic fluid collection; CT (**c**) confirms the pancreatic tail lesion and the peripancreatic collection

15.8 Management

Mortality for pancreatic injuries ranges from 9% to 60%; this variability in ranges depends not only on the severity of the pancreatic injury and on the involving of its duct, but also on the presence of coexisting viscera injuries and covers all types of complications [11].

In fact, many patients with pancreatic injuries have multiple associated injuries including vascular or other intra-abdominal organs (Fig. 15.17); priority must be given to stabilizing the patient before any definitive management of pancreas injuries. When a pancreatic lesion is suspected, it is important to evaluate all the gland, the duct, and the duodenum.

The hemorrhagic lesions of the portal vein, splenic vein, and inferior vena cava are the most responsible for mortality related to pancreatic trauma.

Management of pancreatic trauma depends on [28]:

1. Grade/severity of injuries
2. Location of injuries
3. Other abdominal injuries
4. Time passed after injuries

It is possible to have a conservative or surgical approach which depends on the integrity of the main pancreatic duct, extent of parenchymal damage, location of the injury, and degree of associated organ damages [29].

Once diagnosed it is important to stage pancreatic injuries with CT in accordance with AAST classification [3, 30].

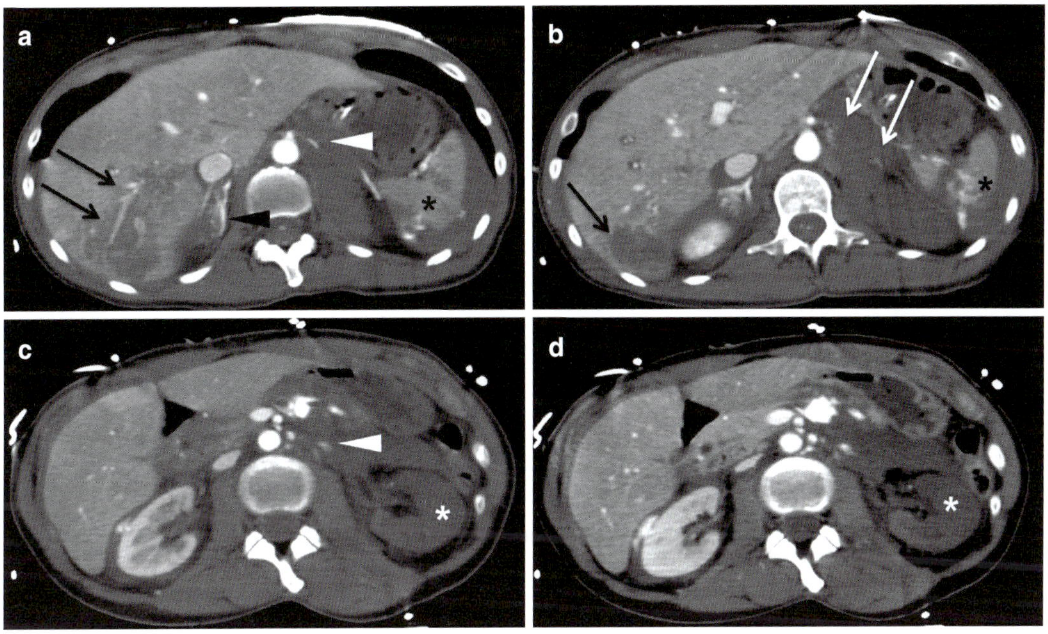

Fig. 15.17 Young girl fallen from great height. (**a–d**) contrast-enhanced CT scans shows traumatic lesion of the body and the tail of the pancreas (*white arrow*), intraglandular (*white arrowhead*) and extraglandular active bleeding. There are other associated organ injuries: liver (*black arrows*), spleen with active bleeding (*black asterisk*), devascularization of the left kidney (*white asterisk*), right adrenal hemorrhage (*black arrowhead*), peritoneal and retroperitoneal free fluid

Grade I injuries allow a conservative treatment, including only patient observation; in some cases, an omental pancreatorrhaphy may be requested. In Grade II, external drainage can be necessary.

Pancreatic injuries with complete transection, from III to V grades, can be sent at surgical treatment.

In grade III, distal pancreatectomy is the standard surgery choice, with or without splenectomy. If the injury occurs at the neck, pancreaticojejunostomy may be done to preserve the entire intact distal pancreas.

For grade IV or V injuries, Whipple's procedure (pancreaticoduodenectomy) may be done at first stage [8, 31]. Other options are: roux-en-Y distal pancreatojejunostomy, pancreatoduodenotomy, anterior roux-en-Y pancreatojejunostomy, endoscopically placed of stent or simple drainage in damage control situations.

ERCP guided stent placement into the major duct has been indicated in selected cases [3].

Endocrine and/or exocrine failure of the pancreas is uncommon if more than 20% of the glandular tissue is conserved and it is more important to conserve as much as possible in cases of young patients.

Medical treatment of traumatic pancreatitis consists of bowel rest, nasogastric suction, and nutritional support [15].

15.9 Complications

In cases of pancreatic traumatic injury, up to a 1/3 of patients develop complications; in many cases, these are the result of missed findings or diagnostic delays or both [10].

Early diagnosis and treatment are associated with better overall outcomes in traumatic pancreas injuries.

In cases of pancreatic duct injury, the leakage of pancreatic juice with its corrosive effect causing inflammation and sepsis is the major reason of morbidity and mortality.

The most frequent complications in pancreatic injury, detected with CT imaging or MRI (when

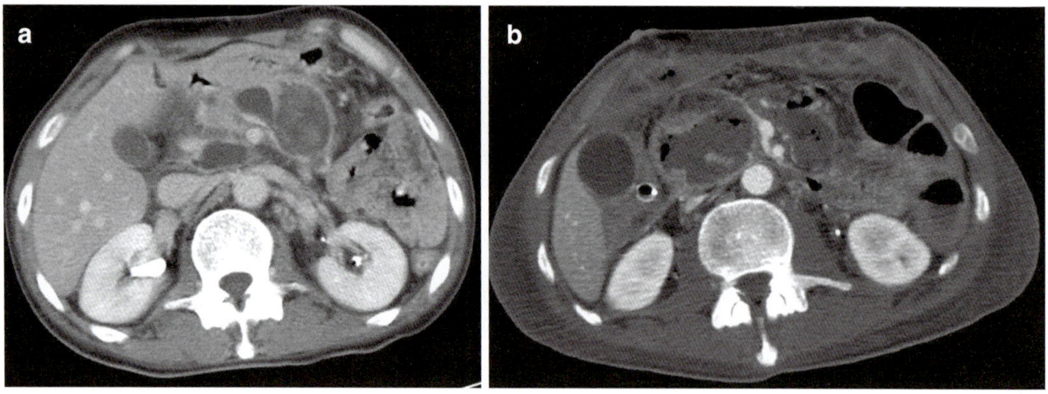

Fig. 15.18 Complication of pancreatic traumatic injury. Contrast-enhanced CT, 6 weeks after trauma (**a**), shows two fluid-corpuscular collections in the region of pancreatic head and in the body and tail of the pancreas. Contrast-enhanced CT, 2 months later (**b**) shows the abscess formation in both collections, with multiple air bubbles within the fluid

patient condition permits to perform MRI), include [32].

Early complications (*48 h*):

- Pancreatic abscess (10–25%) (Fig. 15.18): its frequency increases in the event of ductal lesion and decreases in its absence.
- Traumatic pancreatitis (10% that looks identical to a different cause pancreatitis)
- Pneumonia
- Septicemia

Late complications:

- Pancreatic fistula (10–18%, some report up to 50%) (2–3 weeks later): its frequency increases in the event of ductal lesion and decreases in its absence [33].
- Pancreatic pseudocyst, which appears in 5% of cases around 1 month later. The presence of a pseudocyst is a sign of a ductal lesion.

Other less frequent complications include:

- Peritonitis
- Intestinal obstruction
- Gastrointestinal bleeding
- Endocrine and/or exocrine insufficiency
- Splenic vein thrombosis
- Splenic artery pseudoaneurysm formation or breaking
- Ductal stenosis
- Acalculous cholecystitis
- Multiorgan failure

Active bleeding may occur at any stage (see Fig. 15.2).

The majority of these complications can be managed with conservative therapy and CT follow-up.

If there occur complications, both early or late, the mortality rate significantly increases and it is principally due to sepsis and multiorgan failure.

The mortality in pancreatic trauma is evaluated at 28% in case of head trauma; the death happens generally in the first 48 h. Mortality increases in case of associated vascular/parenchymal/bones or brain lesions. One-third of patients survive with sequelae: pseudocysts, abscesses, bleeding, recurrent pancreatitis, and fistulae.

15.10 Take Home Points

The role of the radiologist is to determinate whether the pancreatic injury is:

1. Is there a traumatic pancreatic injury?
2. Distal or proximal
3. Partial (<50%) or complete (>50%)

4. Signs of ductal injury
5. Pancreatic tissue destroyed is present
6. Other visceral injury that can worsen the situation
7. During the follow-up detection of eventual complications

Contrast-enhanced MDCT is the gold standard technique in the first evaluation of all polytrauma patients [34] and in the assessment of pancreatic involvement. MRI or ECPR are the best techniques for the evaluation of the integrity of the principal duct that can be performed in hemodynamically stable patients and can be used during the follow-up.

If there aren't clinical or laboratory evident signs of pancreas injury but there is high suspect of it, it's important to repeat CT scan after 12 h/24 h from trauma, because radiological CT signs of pancreatic injury often occur late [8].

In children pancreatic damage can happen even in small traumas, due to the lower strength of the abdominal wall.

References

1. Debi U, Kaur R, Prasad KK, et al. Pancreatic trauma: a concise review. World J Gastroenterol. 2013;19:9003–11. doi:10.3748/wjg.v19.i47.9003.
2. Mahadevan V. Anatomy of the pancreas and spleen. Surgery (United Kingdom). 2016;34:261–5. doi:10.1016/j.mpsur.2016.03.014.
3. Menahem B, Lim C, Lahat E, et al. Conservative and surgical management of pancreatic trauma in adult patients. Hepatobiliary Surg Nutr. 2016;5:470–7. doi:10.21037/hbsn.2016.07.01.
4. Rekhi S, Anderson SW, Rhea JT, et al. Imaging of blunt pancreatic trauma. Emerg Radiol. 2010;17:13–9. doi:10.1007/s10140-009-0811-0.
5. Miele V, Di Giampietro I, Ianniello S, et al. Diagnostic imaging in pediatric polytrauma management. Radiol Med. 2015;120:33–49. doi:10.1007/s11547-014-0469-x.
6. Venkatesh SK, Wan JM. CT of blunt pancreatic trauma. A pictorial essay. Eur J Radiol. 2008;67:311–20. doi:10.1016/j.ejrad.2007.07.003.
7. Lahiri R, Bhattacharya S. Pancreatic trauma. Ann R Coll Surg Engl. 2013;95:241–5. doi:10.1308/003588413X13629960045913.
8. Kumar A, Panda A, Gamanagatti S. Blunt pancreatic trauma: a persistent diagnostic conundrum? World J Radiol. 2016;8:159–73. doi:10.4329/wjr.v8.i2.159.
9. Bao W, She G, Duan Y. Diagnosis and management of high-grade pancreatic trauma: report of 14 cases. Indian J Surg. 2015;77:1222–6. doi:10.1007/s12262-015-1258-z.
10. Nanashima A, Imamura N, Tsuchimochi Y, et al. Horizontal traumatic laceration of the pancreas head: a rare case report. Int J Surg Case Rep. 2017;31:119–23. doi:10.1016/j.ijscr.2017.01.030.
11. Linsenmaier U, Wirth S, Reiser M, et al. Diagnosis and classification of pancreatic and duodenal injuries in emergency. Radiographics. 2008;28:1591–602. doi:10.1148/rg.286085524.
12. Panda A, Kumar A, Gamanagatti S, et al. Evaluation of diagnostic utility of multidetector computed tomography and magnetic resonance imaging in blunt pancreatic trauma: a prospective study. Acta Radiol. 2015;56:387–96. doi:10.1177/0284185114529949.
13. Melamud K, LeBedis CA, Soto JA (2015) Imaging of pancreatic and duodenal trauma. Radiol Clin N Am. 53:757–71.viii. doi:10.1016/j.rcl.2015.02.009.
14. Lucey BC, Soto JA. Blunt trauma of the pancreas and biliary tract: a multimodality imaging approach to diagnosis. Radiographics. 2004;24:1381–95.
15. Raghuwanshi S, Gupta R, Vyas MM, et al. CT evaluation of acute pancreatitis and its prognostic correlation with CT severity index. J Clin Diagn Res. 2016;10:TC06–11. doi:10.7860/JCDR/2016/19849.7934.
16. Paspulati RM. Multidetector CT of the pancreas. Radiol Clin N Am. 2005;43:999–1020. doi:10.1016/j.rcl.2005.07.001.
17. Vitellas KM, Keogan MT, Spritzer CE, et al. MR Cholangiopancreatography of bile and pancreatic duct abnormalities with emphasis on the single-shot fast spin-echo technique. Radiographics. 2000;20:939–57.
18. Ansari NA, Ramalho M, Semelka RC, et al. Role of magnetic resonance imaging in the detection and characterization of solid pancreatic nodules: an update. World J Radiol. 2015;7:361–74. doi:10.4329/wjr.v7.i11.361.
19. Tirkes T, Sandrasegaran K, Sanyal R, et al. Secretin-enhanced MR cholangiopancreatography: spectrum of findings. Radiographics. 2013;33:1889–906. doi:10.1148/rg.337125014.
20. Dhaka N, Samanta J, Kochhar S, et al. Pancreatic fluid collections: what is the ideal imaging technique? World J Gastroenterol. 2015;21:13403–10. doi:10.3748/wjg.v21.i48.13403.
21. Halefoglu AM. Magnetic resonance cholangiopancreatography: a useful tool in the evaluation of pancreatic and biliary disorders. World J Gastroenterol. 2007;13:2529–34. doi:10.3748/WJG.V13.I18.2529.
22. Miele V, Piccolo CL, Sessa B, et al. Comparison between MRI and CEUS in the follow-up of patients with blunt abdominal trauma managed conservatively. Radiol Med. 2016;121:27–37. doi:10.1007/s11547-015-0578-1.
23. Pinto F, Miele V, Scaglione M, et al. The use of contrast-enhanced ultrasound in blunt abdominal

trauma: advantages and limitations. Acta Radiol. 2014;55:776–84. doi:10.1177/0284185113505517.
24. Pinto F, Valentino M, Romanini L, et al. The role of CEUS in the assessment of haemodinamically stable patients with blunt abdominal trauma. Radiol Med. 2015;120:3–11. doi:10.1007/s11547-014-0455-3.
25. Sessa B, Trinci M, Ianniello S, et al. Blunt abdominal trauma: role of contrast-enhanced ultrasound (CEUS) in the detection and staging of abdominal traumatic lesions compared to US and CE-MDCT. Radiol Med. 2015;120:180–9. doi:10.1007/s11547-014-0425-9.
26. Miele V, Piccolo CL, Galluzzo M, et al. Contrast-enhanced ultrasound (CEUS) in blunt abdominal trauma. Br J Radiol. 2016;89(1061):20150823. doi:10.1259/bjr.20150823.
27. Miele V, Piccolo CL, Trinci M, et al. Diagnostic imaging of blunt abdominal trauma in pediatric patients. Radiol Med. 2016;121:409–30. doi:10.1007/s11547-016-0637-2.
28. Maeda K, Ono S, Baba K, et al. Management of blunt pancreatic trauma in children. Pediatr Surg Int. 2013;29:1019–22. doi:10.1007/s00383-013-3402-9.
29. Subramanian A, Dente CJ, Feliciano DV, et al. The management of pancreatic trauma in the modern era. Surg Clin North Am. 2007;87:1515–32. doi:10.1016/j.suc.2007.08.007.
30. Wilson RH, Moorehead RJ. Current management of trauma to the pancreas. Br J Surg. 1991;78:1196–202.
31. Martín GM, Morillas PJ, Pino JC, et al. Reconstruction after pancreatic trauma by pancreaticogastrostomy. Int J Surg Case Rep. 2015;9:92–4. doi:10.1016/j.ijscr.2015.02.046.
32. Hughey M, Taffel M, Zeman RK, et al. The diagnostic challenge of the sequelae of acute pancreatitis on CT imaging: a pictorial essay. Abdom Radiol (NY). 2017;42:1199–209. doi:10.1007/s00261-016-0986-2.
33. Lai Y, Wu P, Huang C, Wu C, et al. Hepatobiliary and pancreatic: intra-hepatic arterio-biliary fistula caused by blunt abdomen trauma. J Gastroenterol Hepatol. 2016;31:1672. doi:10.1111/jgh.13433.
34. Soto JA, Anderson SW. Multidetector CT of blunt abdominal trauma. Radiology. 2012;265:678–93. doi:10.1148/radiol.12120354.

Splenic Injuries

16

Giuseppe D'Amico, Diletta Cozzi,
Giovanni Battista Verrone, Gloria Addeo,
Ginevra Danti, and Vittorio Miele

16.1 Epidemiology and Causes

Trauma is the most common cause of death in young people under the age of 45 years, with higher incidence between the ages of 14 and 30 [1]. About 15% of those arriving at the emergency department have intra-abdominal injuries [2] and the spleen is one of the most commonly injured organ in blunt abdominal trauma, in a percentage varying in literature from 37 to 49% [3, 4].

The spleen is very vulnerable in blunt abdominal trauma due to various factors such as its parenchymatous texture and its anatomic position, contiguous to resistant structures like the ribs, spine, and diaphragm. Furthermore, if the patient also suffers from splenomegaly, it increases their susceptibility to traumatic injury. There is an additional risk of splenic injury during childhood due to greater flexibility of the ribs (the ribs break less), the thinner muscles in chest wall, and size of the spleen, which is larger in proportion to the other abdominal organs [3].

Some conditions can underline a spontaneous spleen fracture: some infective diseases (tuberculosis, malaria, mononucleosis), hematological disease (leukemia and lymphoma), and previous splenic infarcts. Splenic lesion can be isolated but often is associated with left hepatic lobe lesions, left adrenal and/or renal lesions, pancreas and diaphragm injuries in 36.5% of cases [3]. Splenic lesion could also be associated with an extra-abdominal lesion in 80% cases.

16.2 Clinical Presentation

The spleen is highly vascular: in fact, a traumatic splenic injury can cause significant bleeding with the risk of hemorrhagic shock and patient death, if it is not identified and treated promptly [5]. Furthermore, in case of early confined spleen injuries or post-traumatic vascular damage (like arteriovenous fistula and pseudoaneurysm), delayed bleeding is common and can result in serious bleeding even a long time after the traumatic event.

G. D'Amico (✉) • D. Cozzi • G.B. Verrone
G. Addeo • G. Danti • V. Miele
Department of Radiology, Careggi University Hospital,
L.go G. A. Brambilla 3, 50134 Florence, Italy
e-mail: giuseppeda70@libero.it;
dilettacozzi@gmail.com;
giovannibattistaverrone@gmail.com;
gloria.addeo@gmail.com; ginevra.danti@gmail.com;
vmiele@sirm.org

V. Miele, M. Trinci (eds.), *Diagnostic Imaging in Polytrauma Patients*,
https://doi.org/10.1007/978-3-319-62054-1_16

Moreover, patients with traumatic splenic injuries have a significantly higher risk of bleeding than those with hepatic ones (5% vs. 1–10%) [6].

Symptoms of a blunt splenic injury are unspecific and change with the severity and type of spleen lesion, from self-limited hemorrhagic effusion to severe hemorrhagic shock. The clinic is represented by upper left quadrant pain radiating to the ipsilateral shoulder (Kehr sign), associated with lower quadrant pain typical of hemoperitoneum, caused by irritation of the serosa; there may also be defensive abdominal signs.

The spleen is one of the most commonly injured solid organs following abdominal trauma. Recognition of its vital role in immune function, especially in children, increased complications and longer hospital stays following splenectomy have led to an increased drive for Non-Operative Management (NOM) of splenic trauma, which is dependent on accurate CT diagnosis and, when necessary, embolization [7, 8].

The clinic and diagnostic imaging always play an important role in grading and diagnosing a splenic injury, but often the symptoms are blurred or missing in more than 40% cases; in fact, these patients with splenic lesion have no sign or clinic symptoms. In addition, the clinic may be masked when there is a state of impaired consciousness, hemorrhagic shock and in case of intoxication (alcohol and narcotics). Therefore, it is necessary to resort to diagnostic imaging to accurately diagnose and classify a splenic injury and it is essential for the prognostic stratification, with the aim of leading the patient into a conservative intervention (NOM) or to a surgical one [9].

16.3 Classification and Grading Systems

During the years, various blunt splenic injuries classifications based on the findings of Computed Tomography (CT) have been proposed. These classifications concern the type of splenic lesions that consist of subcapsular or parenchymatous hematomas, contusions, parenchymal lacerations, and vascular lesions. The CT-based classification system comes from the surgical grading drafted by the American Association for the Surgery of Trauma (AAST) [10]. This classification (Table 16.1) divides splenic trauma in five grades:

- Grade 1 includes subcapsular hematoma and parenchymal lesions involving less than 10% of the surface area or smaller than 1 cm;
- Grade 2 includes subcapsular hematoma involving 10–50% of surface area or parenchymal laceration from 1 to 3 cm without involving intraparenchymal vessels;
- Grade 3 includes subcapsular hematoma involving more than 50% of surface area, ruptured subcapsular or parenchymal hematoma and depth laceration more than 3 cm involving trabecular vessels;
- Grade 4 defines splenic laceration involving segmental or hilar vessels producing a devascularization more than 25% of spleen; at least
- Grade 5 includes complete shattered spleen or a hilar vascular injury with de-vascularized spleen.

However, this surgical classification internationally used is not perfectly comparable to the real CT-findings: the differences could be attributable in some cases to the evolution of the injury by the time of surgery after the CT scanning, but the major limitation of the AAST scaling system was that it has not been reliable in predicting the outcome and guiding the management of blunt splenic injury [11]. In fact, in the last years targeted classification to define a CT-scoring system has been created. The most widely used classification based on CT is the Mirvis' one [12, 13].

Table 16.1 The American Association for the Surgery of Trauma (AAST) spleen injury scale

Grade of injury	Description
I	Hematoma: subcapsular with spleen surface involvement <10%
	Laceration: capsular tear, <1 cm parenchymal depth
II	Hematoma: subcapsular, interest 10–50% of surface area
	Hematoma: intraparenchymal, <5 cm in diameter
	Laceration: capsular injury, 1–3 cm parenchymal depth that does not involve a trabecular vessel
III	Hematoma: subcapsular, interest >50% of surface area or expanding; ruptured subcapsular or parenchymal hematoma
	Hematoma: intraparenchymal, >5 cm or expanding
	Laceration:>3 cm parenchymal depth or involving trabecular vessels
IV	Laceration involving segmental or hilar vessels producing major devascularisation (>25% of spleen)
V	Laceration: complete shattered spleen
	Vascular: hilar vascular injury with devascularized spleen

From Moore EE, Cogbill TH, Jurkovich GJ et al. Organ injury scaling: spleen and liver (1994 revision). J Trauma 1995; 38:323–4. Obtained permission from Wolters Kluwer

This classification includes the distinction in four grades:

- Grade 1 includes capsular avulsion, superficial laceration, and subcapsular hematoma smaller than 1 cm (Fig. 16.1);
- Grade 2 includes parenchymal lesions from 1 to 3 cm, or parenchymal and subcapsular hematoma smaller than 3 cm (Fig. 16.2);
- Grade 3 defines splenic laceration deep more than 3 cm (Fig. 16.3); at least
- Grade 4 defines the fragmentation of the splenic parenchyma ("shattered spleen") or its devascularization, what is called "non-enhanced spleen" (Fig. 16.4).

While severity of splenic injury according to the AAST does correlate with outcome, this classification, with the Mirvis' one, does not take account of active extravasation or contained vascular injury such as arteriovenous fistula or pseudoaneurysm formation (Figs. 16.5 and 16.6). In fact, the last CT-based classification was written by Marmery in 2007 [14] and recalls Mirvis', while adding vascular lesions (Grades 4a–4b), which are predictive of the necessity (or lack thereof) of surgical treatment or splenic embolization (Fig. 16.7).

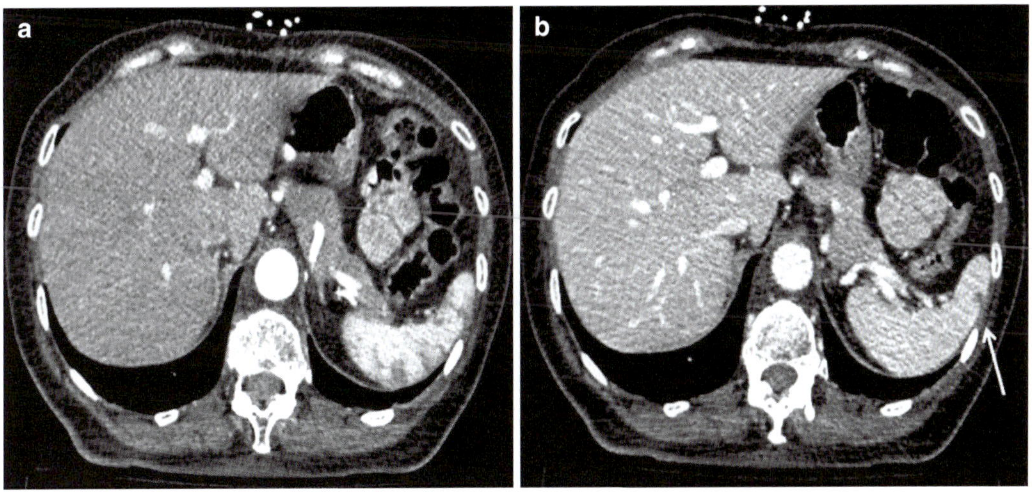

Fig. 16.1 Grade 1. Contrast-enhanced CT scan shows a small splenic laceration: (**a**) arterial and (**b**) venous phase. The portal-venous phase is better for the illustration of parenchymal damage (*arrow*)

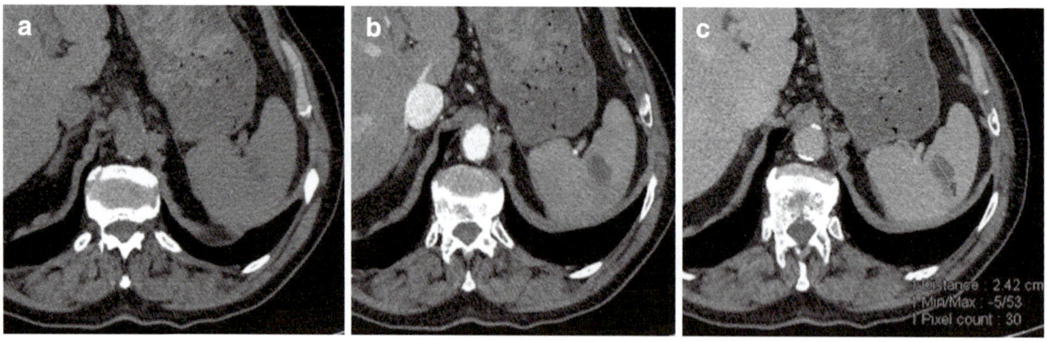

Fig. 16.2 Grade 2: Not replenished parenchymal hematoma (smaller than 3 cm) associated with a small peri-splenic hemoperitoneum. CE-MDCT axial images in baseline (**a**), arterial (**b**), and venous phase (**c**)

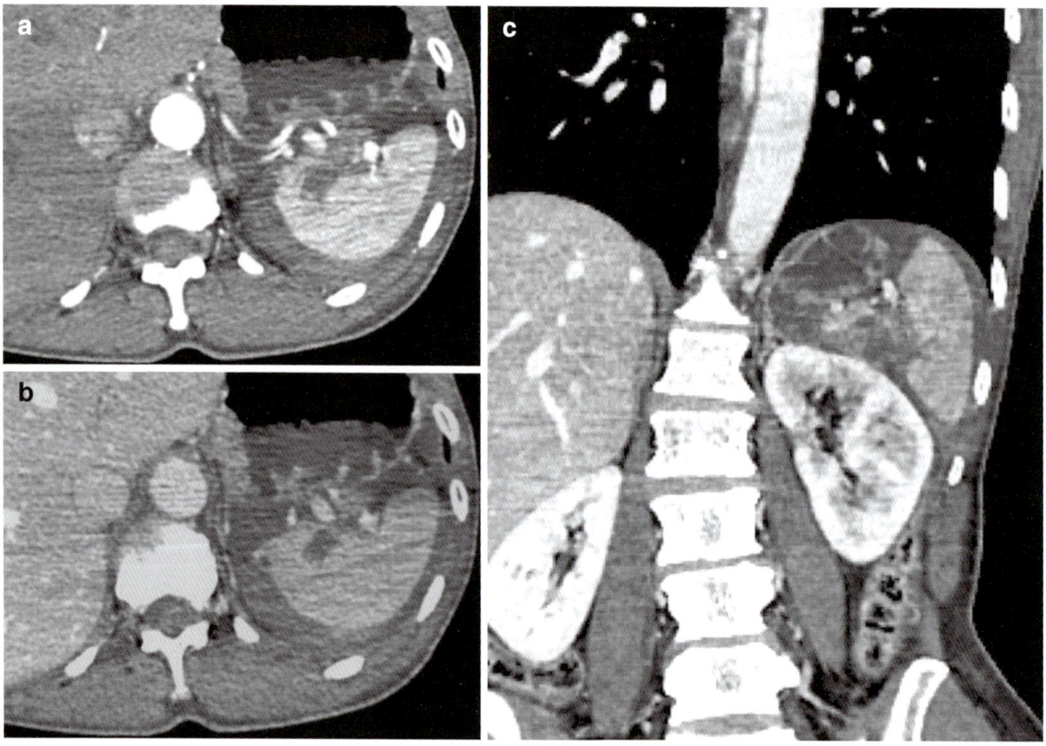

Fig. 16.3 Grade 3: These CT images show a deep hilar splenic laceration with rupture of the capsule. Multiphasic CT scans in arterial (**a**–**c**) and venous phase in (**b**)

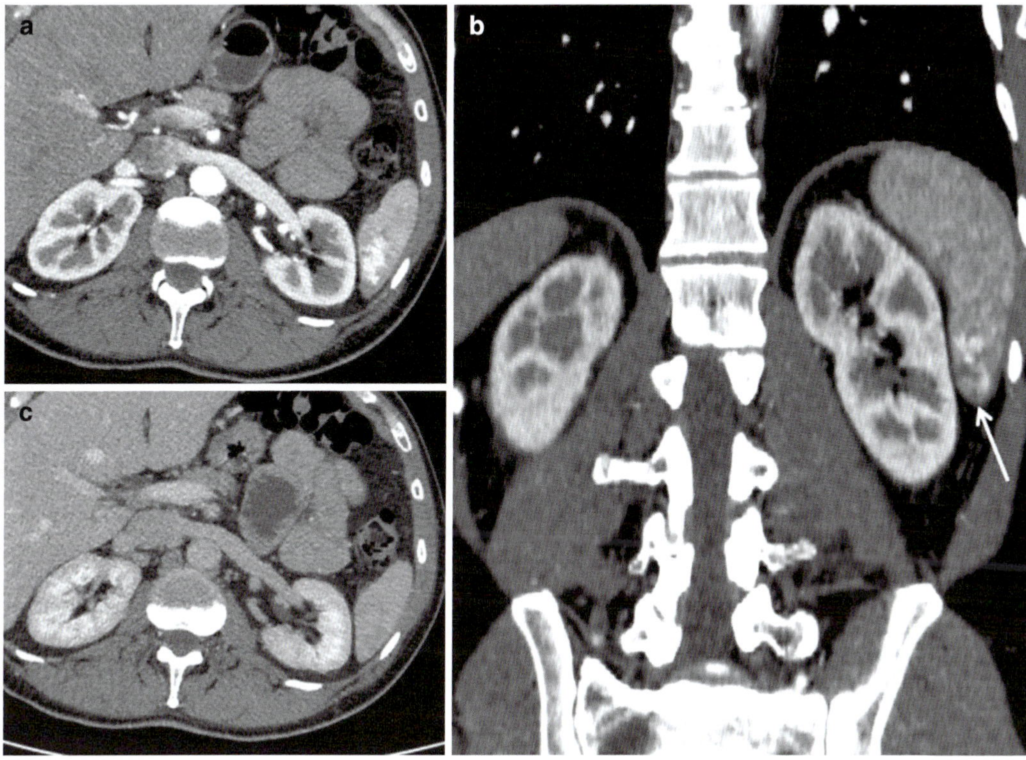

Fig. 16.4 Grade 4: Fragmentation of the splenic upper pole parenchyma, what is called "shattered spleen" (*arrow*). (**a**) Axial CT scan and (**b**) coronal reconstruction of the venous phase

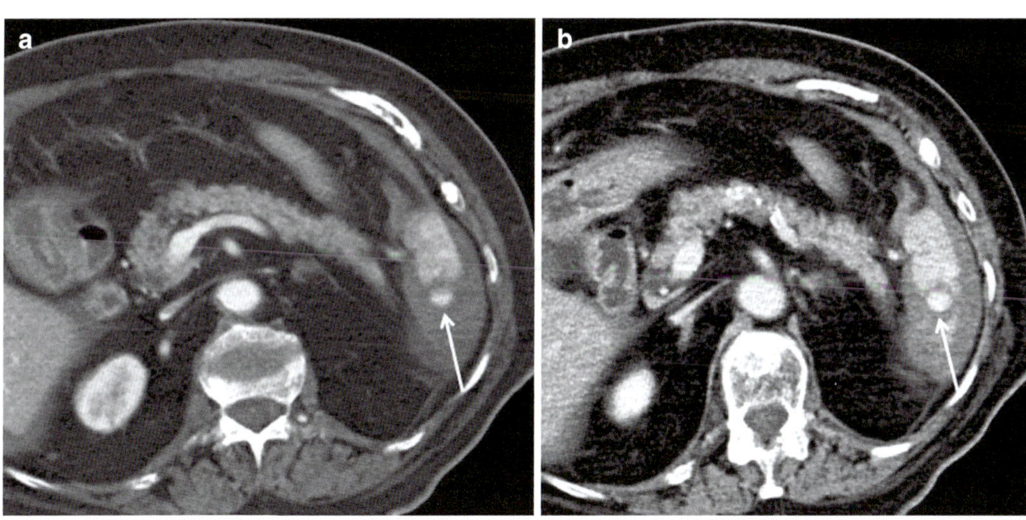

Fig. 16.5 Grade 4a: CE-MDCT in arterial (**a**) and venous (**b**) phases allows to make a diagnosis of lower splenic pole pseudoaneurysm (*arrows*), associated with hemoperitoneum in peri-splenic and peri-hepatic spaces

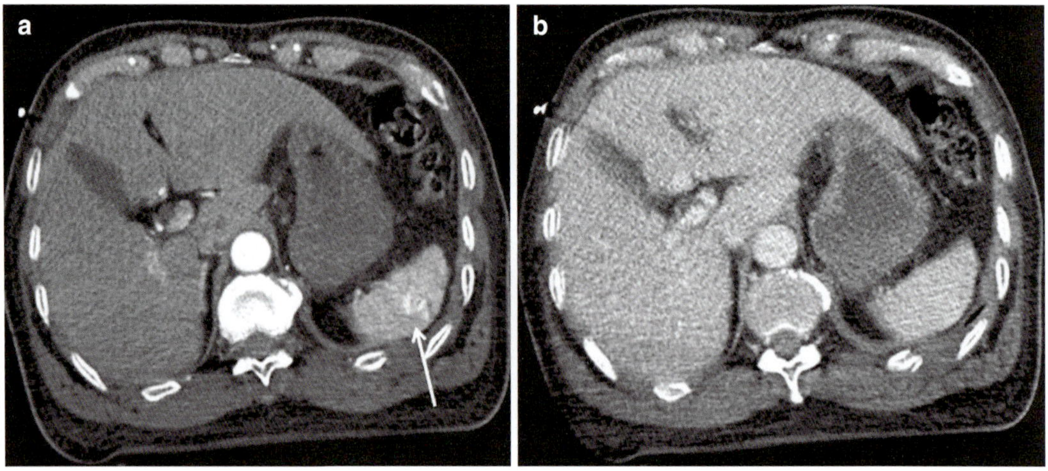

Fig. 16.6 Arteriovenous fistula. Multiphasic CT study shows a small arteriovenous fistula at the upper splenic pole (*arrow*): the dynamic study is essential as it shows the classical sign of a contained vascular lesion that is a focal area of parenchymal hyperdensity in the arterial phase (**a**), followed by a typical "wash-out" isodensity in the portal phase (**b**)

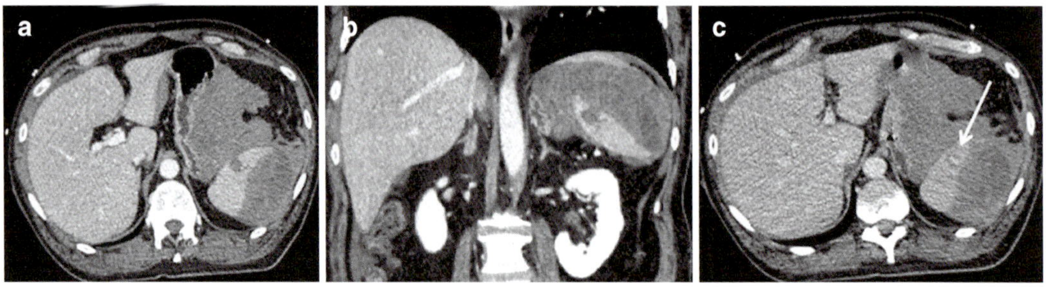

Fig. 16.7 Grade 4a: Subcapsular and parenchymal replenished hematoma associated with "large" hemoperitoneum. CT scan: the venous phase (**a**, **b**) allows to identify the parenchymal lesion and the blood spreading in the abdomen; (**c**) the late phase shows a small blood supply within the lesion (*white arrow*)

16.4 Radiological Diagnosis

The radiologist has the essential task of providing an adequate diagnosis and classification of a splenic injury in order to refer the patient to a conservative treatment or to a surgical one.

The poly-injured patient's radiological study is different according to the dynamics of trauma and their clinical conditions upon arrival at the emergency room.

- Poly-traumatized hemodynamically unstable patient: Basic diagnostic tests are performed (chest and pelvis X-Rays, US e-FAST) to find pneumothorax, hemothorax, and hemoperitoneum. If one of these three is diagnosed and the patient is still hemodynamically unstable, he is directed to the surgical room. In the emergency room, the doctors try to stabilize the patient (with plasma expanders, hemothorax and pneumothorax drainage, pelvis fracture stabilization) and, if they achieve a hemodynamic stability, the patient is subjected to a total-body contrast-enhanced MDCT scan (CE-MDCT).
- Poly-traumatized hemodynamically stable patient: Contrast-enhanced CT scan is always the best choice in major trauma.
- In case of a localized low energy trauma, it is preferred to do an ultrasound exam (US),

possibly complemented with the use of intravenous contrast (Contrast Enhanced UltraSonography—CEUS). If a lesion or free fluid (suspected for hemoperitoneum) are detected, a MDCT exam is requested for a complete evaluation of the patient.

US and CT have a key role in the management of blunt abdominal trauma. Studies have shown that US has sensitivity of 97% and specificity of 100% in predicting the presence of hemoperitoneum: in fact, US is the first choice technique for early screening, allowing to demonstrate the presence of hemoperitoneum in which patients that are hemodynamically unstable, and refer them to embolization or surgery [15]. Ultrasound should be the initial investigation of choice when examining children or in young woman [16]. However, US has low sensitivity in diagnosing an organ injury [17]. Over the last few years, with the introduction of Contrast Enhanced UltraSonography (CEUS) the sensitivity is greatly increased, with 96% sensitivity and 99% specificity rates compared to CT. CEUS shows a high sensitivity both in lesion detection and grading [18, 19] but it has a lower accuracy in the evaluation of prognostic factors; CEUS plays an important role also in blunt abdominal trauma in pediatric patients [20–22]. CT is undeniably the gold standard for the identification, diagnosis, and staging of abdominal organs in trauma patients: CT also shows all non-parenchymal organ lesions that US and CEUS are not capable of detecting. CT must always be performed in CEUS-positive patients to exclude active bleeding [23].

16.5 Computed Tomography

Computed tomography (CT) is the gold standard for patient evaluation in case of blunt injury and for the detection and staging of splenic lesions.

This technique is widely used in Emergency Radiology Departments, due to increasing diffusion of multi-detector CT (MDCT) and because it's able to meet the main targets of Emergency Surgery which are early lesion identification, the assessment of the presence of hemoperitoneum and any further injury in whole body. Computed tomography study, due to its panoramicity, allows to identify any damage to every organ beyond the spleen. The aim of a correct and prompt diagnosis is to refer the patient to a surgical or conservative treatment, already in the acute phase, and avoid the misdiagnosis of the most insidious injuries, that may show signs only hours or days later.

In a patient with left-quadrant isolated trauma, after US and CEUS, CT can be used as a second choice, to clarify any questionable sonographic findings [16]; instead in a polytraumatized hemodynamically stable patient, MDCT is the first choice and helps in differentiation of patients with active splenic bleeding (who risk hemorrhagic shock and which could indicate a need for surgery or embolization) from patients with stable non-bleeding injuries, who are candidates for conservative management, with the valuation of vital parameters and a close follow-up, to reduce surgical morbidity and preserve immune competence [24].

Total-body MDCT is always performed in basal phase and after intravenous administration of contrast, with dual-phase (acquisitions in the arterial and portal-venous phases): it is vital that the amount of contrast is adequate and customized to the patient's weight, and that the flow must be high, because those parameters greatly influence the quality of the examination.

The multiphasic protocol provides a better overall diagnostic tool for the evaluation of the splenic lesions: in particular, the arterial phase is more sensitive for the evaluation of vascular injury including active bleeding and vascular lesions, while the portal-venous phase is better for the illustration of parenchymal damage. Several types of splenic injury can occur: intraparenchymal and subcapsular hematoma, contusion, laceration, active extravasation, and contained vascular injury [25]. Clotted blood has an attenuation of approximately 45–70 Hounsfield Units (HU); it is better seen in basal phase as a slightly hyperdense area, while unclotted blood has an attenuation of 30–45 HU.

- Parenchymal hematoma: At basal exam, a parenchymal hematoma may appear to be an area with defined margins, if it is made up of recent blood it is hyperdense but it can be iso-hypo-hyperdense compared to the surrounding parenchyma in relation to the time elapsed since the blood collected; during the dynamic phases, it is hypodense compared to the remaining parenchyma (Fig. 16.8).
- Subcapsular hematoma: Similarly, at basal exam, subcapsular hematoma has the same semeiotic of a parenchymal hematoma and appears like a peripheral crescent collection that displaces and marks the parenchyma the splenic parenchyma (Fig. 16.9): it can even grow to considerable size, it is always hypodense during dynamic phases, and it can have a multi-stratified appearance due to repeated bleeding.
- Splenic contusion: It is not well defined at baseline; instead at the contrast-enhanced exam, it appears as a small hypodense area with blurred margins caused by perilesional interstitial edema and local blood suffusion.
- Laceration: It appears as a linear lack of parenchymal opacification with an irregular shape that may extend to the capsule (Fig. 16.10). It is important to report the laceration site, which can be superficial, if it interests only the capsule, or deep, involving vascular structures of splenic hilum.
- Severe disruption of splenic parenchyma can result in a "shattered" spleen. Vascular hilum injuries usually result in significant hemorrhage and cardiovascular instability [26].

According to Marmery, the splenic lesion is classified from Grade 1 to Grade 3, and the grade increases according to the depth of the laceration [14, 27]. Concerning vascular lesions, this classification adds grade 4 injury, that is divided into subgroups: 4a and 4b. In fact, a laceration that

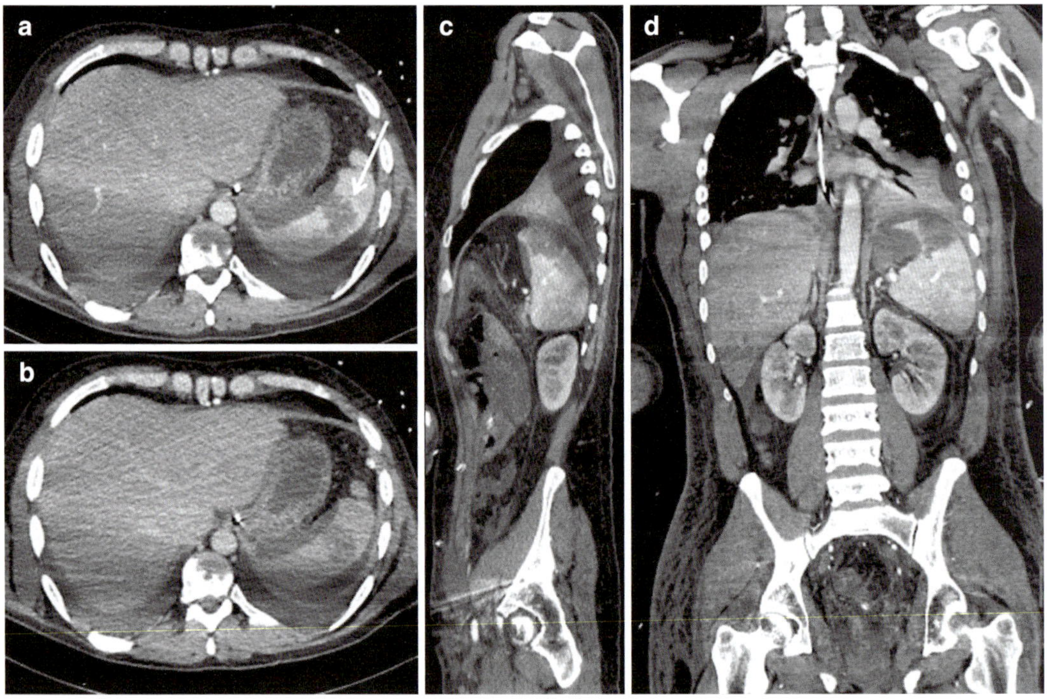

Fig. 16.8 Grade 3: Not replenished parenchymal hematoma of the upper splenic pole associated with a small subcapsular hematoma (*arrow*), as shown in portal-venous phase (**a**, axial scan, arterial phase, **b**, axial scan, late phase, **c**, sagittal and **d**, coronal reconstruction)

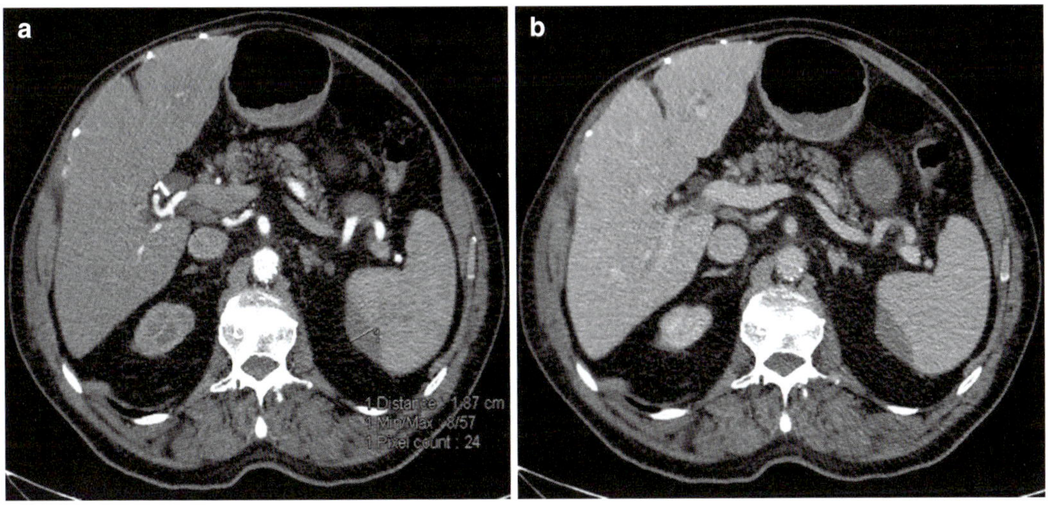

Fig. 16.9 Grade 2: these CT axial pictures show a subcapsular hematoma, smaller than 3 cm, studied in both arterial (**a**) and venous phase, (**b**). The arterial phase is more sensitive for the evaluation of vascular injury including active bleeding and vascular lesions: in fact, it is a not replenished hematoma as we cannot see any sign of active bleeding

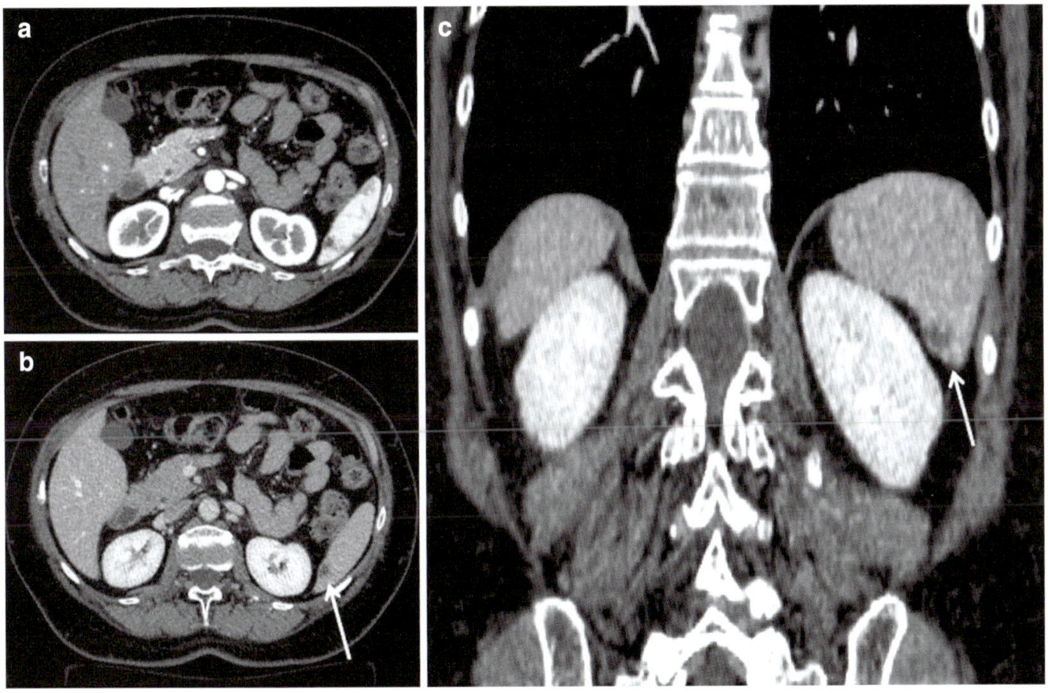

Fig. 16.10 Grade 1. This dual-phase CT shows a small subcapsular laceration to the lower pole of the spleen (*arrows*): axial images in arterial (**a**) and venous phase (**b**). Coronal reconstruction in the venous phase (**c**)

compromises the vascularization of the spleen (vascular hilar damage) coincides with a severe injury (Grade 4). A contrast-medium extravasation is an active sign of bleeding, which can be subcapsular/parenchymal (Grade 4a) (Fig. 16.11) or endo-peritoneal/peri-splenic (Grade 4b) (Fig. 16.12) and almost always requires immediate surgical treatment. When the exam detects a bleeding, a vascular study is essential, as it allows to detect focal areas of high attenuation, which often is evident in the arterial phase and then spreads in portal-venous phase, this change in morphology allows to make a differential diagnosis between active bleeding and a contained vascular lesion (such as pseudoaneurysm and arteriovenous fistula) that does not change in its morphology. On single-phase scanning, it can be difficult to differentiate active extravasation from contained vascular injury; however, on equilibrium phase scans, an area of active extravasation will remain hyperdense and enlarged, whereas a contained vascular injury will typically "wash out" and be isodense or slightly hypodense relative to splenic parenchyma (Fig. 16.13). These contained vascular lesions are recognized as a well-defined margin in intraparenchymal areas, with high attenuation in arterial phase and isodensity in portal-venous phase (Fig. 16.14). The distinction between fistula and post-traumatic pseudoaneurysm is easier to identify with arteriography. In the pseudoaneurysm there is a tear in the artery, but bleeding is typically limited by the arterial adventitia.

Active bleeding increases in size on delayed-phase images unlike a contained vascular lesion [14]. Pseudoaneurysm and arteriovenous fistula are conditions predisposing a late-breaking spleen and typically are managed through embolization. Pseudoaneurysm breaks in a percentage that ranges from 3 to 46% of cases.

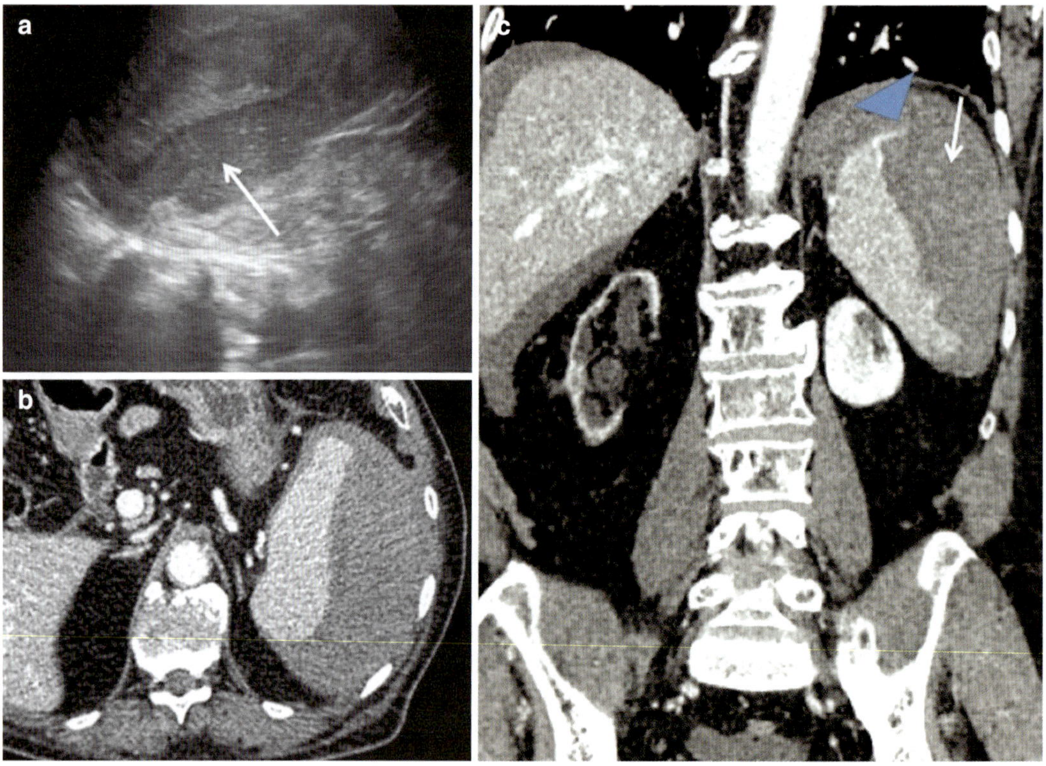

Fig. 16.11 Grade 4a: replenished subcapsular hematoma (*arrows*). (**a**) The US image shows a hematoma that is more hypoechoic than the splenic parenchyma. (**b**) Axial CT scan and (**c**) coronal reconstruction in the venous phase demonstrate a blood spreading at the upper splenic pole (*blue arrowhead*)

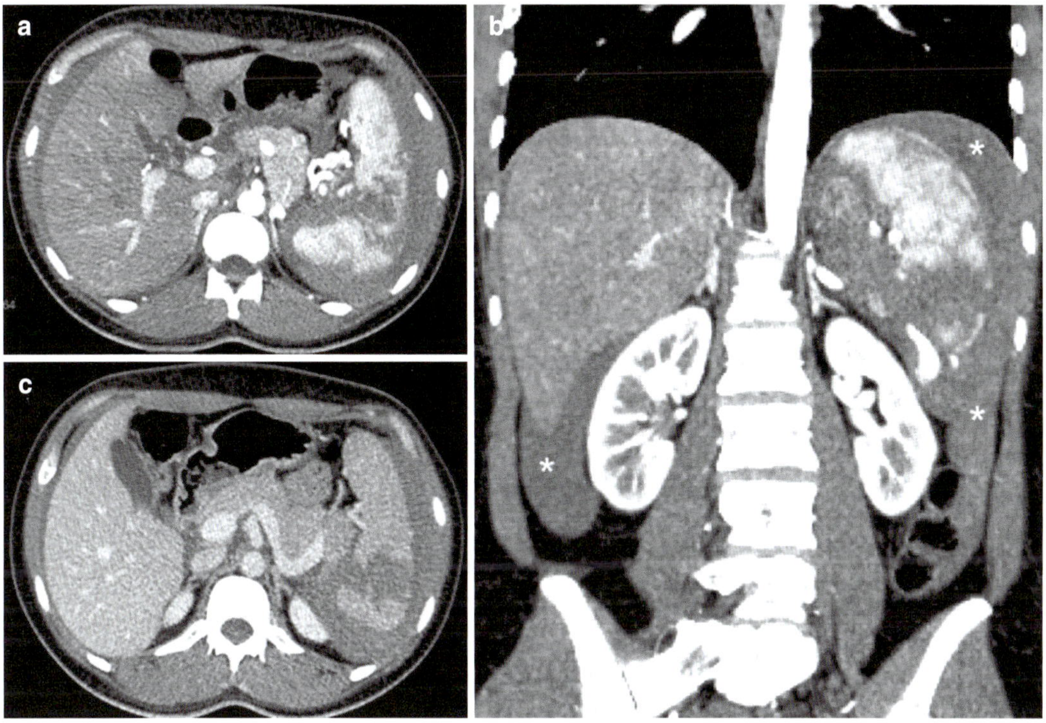

Fig. 16.12 Grade 4b: This vascular CT study shows a splenic fracture associated with "large" hemoperitoneum (*asterisks*) in peri-hepatic, peri-splenic and both parieto-colic spaces. There is no evidence of active blood extravasation: arterial (**a**, **b**) and venous phases (**c**)

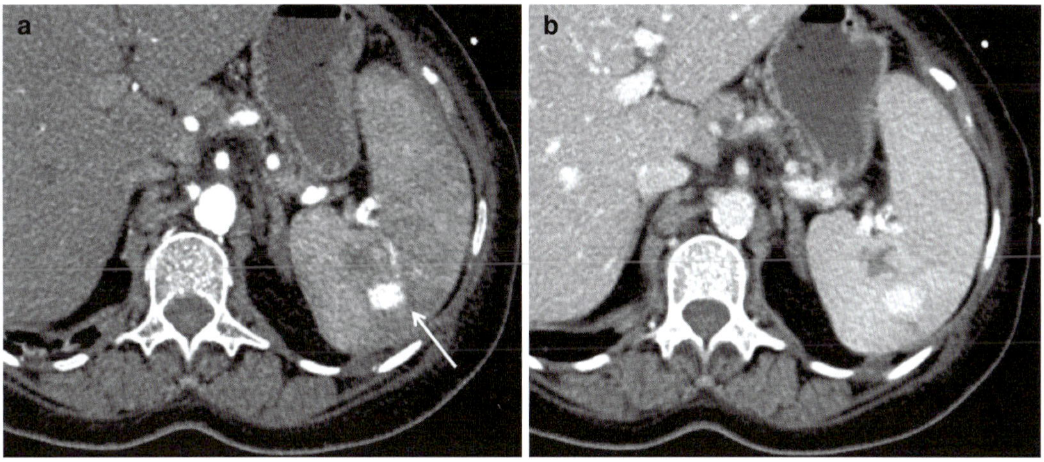

Fig. 16.13 Grade 4a: These arterial (**a**), and venous (**b**), axial CT images show a pseudoaneurysm (*arrow*) associated with a splenic parenchymal laceration: in this case, a vascular study is essential as it allows to make a differential diagnosis between active bleeding and a contained vascular lesion (such as pseudoaneurysm and arteriovenous fistula). On single-phase scanning, it can be difficult to differentiate active extravasation from contained vascular injury; however, on delayed scans, an area of active extravasation will remain hyperdense and enlarged, whereas a contained vascular injury will typically "wash out" and be isodense or slightly hypo/hyperdense relative to splenic parenchyma

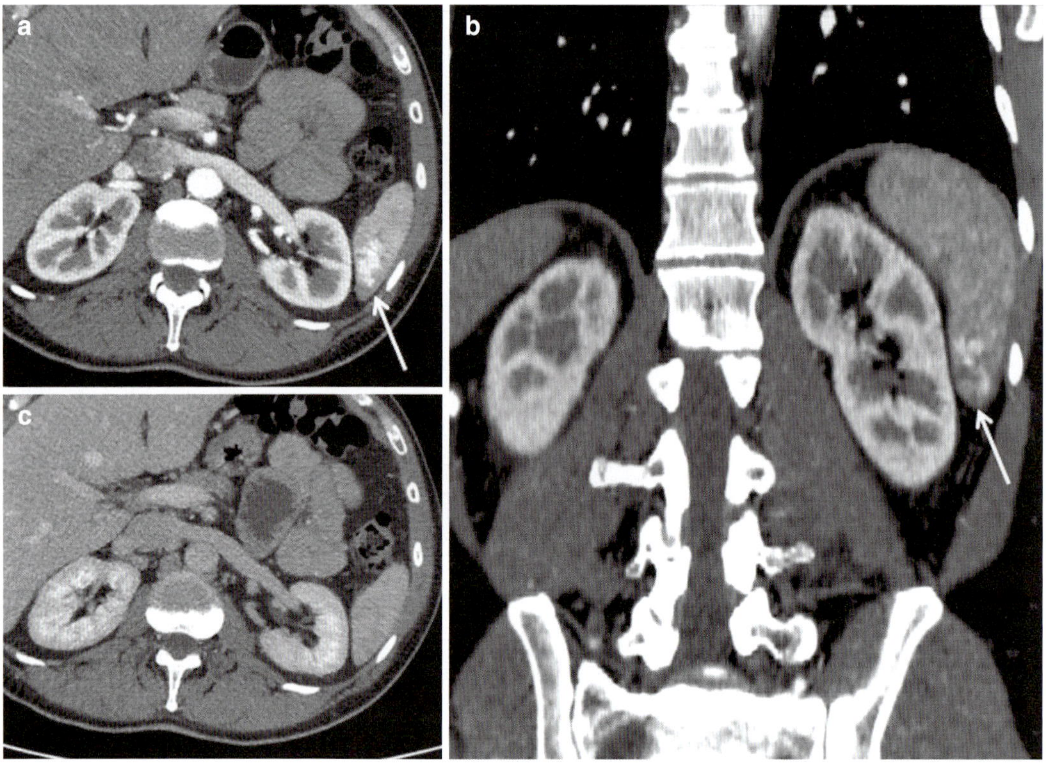

Fig. 16.14 Grade 4a: Arteriovenous fistula of the lower splenic pole: typical hyperdensity in the arterial phase (*arrows*) (**a**, **b**), isodensity in the venous phase (**c**)

When the capsule is break, typically, hemoperitoneum is associated. According to the Federle semi-quantitative scale [28], hemoperitoneum is divided into *small* (when the blood is in only one endo-peritoneal space, as the peri-splenic, perihepatic, in the parieto-colic or Morrison spaces, with an estimated blood loss of about 250–500 mL) or *large* (with blood effusion in two or more endo-peritoneal/pelvic spaces, with blood extravasation greater than 500 mL) (Fig. 16.12).

16.6 Ultrasonography

Ultrasonography is used first in hemodynamically stable patients with minor trauma, because it is easy to perform, quick, affordable, and noninvasive. However, even in expert hands, basic US has too low sensitivity to diagnose organ injuries (no more than 50%) especially in case of spleen injury because the "fresh blood" has similar echogenicity as a recent parenchymal lesion. For this reason, CT was used excessively over the years so as not to miss potentially dangerous splenic injuries [3].

Over the last few years, basic ultrasound limits have been exceeded thanks to the gradual emergence of Contrast Enhanced UltraSonography (CEUS) in the study of blunt abdominal trauma [29, 30]. The use of microbubbles and harmonic imaging has allowed us to increase the diagnostic accuracy of US in the study of parenchymal injuries, avoiding the CT study, especially in pediatric patients and in case of minor trauma. For this reason, CEUS is indicated in low energy abdominal trauma, isolated trauma, and child trauma.

After the injection of the ultrasound contrast agent (USCA), the arterial phase starts at 12–20 s and it has a long duration, responsible for a peculiar irregular enhancement of the organ, called "zebra," because of the movement of the contrast media within the red pulp and the white pulp.

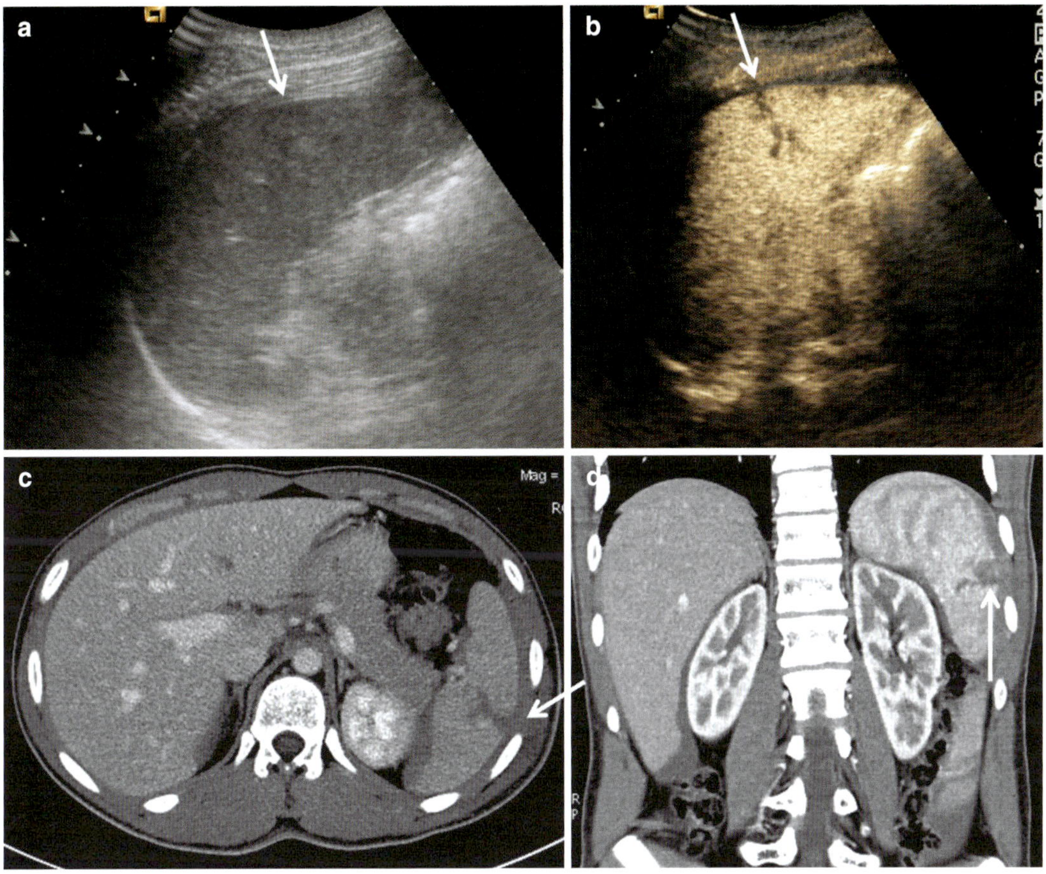

Fig. 16.15 CEUS, Grade 2: (**a**) US image shows a slight parenchymal dishomogeneity which is better clear with the use of contrast (CEUS) in (**b**). The axial (**c**) and coronal (**d**) CT scans better shows the Grade 2 splenic lesion, that extends up to the capsule (*arrows*). Hemoperitoneum is associated

This feature makes difficult to recognize any tissue lesion. The venous phase, starting at 40–60 s after USCA injection, is the most reliable one for the detection of organ injury, because the healthy parenchyma appears as homogeneous enhancing tissue with a long duration (about 5–7 min) [21].

Using CEUS, lacerations and hematomas are represented as non-vascularized hypoechoic areas, compared to adjacent normal parenchyma that is hyper-reflective (Fig. 16.15). The total absence of parenchymal perfusion is a sign of shock or avulsion of the hilum. With CEUS then, it is possible to define the location, the depth and extension of the laceration, the capsule involvement, allowing not only for diagnosis, but also for the staging of the lesion. At CEUS it is possible to detect parenchymal or extracapsular active bleeding, but CEUS has undoubtedly reduced sensitivity as compared to CT in the detection of vascular lesions and high-grade injuries, therefore, in the case of a CEUS examination that is positive for traumatic splenic lesion, CT is indicated as a second choice [30]. The presence of intralesional or extracapsular echoes is suggestive for bleeding. CEUS also has a key role in the follow-up of conservative management or of a lesion known demonstrated at CT.

16.7 Magnetic Resonance

Magnetic Resonance Imaging (MRI) is not a technique usually used in Emergency Departments, because of the long acquisition times and often the lack of patient compliance, making it a method that cannot be easily used in emergencies. It can be used in monitoring and in the follow-up of known injuries, especially in children and in pregnant or young women, due to its low radiobiological invasiveness.

MRI allowed to make a better assessment of injuries because of the improved contrast and soft tissue resolution, allowing also a temporal stage of lesions [31]. MRI is multi-parametric and this feature can be used to enhance the signal inhomogeneity of the splenic parenchyma, caused by the deposition of hemoglobin degradation products (like methemoglobin, deoxyhemoglobin, and other paramagnetic substances) in order to date the bleeding [32]. At MRI, the signal of the hematoma changes in relation with two parameters: the state of hemoglobin oxygenation (which in turn influences the relaxation properties and magnetic susceptibility) and the state of red blood cells membrane (intact or lysed).

During the hyperacute (0–3 h), the acute (4 h–3 days), and the early subacute stage (4 days–4 weeks), red blood cells are intact and the hemoglobin is transformed respectively in oxyhemoglobin, deoxyhemoglobin, and methemoglobin. Subsequently, cell membranes lyse and the methemoglobin become extracellular (late subacute stage).

MRI may have high sensitivity in the diagnosis of splenic hematoma characterized by high signal intensity on both T1- and T2-weighted images [33].

Lacerations are more hyperintense on T2-weighted sequences than normal splenic parenchyma. MRI, compared with contrast-enhanced CT, is also able to better depict subcapsular hematoma, which is an indicator of traumatic injury, appearing as a hyperintense layer on T2-weighted sequences; MRI can also demonstrate vascular lesions, such as pseudoaneurysm, as a nodular hyperintense lesion in arterial phase.

MRI is an excellent imaging technique for diagnosis, evaluation, and characterization of abdominal organ lesions, as liver, spleen, and kidneys. However, MRI has some limits, such as the needs to have compliant patients able to follow breath-hold commands during images acquisition, which is not always simple with pediatric patients; other MR limits are the relatively long exam duration and the impossibility to be performed in cases of pacemaker, cochlea implants and patient's claustrophobia [34].

Today with the many innovations (such as ultrafast sequences with free breath) there will likely be an increase in the widespread use of MRI in Emergency Departments, also due to a surgeons' tendency to prefer a non-operative treatment that requires close follow-up of the patient.

Until now, there is not a standardized protocol for the follow-up of blunt splenic-abdominal trauma conservatively treated, but the follow-up at 1 month can be made by MRI, since MRI, due to its panoramicity and its high contrast resolution, allows a better morphological and temporal trauma staging [32]. The use of MRI is even more important considering that many trauma patients are in childhood; for this reason, the use of this technique in the follow-up, which does not use ionizing radiation, makes it extremely profitable compared to CT.

16.8 Treatment Options

The spleen is an organ that belongs to reticuloendothelial system, and it has a fundamental role in immune defense exerting a mechanism of filtration and phagocytosis on over 90% of arterial blood flowing through it. It also has a key role in hemato-lymphopoiesis, has hemolytic function and is a red blood cell reservoir. Therefore, even if it is not an essential organ for survival, it has its importance and must be preserved as much as possible [3].

Splenic trauma treatment includes an operating and a non-operative management (NOM). The operative management can be conservative (like wrapping) or nonconservative (splenectomy). Urgent splenectomy is generally performed in case of massive hemoperitoneum (more than 1000 mL) with hemodynamically unstable patient, associated with severe intra-abdominal lesions that require surgery with general anesthesia; but actually there are no standardized indications nor written protocols to follow to choose whether to operate or not. Operative management may also become necessary for the treatment of unsuccessful NOM resulting in hemorrhage, necrosis, abscess, fistula, and splenic pseudoaneurysm.

Although it is known from the beginning of the last century that splenectomy increases the risk of infections, however for many decades it has been the preferred treatment for traumatic injuries. Compared with adults, splenic injury in children is less likely to require operative intervention [35].

However, when possible, a non-operative management of splenic traumatic injuries is to be preferred in order to leave the immune function of this organ untouched [36, 37]: this is crucial in pediatric patients, since it is known that splenectomized children undergo many complications, defined as "asplenic syndrome," which involves immunosuppression with increased susceptibility to infections by encapsulated cocci bacteria (Neisseria Meningitidis, Haemophilus Influenzae, Streptococcus Pneumoniae) and an increased risk of septic shock especially in the first 2 years after surgery [38].

From these findings, since the 1970s, an increasingly conservative approach has developed, especially in pediatric patients, thus arriving to the 1980s when a less interventionist and radical approach was proposed even in adults [39]. Since then, the simple observation with clinical and instrumental monitoring and hematic-chemical analysis is increasingly widespread with high success rates.

At present, in qualified centers in hemodynamically stable patients, the preferred treatment of splenic trauma is the non-operative one (about 85%) [40]. Of course, a careful candidate selection is essential for the NOM choice: in fact, hemodynamic stability, non-geriatric age, absence of pre-existing splenic lesions, and the possibility of monitoring in an intensive-care unit are required [41] (Fig. 16.16). There are many related advantages such as preservation of immune function, prevention of immediate and later complications associated with laparotomy and a decline in non-therapeutic explorative laparotomy.

In the event of open abdominal trauma, hemodynamic instability that may evolve into hypovolemic shock, with a diffuse hemoperitoneum and in the presence of serious injury associated with other parenchymal organs, emergency surgery is required. Now there is a dichotomy between observation (NOM) and surgery (splenectomy) because surgical repair therapies or spleen resection are always used less frequently. In the absence of peritoneal irritation, in a patient in stable condition, with grade I-II injuries (and a

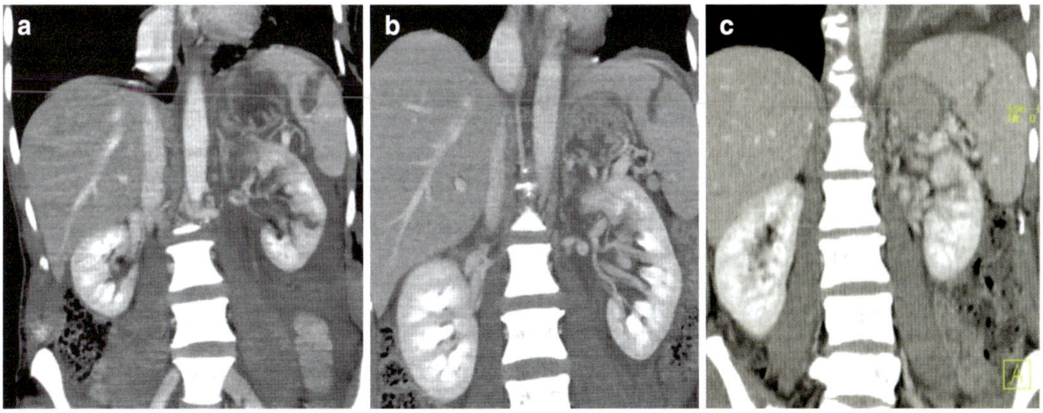

Fig. 16.16 Example of a NOM follow-up: These coronal CT reconstructions show a spontaneous healing of a splenic parenchymal laceration (larger than 3 cm—Grade 3). Figure (**a**) is the early control following the trauma, then after 7 days (**b**), and 14 days (**c**)

careful selection of patients with grade III lesions) [42] according to Mirvis, and the possibility to be monitored in an intensive-care unit, it is better to adopt an attitude of non-operative strict observation that has about a 95% success rate, according to published studies [13, 43].

To avoid complications related also to a possible delayed breaking, it is necessary for all patients initially treated conservatively to be monitored through repeated hemochrome checks, US or CEUS and, at minimum clinical suspect, with a contrast MDCT [11]. Delayed splenic rupture is a rare complication of trauma to the spleen, with relatively high reported mortality rates of up to 15% of cases. Patients usually present around 48 h or more after the initial trauma with symptoms and signs of intraperitoneal hemorrhage due to rupture of a slowly expanding subcapsular hematoma or secondary hemorrhage following dislodgement of a perisplenic hematoma.

The possibility of success of a conservative approach is greatly increased by the use of angiography which has both diagnostic and therapeutic functions [44]. In fact, with this method we have an excellent assessment of vascular lesions and, at the same time, the possibility to embolize the bleeding source, avoiding a splenectomy as often as possible. Splenic embolization is an excellent nonsurgical alternative for the treatment of grade III—IV—V splenic trauma (AAST guidelines) [45] and should be regarded as an additional tool to NOM [46, 47]. The indications to perform arteriography are: hemodynamic stability, the presence of contrast blush on CT exam, progressive decrease in hematocrit, and diagnosis of pseudoaneurysm or post-traumatic arteriovenous fistula [48] (Fig. 16.17). When possible, proximal embolization is preferred, where the embolic material is placed in the main splenic artery (causing permanent occlusion) allowing the development of collateral vessels that maintain an adequate organ perfusion: this method has fewer complications than the distal technique, which presents the highest risk of splenic infarction with necrosis and possible bacterial superinfection [49, 50] (Fig. 16.18). In the event of re-bleeding, re-intervention is possible by angiography only in case of the distal technique, otherwise the patient will be treated with a laparoscopic splenectomy [51].

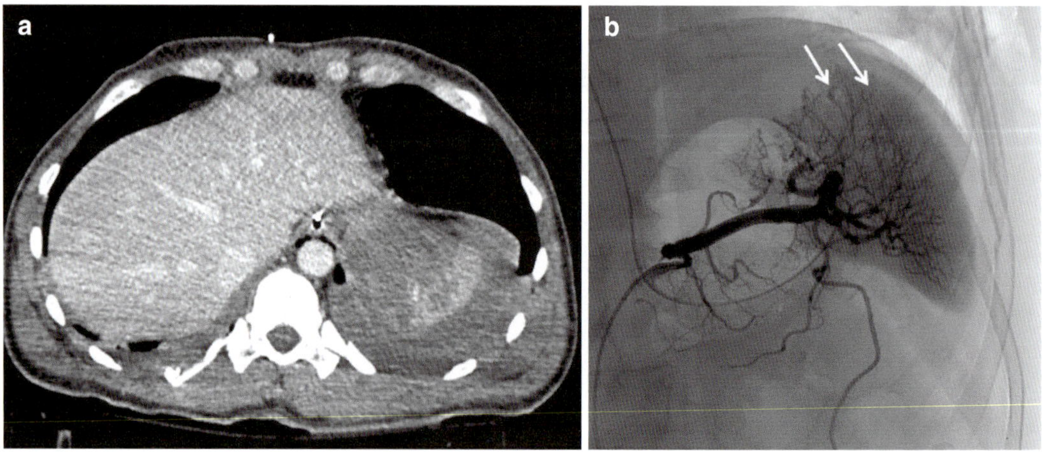

Fig. 16.17 Arteriography: Figure (**a**) shows the fragmentation of the upper splenic pole (shattered spleen). After, selective arteriography of the splenic main artery is performed, (**b**): it is possible to appreciate a de-vascularization of the upper splenic pole associated with small blood leakages (*arrows*)

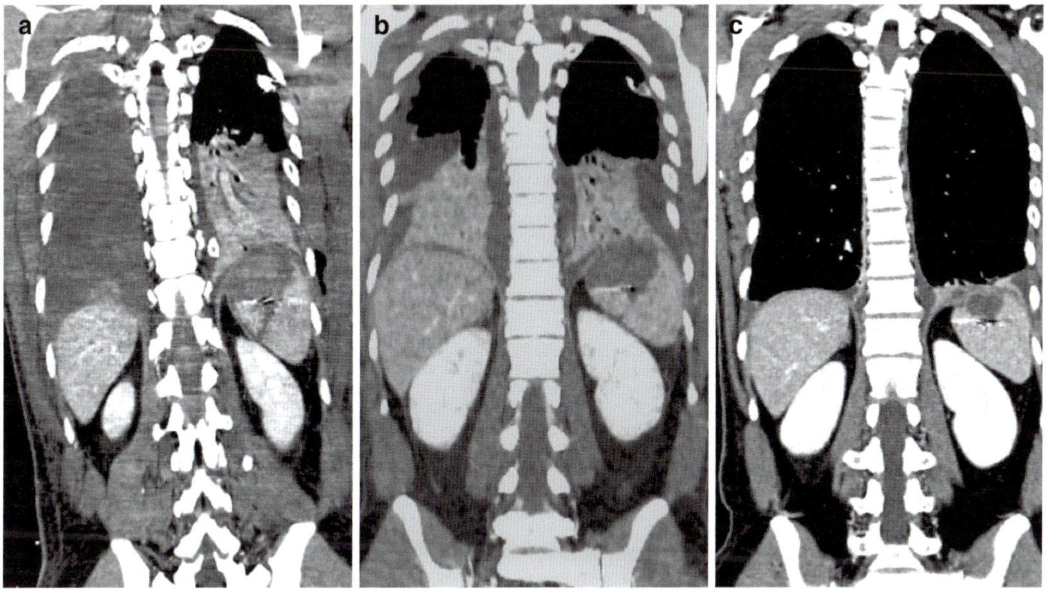

Fig. 16.18 Same case of Fig. 16.17. CT follow-up after treatment with distal embolization of the previous case: the splenic infarct area is spontaneously reduced in size as it can be shown in the CT-control immediately after treatment (**a**), after 7 days (**b**), and 14 days (**c**)

References

1. Rhee P, Joseph B, Pandit V, et al. Increasing trauma deaths in the United States. Ann Surg. 2014;260:13–21. doi:10.1097/SLA.0000000000000600.
2. Poletti PA, Mirvis SE, Shanmuganathan K, Takada T, Killeen KL, Perlmutter D, et al. Blunt abdominal trauma patients: can organ injury be excluded without performing computed tomography? J Trauma. 2004;57:1072–81.
3. Miele V, Errante Y, Galluzzo M, Pieri S, Sessa B, Trinci M. La diagnostica per immagini nelle lesioni traumatiche della milza. Il Giornale Italiano di Radiologia Medica. 2015;2:230–48. doi:10.17376/girm_2-2-03042015-6.
4. Olthof DC, Van der Vlies CH, Gosling JC. Evidence-based management and controversies in blunt splenic trauma. Curr Trauma Rep. 2017;3:32–7. doi:10.1007/s40719-017-0074-2; Epub 2017 Feb 9.
5. Forsythe RM, Harbrecht BG, Peitzman AB. Blunt splenic trauma. Scand J Surg. 2006;95:146–51.
6. Beuran M, Gheju I, Venter MD, et al. Non-operative management of splenic trauma. J Med Life. 2012;22:47–58; Epub: 2012 Mar 5.
7. Wu HM, Kortbeek JB. Management of splenic pseudocysts following trauma: a retrospective case series. Am J Surg. 2006;191:631–4.
8. Singer G, Rieder S, Eberl R, et al. Comparison of two treatment eras sonographic long-term outcome of blunt splenic injuries in children. Eur J Pediatr. 2013;172:1187–90.
9. Clancy AA, Tiruta C, Ashman D, et al. The song remains the same although the instruments are changing: complications following selective non-operative management of blunt spleen trauma: a retrospective review of patients at a level I trauma center from 1996 to 2007. J Trauma Manag Outcomes. 2012;6:4. doi:10.1186/1752-2897-6-4.
10. Moore EE, Cogbill TH, Jurkovic GJ, et al. Organ injury scaling: spleen and liver (1994 revision). J Trauma. 1995;38:323–4. doi:10.1097/00005373-199503000-00001.
11. Raikhlin A, Baerlocher MO, Asch MR, Myers A. Imaging and transcatheter arterial embolization for traumatic splenic injuries: review of the literature. Can J Surg. 2008;51:464–72.
12. Mirvis SE, Whiteley NO, Gens DR. Blunt splenic trauma in adults: CT-based classification and correlation with prognosis and treatment. Radiology. 1989;171:27–32. doi:10.1148/radiology.171.1.2928544.
13. Saksobhavivat N, Shanmuganathan K, Chen HH, et al. Blunt splenic injury: use of a multidetector CT-based splenic injury grading system and clinical parameters for triage of patients at admission. Radiology. 2015;274:702–11. doi:10.1148/radiol.14141060.

14. Marmery H, Shanmuganathan K, Alexander MT, Mirvis SE. Optimization of selection for nonoperative management of blunt splenic injury: comparison of MDCT grading systems. AJR Am J Roentgenol. 2007;189:1421–7. doi:10.2214/AJR.07.2152.
15. Hoffmann L, Pierce D, Puumala S. Clinical predictors of injuries not identified by focused abdominal sonogram for trauma examinations. J Emerg Med. 2009;36: 271–9. doi:10.1016/j.Jemermed.2007.09.035.
16. Miele V, Di Giampietro I, Iannello S, et al. Diagnostic imaging in paediatric polytrauma management. Radiol Med. 2015;120:33–49. doi:10.1007/s11547-014-0469-x.
17. McGrahan JP, Richards J, Gillen M. The focused abdominal sonography for trauma scan pearls and pitfalls. J Ultrasound Med. 2002;21:789–800.
18. Sessa B, Trinci M, Iannello S, et al. Blunt abdominal trauma: role of contrast-enhanced ultrasound in the detection and staging of abdominal traumatic lesions compared to US and CE-MDCT. Radiol Med. 2015;120:180–9. doi:10.1007/s11547-014-0425-9.
19. Valentino M, Serra C, Zironi G, et al. Blunt abdominal trauma: emergency contrast-enhanced sonography for detection of solid organ injuries. AJR Am J Roentgenol. 2006,186:1361–7. doi:10.2214/AJR.05.0027.
20. Menichini G, Sessa B, Trinci M, et al. Accuracy of contrast-enhanced ultrasound (CEUS) in the identification and characterization of traumatic solid organ lesions in children: a retrospective comparison with baseline-US and CE-MDCT. Radiol Med. 2015;120:989–1001. doi:10.1007/s11547-015-0535-z; Epub 2015 Mar 31.
21. Miele V, Piccolo CL, Galluzzo M, et al. Contrast-enhanced ultrasound (CEUS) in blunt abdominal trauma. Br J Radiol. 2016;89:20150823. doi:10.1259/bjr.20150823.
22. Sidhu PS, Cantisani V, Deganello A, et al. Role of contrast-enhanced ultrasound (CEUS) in pediatric practice: an EFSUMB position statement. Ultraschall Med. 2017;38:33–43. doi:10.1055/s-0042-110394.
23. Catalano O, Sandomenico F, Raso MM, Siani A. Real-time, contrast enhanced sonography: a new tool for detective active bleeding. J Trauma. 2005;59:933–9.
24. Anderson SW, Varghese JC, Lucey BC, et al. Blunt splenic trauma: delayed phase CT for differentiation of active hemorrhage from contained vascular injury. Radiology. 2007;243:88–95. doi:10.1148/radiol.2431060376.
25. Hassan R, Abd Aziz A, Md Ralib AR, Saat A. Computed tomography of blunt spleen injury: a pictorial review. Malays J Med Sci. 2011;18:60–7.
26. Uyeda JW, LeBedis CA, Penn DR, et al. Active hemorrhage and vascular injuries in splenic trauma: utility of the arterial phase in multi-detector CT. Radiology. 2014;270:99–106. doi:10.1148/radiol13121242.
27. Marmery H, Shanmuganathan K. Multidetector-row computed tomography imaging of splenic trauma. Semin Ultrasound CT MR. 2006;27:404–19.
28. Federle MP, Jeffrey RB. Hemoperitoneum studied by computed tomography. Radiology. 1983;148:187–92. doi:10.1148/radiology.148.1.6856833.
29. Pinto F, Miele V, Scaglione M, et al. The use of contrast-enhanced ultrasound in blunt abdominal trauma: advantages and limitations. Acta Radiol. 2014;55:776–84. doi:10.1177/0284185113505517; Epub 2013 Sep 23.
30. Pinto F, Valentino M, Romanini L, et al. The role of CEUS in the assessment of the hemodynamically stable patients with blunt abdominal trauma. Radiol Med. 2015;120:3–11. doi:10.1007/s11547-014-0455-3.
31. Gordic S, Alkadhi H, Simmen HP, Wanner G, Cadosh D. Characterization of indeterminate spleen lesions in primary CT after blunt abdominal trauma: potential role of MRI imaging. Emerg Radiol. 2014;21:491–8. doi:10.1007/s10140-014-1227-z.
32. Elsayes KM, Narra VR, Mukundan G, et al. MR imaging of the spleen: spectrum of abnormalities. Radiographics. 2005;25:967–82. doi:10.1148/rg254045154.
33. Robertson F, Leander P, Ekberg O. Radiology of the spleen. Eur Radiol. 2001;11:80–95. doi:10.1007/s003300000528.
34. Miele V, Piccolo CL, Sessa B, et al. Comparison between MRI and CEUS in the follow up of patients with blunt abdominal trauma managed conservatively. Radiol Med. 2016;121:27–37. doi:10.1007/s11547-015-0578-1.
35. Capasso L, Cuomo UM, D'Ambrosio R. Treatment of splenic trauma in paediatric age [article in Italian]. Ann Ital Chir. 2008;79:129–34.
36. Cirocchi R, Boselli C, Corsi A, et al. Is non-operative management safe and effective for all splenic blunt trauma? A systematic review. Crit Care. 2013;17:R185. doi:10.1186/cc12868.
37. Rosito M, Lattarulo S, Pezzolla A, et al. The conservative treatment in the splenic trauma [article in Italian]. Ann Ital Chir. 2009;80:231–6.
38. Sheybany EF, Gonzales-Araiza G, Kousari YM, et al. Pediatric non-accidental abdominal trauma. Radiographics. 2014;34:139–53. doi:10.1148/rg.341135013.
39. Madoff DC, Denys A, Wallace MJ, et al. Splenic arterial interventions: anatomy, indications, technical considerations and potential complications. Radiographics. 2005;25:S191–211. doi:10.1148/rg.25si055504.
40. Tinkoff G, Esposito TJ, Reed J, et al. American Association for the Surgery of Trauma Organ Injury Scale I: spleen, liver and kidney validation based on the national trauma data bank. J Am Coll Surg. 2008;207(5):646–55. doi:10.1016/j.jamcollsurg.2008.06.342.
41. Tartari S, Montalto C, Ferrante Z, et al. Trauma chiuso addominale: indicazioni al trattamento interventistico. Il Giornale Italiano di Radiologia Medica. 2016;3:953–8. doi:10.17376/girm_3-6-11122016-7.
42. Franco F, Monaco D, Volpi A, Marcato C, Larini P, Rossi C. The role of arterial embolization in blunt splenic injury. Radiol Med. 2011;116:454–65. doi:10.1007/s11547-011-0624-y.
43. Schnuriger B, Inaba K, Konstantinidis A, et al. Outcomes of a proximal versus distal splenic artery

embolization after trauma: a systematic review and meta-analysis. J Trauma. 2011;70:252–60. doi:10.1097/TA.0b013e318f2a92e.
44. Gaarder C, Dormagen JB, Eken T, et al. Nonoperative management of splenic injuries: improved results with angioembolization. J Trauma. 2006;61:192–8. doi:10.1097/01.ta.0000223466.62589.d9.
45. Hagiwara A, Fukushima H, Murata A, et al. Blunt splenic injury: usefulness of transcatether arterial embolization in patients with a transient response to fluid resuscitation. Radiology. 2005;235:57–64. doi:10.1148/radiol.2351031132.
46. Miller PR, Chang MC, Hoth JJ, et al. Prospective trial of angiography and embolization for all grade III to V blunt splenic injuries: non-operative management success rate is significantly improved. J Am Coll Surg. 2014;218:644–8. doi:10.1016/j.jamcollsurg.2014.01.040.
47. Van der Cruyssen F, Manzelli A. Splenic artery embolization: technically feasible but not necessarily advantageous. World J Emerg Surg. 2016;11:47. doi:10.1186/s13017-016-0100-7.
48. Farsad K, Ahuja C, Chadha M. An overview of splenic embolization. AJR Am J Roentgenol. 2015;205:720–5. doi:10.2214/AJR.15.14637.
49. Frandon J, Rodière M, Arvieux C, et al. Blunt splenic injury: outcomes of proximal versus distal and combined splenic artery embolization. Diagn Interv Imaging. 2014;95:825–31. doi:10.1016/j.diii.2014.03.009.
50. Ekeh AP, Khalaf S, Ilyas S, et al. Complication arising from splenic artery embolization: a review of a 11-year experience. Am J Surg. 2013;205:250–4. doi:10.1016/j.amjsurg.2013.01.003.
51. Cooney R, Ku J, Cherry R, et al. Limitations of splenic angioembolization in treating blunt splenic injury. J Trauma. 2005;59:926–32.

Bowel and Mesenteric Injury

17

Viola Valentini, Grazia Loretta Buquicchio, Ginevra Danti, Michele Galluzzo, Stefania Ianniello, Margherita Trinci, and Vittorio Miele

17.1 Introduction

Bowel and mesenteric injuries are found in approximately 1.2–5% of patients following blunt abdominal trauma [1–4]. Despite their infrequency, the clinical significance of these lesions cannot be underestimated. The gastrointestinal tract represents the third most commonly involved abdominal organ in blunt trauma, after spleen and liver. Mesenteric injuries are reported to be about three times more frequent than bowel perforations [3, 5, 6].

Clinical diagnosis of blunt and mesenteric injuries is difficult because of scarce specificity of laboratory findings and delayed onset of peritoneal irritation signs. The classic triad of abdominal pain, guarding, and decreased or absent bowel sounds occurs only in one-third of patients [7]. Moreover, physical examination and abdominal assessment may be limited and unreliable in a trauma setting, due to significant neurologic comorbidities.

V. Valentini, M.D. (✉) • G.L. Buquicchio
M. Galluzzo • S. Ianniello • M. Trinci
Department of Emergency Radiology, S. Camillo Hospital, C.ne Gianicolense, 87, 00152 Rome, Italy
e-mail: violavalentini@libero.it

G. Danti • V. Miele
Department of Radiology, Careggi University Hospital, Florence, Italy

Contrary to the trend of nonoperative management of solid intra-abdominal organs, the treatment of choice for significant bowel and mesenteric injuries remains early surgery. A delay in diagnosis and treatment, as little as 5–8 h, results in increased complications and mortality rate [8, 9], with mortality rates as high as 30% if the delay is 24 h or more [3, 9]. A prompt and accurate diagnosis is therefore critical in preventing fatal complications and reducing mortality rates (mostly septic and hemorrhagic) in bowel traumatic injuries, but it is inadequately supported and hardly achieved by clinical examination and other commonly used diagnostic tests, such as diagnostic peritoneal lavage (DPL) and focused assessment with sonography in trauma (FAST scan) [4, 10]. Currently, due to major advancements in technology, multidetector computed tomography (MDCT) has emerged as a critical diagnostic tool, becoming the imaging modality of choice to evaluate abdominal trauma in hemodynamically stable patients.

The role of imaging is, therefore, of great importance: the radiologist is asked not only to detect signs of intestinal and mesenteric traumatic injuries but also to indicate the clinical significance of such lesions, trying to identify those requiring an immediate operative treatment (major injuries), substantially represented by intestinal perforation, active bleeding, and vascular avulsion of the mesentery, that can rapidly result in septic,

V. Miele, M. Trinci (eds.), *Diagnostic Imaging in Polytrauma Patients*,
https://doi.org/10.1007/978-3-319-62054-1_17

hemorrhagic, and ischemic complications [11–14], and to distinguish them from those (minor injuries), such as bowel wall contusion, mesenteric infiltration, and non-bleeding mesenteric hematoma, that can be managed nonsurgically.

17.2 Mechanisms of Blunt Bowel and Mesentery Injury

Mostly due to motor vehicle accidents, bowel and mesentery injuries have registered an increase in incidence after the introduction of seat belts [5, 15, 16]. Other common causes include assaults, occupational accidents, sports, and falls. In general terms, the incidence and significance of gastrointestinal trauma is higher in childhood because of the incomplete development of the abdominal wall musculature.

Three main pathogenic mechanisms have been described to be responsible for causing bowel and mesentery lesions in blunt trauma (Fig. 17.1), which may act isolated or combined:

1. Crush: direct force applied to the bowel wall, causing compression between the spine and the abdominal wall.
2. Shear: rapid deceleration producing a shearing force between fixed and mobile portions of the bowel.
3. Burst: sudden increase in intraluminal pressure causing perforation. The bowel bursts when the intraluminal pressure exceeds the bowel wall tensile strength.

Crushing may determine local lacerations of the bowel wall and mesentery, mural and mesenteric hematomas, localized devascularization, and full-thickness contusions. Susceptibility to crush injuries increases with age, in relation to the relaxation of abdominal musculature. Because of their anatomical features (close contact to the spine), the duodenum and transverse colon are particularly susceptible to this type of injury [17], which are often caused by seat belt, steering wheel or, mostly in pediatric age, bicycle handlebar.

Shearing forces can lead to bowel lacerations, mesenteric tears, and interruption of the mesenteric vessels. Points of anatomical fixity, or intestinal segments close to acquired fixity points, such as bridles and adhesions, are more susceptible to these injuries.

The presence of a "seat belt mark" sign, characterized by patterned ecchymosis or abrasion across the patient's abdominal wall, correspondent to the position of the diagonal or horizontal strap of the seat belt, is considered a reliable predictor of bowel injury [11, 18]. A radiologic seat belt sign, consisting of increased attenuation in the subcutaneous fat over the abdomen, has been described [16]. At impact, the seat belt compression may close off the bowel, causing a sudden increase of the intraluminal pressure in the "closed loop" that may result in bursting injuries. When the intraluminal pressure reaches 120–140 mmHg, either a single perforation or multiple small perforations of the bowel wall can occur, usually on the antimesenteric border of the loop [15, 16]. Requiring less energy to occur than

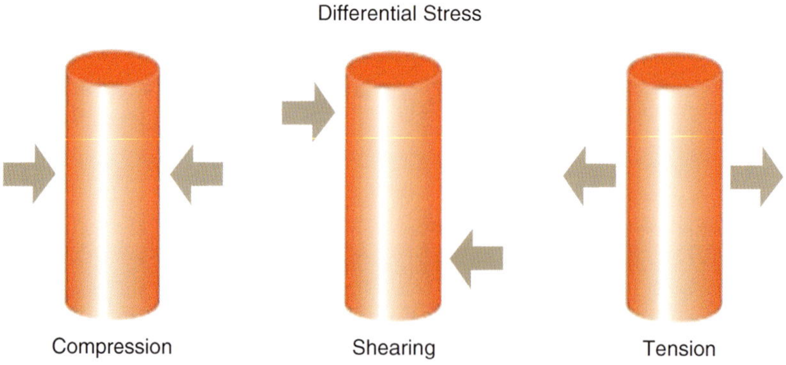

Fig. 17.1 Scheme of the three types of stress that act on bowel and mesentery in abdominal blunt trauma

injuries from the crush and shearing mechanisms, burst lesions are therefore more likely to be isolated (not associated with other injuries) [16]. Pre-existing pathological conditions, such as ileus, Crohn disease, and bowel obstruction, predispose the bowel to this type of injury.

17.3 Anatomo-Pathological Considerations

The small bowel is the most often injured intestinal tract (70%) in blunt abdominal trauma. As already mentioned, intestinal tracts close to fixed point of attachment, such as proximal jejunum near the ligament of Treitz and distal ileum near the ileocecal valve, where mobile and fixed portions of the gut are contiguous, are particularly exposed to damage [19, 20].

The colon accounts for 20% of intestinal traumatic injuries. The ascending and descending colon, fixed and partially retroperitoneal, are generally susceptible to more severe injuries compared to the more mobile transverse and sigmoid colon. Injuries to the right colon are always associated with multiple injuries elsewhere, reflecting the high-energy dissipation required to inflict them [21, 22] (Fig. 17.2). The sigmoid colon is at risk of closed loop perforation. Due to its exposed location, the transverse colon is reported to be the most vulnerable portion of the large bowel, but its relative mobility accounts for the minor entity of most injuries at this site.

Duodenum represents the intestinal tract less frequently involved in blunt trauma (10%). Its anatomical features (mainly retroperitoneal organ, in direct contact with the thoracic spine) explain the peculiarity of diagnostic findings in cases of perforation and the frequent association with pancreatic injury.

Injuries to the appendix, stomach, and rectum are extremely uncommon. Rectum injuries are often associated with major pelvic fractures.

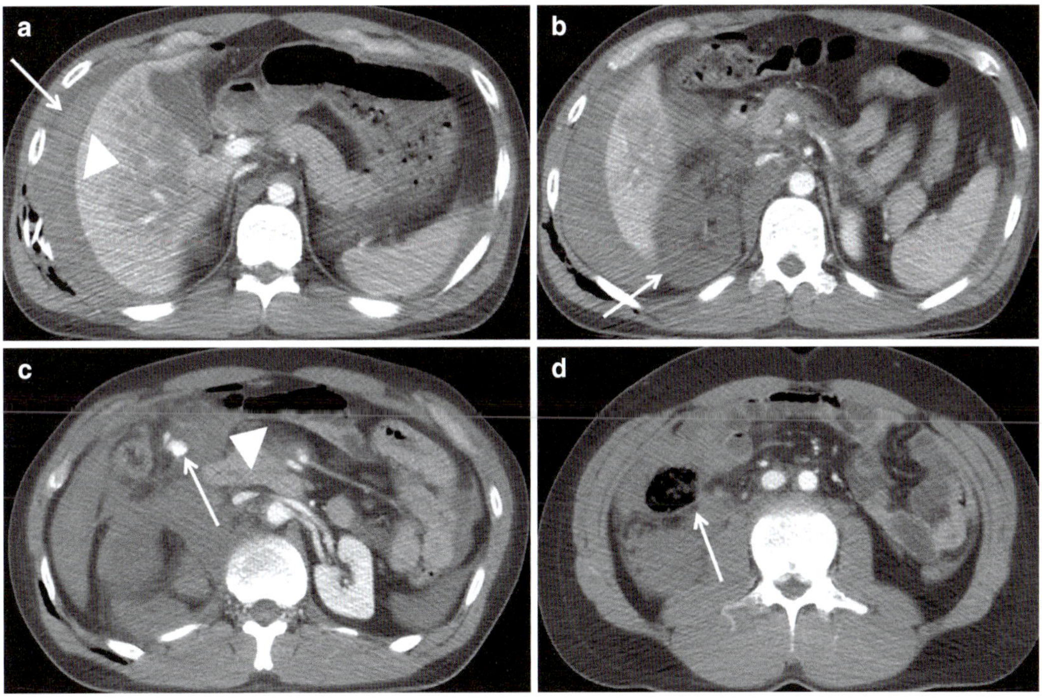

Fig. 17.2 High-energy blunt abdominal trauma. Axial CT images show rib fractures (*curved arrow* in **a**), hemoperitoneum (*arrow* in **a**) and hepatic contusion (*arrowhead* in **a**), devascularization of the right kidney (*arrow* in **b**), mesenteric hematoma (*arrowhead* in **c**) with contrast material extravasation (active bleeding) (*arrow* in **c**), and unenhanced ascendant colon wall (*arrow* in **d**)

Table 17.1 Bowel and mesentery major and minor injuries

Bowel	Mesentery
Significant (major) injuries	
Complete tear of the bowel wall	Active bleeding
Bowel ischemia	Mesentery disruption
	Mesenteric injury with bowel ischemia
Not significant (minor) injuries	
Serosal tear of the bowel wall	Mesenteric hematoma (no bleeding)
Bowel hematoma	Mesenteric stranding

The site of damage correlates well with prognosis, accounting the amount and quality of bowel content, which is less enzymatically active and has low pH and bacterial counts in case of small bowel lesions and more contaminating in case of colonic lesions. Intraperitoneal blood is a minor peritoneal irritant.

Bowel and mesenteric injuries are frequently associated with abdominal solid organ lesions [23] or spine and pelvic bones fractures [24].

The management of bowel and mesenteric traumatic injuries depends on the location and the type of damage. Surgical treatment is not always necessary and depends on the relevance of the lesion: major and minor injuries can be distinguished (Table 17.1). Surgically significant injuries, or "major" lesions, include a complete tear of the bowel, devascularized bowel, active mesenteric bleeding, and mesenteric injury associated with bowel ischemia.

Minor injuries include serosal tear of the bowel wall, bowel hematoma, mesenteric hematoma without active bleeding and mesenteric stranding; these conditions can be managed conservatively.

17.4 The Role of MDCT

Since diagnosis based on clinical findings has low sensitivity and is often unreliable, a set of diagnostic tools has been used to evaluate patients in whom abdominal injury is suspected, including DPL, FAST scan, and CT [4, 25].

DPL, traditionally used in several countries, is fairly sensitive (90%) for the detection of hemoperitoneum, but has several limitations: it is poorly specific in assessing the site and the extent of the damage, it is not reliable in detecting retroperitoneal injuries and, like any invasive procedure, it carries some risk of iatrogenic injuries [4, 10]. The use of results of DPL as the sole indication for surgery has led to a high nontherapeutic laparotomy rate.

FAST scan has a great sensitivity (86%) for the detection of free intra-abdominal fluid, but is nonspecific with regard to organ injury [4].

With a wide range of reported values for sensitivity and specificity (between 80–95% and 48–99%, respectively) [26], the accuracy of CT for detection of intestinal and mesenteric injuries due to blunt trauma has long been controversial. Until the 2000s, surgical literature described CT as unreliable in distinguishing surgical from not-surgical bowel and mesenteric injuries. The recent introduction of MDCT significantly decreased the time taken to perform the examination, decreased the motion artifacts, and improved the blood vessel opacification and solid organ enhancement. Providing a wide spectrum of findings suggestive of bowel and mesenteric injuries, MDCT is more sensitive and specific than DPL, FAST scan, and clinical examination [19]. Owing to the great advances in CT technology and improvement in interpretation, MDCT has currently become the diagnostic tool of choice in the evaluation of blunt abdominal trauma in hemodynamically stable patients [6, 27].

17.5 MDCT Technique

All MDCT examinations must be performed with a high-resolution protocol, with reconstruction interval values equals to 1 mm, and completed with coronal and sagittal multiplanar reconstruction in the post-processing elaboration.

The acquisition of pre-contrast CT abdomino-pelvis scans is useful to identify free air collections, to detect abnormal attenuation of mesenteric fat, and to assess the attenuation values of any fluid collection and/or of the bowel wall.

A biphasic study in arterial and venous phase after the intravenous infusion of 120–150 ml of iodinated contrast material at an adequate rate (≥3 ml/s) is indicated to detect active bleeding and identify perfusion abnormalities in the bowel loops. In suspicious of low-flow vascular active bleeding, a delayed phase (3–5 min) may be added to the examination [11, 28].

Many investigators have proven that administration of oral contrast material is not routinely required in the MDCT evaluation of patients with blunt abdominal trauma [4, 29–31]. Being time-consuming, oral contrast material administration increases the risk of vomiting and aspiration without improvement of diagnostic capability [32].

17.6 MDCT Findings of Intestinal and Mesenteric Injury

According to surgical and prognostic criteria, traumatic injuries of the bowel and mesentery can be classified into "major" and "minor." Major lesions, including bowel perforation, active mesenteric bleeding, and mesenteric injury associated with bowel ischemia, require a surgical treatment. If unrecognized, these injuries may result in high morbidity and mortality, related to sepsis or hemorrhage. Minor lesions, including bowel wall tear limited to the serosa, bowel wall hematoma, and mesenteric hematoma without active bleeding, can be treated conservatively.

Currently, there are several recognized CT features of blunt bowel and mesenteric injury (Tables 17.2 and 17.3). Based on radiological criteria, we distinguish specific (direct) and nonspecific (indirect) bowel and mesenteric injury signs. Getting familiar with the appearance of specific and nonspecific signs is crucial to making a prompt and accurate diagnosis [4].

17.7 MDCT Findings of Bowel Injury

17.7.1 Bowel Wall Discontinuity

Detection of a discontinuous bowel wall is the most specific sign of bowel injury, with 100% specificity [4]. However, this finding is extremely uncommon on MDCT images and it has a very low sensitivity (5–10%) [23]. The relative infrequency of direct visualization of bowel perforation is mainly due to the small size of discontinuities [4]. The type of lesion may also influence the possibility of detection: blowout perforations are harder to identify on CT than lacerations because of the collapsing, cockade shaped, margins of the small hole. Site of perforation is important as well: a lesion occurring on the antimesenteric equatorial border of the loop may be easier to identify on axial scans (Fig. 17.3); lesions involving the superior or inferior wall will be better detected on multiplanar reconstruction. Lesions of the bowel wall are better depicted in the portal venous phase scan [11]. The distribution of free air may be useful in localizing the point of bowel rupture [28].

Table 17.2 MDCT signs of bowel injury

Specific (direct signs)	Nonspecific (indirect signs)
Bowel wall discontinuity	Bowel wall thickening
Extraluminal air	Abnormal bowel wall enhancement
Intramural air	Intraperitoneal/retroperitoneal fluid

Table 17.3 MDCT signs of mesenteric injury

Specific (direct signs)	Nonspecific (indirect signs)
Active bleeding	Mesenteric infiltration
Beading/termination of mesenteric vessels	Intraperitoneal fluid (mesenteric fluid collections)
Mesenteric hematoma	

17.7.2 Extraluminal Air

The presence of extraluminal air has a reported specificity of 95% and a sensitivity of 30–60% for bowel perforation [23]. Pneumoperitoneum or so-called "free air" is not necessarily detectable on CT scans at admission and may be apparent only at later examinations, obtained after 6–12 h. In cases of small bowel perforation, only minimal amount of free air is present.

Pneumoretroperitoneum seems to be a more sensitive finding of perforation of one of the retroperitoneal intestinal tracts: second to fourth portion of duodenum, ascending and descending colon [31].

Although bowel perforation is a major cause of this sign, extraluminal air may also be observed in the absence of bowel perforation [32]. Other possible sources of free air in the abdomen are diffusion of a pneumothorax in patients with diaphragmatic injury, barotrauma, mechanical ventilation, and chest tube placement. Small amounts of air can penetrate through the female genital tract. Intraperitoneal rupture of bladder with Foley catheter in place can cause pneumoperitoneum as well. Mimicking true pneumoperitoneum, the presence of air confined between the inner layer of the abdominal wall and the peritoneum parietal layer, so-called "pseudopneumoperitoneum," represents a potential diagnostic pitfall [4, 11].

However, the presence of free air in association with coexistent ancillary signs, such as bowel wall thickening, abnormalities of parietal enhancement, free fluid, and mesenteric infiltration, is highly predictive of bowel injury.

Using wide window settings (lung or bone windows) to review CT images aids in detecting small amounts of free abdominal air. Free air from bowel rupture commonly tends to extend behind the anterior abdominal wall, under the anterior parietal peritoneal layer, and along the anterior surfaces of liver and spleen (Fig. 17.4). However, foci of air may also be seen at the porta hepatis or in the mesenteric and portal venous system (Fig. 17.5). Extraluminal air can also be seen trapped in the mesentery (Fig. 17.6a), if the bowel wall discontinuity occurs on the mesenteric border, or located in the retroperitoneum, in case of duodenal, ascending and descending colon traumatic perforation (Fig. 17.6b).

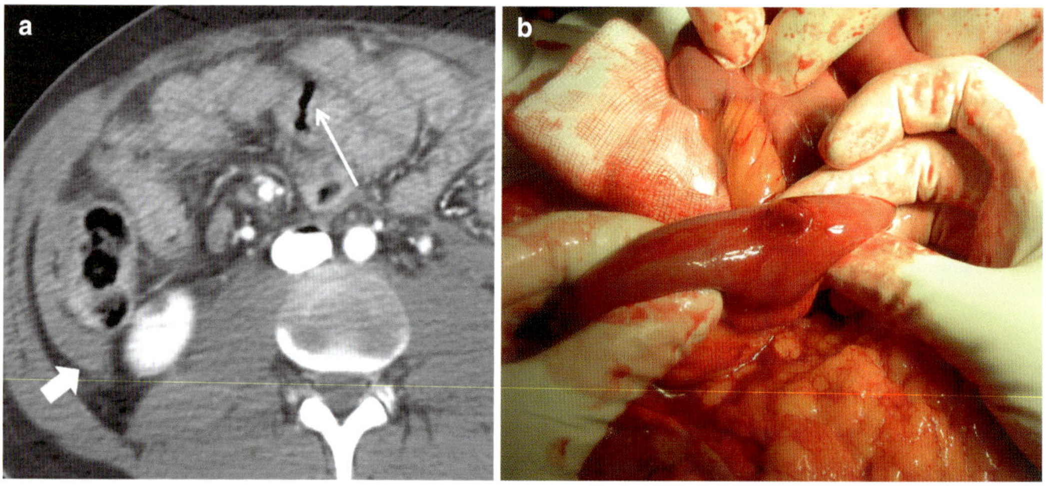

Fig. 17.3 Discontinuous bowel wall. (**a**) Axial CT contrast-enhanced image shows a wall discontinuity (*arrow*) on the anterior, antimesenteric wall of a small bowel loop, with extraluminal air and hemoperitoneum (*thick arrow*). (**b**) Intraoperative photograph of an antimesenteric small bowel wall perforation. Intraoperative image courtesy of Dr. Ennio Adami, MD

17.7.3 Intramural Air

Major and minor bowel injuries have findings of bowel wall thickening and free fluid in common. Along with extraluminal air, the presence of air bubbles confined in the thickness of the bowel wall (Fig. 17.7) increases the probability of a full-thickness injury, a major injury that requires laparotomy, rather a partial thickness injury, which can be treated conservatively [31].

17.7.4 Bowel Wall Thickening

Seen in 75% of transmural injuries, focal bowel wall thickening seems to be more sensitive for

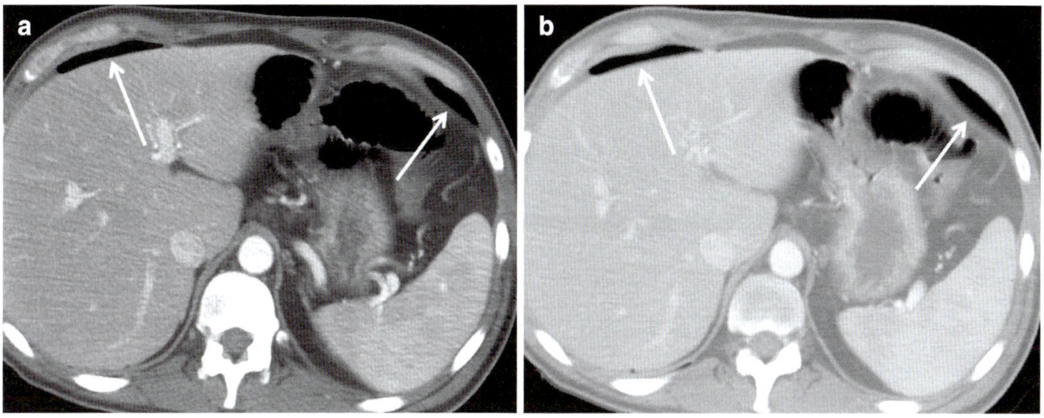

Fig. 17.4 Axial CT contrast-enhanced scan shows free air from bowel rupture laying behind the anterior abdominal wall, along the anterior surfaces of liver and spleen (*arrows* in **a**). Viewing the CT image in a bone window (**b**) better demonstrates the presence of small amounts of extraluminal air collections

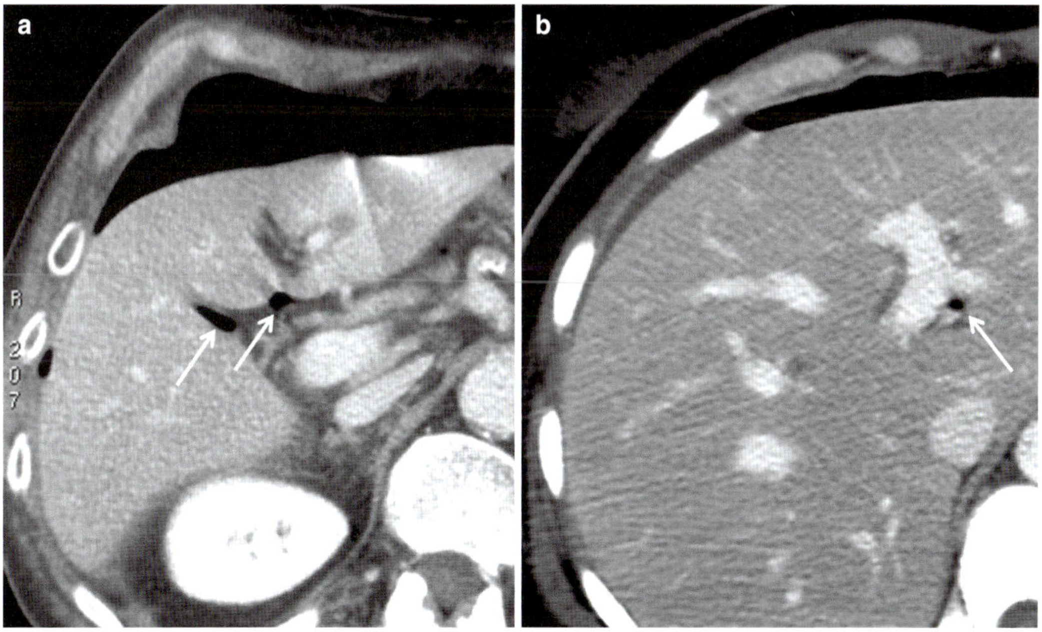

Fig. 17.5 Axial CT scans show air foci at the porta hepatis (*arrows*) (**a**). Axial CT scans show focal air bubble collecting in the portal venous system (*arrow*) (**b**)

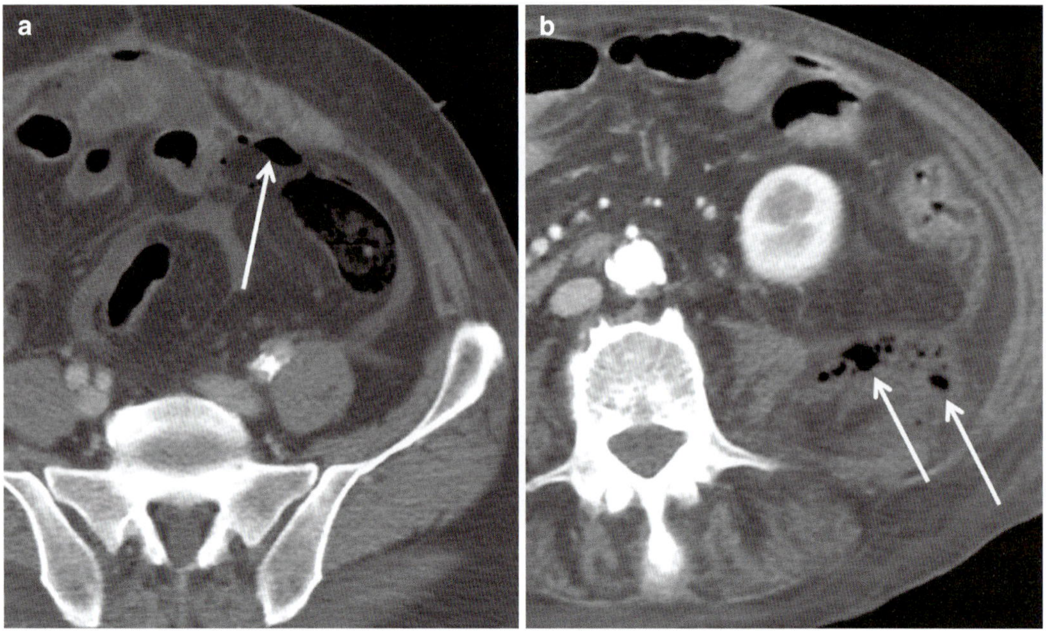

Fig. 17.6 Axial CT contrast-enhanced scans show air foci trapped in the mesentery (*arrow* in **a**). Free air in the retroperitoneum (*arrows* in **b**)

bowel injury than pneumoperitoneum [30–35]. This sign has a reported specificity of 90%, but is relatively insensitive, with reported values ranging 55–75% [36]. To minimize subjectivity in the evaluation of this sign, many authors suggest considering abnormal a disproportionate circumferential thickening of the bowel wall compared with normal appearing segments (Fig. 17.8) or a bowel wall thickness greater than 3 mm for the small bowel and 5 mm for the colon with adequate bowel distension. Focal bowel thickening can also be the expression of a partial thickness bowel injury. Intramural hematoma is a known evidence of blunt traumatic injury. Frequently localized to the duodenum (Fig. 17.9), uncommon in the large bowel, it is generally treated conservatively and tends to spontaneous resolution. Delayed complications such as stricture and obstruction are reported in some cases.

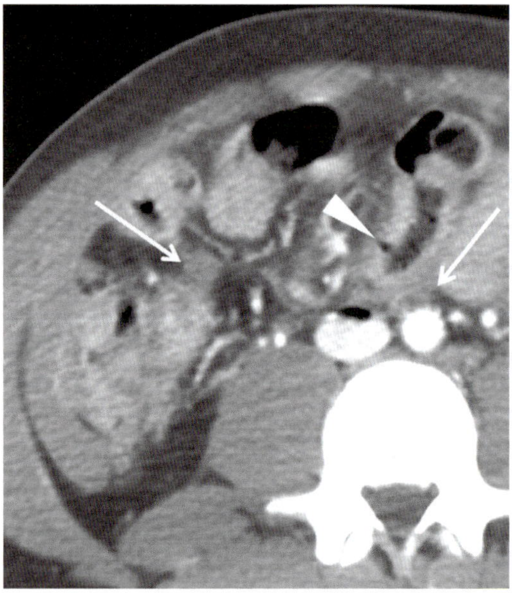

Fig. 17.7 Axial CT contrast-enhanced scan shows foci of intramural air (*arrowhead*) in a thick-walled small bowel loop. Interloop fluid is also seen (*thin arrows*)

Diffuse small bowel wall thickening should not be confused with traumatic bowel injury. It commonly represents bowel edema, secondary to a systemic condition, such as hypoperfusion complex in so-called "shock bowel" (see below) or systemic volume overload from iatrogenic over-resuscitation [10].

17.7.5 Abnormal Bowel Wall Enhancement

Bowel wall enhancement can be evaluated subjectively compared to the enhanced adjacent bowel loops; bowel wall density can be compared to that of the psoas muscle or of the contiguous vessels as well [28].

Focal, patchy areas of increased enhancement of the bowel wall may represent bowel injury with vascular involvement [27]. However, areas of decreased or absent enhancement are indicative of ischemic bowel (Fig. 17.10).

Diffuse increased small bowel wall enhancement in the trauma setting has been described as a consequence of hypovolemic shock, in which intestinal hypoperfusion leads to increased permeability, with interstitial leakage of contrast material [34]. In shock bowel, abnormal parietal enhancement, characterized by intense mucosal enhancement and hypodense submucosal edema, is associated with wall thickening and fluid distension of the whole small bowel, likely related to unsuccessful reabsorption. Intestinal findings are usually associated with other findings of hypovolemic shock, such as increased enhancement of kidneys, adrenal glands and spleen and collapsed inferior vena cava [34] (Fig. 17.11). Hypoperfusion findings cannot be noted in large bowel.

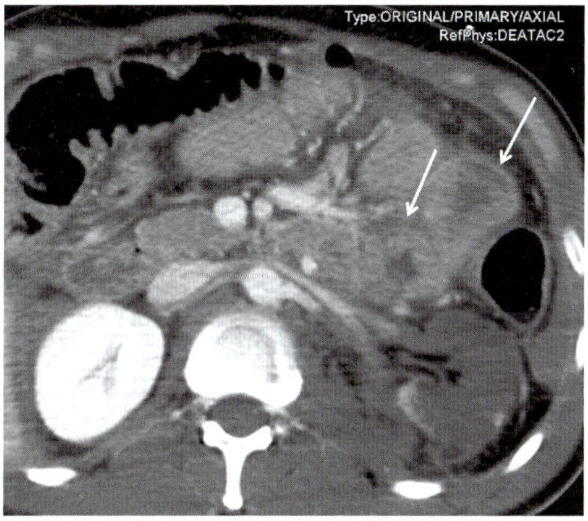

Fig. 17.8 Axial CT image shows small bowel loops with thickened wall and disomogeneous parietal enhancement. Left renal devascularization is also seen

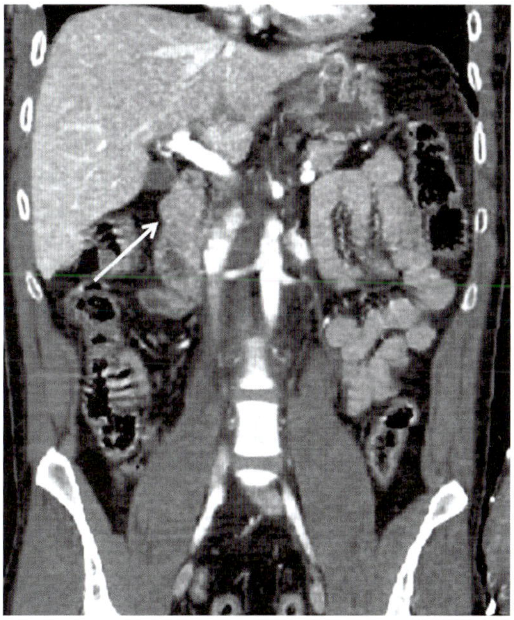

Fig. 17.9 Duodenal hematoma. Coronal reformatted CT image shows a focal thickening of the duodenal wall (*arrow*) in the absence of retroperitoneal fluid or free air

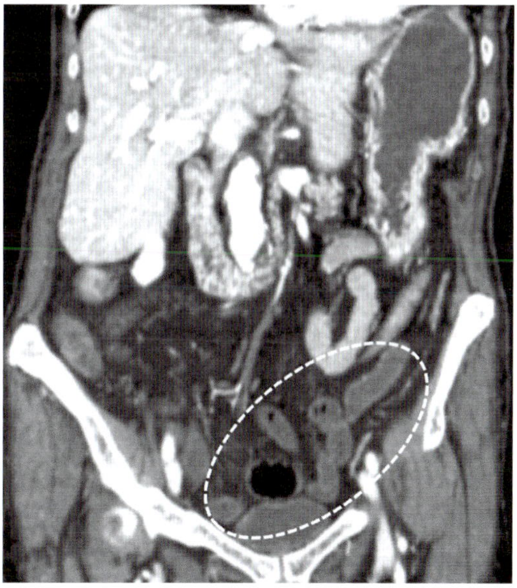

Fig. 17.10 Coronal reformatted CT scan shows reduced parietal enhancement of small bowel ischemic loops in the left lower abdominal quadrant (*oval*)

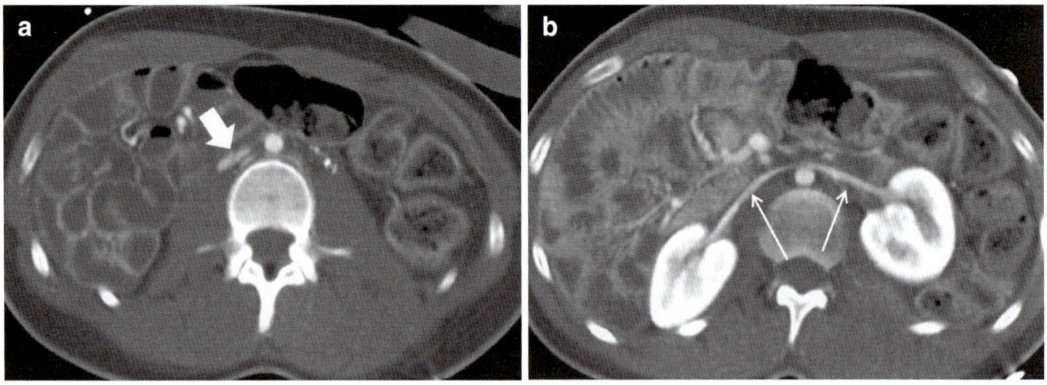

Fig. 17.11 Axial CT contrast-enhanced image shows diffuse hypervascular thickening of small bowel loops, with mucosal feathering, features characteristic of shock bowel. Flattened inferior vena cava (*thick arrow* in **a**) and renal veins (*thin arrows* in **b**) and increased enhancement of the kidneys (**b**) are noted

17.8 MDCT Findings of Mesenteric Injury

17.8.1 Mesenteric Hematoma

Mesenteric hematoma appears as a well-defined inhomogeneous collection of hemorrhagic fluid, with attenuation values varying depending on the degree of degradation of blood components, but, in general, closer to that of the soft tissues than that of fluids. Large mesenteric hematomas may exert mass effect on adjacent vessels and bowel loops. Although specific for mesenteric traumatic injury, in the absence of active extravasation, mesenteric hematoma is not an indication for operative treatment.

"*Sentinel clot sign,*" defined by focal, circumscribed high-density collection of clotted blood, with average CT density greater than 50 HU at basal scans [37], tending to accumulate adjacent to the site of bleeding, has been described as a clue to localize an hemorrhage source (Fig. 17.12).

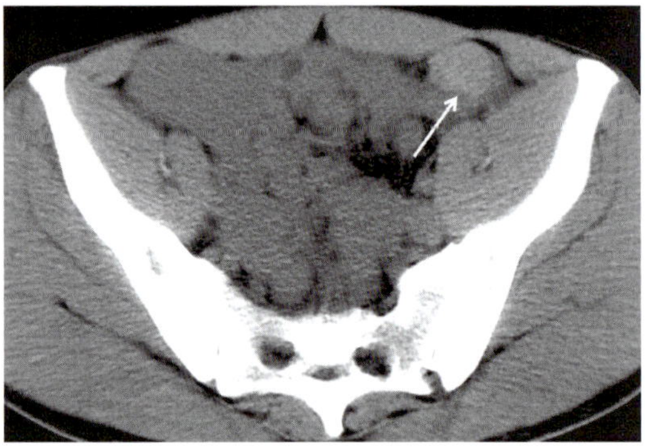

Fig. 17.12 On unenhanced axial CT scan, *"sentinel clot sign"* appears as a focal, circumscribed high-density collection of clotted blood (*arrow*), adjacent to the site of bleeding

17.8.2 Active Bleeding

This finding has 100% specificity for the diagnosis of major mesenteric lesion.

In active mesenteric bleeding, the extravasation appears as high density contrast leak, with attenuation values close to that of an adjacent contrast-enhanced artery, surrounded by lower, disomogeneous attenuation hematoma in the arterial phase (Fig. 17.13); active bleeding usually shows increase in size and decrease in attenuation on delayed phases (Fig. 17.14).

Significant mesenteric bleeding requires urgent surgical exploration, both for stopping the hemorrhage and for investigating the bowel because of the risk of ischemia.

17.8.3 Beading and Termination of Mesenteric Vessels

Most recently recognized, this finding indicates a surgically important mesenteric injury [32].

Vascular beading is defined as focal alteration of the mesenteric vessels size, with the same attenuation of arteries during all the phases of the scan. It represents incomplete lesion of the vascular wall (pseudoaneurysm), contained by the serosa and surrounding tissues. A lack of continuity or tapering of a mesenteric artery or vein indicates irregular contour and abrupt termination of mesenteric vessels. Both signs have high specificity, ranging from 93 to 95%, but low sensibility, ranging from 45 to 50% [1, 4]. Due to the orientation of mesenteric vessels, this CT finding is better appreciated on coronal or sagittal reformatted images [32].

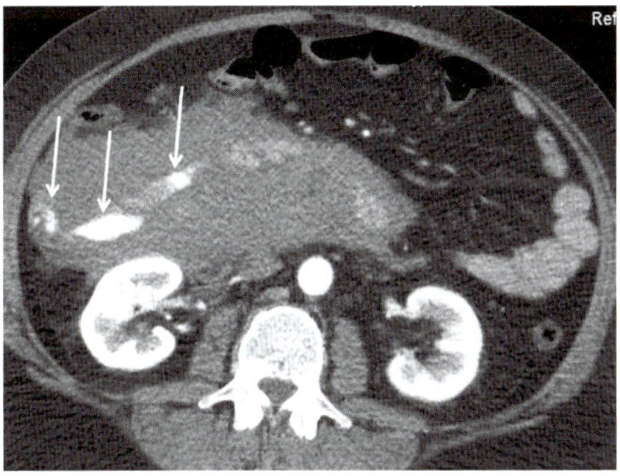

Fig. 17.13 Mesenteric bleeding. Axial CT scan in the arterial phase shows a large, disomogeneous mesenteric hematoma, containing high density contrast leak (*arrows*), with attenuation values close to that of an artery

17.9 MDCT Findings Coincident in Both Intestinal and Mesenteric Injury

17.9.1 Mesenteric Infiltration (Stranding)

Ill-defined, striated soft-tissue infiltration and haziness of mesenteric fat (Fig. 17.15), corresponding to microhemorrhagic foci, is a sensitive, but poorly specific sign, being commonly associated to other findings suggestive of mesenteric injury. Mesenteric stranding may be associated to bowel perforation as well [4, 31].

The coexistence of mesenteric infiltration with increased bowel wall thickness may be highly suggestive for a major intestinal injury, with ischemic sufferance of the bowel.

Pre-existing mesenteric stranding, as in inflammatory panniculitis, may mimic mesenteric traumatic injury. In inflammatory conditions, however, the fat stranding is well defined and multiple lymph nodes are associated.

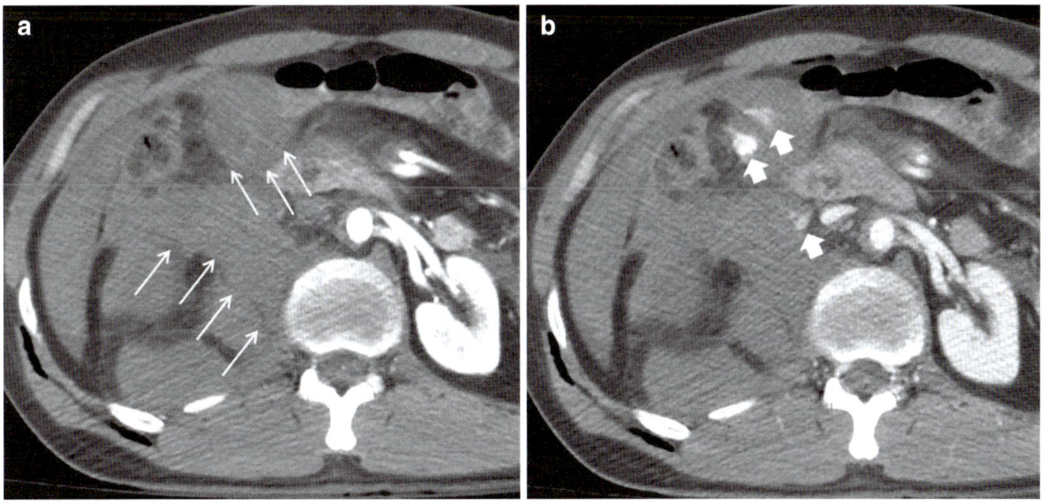

Fig. 17.14 Mesenteric bleeding. Axial CT scan in arterial phase shows multiple large mesenteric hematomas (*arrows* in **a**). Contrast extravasation within the mesenteric hematomas is clearly depicted in the portal phase CT (*thick arrows* in **b**)

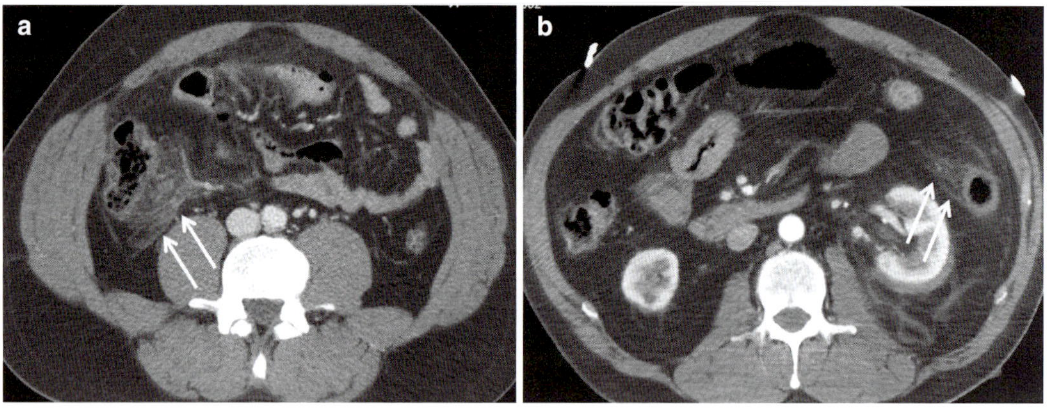

Fig. 17.15 Mesenteric stranding, appearing as ill-defined, striated soft-tissue infiltration of pericecal fat (*arrows* in **a**) and left paracolic gutter (*arrows* in **b**) on axial CT contrast-enhanced scans

17.9.2 Intraperitoneal or Retroperitoneal Fluid

The presence of free fluid is one of the most relevant signs of bowel and/or mesenteric injury.

The evidence of free fluid in the peritoneal/retroperitoneal recesses without concomitant CT scan evidence of traumatic lesion to solid organs seems to be suggestive of bowel or mesenteric injury [31], with a reported sensitivity of about 84% [8]. The combination of free fluid and free air increased the sensitivity for small bowel perforation to 97% [38]. On the other hand, the absence of intra/retroperitoneal fluid substantially rules out a significant bowel and/or mesenteric injury [1].

In the presence of free fluid without signs of any solid organ injury, is mandatory to search for other CT findings predictors of bowel injury.

The fluid may be of low attenuation, representing extravasated bowel contents, or of intermediate to high attenuation (30–50 UH), due to acute hemorrhage (hemoperitoneum).

The presence of a fluid-fluid level, with a dependent layer of high attenuation (sedimented red blood cells), occurring within a few hours, may help confirm the bloody nature of the fluid. Attenuation values should be interpreted with caution: hemoperitoneum may have lower density in a patient with a decreased hematocrit or if the hemorrhage is more than 48 h old.

False positives are possible: a small amount of fluid accumulation in the Douglas patch in a female patient is considered physiologic. Recent studies [32] reported the presence of small amounts of isolated pelvic fluid even in male patients, in the absence of bowel and/or mesenteric injuries. Notice that post-traumatic low-density intraperitoneal fluid may be urine in the case of intraperitoneal bladder rupture.

The location of the fluid may indicate the site of the injury: hemoperitoneum from solid organs injury (liver, spleen) starts near the site of injury and flows along expected anatomic pathways. It collects around the solid organs in the perihepatic and perisplenic spaces and migrates caudally toward the pelvis, passing through the paracolic gutters (Fig. 17.16). Hemorrhage from a bowel or mesenteric injury is typically trapped between the mesenteric leaves that surround intestinal loops (Fig. 17.17). The presence of triangular interloop fluid collections (Fig. 17.18a) should prompt a search for an intraperitoneal bowel and mesentery injury.

Retroperitoneal fluid tends to localize at the site of injury. The presence of fluid in the retroperitoneum commonly indicates injury of duodenum, ascending colon, and descending colon (Fig. 17.18b).

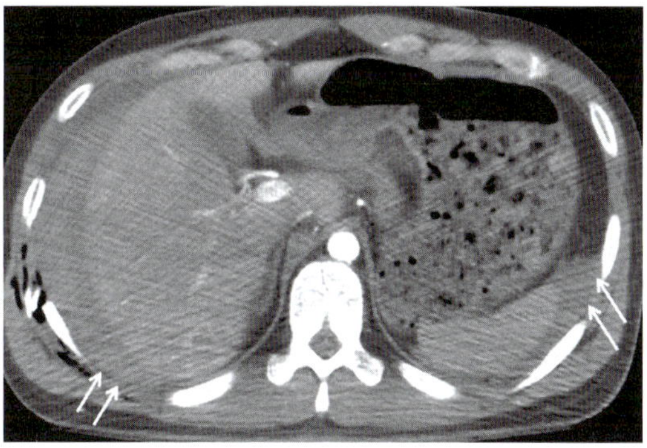

Fig. 17.16 Hemoperitoneum from solid organ injury. Axial contrast-enhanced CT scan shows hemoperitoneum in the perihepatic and perisplenic spaces (*arrows*). A rib fracture is also seen in the right hemithorax

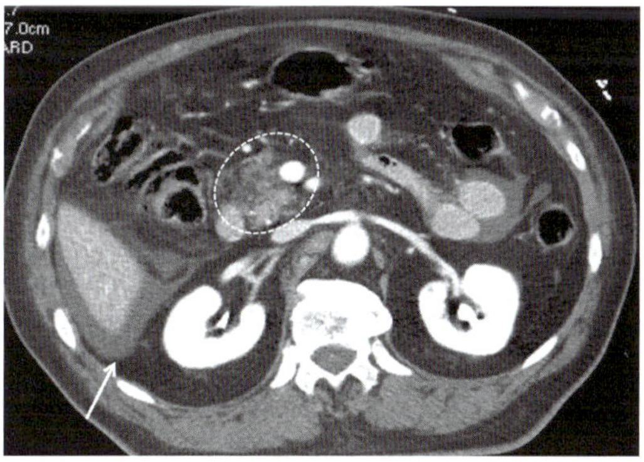

Fig. 17.17 Axial CT contrast-enhanced scan shows interloop fluid (*curved arrow*). Mesenteric stranding (*oval*) and perihepatic fluid (*arrow*) are also seen

17.10 Associated Findings in Patients with Blunt Abdominal and Mesenteric Injury

In one-third of the patients, bowel and mesenteric injuries coexist with solid organs lesions.

As a general rule, the risk of hollow-organ injury increases with an increasing number of injured abdominal solid organs. When three abdominal solid organs are injured, the risk for bowel injury is 34%. The presence of lesions to abdominal solid organs should suggest an accurate detection of the contiguous abdominal territory, searching for additional bowel and mesentery injuries [28].

17.10.1 Pancreatic and Duodenal Injuries

Pancreatic injuries are relatively uncommon, found in 2–12% of patients with blunt abdominal trauma. They most commonly result from the direct impact on the upper part of the abdomen of the steering wheel or the handlebars, with compression of the pancreatic neck and body against the vertebral column. The close duodenopancreatic anatomic relationship explains why pancreatic injuries are associated to duodenal injuries in approximately 20% of cases [39].

Distinguishing among duodenal contusion, duodenal hematoma, and duodenal perforation is

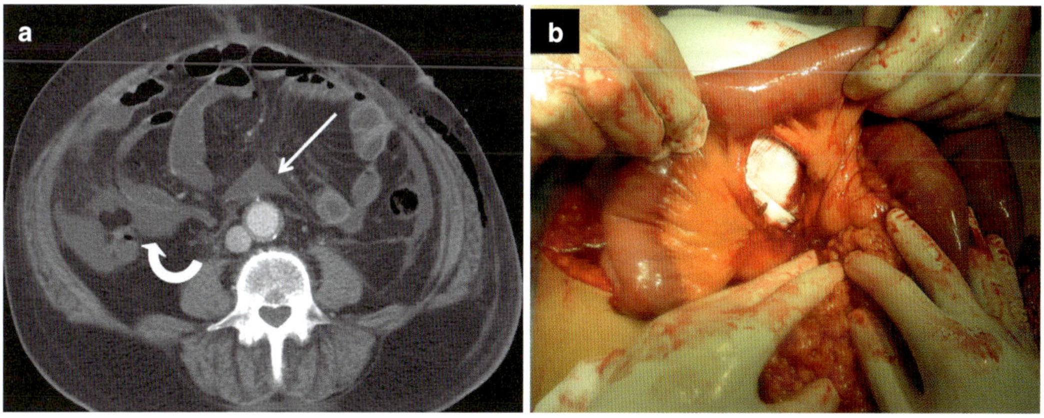

Fig. 17.18 Axial CT contrast-enhanced scan (**a**) shows triangular shaped fluid collection (*arrow*) and interloop fluid (*curved arrows*). Intraoperative image (**b**) shows a focal laceration of the mesentery. Intraoperative image courtesy of Dr. Ennio Adami, MD

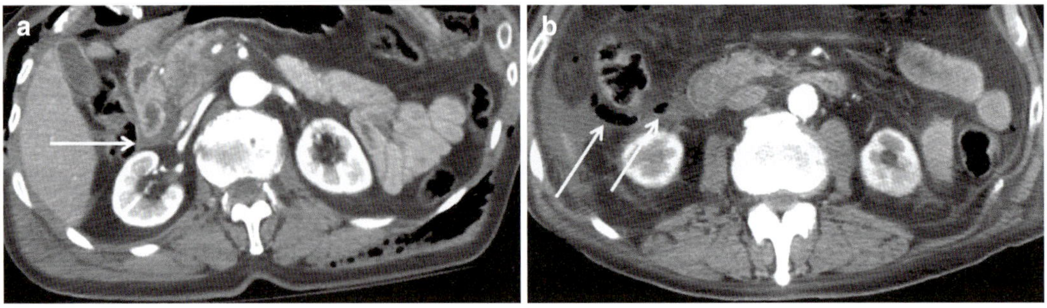

Fig. 17.19 (**a**) Axial CT contrast-enhanced scans show fluid in the right retroperitoneal space (*arrow*) in duodenal contusion. (**b**) The presence of free air in the right retroperitoneal space (*arrows*) suggests a retroperitoneal intestinal perforation

important, because management varies depending on the diagnosis. Whereas duodenal perforation is an acute surgical emergency, hematoma usually resolves in 1–3 weeks with no need of surgical intervention. At CT imaging, a thickening of the duodenal wall associated to retroperitoneal fluid in the right anterior pararenal space may be seen in both duodenal contusion and duodenal perforation. If discontinuity in the duodenal wall is not detected, the presence of extraluminal air in the anterior pararenal space is the most reliable finding for differentiating duodenal perforation from hematoma [40] (Fig. 17.19).

17.10.2 Fractures of the Spine

Often related with seat belt use, Chance fracture is a hyperflexion injury of the lumbar spine that involves distraction of the posterior elements. These unstable transverse fractures, characterized by disruption of the posterior and middle columns, are frequently associated with significant intra-abdominal injuries (40%). Bowel and mesentery, often in association, are the mostly injured abdominal organs in Chance fractures, particularly when the fracture has a burst-type component [41].

Conclusions

During the past decade, conservative management of hemodynamically stable blunt trauma patients, even in the presence of abdominal solid organ injuries, has become the standard of care. The concomitance of significant bowel or mesenteric injury, however, would make conservative treatment inappropriate and necessitate immediate operative treatment. Misdiagnosis of surgical bowel or mesenteric injury, in fact, often results in significant morbidity and mortality. Imaging assessment plays a crucial role for a timely diagnosis of bowel and mesenteric traumatic injuries, allowing a prompt and appropriate management of the injured patients. When specific findings of major bowel and mesenteric injuries are detected on CT, the patient should urgently undergo operative treatment. When only nonspecific findings of bowel and mesenteric injury are found on CT, correlation between radiologic and clinical findings is needed. If the patient is stable, serial clinical examination is needed and a CT scan follow-up at 8–12 h may be recommended [10].

The question of how to manage patients with blunt abdominal trauma who show small amounts of free fluid in the abdomen without evidence of solid organ injury is still a matter of debate [42]. Repeated physical examination and MDCT follow-up at 8–12 h is suggested. In such cases a minimally invasive surgical approach, as diagnostic laparoscopy, should be considered [43, 44].

References

1. Atri M, Hanson JM, Grinblat L, Brofman N, Chughtai T, Tomlinson G. Surgically important bowel and/or mesenteric injury in blunt trauma: accuracy of multidetector CT for evaluation. Radiology. 2008;249(2):524–33.
2. Killeen KL, Shanmuganathan K, Poletti PA, Cooper C, Mirvis SE. Helical computed tomography of bowel and mesenteric injuries. J Trauma. 2001;51(1):26–36.
3. Watts DD, Fakhry SM. Incidence of hollow viscus injury in blunt trauma: an analysis from 275,557 trauma admissions from the east multi-institutional trial. J Trauma. 2003;54(2):289–94.
4. Brofman N, Atri M, Hanson JM, Grinblat L, Chughtai T, Brenneman F. Evaluation of bowel and mesenteric blunt trauma with multidetector CT. Radiographics. 2006;26(4):1119–31.
5. Cox EF. Blunt abdominal trauma. A 5-year analysis of 870 patients requiring celiotomy. Ann Surg. 1984;199:467–74.
6. Scaglione M, de Lutio di Castelguidone E, Scialpi M, et al. Blunt trauma to the gastrointestinal tract and mesentery: is there a role for helical CT in the decision-making process? Eur J Radiol. 2004;50:67–73.
7. Rizzo MJ, Federle MP, Griffiths BG. Bowel and mesenteric injury following blunt abdominal trauma: evaluation with CT. Radiology. 1989;173:143–8.
8. Fakhry SM, Brownstein M, Watts DD, et al. Relatively short diagnostic delays (< 8 hours) produce morbidity and mortality in blunt small bowel injury: an analysis of time to operative intervention in 198 patients from a multicenter experience. J Trauma. 2000;48:408–14.
9. Malinoski DJ, Patel MS, Yakar DO, et al. A diagnostic delay of 5 hours increases the risk of death after blunt hollow viscus injury. J Trauma. 2010;69:84–7.
10. Cinquantini F, Tugnoli G, Piccinini A, et al. Educational review of predictive value and findings of computed tomography scan in diagnosing bowel and mesenteric injuries after blunt trauma: correlation with trauma surgery findings in 163 patients. Can Assoc Radiol J. 2017; doi:10.1016/j.carj.2016.07.003. S0846-5371(16)30091-2 [Epub ahead of print]
11. Iaselli F, Mazzei MA, Firetto C. Bowel and mesenteric injuries from blunt abdominal trauma: a review. Radiol Med. 2015;120:21–32.
12. Tan KK, Liu JZ, Go TS, et al. Computed tomography has an important role in hollow viscus and mesenteric injuries after blunt abdominal trauma. Injury. 2010;41(5):475–8.
13. Yegiyants S, Abou-Lahoud G, Taylor E. The management of blunt abdominal trauma patients with computed tomography scan findings of free peritoneal fluid and no evidence of solid organ injury. Am Surg. 2006;72(10):943–6.
14. Walker ML, Akpele I, Spence SD, et al. The role of repeat computed tomography scan in the evaluation of blunt bowel injury. Am Surg. 2012;78(9):979–85.
15. Christophi C, McDermott FT, McVey I, Hughes ES. Seat belt-induced trauma to the small bowel. World J Surg. 1985;9(5):794–7.
16. Bates DD, Wasserman M, Malek A, et al. Multidetector CT of surgically proven blunt bowel and mesenteric injury. Radiographics. 2017;37(2):613–25.
17. Hughes TMD, Elton C. The pathophysiology and management of bowel and mesenteric injuries due to blunt trauma. Injury. 2002;33:295–302.
18. Borgialli DA, Ellison AM, Ehrlich P, et al. Association between the seat belt sign and intra-abdominal injuries in children with blunt torso trauma in motor vehicle collisions. Acad Emerg Med. 2014;21(11):1240–8.
19. Hawkings AE, Mirvis SE. Evaluation of bowel and mesenteric injury: role of multidetector CT. Abdom Imaging. 2003;28:505–14.
20. Walker ML. Bowel injury. Minerva Chir. 2013;68(3): 233–40.
21. Howell HS, Bartizal JF, Freeark RJ. Blunt trauma involving the colon and rectum. J Trauma. 1976;16: 624–32.
22. Strate RG, Grieco JG. Blunt injury to the colon and rectum. J Trauma. 1983;23:384–8.
23. Castrillon GA, Soto JA. Intestinal and mesenteric trauma. Radiologia. 2011;1:51–9.
24. Anderson PA, Henley MB, Rivara FP, et al. Flexion distraction and chance injuries to the thoracolumbar spine. J Orthop Trauma. 1991;5(2):153–60.
25. Miele V, Di Giampietro I (2014) Diagnostic imaging in emergency. Salute e Società (2EN):127–138. doi: 10.3280/SES2014-002010EN
26. Landry BA, Patlas MN, Faidi S, et al. Are we missing traumatic bowel and mesenteric injuries? Can Assoc Radiol J. 2016;67(4):420–5.
27. Malhotra AK, Fabian TC, Katsis SB, et al. Blunt bowel and mesenteric injuries: the role screening computed tomography. J Trauma. 2000;48(6):991–8.
28. Romano S, Scaglione M, Tortora G. MDTC in blunt intestinal trauma. Eur J Radiol. 2006;59(3):359–66.
29. Allen TL, Mueller MT, Bonk RT. Computed tomographic scanning without oral contrast solution for blunt bowel and mesenteric injuries in abdominal trauma. J Trauma. 2004;56(2):314–22.
30. Stuhlfaut JW, Soto JA, Lucey BC. Blunt abdominal trauma: performance of CT without oral contrast material. Radiology. 2004;233(3):689–94.
31. Lee CH, Haaland B, Earnest A, Tan CH. Use of positive oral contrast agent in abdominopelvic computed tomography for blunt abdominal injury: meta-analysis and systematic review. Eur Radiol. 2013;23(9):2513–21.
32. Pinto A, Miele V, Schillirò ML, Nasuto M, Chianese V, Romano L, Guglielmi G. Spectrum of signs of pneumoperitoneum. Semin Ultrasound CT MR. 2016;37:3–9. doi:10.1053/j.sult.2015.10.008 Epub 2015 Oct 28.
33. Yu J, Fulcher AS, Turner MA, et al. Blunt bowel and mesenteric injury: MDTC diagnosis. Abdom Imaging. 2011;36:50–61.

34. Brody JM, Leighton DB, Murphy BL. CT of blunt trauma bowel and mesenteric injury: typical findings and pitfalls in diagnosis. Radiographics. 2000;20:1525–36.
35. Mirvis SE, Shanmuganathan K, Erb R. Diffuse small-bowel ischemia in hypotensive adults after blunt trauma (shock bowel): CT findings and clinical significance. AJR Am J Roentgenol. 1994;163:1375–9.
36. Levine CD, Gonzales RN, Wachsberg RH. CT findings in bowel and mesenteric injury. J Comput Assist Tomogr. 1997;21:974–9.
37. Faget C, Taourel P, Charbit J, et al. Value of CT to predict surgically important bowel and/or mesenteric injury in blunt trauma: performance of a preliminary scoring system. Eur Radiol. 2015;25(12):3620–8.
38. Shanmuganathan K, Mirvis SE, Sover ER. Value of contrast enhanced CT in detecting active hemorrhage in patients with blunt abdominal or pelvic trauma. AJR Am J Roentgenol. 1993;161(1):65–9.
39. Miller LA, Shanmuganathan K. Multidetector CT evaluation of abdominal trauma. Radiol Clin N Am. 2005;43:1079–95.
40. Linsenmaier U, Wirth S, Reiser M, et al. Diagnosis and classification of pancreatic and duodenal injuries in emergency radiology. Radiographics. 2008;28(6):1591–602.
41. Kukin J, Korobkin M, Ellis J, et al. Duodenal injuries caused by blunt abdominal trauma: value of CT in differentiating perforation from hematoma. AJR. 1992;160:1221–3.
42. Bernstein M, Mirvis SE, Shanmuganathan K. Chance-type fractures of the thoracolumbar spine: imaging analysis in 53 patients. AJR Am J Roentgenol. 2006;187(4):859–68.
43. Rodriguez C, Barone JE, Wilbanks TO, et al. Isolated free fluid on computed tomographic scan in blunt abdominal trauma: a systematic review of incidence and management. J Trauma. 2002;53:79–85.
44. Chersakov M, Sitnikov V, Sarkysian B. Laparoscopy versus laparotomy in management of abdominal trauma. Surg Endosc. 2008;22:228–31.

Adrenal Gland Injuries

18

Margherita Trinci, Federico Greco,
Mariagrazia Ramunno, Diletta Cozzi,
Valeria Saracco, Caterina Maria Trinci,
and Vittorio Miele

18.1 Anatomy

The suprarenal glands, also known as adrenal glands, are a pair of triangular-shaped glands (the right adrenal gland is pyramidal, whereas the left one is more semilunar), that belong to the endocrine system. The right adrenal tends to lie more cephalad than the left. Normal size of adrenal glands ranges from 2 to 6 mm in thickness and from 2 to 4 cm in length. The right adrenal is close to the liver superiorly, the inferior vena cava (IVC) medially, the right kidney laterally and inferiorly, and the diaphragm superiorly and posteriorly. The left adrenal is close to the aorta medially, the stomach, and body of the pancreas anteriorly, the kidney inferiorly, the spleen superiorly, and the diaphragm posteriorly. At age 1 year, each gland weighs approximately 1 g and the weight increases with age until it reaches 4–5 g. Their size in adult is about 2 cm in length and 1 cm in width. They are located on top of the kidneys in the Gerota's fascia deep within the retroperitoneum. The arterial blood supply comes from three sources, with branches arising from the inferior phrenic artery, the renal artery, and the aorta. Venous drainage flows directly into the inferior vena cava on the right side, and into the left renal vein and then into inferior vena cava on the left side. The right adrenal vein is shorter than the left: this anatomical condition makes the right adrenal gland more susceptible to a sudden increase in pressure in the event of compressive phenomena at the inferior cava vein and, for this reason, more susceptible to hemorrhagic lesions as compared to the contralateral. Lymphatics drain medially into the aortic nodes.

Each adrenal gland is formed by two distinct structures: the adrenal cortex and internally the adrenal medulla. The adrenal cortex is divided into three zones that are from outside to inside, the zona glomerulosa, the zona fasciculata, and the zona reticularis (Drawing 18.1).

The suprarenal glands are responsible for the release of hormones that regulate metabolism, immune system function, and the salt-water balance in the bloodstream; they also aid in the body's response to stress.

M. Trinci, M.D. (✉) • F. Greco • M.Ramunno
V. Saracco • C.M. Trinci
Department of Emergency Radiology, S. Camillo Hospital, C.ne Gianicolense, 87, 00152 Rome, Italy
e-mail: margherita.trinci@libero.it

D. Cozzi • V. Miele
Department of Radiology, Careggi University Hospital, Florence, Italy

V. Miele, M. Trinci (eds.), *Diagnostic Imaging in Polytrauma Patients*,
https://doi.org/10.1007/978-3-319-62054-1_18

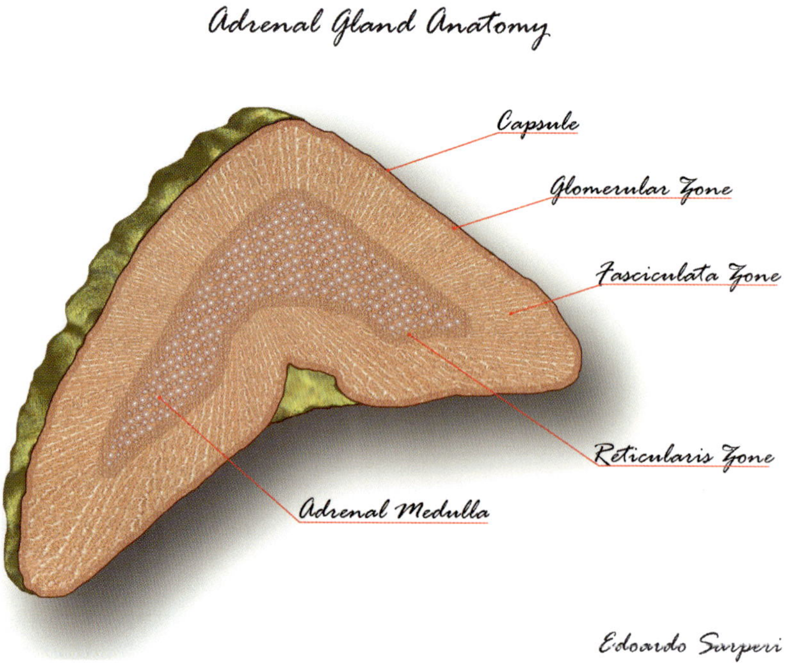

Drawing 18.1 Adrenal gland anatomy

18.1.1 Adrenal Cortex

The adrenal cortex secretes three types of hormones; all adrenocortical hormones are cholesterol-derived steroid compounds:

- Mineralocorticoids, which are secreted by the zona glomerulosa, including aldosterone.
- Glucocorticoids, which are secreted by the zona fasciculata and less from the zona reticularis, as cortisol.
- Adrenal androgen, which is predominantly secreted by the zona reticularis, with small quantities released from the zona fasciculata, as dehydroepiandrosterone (DHEA).

18.1.2 Adrenal Medulla

The adrenal medulla secretes epinephrine (80%) and norepinephrine (20%), with minimal amounts of dopamine. These hormones are responsible for all the physiologic characteristics of the stress response such as increased cardiac output and vascular resistance [1, 2].

18.2 Pathogenesis

The adrenal gland trauma (AGT) occurs rarely in traumatic patients: in several studies, the incidence varies from 0.03% to 4.95% of blunt or penetrating abdominal trauma cases [1–5]. This is because of its deep position within the retroperitoneum and also because it is protected by soft tissue that surrounds it [2–4, 7]. Adrenal gland lesions are more likely in patient with high ISS [4]; in fact, they occur in severe trauma as car, motorbike or pedestrian accident, falling from height, and sport accident. For retroperitoneal organs, the most frequent lesion mechanism is compression against a fixed structure. Male sex is more affected than the female [2, 4, 9, 10]. Non-isolated traumatic lesions of the adrenal gland are more frequent than the isolated lesions

(4%), precisely because they usually occur in severe trauma. In 75–90% of cases, hemorrhages are unilateral and the most affected gland is the right one [2, 3, 6–8, 11, 12].

Bilateral adrenal gland traumatic lesions are still rarer than the monolateral ones and can cause a severe adrenal failure: in literature, there are a few case reports and limited case series [8, 13].

Associated traumatic injuries can affect all organs, by frequency: liver (43%), spleen (23%), lung (19%), and kidney (18%). Pneumothoraces and hemothoraces can be present (80%), as well as, skeletal injuries (46%) to the rib, clavicle, scapulae, pelvis, hip, and spine [2, 4, 6–8, 14] (Figs. 18.1 and 18.2).

The mortality rates are influenced from the presence of one or more associated lesions.

As has just been said, the right adrenal gland is more involved than the left: this is probably due to anatomical reasons and to their complex vascular supply; in fact, adrenal glands (especially the right one) are susceptible to massive intraglandular bleeding.

Among the causes that make the right adrenal gland more involved in trauma compared to the contralateral, there are three principal theories: the direct compression of the gland between the spine and liver by a direct trauma which affects the upper abdomen, the shearing of small vessels that perforate the adrenal capsule due to the deceleration forces, and also a short-term rise in intraadrenal venous pressure due to compression of the inferior vena cava [3, 5–7, 14–17].

It must be remembered that the right adrenal vein is shorter than the left and communicates directly with the IVC: even for this reason the right adrenal gland is more susceptible to trauma than the contralateral one [2, 4, 5]. In case of right adrenal trauma, a thrombosis in IVC may occur, due to compressive effect from adrenal hematoma or hemorrhage (that causes venous stasis and thus promotes thrombosis).

Adrenal lesions are supposed to result from ischemic necrosis caused by an increase in pressure due to a post-traumatic hemorrhage, or for a direct destruction of the adrenal gland or to both mechanisms [2].

Furthermore, the adrenal arterial supply comes through a sinusoidal net of small arterioles, and the stretch mechanism may easily cut these vessels, resulting in vascular compromise.

Even in pediatric patient, blunt adrenal injuries are uncommon (in 1–4%) and often present as part of a multiorgan trauma in which the most frequently associated lesions are those of liver and ipsilateral kidney. It has multifactorial genesis: accident, sports, child abuse, and so on [14]. It must be remembered that the children have adrenal glands relatively large, for this reason they may be more susceptible to injury due to external compressive forces [18]. Instead in adult, adrenal gland injuries are frequently associated with high injury severity [12] and they are a strong indicator of a possible associated blunt visceral lesion [16, 19].

The injury occurs is more likely in males than in females. The right adrenal gland is most commonly involved [13, 18, 20, 21]. When the right adrenal gland is involved, we have to looking for a liver or right kidney lesions; instead, in case of left adrenal gland injury, we have to consider a possible pancreatic or splenic lesion: in both cases we have to search for a lesion of the lower chest. In case of isolated adrenal injuries, child abuse is a possibility to be considered [17, 22].

18.3 Clinical Findings

There are not specific clinical findings in case of adrenal gland trauma especially in case of monolateral involvement because bilateral lesions that would lead to acute adrenal failure are really rare and because usually adrenal lesion occurs in polytrauma patient and the symptoms are due to multiorgan involvement [7]. There may be nonspecific skin wounds, bruises, or abrasions in the thoracoabdominal region. Anyway, in case of unilateral traumatic adrenal hemorrhages, the symptoms are nonspecific and include abdominal pain, vomiting, nau-

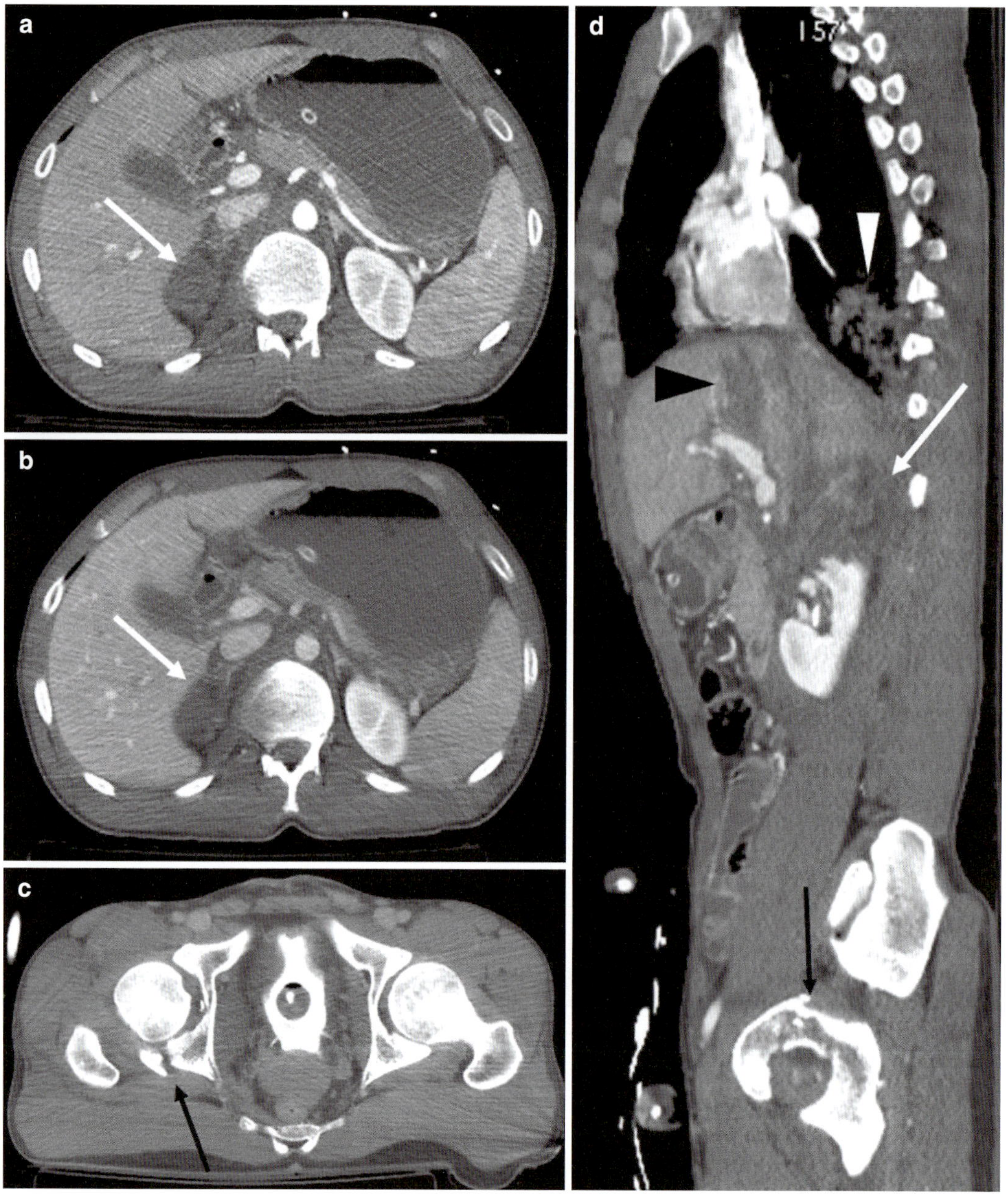

Fig. 18.1 Contrast-enhanced CT. (**a**, **b**, and **c**) Axial scans; (**d**) sagittal reconstruction. The patient has fallen from height. Adrenal hematoma with associated lesions: axial CT scans show hypodense enlarged adrenal gland (*white arrow* in **a** and **b**); note the presence of associated lesions of liver (*black arrowhead* in **d**), upper polar of left kidney (*white arrow* in **d**), hemoretroperitoneum, left acetabulum (*black arrow* in **c** and **d**), and lung contusion (*white arrowhead* in **d**)

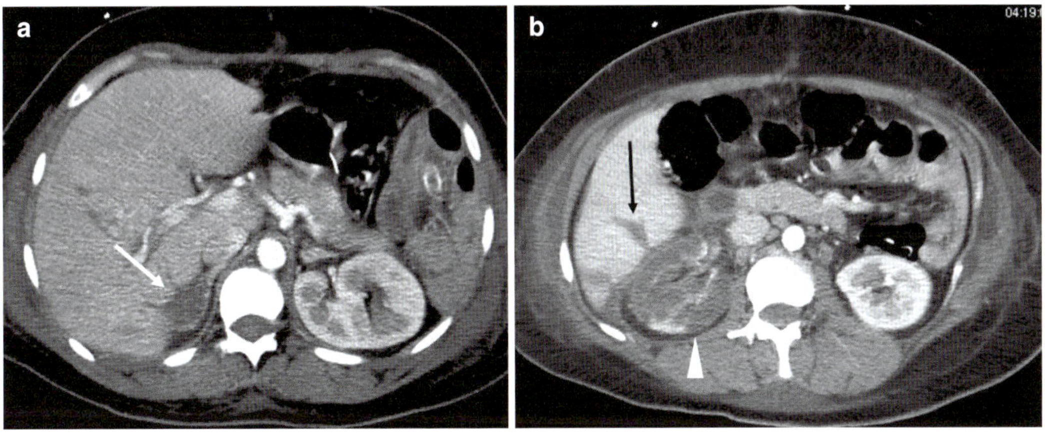

Fig. 18.2 (**a** and **b**) Right adrenal hematoma (*white arrow*), associated with lacerations of the right lobe of the liver (*black arrow*) and devascularization of the ipsilateral kidney (*white arrowhead*)

sea, hypo- or hypertension, and decrease in hematocrit [2, 23]. The lack of specific symptoms causes the diagnosis to be often misunderstood, but we have to consider that the presence of adrenal lesion can lead to retroperitoneal persistent hemorrhage and hematoma that can evolve in abscess [24]. In case of bilateral adrenal gland, hemorrhage can cause adrenal insufficiency with "endocrine-related syndromes" which consists in a sudden decrement production of adrenal steroids that cause a state of shock, typically accompanied by a laboratory triad of hypoglycemia, hyperkalemia, and hyponatremia; acidosis-hypotension and lethargy may be present too. If this condition is left untreated, it can be fatal [2, 6, 17, 23]. There are predisposing factors as thromboembolic disease, coagulopathy, pregnancy, and burns [2, 23]. The lack of specific clinical symptoms of an adrenal lesion causes identification to be carried out by diagnostic imaging.

18.4 Imaging

Whole Body Computed Tomography (WBCT) is the choice for the evaluation of the stable polytrauma patient [7, 25, 26] and for traumatic adrenal lesions too. The management of the high energy trauma patient is essentially based on his hemodynamic values and on CT findings [25]. Ultrasonography (US), Contrast-Enhanced Ultrasound (CEUS), and Magnetic Resonance Imaging (MRI) are methods which evaluate the adrenal gland but, in case of trauma, the CT is the method of choice. CEUS and MRI usually can be employed in stable patient, especially during follow-up and in children, according to the radioprotectional criteria [27–29]. Plain radiographs have no value in the detection of traumatic adrenal lesions [4].

18.5 X-Ray

The diagnosis in adrenal trauma fails with conventional radiology for its insufficient diagnostic capacity. The plain X-ray can show bone fractures as associated sign, but there is no correlation between a specific bone fracture and adrenal lesion. In case of previous trauma, X-ray can show the presence of calcifications located in the adrenal space due to a previous hemorrhage. This finding, however, gets into differential diagnosis with neuroblastoma or chronic granulomatous disease.

18.6 Ultrasonography

For its deep position in the abdominal cavity, the adrenal gland is quite difficult to evaluate with US in adult patient: this imaging technique has more chances in children and/or young or thin patient. It is noninvasive, safe and easy to perform, no needs of sedation, it is easily accessible, and relatively inexpensive. US can differentiate cystic from solid adrenal masses and it is useful to assess for vascular involvement but it is often inadequate in the evaluation of the retroperitoneal organs and for eventual complications (as retroperitoneal bleeding) especially in adult patient. Furthermore, it depends on the operator, on the patient's constitution and his collaboration [23]. In case of severe trauma, US is not the first choice. In case of localized minor trauma, especially in children, CEUS may be used as a valuable method of study [30–32]; furthermore, in case of lesion detection, it must be followed by a complete evaluation performing a contrast-enhanced CT [7]. US and CEUS have high sensibility in detecting even small amount of free fluid in peritoneal space but they are not so able in the evaluation of retroperitoneal free fluid.

US and CEUS can found a role in the follow-up of a lesion previously evaluated with CT or MRI. However, US has specific semeiotics aspects such as the adrenal hematoma and its evolutionary stages over the time [7, 17, 33, 34].

- Acute stage: an enlarged hyperechoic adrenal gland, the gland maintains its triangular shape and a cleavage with the upper kidney pole (Fig. 18.3) [4].
- Intermediate stage: the mass echogenicity is lower than the previous one, the gland reduces its size, and the mass can assume a complex aspect due to the presence of echoes mixed with anechoic zones (Fig. 18.4).
- Chronic stage: the mass is hypo-anechoic with cystic aspect; its size reduces over the time (Fig. 18.5) [4]. The gland can retake its previous morphology and echogenicity or remain with a pseudocystic aspect with a well-defined thin wall [4, 35, 36]; also adrenal atrophy can be seen at the end stage; it is possible to find thin calcifications seen as hyperechoic images in the gland.

Retroperitoneal or peritoneal fluid may be seen, as well as the other associated lesions of solid organs.

At Doppler examination there is no flow signal in the mass but it is possible to see a peripheral signal due to the capsule. The presence of

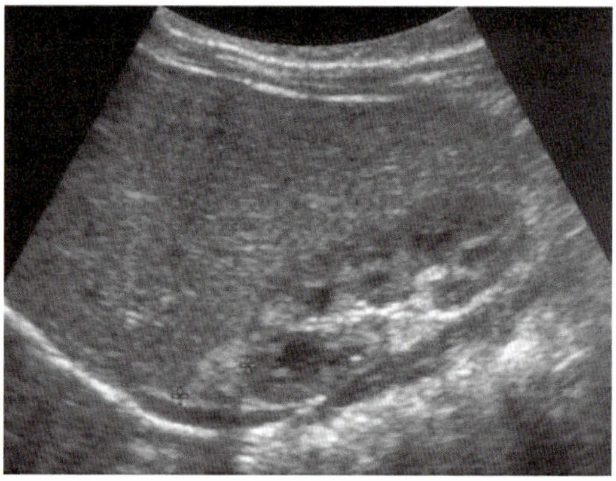

Fig. 18.3 Ultrasound exam shows an acute stage adrenal hematoma: the adrenal gland is hyperechoic (calipers), its maintains its triangular shape and the cleavage with the upper pole of the kidney

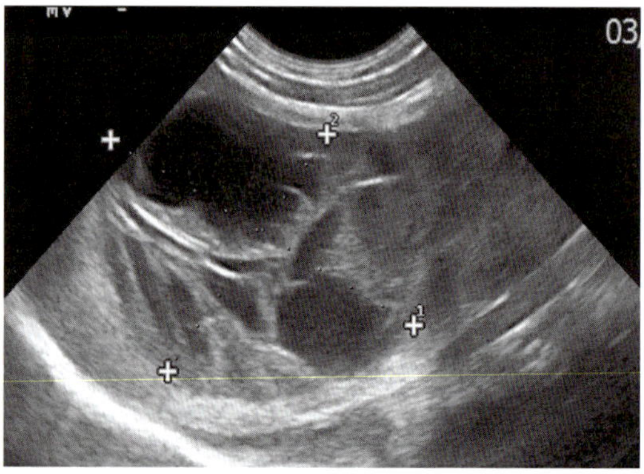

Fig. 18.4 Ultrasound shows an intermediate stage adrenal hematoma: the gland is enlarged (calipers) with complex aspect, due to the presence of echoic mixed with anechoic zones

flow signal within the mass is suspect for a nontraumatic lesion.

The use of contrast medium in US (Contrast Enhancement UltraSonography—CEUS) could easily confirm the absence of contrast enhancement in the adrenal hematoma, delimiting it more accurately than the healthy glandular parenchyma. CEUS may be useful to show the delimitation of the capsule or active bleeding but, about the use of CEUS in adrenal gland traumatic injuries, there are still no scientific data at this time [37–41]. Moreover, CEUS may also be useful in differential diagnosis with other nontraumatic adrenal masses found accidentally and in the follow-up of traumatic and nontraumatic adrenal lesion (Fig. 18.6).

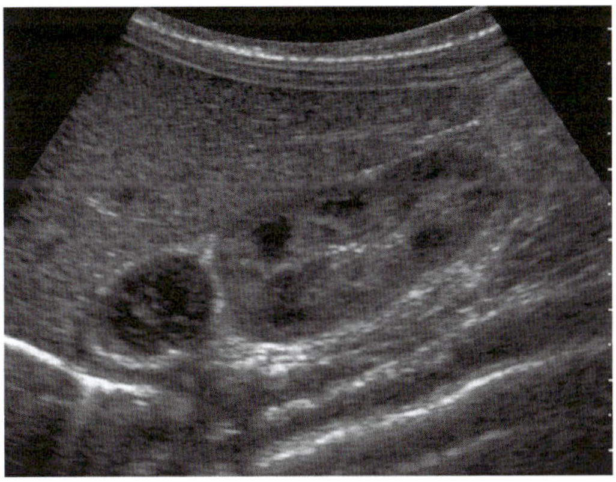

Fig. 18.5 Ultrasound shows a chronic stage adrenal hematoma: the gland is still a little enlarged, its echostructure is predominantly hypo-anechoic, with "pseudocystic aspect"

18.7 Computed Tomography (CT)

CT scan is the best method for evaluating the peritoneum and retroperitoneum especially in emergency conditions, because of its panoramicity, easy accessibility, and rapid scan time [2–5, 7, 23, 42]. In the last years there have been controversies regarding US versus CT in blunt abdominal trauma however, since it is known that US sensitivity is inferior to the CT in detecting all the lesions that can be found in the traumatized patient, US maintains a fundamental role in unstable patient for detecting hemoperitoneum while CT remains the gold standard in stable trauma patient [43, 44].

The most frequent traumatic adrenal gland lesion is hematoma: the gland is enlarged but there is not a disruption of the cortex, often there is periadrenal fat edema or limited hemorrhage [3, 9].

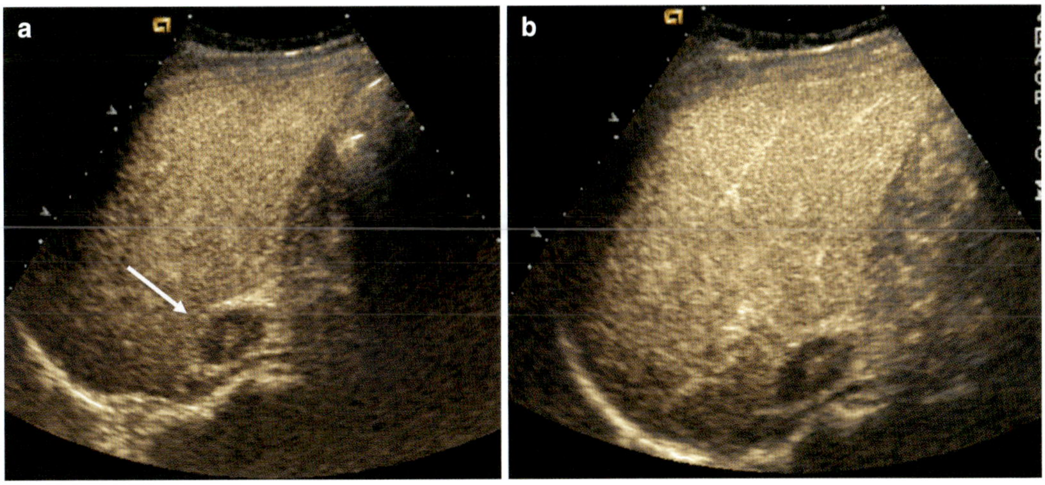

Fig. 18.6 CEUS in patient with blunt abdominal trauma. (**a**) CEUS shows a hypoechoic adrenal lesion (*arrow*), which is indistinguishable from a neoplasm. (**b**) Follow-up, 3 months later: the image is unchanged, demonstrating that it is a little adrenal mass

Some CT findings are diagnostic for adrenal hematoma, although others are not distinguished from adrenal neoplasms. It must be remembered that the prevalence of adrenal incidentalomas is 4% in the general population, percentage that increases with age; it is not always easy to differentiate a traumatic adrenal lesion, a traumatic lesion in a pathologic gland or a gland enlargement not related to the trauma [17]. Multidetector CT (MDCT) accurately defines size, location, and shape of adrenal lesions. In addition, it is useful for assessing local and vascular injury. For clear lesions as simple cysts, myelolipomas and often hemorrhage, CT allows a definitive diagnosis because the image is classic. For solid lesions, CT at baseline or in delayed phase may help in distinguishing benign from malignant lesions by their attenuation values: benign lesions tend to have low attenuation values because of an increased fat content [42].

The CT technique used for the evaluation of an adrenal trauma is the same that is used in polytrauma patient. The CT exam has to be performed from "head to toe" with a first acquisition in basal condition followed by two phases: the first in arterial phase and then a venous phase after 60–70 s the beginning of intravenous infusion contrast material or non-ionic iodinated contrast material [6] with the use of a power injector usually through the antecubital vein. The "split-bolus" technique may be useful in avoiding the double phase scan, allowing a reduction in radioexposure [45]. No oral contrast material should be given before scanning.

After the acquisition in the axial plane, post-processing imaging with multiplanar coronal and sagittal reconstruction has been performed [5].

Along with other abdominal organs, also for the adrenal glands the American Association for the Surgery of Trauma (AAST) has drafted a classification that is divided in grades related to the severity of the glandular lesions [9].

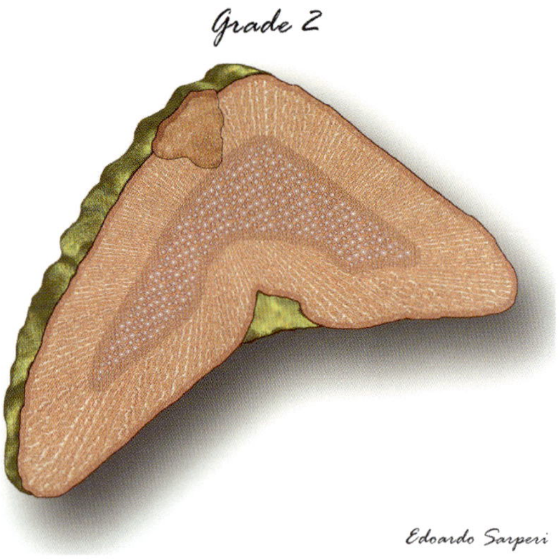

Drawing 18.2 Adrenal injury, grade 2

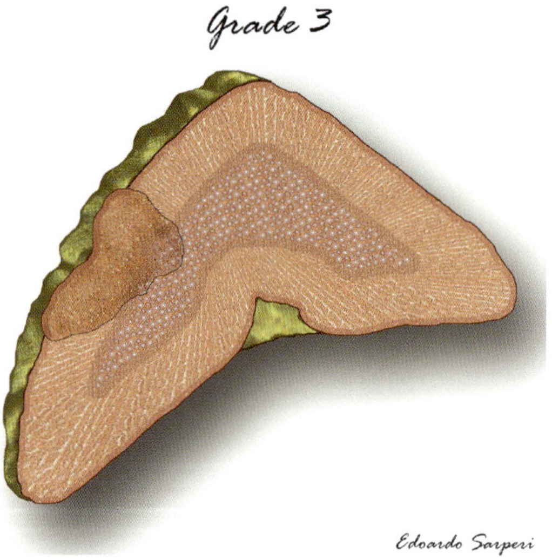

Drawing 18.3 Adrenal injury, grade 3

- Grade I: adrenal enlargement.
- Grade II: adrenal lesion confined to the cortex. (Drawing 18.2)
- Grade III: adrenal lesion extended into the medulla. (Drawing 18.3)
- Grade IV: adrenal lesion involving more than 50% of the gland. (Drawing 18.4)
- Grade V: adrenal lesion involving all the gland or vascular lesion including massive intraparenchymal hemorrhage or avulsion from blood supply. (Drawing 18.5) (Fig. 18.7).

At MDCT exam, it is possible to find specific or nonspecific signs [6, 44].

The specific signs of adrenal injury include [2, 3, 5, 6, 9, 13, 17, 46–49]:

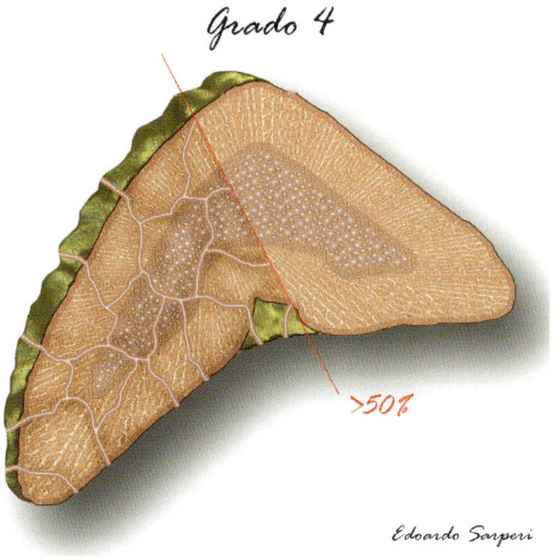

Drawing 18.4 Adrenal injury, grade 4

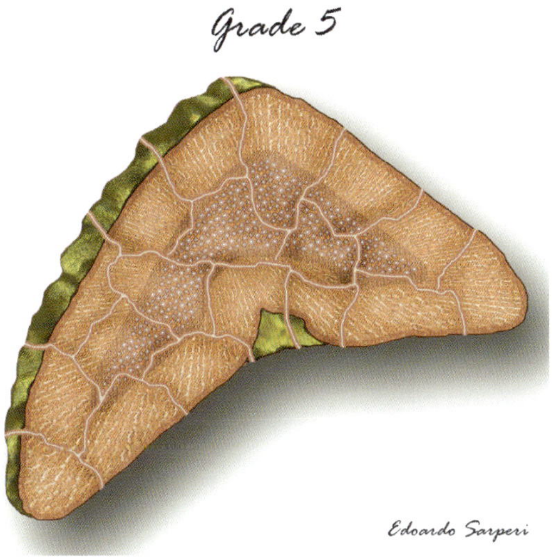

Drawing 18.5 Adrenal injury, grade 5

(a) Round or oval hematoma expanding in the adrenal gland. Oval shape is predominant compared to the round one [4, 7, 14]. At baseline CT, the gland will be enlarged and slightly hyperdense compared to the others abdominal parenchyma. The measured mean attenuation of these lesions are 56 HU ±1 [9, 16, 35]. Instead, in the dynamic phases the gland will be slightly hypodense compared to the others abdominal parenchyma such as liver and spleen [4, 35]: it is possible to see the capsule as a thin hyperdense peripheral rim (Fig. 18.8). The size of the hematoma may vary from 3 cm to more than 10 cm [35]. In case of active bleeding into the hematoma, an hyperdense spot is visible in the enhanced phase (Fig. 18.9).

(b) Irregular hemorrhage obliterating the gland.

(c) Uniform adrenal gland swelling (Fig. 18.10).

(d) Active extravasation of contrast material from the adrenal vessels or hematoma with active bleeding is rare but important pattern: infact, there is an indication for urgent embolization when diagnosed [2, 14, 23, 35] (Figs. 18.11 and 18.12).

(e) Adrenal gland rupture (Fig. 18.12).

Associated CT findings include [1, 3, 5–7, 9, 16, 46, 48, 49]:

(a) Stranding of the periadrenal fat is the most common associated finding in case of adrenal trauma: it is observed in approximately 90% of traumatic adrenal hemorrhage cases. It is due to the blood infiltration through the retroperitoneal fat that causes a nuanced

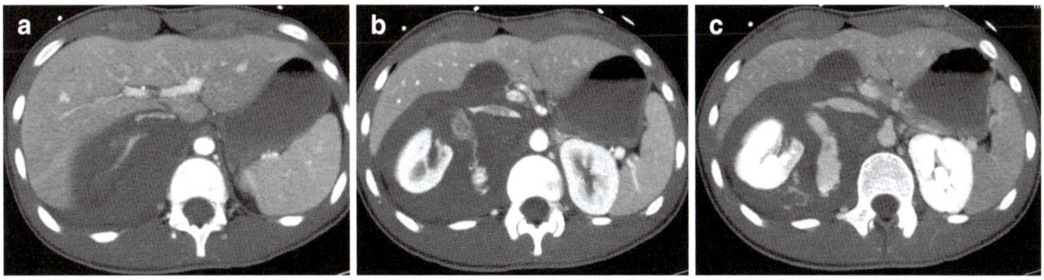

Fig. 18.7 Contrast-enhanced CT, axial scans. (**a** and **b**) Arterial phase; (**c**) venous phase. Widespread hemorrhage of the adrenal loggia, with tearing of the adrenal artery and active bleeding; (**c**) wide pooling in venous phase

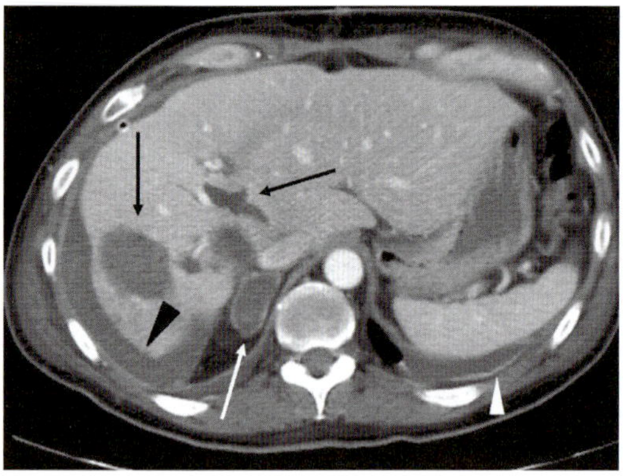

Fig. 18.8 Motorbike accident. Adrenal hematoma: enhanced CT shows hypodense enlarged adrenal gland, the adrenal capsule is expanse and enhanced (*white arrow*). Note the associated lesions in hepatic right parenchyma (*black arrows*), and the presence of perihepatic hemoperitoneum (*black arrowhead*) and a small amount of free right pleural free fluid (*white arrowhead*)

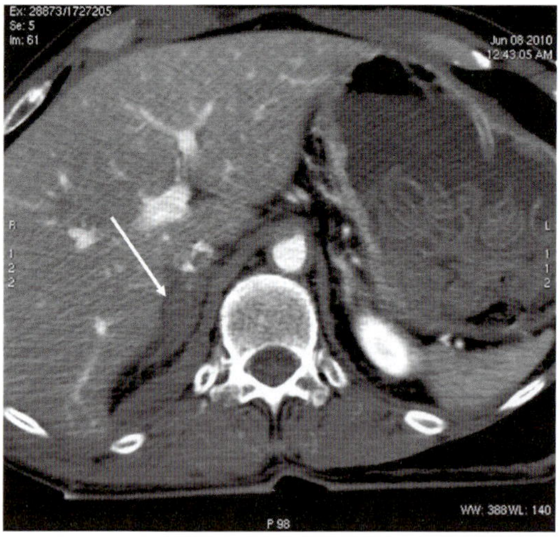

Fig. 18.10 Adrenal hematoma: enhanced CT shows hypodense swelling of the adrenal gland (*white arrow*); note the thickening of the crus of the diaphragm (*white arrowhead*)

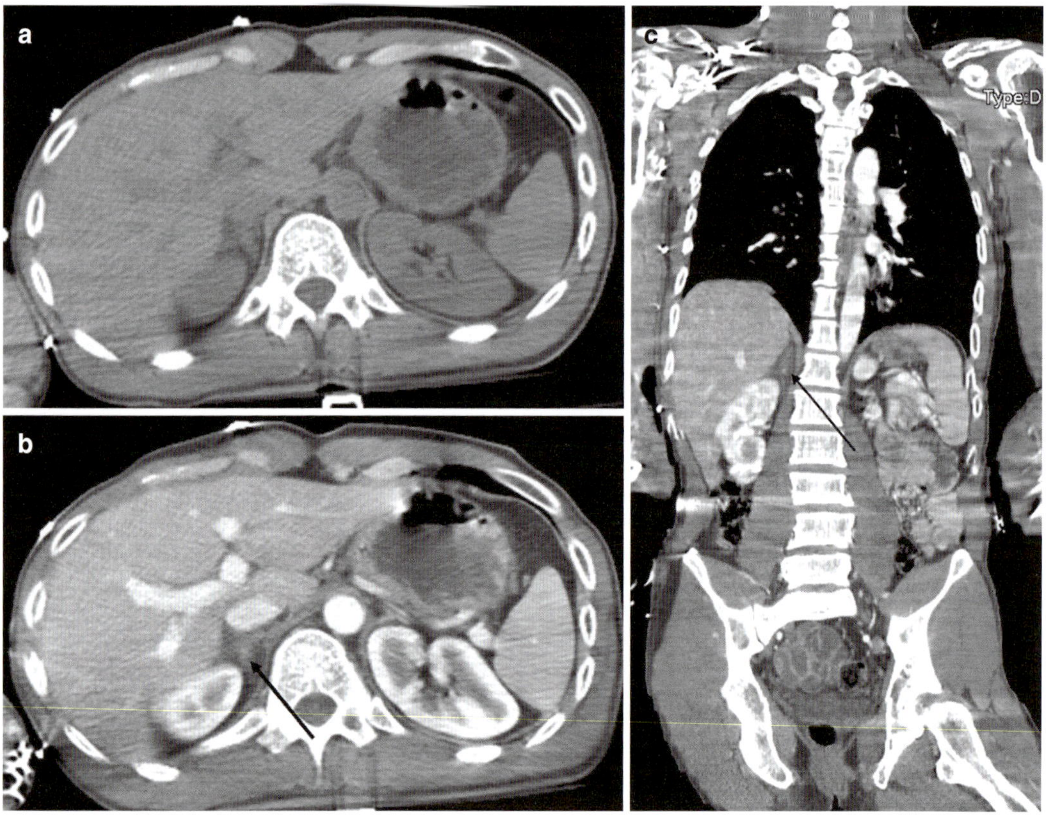

Fig. 18.9 Male, 33 years old, car accident. Unenhanced CT scan (**a**) shows right adrenal hematoma, as a enlarged gland with slight hypodensity; contrast-enhanced CT, in axial scan (**b**) and coronal reconstruction (**c**) show a small slight hyperdensity within the gland (*white arrows*), which represents a small focus of intraadrenal bleeding

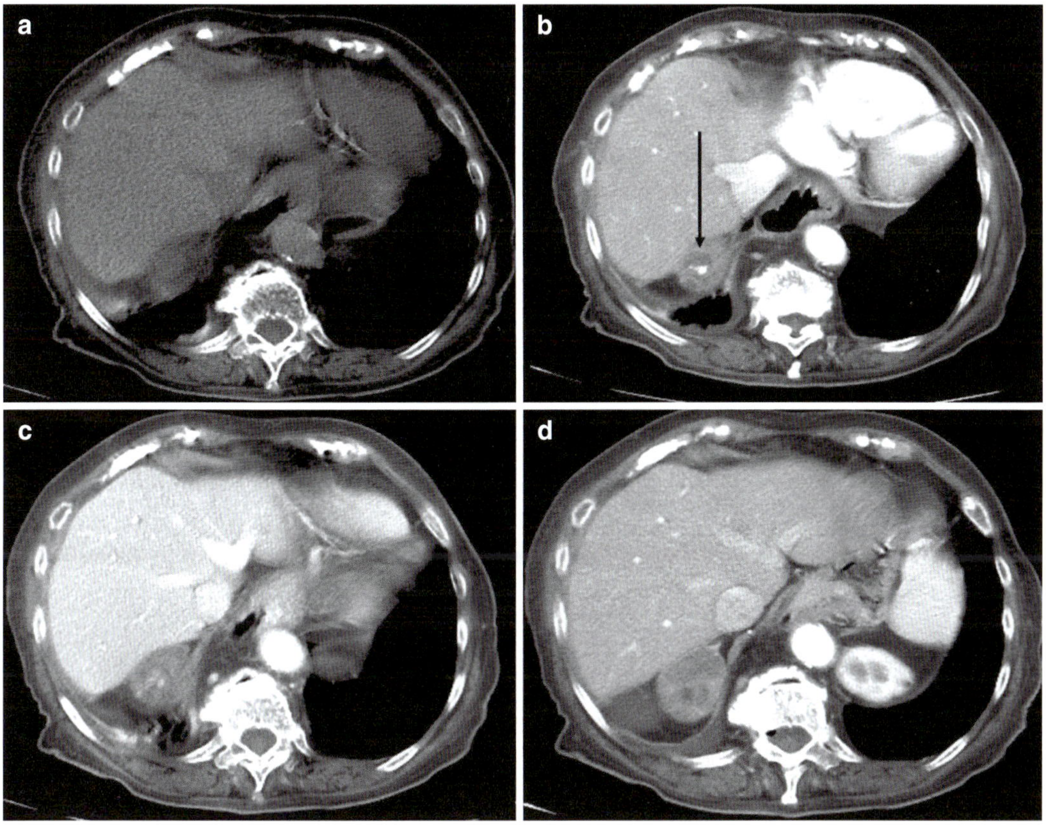

Fig. 18.11 Right adrenal hematoma: CT in (**a**) basal phase (**b** and **c**) arterial phase and (**d**) venous phase: contrast-enhanced CT shows intraglandular active bleeding, with the typical fluid corpuscular level (*arrow*), which happens in recent bleeding

attenuation of the periadrenal fat, contributing to indistinct appearance of the adrenal gland surrounded by it [1, 2, 7–9, 23] (Figs. 18.13 and 18.14).

(b) Diffuse hemorrhage in the adjacent retroperitoneum (20%) and compression of the adrenal gland by adjacent traumatic lesions [9] (see Figs. 18.6, 18.7, 18.8, 18.9, 18.10, 18.11, and 18.12).

(c) Diaphragmatic crural thickening of injured adrenal (10%) [2, 9, 14] (see Figs. 18.10, 18.13, and 18.14).

The differential diagnosis includes the adrenal incidentaloma which represents all those adrenal lesions that are discovered randomly during an investigation and has not yet given any clinical signs of its presence. Incidentaloma is found in 4% of the population, percentage increasing with age [50].

Other lesions must be considered: adenoma, carcinoma, myelolipoma, metastases, pheochromocytoma, and tuberculosis. We have to underline that especially in case of trauma, it is really difficult to discern between a tumor-related adrenal hemorrhage and a non-tumoral adrenal hemorrhage, especially in acute phase [51].

Even if the majority of incidentaloma are benign lesions (like nonfunctioning adrenocortical adenomas), some differential criteria must be known. An hemorrhagic heterogeneous adrenal mass that shows contrast enhancement should be evaluated more carefully considering all the differential diagnoses: adrenal adenoma has a typical attenuation of 60% absolute percent washout (or more than 40% relative washout) after 15-min delay [17, 50].

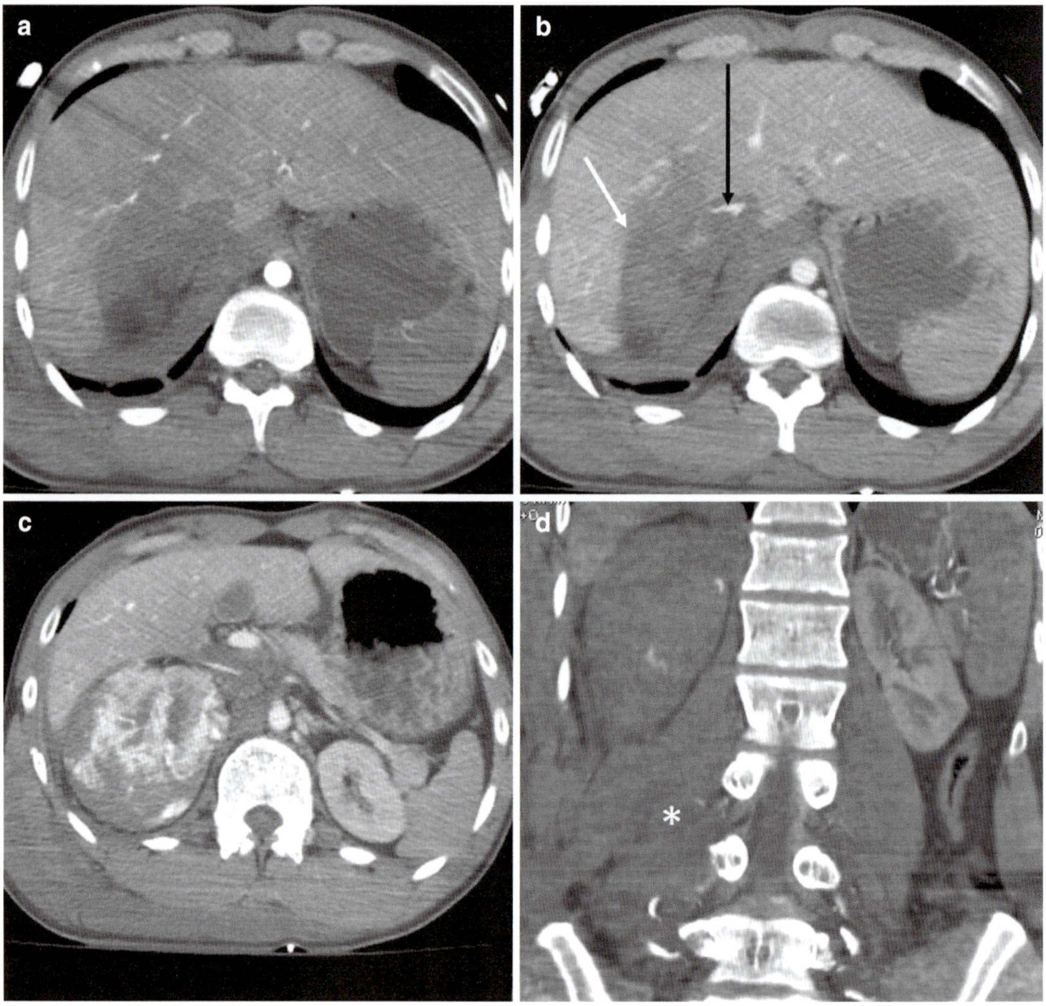

Fig. 18.12 Contrast-enhanced CT: axial scans (**a**–**c**) and coronal reformation (**d**) show adrenal fracture with free active bleeding (*black arrow*) obliterating the gland, associated with traumatic lesion of the liver (*white arrow*) and major kidney injury. Large amount of hemoretroperitoneum (*white asterisk*)

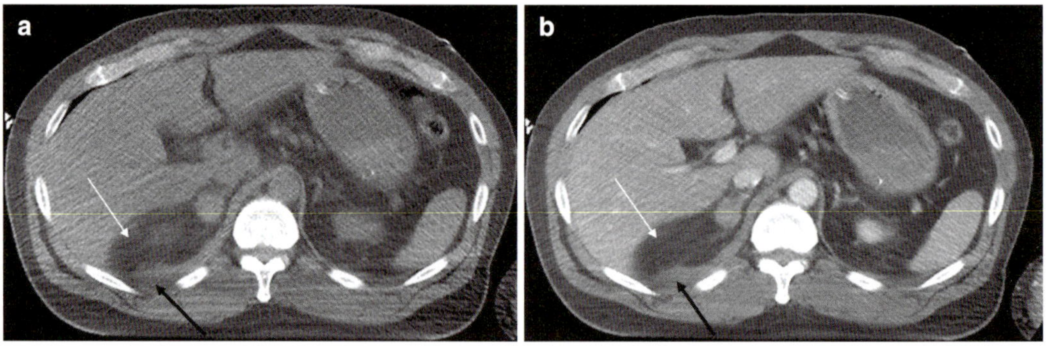

Fig. 18.13 Adrenal hematoma. CT axial images (**a**–**b**) show homogeneous swelling of right adrenal gland, which is slightly hypodense in basal phase (**a**). Periadrenal fat stranding is present (*white arrow*). Note the thickening of the crus of the diaphragm (*black arrow*)

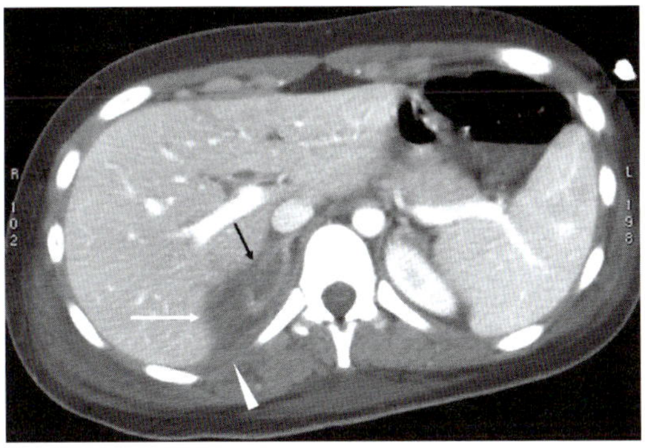

Fig. 18.14 Adrenal hematoma: contrast-enhanced CT, axial scan, shows hypodense enlarged adrenal gland. The adrenal capsule is expanse and enhanced (*black arrow*). Stranding of the periadrenal fat tissue (*white arrow*). Thickening of the crus of the diaphragm (*arrowhead*)

The presence of calcifications is suspected for a tumor-related hemorrhage as well as the hypermetabolic activity on positron emission tomography (PET).

Regarding the size, adrenal metastases or primary tumors may be larger than adrenal hematoma: in fact, it is reported that adrenal carcinoma is large from 4 cm to more than 6 cm in 2% cases. Malignant mass has an early enhancement and a delayed-contrast washout that enlarge over time; lymphadenopathy may be present.

18.8 Magnetic Resonance Imaging (MRI)

Although MRI is the most sensitive and specific modality for diagnosing adrenal hemorrhage, the best imaging technique in detecting adrenal lesions and, in case of incidentaloma, for differentiation between other adrenal masses, MRI is not used in traumatic unstable patient because CT is more feasible and it is a panoramic, quick, and basic technique in case of severe trauma.

In stable patient, MRI with multiplanar axial, coronal, and sagittal acquisition can be used as an alternative imaging method for evaluating the adrenal hemorrhages.

A MRI adrenal study protocol reported in the literature includes the following acquisitions: (1) coronal T2-weighted imaging with half-Fourier rapid acquisition with relaxation enhancement performed during a single breath-hold; (2) axial turbo or fast spin-echo T2-weighted or long-echo-time inversion-recovery sequence performed during a single breath-hold; (3) axial and coronal GRE T1-weighted chemical shift in-phase and out-of-phase imaging in axial-coronal planes during a single breath-hold; and (4) axial and coronal three-dimensional GRE sequence, performed before and after administration of a gadolinium-based contrast agent and with breath-hold [1].

On MRI, we can follow the hematoma changes according to the degradation products of hemoglobin, in accordance with the age of the hematoma [35].

1. Acute phase (less than 7 days): the signal of the hematoma depends on the presence of deoxyhemoglobin. We can see an isointense or hypointense signal with enlarged adrenal gland in T1-weighted images and hypointense signal intensity in T2-weighted images.
2. Subacute phase (7 days to 7 weeks): the signal depends on the presence of methemoglobin and the adrenal gland appears to be hyperintense on T1-weighted images. The T2 signal starts to change in this phase: intracellular methemoglobin will be hypointense on T2-weighted imaging. Then the lysis of the red cells dissipates the methemoglobin homogeneously throughout the hematoma and so we will have a bright signal on T2-weighted imaging.
3. Chronic phasc (lasting more than 7 weeks): the gland is reduced in size. The signal, due to the presence of hemosiderin deposits, will be hypointense on both T1 W and T2 W images.

The hematoma resolution is showed as an area with increase of signal intensity in the central part and a decrease in the peripheral one [4, 23].

At MRI in the chronic phase, the presence of blood products can cause heterogeneous

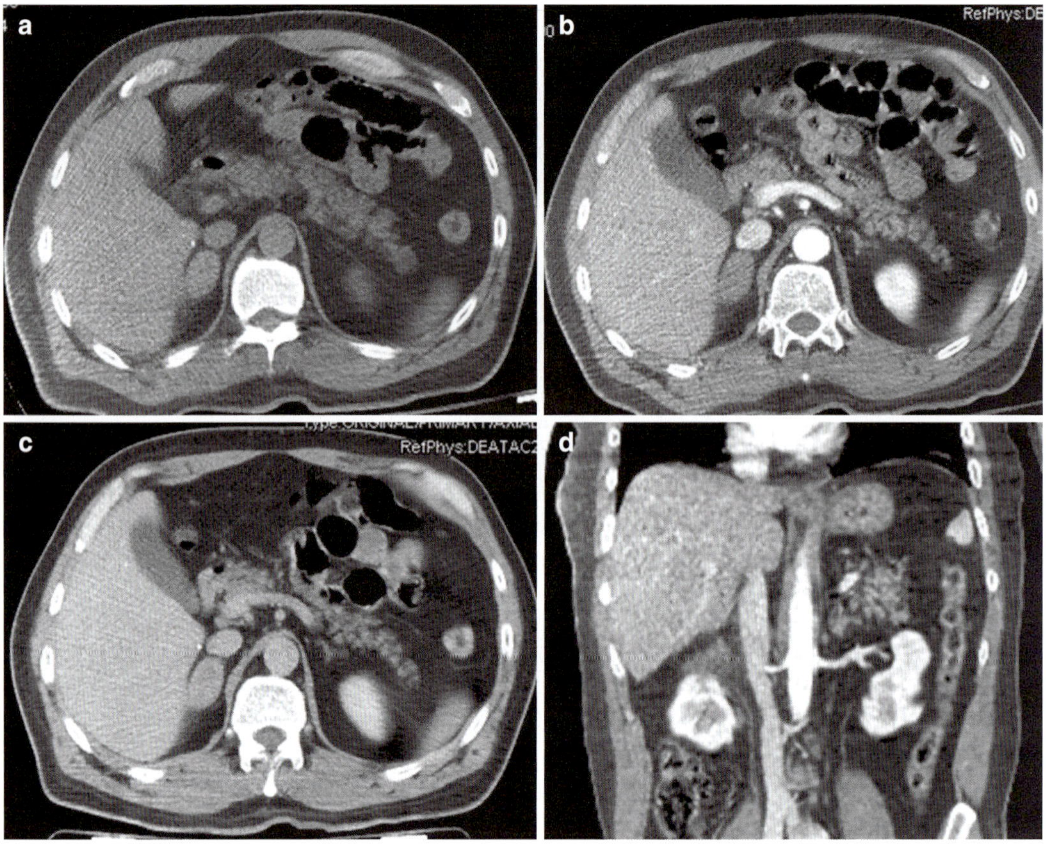

Fig. 18.15 Differential diagnosis in case of incidentaloma in trauma patient. (**a–d**) CT shows an enlarged adrenal gland slightly hyperdense in basal phase which does not enhance in contrast phase

intracystic signal intensity. The peripheral calcifications are not so well appreciated compared to CT, but they are represented as peripheral loss of signal intensity [35].

In case of adrenal hematoma: in-phase/out-of-phase and fat-suppressed sequences do not show suppression in the mass.

Such as CT, MRI is a highly overview method: it can define the total extension of an adrenal lesion, including its relationship to adjacent organs and major vessels, the presence of injuries to others organs. MRI can have a role during the follow-up in the stable patient. MRI with the use of gadolinium or with chemical-shift imaging is superior to CT in distinguishing benign from malignant incidentalomas [23, 42, 52, 53].

It must be remembered that adrenal adenoma is the most common adrenal lesion, found in 3% of cases at autopsy. The presence of intracellular lipid is typical of adrenal adenoma: this presence is well detected with MRI chemical-shift imaging and for this reason the use of in-phase/out-of-phase images is the most reliable technique for diagnosing adrenal adenoma. On out-of-phase images, a decrease in signal intensity more than 20% is considered diagnostic of an adenoma; also an early and uniform enhancement is typical of adenomas. MR imaging findings cannot differentiate from functioning and nonfunctioning adenomas. Rarely, adrenal adenomas may contain hemorrhage foci [1] (Figs. 18.15 and 18.16).

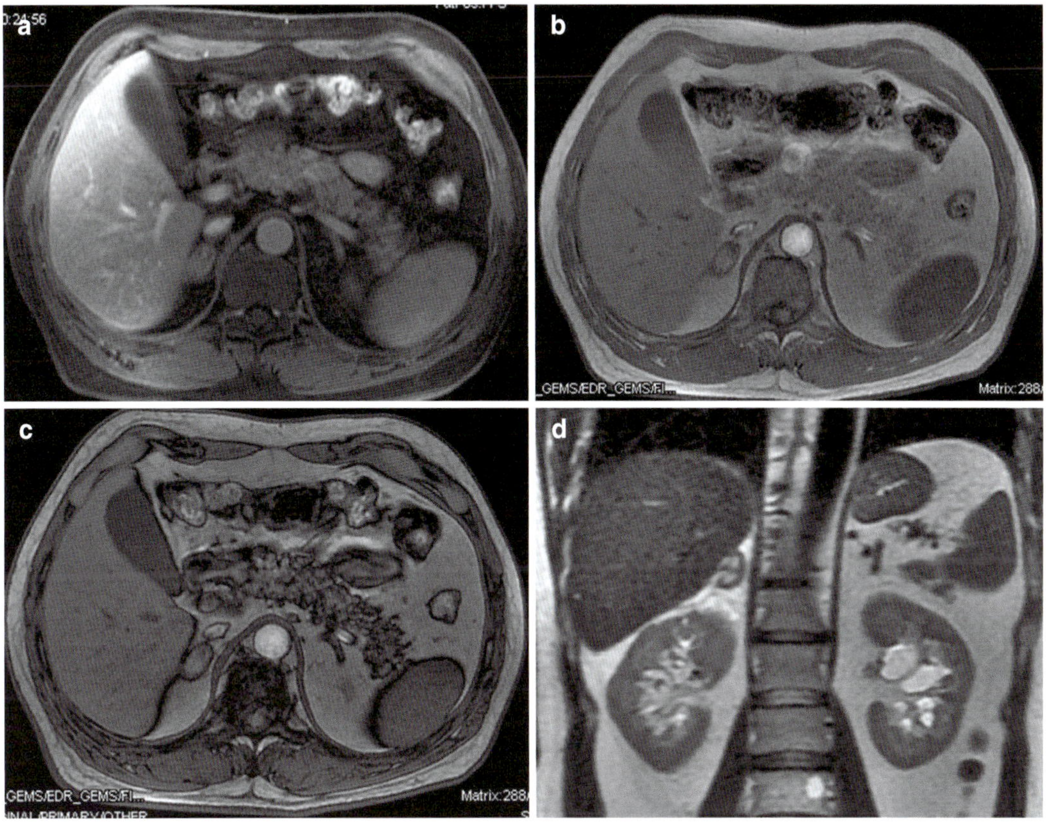

Fig. 18.16 Same patient of Fig. 18.15, 1 month later. MR, axial T1 planes (**a** and **b**), T2 axial (**c**), and coronal (**d**). The gland is always enlarged. Axial and coronal MR scans show the typical fatty signal in the gland, indicating a benign lesion like adenoma

18.9 Management and Prognosis

The management of patient with adrenal gland injury may be operative or nonoperative according to the patients' hemodynamic status, the severity of the adrenal injury, and the presence and severity of the other lesions [4, 47, 49, 54, 55].

Often surgery or interventional embolization is not needed for adrenal hematoma, but it is required because of the associated injuries to other organs [7, 19]. In case of adrenal trauma, often hemorrhage may occur: this is also due to the rich vascularization of the gland. If active bleeding is detected at CT and intractable hypotension occurs, an adrenal embolization or surgery is recommended [24]. Because of the low frequency with the adrenal trauma is found, there is still no unanimous agreement on the procedures to be implemented for its treatment [24]. The literature reports both operative exploration and conservative management. There are also reported some cases of adrenal traumatic hemorrhages management through transcatheter angiographic embolization, both in adult and in pediatric patients [7, 21, 55, 56]. If the patient is under severe general conditions, transcatheter embolization is often chosen to resolve a source of bleeding that could further aggravate the already critical patient condition. Adrenalectomy is rarely performed. However, most of the adrenal traumatic injuries are managed conservatively [2, 3, 15, 21, 24, 56].

Like in the adult population, also in the pediatric patient the management of adrenal injuries generally depends on the concomitant injuries. In pediatric patient, adrenal traumas are typically self-limited and do not need intensive care monitoring or operative intervention: this is due to the typical vasoconstrictive response of the pediatric patient. In the same case, significant adrenal hemorrhage can happen and transfusion or transcatheter embolization is needed [15, 20, 21, 55].

Because of the uncommon nature of isolated adrenal injury, if it occurs in a polytrauma patient, we have to consider and exclude other conditions in the differential diagnosis including adenoma, carcinoma, myelolipoma, metastasis, and pheochromocytoma [8, 43]. Preexisting adrenal disorders can predispose the adrenal gland to injury and hemorrhage even with minor trauma [43]. If comparing the exam with prior images is not possible, it is essential to know the characteristics of any adrenal lesions: it may be useful to subject the patient to an MRI examination and follow-up.

Most of the unilateral adrenal traumatic injuries are managed conservatively [23]. Instead, in case of bilateral adrenal hemorrhage the patient must be treated with corticosteroids, mineralocorticoid and glucocorticoid pharmacological coverage. The administration of fludrocortisone is recommended for mineralocorticoid supplementation. It is important to recognize the clinical signs of adrenal failure and make an early CT-diagnosis because a delayed replacement or misdiagnosis can be fatal for patients. According to the literature, 16–50% of patients with bilateral adrenal hemorrhage have been reported to have life-threatening adrenal insufficiency [49]. Some studies report about monolateral adrenal trauma mortality of 33%, often due to the general clinical patient condition. The day of mortality ranges from 1 to 18 days (median = 6.2), whereas the day of discharge from hospital ranges from 3 to 19 days (median = 7.7) [7].

We know that the trauma of the adrenal gland is associated with a high ISS. In cases of bilateral adrenal injury, the ISS-related morbidity and mortality are higher compared to unilateral adrenal injury. Both in case of unilateral or bilateral trauma, adrenal insufficiency has been hypothesized to play a role in determining worsening prognosis [13, 54, 57–61]. Bilateral adrenal hemorrhage with sepsis has a mortality rate of more than 90% [1, 8, 23].

18.10 Follow-Up

CT signs indicative for hematoma are the presence of a high density at baseline CT scans, the decrease in size or resolution of the lesion over time [23, 42, 48].

There isn't a standard protocol for the follow-up of adrenal lesion in traumatic patients: often it starts early when the patient is still in hospital and it is variable according to the general patient's condition. With routinary use of abdominal CT in the evaluation of trauma patients, adrenal lesions, not only due to the trauma, are increasingly likely to be found. Follow-up of these lesions is variable [6]. When a definitive diagnosis is not possible on the initial CT scan, follow-up imaging in 6–12 weeks is reasonable [13]. If the hematoma does not resolve or decrease in size over several weeks, another disorder should be considered. It must be considered that the distinction between tumoral from non-tumoral hemorrhage is really hard in acute phase, especially when a neoplastic mass is not well appreciable. We have to be careful because it was reported that 7–44% of adrenal pseudocyst (interpreted as due to chronic non-tumoral hemorrhage) was found to be neoplastic at surgery. Imaging findings suspect for underlying tumor as the cause of adrenal hemorrhage are: intralesional calcification (better seen at baseline CT), intralesional enhancement, and hypermetabolic activity at PET, even if it has been reported that most unilocular rim-calcified lesions are benign and can be managed conservatively, with careful follow-up or even resection [35, 36]. According to the radioprotectional criteria, if it is possible, MRI may be the first method of choice for follow-up also because MRI manages to correctly evaluate the hemoglobin degradation and visualizes the evolution of hematoma; in children, US or CEUS may be have a role too.

In some situations, nuclear medicine with radioisotope scanning can be helpful for the differential diagnoses: for example, for detecting primary adrenocortical adenomas, carcinomas, or metastases is used Iodocholesterol.

Dexamethasone suppresses normal ACTH-responsive adrenal tissue. To detect adrenal medullary tumors as pheochromocytomas and neuroblastomas, metaiodobenzylguanidine (MIBG) scans may be used [16].

The role of positron emission tomography (PET) has yet to be fully defined: it has been used in the evaluation of neuroblastoma and recurrent/metastatic adrenal tumors.

For a complete hematoma resolution, it takes about 9 months [7].

If the hematoma is not completely reabsorbed over time, the CT aspects of chronic adrenal hemorrhage may be a non-enhancing, low attenuation adrenal pseudocyst with a well-defined thin wall [14, 35].

Also adrenal atrophy can be seen at the later stage of hemorrhage: it appears on CT images as a shrunken, isodense adreniform structure.

In same cases, it can remain a calcification of the gland: this aspect is easily seen at plain X-ray exam usually as a linear shaped calcification projecting above the renal shadow.

18.11 Take Home Points

1. Adrenal hematoma replacing the whole gland is the most common lesion in case of trauma, followed by a large gland with an internal hematoma.
2. The shape most frequent is oval.
3. Baseline CT scans: a hyperdense solid adrenal mass (50–90 HU) that does not enhance after contrast medium injection associated with periadrenal fat stranding, both of which are diagnostic of adrenal hematoma with fat infiltrating hemorrhage.
4. If the hematoma does not resolve or decrease in size over several weeks, another disorder should be considered.
5. An isointense-hypointense signal in T1-weighted images and hypointense signal in T2-weighted images, that retain an adreniform shape, primarily indicate an acute hemorrhage in a patient with a history of trauma.
6. Bilateral hemorrhage can cause life-threatening adrenal insufficiency.
7. Chronic hemorrhage may appear at imaging as a thin-walled adrenal pseudocyst or adrenal atrophy.
8. The best method for differential diagnosis of high-density adrenal lesions detected on CT in trauma patients is MRI.
9. Imaging findings that are suggestive for a hiding tumor as cause of adrenal hemorrhage are: intralesional foci of calcification, enhancement of the mass, and hypermetabolic activity on PET images.
10. MRI may have a role in the follow-up of stable patient.
11. Especially in pediatric patient, US or CEUS may be considered in the follow-up.

References

1. Elsayes KM, Mukundan G, Narra VR, et al. Adrenal masses: MR imaging features with pathologic correlation. Radiographics. 2004;24(Suppl 1):S73–86.
2. Sinelnikov AO, Abujudeh HH, Chan D, et al. CT manifestations of adrenal trauma: experience with 73 cases. Emerg Radiol. 2007;13:313–8.
3. To'o KJ, Duddalwar VA. Imaging of traumatic adrenal injury. Emerg Radiol. 2012;19:499–503. doi:10.1007/s10140-012-1063-y.
4. Stawicki SP, Hoey BA, Grossman MD. Adrenal gland trauma is associated with high injury severity and mortality. Curr Surg. 2003;60:431–6.
5. Burks DW, Mirvis SE, Shanmuganathan K. Acute adrenal injury after blunt abdominal trauma: CT findings. AJR Am J Roentgenol. 1992;158:503–7.
6. Pinto A, Scaglione M, Guidi G, et al. Role of multidetector row computed tomography in the assessment of adrenal gland injuries. Eur J Radiol. 2006;59:355–8.
7. Kahraman AS, Kahraman B, Ozdemir ZM et al (2016) Traumatic adrenal hematoma: clinical and imaging findings. ECR 2016. Type: Scientific Exhibit, Poster No: C-0193. doi:10.1594/ecr2016/C-0193.
8. Lee MJ, Kim AG, Jang JE, et al. A case of traumatic bilateral adrenal hemorrhage mimicking bilateral adrenal adenomas. Yeungnam Univ J Med. 2012;29:35–7. doi:10.1270/yujm.2012.29.1.35.
9. Mahajan A, Rao V, Thakur M et al (2010) Adrenal injury after blunt abdominal trauma: correlation between CT findings and injury severity score ECR 2010, Poster No.: C-1176. Doi:10.1594/ecr2010/C-1176.

10. Cardia G, Loverre G, Pomarico N, et al. Traumatic retroperitoneal lesions. Ann Ital Chir. 2000;71:457–67.
11. Gabalshehab L, Alagiri M. Traumatic adrenal injuries. J Urol. 2005;173:1330–1.
12. Mehrazin R, Derweesh IH, Kincade MC, et al. Adrenal trauma: Elvis Presley Memorial Trauma Center experience. Urology. 2007;70:851–5.
13. Panda A, Kumar A, Gamanagatti S, et al. Are traumatic bilateral adrenal injuries associated with higher morbidity and mortality? A prospective observational study. J Trauma Manag Outcomes. 2015;9:6. doi:10.1186/s13032-015-0026-1.
14. Sivit CJ, Ingram JD, Taylor GA, et al. Posttraumatic adrenal hemorrhage in children: CT findings in 34 patients. AJR Am J Roentgenol. 1992;58:1299–302.
15. Gomez RG, McAninch JW, Carrol PR. Adrenal gland trauma: diagnosis and management. J Trauma. 1993;35:870–4.
16. Roupakias S, Papoutsakis M, Tsikopoulos G. Adrenal injuries following blunt abdominal trauma in children: report of two cases. Ulus Travma Acil Cerrahi Derg. 2012;18:171–4.
17. Woodruff S, Yeung M, Grodski S, et al. Adrenal injuries and incidentalomas in trauma patients at an urban trauma centre. J Curr Surg. 2012;2:123–9.
18. deRoux SJ, Prendergast NC. Adrenal lacerations in child abuse: a marker of severe trauma. Pediatr Surg Int. 2000;16:121–3.
19. Iuchtman M, Breitgand A. Traumatic adrenal hemorrhage in children: an indicator of visceral injury. Pediatr Surg Int. 2000;16:586–8.
20. Shehab LG, Alagiri M. Traumatic adrenal injuries. J Urol. 2005;173:1330–1.
21. Kim DG, Jung HS, et al. Endovascular treatment of a post-traumatic adrenal hemorrhage in a pediatric patient: a case report. J Korean Soc Radiol. 2016;75:508–11.
22. Nimkin K, Teeger S, Wallach MT, et al. Adrenal hemorrhage in abused children: imaging and postmortem findings. AJR Am J Roentgenol. 1994;162:661–3.
23. Sayit AT, Sayit E, Gunbey HP, et al. Imaging of unilateral adrenal hemorrhages in patients after blunt abdominal trauma: report of two cases. Chin J Traumatol. 2017;20:52–5. doi:10.1016/j.cjtee.2016.05.002.
24. Liao CH, Lin J, Fu CY, et al. Adrenal gland trauma: is extravasation an absolute indication for intervention? World J Surg. 2015;39:1312–9. doi:10.1007/s00268-015-2953-4.
25. Scaglione M. Emergency radiology: state of the art. Radiol Med. 2015;120:1–2. doi:10.1007/s11547-014-0481-1.
26. Sivit CJ, Taylor GA, Bulas DI, et al. Blunt trauma in children: significance of peritoneal fluid. Radiology. 1991;178:185–8.
27. Miele V, Piccolo CL, Sessa B, et al. Comparison between MRI and CEUS in the follow-up of patients with blunt abdominal trauma managed conservatively. Radiol Med. 2016;121:27–37. doi:10.1007/s11547-015-0578-1.
28. Sessa B, Trinci M, Ianniello S, et al. Blunt abdominal trauma: role of contrast-enhanced ultrasound in the detection and staging of abdominal traumatic lesions compared with US and CE-MDCT. Radiol Med. 2015;120:180–9. doi:10.1007/s11547-014-0425-9.
29. Pinto F, Valentino M, Romanini L, et al. The role of CEUS in the assessment of haemodinamically stable patients with blunt abdominal trauma. Radiol Med. 2015;120:3–11. doi:10.1007/s11547-014-0455-3.
30. Miele V, Di Giampietro I, Ianniello S, et al. Diagnostic imaging in pediatric polytrauma management. Radiol Med. 2015;120:33–49. doi:10.1007/s11547-014-0469-x.
31. Menichini G, Sessa B, Trinci M, et al. Accuracy of contrast-enhanced ultrasound (CEUS) in the identification and characterization of traumatic solid organ lesions in children: a retrospective comparison with baseline-US and CE-MDCT. Radiol Med. 2015;120:989–1001. doi:10.1007/s11547-015-0535-z.
32. Miele V, Piccolo CL, Trinci M, et al. Diagnostic imaging of blunt abdominal trauma in pediatric patients. Radiol Med. 2016;121:409–30. doi:10.1007/s11547-016-0637-2.
33. Di Giacomo V, Trinci M, Van der Byl G, et al. Ultrasound in newborns and children suffering from nontraumatic acute abdominal pain: imaging with clinical and surgical correlation. J Ultrasound. 2015;18:385–93. doi:10.1007/s40477-014-0087-4.
34. Trinci M, Trinci CM, Galluzzo M, et al. Neonatal adrenal hemorrhage. In: Miele V, Trinci M, editors. Imaging non-traumatic abdominal emergencies in pediatric patients. Switzerland: Springer International Publishing; 2016. p. 181–92.
35. Jordan E, Poder L, Courtier J, et al. Imaging of nontraumatic adrenal hemorrhage. AJR Am J Roentgenol. 2012;199:W91–8. doi:10.2214/AJR.11.7973.
36. Wedmid A, Palese M. Diagnosis and treatment of the adrenal cyst. Curr Urol Rep. 2010;11:44–50. doi:10.1007/s11934-009-008-1.
37. Cagini L, Gravante S, Malaspina CM, et al. Contrast enhanced ultrasound (CEUS) in blunt abdominal trauma. Crit Ultrasound J. 2013;15:5. doi:10.1186/2036-7902-5-S1-S9.
38. Valentino M, Serra C, Pavlica P, et al. Contrast-enhanced ultrasound for blunt abdominal trauma. Semin Ultrasound CT MR. 2007;28:130–40.
39. Miele V, Piccolo CL, Galluzzo M, et al. Contrast enhanced ultrasound (CEUS) in blunt abdominal trauma. Br J Radiol. 2016;89(1061):20150823. doi:10.1259/bjr.20150823.
40. Cosgrove D. Ultrasound contrast agent: an overview. Eur J Radiol. 2006;60:324–30.
41. Pinto F, Miele V, Scaglione M, et al. The use of contrast-enhanced ultrasound in blunt abdominal trauma: advantages and limitations. Acta Radiol. 2014;55:776–84. doi:10.1177/0284185113505517. Epub 2013 Sep 23
42. Marti JL, Millet J, Sosa JA, et al. Spontaneous adrenal hemorrhage with associated masses: etiology and

management in 6 cases and a review of 133 reported cases. World J Surg. 2012;36:75–82. doi:10.1007/s00268-011-1338-6.
43. Rhea JT, Garza DH, Novelline RA. Controversies in emergency radiology CT versus ultrasound in the evaluation of blunt abdominal trauma. Emerg Radiol. 2004;10:289–95.
44. Pinto A, Scaglione M, Pinto F, et al. Adrenal injuries: spectrum of CT findings. Emerg Radiol. 2003;10:30–3.
45. Scialpi M, Palumbo B, Pierotti L, et al. Detection and characterization of focal liver lesions by split-bolus multidetector-row CT: diagnostic accuracy and radiation dose in oncologic patients. Anticancer Res. 2014;34:4335–44.
46. Lee YS, Jeong JJ, Nam KH, et al. Adrenal injury following blunt abdominal trauma. World J Surg. 2010;34:1971–4. doi:10.1007/s00268-010-0537-x.
47. Daly KP, Ho CP, Persson DL, Gay SB. Traumatic retroperitoneal injuries: review of multidetector CT findings. Radiographics. 2008;28:1571–90. doi:10.1148/rg.286075141.
48. Sacerdote MG, Johnson PT, Fishman EK. CT of the adrenal gland: the many faces of adrenal hemorrhage. Emerg Radiol. 2012;19:53–60. doi:10.1007/s10140-011-0989-9.
49. Ikeda O, Urata J, Araki Y, et al. Acute adrenal hemorrhage after blunt trauma. Abdom Imaging. 2007;32:248–52.
50. Dunnick NR, Korobkin M. Imaging of adrenal Incidentalomas: current status. AJR Am J Roentgenol. 2002;179:559–68.
51. Pinto A, Brunese L, Pinto F, et al. The concept of error and malpractice in radiology. Semin Ultrasound CT MR. 2012;33:275–9. doi:10.1053/j.sult.2012.01.009.
52. Elsayes KM, Mukundan G, Narra VR, et al. Adrenal masses: MR imaging features with pathologic correlation. Radiographics. 2004;1:S73–86.
53. Schultz CL, Haaga JR, Fletcher BD, et al. Magnetic resonance imaging of the adrenal glands: a comparison with computer tomography. AJR Am J Roentgenol. 1984;143:1235–40.
54. Rammelt S, Mucha D, Amlang M, et al. Bilateral adrenal hemorrhage in blunt abdominal trauma. J Trauma. 2000;48:332–5.
55. Igwilo OC, Sulkowski RJ, Shah MR, et al. Embolization of traumatic adrenal hemorrhage. J Trauma. 1999;47:1153–5.
56. Roupakias S, Papoutsakis M, Mitsakou P. Blunt adrenal gland trauma in the pediatric population. Asian J Surg. 2011;34:10310. doi:10.1016/j.asjsur.2011.08.003.
57. Udobi KF, Childs EW. Adrenal crisis after traumatic bilateral adrenal hemorrhage. J Trauma. 2001;51:597–600.
58. Ikekpeazzu N, Bonadies JA, Sreenivas VI. Acute bilateral adrenal hemorrhage secondary to rough truck ride. J Emerg Med. 1996;14:15–8.
59. Castaldo ET, Guillamondegui OD, Greco JA, et al. Are adrenal injuries predictive of adrenal insufficiency in patients sustaining blunt trauma? Am Surg. 2008;74:262–6.
60. Francque SM, Schwagten VM, Ysebaert DK, et al. Bilateral adrenal haemorrhage and acute adrenal insufficiency in a blunt abdominal trauma: a case-report and literature review. J Emerg Med. 2004;11:164–7.
61. Baccot S, Tiffet O, Bonnot P, et al. Bilateral post-traumatic adrenal hemorrhage. Report of a case with acute adrenal insufficiency. Ann Chir. 2000;125:273–5.

Renal Injuries

19

Silvia Lucarini, Alessandro Castellani,
Elena Bertelli, Monica Marina Lanzetta,
Simone Agostini, Margherita Trinci,
and Vittorio Miele

19.1 Introduction

The kidneys are two symmetrical retroperitoneal organs, wrapped in retroperitoneal fat and located at the sides of the lumbar spine; their upper pole is at the level of twelfth dorsal vertebrae, and the lower one is at the third lumbar vertebrae.

The right kidney is slightly moved in lower than the left kidney, for the presence of the liver.

A fibrous capsule wraps the kidney; the parenchyma is formed externally from the cortical part and an inner medulla part. The medial surface of the kidney has a concave incision called hilum, through which arteries, veins, and lymph vessels and ureter enter and exit.

The right kidney is related to the liver, right flexure of the colon, and duodenum. The left kidney gets into relationship with the stomach, pancreas, duodenal-jejunal flexure and spleen, and colon (left flexure). They report, above, with their adrenal gland and posteriorly with the muscles of the back abdomen.

The kidney is involved in 8–10% of abdominal trauma cases, with 245,000 cases/year/world, and it is the most frequently injured organ in genitourinary trauma (80%), followed by external genital organs, bladder, urethra, and ureter. The incidence of renal trauma is about 4.9 per 10,000 of the population [1]. Three quarters of patients with renal trauma are male. In most of the cases, renal involvement occurs in blunt trauma (approximately 90%) [2–4]. The most common causes of blunt trauma are motor vehicle accidents, followed by direct blow to the flank or abdomen during a fight, sport activities or an assault, and a fall from a height [5–7]. Car accidents are associated with renal injuries in 43% of cases, whereas motorcycle accidents are more frequently associated with male external genital organs injuries and urethra; in this latter type of accidents, renal injuries occur in 28% of cases [8]. The incidence of renal injuries due to penetrating trauma, such as gunshot, stab wounds, or iatrogenic injuries during renal biopsies or other medical procedures, is low (approximately 10% of renal traumas) but could be associated with more severe renal damage and is frequently associated with injuries to other organs [9–11].

There are predisposing conditions that can expose a blunt trauma patient to a kidney injury, including hydronephrosis, cystic diseases, horseshoe kidney, and nephroblastoma. Another factor

S. Lucarini, M.D., Ph.D. (✉) • A. Castellani
E. Bertelli • M.M. Lanzetta • S. Agostini • V. Miele
Department of Radiology, Careggi University Hospital,
L.go G. A. Brambilla 3, 50134 Florence, Italy
e-mail: slucarini@iol.it;
lucarinis@aou-careggi.toscana.it

M. Trinci
Department of Emergency Radiology, S. Camillo
Hospital, Rome, Italy

V. Miele, M. Trinci (eds.), *Diagnostic Imaging in Polytrauma Patients*,
https://doi.org/10.1007/978-3-319-62054-1_19

that exposes the kidney to traumatic injuries is its mobility on the pedicle that exposes it to stretching injuries.

In both blunt and penetrating trauma, multiorgan involvement is common (80–90% of patients with penetrating trauma, 75% of those with blunt trauma). The associated lesions by frequency are lung contusion, 46%; splenic injury, 39%; liver injury, 34%; bone damage, 27%; adrenal injury, 7%; and intestinal perforation, 4%. Especially in these cases of multiorgan involvement, contrast-enhanced CT is essential for a complete trauma evaluation.

Isolated renal trauma is rare and is usually classified as a minor injury [6, 12]. While blunt trauma may result in contusion or laceration of the parenchyma or the renal hilum due to sudden deceleration or a crush injury, penetrating ones produce direct damage on the parenchyma, the collecting system, or the vascular structures and involve the peritoneum [10, 13, 14]. Moreover, penetrating injuries are at higher risk of bacterial growth within the hematoma or urine leakage due to the non-sterile condition, and in some cases, a surgical debridement or a nephrectomy could be mandatory [15, 16].

Imaging assessment depends primarily on the hemodynamic status of the patient, because if the patient is hemodynamically unstable, an immediate damage control laparotomy is usually performed. In case of stable patients, the imaging strategy depends on the mechanism of injury and on clinical and laboratory findings.

Renal trauma can occur with a quite wide range of severity; therefore, different kinds of treatment are needed. In the past two decades, important advances have been made in diagnostic imaging and in polytrauma patient management, and therefore the focus has slowly passed from a mainly surgical to a more conservative approach, since urgent surgical exploration often leads to nephrectomy and endovascular embolization is gaining importance in treating ongoing bleeding [17].

Renal trauma management depends widely on lesion type and extension. The radiologist plays an essential role in distinguishing kidney lesions that need surgical or interventional treatment from the ones needing a conservative approach.

Nowadays, two main classifications exist, which are used for the management of traumatic renal injuries: the one developed by the American Association for the Surgery of Trauma (AAST) (Table 19.1), surgical-based, which grades the severity of renal injuries from 1 (minor contusion) to 5 (shattered kidney), and the one proposed by Federle, a CT-based classification, more popular among radiologists, which considers some aspects not included in the AAST grading system (Table 19.2) [18–22].

Of course these two classification systems present several overlaps and don't include all the

Table 19.1 American Association for Surgery of Trauma (AAST) renal injury classification

Grade[a]	Type	Description
I	Parenchyma	Microscopic or gross hematuria; urological studies normal (contusion)
	Hematoma	Non-expanding subcapsular hematoma
II	Parenchyma	Laceration <1 cm in depth, without collecting system rupture
	Hematoma	Non-expanding perirenal hematoma confined to retroperitoneum
III	Parenchyma	Laceration >1 cm in depth without collecting system rupture
IV	Parenchyma	Laceration with collecting system rupture
	Vascular	Main renal artery/vein injury with contained hemorrhage
V	Parenchyma	Shattered kidney
	Vascular	Avulsion of renal hilum that devascularized kidney

Obtained permission from Wolters Kluwer

[a]Advance one grade for bilateral injuries up to grade III

Table 19.2 Federle classification

Category	Type	Injury
I	Minor injury	Renal contusion; intrarenal and subcapsular hematoma; minor laceration with limited perinephric hematoma without extension in the collecting system or medulla; small subsegmental cortical infarct
II	Major injury	Major renal laceration through the cortex extending to the medulla or collecting system with or without urine extravasation; segmental renal infarct
III	Catastrophic injury	Multiple renal lacerations; vascular injury involving the renal pedicle
IV	Ureteropelvic injury	Avulsion (complete transaction); laceration (incomplete tear)

Reproduced with permission from Razali MR, Azian AA, Amran AR, Azlin S (2010) Computed tomography of blunt renal trauma. Singapore Med J 51:468–473; quiz 474

possible conditions; therefore, the communication between radiologist and surgeon is of vital importance to define the grade and severity of the kidney injury.

Moreover, the AAST classification is the most and widely accepted, and it's based on accurate assessment at autopsy, laparotomy, or radiologic study. This grading system is widely used in the urological setting. Increasing grade correlates with the need for nephrectomy and dialysis and with mortality. Grades I through III can be managed conservatively as they heal spontaneously. Grades IV and V with collecting system disruption and vascular injury usually require intervention.

This classification has some limitations, like it does not consider vascular injuries associated with low-grade injuries. There are some proposals for changes, including a sub-stratification of the intermediate-grade injury into low-risk (likely to be managed nonoperatively) and high-risk cases (likely to benefit from angiographic embolization or surgery) [23]. Another suggestion is to comprise all collecting system injuries and segmental arterial and venous injuries in grade IV injuries, while including only hilar injuries (comprising thrombotic events) in grade V injuries [24].

As we have already said, the Federle classification is based on CT findings; however, both classifications, although based on different criteria, have common points and in fact agree that the most serious lesions are those involving the excretory system and/or the vascular one.

Conservative management has become the treatment of choice for the majority of renal injuries, especially in blunt trauma [25, 26]. In particular, a nonoperative approach can be performed in hemodynamically stable patients with:

- Grade I and II injuries
- Most of grade III injuries
- Grade IV with a devitalized fragment or with urinary extravasation
- Grade V with unilateral main arterial injury, comprising unilateral complete blunt arterial thrombosis

In penetrating trauma a selective nonoperative management is generally accepted [27, 28]:

- In stab wounds if the patient is stable and the site of penetration is posterior to the anterior axillary line
- In gunshot injuries if they don't involve the renal hilum or are accompanied by signs of ongoing bleeding, ureteral injuries, or renal pelvis lacerations with a successful outcome in approximately 50% of stab wounds and up to 40% of gunshot wounds [29, 30]

Nowadays angiography and embolization represent essential techniques in the nonsurgical treatment of traumatic kidney lesions. Superselective embolization has shown to increase significantly the chances to preserve the kidney and its function.

Embolization has a fundamental role in the conservative management of active bleeding, arteriovenous fistula, and pseudoaneurysm, and it seems to be most beneficial in the setting of high-grade renal trauma (AAST > 3).

In the management of high-grade renal trauma, embolization can be successful in up to 94.9% of grade III, 89% of grade IV, and 52% of grade V injuries and has decreased significantly nephrectomy [31–33].

Indications to operative management are limited, reserving surgery in case of shuttered kidney. The hemodynamic instability and the unresponsiveness to aggressive resuscitation due to renal hemorrhage are indications for surgical exploration, irrespective of the mode of injury [34, 35].

The exploration aims to control the hemorrhage and to save the kidney. Other indications are the mechanism of trauma; the presence of an expanding perirenal hematoma, identified at exploratory laparotomy performed for associated injuries; and the presence of multiorgan involvement which led the patient to hemodynamic instability.

Endourological techniques are indicated for the management of persistent extravasation or urinoma.

Inconclusive imaging and a preexisting abnormality or an incidentally diagnosed tumor may require surgery even after minor renal injury [36]. The overall exploration rate for blunt trauma is less than 10% [37] and may be even lower, as the conservative approach is increasingly adopted [38].

19.2 Radiological Diagnosis

The purpose of diagnostics imaging is to identify the renal lesion, to evaluate prognostic factors, and to give an indication of the patient's management.

Currently the indications for the different diagnostic imaging modalities are controversial and depend on several things, such as the hemodynamic status of the patient, on the presence of associated lesions, and on the type and locations of the trauma.

Unstable patients are immediately examined with FAST (focused assessment with sonography for trauma), an abdominal ultrasound (US) protocol performed bedside in the emergency room for the detection of free peritoneal fluid [39].

Patients involved in a high-energy accident, in stable condition or whose vital functions have been stabilized, are rapidly examined with a whole-body computed tomography (CT) [40].

The management of patients with mild-/low-energy trauma is controversial: the clinical presentation and the mechanism of injury are fundamental for the decision to immediately perform CT or assess the patient with sonography, conventional radiography, and clinical observation [41–44].

In 2014 the American Urological Association (AUA) released new guidelines, amended in 2017 [45], for management of patients with a suspect of renal trauma.

CT with administration of intravenous contrast material is recommended in adults with blunt trauma and one of the following cases [2, 10, 46, 47]:

- Gross hematuria: represents the main initial indicator of a significant renal lesion, although it is not correlated with the degree of injury
- Microscopic hematuria in the presence of shock (systolic blood pressure < 90 mmHg)
- A mechanism of injury (e.g., rapid deceleration or high-speed collisions)
- A physical examination concerning for renal injury: contusion or flank ecchymosis, fracture of the last ribs or thoracolumbar spine, and open wound of the abdomen, of the flank, or of the lower part of the thorax, in case of expanding mass of the flank that may be a hematoma or urinoma, regardless of the presence or absence of hematuria
- In case of retroperitoneal fluid, nausea, vomit, or paralyzed ileum

A diagnostic evaluation is mandatory also in all cases of penetrating traumas, because in those situations there is a poor correlation between the presence of hematuria and the severity of the injuries [48].

Gross or microscopic hematuria is usually present in 95% of renal trauma, but its absence doesn't preclude the presence of kidney injure, for example, it can be absent in 24% of patients with renal artery thrombosis, and in approximately 30% of urinary tract junction lesions, these lesions, moreover, are major injuries.

Although no exact indications have been given in the AUA 2014 guidelines for patients with penetrating renal trauma, the most accepted one is to perform a CT in the presence of hematuria or in a clinical suspect of a urinary tract lesion.

The Urogenital Trauma guidelines of European Association of Urology (EAU) released in 2013 and updated until 2017 are similar to the AUA ones [2, 46].

Some authors affirm that patients with microscopic hematuria and systolic blood pressure >90 mmHg have a very low risk of major renal injury (incidence of 0.2%) [48], so they could not require a diagnostic imaging evaluation.

Renal injuries, especially high-grade ones, seem to be more frequent in children, and these can also occur for minor trauma [49]; this is because of the anatomy of pediatric patient. In fact, the kidney in children is larger compared to the rest of the body, and it can maintain fetal lobulation that could easier lead to parenchymal disruption; a child's kidney is also less protected because it has less perirenal fat, and the abdominal wall thickness is less than that of the adult [37, 50].

In pediatric patients the diagnostic imaging choice is controverted. Due to the capability of children to maintain their blood pressure, instead of adults, some centers recommend a CT scan in case of suspected renal involvement in pediatric blunt trauma with any degree of hematuria following significant abdominal trauma.

In pediatric blunt renal trauma, CT is indicated when the RBC value in the urine is >50 per HPF and in penetrating trauma when the RBC value in the urine is >5 per HPF [10].

19.2.1 Ultrasonography (US)

Ultrasound, just for its well-known advantages, which consist of low cost, lack of ionizing radiations, and its portability with the possibility to be rapidly performed at patient's bedside, among others, is the most largely available imaging modality in emergency department.

Apart from its use in the emergency room with FAST (focused assessment with sonography for trauma) to highlight the presence of hemoperitoneum, ultrasound is often the first imaging of choice in evaluating a patient with localized low-energy trauma. In fact a standard ultrasound technique is able not only to detect free fluid but also to demonstrate a parenchymal lesion. In the specific case of kidney, the deep retroperitoneal position and the body type of patient can influence the detection of the lesion; moreover, the operator's experience and patient's collaboration are other factors that may affect the outcome of the exam. For these reasons US demonstrates high sensitivity for the detection of free intra-abdominal fluid; in the same study, it is reported more than CT exam for small amount, but fairly low sensitivity (even below 50%) for the detection of abdominal solid organ traumatic lesions [51].

Some studies report that the US, practiced in an emergency environment, has very low sensitivity in the detection of parenchymal renal injury (less than 22% in minor lesion) and perirenal collections [51–55]. The American College of Radiologists (ACR) Renal Trauma guidelines consider US usually not appropriate in renal trauma [46]. It also cannot be a reliable diagnostic tool for major vascular injuries and renal function.

Contrast-enhanced ultrasound (CEUS) in traumatic patients has been shown to be more sensitive than US for the detection of solid organ injuries, improving the identification and grading of traumatic abdominal lesions with levels of sensitivity and specificity similar to CT (up to 95%) [56]. With CEUS is also easier demonstrated even small amount of perirenal fluid and sometimes is possible to detect active bleeding. The principal limit of CEUS is the impossibility to evaluate the excretory phase, because microbubbles are not excreted into the collecting system; therefore, CEUS cannot demonstrate injuries to the urinary system: renal pelvis or ureter [57–60].

For these reasons both basic ultrasound and CEUS may not be the only investigations to evaluate a patient with trauma. Their role, especially that of CEUS, is to identify patients with a positive traumatic injury response and to send them a CT diagnostic completion test, differentiating them from negative traumatic injury patients who, if in agreement with the clinic, cannot continue the radiological diagnostic iter.

In this way it decreases the unnecessary radiation exposure, using the US-CEUS as a screening tool to select patients who require a CT or not.

This is very important especially in selected series of patients, such as pediatric patients, young women in reproductive age, and low-energy trauma patients, or in the follow-up of stable patients with kidney injury [39, 41, 61].

An US exam is performed using a convex-array multifrequency 3.5–8 MHz probe. During the US exam, a parenchymal renal injury can be seen as a slightly hyperechoic area with no defined margins that may be difficult to detect in renal parenchyma. Often even in case of minor trauma a surrounding hematoma is visible, as well as a recent hyperechogeneous hematoma, which sometimes can be confused with renal parenchyma (Fig. 19.1).

Over time, hematoma loses its echogenicity, becoming hypo-anecdotal and decreasing its volume (Fig. 19.2).

Usually CEUS exam, in case of low-energy localized renal trauma or during a follow-up of known injuries, is performed using a convex-

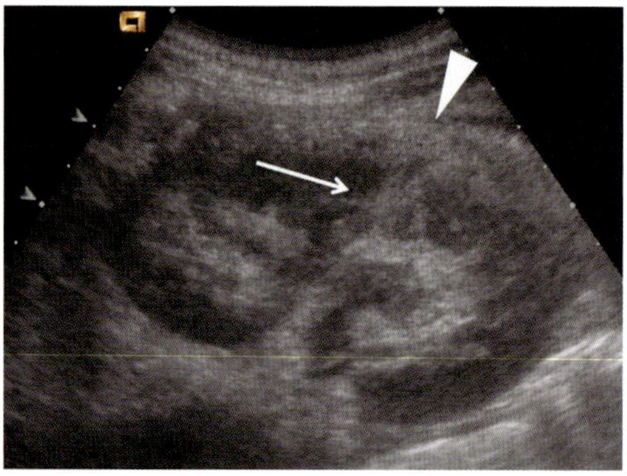

Fig. 19.1 Ultrasound shows injured left kidney, with a hyperechoic parenchymal area at the medium of the kidney, corresponding to the lesion (*arrow*); there is a hyperechoic hematoma surrounding the kidney (*arrowhead*)

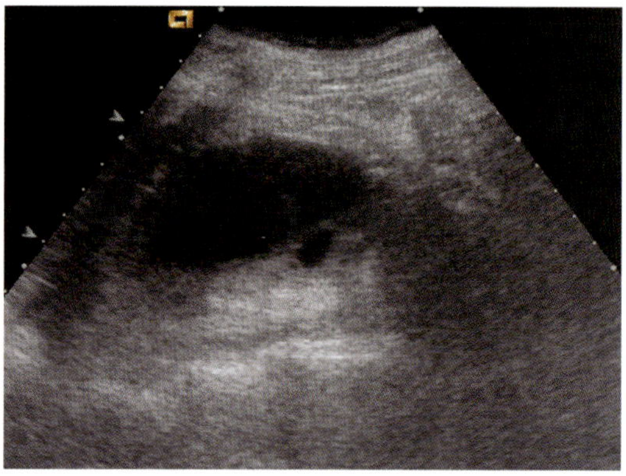

Fig. 19.2 Ultrasound shows a non-recent subcapsular hematoma, which appears as an hypoechoic mass compressing renal parenchyma

array multifrequency 3.5–8 MHz probe after a previous basal ultrasound. CEUS uses second-generation ultrasound contrast agents and needs dedicated software operating at low mechanical index.

Like any contrastographic examination, the informed consent of the patient is required.

After contrast agent administration with quick bolus, the renal cortex enhances immediately in arterial phase (10–30 s), very brightly and evenly, and the pyramids enhance diffusely from the periphery to the center over about 30 s. The homogeneous phase of the kidneys generally lasts 2–2.5 min: this homogeneous phase (venous phase or nephrographic phase) is still the most effective for detection of traumatic injuries. At CEUS exam the injured area is detected as anechoic surrounded by normal strongly hyperechogenic renal parenchyma (Fig. 19.3). Perirenal or subcapsular hematoma is easily seen as perirenal hypo-anechoic zone, in case of subcapsular hematoma, with the typical imprint on the kidney profile (Fig. 19.4). In case of active bleeding, it is possible to detect in the injured area the hyperechoic spots. As we already said, it is impossible evaluate the excretory system [53, 60].

When a renal lesion is detected at US or CEUS complete, the examination of the patient performing a CT with intravenous contrast medium is recommended.

Eco-color-Doppler imaging can be useful in monitoring vascular posttraumatic complications

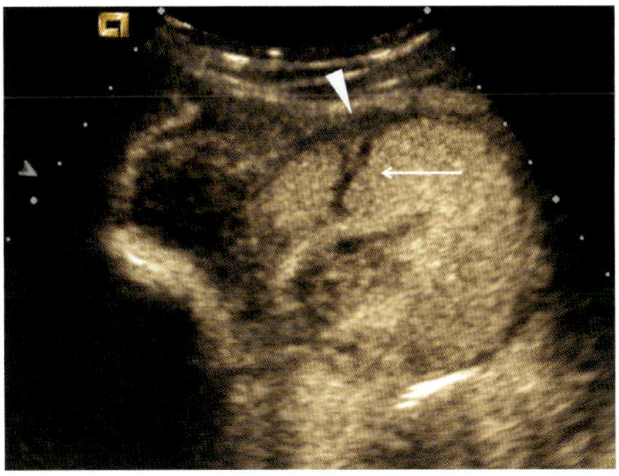

Fig. 19.3 CEUS, axial view of the kidney, shows the renal injury as linear anechoic area. Note the small perirenal hematoma as a subtle fluid collection surrounding the kidney (*arrowhead*)

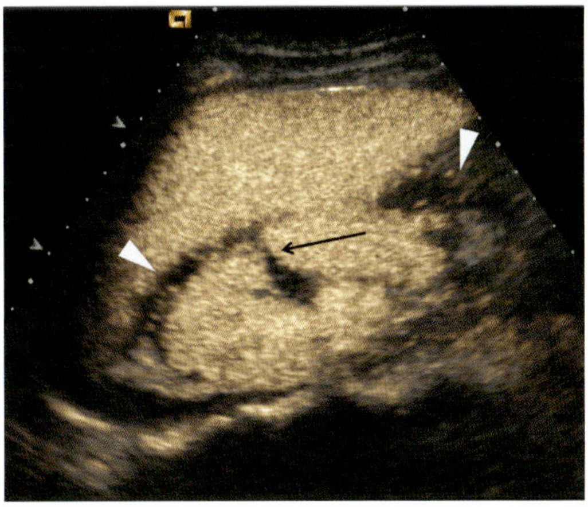

Fig. 19.4 CEUS shows a deep laceration of renal parenchyma (*black arrow*). Perinephric hematoma is seen as a hypoechoic fluid collection surrounding the kidney (*arrowheads*)

such as pseudoaneurysms, arteriovenous fistulas, and arterial or venous renal thrombosis.

19.2.2 Multidetector Computed Tomography (MDCT)

With the technological development in the past two decades, contrast-enhanced MDCT has gained a central role in the evaluation of stable polytrauma patients, becoming the first choice examination. Integration of whole-body CT into the initial management of polytrauma patients significantly increases the probability of survival and a better prognosis [62].

CT can quickly and accurately identify and grade renal injury [63], can establish the condition of the contralateral kidney, and can demonstrate injuries to other organs.

In the setting of renal trauma, multiphase CT allows the most comprehensive assessment of the injured kidney. The standard protocol consists in an abdominal pre-contrast acquisition from the diaphragm to the pubic symphysis, followed by a post-intravenous contrast exam in arterial phase (delay around 40 s) and venous nephrographic phase (delay around 80 s). A pyelographic phase (at 5–10 min or more) is practiced only in the suspected urinary tract injury, e.g., in the presence of collections to differentiate an active bleeding from a urinoma (Fig. 19.5) [64, 65].

A volume of nonionic contrast medium of 100–150 mL is injected at a rate of 2–4 mL/s through an 18–20-gauge needle.

Concerns regarding contrast media worsening outcomes via renal parenchymal toxicity are likely unwarranted, with low rates of contrast-induced nephropathy seen in trauma patients [66].

However, in practice, trauma patients usually undergo standardized whole-body imaging protocols; it may happen that, caused by critical patient's condition, it is not possible to perform an excretory phase; and in this case if there is suspicion that renal injuries have not been fully evaluated, repeating renal imaging when it is possible should be considered.

19.2.3 Magnetic Resonance Imaging

Magnetic resonance imaging (MRI) is not commonly used imaging modality in trauma patients, due to the time needed for examination, the difficulty to manage a traumatized patient in MR room, the limited access to the patient during the acquisition of imaging, the need for MRI-safe equipment, and the logistical challenges of moving a trauma patient to the MRI suite. Anyway the diagnostic accuracy of MRI in renal trauma is similar to that of CT with the benefit due to the

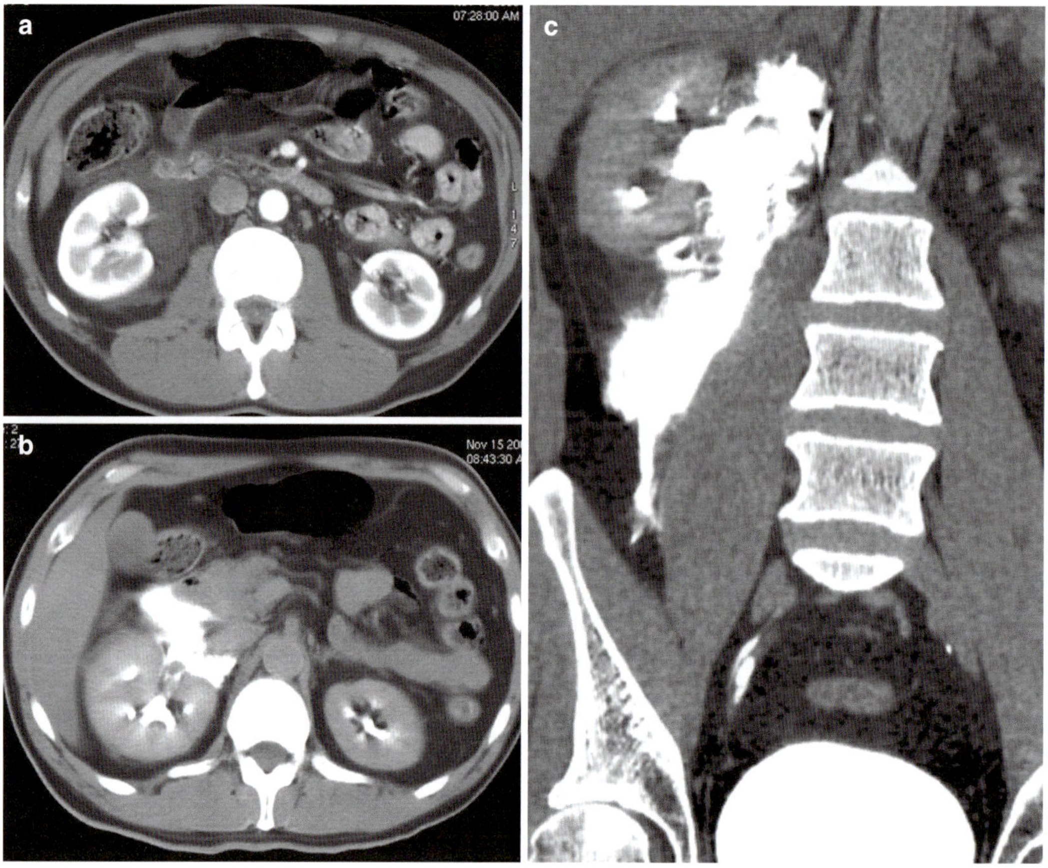

Fig. 19.5 CT exam in a patient with a urine leakage from pyelo-ureteral tract, with huge urinoma. (**a**) Arterial phase and (**b**) axial and (**c**) coronal MPR in excretory phase. Note the importance of the late excretory phase that allows to differentiate a perirenal collection, e.g., hematoma from urinoma

lack of radiations exposure [67, 68]. Due to the lack of radiations, MRI can be useful, especially in the assessment of pediatric patients and young women, in cases in which the use of iodine contrast material is contraindicated or in follow-up of renal and urinary tract lesions, since with the administration of gadolinium the extravasations of urine can be visualized [69–71].

19.2.4 Urography, Angiography, and Scintigraphy

Intravenous urography is nowadays an obsolete imaging modality for the evaluation of renal trauma. It can be used only in rare situations, if the MDCT is not available or in the operating room, in hemodynamically unstable patients taken to the operating room without imaging, to confirm the contralateral renal function if nephrectomy is considered. The technique consists of an injection of intravenous contrast (2 mL/kg) followed by a single plain film taken after 10–15 min [46, 72]. In doubt or positive cases, MDCT is anyway necessary once the patient is stable.

Angiography has only a therapeutic role in renal vascular lesions in stable patients. This topic will be treated in Chap. 22.

Kidney scintigraphy with Tc-99m glucoheptonate, Tc-99m mercaptoacetyltriglycine, or Tc-99m-diethylenetriamine penta-acetic acid can be useful in the follow-up of renal injuries, to counsel the patient on the expected renal function [65].

It can be used also in studying the renal function in patients with contraindications to contrast media or in very selected cases.

19.3 Renal Trauma Classification

Renal trauma management depends widely not only on the detection of renal parenchyma lesion but also on the presence of bleeding parenchymal lesions or direct damage to the vascular peduncle or compromise of the urinary excretory system. The presence of these kinds of injury, detected at CT exam, completely changes management from nonoperative to operative. The CT exam with intravenous contrast medium can show accurately not only the presence of a renal injury and its grade but also can allow the identification of a preexisting renal condition mimicking trauma and can explore the contralateral kidney and the presence of concomitant lesions of other organs.

Therefore the radiologist plays an essential role in the management of traumatic patient and regarding renal trauma distinguishing kidney lesions that need interventional/surgical treatment from the ones needing only a conservative approach.

Since this manuscript is mainly intended for an imaging-based audience, we take into consideration the Federle classification dividing traumatic renal injury in two principal categories of injury: minor and major—anyway the two principal classifications will be considered for the description of the different kidney lesion.

19.3.1 Category I: Minor Traumatic Lesions

This category comprises minor renal contusions and lacerations which don't extend to the collecting system or medulla, subcapsular hematomas with less than 1 cm or more than 1 cm of thickness but without urinary excretal delay, and perinephric hematomas without active bleeding comprised in the perinephric adipose space and small subsegmental cortical infarcts.

Category I corresponds in the AAST renal injury scale to grades I and II. It includes most of kidney injuries (75–85%), which generally are treated conservatively.

19.3.1.1 Imaging Findings

Renal Contusion

Contusion represents a self-limiting blood extravasation (hematoma) in the renal parenchyma (grade I AAST; type I Federle). These minor injuries will spontaneous resolve and follow-up imaging is not required.

At an early US examination (within 1 h from trauma), it can appear as an oval or round hyperechoic area, with margins that after being undefined at the beginning become more and more distinct; rarely it is large enough to lead to a mass effect, alter the cortical profile, or determine a dilatation of nearby chalices (Fig. 19.6). The echogenicity of renal contusions reduces in a few days until becoming isoechoic within 2 weeks, generally without leaving sequelae. Anyway contusion has to be suspected when a trauma patient presents hematuria without significant alterations or abnormalities of the urinary tract at US. On CEUS kidney contusion lesion can appear as a hypoechoic area without clear delimitation [50, 53, 59, 71].

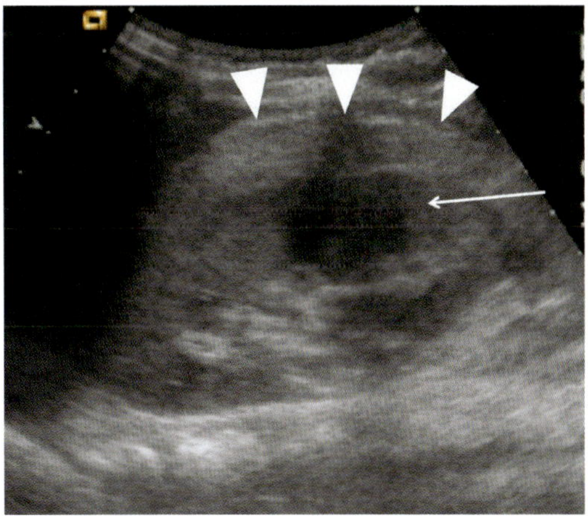

Fig. 19.6 Minor lesion: US shows the lower pole renal contusion as a non-well-defined inhomogeneous parenchymal (*arrow*); note the surrounding perirenal hematoma as a hyperdense collection (*arrowheads*), not compressing the renal profile

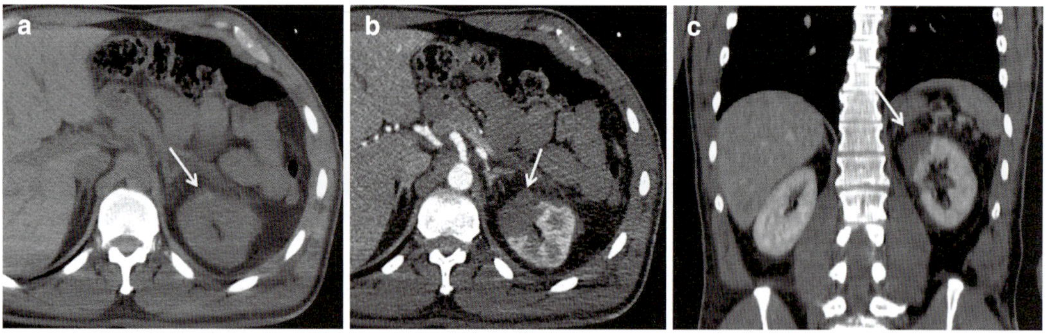

Fig. 19.7 Renal contusion seen on MDCT. Unenhanced CT scan (**a**) shows an iso-hyperdense area, which is better delineated on post-contrast images (**b**) and coronal reconstruction (**c**) as a hypodense area

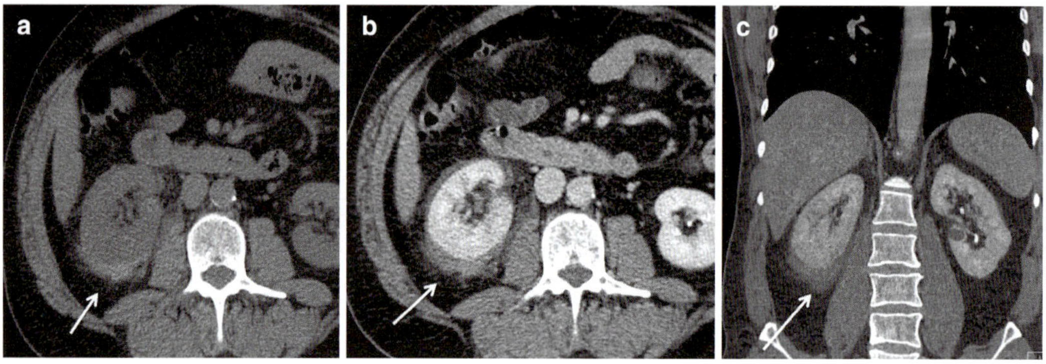

Fig. 19.8 Subcapsular hematoma seen on MDCT unenhanced scan (**a**) as a hyperdense area, without expanding signs on post-contrast images (**b** and **c**)

Compared to US, MDCT is more sensible in detecting renal contusion. On unenhanced images, it may be slightly hyperdense (due to the accumulation of acute blood products); in enhanced phases contusion appears as an ill-defined hypoattenuating lesion. Sometimes renal contusions can be seen as focal areas of striated nephrogram and as hyperdense areas in the excretory phase, due to small iodinated urine extravasations in the intraparenchymal collecting system. These lesions have to be distinct from segmental infarction that is usually linear or wedge-shaped sharply defined non-enhancing areas [21, 64, 65, 73, 74] (Fig. 19.7).

Subcapsular Hematoma

Subcapsular hematoma is a collection of clotted blood situated under the renal capsule. It is quite rare due to the tight adherence of renal capsule and cortex (grade I AAST; type I Federle). On US it is seen at the beginning as hyperechoic lenticular lesion, which is distributed along the external kidney surface, confined between the cortex and the capsule, determining a compressive effect on the renal parenchyma. Over time, it becomes a hypo-/anechoic lesion and reduces its thickness. On CEUS a subcapsular hematoma appears as a nonhomogeneous fluid collection without enhancement surrounding the kidney [41, 43, 53, 59].

On CT, acute hematomas are seen as a round or elliptical fluid hyperdense collection (>35–55 UH) [21, 64] on unenhanced scan, with an oval or crescent shape which imprints the underlying renal parenchyma; if the fluid collection is of greater size, it can have a biconvex shape and causes a delay in the nephrographic phase (Fig. 19.8). The Federle classification, unlike the AAST, evaluates the presence of any delay or reduction of parenchymal vascularity due to hematoma compression. In case of a chronic and prolonged compression and distortion of the renal parenchyma and vessels, a reduction of the blood flow to the kidney occurs resulting in activation of the renin-angiotensin system with development of hypertension, also known as "Page kidney phenomenon." Surgical treatment of the renal compression is indicated in these cases [21, 64].

Superficial and Deep Laceration

Superficial renal laceration (< 1 cm depth) is a tear of the renal parenchyma that involves only the cortical zone, often associated with contusion. Instead a deep laceration (>1 cm depth) passes through the cortical zone extending to the medullary one. A laceration appears as irregular or linear parenchymal defects that may contain clot (grade I–III AAST; type I Federle) [74].

Superficial or deep renal lacerations appear as defects in the renal parenchyma without involvement of the collecting system and typically resolve spontaneously, without the need for follow-up imaging, especially in case of superficial laceration [21]. If it extends only to the renal cortex, it is classified as AAST grade II, and if it goes until the medullar part, without comprising the collecting system, it is classified as AAST grade III and may need follow-up imaging.

On US it is difficult to observe, and it can be suspected if a subcapsular or perirenal hematoma is seen; it can be evident as a hyperechoic line or an undefined area of the kidney profile. On CEUS laceration is seen as a linear or branched hypoechoic streak, perpendicular to the surface of the kidney [59] (Fig. 19.9). The rapid enhancement can generate questions of interpretation that can possibly be solved only with a second injection of contrast agent [75]. An injection of too high a dose of contrast media will have a negative effect due to the intense enhancement, potentially masking the presence of lacerations [61].

On MDCT it is seen as a hypodense linear or irregular streak on unenhanced scan; after contrast material administration, it is visualized as a less or unenhanced area; therefore, sometimes the differential diagnosis with a segmental or subsegmental infarct can be difficult (Fig. 19.10).

Perirenal Hematoma

Perirenal hematoma is a hemorrhagic extravasation in the perirenal adipose tissue, within Gerota's fascia, which normally represents the result of a laceration of the renal capsule. Usually it is not creating a distortion of the kidney's profile (from grade II AAST; type I Federle). This kind of finding is treated conservatively. Sometimes the hematoma can be very large and dislocate the kidney.

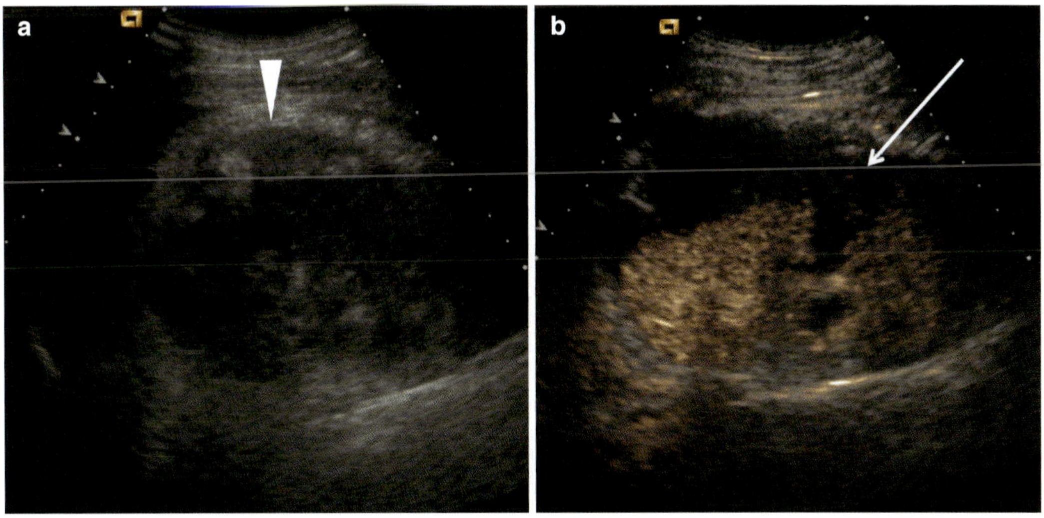

Fig. 19.9 (**a**) US shows a large perirenal hematoma (*arrowhead*); it isn't appreciable the renal parenchymal injury. (**b**) CEUS demonstrates a deep parenchymal laceration at the lower pole of the kidney (*arrow*)

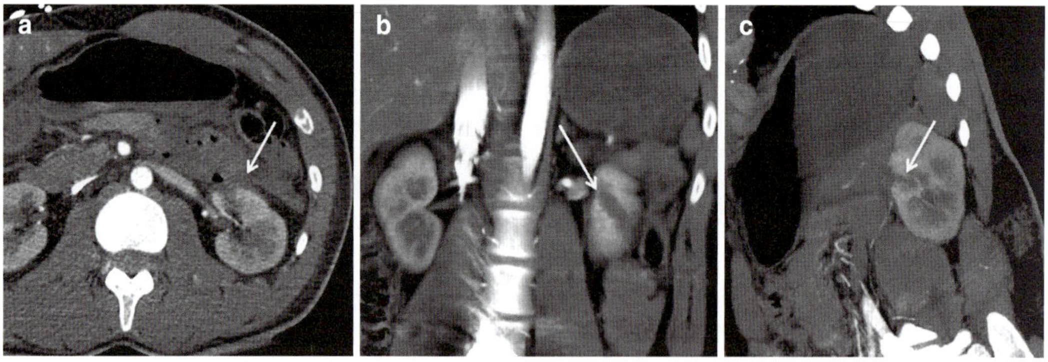

Fig. 19.10 Superficial laceration seen as a hypodense streak on post-contrast images (**a**), better visualized on 3D (**b**) and sagittal (**c**) reconstructions

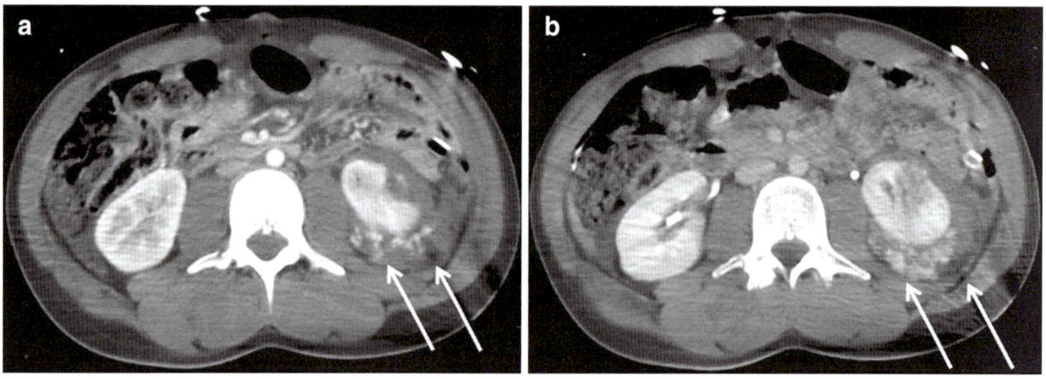

Fig. 19.11 Contrast-enhanced CT scans in arterial phase (**a**) and venous phase (**b**) show the lower pole parenchymal injury, with perirenal hematoma; in both arterial and venous phases, active bleeding is evident (*arrows*)

Ultrasound is not sensible in distinguishing between acute hematoma and the perirenal fat tissue density, since both are hyperechoic. On CEUS the adipose tissue shows a low enhancement and can therefore be differentiated from the non-enhancing fluid collection.

On MDCT in basal phase, an acute perirenal hematoma is seen as a hyperdense collection more irregular in shape than subcapsular hematoma. The perirenal fascia can be thickened if it is infiltrated by the hematic collection [18, 65]. After contrast intravenous medium, the hematoma will be hypodense; in case of active bleeding, hyperdense foci or pooling of contrast medium will be seen in the hematoma (Fig. 19.11).

Subsegmental Kidney Infarct

Subsegmental infarct is caused by traction or stretching and consequent thrombotic occlusion of an accessory, subsegmental, or capsular renal artery; it normally heals with a scar and doesn't require treatment (no AAST grade, type I Federle).

On US examination no distinguishing signs are present. Eco-color Doppler instead can give important information regarding vascularization and can identify the infarcted area. With CEUS a wedge-shaped region of absent vascularization can be identified.

The main imaging technique is MDCT, which shows a small hypo-perfused parenchymal wedge-shaped area and hypodense and with well-delineated margins, more often seen on the

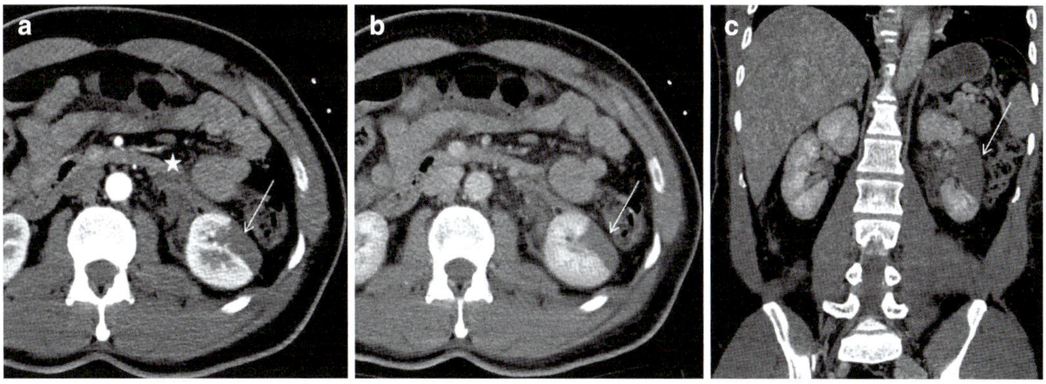

Fig. 19.12 Segmental infarct of the kidney is seen as a wedge-shaped hypodense area on post-contrast images (*arrow*); the infarct is caused by dissection/thrombosis of the renal artery with is never opacified (*star*)

lower polar region, and compared with renal contusions, it is more well defined and demarcated (Fig. 19.12) [18].

19.3.2 Category II: Major Traumatic Injuries

Renal injuries comprised in this category can necessitate an interventional/surgical approach; this category includes vascular injuries and/or deep laceration extending to collecting system or urinary tract injuries with iodate urine extravasation. AAST grade IV comprises lacerations affecting the collector system with urine outflow, renal pelvis laceration or complete ureteropelvic destruction, and arterial lesions or segmental veins; AAST grade V comprises renal vascular peduncle injury, devascularized kidney, venous thrombosis, and shattered kidney.

The management of these lesions is variable, in the majority of cases needing just conservative treatment but occasionally requiring surgical exploration depending on the hemodynamic status and the evolution of the injury. Usually in case of devascularized kidney or shattered one, surgical management is requested.

19.3.2.1 Imaging Findings

Major Laceration

Major laceration of the renal parenchyma or incomplete renal fracture appears as deep cleft which runs through the renal cortex and medulla reaching the collecting system and can be associated to a hematoma and/or a urinary extravasation (urinoma) confined to the perirenal or pararenal fat tissue (grade IV AAST; type II Federle) [76, 77].

Major lacerations appear similar to minor lacerations but are wider, usually more numerous, and larger.

On CT exam multiplanar reconstructions can be useful in better visualizing the extension of the lacerations and their relationship with the collecting system.

Major lesions usually are associated with an extensive perinephric hematoma, a blood collection which infiltrates the perirenal fat tissue and can have a mass effect and dislocation of the kidney, altering the renal contour, the nearby muscle, or the organ shape (such as the psoas muscle or the colon); it can also diffuse toward the abdominal aorta, becoming bilateral. If it trespasses Gerota's fascia, it becomes a paranephric hematoma, with thickening of Gerota's fascia (Fig. 19.13).

When in the case of kidney injury we find peripheral fluid, we must always ask ourselves what kind of fluid is it, blood or urine. An excretory phase should always be performed to exclude an involvement of the collecting system and to demonstrate the presence of a retroperitoneal urinoma, a urine extravasation into the retroperitoneum due to a laceration of the collecting system, or a transection of the ureteropelvic junction,

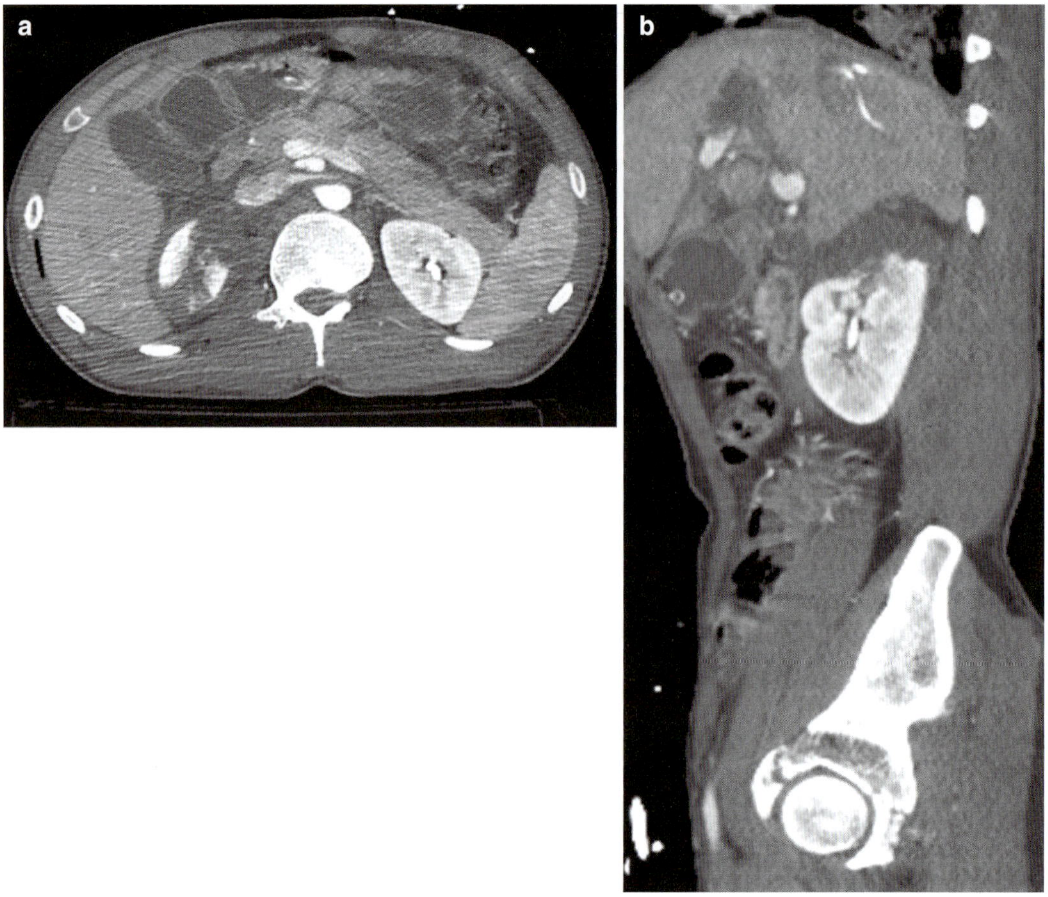

Fig. 19.13 Contrast-enhanced CT, axial scan (**a**), and sagittal reconstruction (**b**) show a deep laceration of the upper pole of the right kidney, associated with retroperitoneal hematoma

causing lipolysis of the surrounding fat with resultant encapsulation of urine. In fact, when the laceration extends into the renal collecting system, extravasation of excreted contrast material will be present on delayed views.

On B-mode US images, urinoma can be seen as a hypo-anechoic area surrounding the kidney, resembling a fluid collection.

On enhanced MDCT, as said before, the retroperitoneal urinoma can be visualized in the excretory phase (at least 4–5 min after contrast media administration) due to the urine extravasation, markedly hyperdense (Fig. 19.14), although often a later scan can be needed (8–15 min from contrast media administration).

The management of this kind of lesions is variable, affected patients are usually treated conservatively, and there may be a need to place a stent, but occasionally require surgical exploration depending on hemodynamic status and the evolution of the injury.

The presence of a voluminous perirenal hematoma or small blood clots can block the urinary extravasation right after trauma, leading to a non-immediate visualization of it; often it is then diagnosed in a CT scan performed after 6–12 h, the time in which the blood clot dissolves permitting the urine to exit. The patient with an expanding perinephric hematoma and a decrease in hematocrit often requires intervention.

When intense contrast enhancement occurs within a laceration or an adjacent hematoma during the early phase of the CT examination, the

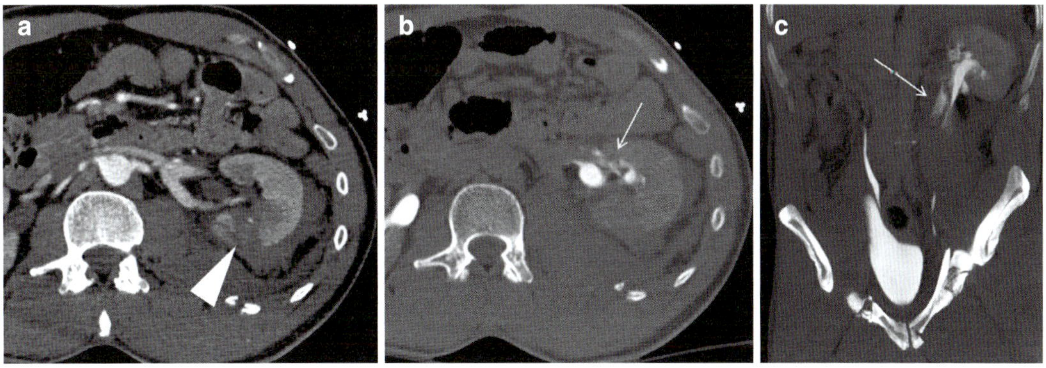

Fig. 19.14 Axial CT scan in arterial (**a**) and excretory (**b**) phase and coronal reconstruction (**c**) show the deep laceration (*arrowhead*) seen as a hypodense cleft on post-contrast images (**a**); the excretory phase on axial (**b**) and better on coronal (**c**) plane show collective system involvement with urine extravasation (*arrows*)

diagnosis of traumatic false aneurysm or active hemorrhage should be considered. Active hemorrhage tends to track into surrounding tissues and has a linear or flame-like appearance, whereas false aneurysms tend to be more focal and rounded. Extravasation of vascular contrast medium appears with attenuation values of 80–370 HU, is typically within 10–15 HU of the aorta or adjacent major artery, and is generally surrounded by lower-attenuation clotted blood. This finding is an important indicator that a patient may be about to pass from hemodynamic stability to decompensation. In one series, 38% of patients with this finding became hypotensive during or immediately after the CT examination. Patients in stable condition with active vascular extravasation should be referred for angiographic embolization [78–80].

The isolated urine extravasation doesn't represent anymore an indication for surgical exploration, reserved only to very extensive lesions, since most of urinary leaks tend to resolve spontaneously and need just a "watch-and-wait" approach. However, in 37% of cases, an endoscopic ureteral stent placement is needed (nephrostomic catheter or ureteral double J); in other cases the urinoma can get infected due to the urinary stasis, needing a percutaneous drainage.

Follow-up CT or MRI may be necessary to assess interval change in the appearance of the injury [21, 71].

Segmental Infarct

Segmental infarct appears as a sharply demarcated, dorsal, or ventral segmental region of decreased enhancement of the parenchyma (type II Federle); it is present in approximately 10% of renal injuries and seen on MDCT as a wedge-shaped, sharply demarcated hypodense lesion involving the renal parenchyma, with a subcapsular basis and the apex toward the hilum; it is caused by a traumatic dissection and/or thrombosis of segmental vessels (AAST V) (see Fig. 19.12). Vascular thrombosis and a segmental area of parenchymal infarction can be seen also with Doppler and with CEUS as feeling defect in the vessel or an area of anechoic parenchyma surrounded by the normally hyperechoic vascular parenchyma.

Management is usually conservatory, but if it involves more than 50% of the renal parenchyma, a surgical debridement is indicated.

19.3.3 Catastrophic Lesions

These lesions (type III Federle) consist in vascular injury involving the vascular pedicle (AAST V); they represent approximately 5% of all renal injuries and thus generally require an interventional intravascular and/or surgical approach.

Part of this group is multiple severe lacerations generating three or more devascularized fragments (shattered kidney) and arterial and/or venous vascular pedicle lesions.

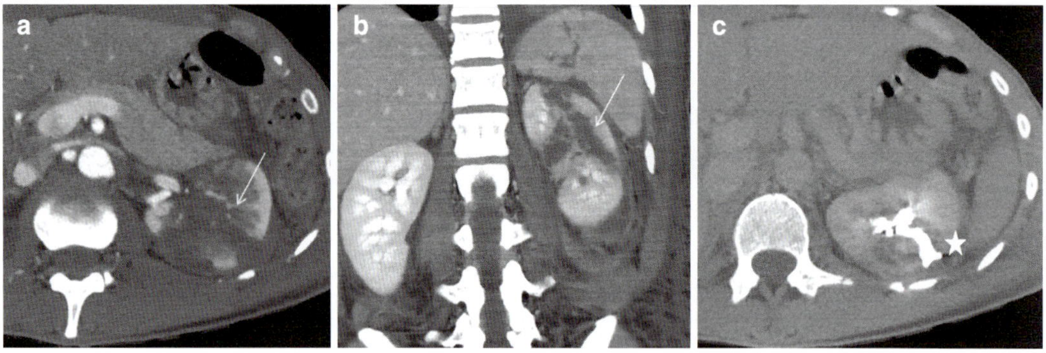

Fig. 19.15 Shattered kidney: multiple deep clefts (*arrow*) are identified on post-contrast images (**a**), (**b**) and (**c**); in the excretory phase in (**c**), an important involvement of the collective system is seen, with abundant urine extravasation trough the clefts (star).

For this category of lesions, the leading imaging modality is MDCT with contrast media administration, due to its capability to visualize the active bleeding differentiating it from urine extravasation.

19.3.3.1 Imaging Findings

Shattered Kidney

The shattered kidney and renal pedicle avulsion represent some of the most severe renal injuries, since they determine a complete devascularization of the kidney, leading to a nephrectomy.

The term shattered kidney refers to gross renal parenchymal disruption by multiple lacerations; these injuries are frequently associated with multiple areas of renal infarction [73].

In rare cases (hemodynamic stability, non-expanding perinephric hematoma, scarce or absent urine extravasation), an interventional approach can be attempted, with a vascular embolization and a percutaneous drainage of the hematoma.

On MDCT in a shattered kidney, the gland has lost its normal morphology and structure, with multiple deep clefts passing through the renal parenchyma and collecting system, creating devitalized fragments due to a lack of vascular supply; these non-enhancing segments may not be depicted because of the presence of a large perinephric hematoma, which appears hypodense (Fig. 19.15). Within this hematoma, often foci of active arterial bleeding can be visualized as a patchy hyperdense area (with a density of 85–370 HU; mean, 132 HU) that is best appreciated at dynamic contrast-enhanced CT.

Vascular Injury Involving the Renal Pedicle

The most significant vascular injury following blunt trauma is thrombosis of the main renal artery. The other vascular injuries comprise vein thrombosis and renal artery avulsion [81].

Deceleration forces dislocate the kidneys in the retroperitoneal adipose space, causing a stretching and tearing of the intima and the formation of an intimal flap, which leads to the formation of blood clots and arterial thrombosis; in blunt trauma, this rarely is complete. More often a segmental or subsegmental infarction occurs. The renal artery occlusion occurs in higher percentage of cases at the proximal-medial third of the kidney with a distal distribution.

On MDCT the non-visualization of the whole kidney, correlated to the absence of perinephric hematoma, should give the suspect of main renal artery thrombosis (Fig. 19.16) although other causes should be excluded, such as renal vascular spasm due to severe contusion, renal pedicle avulsion, or high-grade urinary obstruction. If the thrombus is detectable, it appears as an endovascular filling defect, hyperdense on unenhanced CT images, and hypodense on enhanced scans. A "cortical rim sign" can be rarely observed (it usually is seen after at least 8 h), in which the peripheral cortex and renal capsule show a higher enhancement, as perfusion is maintained by the renal capsular artery (Fig. 19.17).

If this kind of condition is depicted, the treatment decision has to be chosen also keeping in mind a 2 h time limit for revascularization.

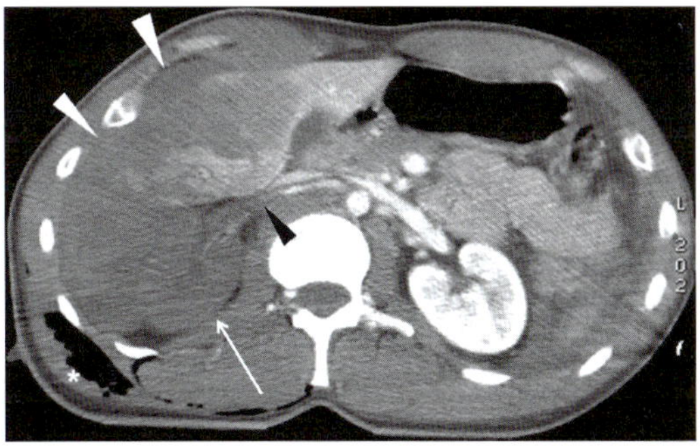

Fig. 19.16 Contrast-enhanced axial CT scan, arterial phase, shows the complete ischemia of the right kidney (*white arrow*), due to renal artery thrombosis (*black arrowhead*). Note the huge intraparenchymal hepatic hematoma (*white arrowheads*) and the subcutaneous emphysema (*asterisk*)

Renal vein thrombosis is a rare condition in blunt trauma; the vein is dilated and not compressible during the ultrasound evaluation; in acute conditions, the thrombus is hypoechoic and difficult to visualize. In case of complete renal vein thrombosis, the eco-color-Doppler examination doesn't show any flow, and several signs can be associated, such as kidney enlargement, the absence of intraparenchymal flow, and the presence of a collateral venous system at the kidney hilum. On MDCT an endovascular filling defect (in case of partial thrombosis) or absent filling (complete thrombosis) of the distended renal vein is seen, associated with nephromegaly, delayed nephrographic progression, reduced nephrogram (Fig. 19.18), or delayed excretion of contrast material into the collecting system due to the acute venous hypertension.

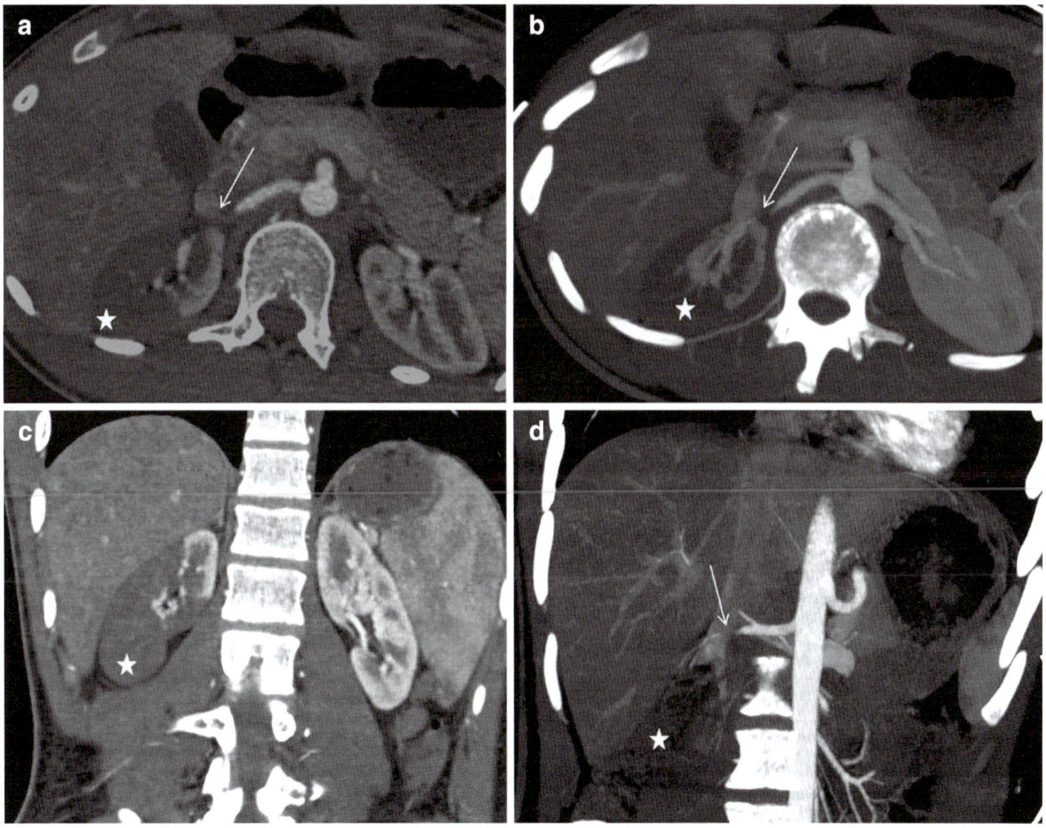

Fig. 19.17 Contrast-enhanced CT (**a–d**) demonstrates the absence of vascularization of most of the right kidney on post-contrast images (*star*), caused by thrombosis of the main renal artery seen as a filling defect (*arrow*) on the arterial phase (**a** and **d**)

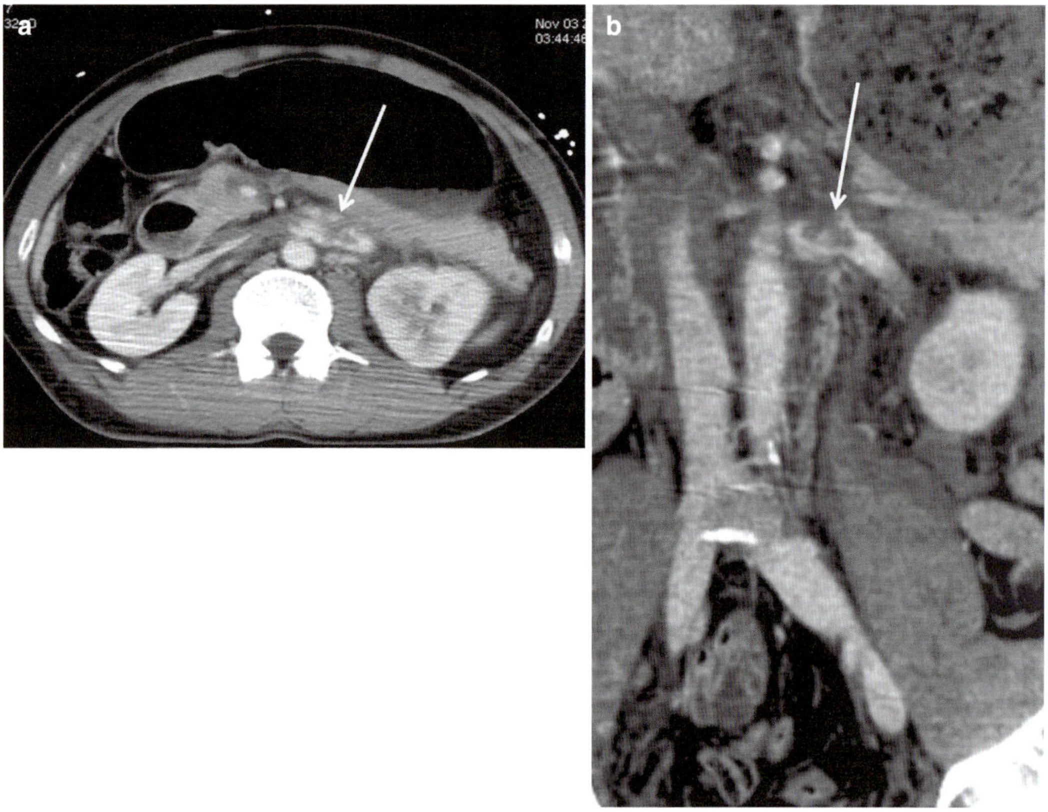

Fig. 19.18 Contrast-enhanced CT, axial scan (**a**), and coronal reconstruction (**b**) show the filling defect in the left renal vein (*arrows*), due to partial thrombosis. The left kidney has a reduced parenchymal enhancement with respect to the right kidney

Avulsion of the renal artery is a rare life-threatening condition in blunt trauma, not often seen on CT, due to the hemodynamical instability of the patient; caused by tearing of the tunica muscularis and adventitia, it is associated with global renal infarction (seen on CT as a completely or largely devascularized kidney) (see Fig. 19.16) and large perinephric hematoma (mainly distributed medially to the renal hilum), with important contrast material extravasation between the kidney and the aorta, which becomes larger in the venous phase, with a higher density than the one of the aorta (active arterial bleeding). In case of renal vein avulsion, the perinephric hematoma is self-limiting due to the compression of the perirenal adipose tissue. Renal enhancement is usually delayed and reduced, but uniformly present. In case of avulsion of the renal hilum, a total absence of parenchymal enhancement is found at MDCT and CEUS [61, 82].

19.3.4 Ureteropelvic Junction Injuries

This group comprises ureteropelvic junction injuries, a rare consequence of blunt trauma. In case of sudden deceleration and hyperextension, the relative mobility in the retroperitoneal space of the kidney compared to the aorta and vertebrae can cause traction and tension on the renal pedicle.

A predisposing condition is congenital or secondary obstructive uropathy, which causes chronic renal pelvis dilatation.

Keep in mind that in 30% of cases, these injuries occur in the absence of hematuria and the diagnosis may be delayed.

This kind of damage is mentioned in Category IV of the Federle classification, corresponding to grade V of the AAST injury scale.

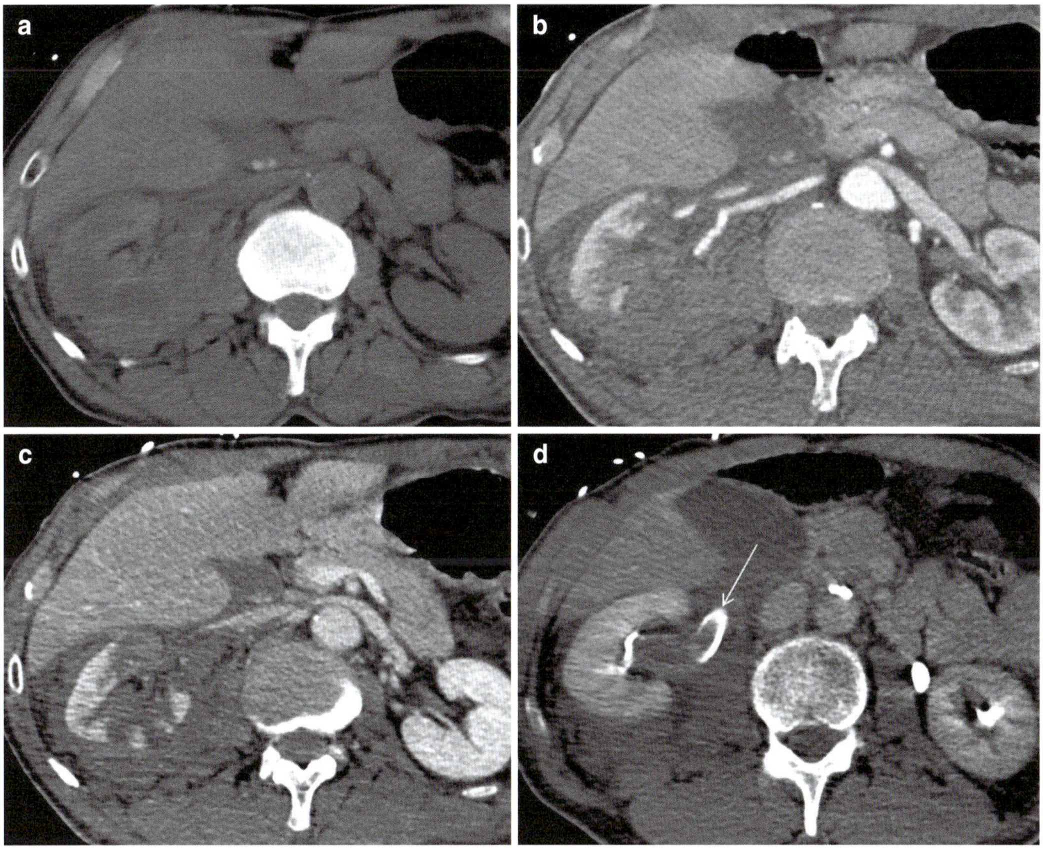

Fig. 19.19 Renal pedicle injury: perirenal hematoma and inhomogeneous parenchyma are already seen on direct scan (**a**); on arterial phase (**b**) an incomplete vascularization of the kidney is seen, with multiple deep clefts, better visualized on venous phase (**c**); in the excretory phase, the urine runs along the renal pelvis toward the ureter, surrounding it (**d**) (*arrow*)

The ureteropelvic junction can be completely transected (avulsion) or incompletely teared (laceration). In these cases an excretory phase imaging is necessary to visualize correctly the injury; in fact in both situations, urine extravasation surrounding the ureteropelvic junction is present (circumrenal urinoma), typically without hematoma, and the presence of contrast material in the ureter distal to the ureteropelvic junction helps differentiate laceration from avulsion (Fig. 19.19). However, when neither CT nor intravenous urography unequivocally demonstrates ipsilateral ureteral filling, retrograde pyelography should be performed [21].

Treatment of avulsion of the ureteropelvic junction is always surgical; laceration can also be treated in some cases conservatively with or without stent placement.

19.4 Other Nonclassified Renal Injuries

Contained vascular lesions such as pseudoaneurysm and arteriovenous fistulae are lesions that can be identified on CT imaging, but are not classified in the AAST or Federle injury scale.

Pseudoaneurysm or false aneurysm occurs when all three layers of the arterial wall (intima, media, and adventitia) are disrupted and the blood pool is external to the vessel, without an own wall but contained by the surrounding connective tissue.

On eco-color-Doppler ultrasound, a pulsatile flow sign is seen within the lesion (with a swirling pattern), and documentation of the to-and-fro flow with spectral Doppler is essential to make diagnosis.

On MDCT it is identified as a round or oval area, with a size between 5 mm and 5 cm, of vascular origin, and hyperdense in the arterial phase, next to the vessel, with a decrease in attenuation in the following post-contrast phases, similar to the aorta. This behavior is useful to distinguish it from active bleeding, which increases in size and retain a higher attenuation than the aorta on delayed imaging.

Pseudoaneurysms of the main renal artery branches may require embolization, in contrast to the ones of the main renal artery that require surgical treatment by stent positioning.

An arteriovenous fistula is an abnormal connection between an artery and a vein, which on eco-color-Doppler imaging may be visualized directly, with an abnormal high-velocity flow.

On MDCT it is seen as an early intensity of the renal vein, which is usually larger in diameter and lower attenuation on the parenchymal phase due to the "stolen effect" of the enhanced blood. Differential diagnosis with pseudoaneurysm can be difficult and only resolved by angiography.

19.5 Traumatic Injuries to Kidneys with Preexisting Abnormalities

A kidney with a preexisting abnormality is at increased risk for injury [83]. An underlying renal disorder may be first brought to medical attention because the severity of the patient's symptoms is disproportionate to the degree of injury suffered.

Trauma to an abnormal kidney occurs more frequently in children than in adults. Such injuries include disruption of the renal pelvis or ureteropelvic junction in patients with hydronephrosis or an extrarenal pelvis intracystic hemorrhage or rupture of a renal cyst with or without communication with the collecting system, rupture of a tumor, laceration of poorly protected ectopic or horseshoe kidneys (Fig. 19.20) [50, 53], and laceration of fragile, infected kidneys.

CT provides more specific and clinically useful information than excretory urography in this context [84].

19.6 Complications

Complication of renal injury mostly occurs within 1 month from the traumatic event with a wide range from 3 to 33% of all kidney injuries. Early complications include urinoma, urinary fistula, infected urinoma or perinephric abscess, pseudoaneurysm, delayed bleeding, persistent hematuria, and hypertension.

Late complications include A-V fistula, hydronephrosis, delayed hypertension, calculus formation, and chronic pyelonephritis.

Low-grade lesions usually resolve completely without complications, and high-grade lesions instead often result in the formation of one or more scars, which can be responsible of obstructive conditions, with urinary stasis, calculi, or infection.

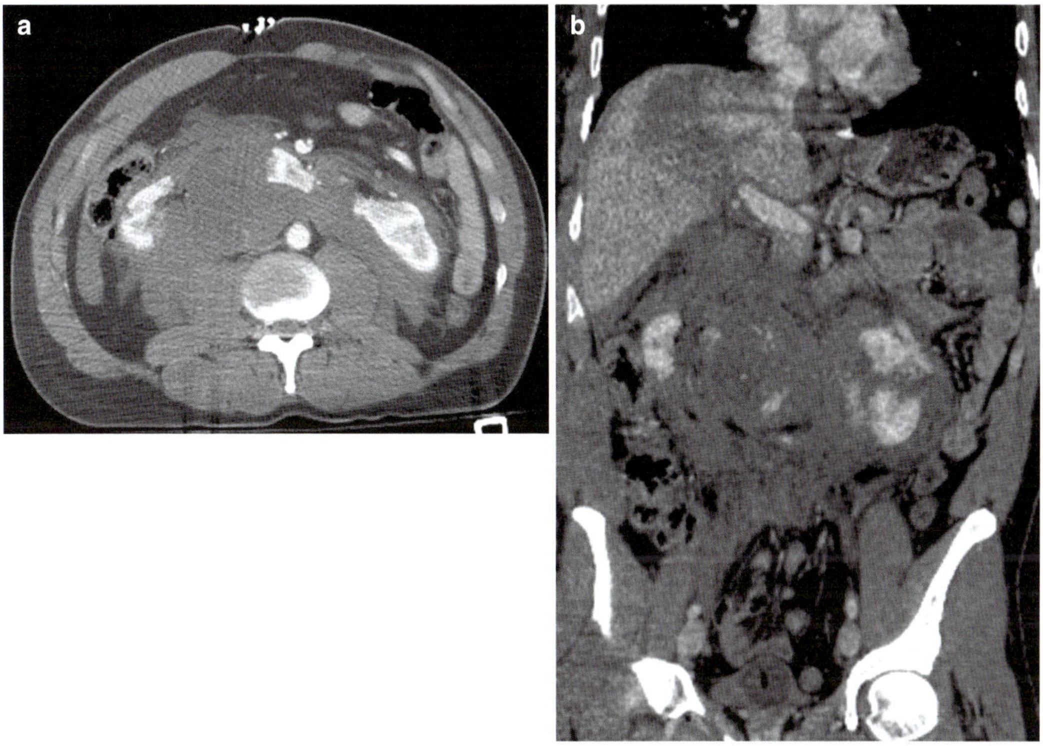

Fig. 19.20 Contrast-enhanced CT, axial scan (**a**), and coronal reconstruction (**b**) show a complete fracture of the middle part of a horseshoe kidney, with huge retroperitoneal hematoma

References

1. Wessells H, Suh D, Porter JR, et al. Renal injury and operative management in the United States: results of a population-based study. J Trauma. 2003;54:423–30. doi:10.1097/01.TA.0000051932.28456.F4.
2. Morey AF, Brandes S, Dugi DD III, et al. Urotrauma: AUA guideline. J Urol. 2014;192:327–35. doi:10.1016/j.juro.2014.05.004. Epub 20 May 2014.
3. Safir MH, McAninch JW. Diagnosis and management of trauma to the kidney. Curr Opin Urol. 1999;9:227–31.
4. Bruce LM, Croce MA, Santaniello JM, et al. Blunt renal artery injury: incidence, diagnosis, and management. Am Surg. 2001;67:550–4; discussion 555–6.
5. Lee YJ, Oh SN, Rha SE, Byun JY. Renal trauma. Radiol Clin North Am. 2007;45:581–92, ix. doi:10.1016/j.rcl.2007.04.004.
6. Park SJ, Kim JK, Kim KW, Cho KS. MDCT findings of renal trauma. AJR Am J Roentgenol. 2006;187:541–7. doi:10.2214/AJR.05.0543.
7. Jankowski JT, Spirnak JP. Current recommendations for imaging in the management of urologic traumas. Urol Clin North Am. 2006;33:365–76. doi:10.1016/j.ucl.2006.04.004.
8. Paparel P, N'Diaye A, Laumon B, et al. The epidemiology of trauma of the genitourinary system after traffic accidents: analysis of a register of over 43000 victims. BJU Int. 2006;97:338–41. doi:10.1111/j.1464-410X.2006.05900.x.
9. Kansas BT, Eddy MJ, Mydlo JH, Uzzo RG. Incidence and management of penetrating renal trauma in patients with multiorgan injury: extended experience at an inner city trauma center. J Urol. 2004;172:1355–60.
10. Santucci RA, Wessells II, Bartsch G, et al. Evaluation and management of renal injuries: consensus statement of the renal trauma subcommittee. BJU Int. 2004;93:937–54. doi:10.1111/j.1464-4096.2004.04820.x.
11. Shariat SF, Jenkins A, Roehrborn CG, et al. Features and outcomes of patients with grade IV renal injury. BJU Int. 2008;102:728–33; discussion 733. doi:10.1111/j.1464-410X.2008.07638.x. Epub 24 Apr 2008.
12. Smith J, Caldwell E, D'Amours S, et al. Abdominal trauma: a disease in evolution. ANZ J Surg. 2005;75:790–4. doi:10.1111/j.1445-2197.2005.03524.x.
13. Sangthong B, Demetriades D, Martin M, et al. Management and hospital outcomes of blunt renal artery injuries: analysis of 517 patients

from the National Trauma Data Bank. J Am Coll Surg. 2006;203:612–7. doi:10.1016/j.jamcollsurg.2006.07.004. Epub 27 Sep 2006.
14. Najibi S, Tannast M, Latini JM. Civilian gunshot wounds to the genitourinary tract: incidence, anatomic distribution, associated injuries, and outcomes. Urology. 2010;76:977–81; discussion 981. doi:10.1016/j.urology.2010.01.092.
15. Goldman SM, Sandler CM. Urogenital trauma: imaging upper GU trauma. Eur J Radiol. 2004;50:84–95. doi:10.1016/j.ejrad.2003.11.018.
16. Broghammer JA, Fisher MB, Santucci RA. Conservative management of renal trauma: a review. Urology. 2007;70:623–9. doi:10.1016/j.urology.2007.06.1085.
17. Santucci RA, Fisher MB. The literature increasingly supports expectant (conservative) management of renal trauma-a systematic review. J Trauma. 2005;59:493–503.
18. Razali MR, Azian AA, Amran AR, Azlin S. Computed tomography of blunt renal trauma. Singap Med J. 2010;51:468–73; quiz 474.
19. The American Association of Surgery for the Surgery of Trauma. Injury scoring scale. http://www.aast.org/Library/TraumaTools/injuryscoringscales.aspx
20. Moore EE, Shackford SR, Pachter HL, et al. Organ injury scaling: spleen, liver, and kidney. J Trauma. 1989;29:1664–6.
21. Kawashima A, Sandler CM, Corl FM, et al. Imaging of renal trauma: a comprehensive review. Radiographics. 2001;21:557–74. doi:10.1148/radiographics.21.3.q01ma11557.
22. Federle MP, Kaiser JA, McAnninch JW, et al. The role of computed tomography in renal trauma. Radiology. 1981;141:455–60. doi:10.1148/radiology.141.2.7291573.
23. Dugi DD III, Morey AF, Gupta A, et al. American Association for the Surgery of Trauma grade 4 renal injury substratification into grades 4a (low risk) and 4b (high risk). J Urol. 2010;183:592–7. doi:10.1016/j.juro.2009.10.015. Epub 16 Dec 2009.
24. Buckley JC, McAninch JW. Revision of current American Association for the Surgery of Trauma renal injury grading system. J Trauma. 2011;70:35–7. doi:10.1097/TA.0b013e318207ad5a.
25. Holmes JF, McGahan JP, Wisner DH. Rate of intra-abdominal injury after a normal abdominal computed tomographic scan in adults with blunt trauma. Am J Emerg Med. 2012;30:574–9. doi:10.1016/j.ajem.2011.02.016.
26. Alsikafi NF, McAninch JW, Elliott SP, Garcia M. Nonoperative management outcomes of isolated urinary extravasation following renal lacerations due to external trauma. J Urol. 2006;176:2494–7. doi:10.1016/j.juro.2006.08.015.
27. Jansen JO, Inaba K, Resnick S, et al. Selective non-operative management of abdominal gunshot wounds: survey of practise. Injury. 2013;44:639–44. doi:10.1016/j.injury.2012.01.023. Epub 15 Feb 2012.
28. Buckley JC, McAninch JW. Selective management of isolated and nonisolated grade IV renal injuries. J Urol. 2006;176:2498–502; discussion 2502. doi:10.1016/j.juro.2006.07.141.
29. Hope WW, Smith ST, Medieros B, et al. Nonoperative management in penetrating abdominal trauma: is it feasible at a Level II trauma center? J Emerg Med. 2012;43:190–5. doi:10.1016/j.jemermed.2011.06.060. Epub 1 Nov 2011.
30. DuBose J, Inaba K, Teixeira PG, et al. Selective nonoperative management of solid organ injury following abdominal gunshot wounds. Injury. 2007;38:1084–90. doi:10.1016/j.injury.2007.02.030.
31. Lanchon C, Fiard G, Arnoux V, et al. High grade blunt renal trauma: predictors of surgery and long-term outcomes of conservative management. A Prospective Single Center Study. J Urol. 2016;195:106–11. doi:10.1016/j.juro.2015.07.100. Epub 6 Aug 2015.
32. Shoobridge JJ, Bultitude MF, Koukounaras J, et al. A 9-year experience of renal injury at an Australian level 1 trauma centre. BJU Int. 2013;112(Suppl 2):53–60. doi:10.1111/bju.12003.
33. van der Wilden GM, Velmahos GC, Joseph DK, et al. Successful nonoperative management of the most severe blunt renal injuries: a multicenter study of the research consortium of New England Centers for Trauma. JAMA Surg. 2013;148:924–31. doi:10.1001/jamasurg.2013.2747.
34. Armenakas NA, Duckett CP, McAninch JW. Indications for nonoperative management of renal stab wounds. J Urol. 1999;161:768–71.
35. Glass AS, Appa AA, Kenfield SA, et al. Selective angioembolization for traumatic renal injuries: a survey on clinician practice. World J Urol. 2014;32:821–7. doi:10.1007/s00345-013-1169-1.
36. Schmidlin FR, Iselin CE, Naimi A, et al. The higher injury risk of abnormal kidneys in blunt renal trauma. Scand J Urol Nephrol. 1998;32:388–92.
37. McAninch JW, Carroll PR, Klosterman PW, et al. Renal reconstruction after injury. J Urol. 1991;145:932–7.
38. Hammer CC, Santucci RA. Effect of an institutional policy of nonoperative treatment of grades I to IV renal injuries. J Urol. 2003;169:1751–3. doi:10.1097/01.ju.0000056186.77495.c8.
39. Valentino M, Ansaloni L, Catena F, et al. Contrast-enhanced ultrasonography in blunt abdominal trauma: considerations after 5 years of experience. Radiol Med. 2009;114:1080–93. doi:10.1007/s11547-009-0444-0.
40. Poletti PA, Wintermark M, Schnyder P, Becker CD. Traumatic injuries: role of imaging in the management of the polytrauma victim (conservative expectation). Eur Radiol. 2002;12:969–78. doi:10.1007/s00330-002-1353-y. Epub 15 Mar 2002.
41. Sessa B, Trinci M, Ianniello S, et al. Blunt abdominal trauma: role of contrast-enhanced ultrasound (CEUS) in the detection and staging of abdominal traumatic lesions compared to US and CE-MDCT. Radiol Med. 2015;120:180–9. doi:10.1007/s11547-014-0425-9. Epub 25 Jun 2014.
42. Catalano O, Aiani L, Barozzi L, et al. CEUS in abdominal trauma: multi-center study. Abdom Imaging. 2009;34:225–34. doi:10.1007/s00261-008-9452-0.

43. Pinto F, Miele V, Scaglione M, Pinto A. The use of contrast-enhanced ultrasound in blunt abdominal trauma: advantages and limitations. Acta Radiol. 2014;55:776–84. doi:10.1177/0284185113505517.
44. Pinto F, Valentino M, Romanini L, Basilico R, Miele V. The role of CEUS in the assessment of haemodynamically stable patients with blunt abdominal trauma. Radiol Med. 2015;120:3–11. doi:10.1007/s11547-014-0455-3. Epub 21 Aug 2014.
45. Morey AF, Brandes S, Dugi DD III, et al. Urotrauma: AUA guideline. Copyright © 2014 American Urological Association Education and Research, Inc.®; (published 2014–amended 2017). http://www.auanet.org/guidelines/urotrauma-(2014-amended-2017)
46. Sheth S, Casalino DD, Remer EM, et al. Appropriateness criteria: renal trauma. American College of Radiology; 2012.
47. McCombie SP, Thyer I, Corcoran NM, et al. The conservative management of renal trauma: a literature review and practical clinical guideline from Australia and New Zealand. BJU Int. 2014;114(Suppl 1):13–21. doi:10.1111/bju.12902.
48. Mee SL, McAninch JW, Robinson AL, et al. Radiographic assessment of renal trauma: a 10 years prospective study of patient selection. J Urol. 1989;141:1095–8.
49. Kurtz MP, Eswara JR, Vetter JM, et al. Blunt abdominal trauma from motor vehicle collisions from 2007 to 2011: renal injury probability and severity in children versus adults. J Urol. 2017;197:906–10. doi:10.1016/j.juro.2016.07.085. Epub 16 Dec 2016.
50. Miele V, Piccolo CL, Trinci M, Galluzzo M, Ianniello S, Brunese L. Diagnostic imaging of blunt abdominal trauma in pediatric patients. Radiol Med. 2016;121:409–30. doi:10.1007/s11547-016-0637-2.
51. Valentino M, Serra C, Zironi G, et al. Blunt abdominal trauma: emergency contrast-enhanced sonography for detection of solid organ injuries. AJR Am J Roentgenol. 2006;186:1361–7. doi:10.2214/AJR.05.0027.
52. Körner M, Krötz MM, Degenhart C, et al. Current role of emergency US in patients with major trauma. RadioGraphics. 2008;28:225–42. doi:10.1148/rg.281075047.
53. Miele V, Piccolo CL, Galluzzo M, et al. Contrast-enhanced ultrasound (CEUS) in blunt abdominal trauma. Br J Radiol. 2016;89:20150823. doi:10.1259/bjr.20150823. Epub 8 Jan 2016.
54. Kitrey ND, Djakovic N, Gonsalves M, et al. EAU guidelines on urological trauma. Updated 2017. uroweb.org/guideline/urological-trauma/
55. Poletti PA, Platon A, Becker CD, et al. Blunt abdominal trauma: does the use of a second-generation sonographic contrast agent help to detect solid organ injuries? AJR Am J Roentgenol. 2004;183:1293–301. doi:10.2214/ajr.183.5.1831293.
56. Regine G, Atzori M, Miele V, et al. Second-generation sonographic contrast agents in the evaluation of renal trauma. Radiol Med. 2007;112:581–587. Epub 11 June 2007. doi:10.1007/s11547-007-0164-2.
57. Valentino M, De Luca C, Galloni SS, et al. Contrast-enhanced US evaluation in patients with blunt abdominal trauma. J Ultrasound. 2010;13:22–7. doi:10.1016/j.jus.2010.06.002. Epub 8 Jul 2010.
58. Mihalik JE, Smith RS, Toevs CC, et al. The use of contrast-enhanced ultrasound for the evaluation of solid abdominal organ injury in patients with blunt abdominal trauma. J Trauma Acute Care Surg. 2012;73:1100–5. doi:10.1097/TA.0b013e31825a74b5.
59. Cagini L, Gravante S, Malaspina CM, et al. Contrast enhanced ultrasound (CEUS) in blunt abdominal trauma. Crit Ultrasound J. 2013;5(Suppl 1):S9. doi:10.1186/2036-7902-5-S1-S9.
60. Menichini G, Sessa B, Trinci M, Galluzzo M, Miele V. Accuracy of Contrast-Enhanced Ultrasound (CEUS) in the identification and characterization of traumatic solid organ lesions in children: a retrospective comparison with baseline-US and CE-MDCT. Radiol Med. 2015;120:989–1001. doi:10.1007/s11547-015-0535-z. Epub 31 Mar 2015.
61. Valentino M, Serra C, Pavlica P, Barozzi L. Contrast-enhanced ultrasound for blunt abdominal trauma. Semin Ultrasound CT MR. 2007;28:130–40.
62. Huber-Wagner S, Lefering R, Qvick LM, et al. Effect of whole-body CT during trauma resuscitation on survival: a retrospective, multicentre study. Lancet. 2009;373:1455–61. doi:10.1016/S0140-6736(09)60232-4.
63. Heller MT, Schnor N. MDCT of renal trauma: correlation to AAST organ injury scale. Clin Imaging. 2014;38:410–7. doi:10.1016/j.clinimag.2014.02.001. Epub 24 Feb 2014.
64. Dane B, Baxter AB, Bernstein MP. Imaging genitourinary trauma. Radiol Clin North Am. 2017;55:321–35. doi:10.1016/j.rcl.2016.10.007. Epub 27 Dec 2016.
65. Gross JA, Lehnert BE, Linnau KF, et al. Imaging of urinary system trauma. Radiol Clin North Am. 2015;53:773–88, ix. doi:10.1016/j.rcl.2015.02.005. Epub 9 Apr 2015.
66. Colling KP, Irwin ED, Byrnes MC, et al. Computed tomography scans with intravenous contrast: low incidence of contrast-induced nephropathy in blunt trauma patients. J Trauma Acute Care Surg. 2014;77:226–30. doi:10.1097/TA.0000000000000336.
67. Ku JH, Jeon YS, Kim ME, et al. Is there a role for magnetic resonance imaging in renal trauma? Int J Urol. 2001;8:261–7.
68. Leppäniemi A, Lamminen A, Tervahartiala P, et al. MRI and CT in blunt renal trauma: an update. Semin Ultrasound CT MR. 1997;18:129–35.
69. Sarani B, Powell E, Taddeo J, et al. Contemporary comparison of surgical and interventional arteriography management of blunt renal injury. J Vasc Interv Radiol. 2011;22:723–8. doi:10.1016/j.jvir.2011.01.444.
70. McAninch JW, Santucci RA. Renal and ureteral injuries. In: Gillenwater JY, Grayhack JT, Howards SS, Mitchell ME, editors. Adult and pediatric urology.

Philadelphia: Lippincott Williams & Wilkins; 2002. p. 451–83.
71. Miele V, Piccolo CL, Sessa B, Trinci M, Galluzzo M. Comparison between MRI and CEUS in the follow-up of patients with blunt abdominal trauma managed conservatively. Radiol Med. 2016;121:27–37. doi:10.1007/s11547-015-0578-1. Epub 8 Jan 2016.
72. Morey AF, McAninch JW, Tiller BK, et al. Single shot intraoperative excretory urography for the immediate evaluation of renal trauma. J Urol. 1999;161:1088–92.
73. Harris AC, Zwirewich CV, Lyburn ID, et al. CT findings in blunt renal trauma. Radiographics. 2001;21:S201-14. https://doi.org/10.1148/radiographics.21.suppl_1.g01oc07s201
74. Ramchandani P, Buckler PM. Imaging of genitourinary trauma. AJR Am J Roentgenol. 2009;192:1514–23. doi:10.2214/AJR.09.2470.
75. Scialpi M, Mazzei MA, Barberini F, et al. Traumi del surrene. In: Miele V, Scaglione M, Grassi R, Rotondo A, editors. Diagnostica per immagini del trauma maggiore. Milano: Elsevier Masson; 2010. p. 193–203.
76. Knudson MM, Maull KI. Nonoperative management of solid organ injuries. Past, present and future. Surg Clin North Am. 1999;79:1357–71.
77. Brandes SB, McAninch JW. Reconstructive surgery for trauma of the upper urinary tract. Urol Clin North Am. 1999;26:183–99, x.
78. Shanmuganathan K, Mirvis SE, Sover ER. Value of contrast-enhanced CT in detecting active hemorrhage in patients with blunt abdominal or pelvic trauma. AJR Am J Roentgenol. 1993;161:65–9. doi:10.2214/ajr.161.1.8517323.
79. Jeffrey RB Jr, Cardoza JD, Olcott EW. Detection of active intraabdominal arterial hemorrhage: value of dynamic contrast-enhanced CT. AJR Am J Roentgenol. 1991;156:725–9. doi:10.2214/ajr.156.4.2003435.
80. Shanmuganathan K, Mirvis SE, Reaney SM. Pictorial review: CT appearances of contrast medium extravasations associated with injury sustained from blunt abdominal trauma. Clin Radiol. 1995;50:182–7.
81. Regine G, Stasolla A, Miele V. Multidetector computed tomography of the renal arteries in vascular emergencies. Eur J Radiol. 2007;64:83–91. doi:10.1016/j.ejrad.2007.06.007.
82. Cokkinos D, Antypa E, Stefanidis K, et al. Contrast-enhanced ultrasound for imaging blunt abdominal trauma—indications, description of the technique and imaging review. Ultraschall Med. 2012;33:60–7. doi: 10.1055/s-0031-1273442. Epub 24 Jan 2012.
83. Pollack HM, Wein AJ. Imaging of renal trauma. Radiology. 1989;172:297–308.
84. Rhyner P, Federle MP, Jeffrey RB. CT of trauma to the abnormal kidney. AJR Am J Roentgenol. 1984;142:747–50. doi:10.2214/ajr.142.4.747.

Pelvic Trauma: Bone

20

Michele Galluzzo, Francesco Gaudino, Gloria Addeo, Grazia Loretta Buquicchio, Ginevra Danti, Margherita Trinci, and Vittorio Miele

20.1 Introduction

The incidence of pelvic ring disruption (PRD) is constantly increasing due to the exponential high number of motor vehicle accidents (60–80% of cases), falls from a height especially at work (10–30% of cases), crush injuries (5–10% of cases), certain sports especially in those disciplines called extremes, and suicide attempts [1–3]. Pelvic fractures represent 2–8% of all skeletal injuries. The incidence and the complexity of trauma caused by high-speed motor vehicle accidents are increased, despite the evolution and the use of sophisticated security and protection vehicle systems [4, 5].

The distribution of this type of trauma is usually bimodal. The first peak is between 30 and 50 years and is often associated with high-energy trauma, and the prevalence is higher in male compared to female with a proportion of 3:1. The second peak is represented by patients older than 65 years, in which also a low-energy trauma, often on a substrate of osteopenia, can cause fracture injuries sometimes with little clinical significance, generally stable, which do not need of surgical treatment. The prevalence in this group is higher in female (elderly women), with a proportion of 1:2 [4, 5].

High-energy trauma is determined by the combined action of one or more vector forces, and these patients are generally polytraumatized (75%), in a significant proportion (2:3), with high index of severity of trauma (ISS), in which occurs the combined presence of one or more life-threatening injuries, and are associated with high morbidity and mortality rates. Overall mortality in patients with pelvic fractures is 5–10%. For unstable pelvic fractures, especially with uncontrolled pelvic-related hemorrhage, the mortality rate is around 40% to 50% [1, 6, 7].

Hemodynamic instability, multiple organ failure (MOF, 20%), as direct consequences of pelvic hemorrhage, and sepsis are the primary causes of mortality after PRD [5].

Complications of pelvic ring are distinct in early, which occur in a percentage higher than 50% of cases (vascular, nervous, and visceral), intermediate, and late [8].

The mortality rate of patients with hypovolemic shock or hemorrhage remains high (7–17%) and challenging, in spite of the progress in the diagnosis and choice of therapeutic treatment to quickly stop the bleeding [9–15].

M. Galluzzo, M.D. (✉) • F. Gaudino
G.L. Buquicchio • M. Trinci
Department of Emergency Radiology, S. Camillo Hospital, C.ne Gianicolense, 87, 00152 Rome, Italy
e-mail: galluzzom@tiscali.it

G. Addeo • G. Danti • V. Miele
Department of Radiology, Careggi University Hospital, Florence, Italy

V. Miele, M. Trinci (eds.), *Diagnostic Imaging in Polytrauma Patients*,
https://doi.org/10.1007/978-3-319-62054-1_20

The pelvic ring fracture, especially when unstable, may be the cause of hemorrhagic shock in patients, excluding those with the presence of abdominal parenchyma injuries.

Vascular complications, generally due to arterial, venous and bone bleeding, single or often multiple, most commonly associated with complex pelvic ring disruption and especially pelvic fractures, may increase the compliance of the pelvic bone. When a significant increase of pelvic compliance happens, If there had been a significant increase in the pelvic compliance, it is important the early identification of potential bleeding sources followed by prompt measures to minimize blood loss.

Soft tissue involvement is cause of acute and late complications and can develop serious infections culminating in septic shock conditions.

Pelvic fractures are defined "open" (2–4% of all pelvic injuries), when there are direct continuous solutions between the skin wound of the perineum or of the genitals and the fracture site. They are most commonly seen in young males involved in traffic accidents and range from small penetrating wounds that are at low risk of fecal contaminations and can be treated with medical therapy and through injury toilette to the complete traumatic hemipelvectomy.

Together with these types of fractures often occurs the disruption of the pelvic floor musculature, leading to the loss of tamponade effect and persistent bleeding. Despite the advances in care and treatment of aggressive fractures, the mortality rate of open pelvic fractures remains as high as 25–50%, if not promptly treated, and this high rate justifies the definition of "ultimate" or "lethal" for the open pelvic fractures [1, 5, 8, 15].

"Late" complications of pelvic bone fractures are predominantly orthopedic (pseudoarthrosis, defects of fracture's consolidation, deformity, or dysmetria of lower limbs) and/or neurological (chronic low back pain, sphincter disorders, sexual dysfunction, and disorders of the birth canal) [14].

Pelvic ring fractures are associated with different types of injuries in other districts generally in relation with the trauma dynamics.

Secondary to high-energy trauma, pelvic ring fractures are commonly associated with injuries to other body systems: brain injuries (35–51%), long bone fractures (48%), peripheral nerve injury (26%), chest trauma (20%), spleen (10%) or liver injuries (7%), urogenital system (kidney, >15%; male urethra or bladder, >15%), bowel trauma (5–18%), mesentery (4%), diaphragm (2%), nerve injuries (>20%), and in more of 2% of cases thoracic aorta injury [5, 10, 11, 15–17].

The incidence of urethra lesions is higher in male for the anatomical differences. In men, due to the anatomical gender differences in the area, the incidence of urethra lesions is higher than in women. In man, the bulbar portion downstream along the urogenital diaphragm is more prone to urethral lesions. The urethra is short in the female, while the male in the bulbous portion downstream of the urogenital diaphragm is more easily susceptible to lesion mechanisms.

20.2 Relevant Anatomy and Biomechanics

It is important to know the anatomy and biomechanical concepts of the bone and ligamentous pelvic structures to understand the general mechanisms of injury, the functions of these structures in pelvic stability, and their influence on the diagnosis and management of different kinds of lesions [18].

The pelvis is a complex structure with a small and rigid cavity that contains important nervous, vascular, gastrointestinal, and genitourinary structures.

The arcuate lines and the sacral promontory determine the outer bony edges so-called pelvic brim: this allows distinguishing the true pelvis from the false pelvis. The superior portion of the pelvis is known as the greater pelvis (or false pelvis): it provides support for the lower abdominal viscera (the ileum and sigmoid colon). The inferior portion of the pelvis is known as the lesser pelvis (or "true" pelvis): within this reside the pelvis viscera and the pelvic diaphragm (the levator ani and coccygeal musculature), which constitute the pelvic floor. The junction between the greater and lesser pelvis is known as the pelvic inlet.

The pelvic bone is a ringlike structure composed of three bones including the sacrum, posteriorly the sacroiliac joints, and laterally and anteriorly the innominate bone which is formed by the fusion of the ilium, the ischium, and the pubis at the triradiate cartilage of the acetabulum at skeletal maturity, which are joined forward together to form anteriorly in the midline the pubic symphysis. At the symphysis the opposite surface is covered with fibrocartilage of fibrous tissue.

The symphysis biomechanically has the main function to stabilize the anterior pelvis, allowing a small degree of movement (up to 2 mm in the craniocaudal direction and up to 3° of rotation during walking), and to prevent the collapse of the pelvis in the upright position, contributing approximately to 40% of the stiffness of the pelvis. The large contact area of the joint allows a uniform distribution of the superior and inferior shear forces generated during walking and running, thus helping protect the joint from injury.

The pubic bones are the most common pelvic bones at risk for fracture due to the anatomical position of the anterior arch and to their thin structure.

The body burden is in fact transferred from the spine to the acetabulum and then to the legs through the so-called posterior sacroiliac complex, formed by the interosseous sacroiliac ligament complex, the posterior portions of the sacrum, and the iliac wings.

The stability of the pelvic ring does not depend exclusively on the osseous components, which do not have an inherent stability, but on the integrity of the ligamentous structures, and particularly these constitute together with the sacroiliac joints the posterior sacroiliac complex [4, 19].

The sacroiliac articulation (SI) is not a true synovial joint, and there is minimal intrinsic motion; the sacral portion is covered in cartilage, whereas the iliac component is with fibrocartilage. The width of the joint space is generally 2–4 mm [5]. In case of articular SI injury, they can generally determine three different conditions: The first is when the front and back parts of the joint are intact, the second is when the lesion is frontal (rotational instability), and the third is when involving both components (rotational and vertical instability).

According to Tile, the posterior sacroiliac complex, also known as the "posterior tension band," is conceptually comparable like a sort of "suspension bridge" where the sacrum represents the horizontal component (the bridge); the interosseous sacroiliac, a very strong ligament, acts as suspension bars; the posterior superior iliac spines behave as pillars; and the iliolumbar ligaments act as additional stabilizing elements that join the iliac crest to the transverse process of the fourth and fifth lumbar vertebrae [7–9, 18–24] (Scheme 20.1).

The pelvic ring rotational stability is possible by ligaments with a transverse-horizontal course (the anterior sacroiliac; the posterior sacroiliac "short" horizontal component; the sacrospinous, a strong ligamentous band extended from the posterior surface of the sacrum to the ischial spines; and the iliolumbar), which are opposed to the external rotation of the pelvis.

The vertical stability is possible by ligaments with a vertical course (the sacrotuberous extended from the posterior surface of the sacroiliac complex to the ischial tuberosity and the posterior sacroiliac "long" vertical component), which are opposed to vertical and multidirectional dislocation.

Conceptually, it is important to remember, because of its particular ring constitution, that for each injury caused by the action of a high-energy force vector in one area, it must always correspond to another bone or ligamentous lesion on the opposite side [9, 25, 26] (Scheme 20.2).

Exceptions to this rule are insufficiency fractures, due to trauma caused by "low-energy" force vectors, as it occurs in osteoporotic patients, in some stress fractures, or in avulsion fractures typical of adolescent sport injuries.

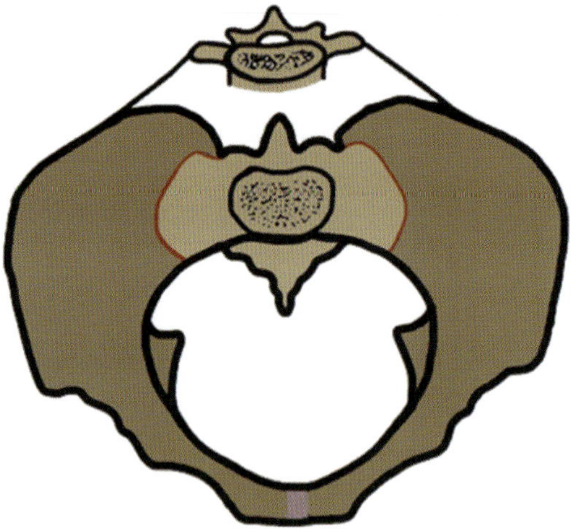

Scheme 20.1 Representation of the "posterior tension band" comparable to a "suspension bridge" where the sacrum represents the horizontal component (*red arrow*) and the iliolumbar ligaments as additional stabilizing elements that join the iliac crest to the transverse process of the fourth and fifth lumbar vertebrae (*black arrow*)

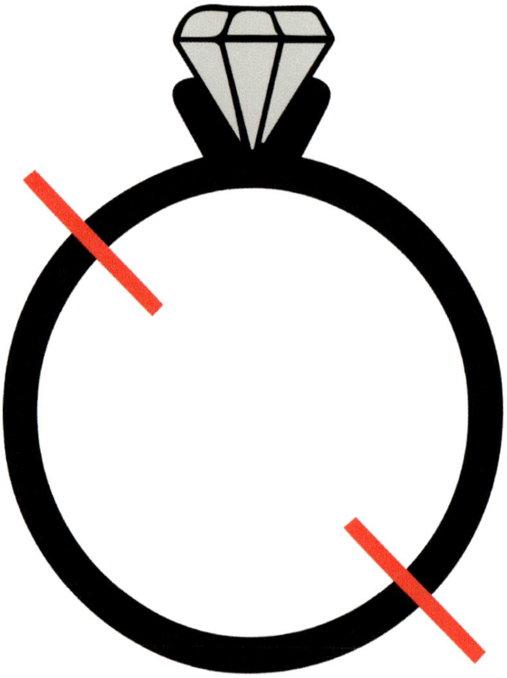

Scheme 20.2 The pelvic ring constitution demonstrates that for each injury caused by the action of a high-energy force vector in one area, it must always correspond another lesion on the opposite side

Avulsion fractures are common in young athletes aged between 11 and 16 years with predominance in males. They usually occur in a *locus minoris resistentiae*, represented by the insertion of the tendons at the level of the apophysis that are secondary ossification centers before the fusion. They are mostly composed by cartilage.

20.3 Classification

Pelvic ring fractures may be classified into two subtypes based on the trauma energy.

Low-energy traumas are represented by stable fractures, which do not interrupt the continuity of the ring and are less frequently associated with complications.

High-energy traumas determine a significant anatomical alteration and are therefore potentially associated with severe complications, representing one of the fundamental challenges in the clinical and therapeutic management of major polytraumatized patients.

The PRD represents historically an important dilemma, both clinically and diagnostically, and for the therapeutic decision. The fractures are characterized by a great variety of very different kinds of injuries from anatomical and clinical point of view, as a "grayscale," which may include at one end of the spectrum a stable intact pelvic ring and at the other part a completely unstable pelvis.

The radiologist will assess which part of the spectrum will place the single type of fracture.

The management of a polytrauma patient with pelvic fracture is based on clinical and hemodynamic conditions and on the degree of pelvic instability, which can be well understood through the analysis of the injury mechanism [8].

If the stability is the key, analyzing the combination of individual anterior and posterior injuries, with a particular focus to the posterior one, will carryout an accurate radiological evaluation. The instability condition depends essentially on the degree of involvement of the posterior tension band.

There are historically known different classification systems proposed by many authors [27], often articulated in different and poorly standardized modality.

The technological revolution determined by the use and the increasing availability of CT and then the spiral and spiral multi-slices scans, in addition to the evolution of surgical and orthopedic instruments, has profoundly changed the treatment approach with a higher number of surgical operations compared to conservative therapy.

Classification systems should be used as tools to help determine prognosis, to direct the search of complications, and to guide for the most appropriate treatment.

The traditional classification systems are based mainly on the definition of the degree of instability of the pelvic ring. The fundamental assumption was that the more unstable the fracture, the greater the risk of complications, especially hemorrhagic [19]. This undoubtedly logical and correct principle was subsequently dismissed by some authors [28] because of the poor diagnostic impact of the principal classification system especially on the search of vascular complications, which could not be present in fractures with an important dislocation of osseous components, often occuring in other less significant fractures.

The modern history of pelvic fracture management begins with iliac wing fracture reported by Duverney in 1751 (Duverney's fracture), from the French surgeon Joseph-François Malgaigne in 1859, with the clinical description of "double vertical" and shear shaped, known as "Malgaigne's fracture," as a combination of pubic rami and iliac wing fractures [5].

Watson-Jones, in 1937, first defined and classified the fractures based on the location of the fracture.

Connoly and Hedberg, in 1969, focused on the concept of stability and the importance of the biomechanical integrity of the posterior pelvis.

Bucholz clarifies the concepts based on the importance of the anterior pelvic ring than the posterior and on the search of the no detectable injuries of the posterior side.

He provides pathological demonstration that double injury to the pelvic ring is the rule confirming the presence of a posterior lesion in all his victims of fatal motor vehicle accidents at the time of medicolegal autopsy; lesions are graded as type I, type II, or type III depending on the degree of instability [29].

Huittinen and Slatis study pelvic pathoanatomy and are the first who note the relationship between the force energies of impact (high- versus low-energy injuries).

The Looser and Crombie classification takes into consideration both anterior and posterior components of pelvic injury.

Trunkey introduces the concept of stability, adding the terms "comminuted," "stable," and "unstable" in grading pelvic fracture.

Classic anatomic and biomechanical studies in pelvic disruption, performed during the mid-twentieth century by a Canadian surgeon George Pennal, are a fundamental contribution, and he is the first one who analyzes in detail the basic mechanism of pelvic injury. The classification system recognizes three mechanisms of direction of force action, which determine injuries: anterior-posterior compression (APC), lateral compression (LC), and "vertical shear" (VS) [5, 9].

During this period, the management of pelvic fracture is generally nonoperative with poor clinical outcome and post-traumatic secondary orthopedic and neurological complications.

Tile classification greatly appreciated by orthopedists uses an alphanumeric criterion based on the assessment of stability of the posterior arch (sacroiliac complex) with the purpose of harmonizing the therapeutic and prognostic management of fractures. It divides the pelvis into the posterior arch (posterior to the acetabulum) and the anterior arch (anterior to the acetabulum), with a spectrum ranging from stable injuries to unstable fractures; each type is divided into three types [1–4]:

Type A [1–3]: Stable and the posterior part of the ring is intact; generally nonoperative management—NOM (avulsion fractures, iliac wing fractures, fractures of the sacrum or coccyx).

Type B [1–3]: Vertically stable but rotationally unstable or partially stable, secondary to an incomplete disruption of the posterior arch structures; these include an external rotation of so-called open-book-type fractures (APC) with disruption of the anterior pelvic arch through the symphysis pubis or through the rami and internal rotation LC injuries with a combination of anterior and posterior arch fractures.

Type C [1–3]: Vertically and rotationally unstable with complete disruption of the anterior arch, posterior arch (sacroiliac complex), and pelvic floor.

Acetabular fractures are considered separately in the classifications of Tile [30].

A fundamental concept both in clinical and radiological management is to speak generally of pelvic fracture but to distinguish a PRD from an acetabulum fracture.

The polytraumatized patient with a pelvic ring fracture, for the complex clinical problems and consequently more complex management issues, is profoundly different from an acetabular fracture patient, whose problems are mainly orthopedic.

A fracture of the acetabulum is even so associated with pelvic ring fracture in a variable percentage from 15 to 20% of cases.

The American Orthopedic Trauma Association (OTA)/AO (Association for Osteosynthesis) pelvic fracture classification is an alphanumerical and more comprehensive classification system designed to standardize and more accurately report various fracture patterns.

The AO/OTA classification of pelvic ring fractures is divided in three groups (A, B, C) and in relative subgroups [1–3] with increased instability.

Type A fractures are lesion sparing (avulsion fractures of the innominate bone, fractures of the sacrum and coccyx). Type B fractures, with incomplete, unilateral disruption of the posterior arch, are partially stable (external rotation, APC with open-book-type injury; internal rotation, LC injury). Type C fractures are totally unstable, secondary to complete disruption of the posterior arch, and are more commonly seen in the younger patient population.

This classification describes accurately specific fracture patterns and is useful for research purposes but relatively less practical for routine use [5, 31].

The classification of Young revisited by Burgess combines the concepts of the two classifications of Tile and Pennal and is therefore extremely useful in finding the associated complications. Tile's criteria concern the stability, while Pennal's criteria concern comprehension of the mechanism of action. It is currently the most widely used system reported in the orthopedic literature.

These criteria, through the stratification of the grade of force vector of injury, represent a valid tool in the management of the patient in the emergency room.

The classification of Young revisited by Burgess is based on the direction and on the grade of force vector energy of the lesion, determining a gradual severity on the compression fractures that are classified in four types with growing instability: lateral compression, LC; anterior-posterior compression, APC; vertical shear, VS; and combined mechanism injury, CM [1, 4, 7, 9, 24, 30–35].

Lateral compression (LC) fractures: The "implosion type" (LC1, LC2, LC3).

The most frequent. Represent 59% of fractures. The force vector acts in lateral direction, resulting in an internal rotation of the injured hemi-pelvis. The ilium rotates medially.

In these fractures the sacrospinous and sacrotuberous ligaments are shortened determining a reduction of the transverse diameter of the entire pelvis and a possible overlap of the pubic branches with the appearance of blocked sym-

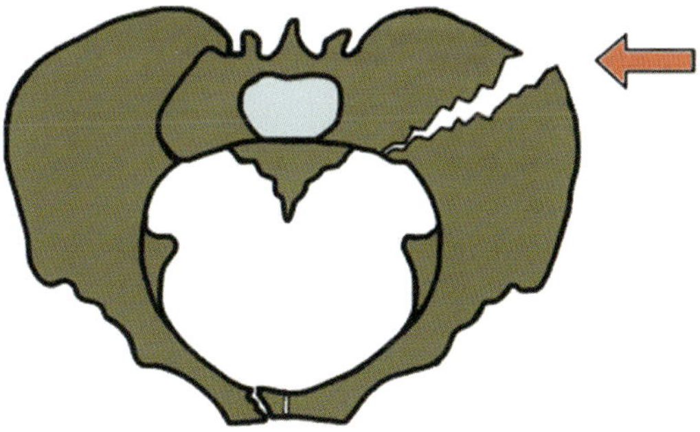

Scheme 20.3 Figure of lateral compression fracture (LC) with force vector that acts in lateral direction, resulting in an internal rotation of the injured hemi-pelvis and the possibility of overlap of the pubic branches with the appearance of blocked symphysis ("locked symphysis")

physis classically defined as a "lock" ("locked symphysis") (Scheme 20.3) (Fig. 20.1).

Usually you can find a transverse fracture of pubic rami ipsilateral or contralateral to the posterior injury.

Four different combinations of the anterior pelvic ring fractures are described (unilateral of both branches, unilateral of both branches + symphysis, both branches bilateral, both branches bilateral + symphysis).

The reduction of the pelvis' transverse diameter, with a consequent reduction of compliance, justifies its potential association with vascular complications, even if severe vascular lesions can

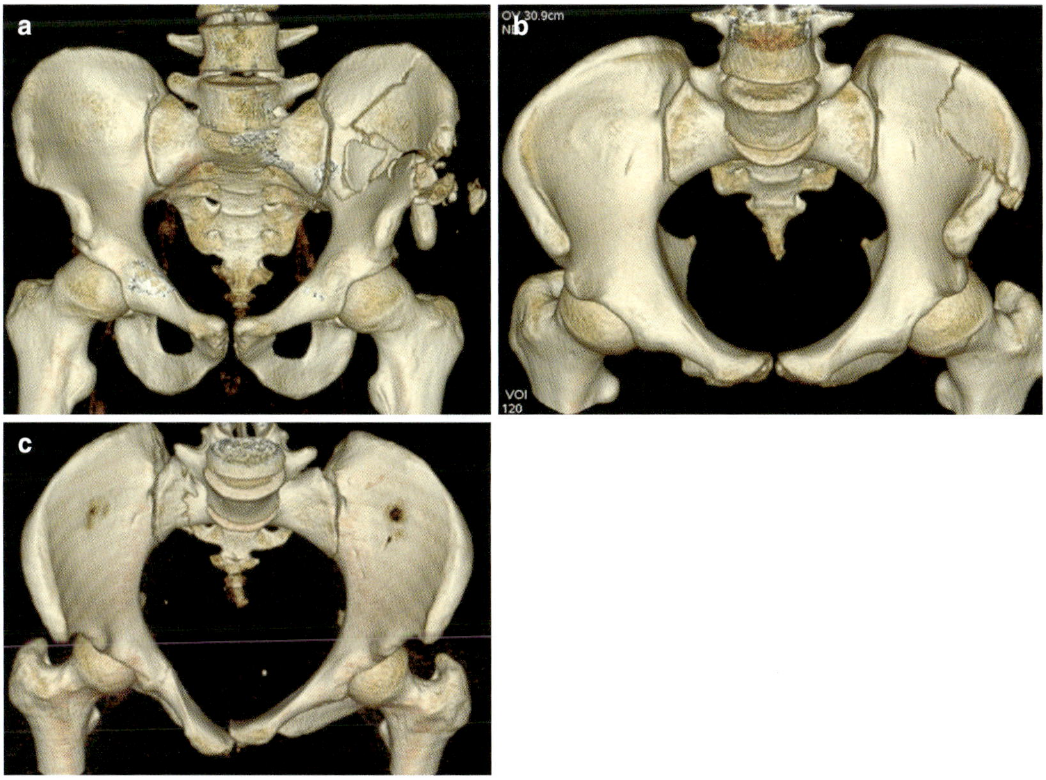

Fig. 20.1 (**a**–**c**) Lateral compression fractures (LC), type I. (**a**, **b**) CT 3D (VR) reconstruction AP and inlet view show lateral force vector, resulting in fracture of the left iliac wing on the side of the impact. (**c**) CT 3D (VR) reconstruction inlet view shows a "locked symphysis" fracture due to the overlap of the pubic branches with appearance of blocked symphysis. In these fractures the lesions of sacrospinous and sacrotuberous ligaments determine a reduction of the transverse diameter of the entire pelvis

result in direct action of a fragment that acts on vascular structures.

Visceral lesions, especially of the bladder, frequently complicate fractures for direct action of pubic disassembled and dislocated element fragments on the anterior wall.

In higher degrees of injury (LC1 + APC or LC2 + APC), the lateral compression force on the impact site is associated with a destructive force by anterior-posterior contralateral compression with a type of mechanism of "rollover," resulting in a multidirectional instability ("windswept pelvis").

LC1: Internal rotation. Stable. Associated sacral compression fracture on side of impact. Intact tension bands. Transverse fractures of the pubic rami. It is the most common pelvic fracture pattern, often associated with lower-energy injury mechanism (Fig. 20.2).

LC2: Internal rotation. Unstable internal rotation. Crescent posterior iliac wing fracture on the side of impact and posterior diastasis of the sacroiliac joint (Fig. 20.3).

LC3: Internal rotation ("windswept pelvis"). Multidirectional unstable. LC1 or LC2 injury

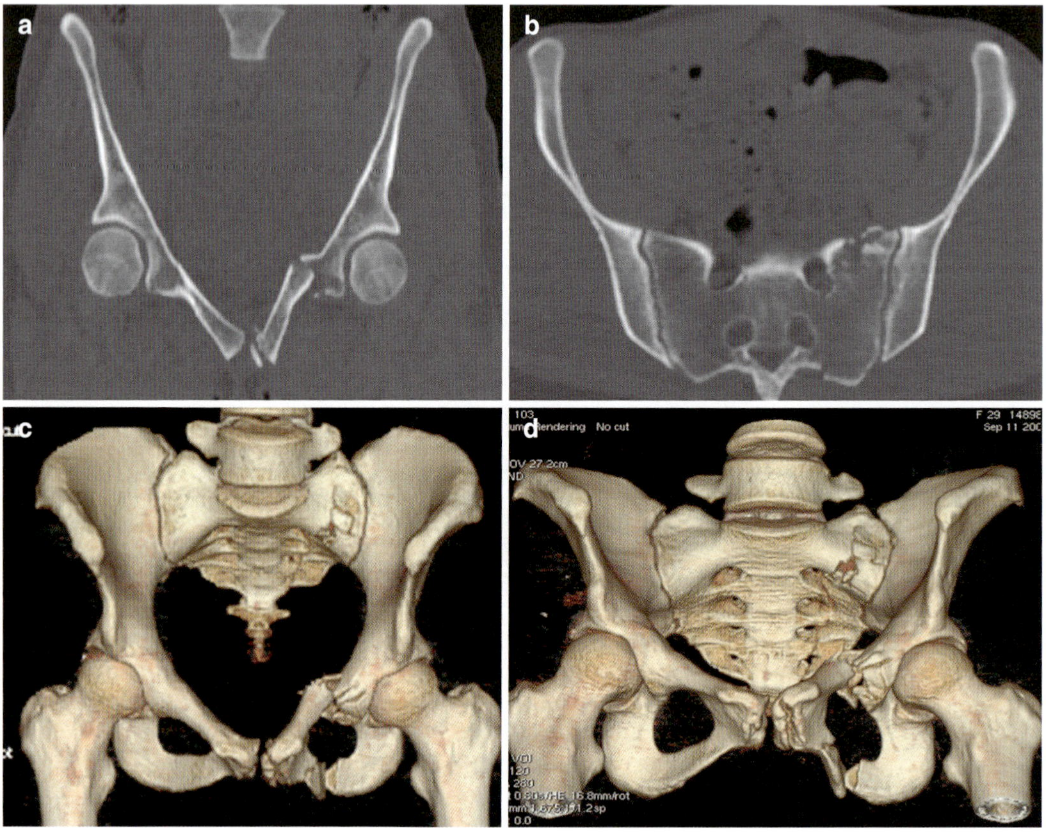

Fig. 20.2 (**a–d**) Lateral compression fractures (LC), type I stable. (**a**) CT coronal view shows the horizontal fracture of the left pubic branch on the side of the impact; (**b**) CT axial view depicts the omolateral compression fracture of the sacrum. (**c**) CT 3D (VR) reconstruction AP view shows the fracture of left pubic branch; (**d**) CT 3D (VR) reconstruction outlet view demonstrates the omolateral fracture of the sacrum

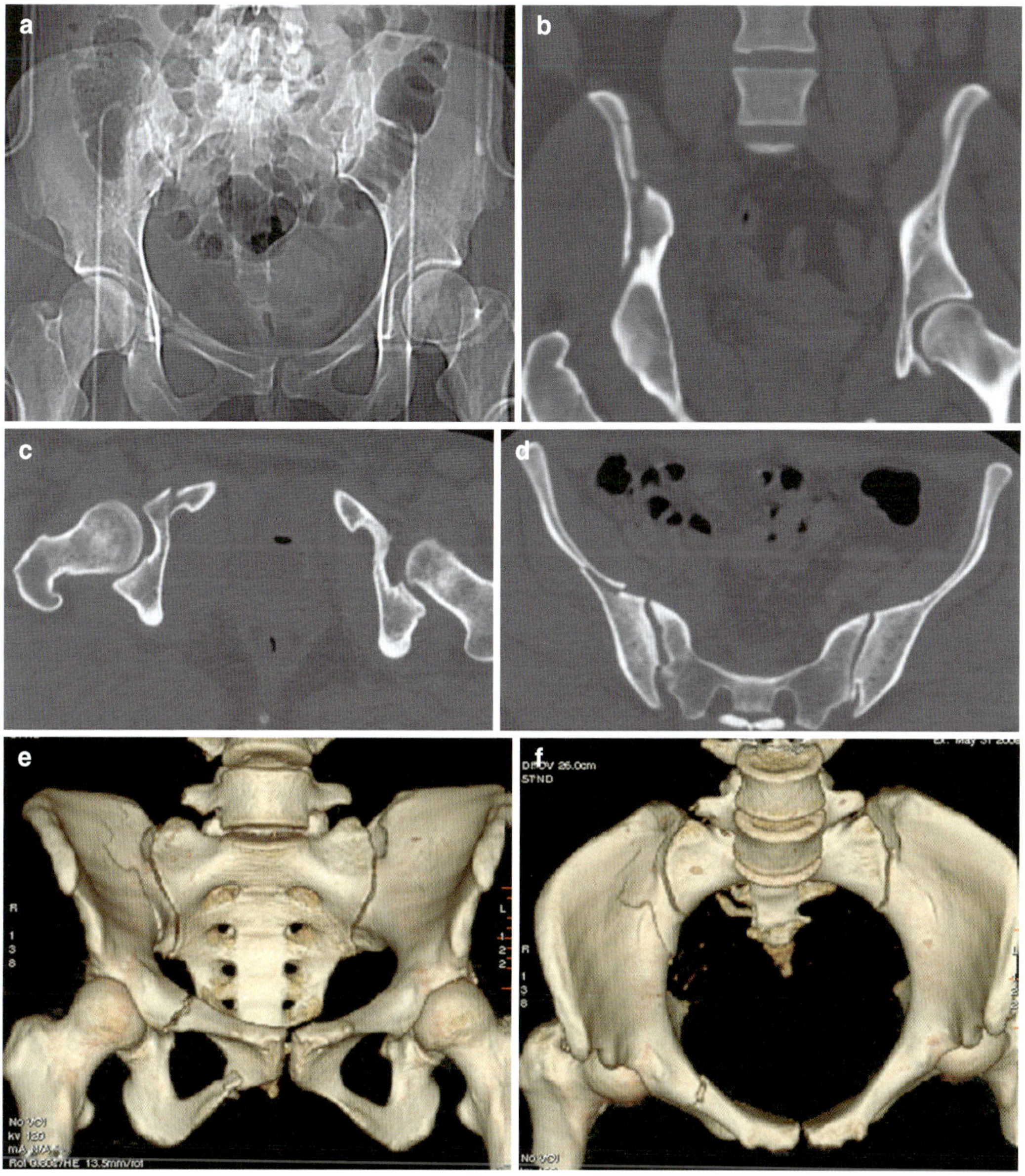

Fig. 20.3 (**a**–**f**) Lateral compression fractures (LC), type II unstable. (**a**) Scout view, CT scan MPR coronal view (**b**), and CT axial view show posterior iliac wing fracture (**b**, **d**) on the side of the impact and posterior diastasis of the sacroiliac joint (**d**). CT 3D (VR) reconstruction AP view (**c**) and inlet view (**d**) well depicting fractures of the right pubic branch, right iliac wing, and the posterior diastasis of the homolateral sacroiliac joint

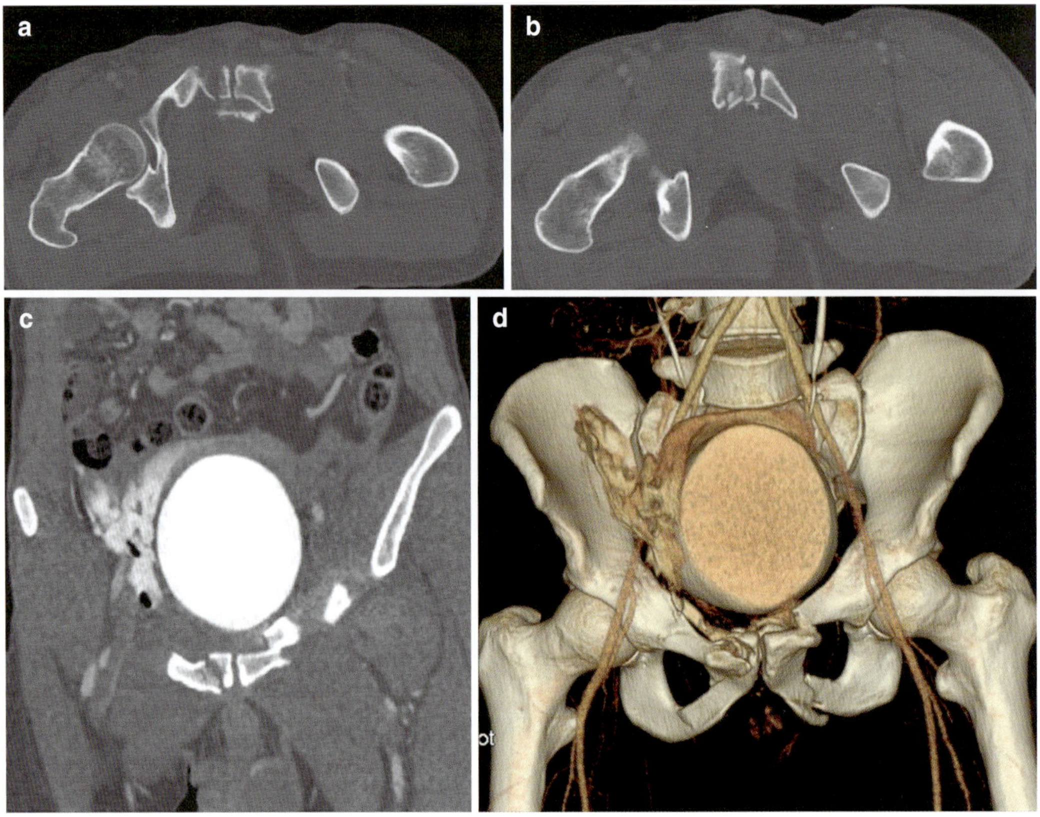

Fig. 20.4 (**a–d**) Lateral compression fractures (LC), type III unstable. (**a**, **b**) CT coronal view shows the fractures of the pubic branches on the impact side and the lateral compression fracture on the opposite side. (**c**) CT coronal view shows the dislocation of a fragment of the left pubic branch (*white arrow*) that results in a direct lesion on the bladder with evident iodinated urinary extravasations

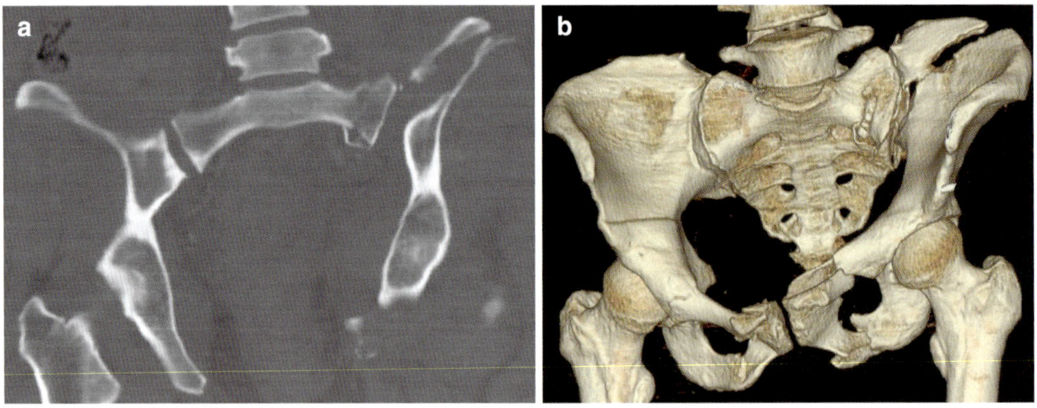

Fig. 20.5 (**a–b**) Lateral compression fracture (LC), type III. "Windswept pelvis." CT scan MPR coronal view (**a**) and CT 3D (VR) reconstruction AP view (**b**) show pubic branch fractures on the impact side and lateral compression fracture on the opposite side. In these fractures a complete destruction of the back tension band occurs, resulting in both rotational and vertical instability

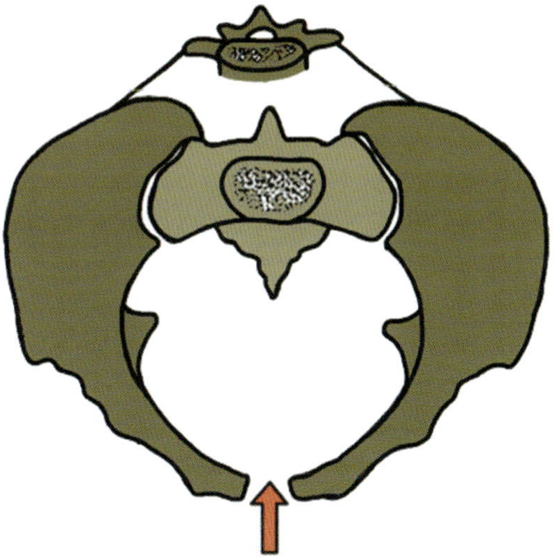

Scheme 20.4 Figure of an anterior-posterior compression fracture (APC) with force vector that acts in anterior-posterior direction on the pubic symphysis and the anterior or posterior superior iliac spines, resulting in an external rotation of the pelvis with diastasis of the pubic symphysis and the sacroiliac joints

on the side of impact and associated contralateral open-book (APC) injury (Figs. 20.4 and 20.5).

Anterior-posterior compression (APC) fractures: The so-called open-book fractures (APC1, APC2, APC3). Represent 21% of fractures.

The force vector acts in anterior-posterior direction on the anterior pelvis, the pubic symphysis, and the anterior or posterior superior iliac spines, determining an external rotation of the pelvis.

It is divided into three subgroups with a growing instability, which depends on energy force trauma and on the degree of involvement of the posterior sacroiliac complex and of the sacrospinous and sacrotuberous ligaments (Scheme 20.4).

The true pelvis can be compared to a conical sphere. The compression fracture can theoretically increase the radius of the sphere and consequently the pelvic volume, up to tripling or quadrupling consequently the compliance. This is the reason why the so-called open-book fractures must be promptly treated with circumferential compression by tensile strength, even the simplest (pelvic sheet wrap), to normalize the pelvic diameter and consequently the compliance, because hemorrhage is a threatening risk for life.

External rotation of the hemi-pelvis can increase the volume of the pelvic cavity, up to tripling the compliance, with possible potential serious hemodynamic complications from occult bleeding if not identified and promptly treated.

They can determine, due to the diastasis, bladder lesions or specifically of the urethra (straddle fracture) and alterations of the penile shaft vasculature and its innervations with impotence (37% of patients) as the result of nervi erigentes injury. Basta and associates [5, 36] have observed that the probability of urethra lesion becomes higher with increasing of the pubic diastasis: each millimeter of pubic diastasis or inferomedial pubic bone fracture fragment displacement is associated with a 10% increased risk.

Pathognomonic findings of these fractures are represented by the pubic symphysis diastasis, expression of instability if greater than 1 cm, and expression of the contemporary lesion of the sacroiliac synchondrosis when greater than 2.5 cm.

Vertical fracture lines are evident at the level of the pubic rami.

APC1: External rotation. Stable. Little widening (>1 < 2.5 cm) of the pubic symphysis, stretched but intact anterior component of sacroiliac joint, intact posterior ligamentous complex, sometimes minimal diastasis of the sacroiliac synchondrosis, and vertical fracture of one or more pubic rami (Fig. 20.6)

APC2: External rotation. Rotational instability. Widening (>2.5 cm) of the pubic symphysis; diastasis of the anterior component of sacroiliac joint with disrupted sacrotuberous and sacrospinous ligaments; intact poste-

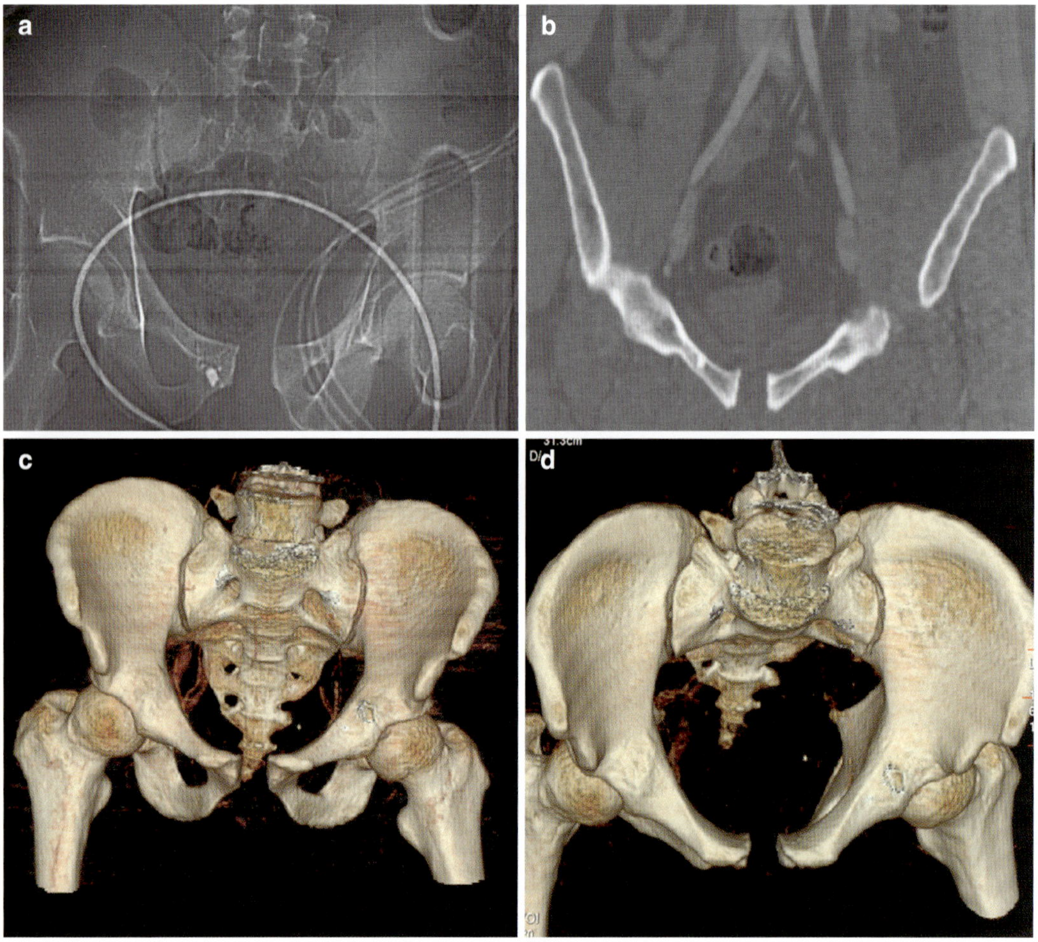

Fig. 20.6 (**a–d**) Anterior-posterior compression (APC) fracture, type I. (**a**) Scout view and CT scan MPR coronal view (**b**); CT 3D (VR) reconstruction AP view (**c**) and inlet view (**d**) demonstrate pubic symphysis diastasis <2.5 cm. These fractures are stable; the back tension band is intact

rior ligamentous complex, which maintains a residual condition of stability, like the binding of the book. Unilateral or bilateral. Vertical fracture of one or more pubic rami (Fig. 20.7)

APC3: External rotation with so-called open book. Complete rotational instability. Diastasis (>2.5 cm) of the pubic symphysis; uni- or bilateral sacroiliac dislocation; disrupted posterior ligamentous complex, dissociated from the sacrum, determining the condition of instability with splaying of the anterior arch. Vertical fracture of one or more pubic rami

In this type of fracture, when posterior sacroiliac joint is disrupted, instability is determined.

In these kinds of patients, the association with vascular (and neural) complications is very frequent (Figs. 20.8 and 20.9).

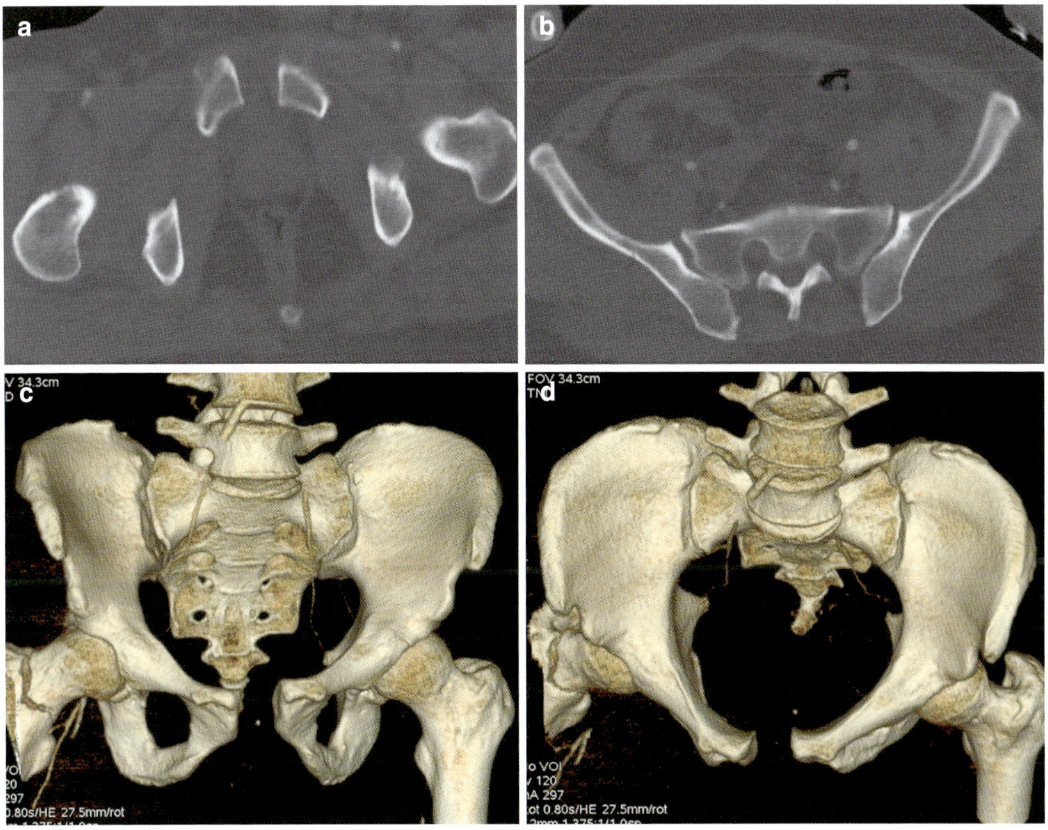

Fig. 20.7 (**a**–**d**) Anterior-posterior compression (APC) fracture, type II. (**a**–**c**) CT axial view (**a**) and CT 3D (VR) reconstruction AP view (**c**) show diastasis of the pubic symphysis >2.5 cm; (**b**, **d**) axial view (**b**) and CT 3D (VR) reconstruction inlet view well depicting the widening of the right sacroiliac joint. These fractures are rotationally unstable

Vertical shear (VS): Malgaigne's or straddle fracture.

Highly unstable. Represent 7% of lesions.

The vector acts in vertical direction (shearing forces), resulting in the destruction of the pelvic ring and of the posterior tension band with dislocation of sacroiliac complex (Scheme 20.5).

Their main characteristic is the involvement of the posterior pelvic elements, represented by vertically oriented sacral fractures (Wallnerfractures), transforaminal or lateral to the foramina; sacroiliac fractures/dislocations; the typical fracture of Malgaigne, in which the posterior fractured element is the iliac wing; or straddle fracture with fracture of both superior and inferior pubic rami (often there is 40% injuries of the genitourinary tract) [29].

The pathognomonic finding is the cranial dislocation of the injured hemi-pelvis, which frequently is associated with an avulsion fracture of the homolateral transverse process of the fifth lumbar vertebrae.

On the front side, there are evident vertical fractures of the pubic rami and/or diastasis of the pubic symphysis as in AP compression fractures.

The sign that allows to distinguish these fractures than those from AP compression is the

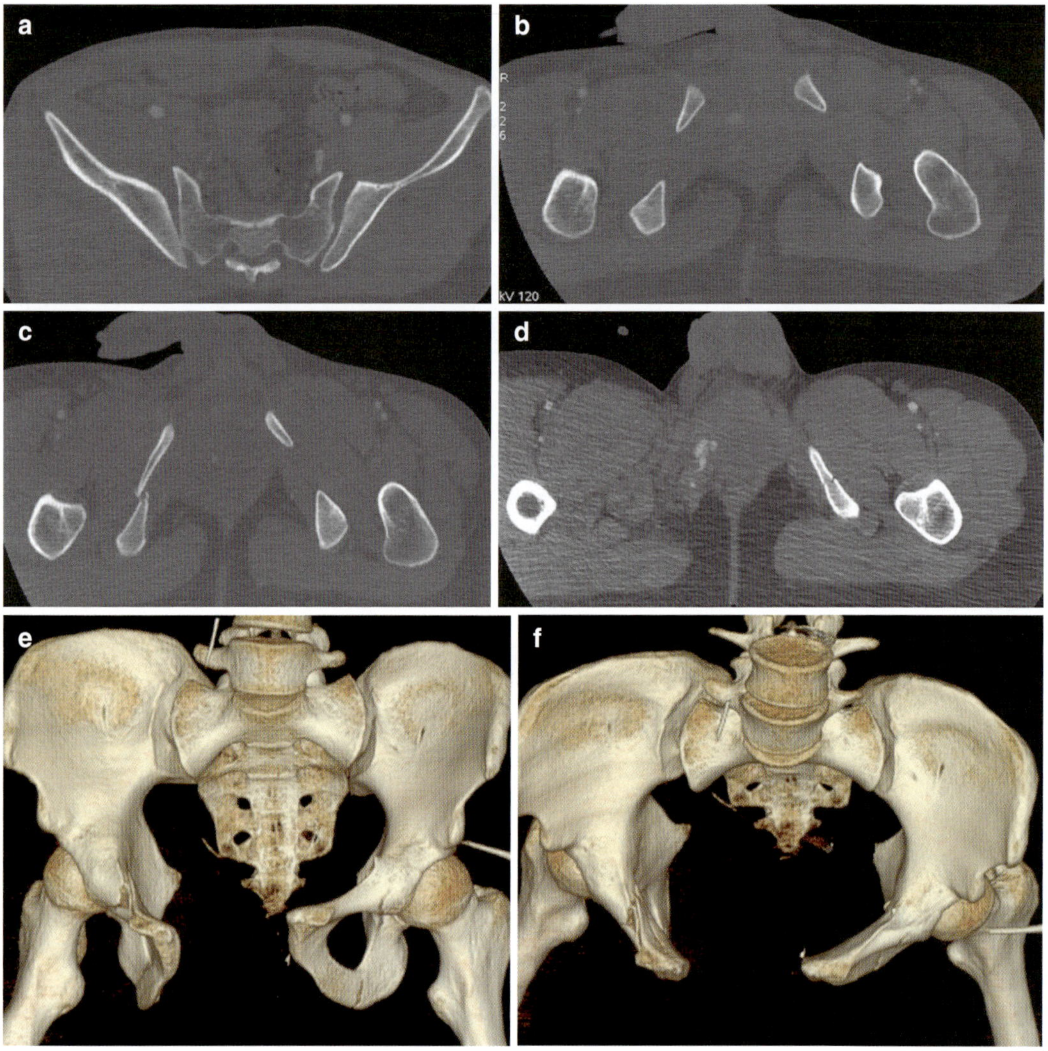

Fig. 20.8 (**a**–**f**) Anterior-posterior compression (APC) fracture, type III. "Open-book" fracture with instability condition. (**a**–**d**) CT axial view demonstrates widening of both sacral-iliac joints (**a**), pubic symphysis diastasis >2.5 cm, (**b**) and vertical fractures of both pubic rami (**c**, **d**); (**e**) CT 3D (VR) reconstruction AP view and CT 3D (VR) reconstruction inlet view (**f**) show better the diastasis of the pubic symphysis >2.5 cm and the widening of both sacroiliac joints

cranial dislocation of the hemi-pelvis (Figs. 20.10, 20.11, 20.12, 20.13, and 20.14).

Complex fractures (CF)

Generally unstable. Represent 14% of injuries.

They are the result of simultaneous actions and by combining force vectors by AP compression and vertical compression or by lateral and vertical compression (LC + APC or LC + VS) (Fig. 20.15).

The sacrum fractures should always be remembered, because they are rarely isolated and therefore in the most of cases part of pelvic ring fractures.

Several fracture classification systems have been proposed with the aim to predict possible

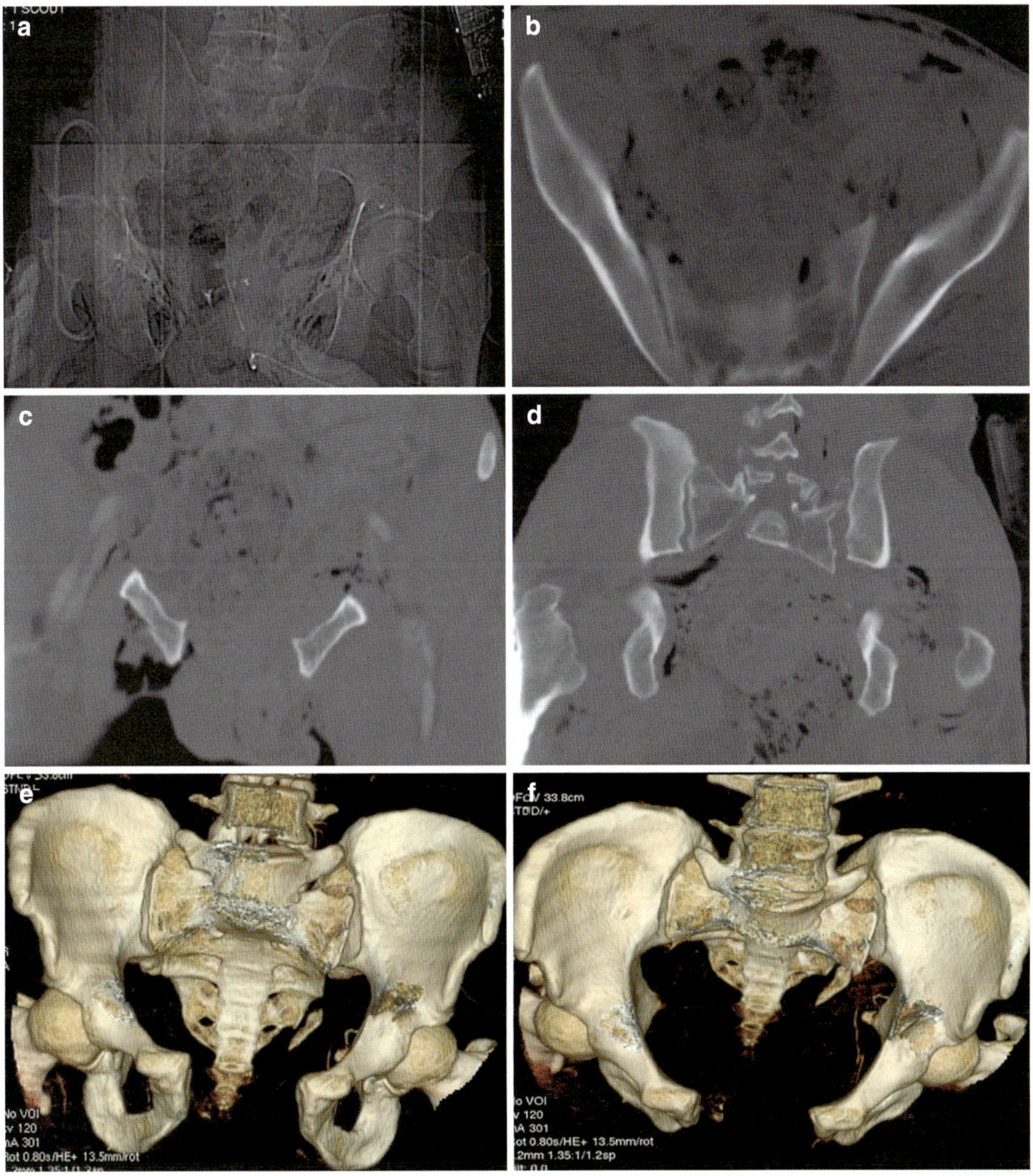

Fig. 20.9 (**a**–**f**) Anterior-posterior compression (APC) fracture, type III. (**a**) CT scout view; (**b**) CT axial view; (**c**, **d**) CT coronal view. Pubic symphysis diastasis >2.5 cm (**a**, **c**) and widening of both sacroiliac joints with dislocation of the left sacroiliac joint are evident (**b**, **d**). "Open-book" fracture with instability condition. These fractures are called "open" when they exist in a continuous solution between the fracture site and the skin with soft tissue involvement (**b**–**d**). CT 3D (VR) reconstruction AP view (**e**) and CT 3D (VR) reconstruction inlet view (**f**) well depicting pubic symphysis diastasis, vertical fractures of both pubic rami, and dislocation of the left sacroiliac joint. Instability condition is due to a complete destruction of the back tension band, resulting in both rotational and vertical instability

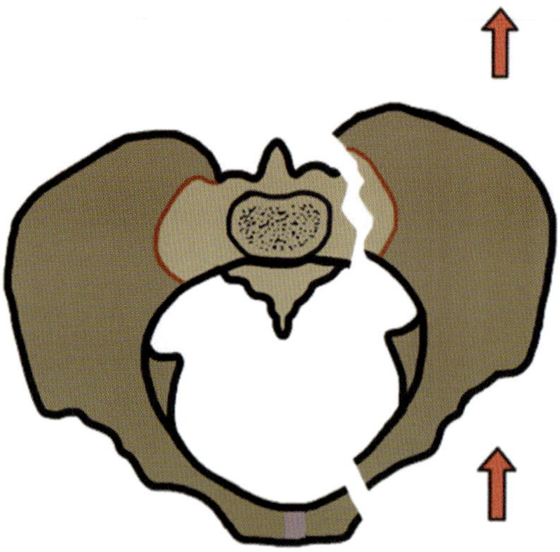

Scheme 20.5 Figure of a vertical shear fracture (VS) with force vector that acts in vertical direction, resulting in the disruption of the pelvic ring and of the posterior tension band with cranial dislocation of the injured hemi-pelvis

neurological injuries and to guide for the best therapeutic choice.

The best-known classification system was introduced by Denis, which divides the sacrum into three different zones (I, II, III), with a scheme elaborated in a retrospective study based on fracture location relative to the neuroforamen (Scheme 20.6):

Zone I fracture: Vertical orientation involves the sacral wing, positioned laterally to the course of the foramina, and generally is not associated with neurological problems (6%—L5/S1 radiculopathy).

Zone II fracture: Denis fracture type II generally from LC compression is localized along the course of the foramina but does not involve the spinal canal and may be associated in some conditions with homolateral neurological lumbar disorders or sacral

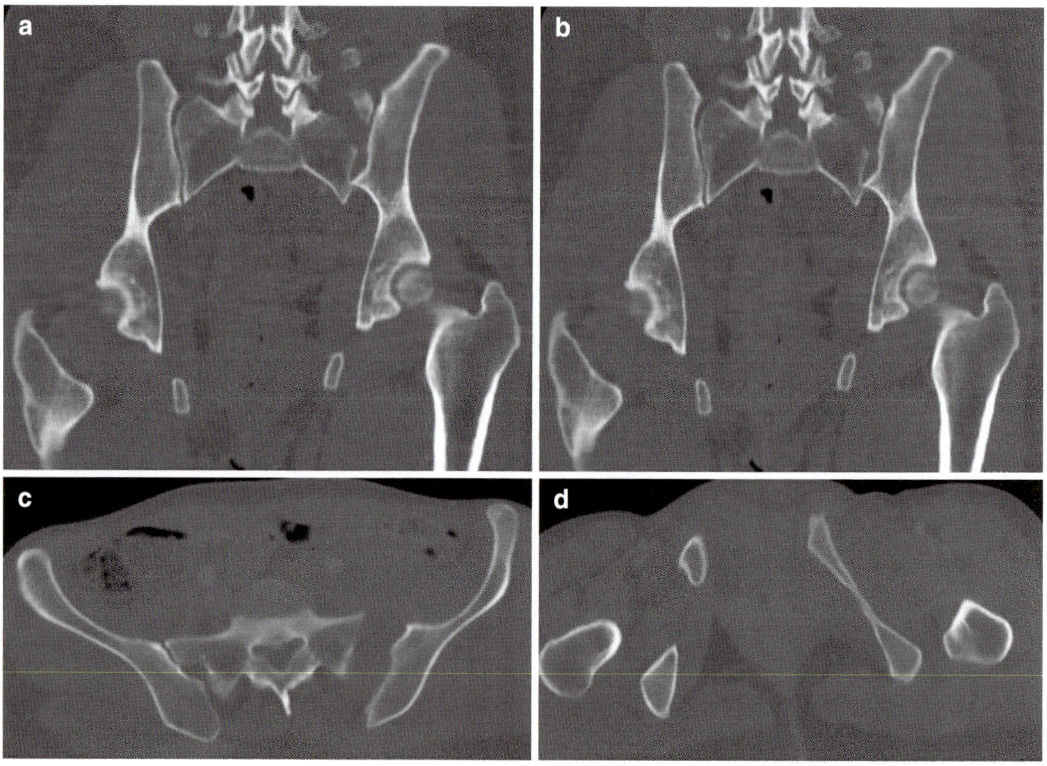

Fig. 20.10 (**a–d**) "Vertical shear" (VS) fracture. (**a**, **b**) CT scan MPR coronal view (**a**, **b**) and CT axial view (**c**, **d**) show the involvement of posterior pelvic elements. The vertical vector forces result in the destruction of the pelvic ring and of the posterior tension band with dislocation of sacroiliac complex. In (**a**) and (**b**), the cranial dislocation of the injured hemi-pelvis is evident

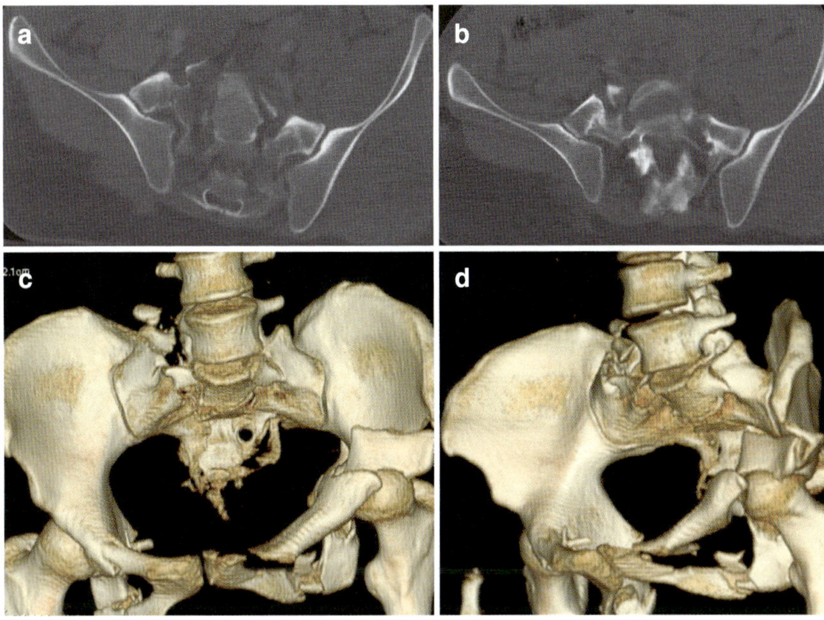

Fig. 20.11 (**a–d**) Precipitated patient. "Vertical shear" (VS) fracture; condition of high instability. (**a**, **b**) CT axial view shows bilateral fractures of the sacrum along the course of the foramina, with diastasis of the sacroiliac joint and fracture of the transverse process of the fifth lumbar vertebrae. (**c**, **d**) CT 3D (VR) reconstruction AP view shows bilateral fractures of pubic branches (horizontal force component)

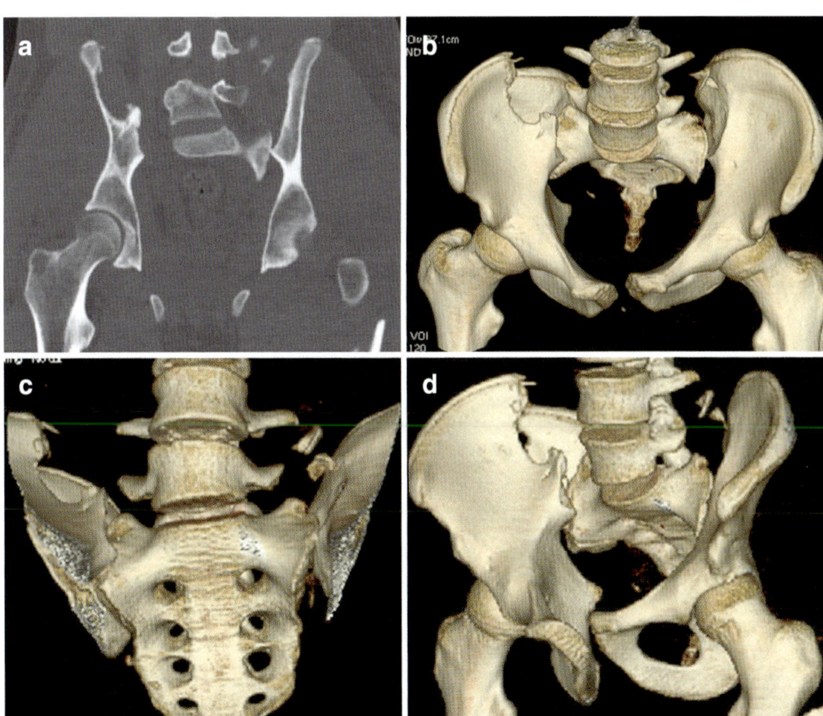

Fig. 20.12 (**a–d**) "Vertical shear" (VS) fracture. (**a**) CT MPR coronal view demonstrates bilateral sacroiliac fractures; CT 3D (VR) reconstruction AP view (**b**) and lateral view (**d**) show better sacroiliac fractures and dislocation; CT 3D (VR) reconstruction posterior view well depicting sacroiliac diastasis and avulsion fracture of the transverse process of the fifth lumbar vertebrae

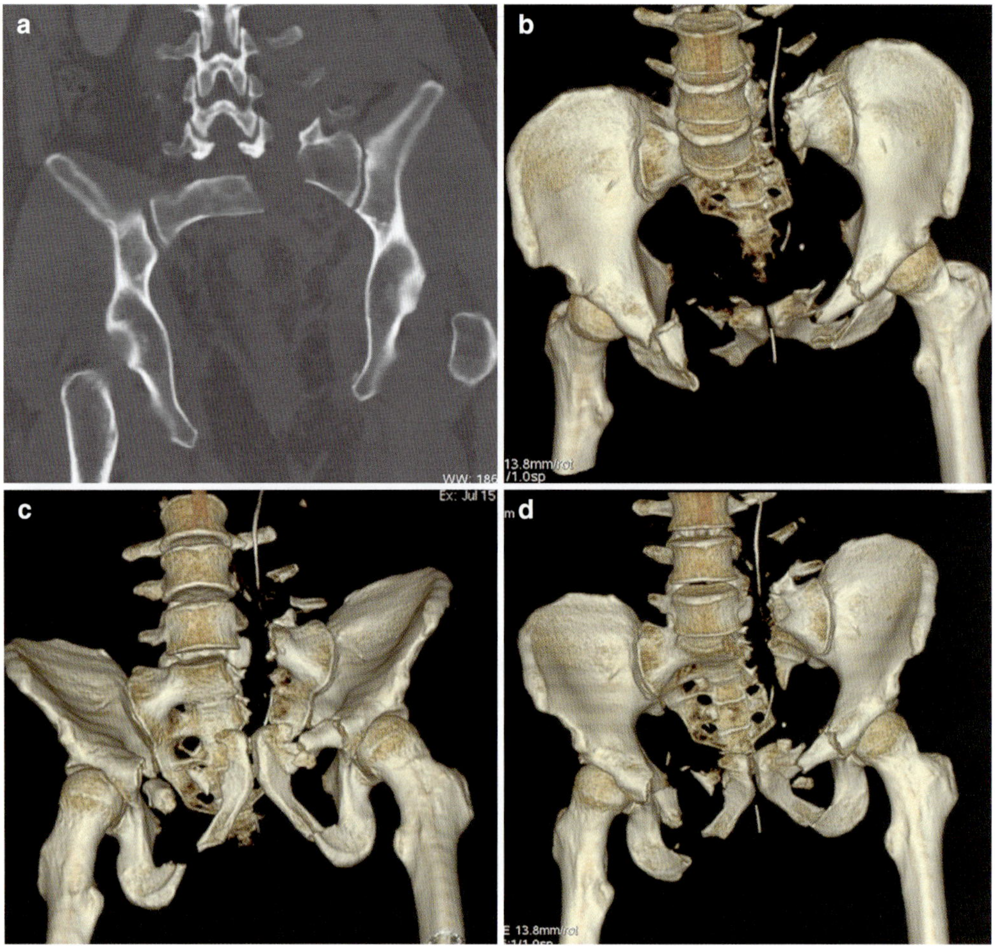

Fig. 20.13 (**a–d**) "Vertical shear" (VS) fracture. (**a**) CT MPR coronal view; CT 3D (VR) reconstruction AP view (**b**, **d**) and posterior view (**c**) show bilateral fractures of pubic rami (horizontal force component), sacroiliac fractures, and dislocation with consequent cranial dislocation of the injured hemi-pelvis; fractures of the transverse process of the fourth and fifth lumbar vertebrae. These fractures are the result of simultaneous force vectors and are highly unstable

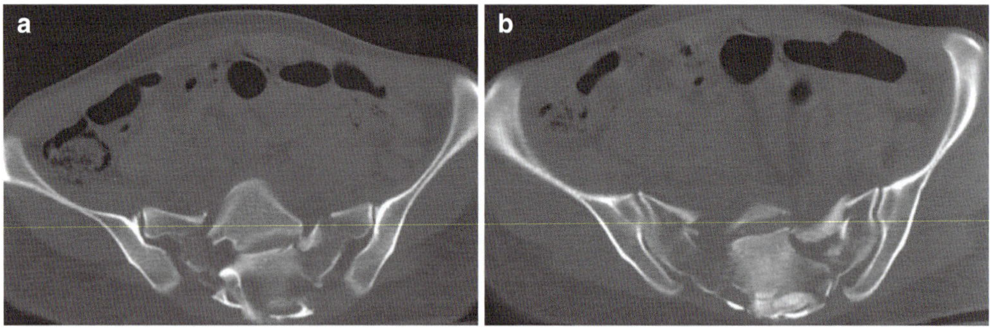

Fig. 20.14 (**a–e**) Precipitated patient. "Vertical shear" (VS) fracture; condition of high instability. (**a**, **b**) CT axial view shows bilateral fractures of the sacrum along the course of the foramina, with diastasis of the sacroiliac joint (double vertical force component). CT MPR sagittal view (**c**) and CT 3D (VR) reconstruction AP view (**d**) show the instability of the sacrum with the back of the coccyx. (**e**) X-ray of the ankle shows the complex associated ankle fracture

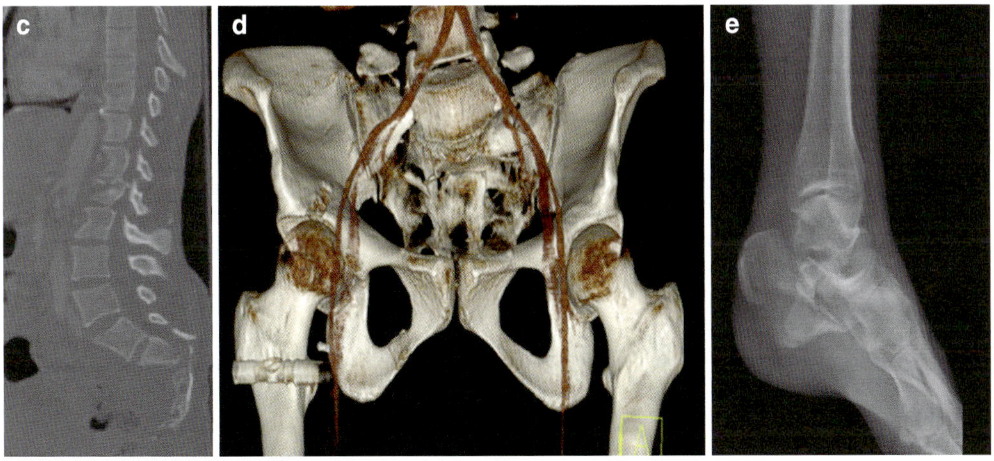

Fig. 20.14 (continued)

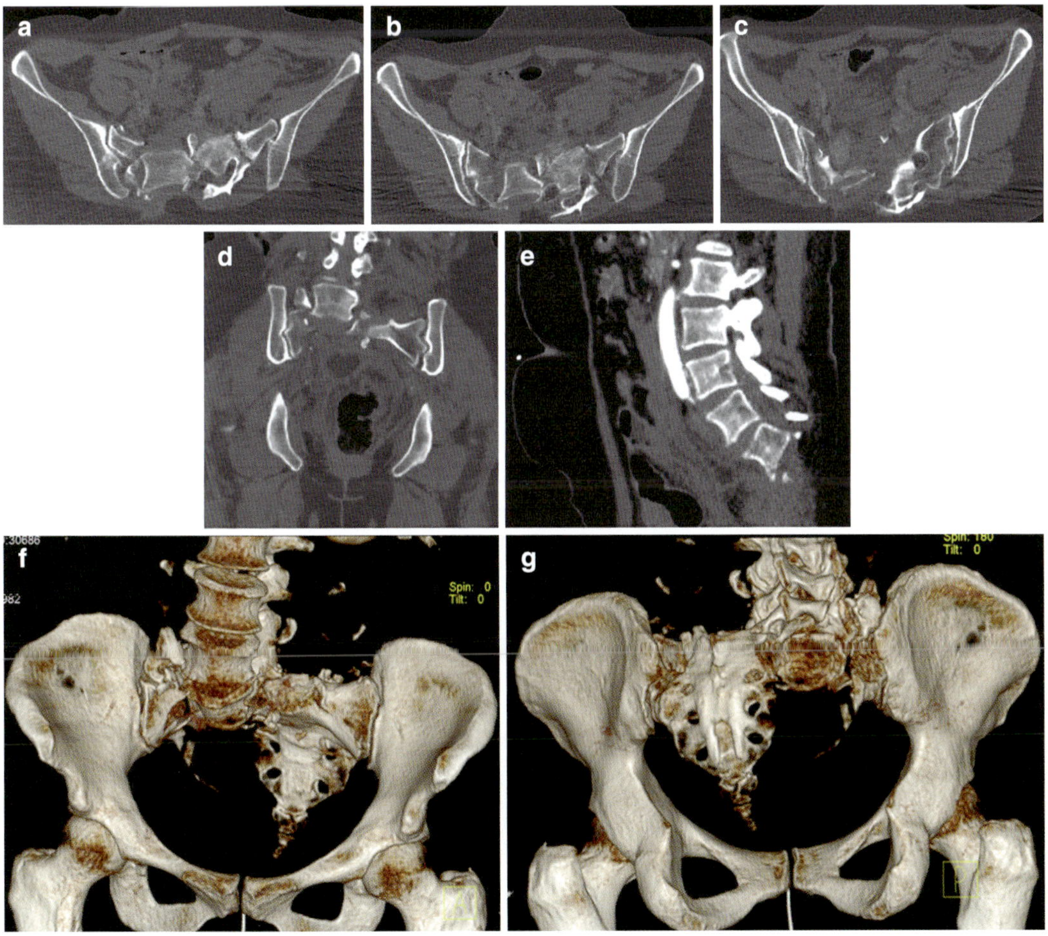

Fig. 20.15 (**a**–**g**) Precipitated patient in attempted suicide. Complex fracture (CM); condition of high instability. (**a**–**c**) CT axial view; (**d**) CT MPR coronal view; (**e**) CT MPR sagittal view shows fracture and dislocation of the sacrum, fracture of the right sacral wing, and avulsion of bilateral transverse apophysis of the fourth and fifth lumbar vertebrae. (**f**, **g**) CT 3D (VR) reconstruction AP view demonstrates the complete dislocation of the sacrum with lumbar-sacral dissociation

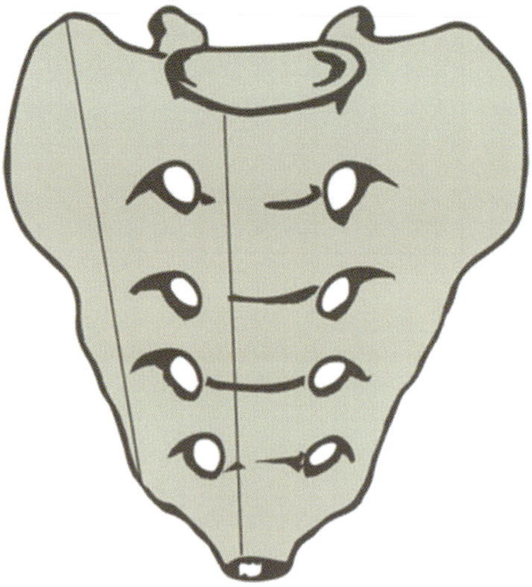

Scheme 20.6 Figure of Denis' classification system, which divides the sacrum with two vertical lines into three different zones (1, 2, 3)

radiculopathy (28%—L5, S1 and S2 nerve roots) (Fig. 20.16).

Zone III fracture: Frequently transverse orientation, these fractures are positioned medially on the foramina lines and involve the spinal canal. In relation to the fact that the central part is involved, neurological disorders, often bilateral, but also intestinal and bladder incontinence or alteration of the sexual function, are present (56%).

Medial fractures may have a transverse or longitudinal course and are classified into four additional groups in relation to the simple angle without translation (type 1), the angle with the translation of the distal portion of the sacrum (type 2), the angle with complete offset fracture elements (type 3), and comminuted S1 segment (type 4).

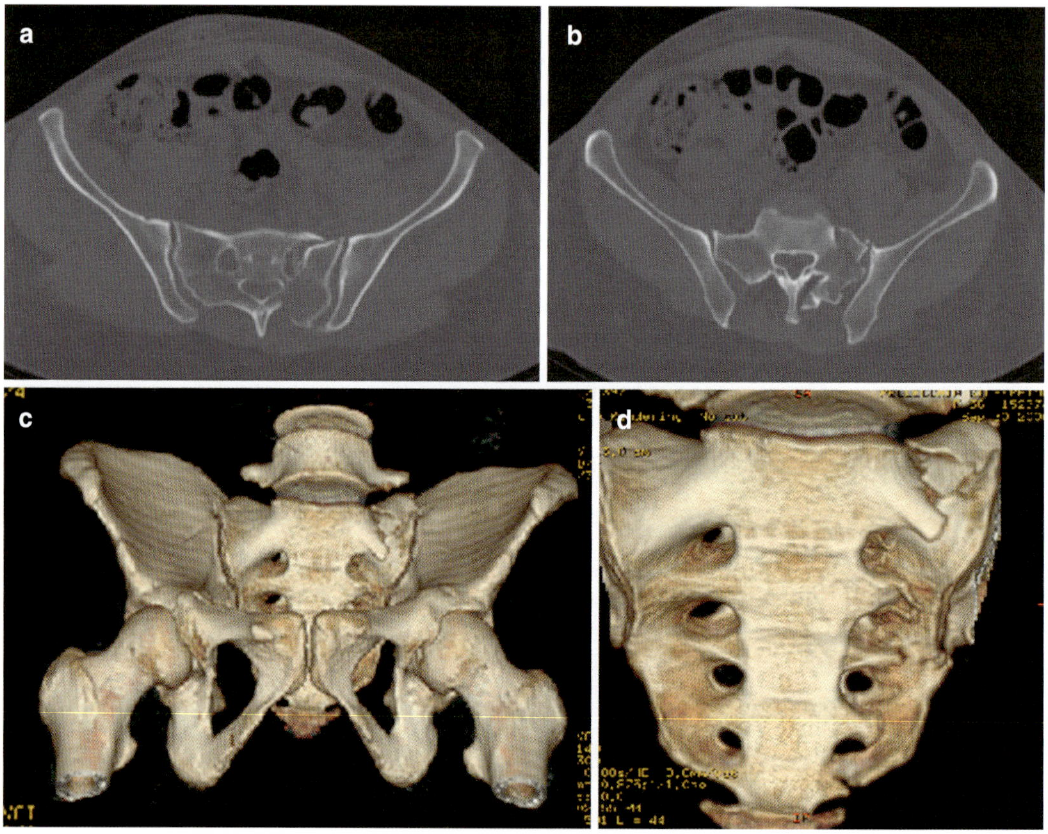

Fig. 20.16 (**a–d**) Fracture of the sacrum. CT axial view (**a**, **b**) and CT 3D (VR) reconstruction AP (**c**) and posterior view (**d**) show fracture of the sacrum along the course of the foramina, without involving the spinal canal

Morphologic injury patterns of zone III fractures are "H," "U," "lambda," and "T" shaped.

Sacral fractures could also occur without a fracture of the pelvic ring with a biomechanics different than that of the other pelvic ring fractures [37].

20.4 Imaging Evaluation of Pelvic Ring Fractures

The pelvic ring stability therefore depends on the integrity of the osseous but also of the ligamentous components.

The radiological assessment is to provide accurate information on the extension of the fracture lines, the possible dislocation or rotation of the injured hemi-pelvis, and the number and size of the bone fragments, on the three planes of space.

The radiologist is an integral part of the multidisciplinary team and must be able, through the interpretation of the morphology of the fracture, to hypothesize the presence of possible associated complications and to communicate in a rapid and incisive way possible clinical events both to other team's specialists but also to his collaborators.

The radiologist, through the interpretation of the fracture type and the degree of instability, helps the orthopedic surgeon to manage and to choose the most appropriate therapeutic treatment [38, 39].

20.4.1 X-rays

The routine radiographic examination is the anterior-posterior (AP) projection; it is fundamental in the evaluation of pelvic trauma, and it is part of Advanced Trauma Life Support (ATLS) protocol.

The radiogram execution is generally following the clinical evaluation for stability assessment and should be performed to avoid in case of "open pelvis" the risk of hemorrhagic complications.

It is important to remember that a PRD could be the cause of hypotension, in patients with a negative focused assessment with sonography for trauma (E-FAST) [1].

The radiogram can be performed in the emergency room, during the primary survey. A radiograph performed according to the correctness criteria should include iliac crests, coxofemoral joints, and proximal femoral portions.

The pelvic ring is the round-shaped plane passing through the prominence of the sacrum, the inferior margins of the sacroiliac joints extending to the upper margin of the pubic symphysis.

PRD is defined as an interruption of the normal contour of the true pelvis on the "inlet" plane, into two or more opposite points.

An ideal line passing through the ischial spines allows to consider an anterior and posterior pelvic arch.

The standard AP view provides the greatest number of diagnostic information and can identify the morphology and the extent mechanism of injury, but it is often insufficient. It allows to accurately assessing some fundamental landmarks like the ilioischial and the iliopectineal line. Anteriorly it allows identifying the presence and extent of diastasis of the symphysis pubis and/or the obturator ring fracture and posteriorly the presence and extent of dislocation of the injured hemipelvis, dislocations of the sacroiliac joint, or fractures of the transverse processes of L5.

However, this projection does not allow defining the real extension of the lesion, especially in its posterior component.

The anatomical complexity of the pelvic ring in its three-dimensional geometry implies that, in the AP projection, the incident beam is perpendicular only to some portions of the various skeletal segments and, oblique or parallel, to many others. For this reason, the radiological protocol should include other projections, in particular the Pennal's oblique pelvic inlet and outlet views (Fig. 20.17).

The pelvic inlet (cephalo-caudad beam) view is obtained directing the x-ray beam from the head with the ray centered between the navel and the pubic symphysis with an angle of 35° to the

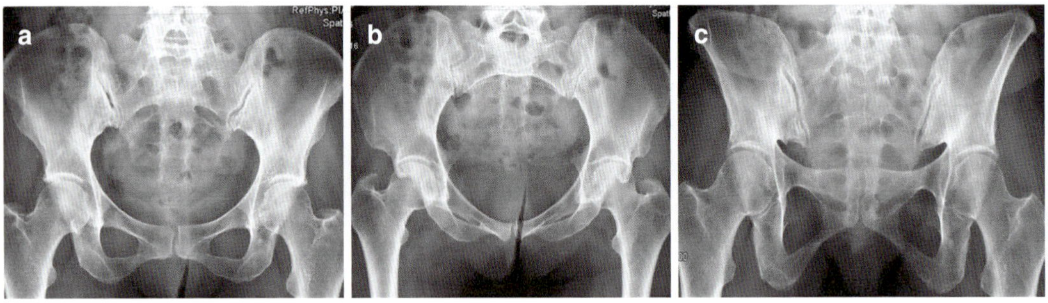

Fig. 20.17 (**a–c**) X-ray AP, inlet, and outlet view. The AP projection (**a**) allows identifying the presence and the extent of diastasis of the symphysis pubis and/or the obturator ring fracture. The inlet view, or descending oblique projection, (**b**) is fundamental to understand the entity of the diastasis and the degree of posterior displacement of the fracture. The outlet view or ascending oblique projection (**c**) is the best way for disclosing true cranial displacement of the innominate bone and determining vertical displacement of the posterior pelvis

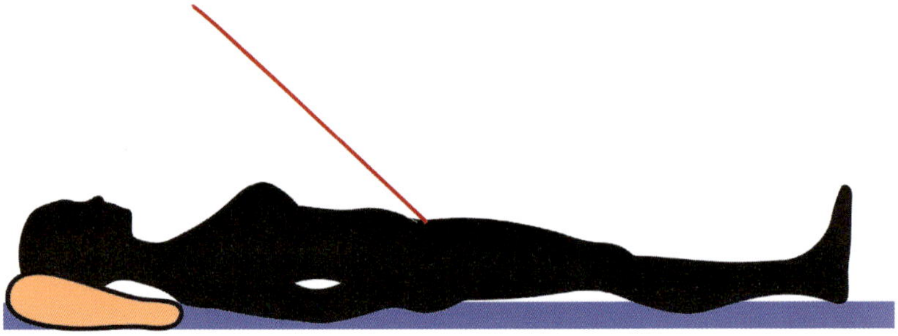

Scheme 20.7 Figure shows the orientation of the x-ray beam from the head with the ray centered between the navel and the pubic symphysis with an angle of 35° to the x-ray table, to obtain the right pelvic inlet view

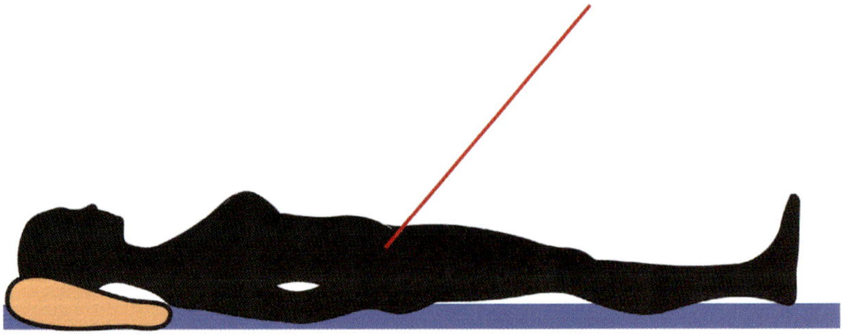

Scheme 20.8 Figure shows the orientation of the x-ray beam 35° cephalad on the symphysis, to obtain the right pelvic outlet view

x-ray table (Scheme 20.7). This view, perpendicular to the pelvic brim, allows to document, through the plane of the real pelvis, the anterior and posterior margin of the sacroiliac joints, the referent of the ilioischiatic line, and the alignment of the pubic symphysis plane. It is fundamental to understand the entity of the diastasis and the degree of posterior displacement of the fracture and internal or external rotation of anterior aspect of the pelvis. In the case of pelvic trauma, the radiographic evaluation of the pelvic ring with an inlet view is helpful in determining the opening of the symphysis, any posterior displacement, as well as overall ring deformity produced by lateral or anterior-posterior compression forces.

The outlet (caudocephalad beam) view is obtained directing the x-ray beam 35° cephalad on the symphysis and is the best way for disclosing true cranial displacement of the innominate bone (Scheme 20.8). The outlet or transverse view is helpful to visualize the entire sacrum, the wing including both sacroiliac joints, the ilioischial line, and, in a different projection, the pubic symphysis plane, determining vertical displacement of the posterior pelvis secondary to a vertical shear injury.

Once the type of fracture is identified, the radiologist should indicate exactly the pathology that has been created in order to define the degree of instability of the fracture.

From a radiographic point of view, there are three signs of instability:

- The first one is a displacement of the posterior sacroiliac complex greater than 0.5 cm; the inlet view, showing a break of the innominate line, is the best for disclosing this sign.
- The second sign is a posterior fracture gap, rather than impaction, or sacroiliac joint dislocation, which must be unstable, since the interosseous sacroiliac ligament must be disrupted.
- The third sign is avulsion of a fifth lumbar transverse process or sacral or ischial ends of the sacrospinous or sacrotuberous ligaments; avulsion fracture of the fifth lumbar transverse process is a sign of instability because it, usually, results from cranial displacement of the underlying hemi-pelvis [5, 9, 15, 24, 30, 40–43].

20.4.2 Multi-detector Computed Tomography (MDCT)

It is known that the multi-slice computer tomography (MSCT) is the "gold standard" method in the study of polytrauma and in fractures of the pelvic ring; it can rapidly generate large volumetric data sets of the body, allowing panoramic exploration, and also providing great anatomical details [3, 5, 43–48]. The speed of a CT equipment produces several advantages allowing, amongst others, i) patients to spend less time in the exam room, ii) a more efficient use of contrast medium dose iii) to speed up the decision-making processes by searching for associated injuries and complications, iv) to assess basic prognostic factors such as staging of parenchymal lesions, v) relief of hemoperitoneum and hemoretroperitoneum, vi) involvement of vascular structures, and vii) presence or absence of "active bleeding" within the site of bleeding. Compared with angiographic gold standard, MSCT has been shown to be both sensitive (84%) and specific (85%) for detection of active pelvic bleeding in pelvic trauma [16, 49]. The information will be crucial in view of the subsequent vascular treatment.

Rapid image acquisition with reduction of motion artifacts allows multi-planar (MPR), maximum intensity projection (MIP), and three-dimensional (3D) with volume-rendering (VR) reconstructions with highest quality. In the study of polytraumatized patients, the integration between axial, coronal, and sagittal MPR and 3D-VR reconstructions represents the "reference standard" in the evaluation of pelvic fractures and its complications.

In the literature it is described that in patients with pelvic fractures seen on axial CT images, treatment decisions have been shown to be altered in up to 30% of cases; in general this change in treatment resulted when MPR or VR images reveal a more severe injury than was seen on conventional axial images. Those reconstructions allow to define in detail the morphology of the fracture, to evaluate the extent of any dislocations, and, in case of acetabulum, femoral head, and neck fractures, to assess the degree of involvement of the articular surface and the presence of articular fragments, imprisoned and/or impacted, to exclude the involvement of the femoral head, of the acetabular roof, and of the quadrilateral surface.

MPR images generally provide superior anatomic detail, while surgeons tend to prefer 3D-VR images for surgical planning, especially in determining surgical approach and screw placement. Complex spatial relationships among fracture fragments are well delineated on 3D-VR images, and generation of these images can facilitate communication of this complicated anatomic information from the radiologist to the surgeon [50].

Using 3D-VR imaging, it is possible a better understanding of the pelvic anatomy, whose interpretation is much more difficult having the frontal view alone. It allows reproducing the principal classical radiological projections, the panoramic anterior-posterior (and posterior-anterior) view, and the oblique inlet and outlet views of Pennal, to understand the morphology of fracture and the possible degree of destruction.

Sacral fractures are of great clinical significance for possible sequels and often underestimated in the standard radiological examination, even if performed under the most suitable conditions.

This side has also frequent anatomical variants, in particular at the lumbar-sacral hinge.

MSCT also allows to easily demonstrate sacral fractures, present in a variable percentage between 7 and 75% of the pelvic ring fractures and unrecognizable in the first radiographic examination in varying percentages up to 70% of cases for soft tissue overlay or for the obstacle caused by the presence of intestinal gas. A delay in the diagnosis of these fractures can be clinically very significant, as they may hesitate in deformation of bone components, and cause neurological disorders and bowel, bladder, and sexual dysfunctions [37]. CT through scans acquired on the axial images, and coronal- and sagittal-oriented images, allows understanding the degree of involvement of foramina to characterize the different morphologies of complex fractures with deformation and dislocation of the sacrum [9, 30, 40, 42, 43].

Complex fractures with dislocation of the fragments are associated with severe PRD with a potential higher mortality rate. In addition to knowing the fracture morphology, it is extremely useful in the therapeutic decision, if necessary the stabilization with screws, particularly in the presence of anatomical variants.

Finally, the CT allows identifying and typifying a possible, associated fracture and/or dislocation of the lumbosacral junction. The most frequent complication of chronic pelvic fractures is certainly a low back pain, often highly debilitating. The main cause of this low back pain, even in the presence of an optimal reduction and stabilization of pelvic fracture, is precisely an involved lesion of the lumbosacral junction, underestimated or misunderstood in the diagnostic phase.

The role of this method in the study of acetabular fractures should also be mentioned. The acetabular fracture can be isolated or complicate a pelvic ring fracture. These fractures need a rigorous evaluation for a correct anatomic-pathologic diagnosis and for an orthopedic treatment planning, which in the last decades has profoundly changed, now more often surgical than conservative. The number of patients with surgically treated acetabular fractures is increased in relation to advantages compared to a conservative treatment, which can be obtained if the surgery is performed by a specialized surgical team in this area. The treatment of acetabular fractures is aimed to obtain the *restitutio ad integrum* of the normal articulation anatomy, the congruity of joint interface, a rapid patient mobilization, and a reduction of painful symptoms and of serious complications often associated with a prolonged state of inactivity. The anatomical fracture reduction is statistically correlated to a high percentage of good results, which determine a less incidence of osteoartrosis. For this purpose, the diagnostic imaging has the role to correctly define the site and the morphology of fracture. In the decision for treatment and for surgical approach, knowledge of the anatomical situation and the location, course, and morphology of the fracture is of crucial importance. The surgical objective is to obtain an anatomical reduction through a single surgical route.

The Letournel and Judet classification criteria are morphological, and they are obtained through the comparison between surgical observation and radiographic projections of Judet (AP frontal centered on the affected hip, iliac oblique view, and obturator oblique view) (Fig. 20.18).

In the phase of post-processing of the images we will be able to faithfully reproduce the Judet oblique projections, iliac and obturator oblique views, through which is possible the accurate analysis of the landmarks required for the classification of fractures. The classification system divides fractures into two main types: elementary (isolated) fractures and associated fractures in which a combination of at least two elementary

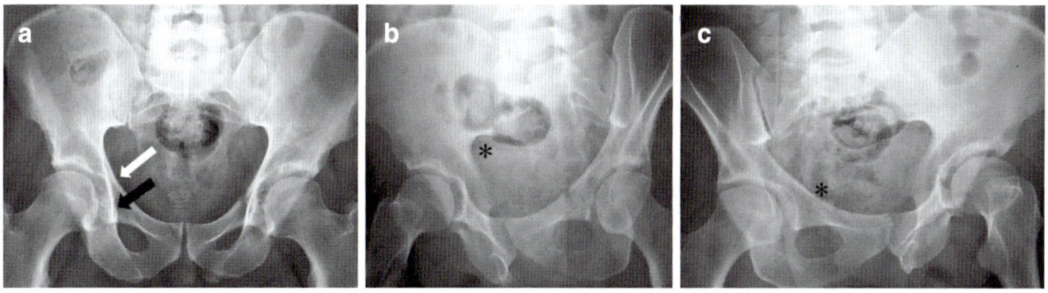

Fig. 20.18 (**a**–**c**) X-ray AP projection (**a**), iliac oblique view (**b**), and obturator oblique view (**c**) (projections of Judet). These three projections allow to identify the radiographic references of the two columns that are the iliopubic line as anterior column landmark (*white arrow* in **a**) and the ilioischiatic line as posterior column repere (*black arrow* in **a**) and the front and back acetabular edges that correspond to the anterior (*black arrow* in **b**) and posterior (*black arrow* in **c**) acetabular walls. The iliopubic line is best seen in the iliac oblique projection (*asterisk* in **c**); the ilioischiatic line is best seen in the obturator oblique projection (*asterisk* in **b**)

fractures is realized. The most commonly known is the fracture of the posterior wall (dashboard fracture), which can be complicated by the posterior limb of the femoral head. These images, though allow defining the fracture site and extension, do not always allow diagnosing composed or occult fracture lines and intra-articular fragments. CT has the possibility to evaluate the anatomy of the acetabulum, which looked like in front an overturned "Y" or "lambda" composed from the anterior (longer) and the posterior (smaller) columns which join on the supra-acetabular region; this is difficult to do with traditional radiographic methods for the particular "helix" configuration of the pelvis.

The surgical anatomy of the acetabulum described from Emile Letournel allows to distinguish the anterior (iliopubic) column which descends down from the iliac crest to the pubic symphysis and the posterior (iliopectineal) column extending from the incision of the great sciatic cranial to the ischiatic tuberosity.

Furthermore, CT allows the accurate diagnosis of the site and the morphology of the fracture, the precise evaluation of its extension and course, the definition of joint relationships, and the detection of free endo-articular or impact fragments. It also helps to diagnose roof and medial column fractures, which are often difficult to see. A working scheme suggested is to revive the conventional radiological AP, inlet, and outlet views of acetabular fractures with 3D reconstruction techniques at MSCT console. This allows us to no longer use the classical radiological semeiotics, thus overcoming the past with the new technological advances (Fig. 20.19).

It should also be remembered that, especially in the case of young subjects, the CT studies should be replaced, when possible, by alternative conventional radiological techniques in order to minimize the radiation dose. of the patient compared with conventional CT, using techniques that reduce the dose to the patient.

In conclusion, MSCT is a valid tool, is gaining an increasing role in the management of polytrauma patients, and is a powerful modality in the evaluation of skeletal trauma. MSCT with the use of MPR and 3D images is the technique of choice for evaluation of skeletal trauma.

20.4.3 Magnetic Resonance Imaging (MRI)

MRI is a second-level investigation dedicated to a selected case in which the first-instance methods are not sufficient. The use of MRI can obtain useful information in the research of radiographically occult fractures and in the study of bone lesions by impact or stress fractures. In

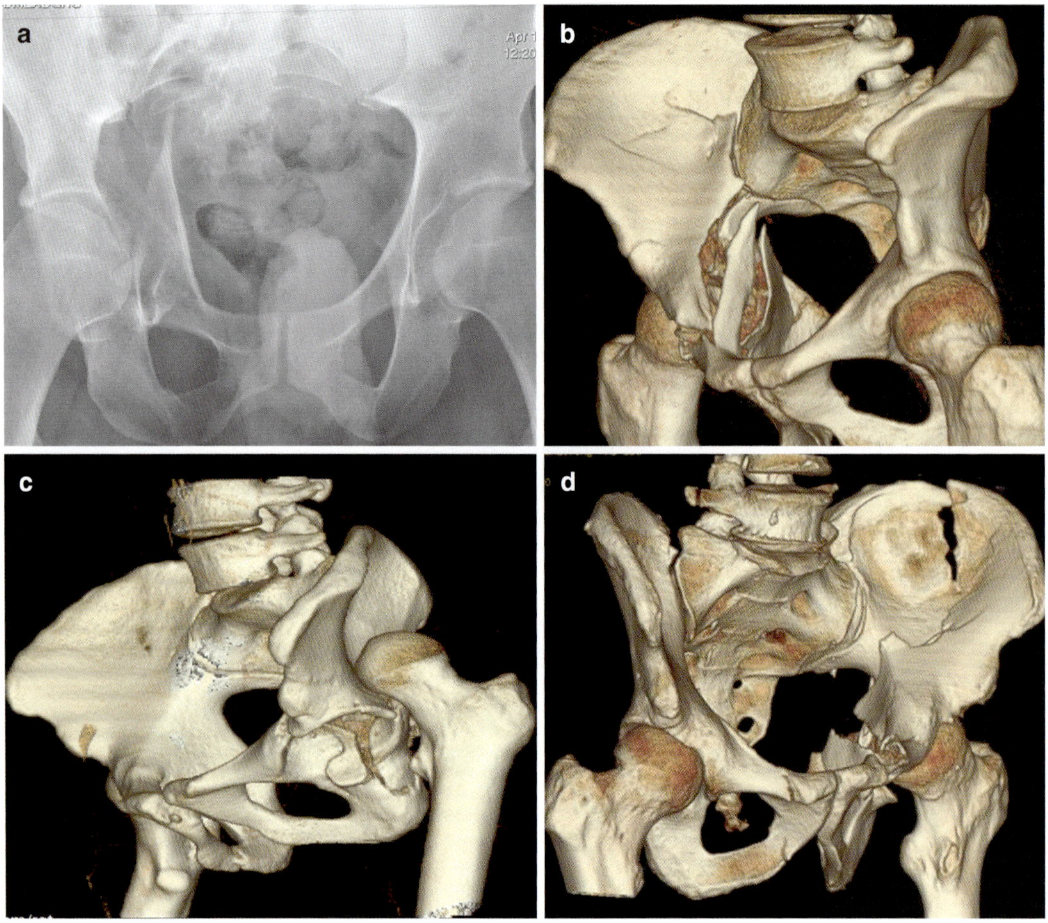

Fig. 20.19 (**a–d**) (**a**) X-ray AP projection: complex acetabular fracture; (**b**) CT 3D (VR) reconstructions show the involvement of the medial wall of the acetabulum; (**c**) CT 3D (VR) reconstruction iliac oblique view shows the posterior wall fracture associated with the posterior dislocation of the femoral head. (**d**) CT 3D (VR) reconstruction obturator oblique view demonstrates fracture of the two columns. 3D reconstruction shows the anterior fracture, with the fracture of the iliac crest and the complete detachment of the posterior column

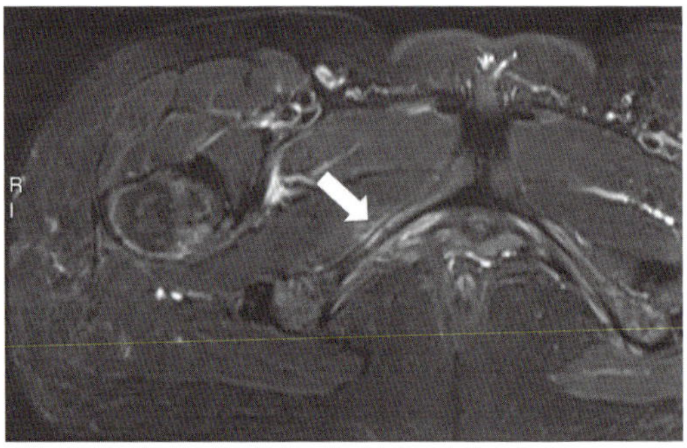

Fig. 20.20 STIR-weighted MRI axial view of the pelvis shows bone marrow edema of the right pubic branch and around soft tissues (*white arrow*), which is a sign of a radiographically occult fracture

stress fractures, in almost all of these situations, the characteristic symptom is pain, of varying degrees, which can be accompanied by functional impairment.

Early research and early diagnosis of stress fracture in the athlete, and in particular young people, avoid the possible dire consequences of failure to diagnose. Awareness of the possibility of a stress injury by knowing which athletic gesture can determine it is crucial. Early diagnosis allows the most appropriate therapeutic choice and is useful in reducing the recovery time of the patient and then initiating it safely in the recovery of the activity.

When the radiograph, first-instance examination, does not provide enough information to diagnose and clinical suspicion is grounded, MRI examination is appropriate and should be performed with T1- and T2-weighted sequences but also with STIR weighted that is of fundamental importance in the research and demonstration of bone marrow edema (Fig. 20.20).

In avulsion fractures, x-ray of the pelvis is usually sufficient to diagnose and to assess the extent of the lesion. MRI examination can better characterize the injury by showing the bone edema with long TR-weighted and STIR images and the focal extension in the unmineralized cartilage.

With MRI, it is also possible to estimate the extent of involvement of growth nuclei to direct the selection of those patients who need surgical treatment compared to those in which the conservative is sufficient. It is useful in completing the preoperative study of some complex sacral bone fractures.

Also in doubtful cases, the method can reduce the number of errors in diagnosis by improving patient outcomes and thus reducing the potential for medical-legal disputes resulting from failure to diagnose [51–56].

References

1. Flint L, Cryer HG. Pelvic fracture, the last 50 years. J Trauma. 2010;69:483–8.
2. Leone A, Galluzzo M, Miele V. Traumi del bacino. In: Miele V, Scaglione M, Grassi R, Rotondo A, editors. Diagnostica per Immagini nel trauma maggiore. Milano: Elsevier Editore; 2010. p. 231–40.
3. Galluzzo M, Buquicchio GL, Gaudino F, et al. Traumi del cingolo pelvico: pictorial essay. Il Giornale Italiano di. Radiol Med. 2016;3:46–57. doi:10.17376/girm_3-1-01022016-7.
4. Trainham L, Rizzolo D, Diwan A, Lucas T. Emergency management of high-energy pelvic trauma. JAAPA. 2015;28:28–33.
5. McCormak R, Strauss EJ, Alwatter BJ, Tejwani NC. Diagnosis and management of pelvic fractures. Bull NYU Hosp Jt Dis. 2010;68:281–91.
6. Burgess AR, Eastridge BJ, Young JW, et al. Pelvic ring disruptions: effective classification system and treatment protocols. J Trauma. 1990;30:848–56.
7. Hak DJ, Smith WR, Suzuki T. Management of hemorrhage in life threatening pelvic fracture. J Am Acad Orthop Surg. 2009;17:447–57.
8. Tile M. Acute pelvis fractures – I. Causation and classification. J Am Acad Orthop Surg. 1996;4:143–51.
9. Pennal GF, Tile M, Waddell JP, et al. Pelvic disruption: assessment and classification. Clin Orthop Relat Res. 1980;(151):12–21.
10. Riemer BL, Butterfield SL, Diamond DL, et al. Acute mortality associated with injuries to the pelvic ring: the role of early mobilization and external fixation. J Trauma. 1993;35:671–5.
11. McMurtry R, Walton D, Dickinson D, et al. Pelvic disruption in the polytraumatized patient: a management protocol. Clin Orthop. 1980;151:22–30.
12. Ward RE, Clark DG. Management of pelvic fractures. Radiol Clin North Am. 1981;19:167–70.
13. Agnew SG. Hemodynamically unstable pelvic fractures. Orthop Clin North Am. 1994;25:715–21.
14. Tile M. Pelvic fractures: operative versus nonoperative treatment. Orthop Clin North Am. 1980;11:423–64.
15. Stephen DJG. Understanding high-energy pelvis fractures. Can J CME. 2004;75–8.
16. McCort JJ, Mindelzum RE. Bladder injury and pelvic fractures. Emerg Radiol. 1994;11:47–51.
17. Rothenberger DA, Fischer RP, Strare R, et al. The mortality associated with pelvic fractures. Surgery. 1978;84:356–61.
18. Khurana B, Sheehan SE, Sodickson AD, Weaver MJ. Pelvic ring fractures – what the orthopaedic surgon wants to know. Radiographics. 2014;34:1317–33.
19. Woodley SJ, Kennedy E, Mercer SR. Anatomy in practice: the sacrotuberous ligament. N Z J Physiother. 2005;33:91–4.
20. van Wingerden J-P, Vleeming A, Snijders CJ, Stoeckart R. A functional-anatomical approach to the spine-pelvis mechanism: interaction between the biceps femoris muscle and the sacrotuberous ligament. Eur Spine J. 1993;2:140–4.
21. Pool-Goudzwaard AL, Kleinrensink GJ, Snijders CJ, et al. The sacroiliac part of the iliolumbar ligament. J Anat. 2001;199:457–63.
22. Gamble JG, Simmons SC, Freedman M. The symphysis pubis. Anatomic and pathologic considerations. Clin Orthop Relat Res. 1986;203:261–72.
23. Salari P, Moed BR, et al. Supplemental S1 fixation for type C pelvic ring injuries: biomechanical study of a long iliosacral versus a transsacral screw. J Orthop Traumatol. 2015;16:293–300.
24. Chenoweth DR, Cruickshank B, Gertzbein SD, et al. A clinical and experimental investigation of occult injuries of the pelvic ring. Injury. 1980;12:59–65.
25. Gertzbein SD, Chenoweth DR. Occult injuries of the pelvic ring. Clin Orthop Relat Res. 1977;128:202–7.
26. Stahel PF, Hammerberg EM. History of pelvic fracture management – a review. World J Emerg Surg. 2016;11:18.
27. Sarin EL, Moore JB, Moore EE, et al. Pelvic fracture pattern does not always predict the need for urgent embolization. J Trauma. 2005;58:973–7.
28. Ben-Menachem Y, Coldwell DM, Young JW, Burgess AR. Hemorrhage associated with pelvic fractures:

causes, diagnosis, and emergent management. AJR Am J Roentgenol. 1991;157:1005–14.
29. Bucholz RW. The pathological anatomy of Malgaigne fracture-dislocations of the pelvis. J Bone Joint Surg Am. 1981;63:400–4.
30. Gorczyca JT, Powell JN, Tile M. Lateral extension of the ilioinguinal incision in the operative treatment of acetabulum fractures. Injury. 1995;26:207–12.
31. Langford JR, Burgess AR, Liporace FA, Haidukewych GJ. Pelvic fractures, Part 1 – evaluation, classification and resuscitation. J Am Acad Orthop Surg. 2013;21:448–57.
32. Young JW, Burgess AR, Brumback RJ, Poka A. Pelvic fractures: value of plain radiography in early assessment and management. Radiology. 1986;160:445–51.
33. Young JWR, Resnik CR. Fractures of the pelvis: current concepts of classification. AJR. 1990;155:1169–75.
34. Langford JR, Burgess AR, Liporace FA, Haidukewych GJ. Pelvic fractures: part 2. Contemporary indications and techniques for definitive surgical management. J Am Acad Orthop Surg. 2013;21:458–68.
35. Huitten VM, Slatis P. Fractures of the pelvis: trauma mechanism, types of injury and principles of treatment. Acta Chir Scand. 1972;138:563–9.
36. Basta AM, Blackmore CC, Wessells H. Predicting urethral injury from pelvic fracture patterns in male patients with blunt trauma. J Urol. 2007;177:571–5.
37. Beckmann N, Cai C. CT characteristics of traumatic sacral fractures in association with pelvic ring injuries: correlation using the Young-Burgess classification system. Emerg Radiol. 2016;24:255–62.
38. Daffner RH, Sciulli RL. CT-guided iliosacral screw placement. Semin Musculoskelet Radiol. 2013;17:407–15.
39. Hakim RM, Gruen GS, Delitto A. Outcomes of patients with pelvic-ring fractures managed by open reduction internal fixation. Phys Ther. 1996;76:286–95.
40. Hunter JC, Brandser EA, Trank KA. Pelvic and acetabular trauma. Radiol Clin North Am. 1997;35(3):559–90.
41. Resnik CS, Stackhouse DJ, Shanmuganathan K, et al. Diagnosis of pelvic fractures in patients with acute pelvic trauma: efficacy of plain radiographs. AJR Am J Roentgenol. 1992;158:109–12.
42. Mears DC, Ward AJ, Wright MS. The radiological assessment of pelvic and acetabular fractures using three-dimensional computed tomography. Int J Orthop Trauma. 1992;2:196–209.
43. Tile M. Acute pelvic fractures – II. Principles of management. J Am Acad Orthop Surg. 1996;4:152–61.
44. Chaumòitre K, Portier F, Petit P, et al. CT imaging of pelvic injuries in polytrauma patients. J Radiol. 2000;81:111–22.
45. Gill R, Bucholz RW. The role of computerized tomographic scanning in the evaluation of major pelvic fractures. J Bone Joint Surg. 1984;66:34–9.
46. Pretorius ES, Fishman EK. Volume-rendered three-dimensional spiral CT: musculoskeletal applications. Radiographics. 1999;19:1143–60.
47. Rafii M, Firooznia H, Golimbu C, et al. The impact of CT in clinical management of pelvic and acetabular fractures. Clin Orthop. 1983;178:228–35.
48. Rommens P, Hartvig T, Wissing H, et al. Diagnosis and treatment of unstable fractures of the pelvic ring. Acta Chir Belg. 1986;6:352–9.
49. Yoon W, Kim JK, Jeong YY, et al. Pelvic arterial hemorrhage in patients with pelvic fractures: detection with contrast-enhanced CT. Radiographics. 2004;24:1591–605.
50. Dunn EL, Berry PH, Connoly PJ. Computed tomography of the pelvis in patients with multiple injuries. J Trauma. 1983;23:378–83.
51. Benedetti PF. MR imaging in emergency medicine. Radiographics. 1996;16:953–62.
52. Eustace S, Adams J, Assaf A. Emergency MR imaging of orthopedic trauma. Current and future directions. Radiol Clin North Am. 1999;37:975–94.
53. Elsayes KM, Lammle M, Shariff A, et al. Value of magnetic resonance imaging in muscle trauma. Curr Probl Diagn Radiol. 2006;35:206–12.
54. Piccolo C, Galluzzo M, Ianniello S, et al. Pediatric musculoskeletal injuries: role of ultrasound and magnetic resonance imaging. Musculoskelet Surg. 2017;101(Suppl 1):85–102.
55. Piccolo CL, Galluzzo M, Trinci M, et al. Upper limbs trauma in pediatrics. Semin Musculoskelet Radiol. 2017;21:167–74. doi:10.1055/s-0037-1602416.
56. Piccolo CL, Galluzzo M, Trinci M, et al. Lower limbs trauma in pediatrics. Semin Musculoskelet Radiol. 2017;21:175–83. doi:10.1055/s-0037-1602417.

Pelvic Trauma: Vascular/Visceral

21

Stefano Giannecchini, Valentina Caturano, Carmelo Rende, Viola Valentini, Margherita Trinci, and Vittorio Miele

21.1 Introduction

Over the past few years, trauma has become one of the leading causes of morbidity and mortality. Trauma is the fourth cause of all life years lost in the United States and abdominal and pelvis trauma contributes to a large number of these deaths [1]. Injuries of the pelvis are the result of high-energy impact force and are often associated with serious hemorrhage with high risk of fatal events. Pelvis trauma are also associated with a number of other acute and chronic complications, such as urological and neurological injuries, urinary and pulmonary infection, coagulopathies and chronic pains, leading to an high morbidity and long-term disability. In these patients, considerable resources are used and the socioeconomic implication is substantial. Therefore, a ready and accurate diagnosis is crucial, and it is still a great challenge for the radiologist.

S. Giannecchini (✉) • V. Caturano • C. Rende
V. Valentini • M. Trinci
Department of Emergency Radiology, S. Camillo Hospital, Rome, Italy
e-mail: giannecchinis@gmail.com

V. Miele
Department of Radiology, Careggi University Hospital, Florence, Italy

21.2 Mechanism of Injury and Pathophysiology

Fractures and injuries of solid and hollow viscera of the pelvis result from high-energy traumatic events as motor vehicle accident, falls from height, assaults, and sport accident. External compression and crushing injuries can explain the damage to the pelvic organs and several biomechanical studies have demonstrated the importance of the force vector in determining fracture pattern. The consequent possible instability of the pelvic ring has the effect of increasing the internal volume with a much higher incidence of soft tissue and vascular rupture and acute hemorrhage because of the reduced staunch effect. Most of the blood loss is derived from injured retroperitoneal veins and osseous fractures but discontinuity of pelvic arteries—commonly the superior gluteal and internal pudendal arteries—can cause uncontrolled bleeding with an alteration in hemodynamic status.

21.3 Morbidity and Mortality

Although pelvic fractures are relatively uncommon injuries, morbidity and mortality rates remain high and intrapelvic bleeding is the major determining factor of mortality. Mortality rates vary widely within the literature—ranging from 5% up to 60% [2, 3]—since pelvic fracture is usu-

V. Miele, M. Trinci (eds.), *Diagnostic Imaging in Polytrauma Patients*,
https://doi.org/10.1007/978-3-319-62054-1_21

ally associated with multisystem injuries as head trauma, liver and spleen trauma, chest trauma, and genitourinary trauma. However, up to 40% of pelvic fractures are complicated by intrapelvic bleeding [4] and hemodynamic instability and multiple organ failure as direct consequences are considered the primary cause of death.

Besides potentially life-threatening injuries, pelvic fractures are also associated with several acute lesions and chronic complications, leading to high morbidity and long-term disabilities [5].

21.4 Principles of Management

In these trauma, a punctual diagnosis and efficacious management is essential and despite the great efforts made to improve treatment of pelvic fracture and its complications, pelvic injuries continue to pose difficult management problems. Details of the mechanism of trauma and patient presentation at the emergency room may be useful to raise suspicion a pelvic fracture and possible associated injuries. The anatomical description of pelvic ring lesion is not crucial in the management of pelvic injuries and the first decisions are based mainly on the clinical conditions and associated injuries according to the guidelines of the Advanced Trauma Life Support (ATLS) protocol (Committee of Trauma of ACS.2012). Hemodynamic stabilization is the first and main aim. Focused assessment sonography for trauma (E-FAST) and pelvic X-ray should be utilized in hemodynamic and unstable patient in order to identify injuries that require temporary pelvic stabilization, immediate laparotomy, and angiography. A negative E-FAST does not exclude intraperitoneal hemorrhage and stable and stabilized patients must undergo further diagnostic study with a whole body continuous panoramic scan with intravenous contrast medium (c.m.) to locate quickly a possible primary source of hemorrhage and early identify other organ injuries. The frequent presence of other body lesions and the complexity of pelvic injuries impose a standardization of the diagnostic strategies at the emergency room in order to avoid wasting time, complicating the management, and compromising the outcome [6].

21.5 Major Vascular Injuries

Intrapelvic bleeding is the major determining factor of mortality in patients with pelvic fractures [4] with an overall mortality up to 17% [7]. Hemorrhage can occur from veins (80%) or arteries (20%) [8], and it can be difficult to determine whether the source of bleeding is arterial or venous. Laceration of branches of internal iliac artery alone accounts for about 25% of hemodynamically unstable pelvic fractures [3] but common sources of bleeding are also cancellous bone and retroperitoneal veins.

21.6 MDCT Imaging Findings

The imaging findings at CT may be classified as direct or indirect. Direct signs, which often need immediate endovascular procedure or surgery, are more specific but less sensitive and include abnormalities of the vessel wall such as laceration and active hemorrhage, intimal tear, dissection, occlusion, pseudoaneurysm, focal stenosis, and arteriovenous fistulas. Indirect signs, which tend to be more sensitive but less specific, are represented by muscle hematoma and pelvic extraperitoneal spaces hematoma.

21.6.1 Active Hemorrhage

Among vascular injuries of the pelvis, active arterial hemorrhage is the most significant cause of morbidity and mortality [4] and active extravasation of contrast media accounts for 50% of all pelvic vascular injuries identified at pelvic MDCT in severe blunt trauma patient [7]. Acute bleeding appears as extravascular hyperattenuating focus because of the contrast-enhanced blood extending beyond the vessel lumen. This focus expands in the following phases of acquisition but on arterial phase images, any area of hyperattenuation, regardless of the size, must be considered an arterial hemorrhage. Given the potential difference in management though, it is important to understand if the source of bleeding is arterial or venous [9]. Commonly an arterial injury appears as extravascular pooling of contrast material, with attenuation similar to or greater than that of the aorta in the arterial phase. Areas of active extravasation enlarge and have a greater attenuation value than the aorta in subsequently portal venous and delayed phase images (Fig. 21.1). Conversely, venous bleeding has later and less intense enhancement and it is seen only in the portal venous phase as a focus of extravascular hyperattenuation, also enlarging during the portal and capillary phase (Fig. 21.2). Most of venous vessel lesions are treated conservatively since hematoma is often self-limited but in a prefund hypotensive patient, also an arterial bleeding may be seen only in the portal or delayed phase.

Fractures involving the lesser sciatic foramen and mostly the greater sciatic foramen, common pathway for many pelvic vessels, have a great risk of bleeding, especially from the superior gluteal and the internal pudendal arteries. Therefore, the fracture location can be used to presume the injured artery [10, 11] but a readily and certain identification can only be obtained by a CT angiography.

There are a host of factors that influence the diagnostic quality of a CT examination and lead to a misinterpretation [12] but a careful attention to technique is crucial. For the purposes of this review, we will not discuss about contrast media CT protocol but it should be noted that a preliminary unenhanced scan must be obtained to differentiate active extravasation from other high-attenuation entities, such as bone fragments, foreign bodies, or drugs [13] (Fig. 21.3). Once ongoing hemorrhage is identified as focal area of high attenuation (greater than 90UH), equally important are coronal maximum intensity projection (MIP) reformatted images, useful

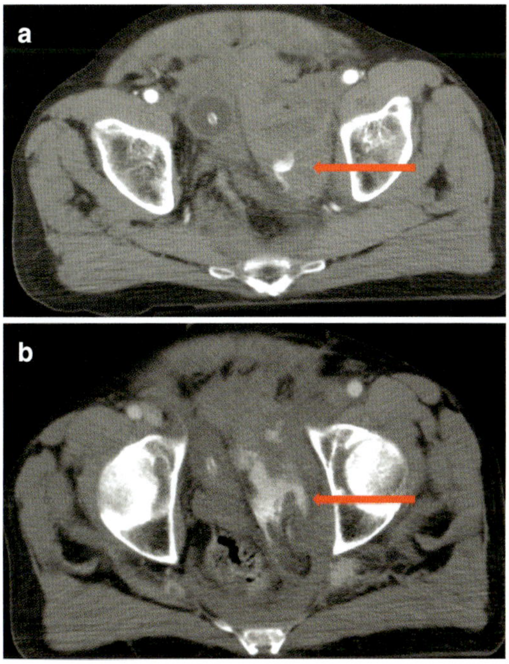

Fig. 21.1 Acute arterial bleeding; axial CT image of the pelvis on arterial (**a**) and venous (**b**) phases. Extravascular hyperattenuating focus with attenuation similar to that of the iliac arteries in the extraperitoneal left pelvic space (*arrow*) (**a**) enlarging (*arrow*) in the following phase of acquisition (**b**)

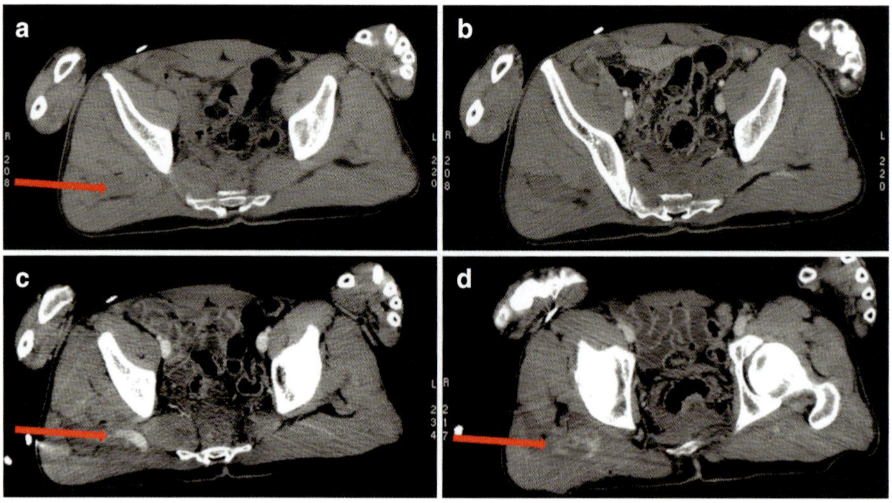

Fig. 21.2 Venous bleeding; axial CT image of the pelvis without c.m. (**a**) and with c.m. on arterial (**b**), venous (**c**), and capillary late (**d**) phases. Extrapelvic hematoma seen as an iso-hypoattenuating area in the right gluteal region (**a**) has the same attenuation values in the arterial phase (**b**). In the portal venous phase (**c**), a late focus of extravascular hyperattenuation appears into the hematoma (*arrow*), enlarging during capillary late phase (*arrow*) (**d**)

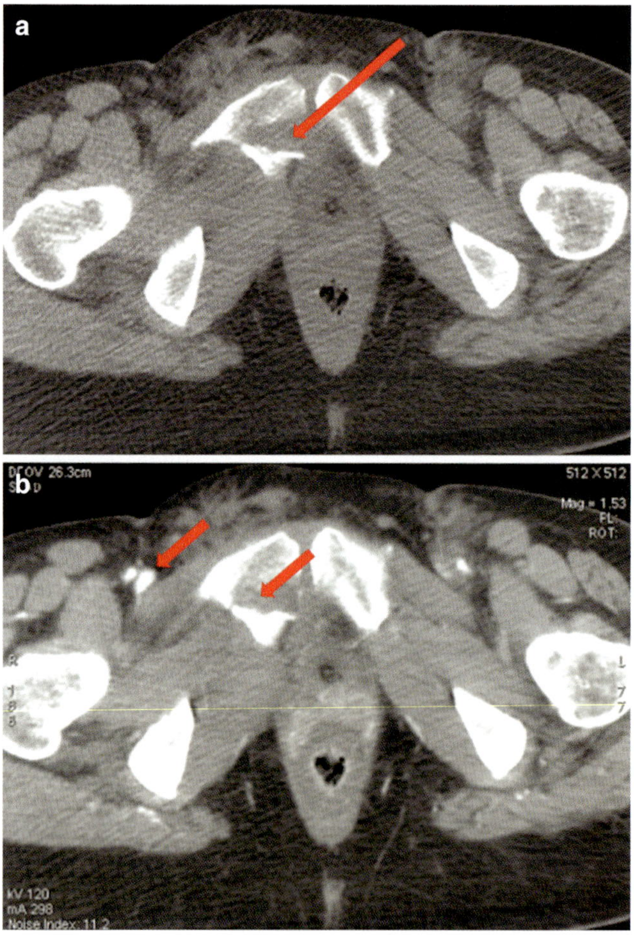

Fig. 21.3 Unenhanced (**a**) and post-contrast arterial phase (**b**) axial CT image. Hyperdense area close to the right ischio-pubic branche (*long arrow*) showing an attenuation higher than that of the iliac arteries (*short arrows*) (**b**) but equal in both unenhanced (**a**) and arterial (**b**) phases, corresponding to a bone fragment

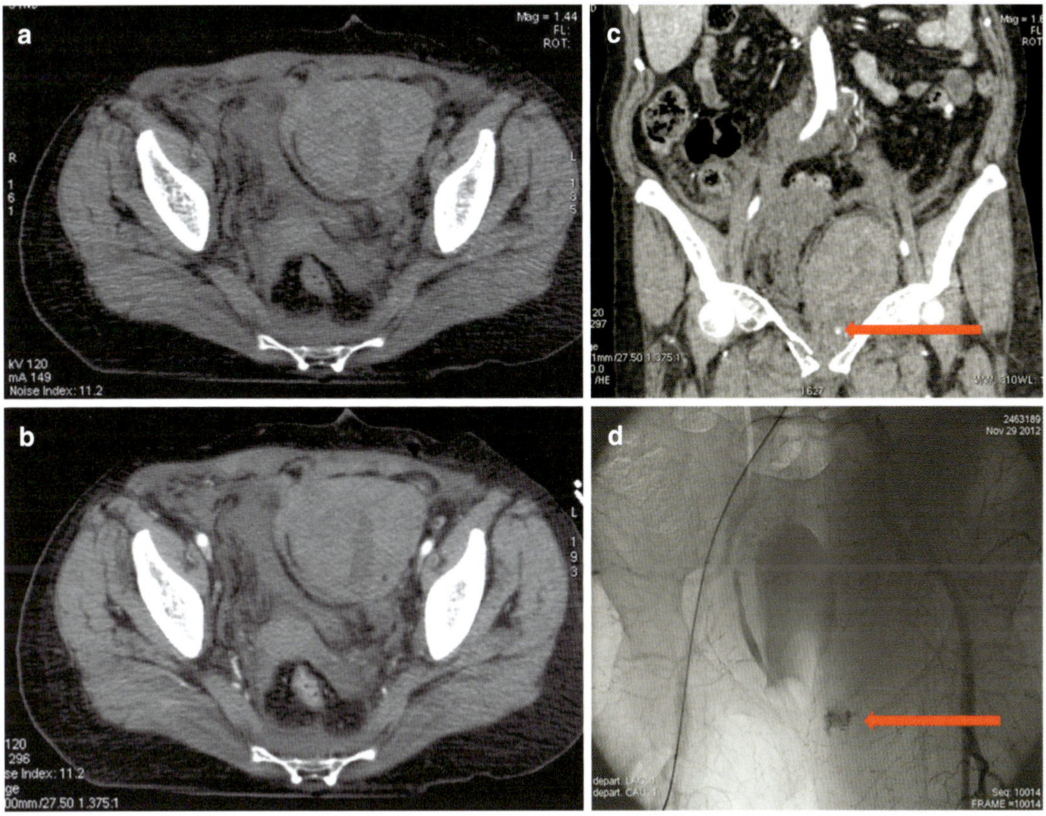

Fig. 21.4 Axial unenhanced (**a**) and arterial phase (**b**) CT image, coronal reformatting (**c**) and angiography (**d**) of the pelvis. Large extraperitoneal hematoma in the left pelvic side wall, appearing as an hyperattenuating collection in the unenhanced (**a**) and arterial axial images (**b**); the coronal reformatting of the arterial phase (**c**) shows a minute focus of enhancement (*arrow*), corresponding to an active arterial bleeding. Selective angiography (**d**) confirmed blood extravasation and the exact site (*arrow*)

to detect the exact site of extravasation [5]. Finally, multiplanar reformation (MPR), viewed in combination with axial images, may be used to evaluate vessel along its long axis and reveal subtle injuries [1] (Fig. 21.4).

21.6.2 Other Form of Vascular Injuries

Vessel injuries may be present in the absence of active hemorrhage [5]. These lesions must be known and accurately identified since can be a source of emboli, occlusion, or progress to complete rupture with a concomitant active hemorrhage. Vessel wall injuries have a spectrum of imaging more subtle at CT, ranging from irregular narrowing and outpouching to complete occlusion.

21.6.2.1 Intimal Tear and Arterial Dissection

At imaging, the separation of the intima from the adjacent media leads to a segmental, linear, or curvilinear hypoattenuating filling defect originating from the vessel wall in the enhanced arterial lumen. In the case of dissection, blood is interposed between the intima/inner media and the outer adventitia by forming a true and false lumen. Arterial dissection may be caused by mechanical forces from trauma often in combination with underlying arteriopathies. Dissection may cause thromboemboli that may occlude the arterial lumen. With thrombosis an arterial dissection may manifest at CT as a crescent focal region of vessel narrowing. Traumatic dissection can also be the cause of an intermittent ongoing bleeding, not evident on CT, and therefore it requires an angiographic study [4, 7, 13].

21.6.2.2 Pseudoaneurysm

A pseudoaneurysm occurs secondary to a complete or partial disruption of the wall vessel with blood contained by the adventitia or perivascular tissues through formation of a fibrous capsule (Fig. 21.5). Pseudoaneurysm are unstable and at increased risk for rupture or partial thrombosis and cause emboli to distal organ. At imaging, a focal well-circumscribed arterial outpouching of contrast-enhanced blood is seen adjacent to the vessel lumen. On portal veins and delayed phase images, pseudoaneurysm does not enlarge and reflect the attenuation of the blood pool, showing a hypoattenuating values over time as arterial enhancement washes out [4, 7, 13] (Fig. 21.6).

21.6.2.3 Occlusion

Occlusion of a major vessel may result from intimal disruption with subsequent platelet aggregation, leading to thrombosis. A full-thickness injury with spasm also can cause a vessel occlusion and in these cases the possibility of hemorrhage should be taken seriously, even if there is no extravasation of c.m. when CT is performed. Occlusion appears as abrupt cutoff of a contrast-enhanced vessel [4, 13].

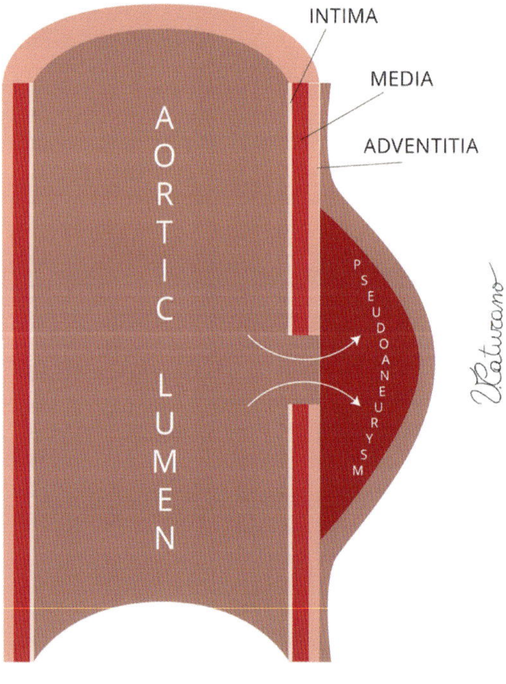

Fig. 21.5 Pseudoaneurysm: a complete or partial disruption of the wall vessel leads to an outpouching blood collection delimited by adventitia or fibrous capsule

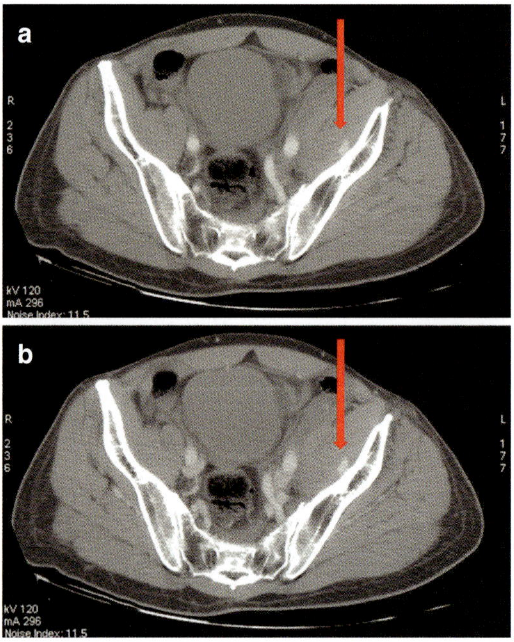

Fig. 21.6 Pseudoaneurysm on axial CT image on arterial (**a**) and venous (**b**) phases. A focal well-circumscribed arterial outpouching of contrast-enhanced blood is seen inside left iliac muscle (*arrow*) in the arterial phase (**a**). On portal venous phase (**b**), the area does not enlarge and it reflects the attenuation value of the blood pool

21.6.2.4 Focal Stenosis

Intra- or extramural hematoma, intimal injuries with partial thrombosis, and spasms are all potential causes of focal areas of narrowing and irregularity of the arterial lumen. On CT images, generally, it can be hard to differentiate a spasm from a true injured vessel and although an arterial spasm generally appears as concentric smoothly tapered traits of narrowing adjacent or even distal to the site of injury, imaging findings are not specific and cannot be used to exclude other type of vessel injuries. Nevertheless, vasospasm should remain in the differential diagnosis because, although it may resolve spontaneously, it can also mask an intraluminal thrombosis [7].

21.6.2.5 Arteriovenous Fistula

Arteriovenous fistulas, a direct communication between an artery and a vein, are rare in blunt trauma and difficult to detect and the diagnosis often delayed. Although infrequent, immediate diagnosis of this injury is important due to high risk of rupture. The typical finding on MDCT is an early filling of a pelvic vein with contrast material in the arterial phase when c.m. should only be visible within the pelvic artery. It is important to look through contralateral anatomic equivalent of the pelvis veins because an asymmetric early filling can also be diagnostic [4, 7, 13].

21.7 Urological Injuries After Pelvic Trauma (Urinary Bladder and Urethra)

Genitourinary injuries are well-identified complications and occur in as many as 15–20% of pelvic fractures cases, especially if pubic symphysis is involved (3,8). Pelvic fracture pattern, as shown by the pelvic X-ray eventually performed at emergency room, may predict the risk of genitourinary injury and the presence of blood at the urethral meatus and gross hematuria [14], should raise the suspicion for a genitourinary injury. In patients with blunt trauma pelvic fracture associated with bladder injury, it was demonstrated that pelvic injuries included diastasis of the pubic symphysis greater than 1 cm and fracture of obturator ring, with a displacement greater than 1 cm [15]. In the western world, the most common cause of urological injuries are wide-impact blunt abdominal traumas in road accidents, but the incidence of penetrating trauma is increasing [16, 17]. Whether the trauma is blunt or penetrating, associated multiorgan injuries are common and affect frequently the liver and the spleen [18].

21.7.1 Urinary Bladder Trauma

Motor vehicle crashes, falls, and crush injuries are the most frequent cause of bladder trauma [19] and major mechanisms of injuries are blunt trauma or penetrating trauma by fracture fragments. In any case, 60–90% of patients suffering from a blunt trauma bladder injury have associated pelvic fractures [19] and 25% of intraperitoneal bladder lesions occur without a pelvic fracture [20]. Injuries range from contusions to rupture and most of the ruptures result from a blunt trauma with distended bladder. In effect the type and the extent of lesion depend not only on external mechanism but also on the state of bladder relaxation at the time of trauma. Beyond contusion lesions, limited to the mucous membrane with no imaging finds [21], intraperitoneal rupture occurs when a strong compression on the lower abdomen causes sudden increase in pressure in a distended lumen bladder. The rupture affects the dome which is the weakest portion of the bladder and covered by peritoneum, causing an intraperitoneal extravasation which outline peritoneal structures, such as the bowel and the mesentery. Yet most frequent bladder injuries are extraperitoneal rupture (accounting for 80–90% of cases) and generally associated with pelvic fractures [14]. Urine extravasation can be restricted in the pelvic extraperitoneal space (simple extraperitoneal rupture) or reach distant locations, as the anterior abdominal wall, the penis, the scrotum, and the perineum since the injury may cause a disruption of the fascial planes of the pelvis (complex extraperitoneal rupture). Combined intraperitoneal and extraperitoneal bladder injuries occur in as many as 5% of major bladder trauma [14].

21.7.1.1 Classification

The American Association for the Surgery of Trauma (AAST) classified bladder injuries according to five grades scale, while the Societé Internationale d'Urologie (SIU) uses a classification into four types (type 1 bladder contusion, type 2 intraperitoneal rupture, type 3 extraperitoneal rupture, type 4 combined injury). The latter classification does not take into account the length and extent of the wall laceration but it simply aims to determine the presence of the injury as assessed by contrast extravasation on CT cystography [14].

21.7.1.2 Imaging

Diagnosis of bladder injury on MDCT may be challenging if bladder is not well distended. On the other hand, polytrauma patients are catheterized and bladder is empty when they are examined. Decision to performing a CT cystography is taken on the basis of clinical and radiological basis. The finding of pelvic fractures may be determinant but if associated with gross hematuria, the indication for evaluation of bladder is absolute. Relative indications are also gross hematuria without pelvic fracture, microhematuria with pelvic fracture, and isolated microhematuria. The only reliable method for filling the bladder is the retrograde active distension with c.m [14]. The passive distension of the bladder during the abdominal CT cannot be considered reliable on to diagnose bladder rupture, even with bladder catheter clamped or acquisition of a delayed scan, no matter if bladder appears distended. Indeed, the antegrade approach may detect intra- or extraperitoneal fluid but is not capable to differentiate urine from ascites. 300 ml of diluted water-soluble iodinated radiopaque c.m. is introduced into the bladder through a urethral catheter, and a CT scan performed before the infusion of intravenous c.m. for routine next abdominal CT [22]. Typically, a CT cystography shows a contrast extravasation into perivesical fat and occasionally into anterior abdominal wall, allowing a distinction between intra- and extraperitoneal rupture (Figs. 21.7 and 21.8). This distinction has a paramount importance and immediate therapeutic implications because intraperitoneal rupture requires surgical management while extraperitoneal rupture can be treated conservatively [23].

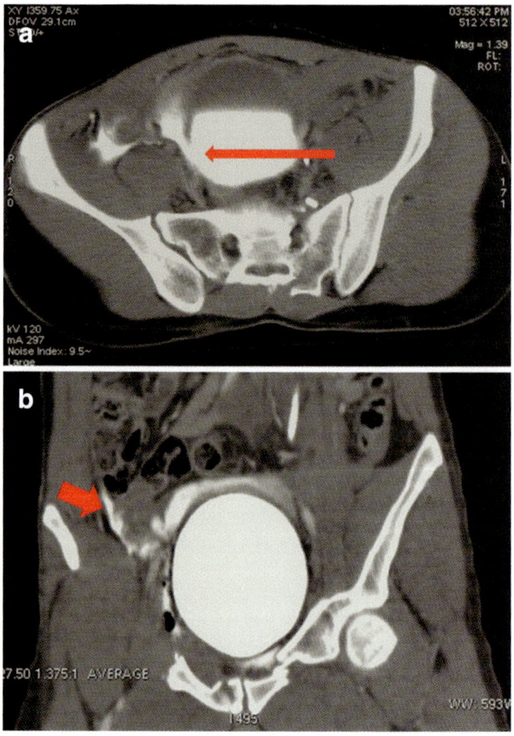

Fig. 21.7 Urinary bladder intraperitoneal rupture; axial (**a**) and coronal (**b**) reformatting image of a CT cystography. Laceration of the left bladder wall seen as a defect in wall contour (*long arrow*) and contrast extravasation outlining peritoneal space (*short arrow*)

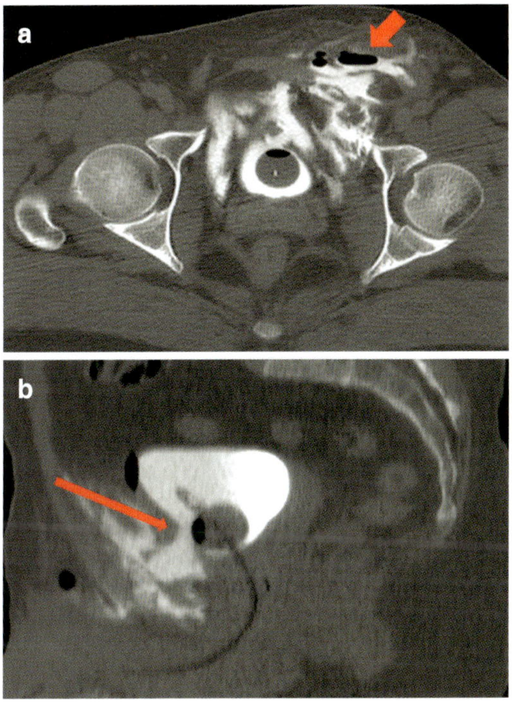

Fig. 21.8 Urinary bladder extraperitoneal rupture; axial image (**a**) and sagittal reformatting (**b**) of a CT cystogram. Focal disruption of bladder floor in the anterior site (*arrow*) with diffuse contrast extravasation into the perivesical extraperitoneal space and in the anterior abdominal wall (*short arrow*); note the presence of gas bubbles

21.7.2 Urethral Trauma

While isolated urethral injury is rare, urethral injury is a common complication of pelvic trauma associated with pelvic fracture and occurs in as many as 24% of these adult patients [24]. 10–29% of males with pelvic trauma may be affected by simultaneous rupture of bladder and prostatomembraneous urethra [14] and except for these cases, urethral injuries are rarely life-threatening in the acute phase. Nevertheless these lesions must be promptly suspected and appropriately treated since they are often cause of late complications, as strictures, impotence, incontinence, that result in significant long-term morbidity [25]. Although retrograde urethrography should be the diagnostic procedure of choice to evaluate patients with suspected urethral injury (Fig. 21.9), in polytrauma patients a Foley catheter is immediately placed for the purpose of monitoring fluid intake and output, so that CT does play a primary role and becomes the main diagnostic modality. And since urethral injury is mainly suspected on the basis of indirect findings on CT scan, the radiologist plays a key role in advancing the suspect of lesion to be accurate identified with further subsequent urethrography [14, 25].

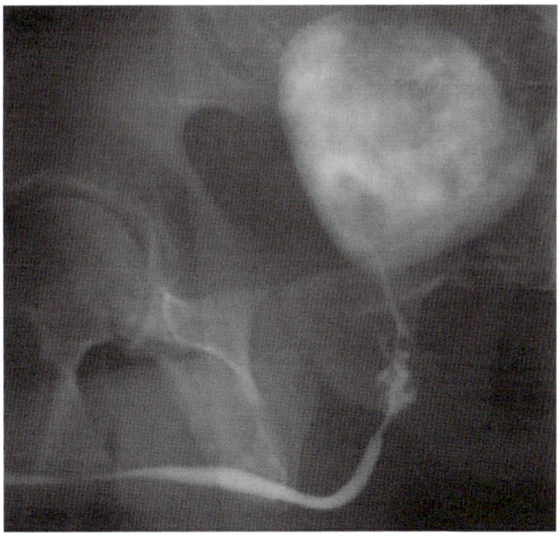

Fig. 21.9 Retrograde urethrography performed to assess site and extension of the urethral laceration

21.7.2.1 Anatomy

Male urethra is divided into two main parts: the posterior urethra and the anterior urethra, respectively, divided into prostatic and membranous segments and bulbous and penile segments. The two main portions are anchored to the anterior pubic arch by puboprostatic ligaments and separated by the urogenital diaphragm (Fig. 21.10). The female urethral anatomy is simpler because of its small size, internal location in the distal anterior vaginal wall, and the absence of a firm attachment to the pubic bone [14, 25].

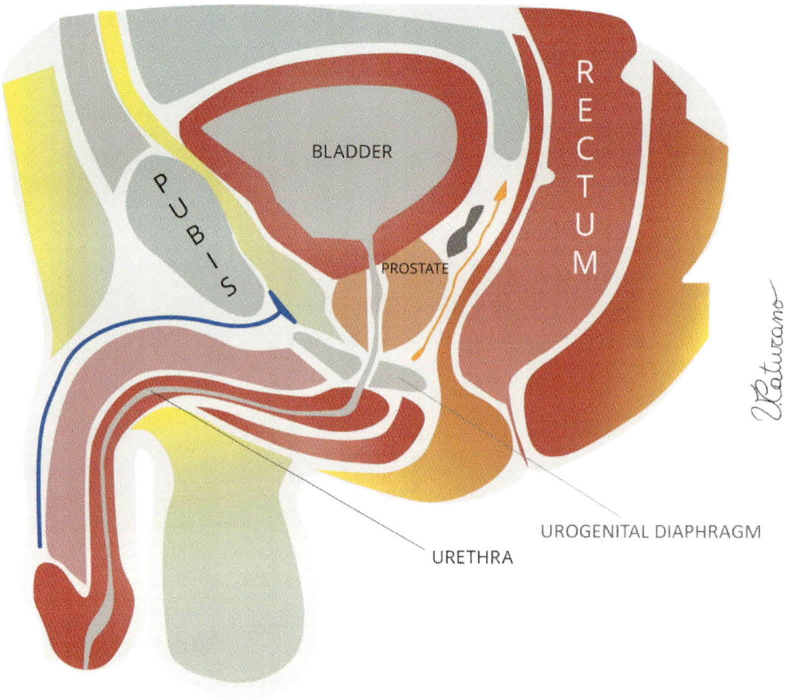

Fig. 21.10 Normal male urethral anatomy in the sagittal plane. Urogenital diaphragm is a key anatomic landmark in urethral traumas

21.7.2.2 Mechanism and Classification

The most common causes of urethral injury are motor vehicle crashes and fall from height. 3–25% of patients have pelvic fracture [25] and the most frequent injury affects the posterior portion of urethra due to the frequent involvement of the pubic bones and the puboprostatic ligaments. 20% of patients suffering from a urethral injury have associated bladder laceration [26]. The anterior urethra is inserted into a less rigid system than the posterior portion and injuries are less frequent and account for about 33% of patients. This type of lesion results from the crushing of the urethra against the pubis (straddle injury), which directly injuries the bulbous urethra. Commonly, urethra is compressed between an external hard object, blown to the perineum, and the lower margin of the symphysis pubic. Generally, there are no associated pelvic fractures. Lesions of female urethra are uncommon (less than 6% of female pelvic fractures) and often part of severe pelvic trauma and frequently accompanied by vaginal and rectal injuries [25].

The unified classification system proposed by Goldman marks the anatomic location of the lesion, and it is commonly used to classify the urethral injuries [26]. However, urethrography remains the gold standard for a correct injury classification and before it can be executed in a polytrauma patient, days may pass. It is therefore crucial to know clinical signs of urethral injury and recognize findings on CT, related to posterior urethral injuries [14].

21.7.2.3 Imaging

When a patient with pelvic trauma presents with gross hematuria blood at the meatus, hematoma, and swelling of the perineum, urethral injury must be suspected. As already pointed out, on CT scan urethral injury can only be diagnosed or suspected based on indirect signs. Major findings include obscuration of the urogenital diaphragmatic fat plane, swollen and increased volume

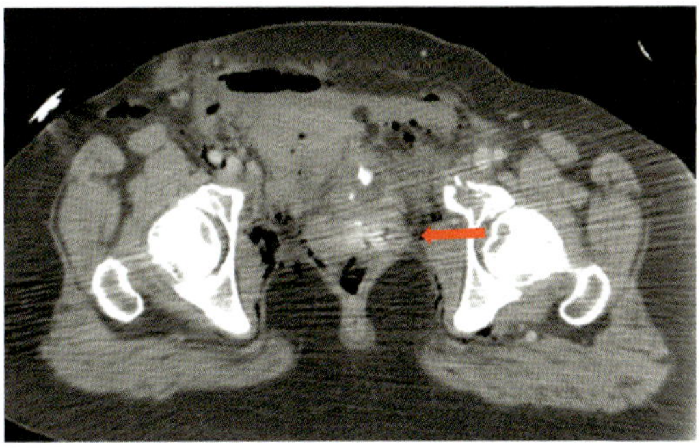

Fig. 21.11 Delayed axial CT cystographic image. Hematoma causes obscuration of the urogenital diaphragmatic fat plane (*short arrow*) and loss of prostatic contour. These findings are suggestive for urethral laceration

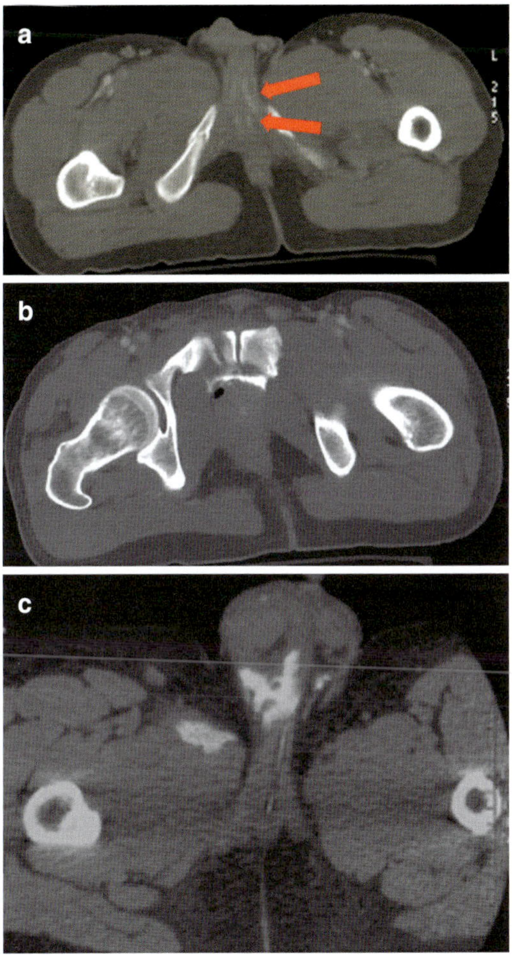

Fig. 21.12 Unenhanced axial CT image (**a**), delayed axial CT cystographic image (**b** and **c**). A mural hematoma causes ischiocavernosus and bulbocavernosus muscle high attenuation (*short arrows*) (**a**). Extravasation of iodinated c.m. is associated in the periprostatic space (**b**) and along the bulbar tract of the urethra (**c**)

ischiocavernosus and obturator internus muscles due to mural hematoma, loss of prostatic contour and obscuration of the bulbocavernosus muscle (Figs. 21.11 and 21.12). Among these signs, the most significant are obscuration of the urogenital diaphragmatic fat plane and hematoma of the ischiocavernosus muscle, both seen in 88% of patients with urethral injury. Loss of prostatic contour and obscuration of the bulbocavernosus muscle are present, respectively, in 59% and 47%, and hematoma of the obturator internus muscles is seen in 53% of patients with urethral injury [14].

21.8 Neurological and Bowel Injuries

21.8.1 Nervous Structure Trauma

21.8.1.1 Mechanism

Neurological injuries can be difficult to be detected, and they are often overlooked during the initial complex trauma management. The risk and nature of neurological injury is closely related to the fracture pattern. The extension to the posterior portion of pelvic ring and mostly the presence of a sacral fracture [27] are very significant signs for suspecting the involvement of nerve structures in the pelvic floor (Fig. 21.13).

Commonly, these are high-energy traumas, as it happens in motor vehicle crashes, fall from height and crushing trauma, though most pelvic fractures involving the sacral region the elderly are caused by low-energy trauma.

The neurological lesions associated with pelvic or sacral fractures may affect a single nerve, multiple nerve roots, or a whole nervous plexus with different clinical presentations and symptoms. Pain in the affected region, urinary disorders such as bladder incontinence, genital disorders such as erectile dysfunction, fecal incontinence and poor anal tone, loss of sensitivity, and the absence of reflections are some of the possible signs and symptoms of a neurological injury with often permanent consequences.

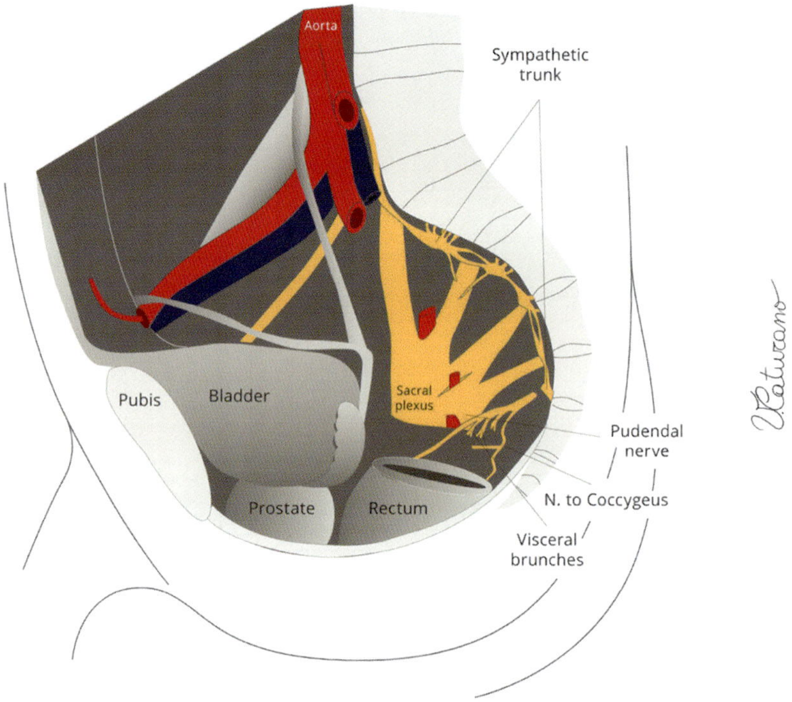

Fig. 21.13 The strict relationship between posterior portion of pelvic ring and sacral bone and sacral plexus

21.8.1.2 Imaging

The fracture location can be used to presume the injured nervous structure but a readily and certain identification in emergency is quite difficult since CT has limited sensitivity in soft tissue contrast. Lesions of nerve roots nervous are only detected in 30% of cases during the early assessment after the trauma and frequently the diagnosis may be delayed up to 1 year after the traumatic event [28].

So the radiologist, along clinical signs, must consider the pattern of fracture where a sciatic nerve injury may occur in fracture involving the greater sciatic foramen while a transverse sacral fracture can be the cause of intraspinal nerve root injury (Fig. 21.14).

Once the suspect of a neurological injury has been placed, it will be accurately identified with further subsequent MRI which has no role in the acute setting.

21.8.2 Lower Gastrointestinal Trauma

21.8.2.1 Mechanism

Traumatic injuries of the bowel following pelvic fractures are relatively common, [29] and it can be easily diagnosed because of the typical symptoms and signs, such as peritoneal irritation, free abdominal air and fluid, and severe sepsis. Conversely, bowel entrapment at the pelvic fracture site is a rare complication in pelvic fracture, and it can be fatal because of its clinical complexity. It is also difficult to distinguish from adynamic ileus, a more benign condition that occurs in up to 5–18% of pelvic fractures [3].

Disruption of the bowel is seen in the setting of severe pelvic fractures, and it is often associated with serious injuries of other organs. Colorectal and anus injuries are usually due to high-energy trauma though no penetrating rectum

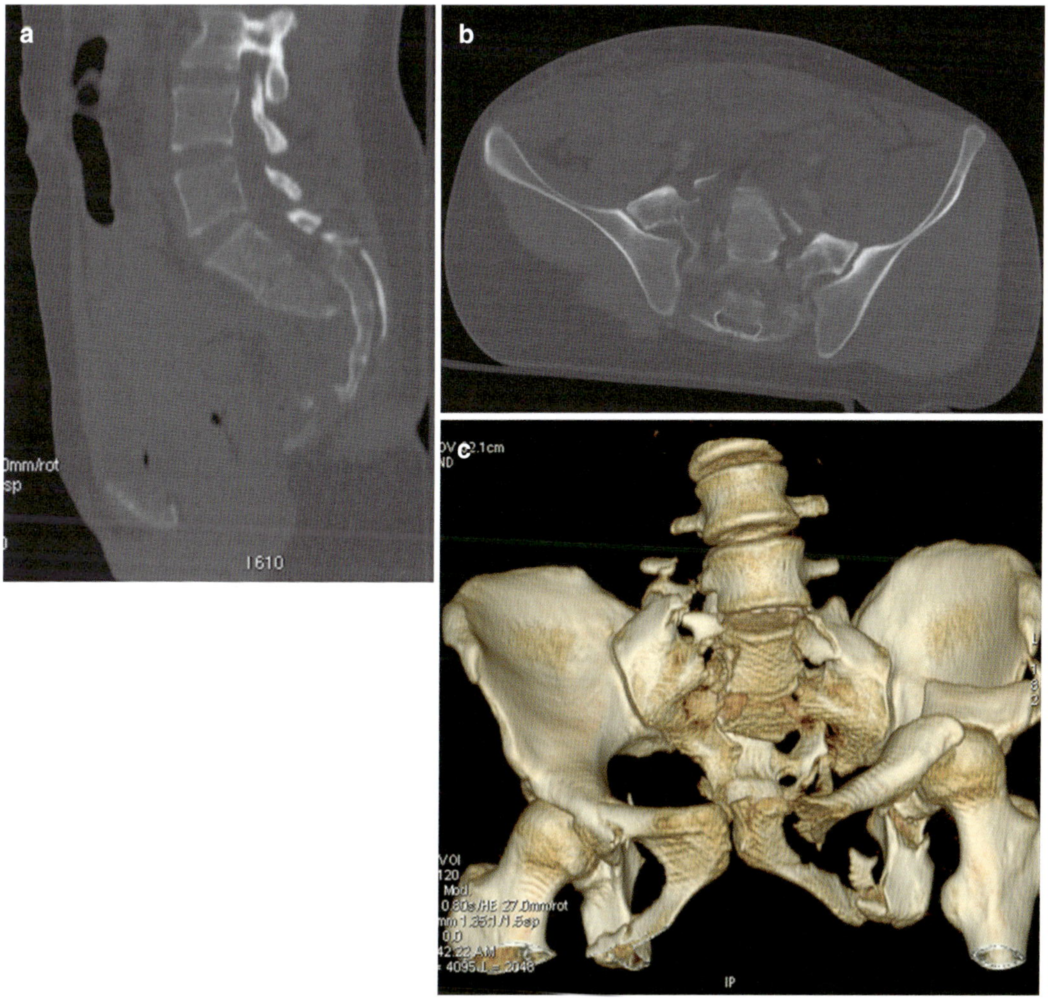

Fig. 21.14 Unenhanced CT scan; sagittal (**a**), axial (**b**) images, and 3D volume rendering (**c**). A complex fracture of the sacrum and ileus involving the ischiatic foramen currently causes sciatic nerve injury and intraspinal nerve root injury

injuries are uncommon (from 1% to 5% of patients with blunt abdominal trauma) [30] due to the anatomical protection offered from the bone pelvis.

21.8.2.2 Imaging

CT is considered a very sensitive imaging modality for both the diagnosis of colorectal and anus disruptions [31] and the diagnosis of bowel entrapment. Free abdominal air is a strongly suggestive direct sign of hollow viscus injury but free intraperitoneal or retroperitoneal fluid has a high predictive value for bowel disruption. An indirect sign of colorectal or anus injury is a focal bowel wall thickening (intestinal contusion). Finally, focal increased density of intestinal wall can mean an arterial or venous ischemia, a strong indication for a prompt laparotomy [32].

Careful monitoring and awareness should be instead the main attitude to exclude and possibly diagnose a bowel entrapment. Patients with pelvic fractures and a persistent progressive ileus should undergo a CT with combined use of oral and IV contrast to rule out entrapment at the fracture site [3, 33].

References

1. Soto JA, Anderson SW. Multidetector CT of blunt abdominal trauma. Radiology. 2012;265(3):678–93.
2. Papakostidis C, Kanakaris N, Dimitriou R, Giannoudis PV. The role of arterial embolization in controlling pelvic fracture haemorrhage: a systematic review of the literature. Eur J Radiol. 2012;81(5):897–904.
3. McCormack R, Strauss EJ, Alwattar BJ, et al. Diagnosis and management of pelvic fractures. Bull NYU Hosp Jt Dis. 2010;68(4):281–91.
4. Kertesz JL, Anderson SW, Murakami AM, et al. Detection of vascular injuries in patients with blunt pelvic trauma by using 64-channel multidetector CT. Radiographics. 2009;29(1):151–64.
5. Galluzzo M, Buquicchio GL, Gaudino F, Ianniello S, Leone A, Trinci M, Miele V. Traumi del cingolo pelvico: Pictorial essay. Il Giornale Italiano di. Radiol Med. 2016;3:46–57. doi:10.17376/girm_3-1-01022016-7.
6. Miele V, Di Giampietro I (2014) Diagnostic Imaging in Emergency. Salute e Società (2EN):127–38. doi:10.3280/SES2014-002010EN.
7. Romano L, Pinto A, Niola R, et al. Bleeding due to pelvic fractures in female patients: pictorial review of multidetector computed tomography imaging. Curr Probl Diagn Radiol. 2012;41(3):83–92.
8. Coccolini F, Stahel PF, Montori G, et al. Pelvic trauma: WSES classification and guidelines. World J Emerg Surg. 2017;12:5.
9. Baghdanian AH, Armetta AS, Baghdanian A, et al. CT of major vascular injury in blunt abdominopelvic trauma. Radiographics. 2016;36(3):872–90.
10. Slater SJ, Barron DA. Pelvic fractures-a guide to classification and management. Eur J Radiol. 2010;74(1):16–23.
11. Pieri S, Agresti P, Buquicchio GL, DI Giampietro I, Trinci M, Miele V. Endovascular management of the rectus muscle hematoma. Radiol Med. 2015;120(10):951–8. doi:10.1007/s11547-015-0516-2.
12. Patlas MN, Dreizin D, Menias CO, et al. Abdominal and pelvic trauma: misses and misinterpretations at multidetector CT: trauma/emergency radiology. Radiographics. 2017;37(2):703–4.
13. Hamilton JD, Kumaravel M, Censullo ML, et al. Multidetector CT evaluation of active extravasation in blunt abdominal and pelvic trauma patients. Radiographics. 2008;28(6):1603–16.
14. Ramchandani P, Buckler PM. Imaging of genitourinary trauma. AJR Am J Roentgenol. 2009;192(6):1514–23.
15. Avey G, Backmore CC, Wessells H, et al. Radiographic and clinical predictors of bladder rupture in blunt trauma patients with pelvic fracture. Acad Radiol. 2006;13(5):573–9.
16. Baverstock R, Simons R, McLoughlin M. Severe blunt renal trauma: a 7-year retrospective review from a provincial trauma centre. Can J Urol. 2001;8(5):1372–6.
17. Smith J, Caldwell E, D'Amours S, et al. Abdominal trauma: a disease in evolution. ANZ J Surg. 2005;75(9):790–4.
18. Yao DC, Jeffrey RB Jr, Mirvis SE, et al. Using contrast-enhanced helical CT to visualize arterial extravasation after blunt abdominal trauma: incidence and organ distribution. AJR Am J Roentgenol. 2002;178(1):17–20.
19. Gomez RG, Ceballos L, Coburn M, et al. Consensus statement on bladder injuries. BJU Int. 2004;94(1):27–32.
20. Sandler CM, Goldman SM, Kawashima A. Lower urinary tract trauma. World J Urol. 1998;16(1):69–75.
21. Kane NM, Francis IR, Ellis JH. The value of CT in the detection of bladder and posterior urethral injuries. AJR Am Roentgenol. 1989;153(6):1243–6.
22. Quagliano PV, Delair SM, Malhotra AK. Diagnosis of blunt bladder injury: a prospective comparative study of computed tomography cystography and conventional retrograde cystography. J Trauma. 2006;61(2):410–21.
23. Fu CY, Teng LH, Liao CH, et al. The diminishing role of pelvic stability evaluation in the era of computed tomographic scanning. Medicine (Baltimore). 2016;95(16):e 3421.
24. Koraitim MM. Pelvic fracture urethral injuries: evaluation of various methods of management. J Urol. 1996;156:1288–91.
25. Ingram MD, Watson SG, Skippage PL, et al. Urethral injuries after pelvic trauma: evaluation with urethrography. Radiographics. 2008;28(6):1631–43.
26. Goldman SM, Sandler CM, Corriere JN Jr, et al. Blunt urethral trauma: a unified, anatomical mechanical classification. J Urol. 1997;157(1):85–9.
27. Schmidek HH, Smith DA, Kristiansen TK. Sacral fractures. Neurosurgery. 1984;15(5):735–46.
28. Garozzo D, Zollino G, Ferraresi S. In lumbosacral plexus injuries can we identify indicators that predict spontaneous recovery or the need for surgical treatment? Results from a clinical study on 72 patients. J Brachial Plex Peripher Nerve Inj. 2014;9(1):1.
29. Kekez T, Augustin G. Small bowel entrapment associated with pelvic fracture: a case report with review of the literature and differentiation of clinical picture. Eur J Emerg Med. 2012;19(1):60–1.
30. Cleary RK, Pomerantz RA, Lampman RM. Colon and rectal injuries. Dis Colon Rectum. 2006;49(8):1203–22.
31. Bondia JM, Anderson SW, Rhea JT, Soto JA. Imaging colorectal trauma using 64-MDCT technology. Emerg Radiol. 2009;16(6):433–40.
32. Atri M, Hanson JM, Grinblat L, et al. Surgically important bowel and/or mesenteric injury in blunt trauma: accuracy of multidetector CT for evaluation. Radiology. 2008;249(2):524–33.
33. Zong ZW, Bao QW, Liu HY, et al. Diagnosis and treatment of rare complications of pelvic fractures. Chin J Traumatol. 2016;19(4):199–205.

Abdominal Trauma: Interventional Radiology

22

Germano Scevola, Marco Rastelli, Giorgio Loreni, Claudio Raspanti, Gloria Addeo, and Vittorio Miele

22.1 Introduction

Over the last decades, as well as diagnostic radiology, interventional radiology techniques have been improved thanks to technological evolution, mostly related to the production of new devices enabling the interventional radiologist to reach anatomical districts not accessible before. As a result of this technological improvement, it was observed an increase of procedures around the world in both vascular and extravascular interventions in terms of numbers and variability, and this was associated with a change in treatment strategies for traumatic patients with the willing of surgeons to prefer, when possible, a Non-Operative Management (NOM).

The numerical growth of interventional radiology procedures and the evolution of the treatment options that have occurred in the last decades represent the result of a combination of several factors, among which are the progressive miniaturization of devices that allow a greater number of conservative treatments.

Non-Operative Management (NOM) can be associated at mini-invasive techniques such as arterial embolization for active bleeding, stent-graft positioning to repair vessels tears and temporary occlusion balloon catheters positioning as a bridge to surgical repair. In the non-operative management, interventional radiology techniques allow a quicker and less invasive treatment if compared with surgery in the management of haemorrhages [1, 2], especially in blunt abdominal trauma with solid organs injuries and active bleeding suspected on the basis of clinical assessment and confirmed at the Contrast Enhanced Computed Tomography (CECT) study. Some authors argue that even patient with severe traumatic lesions of solid abdominal organs (degree IV, the American Association for the Surgery of Trauma injury scoring scale, AAST) may benefit from an interventional treatment if in stable haemodynamic conditions, and that in more severe cases (degree V) a combined surgical and interventional treatment can be performed in a hybrid operatory theatre. In this regard, interventional radiology techniques are considered the standard of care for haemodynamically stable patients with blunt abdominal trauma in the Emergency Department [3, 4].

All this factors, along with the availability of the most powerful digital angiographers with cone-beam technology, have contributed to move

G. Scevola (✉) • M. Rastelli • G. Loreni
Department of Interventional Radiology, Sandro Pertini Hospital, Rome, Italy
e-mail: germano.scevola@gmail.com

C. Raspanti
Department of Interventional Radiology, Careggi University Hospital, Florence, Italy

G. Addeo • V. Miele
Department of Radiology, Careggi University Hospital, Florence, Italy

V. Miele, M. Trinci (eds.), *Diagnostic Imaging in Polytrauma Patients*,
https://doi.org/10.1007/978-3-319-62054-1_22

good part of surgery treatments in interventional radiology treatments [4].

Following this evolution, the hospital structures are equipping themselves with new angiographic suite, usually located in the Radiology department but in the majority of cases far away from the Emergencies Department (ED). With the increasing use of interventional radiology procedures in traumatic patients, in the organization of new hospitals it has to be reconsidered the collocation for these equipment closer to the A&E department, moreover with the creation of hybrid operatory theatres.

Angiographic Suites or Hybrid Operation Theatres are multifunctional rooms that integrate the structural, technological and organizational features of the operating room with the interventional angiography, in order to instantly convert a percutaneous procedure into a surgical one [5]. The creation of an angiographic suite or a hybrid theatre placed in general operatory blocks or operatory blocks dedicated to Emergency Departments contributes to a better management of time-dependent conditions such as traumatic injuries, providing a fast, effective and efficient treatment for blunt abdominal trauma. Furthermore, the availability of a sliding CT in the operatory block enables a modern approach to traumatic patients by allowing a simultaneous onset of different operating figures in only one venue.

Inside the hybrid operating theatre several specialists coexist and operate simultaneously and in sequence. The organization of the hybrid operating theatre requires a clear team leadership assignment in relation to the clinical priorities of the polytraumatized patient: the team leader has a dynamic, interchangeable role. Although in most cases the surgeon has the role of the team leader, it can switch to anaesthetist or orthopaedic surgeon or interventional radiologist in relation to clinical situation. There are no data in literature that can suggest the benefit of a second surgeon who may be a leading subject, not directly involved in the operation but coordinating the various figures involved in monitoring, resuscitation and treatment (surgical or interventional). Some authors hypothesize in the near future a new figure in this new scenario (the hybrid operating theatre) with a specific role of supervisor [4].

22.2 State of Art in Diagnosis of Abdominal Bleeding for Trauma

Currently, the abdominal diagnostic angiography, used in the past to highlight abdominal bleeding, is no longer used with this purpose and its prevalent role is included in the interventional treatments in NOM as the preliminary phase of localization of the segment to be treated. Its role has been completely replaced by Contrast Enhanced multidetector Computed Tomography (CE-MDCT), which today is the gold standard diagnostic method in the identification and classification of traumatic lesions and bleeding in haemodynamically stable or stabilized patients. This diagnostic technique is able to offer a fast, complete and accurate description of localization, extension and severity of traumatic injuries, allowing a complete and adequate treatment plan.

Thanks to its ability to simultaneously investigate extra-abdominal organs, CE-MDCT can also provide information on other structures eventually involved in trauma, such as spinal cord or retroperitoneal space. However, despite the fact that CE-MDCT is now considered the gold standard for abdominal trauma, a study on patients with pelvic trauma reiterated the importance of diagnostic angiography in pelvic trauma. In a retrospective study conducted on a group of 327 patients to evaluate factors that required arterial embolization for treatment of patients with pelvic bones fractures,

Bozeman et al. [6] reported that patients over 55 years having systolic blood pressure lower than 90 mmHg and with evidence of active bleeding on CECT were significantly associated with the need for angio-embolic treatment. On the other hand, active contrast medium extravasation on CT-scan was absent in 25% of patients who needed therapeutic angioembolization [6]. The clinical results of this study are important because they attest that in specific clinical situations CECT angiography may not be as sensitive as

Digital Subtraction Angiography (DSA) to identify haemodynamically significant bleeding. Therefore, patients with clinical evidence of continuous bleeding should also be considered to be subjected to therapeutic angiography although if it was not observed any active contrast extravasation on CECT, especially with regard to the bleeding of the pelvis [4].

22.3 Liver

The liver is a vital organ located in the upper right quadrant of the abdomen, below the diaphragm. Due to its position and its size, the liver is one of the most frequently injured abdominal organs and hepatic involvement in abdominal trauma is frequent (10–15% blunt trauma, 20–25% open trauma), often associated with splenic injury. Usually sustained during motor vehicle collisions, the possibility of uncontrolled haemorrhage and a myriad of delayed complications contribute to a high morbidity and mortality rate [7, 8].

Hepatic injuries include capsular laceration, parenchymal tear or rupture, subcapsular or intraparenchymal haematoma and partial devascularization for parenchymal damage; when, in addition to the parenchyma, the portal vein, the vena cava or the biliary tract is involved, the mortality and morbidity rate are increased. The management of hepatic trauma is a dynamic field with significant paradigm shifts over the past several decades, with a central role of surgical repair [8].

During the early 1980s, the rapid development of new diagnostic techniques as angiography and CT supported the rising of interventional radiology and opened new quicker diagnostic options and therapeutic mini-invasive techniques for the management of patients with hepatic trauma.

The earliest reports of angioembolizations of liver bleedings occur in the early 1970s: Rosch and Dotter, fathers of Interventional Radiology, in 1972 published "Selective Arterial Embolization", in which they described this new technique for stopping gastrointestinal active bleeding [9]. A year later, Bookstein described the embolization of a hepatic arteriovenous fistula [10]. During the mid 1990s, the mini-invasive endovascular techniques enter definitely in the diagnostic and therapeutic guidelines for liver trauma. At the same time, good results from NOM of paediatric patients with hepatic trauma, as well as the ever-increasing medical options, have pushed a part of the academic-surgical world to review the immediate operative approach, especially in haemodynamically stable patients [11, 12].

Angioembolization, associated with advances in non-surgical intervention, has allowed a significant decrease in mortality and morbidity from liver injuries. Today the attitude in hepatic trauma with haemodynamic stability is the NOM, even with extensive parenchymal injury (IV-V AAST degree), with significant decrease in mortality rates [7, 12, 13].

The development and improvement of imaging techniques have provided significant impetus to the success of the NOM: ultrasound, CEUS and CECT represent the gold standard in the diagnostic algorithm of patients with abdominal trauma, especially for the liver in which CECT usually identifies the site and extent of parenchymal damage, as well as the presence of active bleeding (Fig. 22.1) [13].

In literature several authors highlighted good results with treatment of bleeding even in haemodynamically unstable patients: in particular Monnin et al., with a multidisciplinary approach including embolization, has achieved a 93% success also with haemodynamically unstable patients [14]. Furthermore, in trauma patients who respond to resuscitation treatment, the guidelines of the Eastern Association for the Surgery of Trauma (EAST) in first instance recommend (level 2) arterial embolization, possibly in addition to surgery [15]. Indications for conventional hepatic angiography include active contrast extravasation identified by CECT, evidence of ongoing bleeding despite conservative resuscitative measures, haemobilia and control of continued haemorrhage after surgery. Active bleeding is the leading indication for interventional radiology procedures, in particular as a valid support to the NOM; hepatic angioembolization is usually performed in a dedicated angiographic suite and starts with a retrograde common femoral approach: the goal is to selec-

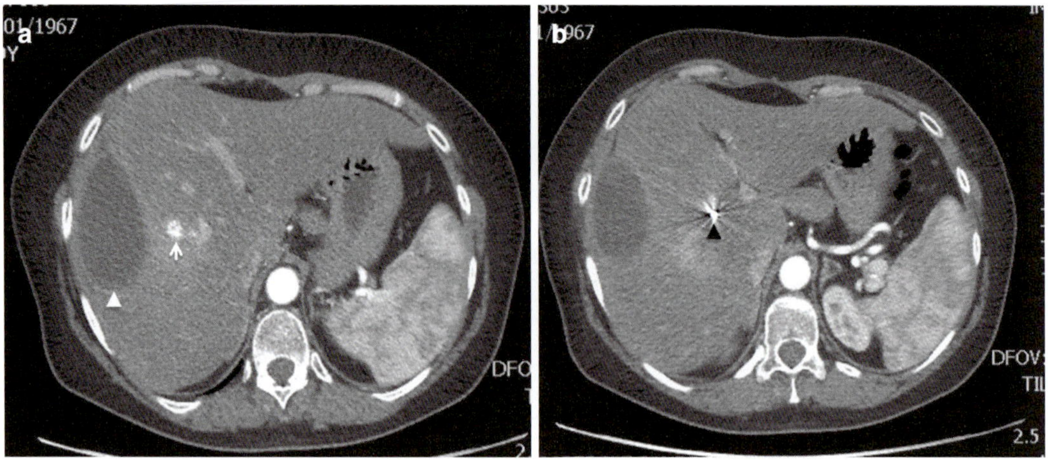

Fig. 22.1 Liver CECT scan before and after angioembolization, arterial phase: (**a**) evidence of active bleeding (*white arrow*) and subcapsular fluid collection (*white arrowhead*); (**b**) presence of metallic coils (*black arrowhead*) and absence of bleeding

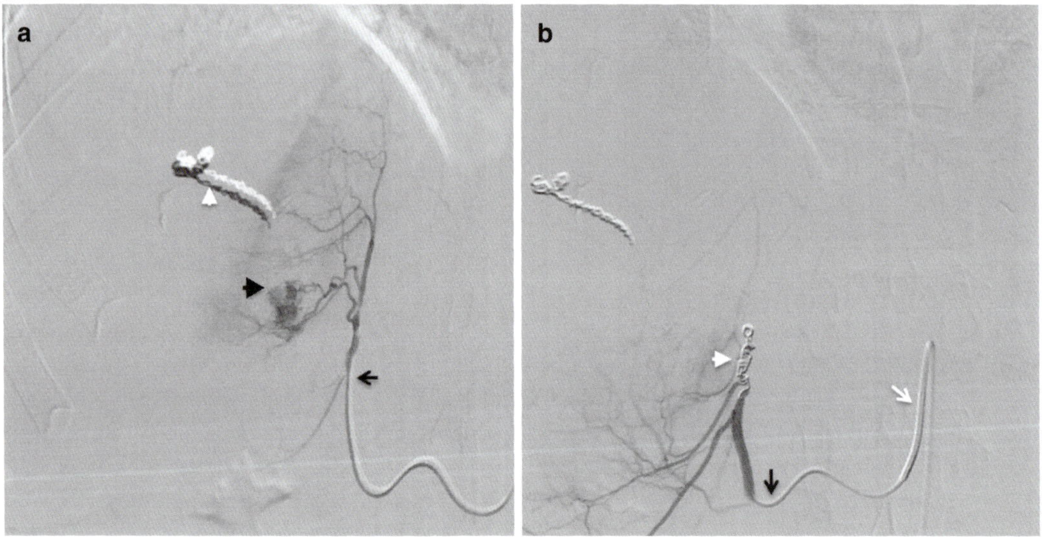

Fig. 22.2 Angioembolization of hepatic bleeding arteries (*black arrowhead*) by the selective catheterism of the celiac trunk using a Simmons 1 shaped macrocatheter (*white arrow*), super selective microcatheterism of the bleeding artery (*black arrows*) and microcoils deployment (*white arrowheads*)

tively catheterize the hepatic artery and after superselective catheterization reaching up to the site of vascular disease (extravasation, pseudoaneurysm or arteriovenous fistula) to embolize using coils or embolic agents (liquid agents such as Glue and Onyx, gelfoam) (Fig. 22.2).

The most common vascular catheter used for the celiac trunk is Cobra or Simmons shaped; the external size of microcatheters used for superselective catheterization usually has a range from 2.0 to 2.8 French (3 Fr = 1 mm). In case of pre-procedural CT with extensive liver injury, some authors suggest to release embolizing agents such as gelfoam or Spongostan from the hepatic artery of affected lobe even in the absence of angiographic evidence of active bleeding: this however may help in achieving haemostasis and haemodynamic stabilization of the patient; however, it is controversial [16]. In the setting of trauma, the technical success rate of hepatic angioembolization ranges from 88% to 100%, but in cases following surgical packing owing to distorted anatomy and manipulation, technical success rate drops to 60–70% [14]. Usually technical difficulties are related to vascular tortuosity, artery stenosis, most commonly of the celiac trunk, and vessel spasm. In case of complex vascular anatomy, it may help to use smaller size and more navigable microcatheters; similarly, in case of vasospasm, the use of microcatheter and delicate catheter manipulation will help to reach the site of hepatic injury [16]. Lee et al. reported 11 cases of incomplete embolization: ten of these cases were secondary to a persistent contrast blush without an identifiable vessel or a blush supplied by multiple collaterals that could not be embolized, and one reported failure secondary to a stenotic celiac artery [17]. Both Lee et al. and Hagiwara et al. reported failures of NOM despite technical success of angioembolization [18]. Often, the failure of conservative management despite successful angioembolization is related to venous bleeding, that can be difficult to identify during angiography and even harder to treat.

Late liver bleeding is an uncommon (3% of liver trauma) possible complication of NOM [19]. The number of complications is higher in patients with higher degree liver injuries; the most common complications of a hepatic angioembolization include hepatic necrosis, abscess formation and non-target embolization [20]. Due to its vascular conformation, the liver receives constant inflow from both portal and arterial venous vessels. However, despite this robust dual supply, the combined insult of trauma and embolization has been shown to cause significant hepatic necrosis that ranged from 0 to 42% with a weighted mean rate of 15% and was associated with longer hospital stay and increased transfusion requirement [8]. It is evident that liver trauma and subsequent liver devascularization play a major role in hepatic necrosis compared to angioembolization, in particular with a superselective embolization. Green et al. reported that a major degree of arterial selectivity during embolization was generally related to a lower necrosis rate [8].

The next two common complications are abscess formation and bile leak/biloma [21, 22]. These complications are not clearly related to angioembolization and, in literature, they are reported both in operative and non-operative management of hepatic trauma [23, 24]. Probably, hepatic injury and death of a large number of hepatocytes together create a combined state of parenchymal flogosis and tissue necrosis, increasing the risk of abscess formation independently from angioembolization.

Even in the management of complications, interventional radiology through the positioning of percutaneous drainage on abscess sites plays a key role. In a multidisciplinary approach, today the conservative management in patients with liver injury appears a successful algorithm in order to reduce mortality and morbidity rate: angiography and angioembolization are essential components of successful NOM of hepatic trauma patients, as well as a critical component of haemorrhage control following laparotomy [25, 26]. In particular, despite there are no consensus guidelines on appropriate patient selection criteria for those who would benefit from angiography and angioembolization, several articles have suggested that early angiography and embolization improve outcomes in patients with high-grade hepatic injuries [12, 26–30].

In summary, hepatic angioembolization is an effective and important component in the management of traumatic hepatic haemorrhage, also in an operative or non-operative management. Hepatic necrosis is the most important complication and can occur following embolization, but this risk can be safely managed by medical therapy without serious sequelae.

Today interventional radiologists, as real "playmakers" of the multidisciplinary team, play a central role in the treatment of hepatic trauma.

22.4 Aorta

Traumatic aortic injury, a consequence of penetrating injuries or blunt trauma, is a life-threatening condition, which requires prompt diagnosis and management: the vast majority of patients die before they can receive medical care; furthermore, the mortality rate for patients with aortic rupture who survive until they reach the hospital is estimated to be 41–50% [31]. Traumatic aortic injury commonly occurs at the sites of aortic tethering that is the aortic root, the isthmus and at the diaphragmatic hiatus; although it is rare in the abdomen, the most common site of injury is the infrarenal abdominal aorta [32].

Abdominal vascular injuries can be caused by penetrating or blunt trauma. Blunt Abdominal Aortic Injuries (BAAIs) are caused by traffic accidents commonly referred to as the "seat belt aorta" [33, 34]. These injuries are rare in the current reported world literature because the thoracic aorta is fairly well protected by the bony thoracic cage [35]. Starnes et al. proposed a CT-based management classification system for BAAI [36]: he classified BAAI into 4 types based on aortic external contour abnormality, intimal tear and contrast extravasation. Most patients with BAAI rarely reach the hospital alive and those who do have a reported 24% mortality. Most abdominal aortic injuries have been repaired via an open surgical approach, with endovascular stent graft as an alternative. Despite significant improvements in critical care support, non-invasive diagnosis, anaesthesia and surgery over the last few decades, the conventional open surgical repair of an aortic rupture still carries a significant risk of serious complications and mortality, and in patients with concomitant injuries and comorbidities is associated with high morbidity and mortality [37–39]. Therefore, endovascular repair techniques have emerged as a promising alternative in these patients [40]. Several case reports and case series evaluating the technical feasibility and safety of endovascular treatment for ruptured abdominal aortic aneurysm (rAAA) or a thoracic aortic injury (TAI) suggest that between 40% and 80% of rAAAs are suitable for endovascular aortic repair (EVAR), with a perioperative mortality rate of 10%–29% for endovascular repair of rAAA [41–44].

Both conventional open surgical and endovascular treatment options for aortic ruptures are available in referral centres; however, the transferring of patients who need emergency treatment to a referral centre is usually not possible. Therefore, the widespread use of endovascular techniques is important for the rapid and adequate treatment of these patients [45]. A key role in the success of endovascular approach is an accurate patient selection by an early Angio-CT examination assessing the feasibility of the endovascular procedure (aneurysm neck, iliac axes involvement, etc.) as well as the evaluation of haemodynamic and vital signs; so, an optimal patient selection for EVAR requires a multidisciplinary approach including interventional radiologists, vascular surgeons, emergency doctors and anaesthetists.

In conclusion, in cases of abdominal aorta ruptures from blunt trauma, endovascular aortic repair is evolving and offers the potential to improve mortality rates in acute aortic injuries: therefore, interventional radiology can play a crucial role in trauma centres.

22.5 Spleen

The spleen is the second abdominal organ most commonly involved in closed abdominal trauma after the liver. Splenic injuries, occurring in 32% of abdominal injuries, most often are observed in blunt abdominal trauma such as in traffic accidents, assaults, fall from height and sports. Spleen damage is a serious and fearful consequence of abdominal trauma; as it is a highly vascularized organ, splenic injuries can result in prolonged bleeding with the risk of a threat to the life of the patient if not recognized and treated correctly.

In addition to the immediate danger caused by intraperitoneal bleeding with haemorrhagic shock potential, delayed bleeding may occur in capsular lesions or post-traumatic vascular lesions (artery venous fistula, pseudoaneurysms), that may cause severe bleeding even after discharge from the hospital [46].

The method of choice for rapid evaluation of the abdomen to early identify the presence of abdominal free fluid is the Focused Abdominal Sonography for Trauma (FAST), that can be performed simultaneously with resuscitation efforts during the initial trauma management. For this reason it is also useful in haemodynamically unstable patients. However, FAST has a low sensitivity for detecting and grading splenic injuries and is unable to detect the presence of active haemorrhage.

CT is the imaging modality of choice for haemodynamically stable patients with blunt abdominal trauma [47], being the most accurate test to assess the grade of injury, and it can give a relatively accurate evaluation of the volume of haemoperitoneum. It can also detect the presence and location of active arterial bleeding as well as the presence of pseudoaneurysms or arteriovenous fistulas in the spleen (Fig. 22.3).

Splenic injuries can be radiologically classified using The American Association for the Surgery of Trauma (AAST) grading system (see table in Chap. 16) [48, 49]. This grading system is based on the anatomic extension of disruption of the spleen, as shown on CECT scans or during laparotomy. However, this grading system is not reliable for the prediction of the outcome of splenic injuries and not decisive about whether surgery or conservative treatment should be applied.

Historically a large proportion of patients with bleeding splenic trauma were subjected to emergency splenectomy to avoid the risk of fatal haemorrhage. However, 45–49% of patients undergoing surgery for splenic lesions present post-operative complications including pneumonia, bacteraemia, urinary tract infections and abscesses. Surgical splenectomy is associated with a mortality of 8–10% [50]. NOM of blunt splenic injury by clinical observation alone has a reported failure rate of 34–52% with these patients often requiring subsequent splenectomy.

In 1981, Sclafani published the first case report of arterial embolization for traumatic splenic injury as an alternative to surgery. The development of advanced endovascular interventional techniques has led to greater consideration of NOM for haemodynamically stable patients. Splenic artery angiography and either selective embolization for active haemorrhage or proximal splenic arterial embolization can be used to reduce the risk of delayed haemorrhage. Worldwide the majority of trauma centres now prefer NOM in haemodynamically stable patients with blunt splenic injury. As a result, splenic artery embolization (SAE) is increasingly performed reducing the need for operative intervention [51]. Wait-and-see approach has been

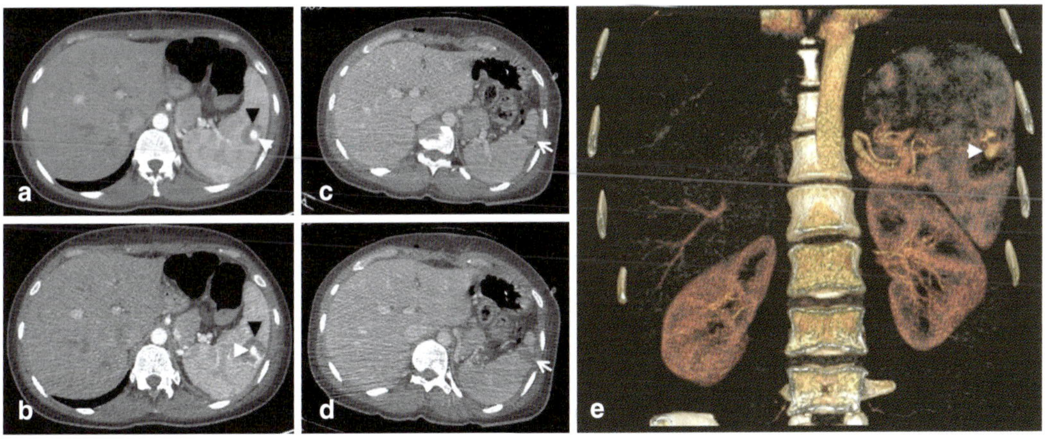

Fig. 22.3 CECT scan, arterial (**a** and **b**) and portal (**c** and **d**) phases: splenic subcapsular laceration (*white arrows*) and parenchymal haematoma (*black arrowheads*) with pseudoaneurysm (*white arrowheads*); (**e**) arterial phase 3D Volume Rendering

reported to have a failure rate as high as 34%; the rate is even higher among patients with high-grade splenic injury (AAST grade III–V) [52–55].

Splenic arterial catheterization is commonly performed using common femoral artery access. Placement of a 5–6 French introducer sheath is sufficient in most cases. Selective angiography of splenic artery should always be performed to evaluate arterial injury type and extension. Diagnostic series of the splenic artery can be obtained using a macrocatheter, but for selective catheterization of the splenic artery branches coaxial microcatheters and micro-guidewires may be required. Technique and materials used for embolization depend on anatomical considerations, the haemodynamic situation of the patient, and the type and distribution of vascular injuries. Coils are usually the embolic agents of choice, and gelfoam may be used in some critical situations requiring quick and massive arterial occlusion (Fig. 22.4). Occasionally, the use of an Amplatzer vascular plug may be useful [56].

Haemostasis after coil embolization usually occurs as a result of coil-induced thrombosis rather than mechanical occlusion of the lumen by the coil; therefore, this technique works best when the coagulation profile of the patient is normal or only mildly abnormal. In case of serious clotting disturbances, addition of another embolic agent, such as gelfoam, is indicated. Gelfoam is a sterile gelatine sponge intended for use as a temporary intravascular embolic material and it can be used in the shape of a "torpedo" or as pledgets. The major advantage of coils compared with gelfoam is the ability to improve permanent embolization, which is most desirable in treating vascular injuries. In fact, temporary occlusive agents such as gelfoam seem to have a higher failure rate (50%) compared with coil embolization (23%) [57].

There are two angiographic techniques to achieve splenic haemostasis [58]: Proximal Splenic Artery Embolization (PSAE) and selective distal splenic embolization. Proximal embolization of the splenic artery is the surgical equivalent of the arterial ligature and is based on the concept that decreasing the flow and splenic pressure the bleeding should consensually stop; rescue of the organ is ensured by sufficient perfusion through collateral gastric and pancreatic arteries. Coils are generally used for proximal embolization and, in some specific situations, also Amplatzer vascular plugs can be deployed to achieve PSAE. Proximal embolization is used in cases of widespread spleen bleeding, i.e. when there are multiple focal bleeds, and/or when the haemodynamic conditions of the patient require fast treatment; moreover, it can be performed when the splenic artery tortuosity prevents selective distal embolization. It is also used in those situations where the haemorrhage site is not identifiable at angiography but the clinical situation of the patient suggests active splenic bleeding. A potential disadvantage of proximal embolization of splenic artery may be that in the event of a bleeding recurrence it may be difficult to repeat the embolization as the catheterism of splenic artery could not be possible anymore.

Selective distal embolization only concerns damaged arterial blood vessels, usually in their distal part within the splenic parenchyma; generally, this type of embolization requires the use of a microcatheter. A potential complication of selective distal embolism is the possibility of splenic infarction with superinfection and abscess formation, which rarely lead to clinical consequences and are generally treated percutaneously by the positioning of a drainage catheter.

Follow-up is usually clinical but in some selected cases, when distal embolization is per-

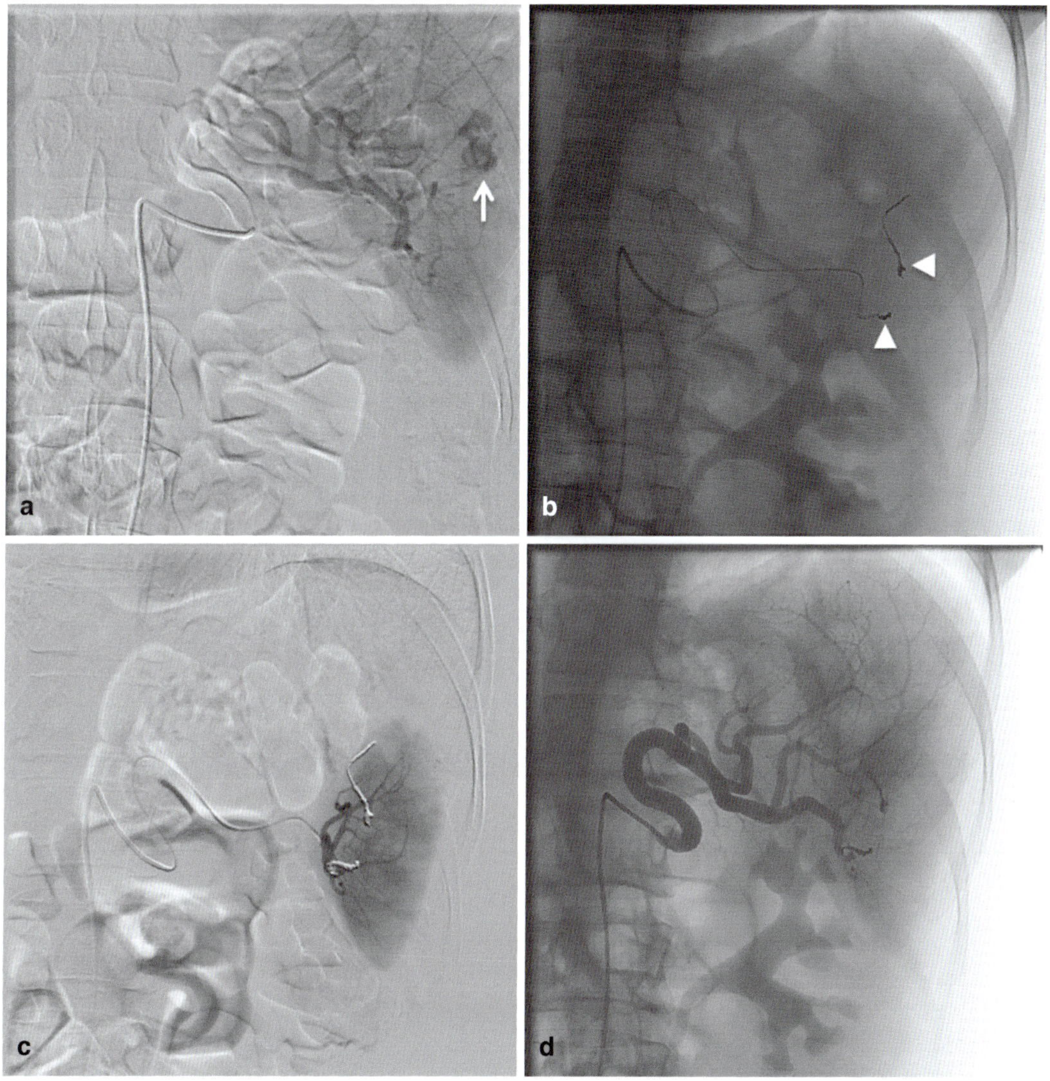

Fig. 22.4 Angioembolization procedure: (**a**) diagnostic angiogram showing a peripheral vascular lesion of the spleen (*white arrow*), (**b**) microcatheterism of the bleeding vessel and coils positioning (*white arrowheads*), (**c** and **d**) post-embolization angiograms showing complete haemostasis

formed to exclude some unstable lesions of the splenic artery as pseudoaneurysms or arteriovenous fistulas, a CECT scan could be repeated to assess the complete exclusion of the treated lesion (Fig. 22.5).

In conclusion, splenic artery embolization is a safe and effective procedure for the NOM of splenic trauma in haemodynamically stable patients, with low rates of complications and need for re-interventions.

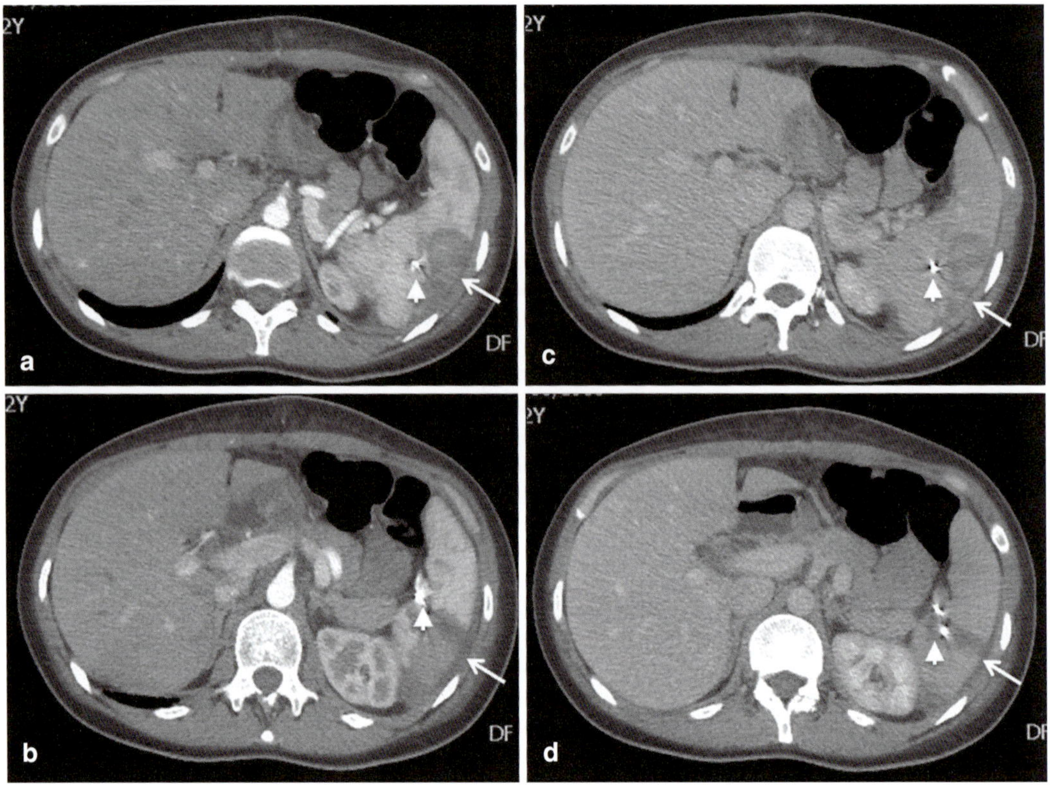

Fig. 22.5 Post-embolization CECT scan of the spleen, arterial (**a** and **b**) and portal (**c** and **d**) phases. Subcapsular haematoma (*white arrows*) is still present and the parenchymal pseudoaneurysm (Fig. 22.3a, b) is completely excluded by coils (*white arrowheads*)

22.6 Kidney

After severe trauma, acute kidney injury (AKI) is a frequent and severe complication leading to increased morbidity and mortality. After renal trauma, additional risks have been identified due to direct parenchymal or vascular injuries [59].

Renal injuries are identified in approximately 1–5% of all polytraumatized patients, and they can be secondary to multiple mechanisms such as penetrating, blunt, and iatrogenic trauma. 80–90% of injuries are caused by blunt trauma, with the most common mechanism being traffic accidents.

After FAST assessment of the presence of solid abdominal organs injuries, diagnosis and extension of renal injuries is usually based on CECT imaging and graded according to the American Association for the Surgery of Trauma (AAST) organ injury scale (see Table 1 in Chap. 19). CECT is in fact considered the gold standard diagnostic method for the radiographic assessment of patients with renal trauma. With a short examination time, it can provide all the information related to the degree of renal injury, the eventual involvement of pyelo-caliceal system and the presence and type of vascular injuries; furthermore, CECT can also provide information about the renal functional status [60, 61].

Operative vs. non-operative management of traumatic renal injuries has been debated for many years. Traditionally, surgical exploration or nephrectomy represents the gold standard approach for high-grade renal injuries. However, on the basis of the advances in diagnostic imaging and the rise of minimally invasive techniques, NOM has become the standard of care. The majority of renal injuries are low-grade (grades 1–3 AAST organ injury scale) and can be conservatively treated. However, intervention may be needed in the presence of active arterial bleeding: surgery is usually reserved to haemodynamically unstable patients while for stable patients Renal Artery Embolization (RAE) should be considered [61].

Indications for RAE following trauma are debated. In cases of penetrating trauma, RAE is often a first-line alternative to surgery. For blunt trauma, the relative role of wait-and-see, RAE and surgical management may depend upon the grade of injury and patients' haemodynamic conditions. Typically, RAE is indicated in the management of lower-grade renal injuries and penetrating injuries previously identified on CECT imaging [62]. However, Sarani and colleagues in a retrospective study compared angioembolization to surgery for the treatment of high-grade renal injuries (≥ grade III) concluding that RAE was a safe and effective technique to stop the bleeding and arrest haemorrhage [63].

There are two ways RAE can be performed: selective and non-selective embolization. The only indication for non-selective embolization is in case of shattered kidney from trauma when a surgical nephrectomy could be life-threatening because of comorbidities, while selective embolization is the treatment of choice for focal vascular injuries in haemodynamically stable patients. When right or left common femoral artery vascular access is obtained under ultrasound or fluoroscopic guidance, a macrocatheter is used to gain the main renal artery and a diagnostic angiogram is then performed. In case of iliac arteries occlusion or unfavourable angle at the origin of the main renal artery, a radial or brachial artery approach can be used. Non-selective embolization can be obtained with polyvinyl alcohol (PVA), microspheres or gelfoam, and metallic coils could be eventually deployed at the end of the procedure to achieve complete exclusion of the renal artery; however, this could make clamping the main renal artery tricky, so this possibility should be discussed with the surgeon prior to the procedure. Selective embolization, that represents the treatment of choice in most of cases because it permits to maintain viable functioning kidney, is usually achieved through the superselective microcatheterism of the vascular lesion and the deployment of microcoils to achieve haemostasis (Fig. 22.6) [62].

Despite its efficiency in active bleeding control, RAE can be followed by some complications such as renal parenchymal infarction and contrast medium nephrotoxicity, with consequent transient or definitive renal function impairment [59].

In conclusion, RAE can be considered to be an effective technique to increase the chances of success of NOM in haemodynamically stable patients with traumatic renal injuries.

22.7 Pelvic Trauma

Three percent of all skeletal fractures are represented by pelvic fractures, ranging in severity from low-energy stable bone injuries to high-energy unstable fractures, often associated with haemodynamic instability due to active bleeding that is arterial in 10–20% of cases [64]. Arterial haemorrhage represents the first cause of death associated to pelvic fracture [65]. The rate of mortality among patients with all types of pelvic fracture is approximately 16%, and the percentage rises to approximately 27% in patients with closed pelvic fractures, and moreover to approximately 55% in those who report open pelvic fractures with haemodynamic instability [66].

Haemorrhage represents the major reversible cause of death of pelvic trauma patients, with a reported overall mortality of around 42%, due to pelvic haemorrhage in 62% of cases and associated to intrathoracic and intraabdominal bleedings in the remaining proportion [66]. Bleeding can be bone-related or can be secondary to arterial and/or venous injuries. Arterial injuries, representing as mentioned above the first cause of death in these patients, are mainly associated to instability of pelvic bone fractures, and usually

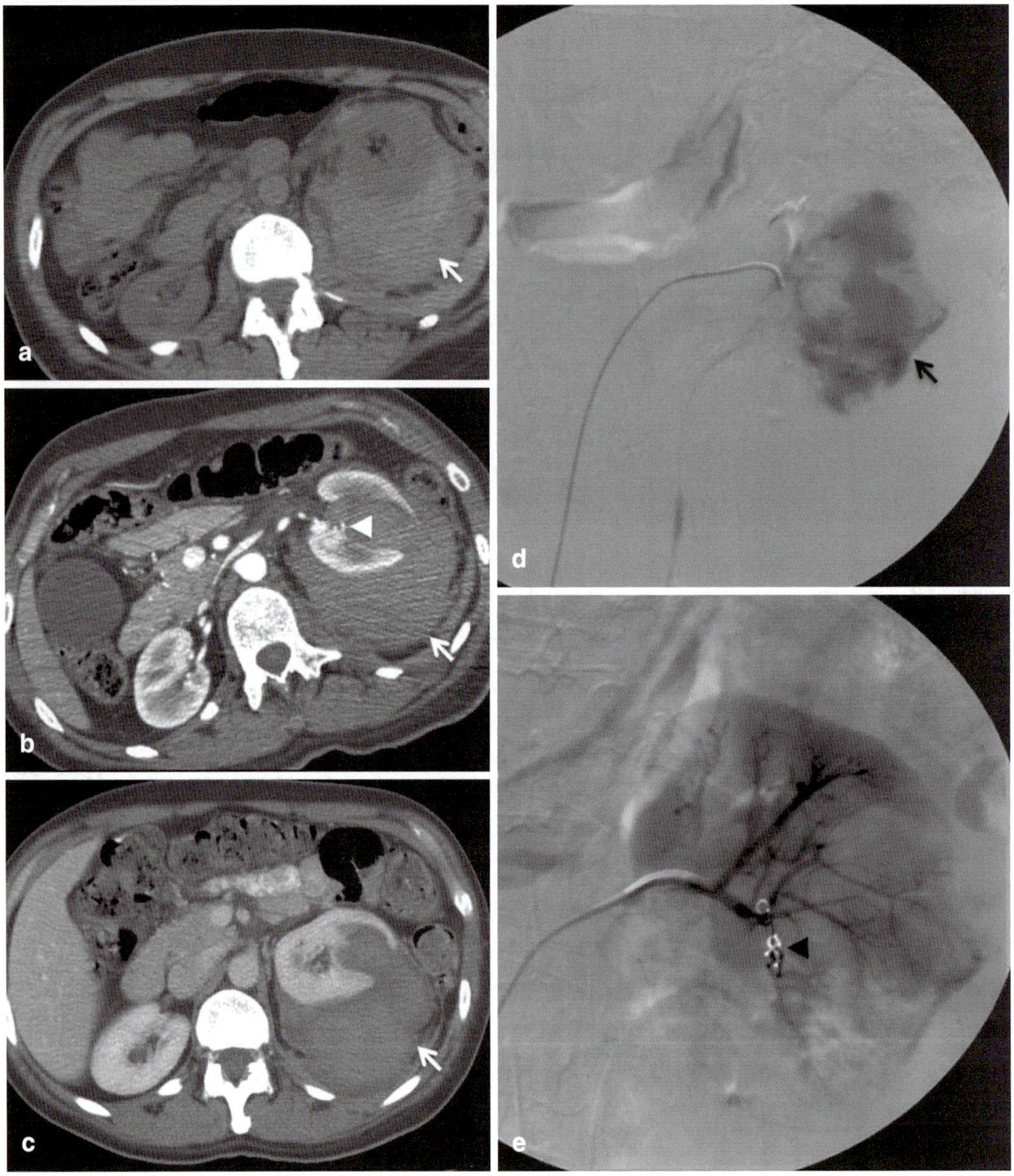

Fig. 22.6 Traumatic rupture of the kidney in haemodynamically stable patient: (**a–c**) CECT scan showing the presence of a massive extra-renal haematoma (*white arrows*) and a bleeding arterial lesion (*white arrowhead*); (**d** and **e**) angioembolization procedure confirming the active extravasation of contrast medium (*black arrow*) and the effective haemostasis obtained through selective microcoils deployment (*black arrowhead*)

require haemostatic embolization and orthopaedic fixation [67].

CE-MDCT has been reported to be the most sensitive non-invasive technique for bleeding identification in the trauma centre, providing at the same time information about skeletal injuries and the presence, type and location of bleeding [66]. As reported in several studies, transcatheter angioembolization represents a quick and effective mini-invasive technique

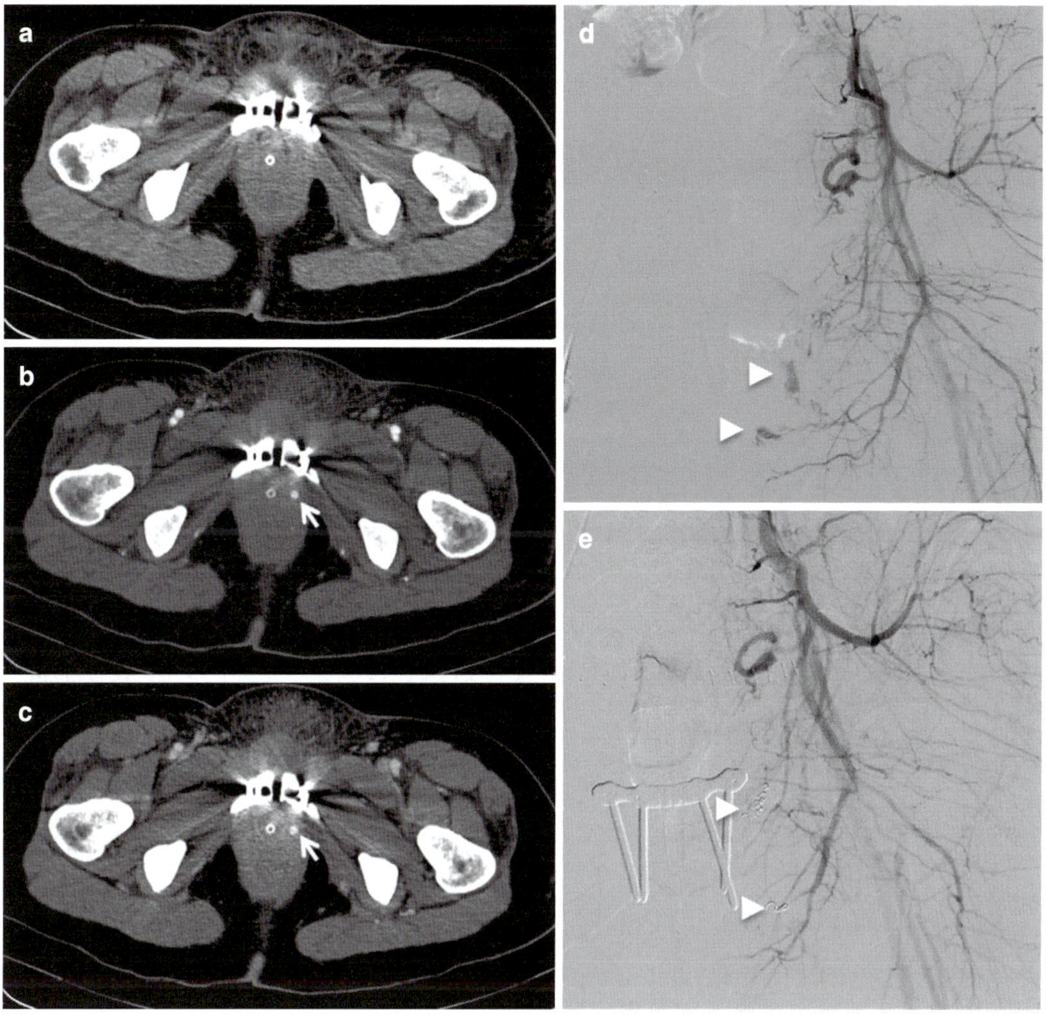

Fig. 22.7 After orthopaedic fixation of a post-traumatic pubic symphysis diastasis (**a**), there is persistence of active bleeding (**b** and **c**) (*white arrows*) treated by angioembolization with coils (**d** and **e**) (*white arrowheads*)

to control haemorrhage before orthopaedic fixation of pelvic fractures [68]. As described for the embolization of other bleeding sites, angioembolization of bleeding lesions associated to pelvic trauma is performed through a 5- or 6-Fr common femoral access, usually contralateral to the site of active contrast extravasation identified at CE-MDCT. After selective catheterism of the internal iliac artery, an angiogram is performed and any site of contrast extravasation or unstable vascular lesion (such as pseudoaneurysms or AV fistulas) is embolized more selectively as possible, usually by the usage of a microcatheter (Fig. 22.7). Most commonly used embolizing materials are metallic coils and resorbable liquid agents like gelfoam.

Some authors have recently proposed non-selective embolization of the internal iliac arteries of patients with pelvic fractures also when arterial bleeding is not visible at the CE-MDCT scan [6]. However, the argument is still debated, and some authors suggest that the usage of this technique should be limited to those patients with unstable pelvic fractures requiring resuscitation and blood transfusion, and that selective occlusion of more distal vessels rather than of the main internal iliac artery should be performed [69].

In conclusion, in any patient presenting at the A&E department with pelvic fractures and haemodynamic instability the angioembolization procedure may be useful to control active bleeding or even to stabilize patient's haemodynamics as a bridge to orthopaedic fixation, being a safe and effective, time-saving mini-invasive technique more and more available in the trauma centres.

References

1. Sclafani SJA. Diagnostic and interventional radiology. In: Mattox KL, Moore EE, Feliciano DV, editors. Trauma. New York: McGrawHill; 2013. p. 251–300.
2. Hoffer EK, Borsa JJ, Bloch RD, et al. Endovascular techniques in the damage control setting. Radiographics. 1999;19:1340–8. doi:10.1148/radiographics.19.5.g99se051340.
3. Chakraverty S, Zealley I, Kessel D. Damage control radiology in the severely injured patient: what the anaesthetist needs to know. Br J Anaesth. 2014;113:250–7. doi:10.1093/bja/aeu203.
4. D'Amours SK, Rastogi P, Ball CG. Utility of simultaneous interventional radiology and operative surgery in a dedicated suite for seriously injured patients. Curr Opin Crit Care. 2013;19:587–93. doi:10.1097/MCC.0000000000000031.
5. Scevola G, Orlacchio A. et al. (2012) Criteria for Clinical, Structural and Technological appropriateness of Interventional Radiology. Quaderni della salute n. 12 – nov 2012. www.quadernidellasalute.it
6. Bozeman MC, Cannon RM, Trombold JM, et al. Use of computed tomography findings and contrast extravasation in predicting the need for embolization with pelvic fractures. Am Surg. 2012;78:825–30.
7. Gourgiotis S, Vougas V, Germanos S, et al. Operative and nonoperative management of blunt hepatic trauma in adults: a single-center report. J Hepato-Biliary-Pancreat Surg. 2007;14:387–391. Epub 2007. doi:10.1007/s00534-006-1177-2.
8. Green CS, Bulger EM, Kwan SW. Outcomes and complications of angioembolization for hepatic trauma: a systematic review of the literature. J Trauma Acute Care Surg. 2016;80:529–37. doi:10.1097/TA.0000000000000942.
9. Rösch J, Dotter CT, Brown MJ. Selective arterial embolization. A new method for control of acute gastrointestinal bleeding. Radiology. 1972;102:303–6.
10. Bookstein JJ, Goldstein HM. Successful management of postbiopsy arteriovenous fistula with selective arterial embolization. Radiology. 1973;109:535–6.
11. Oldham KT, Guice KS, Ryckman F, et al. Blunt liver injury in childhood: evolution of therapy and current perspective. Surgery. 1986;100:542–9.
12. Carrillo EH, Platz A, Miller FB, et al. Non-operative management of blunt hepatic trauma. Br J Surg. 1998;85:461–8.
13. Velmahos GC, Toutouzas K, Radin R, et al. High success with nonoperative management of blunt hepatic trauma: the liver is a sturdy organ. Arch Surg. 2003;138:475–480.; discussion 480–1. doi:10.1001/archsurg.138.5.475.
14. Monnin V, Sengel C, Thony F, et al. Place of arterial embolization in severe blunt hepatic trauma: a multidisciplinary approach. Cardiovasc Intervent Radiol. 2008;31:875–82. doi:10.1007/s00270-007-9277-1. Epub 2008 Feb 5
15. Stassen NA, Bhullar I, Cheng JD, et al. Nonoperative management of blunt hepatic injury: an eastern Association for the Surgery of trauma practice management guideline. J Trauma Acute Care Surg. 2012;73:288–93. doi:10.1097/TA.0b013e318270160d.
16. Gamanagatti S, Rangarajan K, Kumar A, et al. Blunt abdominal trauma: imaging and intervention. Curr Probl Diagn Radiol. 2015;44:321–36. doi:10.1067/j.cpradiol.2015.02.005.
17. Lee YH, Wu CH, Wang LJ, et al. Predictive factors for early failure of transarterial embolization in blunt hepatic injury patients. Clin Radiol. 2014;69:505–11. doi:10.1016/j.crad.2014.08.013.
18. Hagiwara A, Murata A, Matsuda T, et al. The efficacy and limitations of transarterial embolization for severe hepatic injury. J Trauma. 2002;52:1091–6.
19. Tartari S, Montalto C, Ferrante Z, et al. Trauma chiuso addominale: indicazioni al trattamento interventistico. Il Giornale Italiano di. Radiol Med. 2016;3:953–8. doi:10.17376/girm_3-6-11122016-7.
20. Dabbs DN, Stein DM, Scalea TM. Major hepatic necrosis: a common complication after angioembolization for treatment of high-grade liver injuries. J Trauma. 2009;66:621–627. discussion 627–9. doi:10.1097/TA.0b013e31819919f2.
21. Kozar RA, Moore JB, Niles SE, et al. Complications of nonoperative management of high-grade blunt hepatic injuries. J Trauma. 2005;59:1066–71.
22. Bala M, Gazalla SA, Faroja M, et al. Complications of high grade liver injuries: management and outcomewith focus on bile leaks. Scand J Trauma Resusc Emerg Med. 2012;20:20. doi:10.1186/1757-7241-20-20.
23. Hsieh CH, Chen RJ, Fang JF, et al. Liver abscess after non-operative management of blunt liver injury. Langenbeck's Arch Surg. 2003;387:343–7. Epub 2002 Dec 12
24. Krige JE, Bornman PC, Terblanche J. Therapeutic perihepatic packing in complex liver trauma. Br J Surg. 1992;79:43–6.
25. Tinkoff G, Esposito TJ, Reed J, et al. American Association for the Surgery of Trauma organ injury scale I: spleen, liver, and kidney, validation based on the national trauma data bank. J Am Coll

Surg. 2008;207:646–55. doi:10.1016/j.jamcollsurg. 2008.06.342. Epub 2008 Aug 30
26. Asensio JA, Roldán G, Petrone P, et al. Operative management and outcomes in 103 AAST-OIS grades IV and V complex hepatic injuries: trauma surgeons still need to operate, but angioembolization helps. J Trauma. 2003;54:647–53. discussion 653–4
27. Gaarder C, Naess PA, Eken T, et al. Liver injuries: improved results with a formal protocol including angiography. Injury. 2007;38:1075–83. Epub 2007 Aug 13
28. Wahl WL, Ahrns KS, Brandt MM, et al. The need for early angiographic embolization in blunt liver injuries. J Trauma. 2002;52:1097–101.
29. Carrillo EH, Richardson JD. Delayed surgery and interventional procedures in complex liver injuries. J Trauma. 1999;46:978.
30. Mohr AM, Lavery RF, Barone A, et al. Angiographic embolization for liver injuries: low mortality, high morbidity. J Trauma. 2003;55:1077–81. discussion 1081–2
31. Bown MJ, Sutton AJ, Bell PR, Sayers RD. A meta-analysis of 50 years of ruptured abdominal aortic aneurysm repair. Br J Surg. 2002;89:714–30.
32. De Mestral C, Dueck AD, Gomez D. Associated injuries, management, and outcomes of blunt abdominal aortic injury. J Vasc Surg. 2012;56:656–60. doi:10.1016/j.jvs.2012.02.027. Epub 2012 Jul 12
33. Tucker S Jr, Rowe VL, Rao R, et al. Treatment options for traumatic pseudoaneurysms of the paravisceral abdominal aorta. Ann Vasc Surg. 2005;19:613–8. doi:10.1007/s10016-005-4652-3.
34. Yeh MW, Horn JK, Schecter WP, et al. Endovascular repair of an actively hemorrhaging gunshot injury to the abdominal aorta. J Vasc Surg. 2005;42:1007–9. doi:10.1016/j.jvs.2005.06.007.
35. Dajee H, Richardson IW, Iype MO. Seat belt aorta: acute dissection and thrombosis of the abdominal aorta. Surgery. 1979;85:263–7.
36. Starnes BW, Lundgren RS, Gunn M, et al. A new classification scheme for treating blunt aortic injury. J Vasc Surg. 2012;55:47–54. doi:10.1016/j.jvs.2011.07.073. Epub 2011 Nov 29
37. Garzón G, Fernández-Velilla M, Martí M et al (2005) Endovascular stent-graft treatment of thoracic aortic disease. Radiographics 1:229–244. DOI: 10.1148/rg.25si055513.
38. Kasirajan K, Heffernan D, Langsfeld M. Acute thoracic aortic trauma: a comparison of endoluminal stent grafts with open repair and nonoperative management. Ann Vasc Surg. 2003;17:589–595. Epub Oct 23. doi:10.1007/s10016-003-0066-2.
39. Saratzis NA, Saratzis AN, Melas N, et al. Endovascular repair of traumatic rupture of the thoracic aorta: single-center experience. Cardiovasc Intervent Radiol. 2007;30:370–5.
40. Watanabe K, Fukuda I, Asari Y. Management of traumatic aortic rupture. Surg Today. 2013;43:1339–46. doi:10.1007/s00595-012-0471-7. Epub 2013 Jan 23
41. Reichart M, Geelkerken RH, Huisman AB, et al. Ruptured abdominal aortic aneurysm: endovascular repair is feasible in 40% of patients. Eur J Vasc Endovasc Surg. 2003;26:479–86.
42. Alsac JM, Desgranges P, Kobeiter H, Becquemin JP. Emergency endovascular repair for ruptured abdominal aortic aneurysms: feasibility and comparison of early results with conventional open repair. Eur J Vasc Endovasc Surg. 2005;30:632–9. Epub 2005 Aug 1
43. Resch T, Malina M, Lindblad B, et al. Endovascular repair of ruptured abdominal aortic aneurysms: logistics and short-term results. J Endovasc Ther. 2003;10:440–6. doi:10.1177/152660280301000307.
44. Franks S, Lloyd G, Fishwick G, et al. Endovascular treatment of ruptured and symptomatic abdominal aortic aneurysms. Eur J Vasc Endovasc Surg. 2006;31:345–50. Epub 2006 Jan 24
45. İslim F, Erbahçeci Salık A, Güven K, et al. Endovascular repair of thoracic and abdominal aortic ruptures: a single-center experience. Diagn Interv Radiol. 2014;20:259–66. doi:10.5152/dir.2013.13165.
46. Miele V, Errante Y, Galluzzo M, et al. La diagnostica per immagini nelle lesioni traumatiche della milza. Il Giornale Italiano di. Radiol Med. 2015;2:230–48. doi:10.17376/girm_2-2-03042015-6.
47. Federle MP, Crass RA, Brooke Jeffrey R, Trunkey DD. Computed tomography in blunt abdominal trauma. Arch Surg. 1982;117:645–50.
48. The American Association of Surgery for the Surgery of Trauma. Injury Scoring Scale. Available at http://www.aast.org/Library/TraumaTools/injuryscoringscales.aspx
49. Moore EE, Cogbill TH, Jurkovich GJ, et al. Organ injury scaling; spleen and liver (1994 revision). J Trauma. 1995;38:323–4.
50. Wiseman J, Brown CV, Weng J, et al. Splenectomy for trauma increases the rate of early postoperative infections. Am Surg. 2006;72:947–50.
51. Gauer JM, Gerber-Paulet S, Seiler C, Scheweizer WP. Twenty years of splenic preservation in trauma: lower early infection rate than in splenectomy. World J Surg. 2008;32:2730–5. doi:10.1007/s00268-008-9733-3.
52. Hann JM, Bochicchio GV, Kramer N, Scalea TM. Non-operative management of blunt splenic injury: a 5-years experience. J Trauma. 2005;58:492–8.
53. Brasel KJ, DeLisle CM, Olson CJ, Borgstrom DC. Splenic injury: trends in evaluation and management. J Trauma. 1998;44:283–6.
54. Cogbill TH, Moore EE, Jurkovich GJ, et al. Non-operative management of blunt splenic trauma: a multicenter experience. J Trauma. 1989;29:1312–7.
55. Velmahos GC, Toutouzas KG, Radin R, Chan L, Demetriades D. Non-operative treatment of blunt injury to solid abdominal organs: a prospective study. Arch Surg. 2003;138:844–51. doi:10.1001/archsurg.138.8.844.
56. Ng EH, Comin J, David E, Pugash R, Annamalai G. Amplatzer vascular plug 4 for proximal splenic artery embolization in blunt trauma. J Vasc Interv Radiol. 2012;23:976–9. doi:10.1016/j.jvir.2012.04.009.

57. Smith HE, Biffl WL, Majercik SD, et al. Splenic artery embolization: have we gone too far? J Trauma. 2006;61:541–544.; discussion 545–6. doi:10.1097/01.ta.0000235920.92385.2b.
58. Schnüriger B, Inaba K, Konstantinidis A, et al. Outcomes of proximal versus distal splenic artery embolization after trauma: a systematic review and meta-analysis. J Trauma. 2011;70:252–60. doi:10.1097/TA.0b013e3181f2a92e.
59. Saour M, Charbit J, Millet I, et al. Effect of renal angioembolization on post-traumatic acute kidney injury after high-grade renal trauma: a comparative study of 52 consecutive cases. Injury. 2014;45:894–901. doi:10.1016/j.injury.2013.11.030.
60. Regine G, Stasolla A, Miele V. Multidetector computed tomography of the renal arteries in vascular emergencies. Eur J Radiol. 2007;64:83–91. doi:10.1016/j.ejrad.2007.06.007.
61. Dayal M, Gamanagatti S, Kumar A. Imaging in renal trauma. World J Radiol. 2013;5:275–84. doi:10.4329/wjr.v5.i8.275.
62. Ramaswamy RS, Darcy MD. Arterial embolization for the treatment of renal masses and traumatic renal injuries. Tech Vasc Interv Radiol. 2016;19:203–10. doi:10.1053/j.tvir.2016.06.005. Epub 2016 Jun 3
63. Sarani B, Powell E, Taddeo J, et al. Contemporary comparison of surgical and interventional arteriography management of blunt renal injury. J Vasc Interv Radiol. 2011;22:723–8. doi:10.1016/j.jvir.2011.01.444.
64. Niola R, Pinto A, Sparano A, et al. Arterial bleeding in pelvic trauma: priorities in angiographic embolization. Curr Probl Diagn Radiol. 2012;41:93–101.
65. Gansslen A, Giannoudis P, Pape HC. Hemorrhage in pelvic fracture: who needs angiography? Curr Opin Crit Care. 2003;9:515–23.
66. Heetveld MJ, Harris I, Schlaphoff G, et al. Guidelines for the management of haemodynamically unstable pelvic fracture patients. ANZ J Surg. 2004;74:520–9.
67. Ierardi AM, Piacentino F, Fontana F, et al. The role of endovascular treatment of pelvic fracture bleeding in emergency settings. Eur Radiol. 2015;25:1854–64.
68. Pieri S, Agresti P, Morucci M, et al. Percutaneous management of hemorrhages in pelvic fractures. Radiol Med. 2004;107:241–51.
69. Hymel A, Asturias S, Zhao F, et al. Selective vs nonselective embolization vs no embolization in pelvic trauma: a multicenter retrospective cohort study. J Trauma Acute Care Surg. 2017; doi:10.1097/TA.0000000000001554.

The Follow-Up of Patients with Thoracic Injuries

23

Stefania Ianniello, Maria Gabriella Merola, Matteo Pignatelli, Riccardo Ferrari, Margherita Trinci, and Vittorio Miele

23.1 Introduction

Thoracic trauma represents today the second cause of death by trauma, with a specific mortality rate of about 10% and a global mortality of 25%.

Blunt chest trauma affects predominantly the male sex in the middle age and is usually caused by several different trauma dynamics like road accidents, falls, sports injuries, crushing, or weapons.

Moreover chest injuries, especially in polytrauma patients, are often associated with other intra- or extra-thoracic injuries as, respectively, lung contusions, pneumothorax and pleural effusions with rib fractures or injuries to extremities or pelvic bones or head injuries too.

90.9% of patients with lethal outcome, in fact, has associated thoracic injuries; these numbers depend on the impairment of respiratory function that can result in chest injuries, such as hypoxia, hypercapnia, acidosis and hypotension up to shock.

The ATLS recommendations underline the main diagnostic role of imaging [1–4], to recognize the "immediate" or "potentially" life-threatening traumatic conditions to ensure an intensive treatment, often including mechanical ventilation if necessary.

Although plain chest radiography is the first-line modality to screen the traumatized patient, Multidetector Computed Tomography (MDCT) is actually considered the gold standard technique, essential to identify otherwise occult injuries, especially lung parenchymal or pleural injuries.

Follow-up of patients with blunt thoracic trauma is very important to ensure the complete resolution of the clinical conditions and monitor the results of the therapeutic strategies. Repeated lung diagnostic evaluations are primarily carried out by clinical evaluation and serial measurements of respiratory variables, then with periodic bedside radiography. Nevertheless, a daily chest X-ray is not more recommended, but actually required only on clinical indications or changing in clinical condition. Another imaging modality, which is nowadays increasingly considered in many stages of trauma care [5, 6], including follow-up, is lung ultrasound, even though with accurate definition of indications [7].

S. Ianniello, M.D. (✉) • M.G. Merola • M. Pignatelli
R. Ferrari • M. Trinci
Department of Emergency Radiology, S. Camillo Hospital, Rome, Italy
e-mail: stefianni66@gmail.com

V. Miele
Department of Radiology, Careggi University Hospital, Florence, Italy

V. Miele, M. Trinci (eds.), *Diagnostic Imaging in Polytrauma Patients*,
https://doi.org/10.1007/978-3-319-62054-1_23

The main features of each imaging modality are detailed in the text in relation to individual clinical conditions with the aim of ensuring the best clinical management of the traumatized patient, assessing their outcome and preventing or identifying the possible occurrence of complications.

23.2 The Follow-Up of Contusions

Contusions are a common finding after trauma, occurring in approximately 17–20% of patients with multiple injuries (ISS >15 Yale Trauma Registry). Contusion achieves its maximum in the 24–48 h followed by absorption, which takes 1–2 weeks. They are considered an independent risk factor for Pneumonia and Acute Respiratory Distress Syndrome (ARDS) with an associated mortality rate ranging between 10 and 25% [8–10]. Because these complications may appear after a free interval of 24–48 h, early detection of patients at risk is essential.

Many scoring systems have been developed in recent years to define injury severity in cases of blunt thoracic trauma and pulmonary contusion to predict respiratory impairment [11].

Exact quantification of lung contusions by computed tomography may help clinicians identify high-risk populations: a reconstructed 3D view of pulmonary contusion volume can be calculated and correlated to outcome. Patients who have contusion volume greater than 20% are at risk for developing pneumonia, prolonged hospital stay, and prolonged mechanical ventilation [12–14].

Also Acute Respiratory Distress Syndrome (ARDS) can be a life-threatening complication of lung trauma, that is treated by intubation and positive pressure ventilation. The acute phase of ARDS is associated with diffuse alveolar damage and lung capillary endothelial injury that lead to diffuse pulmonary edema that extend into the alveoli, reducing both gas exchange and lung compliance.

In 2011, a Joint European and American Team attempted to redefine ARDS in what became known as the Berlin Definition, that divides patients into three stages of mild, moderate, and severe based on the degree of hypoxia in the patient; every stage is associated with increased mortality [15].

23.2.1 Radiological Features

On plain chest radiography contusions appear like indistinct opacification (Fig. 23.1), with blurred margins: in many cases of limited contusions, chest X-rays appears totally negative.

But when a precise evaluation for the first diagnosis is needed, referral to CT is mandatory [16] (Fig. 23.2).

Instead at the stage of follow-up, the development of a bedside noninvasive method is desirable.

Ultrasound could be such a method, but the lungs are traditionally deemed to be inaccessible [17].

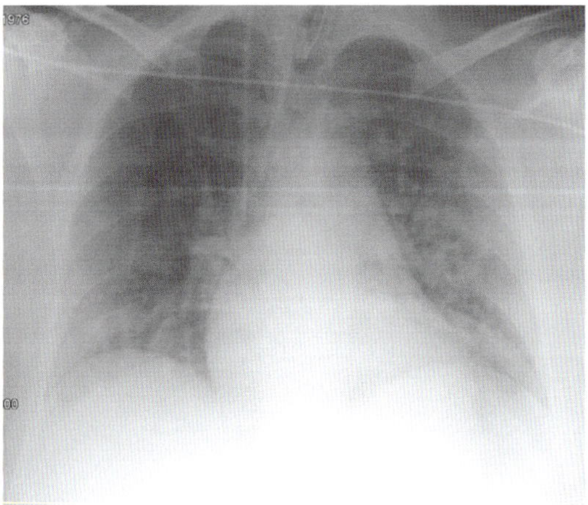

Fig. 23.1 Pedestrian-invested: bilateral, inhomogeneous, ground-glass opacification for lung contusions

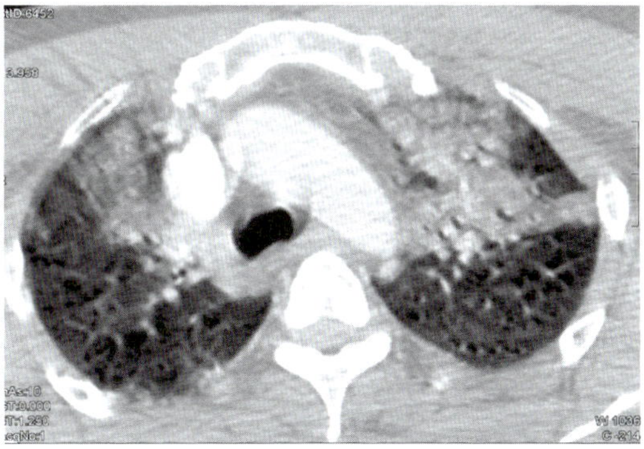

Fig. 23.2 Car crush: at MDCT, wide, dense, confluent anterior consolidations, for lung contusions. Typically, contusions are distributed according to impact force, as in this case anteriorly

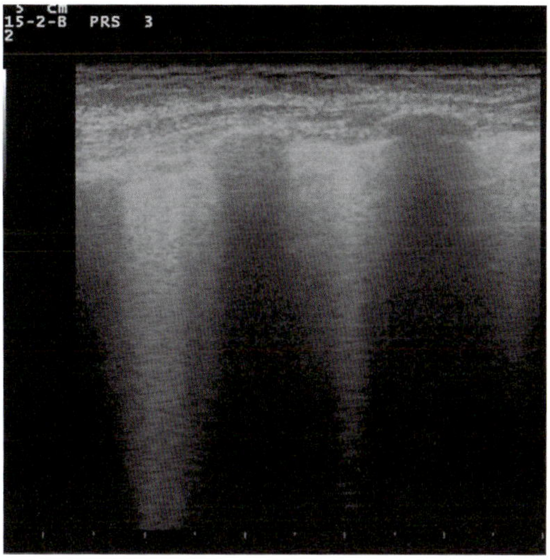

Fig. 23.3 Car crush: at lung ultrasound, anterior, bilateral, confluent B-Lines. The B-lines are "ring-down" artifacts that originate from the pleural line with vertical propagation

However, it has been shown that a whole ultrasound semiology is available at the lung level if one takes care to analyze the artifacts [18]. Although indications for ultrasound of the lungs are increasingly numerous in ICUs, its clinical use is not yet fully developed.

By ultrasonography, lung contusions were defined as:

(a) A moderately hypoechoic blurred consolidation, with indistinct margins, whose dimensions remained unchanged during the inspiration phase. Internal hyperechoic punctiform images represent air bronchograms.
(b) Multiple (at least three) vertical hyperechogenic lines (B-lines) arising from and perpendicular to the pleural surface representing the involvement of interstitial spaces (Fig. 23.3). The distance between the B-lines can be 7 mm or 3 mm corresponding to the thickened interlobular septa and the ground glass areas, respectively.

During follow-up, bedside chest radiography was a poor predictor of the extent of lung contusions compared with lung ultrasonography; CXR is less accurate and with a less sensitivity than LU (Accuracy CXR about 60–70% vs. LU about 80–90%). These data support the routine use of lung ultrasound (eventually in association with CXR) in the management and follow-up of thoracic trauma patients in the ICU. The information obtained from LU, that can show reduction/increase of B-lines and/or consolidations, was adequate to support therapeutical decisions in those patients, suggesting the possibility for a reduced need for further CT scans. However, we must recall the impossibility of a complete chest exploration with US probe, owing to the presence of tubes and wound medications was the main disadvantage of this method.

Limitations of ultrasound should be considered, for example in cases of small consolidations, if care is not taken to scan the entire lung surface, or by consolidations which do not reach the pleural surface, a rare finding, or by a poor echogenicity of the patient. Parietal emphysema, pleural calcifications, or dressings will prevent analysis. Furthermore, alveolar consolidations and B-lines are present in ARDS too, with the same semiotic aspects of lung contusions; only clinical background can differentiate the two different diseases.

Obviously, CT is considered the best imaging technique for visualizing the pulmonary interstitium involvement and alveolar consolidations in lung contusions; but while in less severe cases, repeated CT scans can be performed without major risks, the transporting of mechanically ventilated trauma patients to the CT room can be dangerous: several studies suggest that even intrahospital transfers of critically ill patients are associated with complications [19, 20], the most common and harmful being are hypoxemia and hypotension.

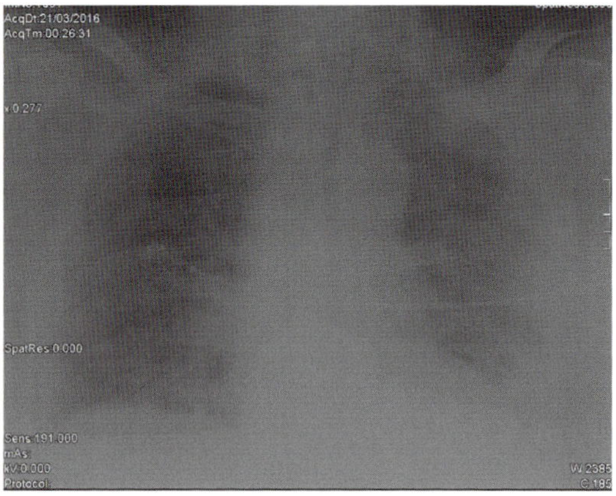

Fig. 23.4 Car crush: 3 days later, at Chest-XR, appearance of bilateral, inhomogeneous, patchy opacifications suggestive of ARDS

23.3 The Follow-Up of ARDS

The most difficult differential diagnosis is between cardiogenic pulmonary edema; the lung in acute respiratory distress syndrome is characterized by a marked increase in lung tissue and a massive loss of aeration. The former is homogeneously distributed, although with a slight predominance in the upper lobes, whereas the latter is heterogeneously distributed.

The lower lobes are essentially non-aerated, whereas the upper lobes may remain normally aerated, despite a substantial increase in regional lung tissue.

The overall lung volume and the cephalocaudal lung dimensions are reduced primarily at the expense of the lower lobes, which are externally compressed by the heart and abdominal content when the patient is in the supine position.

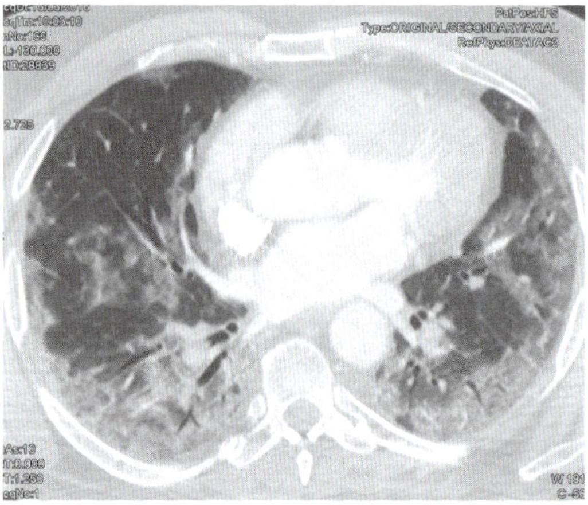

Fig. 23.5 Car crush: 3 days later, MDCT showed clearly appearance of bilateral, inhomogeneous, patchy opacifications suggestive of ARDS; within the areas of consolidation is also visible the air bronchogram. Asymmetric distribution of opacifications is characteristic of ARDS

23.3.1 Radiological Features

Two opposite radiologic presentations, corresponding to different lung morphologies, can be observed.

In patients with focal computed tomographic attenuations, frontal chest radiography generally shows bilateral opacities in the lower quadrants and may remain normal, particularly when the lower lobes are entirely atelectasis (Fig. 23.4).

In patients with diffuse computed tomographic attenuations (Fig. 23.5), the typical radiologic presentation of "white lungs" is observed. If these patients lie supine, lung volume is preserved in the upper lobes and reduced in the lower lobes, although the loss of aeration is equally distributed between the upper and lower lobes.

In fact, interstitial edema, alveolar flooding, or both, not collapse, are histologically present in all regions of the lung in acute respiratory distress syndrome. Compression atelectasis is observed only in caudal parts of the lung, where external forces (such as cardiac weight, abdominal pressure, and pleural effusion) tend to squeeze the lower lobes.

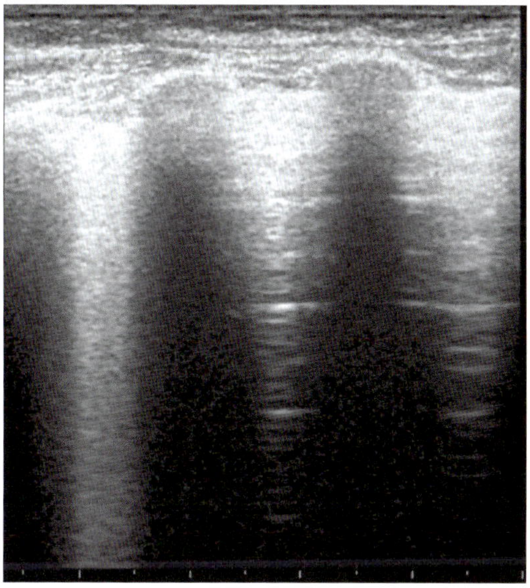

Fig. 23.6 Car crush: 3 days later, lung ultrasound confirmed alternance of B-lines and A-lines, named spared areas; signs suggestive of ARDS; the ultrasound imaging is similar to TC

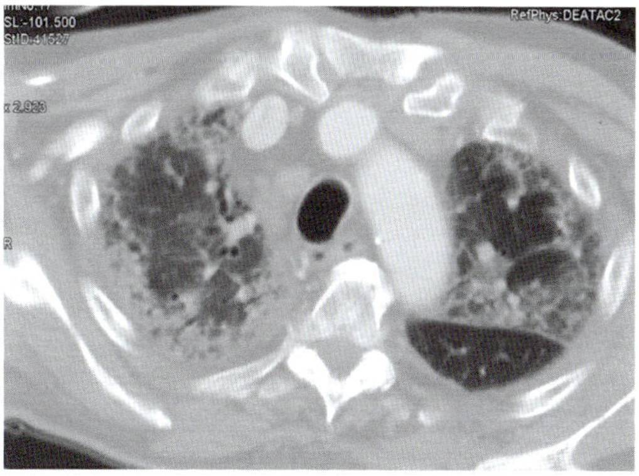

Fig. 23.7 Car crush: 15 days later, MDCT showed early signs of subpleural interstitial thickening, bronchial dilatations, suggestive of fibrosal evolution of ARDS

Ultrasound can visualize a succession of B-lines, sign of interstitial involvement, with spared areas, and posterobasal consolidations for atelectasis areas (Fig. 23.6).

When a positive intrathoracic pressure is applied to patients with focal acute respiratory distress syndrome, poorly aerated and non-aerated lung regions are recruited, whereas lung regions that are normally aerated at zero end-expiratory pressure tend to be rapidly overinflated, increasing the risk of ventilator-induced lung injury, like pneumothorax.

Selection of the optimal positive end-expiratory pressure level should not only consider optimizing alveolar recruitment, it should also focus on limiting lung overinflation and counterbalancing compression of the lower lobes by maneuvers such as appropriate body positioning. Prone and semirecumbent positions facilitate the reaeration of dependent and caudal lung regions by partially relieving cardiac and abdominal compression and may improve gas exchange.

For these reasons, CT is essential to monitoring all exchanges [21] (Fig. 23.7); computed tomography allows an accurate assessment of the volumes of gas and lung tissue, respectively, and lung aeration. If computed tomographic sections are contiguous from the apex to the lung base, quantitative analysis can be performed either on the whole lung or, regionally, at the lobar level.

Analysis requires a manual delineation of lung parenchyma and is facilitated by software, including a color-coding system that allows direct visualization of overinflated, normally aerated, poorly aerated, and non-aerated lung regions.

In addition, lung recruitment can be measured as the amount of gas that penetrates poorly aerated and non-aerated lung regions after the application of positive intrathoracic pressure.

In ARDS, the radiographic abnormalities follow a sequence by tending to mirror the histopathological changes; in the first 24 h following insult, when there is a little alveolar edema, the chest X-ray is generally normal. As ARDS evolves, widespread ground-glass opacification invariably becomes apparent and, during the next 36 h, there is a frank consolidation on the chest radiograph (Fig. 23.8); obviously this is a non-specific radiological sign.

The radiographic changes of uncomplicated ARDS usually plateau after initial catastrophic burst and remain unchanged for a variable time thereafter. Knowledge of this radiographically stable phase can be of practical value to the radiologist; any significant change in serial radiographic appearances like the development of new focal areas of air space opacification may be the harbinger of nosocomial pneumonia.

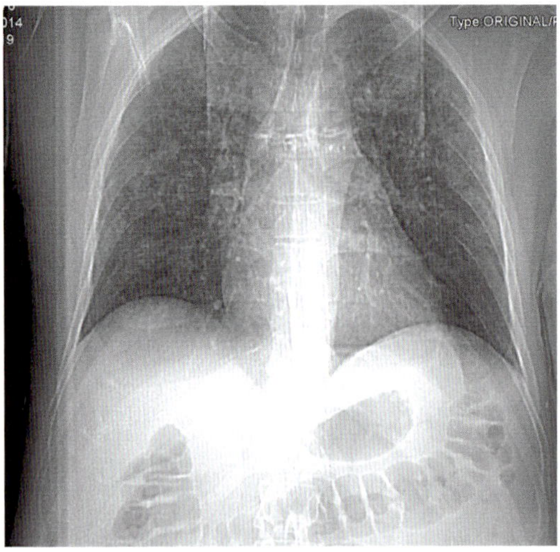

Fig. 23.8 Pedestrian-invested: after 3 days, most evidence of bilateral, inhomogeneous, ground-glass opacification, with appearance of fine micronodular opacities, suggestive for adipose embolism in ARDS

In the final phase, the chest radiographic abnormalities begin to resolve. Although the lungs may revert to normal, there may be coarse reticular opacities and cysts, likely to be a consequence of the effects of both lung repair and barotrauma; this phase will already start after 8–10 days and requires CT for diagnosis and follow-up [22].

Interstitial emphysema, pneumothorax, and pneumomediastinum may be relatively frequent iatrogenic complications of mechanical ventilation support; thoracic ultrasound permits an accurate and early diagnosis of pneumothorax but not of the two other conditions that require CT.

An important finding of earliest CT studies was that lung involvement in ARDS is totally inhomogeneous, a "patchy" distribution intermittent with normally aerated lung (Fig. 23.9); furthermore the dependent (dorsal) region are more densely opacified than the nondependent (ventral) lung, with a gradient of density [23].

It's a common thinking that appearance of nondependent opacities may represent foci of organizing pneumonia. ARDS appears to have a far more diffuse opacity than that associated with congestive heart failure; there are many signs to differentiate the two conditions and the principle is pulmonary picture really inhomogeneous in ARDS.

Bronchial dilatation is seen frequently on CT in patients with ARDS; airway dilatation persists in the majority of survivors and is generally associated with ground-glass opacification. The most common abnormality on CT in survivors is a reticular pattern seen in about 85% of patients [24]. The extent of the reticular pattern, that has a predilection for nondependent lung, at follow-up was negatively correlated with the extent of dense parenchymal opacification (in dependent lung) during acute phase; maybe, atelectasis somehow

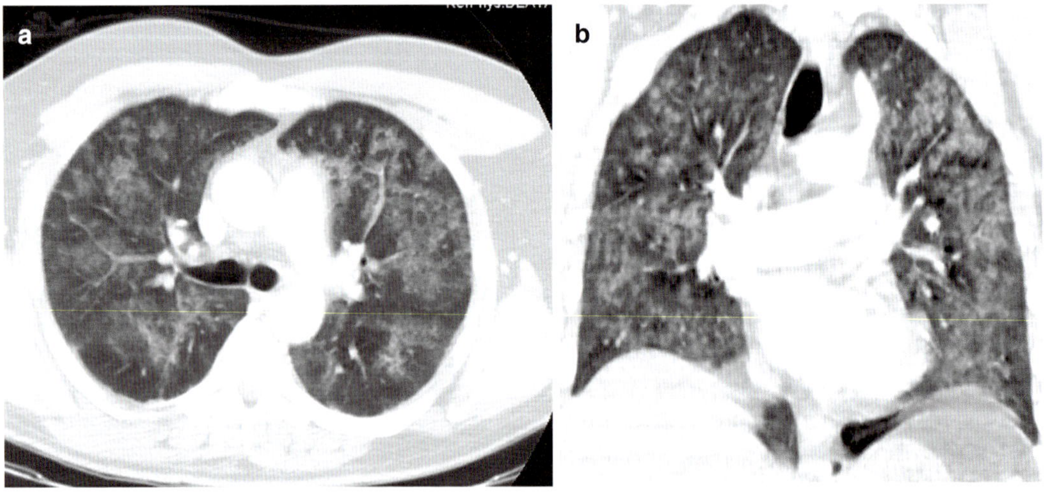

Fig. 23.9 (**a**) Axial CT scan; (**b**) coronal reconstruction. Pedestrian-invested: after 3 days, "cottony" opacifications with spared subpleural regions; signs suggestive of adipose embolism in ARDS

protects dependent regions from the long-term effects of barotrauma (see Fig. 23.5).

One of the principal advantages of CT is that the global extent of parenchymal abnormalities can be quantified accurately and followed-up; furthermore, the effects of PEEP (Positive End-Expiratory Pressure), of recruitment maneuvers, of prone positioning, can be studied using CT.

23.4 The Follow-Up of Pneumothorax

Pneumothorax is one of the most common injuries in thoracic trauma resulting in an abnormal accumulation of gas within the pleural space [25]. This is a virtual space normally filled with a few milliliters of fluid with a negative intrapleural pressure, usually about −5 cmH_2O. In case of pneumothorax, the entry of air into the pleural space compromises the normal dynamics of airflow by compressing the lung that collapses.

Post-traumatic pneumothorax can happen in several chest traumas, like blunt or penetrating trauma, as isolated lesion or in polytrauma patient, with an incidence of 30–40% [26].

Often the presence of pneumothorax, especially if greater than 20%, requires a chest tube insertion to ensure the drainage of air from the pleural space and allow the lung re-expansion [27].

Follow-up of pneumothorax is required after chest tube placement by chest radiographs or, sometimes, by MDCT, to monitor the clinical condition and to identify the etiology of a persistent air leak [28] (Fig. 23.10).

A persistent pneumothorax, in fact, is a condition in which a continued bubbling of air from an in situ chest drain, for more than 48 h after its insertion [29], that can make several difficulties in diagnostic iter, aimed at its recognition and at the identification of potentially treatable etiologies. The most common etiologies may be chest tube related, like malposition or kinking or obstructing (Fig. 23.11), requiring a simple repositioning of the chest tube/drain, whereas lung parenchymal disease, bronchopleural fistula (BPF), alveolar-pleural fistula (APF) or, rarely, esophageal-pleural fistula, especially in penetrating thoracic injury, sometimes not immediately or easily discernible, requires a careful interpretation of imaging studies to make the right diagnosis and to guarantee an optimal therapeutic management.

In these cases, in fact, although radiographs remain the mainstay for diagnosis and follow-up of pneumothorax, able to identify chest tube-related causes of persistent pneumothorax, the use of MDCT is essential to lead to early and proper diagnosis and treatment of non-chest tube-related cases.

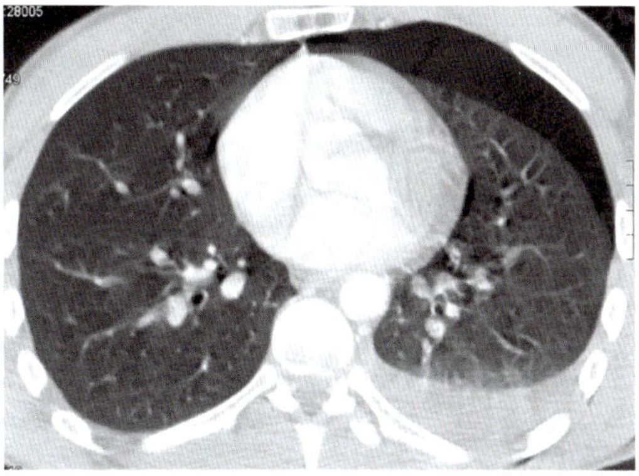

Fig. 23.10 Moto-car crush: at MDCT wide left anterior pneumothorax. Left posterior hemothorax is associated in this patient

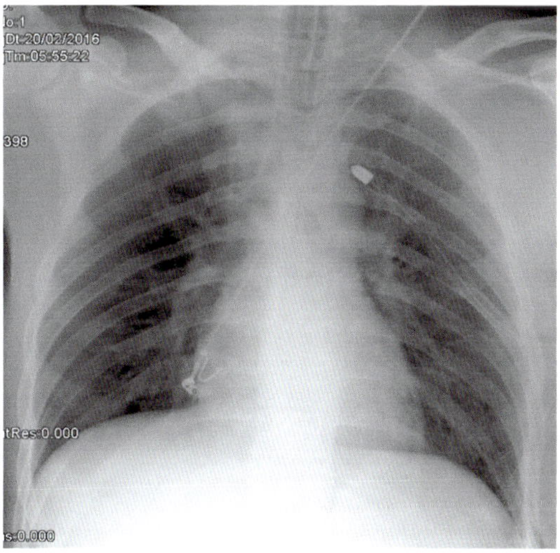

Fig. 23.11 Moto-car crush: kinking of left pleural drainage; residual basal hyperlucency and minimal deep sulcus sign, suggestive of residual left anterior pneumothorax

The radiologic features of pneumothorax are encoded and represented by typical characteristics on RX, US, and TC imaging.

In fact, in trauma patients, usually chest radiograph is the primary modality imaging performed in emergency department, able to identify pneumothorax as a pathological lucency and a visceral pleural line separating the lung, occasionally completely collapse, from the chest wall; in supine chest radiographs, presence of a deep sulcus sign is useful to make the right diagnosis [30].

However, sensitivity of supine chest radiography in traumatized patients, especially in the presence of subcutaneous emphysema along chest wall, is very low, showing low accuracy in the assessment of pneumothorax during the primary survey in the emergency room [31, 32] because free air collects anteriorly, medially, and basally, therefore difficult to identify on supine chest radiographs [33].

Nowadays, however, the use of thoracic ultrasound is been approved; in fact, it has gained a main role in unstable patients with chest trauma during the primary survey in the emergency room for diagnosis of PNX, with high sensitivity (77%) and specificity (99.8%), positive predictive value 98.5%, negative predictive value 97%, accuracy 97.2% [6], useful to guide the chest drainage and in follow-up of persistent pneumothorax too [34, 35].

In healthy patient, there is a movement due to sliding of the two pleural sheets during breathing. This movement is precisely called "sliding or gliding." The of loss of sliding movement due to the presence of air in pleural space, in fact, indicates the presence of pneumothorax [36], but nevertheless it isn't adequate to identify the etiology of pneumothorax, nor even of a persistent pneumothorax (Fig. 23.12).

In these conditions, in fact, computed tomography (MDCT) is the best choice in detecting the main features of a persistent pneumothorax because, although the other imaging techniques consent to make diagnosis of PNX, only CT, thanks to its high sensitivity and specificity, its rapidity and its post-processing potentiality as Multiplanar reconstruction (MPR), maximum

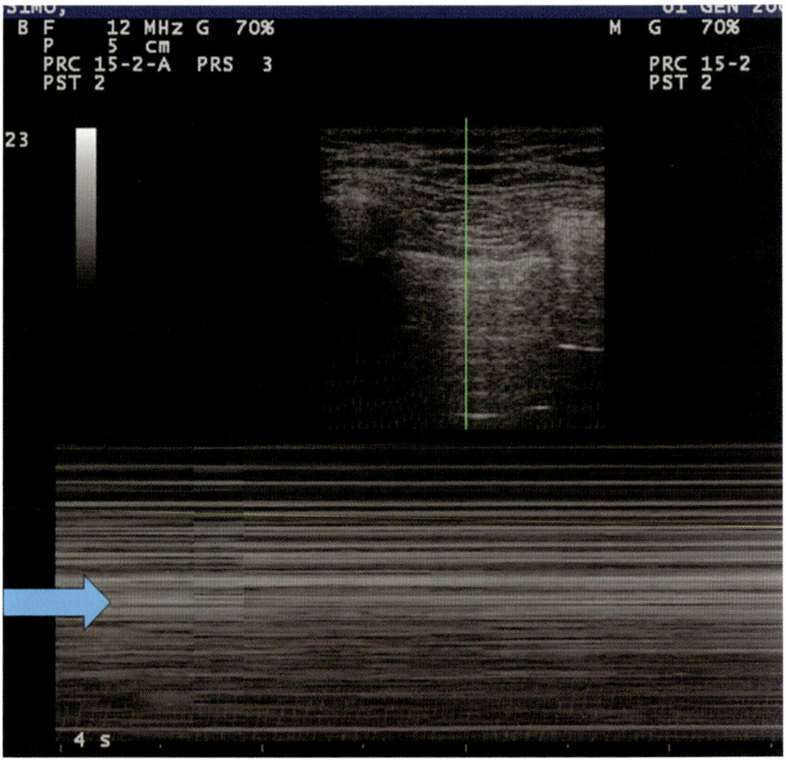

Fig. 23.12 Moto-car crush: at lung ultrasound, with M-Mode, "stratosphere sign" and absence of pleural sliding suggestive of residual left anterior pneumothorax

intensity projections (MIP), minimum intensity projection (minIP), volume rendering, and virtual bronchoscopy, is useful to identify other chest trauma related pathologies as contusion or the etiology of a persistent air leak [37, 38], allowing surgical planning too.

In case of persistent pneumothorax, in fact, follow-up CT, usually employing intravenous contrast, consents to evaluate and to distinguish the possible causes as malposition of chest tubes, or an air leak due to mediastinum or pleural laceration or, even rarely, an esophago-respiratory fistula, usually detected after ingestion of positive oral water-soluble contrast [39].

23.4.1 Chest Drains/Tubes

One of the most frequent etiologies of non-resolving PNX is chest drains/tubes related, as its malposition or its obstruction. These conditions occur usually in emergency department, especially in traumatized patients in which the chest tube placement can be difficult and incomplete, determining a poor drainage of the air from the pleural space [40].

Nowadays, in fact, chest tube placement represents a cornerstone in acute chest trauma management, usually performed as a primary diagnostic procedure, often life-treating decompressing pneumothorax and the underlying collapsed lung, with a success rate ranging between 79 and 95% [41].

The British Thoracic Surgery (BTS) guidelines [42] have described the correct placement of a chest drain in a standardized technique preferably performed by surgeons or emergency physicians, after a prior physical and radiological basic examination with RX or e-FAST or, rarely, CT scan.

Although in emergency care could be difficult,, the chest drain should be inserted, in supine patient's position, within the "safe triangle," namely a thoracic area characterized by a low risk of complications like vascular injuries, circumscribed between the pectoralis major and the latissimus dorsi muscle, with the apex of triangle localized below the axilla and the basis as a superior line passing through the nipple; furthermore, it's also preferable to avoid incisions below the level of the nipple, because of the high risk of intra-abdominal malposition or intra-abdominal organ injuries.

Chest tube should be inserted, after a transverse skin incision, in the 4th–6th intercostal space in the mid-axillary line [43], although, in case of anterior or apical pneumothorax, the 2nd–3rd intercostal space in the medial clavicular line is suitable for chest tube placement, always on the superior rib margin to avoid intercostal neurovascular bundle.

The chest drain insertion in emergency is usually performed percutaneously and requires the correct progression in the pleural space, so that its most peripheral hole, called "sentinel hole," results all inside the pleural space, to avoid false position or insufficient drainage, and its attachment to the skin with a stitch, to avoid its dislodgement and its inefficiency.

After chest drain placement, it's important to check its correct position through the execution of a chest radiograph, as well as rule out any complications, occurring between 2% and 10% [44], or iatrogenic injuries, especially in case of residual PNX, or pleural/mediastinal abnormalities.

An incorrect placement of chest tube, as false position or inadequate drainage, in fact, can occur and, sometimes, requires another chest drain to insert. A suboptimal drainage can occur, in fact, in case of kinking of the chest tube involving the intra- or extra-thoracic portion. The incomplete insertion of the chest drainage, detected with a chest radiograph performed after its placement to ensure the correct positioning, or with computed tomography scan during follow-up of a persistent air leak, is a typical etiology of non-resolving PNX, usually characterized by an abnormal seating of the tube, as outside the pleural cavity or even the chest wall; in the first case, the evacuation of air is inadequate; in the second case, instead, a backflow of atmospheric air into the pleural space can lead to suboptimal drainage and persistent PNX.

Risk factors for improper chest drainage placement, as in the chest wall outside the pleural cavity, are, especially in emergency department in traumatized patients, the presence of chest wall emphysema, or obesity or chest habitus like anomalies or deformities too, as well as the presence of scars of previous chest surgeries suggesting extensive intrathoracic adhesions and the risk of complications, especially if performed without any imaging guide.

Also a wrong seal of tissue around the chest tube insertion site could cause a persistent air leak because of the backflow of atmospheric air into the pleural space.

Other malposition or obstruction etiologies are due to intraparenchymal placement of the chest drain, usually due to traumatic pleuro-parenchymal injury or to a wrong and forced insertion, causing pleuro-parenchymal lesions too.

A more rare occurrence is the mediastinal placement of chest drainage, with high risk of severe complications as cardiovascular injuries or esophagus perforation.

Likewise, intrafissural positioning of the chest tube could lead to inadequate evacuation of air from pleural space.

The radiological features of chest drains/tubes malposition are several and detectable on RX or CT scan [29, 45].

Sometimes chest radiographs show an abnormal seating of the tube, as outside the pleural cavity or even the chest wall, leading to inadequate drainage of air and persistent PNX.

If the tube is displaced across the lateral chest wall, chest radiograph is able to identify its abnormal seating, while in case of anterior or posterior chest wall dislocation of drainage, RX is not satisfactory, requiring a CT evaluation.

In case of intraparenchymal tube placement, chest radiograph and/or chest CT identify the etiology of non-resolving PNX; the first modality imaging, in fact, although it could be unremarkable, usually reveals the presence of an opacity along the course of the intrathoracic portion of the chest tube, due to the formation of a hematoma.

CT scan, instead, especially with post-processing modality, as multiplanar reconstruction (MPR), is able to demonstrate the chest tube crossing the lung parenchyma, usually affected by contusive or lacerative injuries too.

CT, in fact, can demonstrate not only an abnormal seating of chest tube, as outside the pleural cavity or the chest wall or within the lung parenchyma or the mediastinum, or a pathological kinking of the chest drain involving the intra- or extra-thoracic portion, or an incomplete seal, often difficult to identify especially in case of subcutaneous emphysema along chest wall. In case of major subcutaneous emphysema, in fact, CT is able to identify correctly a minimum PNX too, which, instead, is very difficult with the RX scan.

CT can also detect any pleuro-parenchymal complications as lung contusions or lacerations, resulting in persistent tubular opacities along the course of the chest drain or any pathological air leak as a bronchopleural or esophageal-pleural fistula or even any cardiovascular injuries.

23.4.2 Bronchopleural Fistula (BPF)

Bronchopleural fistula (BPF) or persistent air leak (PAL) is an abnormal communication between the bronchial tree, usually a main stem, lobar, or segmental bronchus, or lung parenchyma and the pleural space [46] classified as either central or peripheral, the latter described by some authors as alveolar-pleural fistula (APF), potentially incurring in chest trauma [33].

Another, although more rare entity, is a fistula developing between the esophagus and the pleural space, named esophageal-pleural fistula.

Luckily BPF is not a common entity as it is an important cause of significantly increased morbidity, prolonged hospitalization and mortality, reaching between 18% and 50%, because of the high risk of aspiration pneumonia and acute respiratory distress syndrome, therefore requiring an early diagnosis and a proper management.

BPF can recognize several etiologies, including lung infection (as abscess, tuberculosis, etc.), traumatic injury, neoplastic invasion or iatrogenic causes (as lung biopsy or chest tube insertion or surgery) [46]. Our attention is focused on traumatic bronchopleural fistulae; the reported incidence of BPF after chest trauma, in fact, is extremely variable with a changeable time of onset distinguishable as early (1–7 days), in which the clinical condition is often very unstable needing a timely management with surgical repair and assisted ventilation, or intermediate (8–30 days), or late (more than 30 days), mainly caused by impaired healing of the bronchial leak, often associated with empyema, therefore requiring a pleural drainage too.

Major thoracic trauma, in fact, especially in presence of displaced fractured ribs, can easily cause pleuro-parenchymal injuries as pulmonary lacerations or BPF, because the elastic return of the lungs.

The presence of a bronchopleural fistula would be suspected by clinical signs and confirmed by imaging or endoscopic visualization. Nowadays, in fact, multidetector computed tomography (MDCT) is not only able to detect the fistula tract, but it can also evaluate the number, size, and location of the fistulas as well as identify any underlying traumatic diseases, sometimes avoiding further invasive diagnostic procedure such as bronchoscopies, whose role seems limited to therapy.

The radiological findings suggestive of BPF are aspecific on a plain chest radiograph, usually used as screening modality; in fact, BPF can be suspected in presence of an increased pneumothorax, or an increased opacity of the chest, usually due to pleural effusion or other pleuro-parenchymal complication, like hemo- or pyothorax.

CT scans, in fact, is the best choice in detecting BPF because it can demonstrate the airway injury and the site and the size of fistula as well as help in the surgical planning [47, 48].

CT is an effective noninvasive tool, considered superior to bronchoscopy [47], identifying, on thin slices and by image reconstruction algorithms, the defect of visceral pleura, usually recognized thanks to the presence of extraluminal air bubbles adjacent to a dehiscent bronchial stump.

CT images can demonstrate the direct communication between the bronchial tree, usually a main stem, lobar, or segmental bronchus, or lung parenchyma and the pleural space, as a dehiscent bronchial stump, distinguishing as either central or peripheral BPF.

Sometimes, nevertheless, especially in differential diagnosis with esophageal-pleural fistula, a contrast-enhanced CT with positive oral contrast [39] is required to help in defining the persistent air leak showing, not only esophageal wall thickening or presence of a fluid collection in pleural space, but also the abnormal passage of the positive water-soluble contrast, with clear evidence of a fistula.

Then bronchoscopy finally can demonstrate the air leak and the relation with the airway district and can delineate the extent of fistula, in addition to allowing the treatment of BPF by endoscopic closure.

Nowadays, the BPF management is characterized by several therapeutic options ranging from conservative nonsurgical treatment to aggressive surgical procedures, in relation to the size of fistulas, because while in case of small and peripheral fistulas it is advisable to use prolonged chest tube placement for pleural drainage and transbronchial injection, for large or more proximal fistulas or cases with pleuro-parenchymal complication, like hemo- or pyothorax, an endoscopic or a surgical approach is essential to close the persistent air leak.

Today, furthermore, flexible bronchoscopy is considered as the best diagnostic and therapeutic choice, especially in high-risk surgical patients, ensuring an effective obliteration of the bronchopleural defect using several different biological or artificial materials, including fibrin or tissue glue, spigots, vascular metallic coils, stents, gel foam, silver nitrate, and autologous endobronchial blood patch [49].

The first step in management of BPF is a simple method consisting in the endoscopic injection of glue for bronchoscopic closure of bronchopleural fistula [50]. Glue, in fact, as soon as comes in contact with the mucosa, solidifies, closing the BPF by mechanical sealing; then, the granulation tissue and the following fibrous tissue consent the permanent fistula closure.

In case of middle and large size BPF, endobronchial embolization using EWSs is able to control air leakage [51].

The use of one-way endobronchial valves for management of BPF is indicated in the critical care setting with high efficacy and tolerability, and low complication rate [52].

One of the new trends in the management of BPF, in fact, is a safe, effective, and minimally invasive bronchoscopic procedure consisting in endoscopically injection into the de-epithelialized area and fistulous tract of autologous adipose-derived stem cells [53].

However, a transposition of vascularized flap repair (muscle, diaphragm, omentum, or pericardium), usually a chest wall muscles, like the latissimus dorsi muscle flap [54] in association with an open pleural drainage, is a proper therapeutic option for management of biggest and proximal BPF, effective in obliteration of the pleural cavity with complete BPF repair upon resolution of air leakage from the chest drainage system, actually performed minimal-invasively by video-assisted thoracoscopic surgery (VATS), guaranteeing a better visible and therefore more secure fixation of the muscle flap on the BPF with a successful patient's outcome.

Follow-up imaging with RX and CT after conservative or operative treatment is needed to evaluate the evolution until resolution of BPF.

23.5 The Follow-Up of Hemothorax

Hemothorax is defined as a collection of blood in the pleural space [55], usually due to injuries of the lung parenchyma, pleura, chest wall, diaphragm, or mediastinum [56]. The primary cause of hemothorax is sharp or blunt trauma to the chest. Iatrogenous (complication of cardiopulmonary surgery, placement of subclavian or jugular catheters, lung biopsies, etc.) and spontaneous hemothorax occurs less frequently.

Hemothorax occurs in 30–50% of patients who suffer blunt chest trauma [57, 58]. This lesion along with pneumothorax is present in 83% of thoracic traumas [59] (Fig. 23.13).

Massive hemothorax is defined as a collection of blood exceeding 1 l with clinical signs of shock [60].

Hemothorax may also be defined as pleural fluid with a hematocrit greater than 50% of the patient's blood hematocrit, although hematocrit may be somewhat lower in patients with long-standing hemothorax [61].

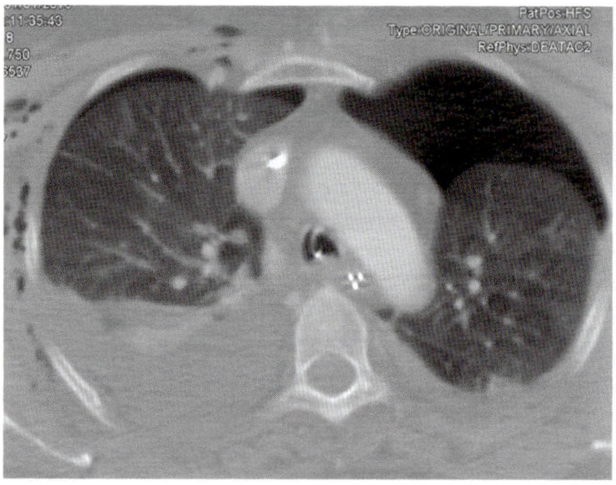

Fig. 23.13 Defenestration: at MDCT, bilateral pneumothorax, wider on left side. On right side, significant hemothorax, lung atelectasis, and subcutaneous emphysema

23.5.1 Radiological Features

Chest radiography is the first-line imaging examination in patients with thoracic polytrauma. Upright chest radiography is a standard part of thoracic trauma evaluation. However, trauma patients often must be imaged in the supine position. Chest radiographic appearance of a large hemothorax may be similar to that of pleural effusion. It can be almost impossible to differentiate a hemothorax from other causes of pleural effusions. When the size of a hemothorax reaches approximately 200 mL, an upright chest radiograph demonstrates blunting of the costophrenic angle. With progressive increase in size, a "meniscus" sign will be seen: a concave upward sloping of fluid in the costophrenic angle. In contrast, a straight air–fluid level on the upright chest radiograph indicates a hemopneumothorax [33]. On a supine chest radiograph, blood will layer in the pleural space and may appear as little more than haziness in one hemithorax relative to the contralateral side; this is appreciated best with a unilateral hemothorax. A large hemothorax may opacify an entire hemithorax or cause mediastinal shift and tension physiology (hypertensive

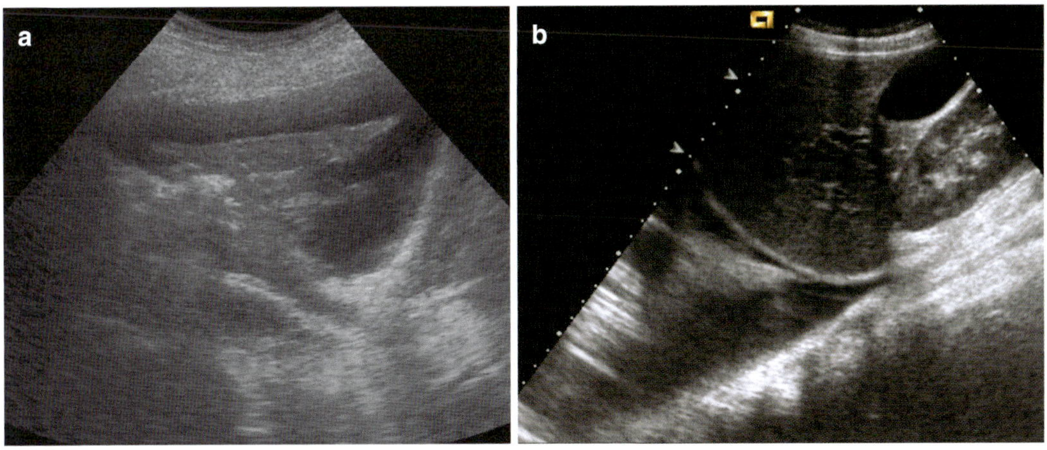

Fig. 23.14 (**a** and **b**) Lung US. Defenestration: on right side, significant hemothorax and lung atelectasis

hemothorax) [62]. These findings require immediate intervention.

Computed tomography (CT) has become common place in the evaluation of the injured patient, and allows for detection of much smaller amounts of fluid than chest radiography. Fluid in the pleural space is assumed to be blood until proved otherwise. However, CT is useful in determining the nature of pleural fluid in the setting of trauma by assessing the attenuation value. An attenuation lower than 15 HU is indicative of serous effusion. Blood in the pleural space typically has an attenuation of 35–70 HU, and clotted blood is 50–90 HU; a mixture of both can present a layered appearance called "hematocrit sign" [63]. Arterial hemorrhage, as opposed to venous bleeding (self-limiting because of the tamponade effect from the lung parenchyma), is characterized by progressive increase in hemothorax volume, with active arterial bleeding having density similar to that of the adjacent contrast-enhanced arterial vessels. This situation needs an urgent intervention.

In the past decade, the use of ultrasonography has become a mainstay in emergency department and trauma evaluation. Ultrasonography is often more readily attainable than CT and can be used in patients who are not stable enough for transport. In most cases, the ultrasonography result was available to the trauma team before the CT results [64]. Regarding hemothorax, a supine or upright CXR requires up to 175 or 50–100 mL of fluid in order to be visualized, compared to e-FAST which can detect as little as 20 mL of fluid in the pleural space [65] (Fig. 23.14).

23.5.2 Complications

Retained hemothorax complicates 2–20% of post-traumatic hemothorax [66] and it occurs when clotted or loculated collections of blood aren't evacuated by single or even multiple chest tubes (Fig. 23.15).

Under normal conditions, a clot in the pleural cavity undergoes fibrinolysis, but for unknown reasons, this process does not always happen. Retained clots in the pleural space may cause adhesion of lung segment, which results in fibrothorax, decreased lung function, and an increased risk of infection and empyema. The diagnosis and management of retained hemothorax after thoracic trauma remains controversial and has been the subject of several recent investigations in the trauma literature [67].

Post-traumatic retained hemothorax complications may result in higher mortality rate and hospital costs, prolonged absence from work, and reduced lung function.

Four risk factors are involved in the development of post-traumatic retained hemothorax: three related to treatment (requiring more than tube thoracostomy, the need for mechanical ventilation, and the length of time with the tube in

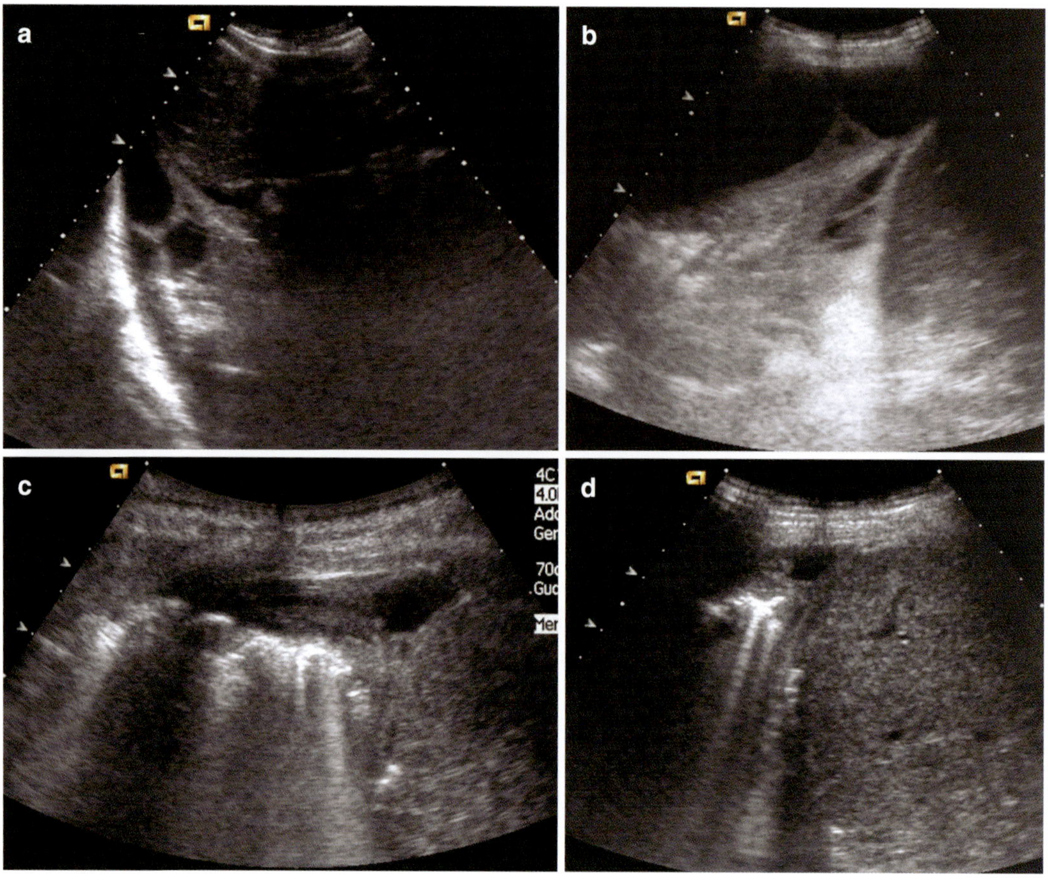

Fig. 23.15 Lung ultrasound. Defenestration, follow-up examinations: (**a**) and (**b**) sonographic signs of septations and pluri-concamerated anechoic areas, suggestive of retained hemothorax; (**c**) and (**d**) after 1 month, resolution

place), and one related to trauma (initial blood drainage volume). Regarding treatment, the incidence of clotted hemothorax may be modified by carefully monitoring patients with risk factors and early intervention. Regarding initial drainage, in hemodynamically stable patients in whom 400 mL or more of blood are drained through the tube thoracostomy, an early thoracoscopy, within the first 24 h, can be used to drain blood and for hemostasis.

23.5.3 Treatment and Management

Tube thoracostomy is the first-line treatment of most hemothoraces. Appropriate placement of the tube is critical for effective drainage of the pleural space. Placement should be directed posteriorly, in the sixth or seventh intercostal space at the mid-axillary line, to allow for dependent drainage in the supine patient. The Advanced Trauma Life Support protocol calls for use of a 36F chest tube in educational materials [68]. However, a recent prospective analysis of size tubes (28Fr until 40Fr) demonstrated no difference in outcomes based on size of chest tube placed [69].

Antibiotic treatment following hemothorax reduces the rate of infectious complications [70, 71]. The guidelines recommend the use of first-generation cephalosporin during the first 24 h in patients treated with thoracostomic drainage tube. When empyema occurs during chest tube drainage, antibiotic treatment should be directed to Staphylococcus aureus and Streptococcus species [72].

Surgical intervention in acute traumatic hemothorax is needed in case of:

- Initial evacuation of more than 1500 mL by thoracostomic tube.
- Persistent bleeding from chest, defined as drainage of more than 200 mL per hour for 4 h.
- Persistent blood transfusion is required to maintain hemodynamic stability.

Despite this, the physiologic parameters and overall condition of the patient must be the primary guide for surgical treatment, rather than these abovementioned parameters.

Patients with active bleeding but with stable hemodynamics can be treated with Video-Assisted Thoracoscopic Surgery (VATS), not only to stop the bleeding but also to evacuate blood clots and breakdown adhesions. Its use, however, should be reserved for experienced operators and limited indications.

Thoracotomy is the procedure of choice in patients with hemodynamic instability due to active blood loss. Surgical exploration permits control of the source of bleeding and evacuation of the intrathoracic blood.

Intrapleural fibrinolytic therapy (IPFT) can be applied to evacuate residual blood clots and breakdown adhesions when initial chest tube drainage is not adequate. Retention of blood in the pleural cavity may cause lung entrapment, chronic fibrothorax, impaired lung function and infection. In most cases, treatment with IPFT leads to complete resolution of radiographic abnormalities, through evacuation of blood clots and loculated effusions. Less than 10% of cases need a more aggressive treatment by means of surgical decortication [73, 74] with VATS or thoracotomy.

23.6 Flail Chest

Flail chest is defined as three or more adjacent ribs fractured in two or more places, creating a chest wall segment that moves paradoxically from the chest wall during the respiration. This condition occurs in up to 15% of wall chest injuries [75] and is a life-threatening complication of severe chest trauma: the paradoxical movement hinders the creation of negative intrathoracic pressure during inspiration and positive airway pressure during expiration causing impairment of breathing mechanics resulting in poor oxygenation and potential asphyxia. Furthermore, the less efficiency of breathing may promote atelectasis, respiratory distress syndrome, and pneumonia [76, 77].

Frequently flail chest is associated with other intrathoracic injuries (pulmonary contusion, pneumothorax, hemothorax, mediastinal injuries) and extra-thoracic injuries (brain, abdominal, and skeletal injuries) [78, 79].

Flail chest itself is an independent predictor of poor outcomes in patients with blunt chest trauma, and its mortality rate is variable and depends on the presence of other abovementioned injuries.

23.6.1 Radiological Features

The standard chest X-ray is still an important initial study because it can quickly diagnose life-threatening intrathoracic pathology like tension pneumothorax or massive hemothorax; however, it commonly underestimates the number of rib fractures. CT scan is more reliable for the detection of rib fractures. Chest CT scan gives more detailed information about the number and location of fractured ribs and the magnitude of dislocation and it has become the standard practice to detect and characterize all of chest and intrathoracic injuries [79], as well as to evaluate whether surgical rib fixation is needed.

23.6.2 Treatment and Management

Chest wall injuries itself may unfrequently be the primary cause of death; however, they influence the management, the survival, and long-term disability.

The management of patients with flail chest consists of the pain control, the management of pulmonary dysfunction, and potentially surgical rib fixation.

The pain control may be achieved using parenteral or oral opioids, or through the employment of locoregional treatment like thoracic epidural anesthesia, intercostal nerve block, or lidocaine patches [80, 81].

The management of pulmonary dysfunction is realized using appropriate ventilation therapies: mechanical ventilation in patient with hypoxemic or hypercapnic respiratory failure. Positive end-expiratory pressure should be used in endotracheally intubated patients to increase alveoli's recruitment as well as continuous positive airway pressure in patients without endotracheal tube [82]. Despite this there is no single mode of ventilation that has been found to be best for patients with flail chest or pulmonary contusion [83].

Although the nonsurgical management is considered the benchmark of care, several recent studies have demonstrated that surgical intervention decreases number of ventilator days, intensive care unit and hospital stays, as well as incidence of pneumonia and hospital costs [84]. Nevertheless the surgical stabilization of ribs fractures is performed in less than 1% of patients with flail chest [85].

References

1. Miele V, Di Giampietro I (2014) Diagnostic imaging in emergency. Salute e Società (2EN):127–138. doi:10.3280/SES2014-002010EN.
2. Miele V, Di Giampietro I, Ianniello S, et al. Diagnostic imaging in pediatric polytrauma management. Radiol Med. 2015;120:33–49. doi:10.1007/s11547-014-0469-x.
3. Ianniello S, Di Giacomo V, Cuneo G, et al. Pediatric thoracic trauma. In: Miele V, Trinci M, editors. Imaging trauma and polytrauma in pediatric patients. Cham: Springer International Publishing; 2015. p. 43–64.
4. Ianniello S, Merola MG, Trinci M, et al. Priorità diagnostiche nel management del trauma maggiore: ruolo dell'E-FAST e della TCMD. Il Giornale Italiano di. Radiol Med. 2015;2:715–20. doi:10.17376/girm_2-4-07082015-19.
5. Kirkpatrick AW, Sirois M, Laupland KB, et al. Hand-held thoracic sonography for detecting post-traumatic pneumothoraces: the extended focused assessment with Sonography for trauma (EFAST). J Trauma. 2004;57:288–95.
6. Ianniello S, Di Giacomo V, Sessa B, et al. First-line sonographic diagnosis of pneumothorax in major trauma: accuracy of e-FAST and comparison with multidetector computed tomography. Radiol Med. 2014;119:674–80. doi:10.1007/s11547-014-0384-1.
7. Volpicelli G, Elbarbabary M, Blaivas M, et al. International evidence-based recommendations for point-of-care lung ultrasound. Intensive Care Med. 2012;38:577–91.
8. Croce MA, Fabian TC, Davis KA, et al. Early and late acute respiratory distress syndrome: two distinct clinical entities. J Trauma. 1999;46:361–8.
9. Antonelli M, Moro ML, Cappelli O, et al. Risk factors for early onset of pneumonia in trauma patients. Chest. 1994;105:224–8.
10. Hoff SJ, Shotts DS, Eddy VA, et al. Outcome of isolated pulmonary contusion in blunt trauma patients. Am Surg. 1994;60:138–42.
11. Daurat A, Millet I, Roustan JP, et al. Thoracic trauma severity score on admission allows to determine the risk of delayed ARDS in trauma patients with pulmonary contusion. Injury. 2015;47:147–53.
12. Strumwasser A, Chu E, Yeung L, et al. A novel CT Volume Index Score correlates with outcomes in polytrauma patients with pulmonary contusion. J Surg Res. 2011;170:280–5.
13. Ianniello S, Piccolo CL, Buquicchio GL, et al. First line diagnosis of paediatric pneumonia in emergency: lung ultrasound (LUS) in addiction to chest-X-ray (CXR) and its role in follow-up. Br J Radiol. 2016;89:20150998. doi:10.1259/bjr.20150998.
14. Miele V, Buquicchio GL, Piccolo CL, et al. Lung injuries. In: Scaglione M, Linsenmaier U, Scheller G, Berger F, Wirth S, editors. Emergency radiology of the chest and cardiovascular system. Heidelberg: Springer; 2017. p. 3–12.
15. ARDS Definition Task Force, Ranieri VM, Rubenfeld GD, et al. Acute respiratory distress syndrome: the Berlin definition. JAMA. 2012;307:2526–33. doi:10.1001/jama.2012.5669.
16. Wyncoll DL, Evans TW. Acute respiratory distress syndrome. Lancet. 1999;354:497–50.
17. Weinberger SE, Drazen JM. Disturbances of respiratory function. In: Braunwald E, Fauci AS, Kaspar DL, Hauser SL, Longo DL, editors. Harrison's principles of internal medicine. 15th ed. New York: McGraw-Hill; 2001. p. 1454.
18. Lichtenstein D. Lung ultrasound in the intensive care unit. Recent Res Dev Resp Crit Care Med. 2001;1:83–93.
19. Meade M, Guyatt G, Cook D, et al. Predicting success in weaning from mechanical ventilation. Chest. 2001;120:400S–24S.
20. Covelli HD, Nessan VJ, Tuttle WK 3rd, et al. Oxygen derived in acute respiratory, failure. Crit Care Med. 1983;11:646–9.

21. Nieszkowska A, Lu Q, Vieira S, et al. Incidence and regional distribution of lung overinflation during mechanical ventilation with positive end-expiratory pressure. Crit Care Med. 2004;32:1496–503.
22. Scialpi M, Cappabianca S, Rotondo A, et al. Pulmonary congenital cystic disease in adults. Spiral computed tomography findings with pathologic correlation and management. Radiol Med. 2010;115:539–50. doi:10.1007/s11547-010-0467-6.
23. Gattinoni L, Presenti A, Torresin A, et al. Adult respiratory distress syndrome profiles by computed tomography. J Thorac Imaging. 1986;1:25–30.
24. Desai SR, Wells AU, Rubens MB, et al. Acute respiratory distress syndrome: computed tomography abnormalities at long-term follow-up. Radiology. 1999;210:29–35.
25. MacDuff A, Arnold A, Harvey J. Management of spontaneous pneumothorax: British thoracic society pleural disease guide-line. Thorax. 2010;65:ii18–31. doi:10.1136/thx.2010.136986.
26. Lomoschitz FM, Eisenhuber E, Linnau KF, et al. Imaging of chest trauma: radiological patterns of injury and diagnostic algorithms. Eur J Radiol. 2003;48:61–70.
27. Weissberg D, Refaely Y. Pneumothorax: experience with 1,199 patients. Chest. 2000;117:1279–85.
28. Miele V, Buquicchio GL, Piccolo CL, et al. Injuries of the pleural spaces. In: Scaglione M, Linsenmaier U, Scheller G, Berger F, Wirth S, editors. Emergency radiology of the chest and cardiovascular system. Heidelberg: Springer; 2017. p. 13–23.
29. Chaturvedi A, Lee S, Klionsky N, et al. Demystifying the persistent pneumothorax: role of imaging. Insights Imaging. 2016;7:411–29.
30. Rhea JT, van Sonnenberg E, McLoud TC. Basilar pneumothorax in the supine adult. Radiology. 1979;133:593–5.
31. Tocino IM, Miller MH, Fairfax WR. Distribution of pneumothorax in the supine and semirecumbent critically ill adult. AJR Am J Roentgenol. 1985;144:901–5.
32. Collins JA, Samra GS. Failure of chest X-rays to diagnose pneumothoraces after blunt trauma. Anaesthesia. 1998;53:74–8.
33. Miller LA. Chest wall, lung, and pleural space trauma. Radiol Clin N Am. 2006;44:213–24.
34. Blaivas M, Lyon M, Duggal S. A prospective comparison of supine chest radiography and bedside ultrasound for the diagnosis of traumatic pneumothorax. Acad Emerg Med. 2005;12:844–9.
35. Soldati G, Testa A, Sher S, et al. Occult traumatic pneumothorax: diagnostic accuracy of lung ultrasonography in the emergency department. Chest. 2008;133:204–11.
36. Lichtenstein DA, Mezière G, Lascols N, et al. Ultrasound diagnosis of occult pneumothorax. Crit Care Med. 2005;33:1231–8.
37. Toombs BD, Sandler CM, Lester RG. Computed tomography of chest trauma. Radiology. 1981;140: 733–8.
38. Trupka A, Waydhas C, Hallfeldt KK, et al. Value of thoracic computed tomography in the first assessment of severely injured patients with blunt chest trauma: results of a prospective study. J Trauma. 1997;43:405–11.
39. Paspatis GA, Dumonceau JM, Barthet M, et al. Diagnosis and management of iatrogenic endoscopic perforations: European Society of Gastrointestinal Endoscopy (ESGE) position statement. Endoscopy. 2014;46:693–711.
40. Gayer G, Rozenman J, Hoffmann C, et al. CT diagnosis of malpositioned chest tubes. Br J Radiol. 2000;73:786–90.
41. Peters S, Wolter D, Schultz JH. Dangers and risks of thoracic drainage at the accident site. Unfallchirurg. 1996;99:953–7.
42. Laws D, Neville E, Duffy J. Pleural Diseases Group, Standards of Care Committee, British Thoracic Society BTS guidelines for the insertion of a chest drain. Thorax. 2003;58:ii53–9.
43. Tomlinson MA, Treasure T. Insertion of a chest drain: how to do it. Br J Hosp Med. 1997;58:248–52.
44. Harris A, O'Driscoll BR, Turkington PM. Survey of major complications of intercostal chest drain insertion in the UK. Postgrad Med J. 2010;86: 68–72.
45. Heim P, Maas R, Tesch C, et al. Pleural drainage in acute thoracic trauma. Comparison of the radiologic image and computer tomography. Aktuelle Radiol. 1998;8:163–8.
46. Stern EJ, Sun H, Haramati LB. Peripheral bronchopleural fistulas: CT imaging features. AJR Am J Roentgenol. 1996;167:117–20.
47. Seo H, Kim TJ, Jin KN, et al. Multi-detector row computed tomography evaluation of bronchopleural fistula: correlation with clinical, bronchoscopic, and surgical findings. J Comput Assist Tomogr. 2010;34:13–8.
48. Ricci ZJ, Haramati LB, Rosenbaum AT, et al. Role of computed tomography in guiding the management of peripheral bronchopleural fistula. J Thorac Imaging. 2002;17:214–8.
49. Sarkar P, Chandak T, Shah R, et al. Diagnosis and management bronchopleural stula. Indian J Chest Dis Allied Sci. 2010;52:97–104.
50. Takanami I. Closure of a bronchopleural fistula using a fibrin-glue coated collagen patch. Interact Cardiovasc Thorac Surg. 2003;2(3):2387–8.
51. Uchida S, Igaki H, Izumo T, et al. Effective treatment of empyema with bronchopleural fistula after esophagectomy by endobronchial embolization using endobronchial Watanabe Spigots. Int J Surg Case Rep. 2017;33:1–3.
52. Giddings O, Kuhn J, Akulian J. Endobronchial valve placement for the treatment of bronchopleural fistula: a review of the current literature. Curr Opin Pulm Med. 2014;20:347–51.
53. Díaz-Agero Álvarez PJ, Bellido-Reyes YA, Sánchez-Girón JG, et al. Novel bronchoscopic treatment for

bronchopleural fistula using adipose-derived stromal cells. Cytotherapy. 2016;18:36–40.
54. Villa MT, Chang DW. Muscle and omental flaps for chest wall reconstruction. Thorac Surg Clin. 2010;20:543–50.
55. Sangster GP, Gonzalez-Beicos A, Carbo AI, et al. Blunt traumatic injuries of the lung parenchyma, pleura, thoracic wall, and intrathoracic airways: multidetector computer tomography imaging findings. Emerg Radiol. 2007;14:297–310.
56. Mirvis SE. Imaging of acute thoracic injury: the advent of MDCT screening. Semin Ultrasound CT MRI. 2005;26:305–31.
57. Shanmuganathan K, Mirvis SE. Imaging diagnosis of nonaortic thoracic injury. Radiol Clin N Am. 1999;37:533–51.
58. Mayberry JC. Imaging in thoracic trauma: the trauma surgeon's perspective. J Thorac Imaging. 2000;15:76–86.
59. Meyer DM. Hemothorax related to trauma. Thorac Surg Clin. 2007;17:47–55.
60. Kaewlai R, Avery LL, Asrani AV, et al. Multidetector CT of blunt thoracic trauma. Radiographics. 2008;28:1555–70. doi:10.1148/rg.286085510.
61. Broderick SR. Hemothorax etiology, diagnosis, and management. Thorac Surg Clin. 2013;23:89–96. doi:10.1016/j.thorsurg.2012.10.003.
62. Ho ML, Gutierrez FR. Chest radiography in thoracic polytrauma. AJR Am J Roentgenol. 2009;192: 599–612. doi:10.2214/AJR.07.3324.
63. Thoongsuwan N, Kanne JP, Stern EJ (2004) Imaging of blunt chest trauma. RSNA Syllabus 71–79.
64. Brooks A, Davies B, Sethhurst M, et al. Emergency ultrasound in the acute assessment of haemothorax. Emerg Med J. 2004;21:44–6.
65. Ma OJ, Mateer JR. Trauma ultrasound examination versus chest radiography in the detection of hemothorax. Ann Emerg Med. 1997;29:312–5.
66. Villegas MI, Hennessey RA, Morales CH, et al. Risk factors associated with the development of post-traumatic retained hemothorax. Eur J Trauma Emerg Surg. 2011;37:583–9. doi:10.1007/s00068-010-0064-3.
67. DuBose J, Inaba K, Demetriades D, et al. Management of post-traumatic retained hemothorax: a prospective, observational, multicenter AAST study. J Trauma Acute Care Surg. 2012;72:11–22.
68. American College of Surgeons. Committee on trauma. ATLS: advanced trauma life support for doctors. 8th ed. Chicago: American College of Surgeons; 2008.
69. Inaba K, Lustenberger T, Recinos G, et al. Does size matter? A prospective analysis of 28-32 versus 36-40 French chest tube size in trauma. J Trauma. 2012;72:422–7.
70. Gonzalez RP, Holevar MR. Role of prophylactic antibiotics for tube thoracostomy in chest trauma. Am Surg. 1998;64:617–20.
71. Wilson RF, Nichols RL. The EAST practice management guidelines for prophylactic antibiotic use in tube thoracostomy for traumatic hemopneumothorax: a commentary. J Trauma. 2000;48:758–9.
72. Luchette FA, Barrie PS, Oswanski MF, et al. Practice management guidelines for prophylactic antibiotic use in tube thoracostomy for traumatic hemopneumothorax: the EAST practice management guidelines work group. J Trauma. 2000;48:753–7.
73. Kimbrell BJ, Yamzon J, Petrone P, et al. Intrapleural thrombolysis for the management of undrained traumatic hemothorax: a prospective observational study. J Trauma. 2007;62:1175–8.
74. Skeete DA, Rutherford EJ, Schlidt SA, et al. Intrapleural tissue plasminogen activator for complicated pleural effusions. J Trauma. 2004;57:1178–83.
75. Ciraulo DL, Elliott D, Mitchell KA, et al. Flail chest as a marker for significant injuries. J Am Coll Surg. 1994;178:466–70.
76. Wanek S, Mayberry JC. Blunt thoracic trauma: flail chest, pulmonary contusion, and blast injury. Crit Care Clin. 2004;20:71–81.
77. Collins J. Chest wall trauma. J Thorac Imaging. 2000;15:112–9.
78. Besson A, Segesser F. Blunt trauma of the chest wall. A colour atlas of chest trauma and associated injuries, vol. 1. Weert, Netherlands: Wolfe Medical Publications Ltd; 1982. p. 153–98.
79. Majercik S, Pieracci FM. Chest wall trauma. Thorac Surg Clin. 2017;27:113–21.
80. Zink KA, Mayberry JC, Peck EG, et al. Lidocaine patches reduce pain in patients with rib fractures. Am Surg. 2011;77:438–42.
81. Britt T, Sturm R, Ricardi R, et al. Comparative evaluation of continuous intercostal nerve block or epidural analgesia on the rate of respiratory complications, intensive care unit, and hospital stay following traumatic rib fractures: a retrospective review. Local Reg Anesth. 2015;8:79–84.
82. Schweiger JW, Downs JB, Smith RA. Chest wall disruption with and without acute lung injury: effects of continuous positive airway pressure therapy on ventilation and perfusion relationships. Crit Care Med. 2003;31:2364–70.
83. Simon B, Ebert J, Bokhari F, et al. Management of pulmonary contusion and flail chest: an Eastern Association for the Surgery of Trauma practice management guideline. J Trauma Acute Care Surg. 2012;73:s351–61. doi:10.1097/TA.0b013e31827019fd.
84. Fowler TT, Taylor BC, Bellino MJ, et al. Surgical treatment of flail chest and rib fractures. J Am Acad Orthop Surg. 2014;22:751–60. doi:10.5435/JAAOS-22-12-751.
85. Slobogean GP, MacPherson CA, Sun T, et al. Surgical fixation vs nonoperative management of flail chest: a meta-analysis. J Am Coll Surg. 2013;216:302–11.e1.

The Follow-Up of Patients with Abdominal Injuries

24

Grazia Loretta Buquicchio, Gavina Cuneo, Stefano Giannecchini, Riccardo Palliola, Margherita Trinci, and Vittorio Miele

24.1 Introduction

Abdominal trauma is very frequent in the population, both adult and pediatric, because such trauma may occur during normal daily activities, during sports, in a car accident as driver or passenger, as a pedestrian, or in a scholastic activity.

Conservative management of abdominal trauma is increasing in both children and adults, but this approach requires close patient monitoring [1, 2]. During the past 20 years this increasing tendency to treat patients with trauma of abdominal organs conservatively has caused much debate whether to use ultrasonography (US) or contrast-enhanced computed tomography (CE-CT).

Contrast-enhanced CT is considered the gold standard technique. It is the most accurate diagnostic method for assessing a traumatic patient. As CT requires the patient to move and needs time to be performed, in recent years US has become increasingly important in the evaluation of patients with abdominal trauma. In fact, US may be performed at the bedside of the traumatized patient without interrupting first-aid procedures [3].

In recent years, the applications of diagnostic US are much improved with the use of the new generation of contrast media, which allows performing contrast-enhanced ultrasound (CEUS). CEUS is a reliable, safe, and highly effective diagnostic method with sensitivity and specificity values close to those of CT for trauma lesions of the solid abdominal organs [4–7].

In consideration of the use of ionizing radiation and contrast medium, nowadays the use of CEUS is reported for the follow-up of those patients who need to undergo a massive amount of monitoring until their traumatic injuries can be completely resolved. CEUS could perhaps be the ideal method, at least allowing us to reduce the number of CT examinations for follow-up in patients who often are of young age. Recent guidelines have reported the use of CEUS when CT is not available or is not indicated for reasons of previous allergic reactions to iodate contrast agents. CEUS is also used to monitor known traumatic injuries or to evaluate minor traumas, especially in pediatric-age patients [8].

G.L. Buquicchio (✉) • G. Cuneo • S. Giannecchini
R. Palliola • M. Trinci
Department of Emergency Radiology, S. Camillo Hospital, Rome, Italy
e-mail: graziabuquicchio@gmail.com

V. Miele
Department of Radiology, Careggi University Hospital, Florence, Italy

V. Miele, M. Trinci (eds.), *Diagnostic Imaging in Polytrauma Patients*,
https://doi.org/10.1007/978-3-319-62054-1_24

Because CEUS has limitations and CT requires the use of ionizing radiation, recent studies have begun to assess the possibility of using magnetic resonance imaging (MRI) in the follow-up of patients with low-energy isolated abdominal trauma injuries as an alternative to the CEUS and CT techniques [9].

In major emergency centers, abdominal US is the first examination in trauma patients and must be performed before the CT study. In these cases, however, the use of abdominal ultrasonography is not aimed at detecting parenchymal lesions but is used to evaluate the presence of peritoneal free fluid, for which detection US has high sensitivity. This examination is called focused assessment with sonography for trauma (or, focused abdominal sonography for trauma) (FAST) and its purpose, in hemodynamically unstable patients, is to document the presence of hemoperitoneum that requires immediate surgical intervention [10, 11].

A patient arriving in an emergency department is managed differently depending on hemodynamic stability. If the patient is stable but has had a high-energy trauma, whole-body CE-CT, which is the best technique for assessing the involvement of all organs, is necessary. In a low-energy focalized injury, the patient can be evaluated directly by CEUS. In either case, known parenchymal lesions can be monitored with CEUS. If the patient is in critical condition and is not hemodynamically stable, that person is evaluated in the emergency room and then, when causes of instability have been identified, undergoes a surgical exploration [12].

In clinical practice, the finding of free abdominal fluid in polytrauma patients requires a CE-CT scan to exclude organ lesions and to evaluate the presence of vascular or omental lesions with active bleeding [3].

In accordance with the advanced trauma life support (ATLS) guidelines, many centers in Europe and in the USA have adopted a standardized protocol for polytrauma patients. For the initial evaluation of all traumatized patients, abdominal ultrasound (FAST) and radiographs are recommended. When the hemodynamic condition of the patient has been stabilized, the patient should then undergo total-body CT examination, which allows evaluating the presence of multiple simultaneous lesions of the abdominal organs, even those poorly visualized with US, and detecting the presence of any active bleeding, better than CEUS.

In unstable patients, US (FAST) allows immediate detection of the presence of hemoperitoneum, which is an indication for immediate surgery [13, 14]. However, many organ injuries are not correctly detected at the US baseline examination. The recent introduction of contrast-enhanced US has increased the accuracy of ultrasound, allowing the execution of a real-time examination directly in the region of interest.

CEUS is particularly important in children, for whom it is now accepted as conservative treatment in hemodynamically stable trauma [15–19]; however, in recent years, attention is being given to the use of MRI, which is an excellent technique for diagnosis, characterization, and evaluation of abdominal organ lesions.

Because patients treated conservatively require close clinical and laboratory monitoring, radiological monitoring can be carried out with US, CEUS, and, lately, with MRI [13, 20]. CEUS has proven effective in detecting and evaluating lesions of solid organs, potentially avoiding the need for CT and thus reducing exposure to radiation and iodinated contrast agents. CEUS has sensitivity and specificity up to 95% in the detection of low-energy abdominal trauma [21].

There are still many studies on this matter, but MRI shows greater panoramic flexibility than CEUS, helps to identify more accurately even small lesions of the abdominal organs, and allows the assessment of any injuries of organs poorly visualized on ultrasound (such as the adrenal glands). MRI also allows the evaluation of the urinary tract, which is not possible with US, and the presence of possible vascular complications.

The use of these techniques is therefore very important, especially for pediatric patients [15].

Introduction of the use of second-generation contrast agents has increased the accuracy of CEUS, which has proved almost as sensitive as CT in the detection of traumatic abdominal organ injuries, in the definition of the extent of the lesion, its margins, and the relationship between the lesion and the capsule of the involved organ [22, 23].

CEUS can be performed at the patient's bedside, without moving the traumatized patient to the radiology department, which makes it an ideal technique in the follow-up of patients with injuries that do not require surgery.

24.2 Technique

First, all patients must be subjected to an accurate baseline US examination. Written informed consent is obtained from all conscious patients and from parents who are present during the examination of minor patients.

Before performing CEUS, an antecubital vein is cannulated with a 20-gauge needle and an intravenous bolus injection of a second-generation blood-pool contrast agent is administered. The contrast agent consists of microbubbles containing an inert gas, sulfur hexafluoride, which resonates at low acoustic pressure ranges (mechanical index, <0.2), emitting a specific signal.

The ultrasound scanner is equipped with software that detects the response of the microbubbles, with continuous low mechanical index (MI, 0.15–0.19), and real-time tissue harmonic imaging allows real-time grey-scale imaging and identifies both the macro- and microcirculation to obtain a dynamic exploration of organ perfusion. A convex array 3.5-MHz probe is used.

The bolus of contrast agent is administered in 1–2 s, followed by 5–10 ml saline solution (0.9% NaCl); this also is a very rapid injection, to prevent any contrast material remaining in the cannula and to flush the contrast material into the peripheral circulation [24, 25]. The contrast agent is completely eliminated through the respiration after about 10 min.

The dynamic study of the parenchyma starts immediately after contrast administration. The kidneys are examined in the first 2 min, because of the intense arterial flow; then, the liver is examined (3–4 min), and finally the spleen (after 5 min). The complete contrast-enhanced US examination requires no more than 6 min, until the progressive extinction of enhancement.

The kidneys are evaluated first, because they have an intense but precocious and fleeting perfusion, then the liver and last the spleen, because the physiological heterogeneity of the CEUS signal in the earliest images is such as to induce false-positives, whereas after the first minutes after injection a homogeneous and very persistent enhancement is seen.

Compared to the baseline US, there is an undoubted loss of image quality, very grainy, but largely offset by the possibility of evaluating the area of interest in real time. These real-time images allow identification of any solid organ lesion in a manner similar to CT or MRI but with the advantage of continuous exploration.

Because CEUS is a technique that is noninvasive, versatile, easy to perform, and repeatable, it appears to be particularly suited to the follow-up of traumatic abdominal lesions. If needed, CT examination is performed within 1 h of CEUS using a standard arterial (40–50 s) and venous (80–100 s) phase protocol, and only in patients with abdominal free liquid is a late phase protocol (3–10 min) performed to detect the presence of any active bleeding or urinary complications. A nonionic contrast medium volume of 100–150 ml is injected at a rate of 2–4 ml/s [14].

Regarding MRI, there is still no standardized protocol for the follow-up of patients with blunt trauma treated conservatively. In a recent study, Miele et al. [9] have proposed performing such examinations in a supine position, and the images were acquired on multiple planes with breath-hold HASTE T_2-weighted sequences (TR, 1500 ms; TE, 95 ms; ST, 6 mm; matrix, 384 × 156), T_1 in phase and out of phase (TR,

120 ms; TE, 2.38 ms; ST, 6 mm; matrix, 384 × 164), and fat-sat VIBE T_1-weighted images (TR, 4.75 ms; TE, 2.39 ms; ST, 3 mm; matrix, 352 × 154) before and after IV administration of paramagnetic contrast media.

The use of MRI in follow-up is even more important considering that most trauma patients are young persons; for this reason, the use of MRI is preferred to CT because MRI can be repeated until complete resolution of the lesions. Another advantage of MRI is the opportunity to study any lesions of the urinary tract, which are not evaluable by CEUS, and the ability to detect small lesions in other organs poorly explored by US (e.g., the adrenal glands).

However, MRI has limitations: compliant patients must follow the instructions on breathing during the examination, the long duration of the examination, the need to move the patients to perform the examination, and finally the examination cannot be performed in the presence of a pacemaker, cochlear implants, or patient claustrophobia. Therefore, follow-up protocol includes CEUS at 24 and 72 h after trauma, CEUS and MRI at 1 month later, and, in the event of persistent structural parenchymal alterations related to the trauma, MRI can be repeated after 3 months and until complete resolution.

24.3 Semeiotic Aspects of Parenchymal Lesions

The most common traumatic alterations of the abdominal organs are hematomas, bruising, lacerations, bleeding, and arteriovenous fistulas. All these lesions are difficult to visualize and characterize with baseline US, in fact, they appear as a hypo- or slightly hyperechoic alteration within the organ being studied (Fig. 24.1).

The findings of abdominal lesions on CEUS are similar to those of CE-CT. On CEUS images, parenchymal traumatic lesions appear as a perfusion defect represented by a hypoechoic area, which persists unchanged during all the acquisition phases, with poorly defined or well-defined margins with or without interruption of the anatomic profile of the capsule of a solid organ [14].

(a) Parenchymal hematomas appear as a hypoechoic image without perfusion; in the case it is subcapsular, the hematoma will have the typical lenticular shape (Figs. 24.2, 24.3, 24.4, 24.5, 24.6, 24.7, 24.8, 24.9, and 24.10).
(b) Bruising appears usually as an inhomogeneous hypoechoic area with poorly defined contours with a poor definition of vessels within it (Figs. 24.11, 24.12, 24.13, and 24.14).

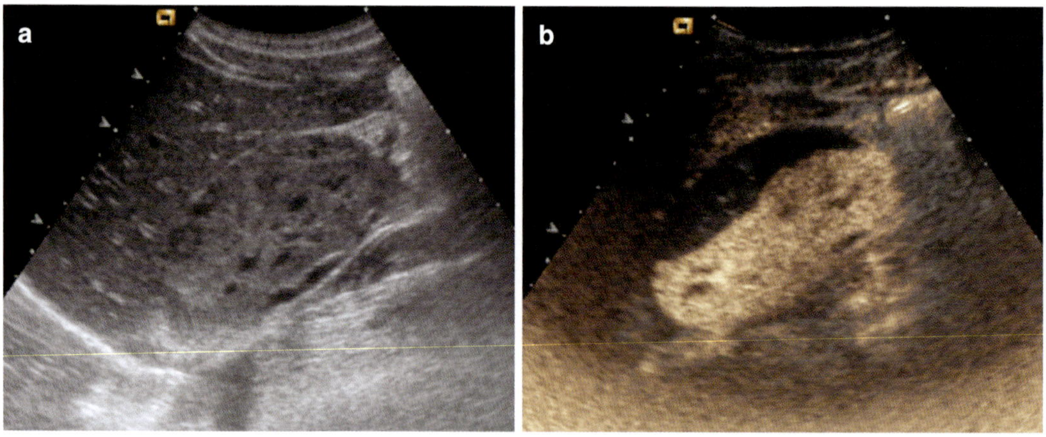

Fig. 24.1 Young male. Kick on left flank, subcapsular renal hematoma. (**a**) Baseline ultrasound (US) shows a hyperechoic oval pseudo-mass imprinting the renal profile. (**b**) Contrast-enhanced ultrasound (CEUS) depicts subcapsular hematoma well

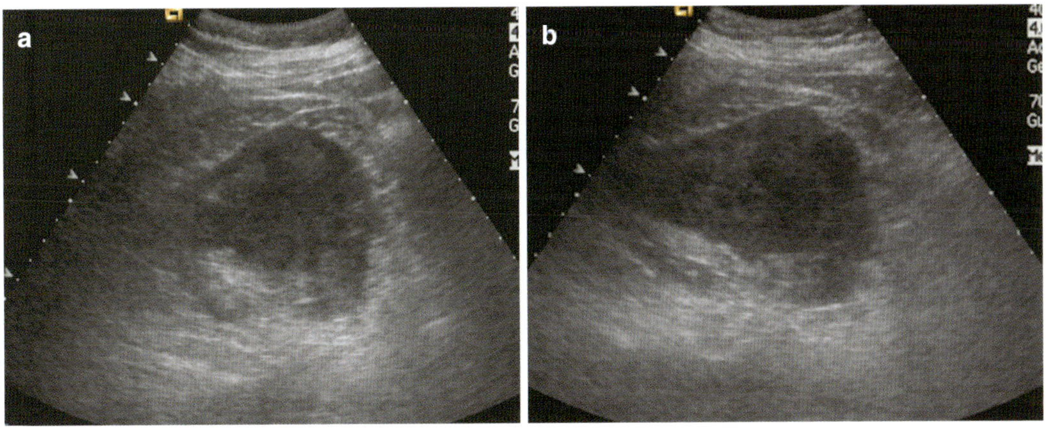

Fig. 24.2 Car accident. (**a**, **b**) Patient with acute urinary retention. On baseline US, in the left kidney there is a solid hypoechoic mass, non-homogeneous, of approximately 8 cm, which compresses the renal profile

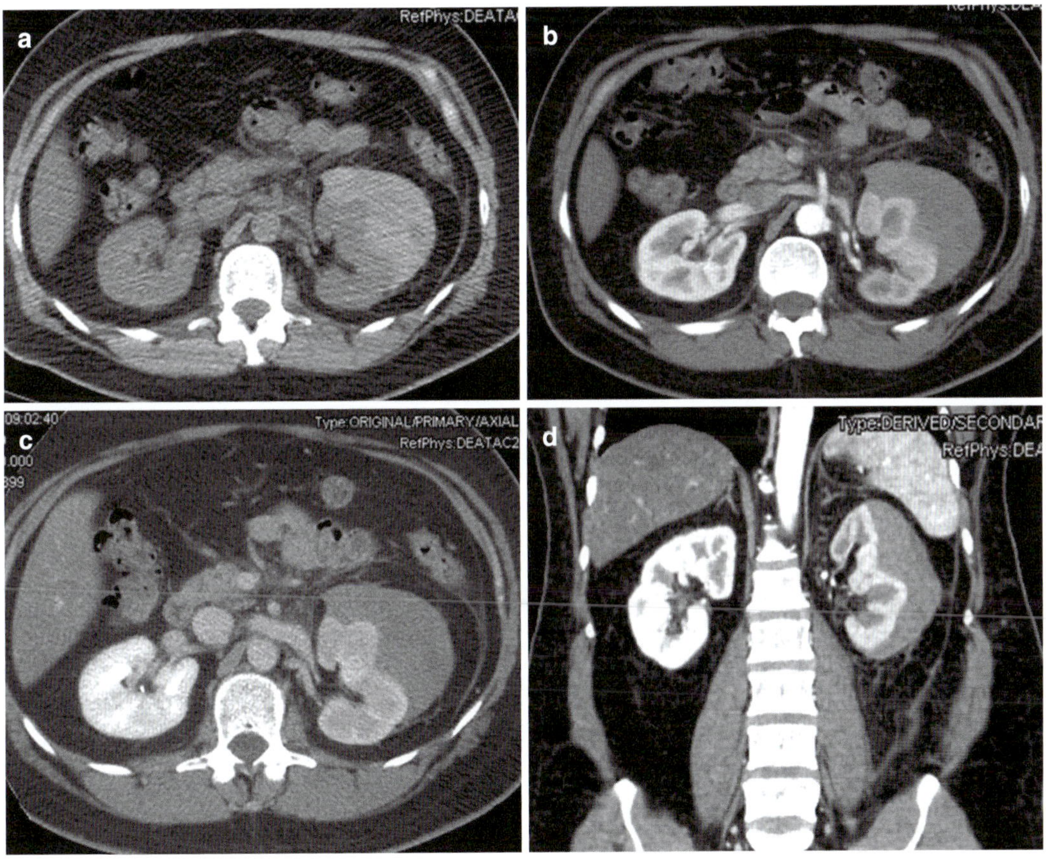

Fig. 24.3 Same patient as Fig. 24.2. Multi-detector computed tomography (MDCT) performed on same day shows a large subcapsular hematoma in the left kidney, with parenchymal compression and delayed contrast medium elimination. There are no signs of active vascular disease. (**a**) Nonenhanced CT shows hyperdense mass compressing the renal profile. (**b–d**) Contrast-enhanced CT scan shows a renal hematoma that appears hypodense as well as the contiguous renal parenchyma

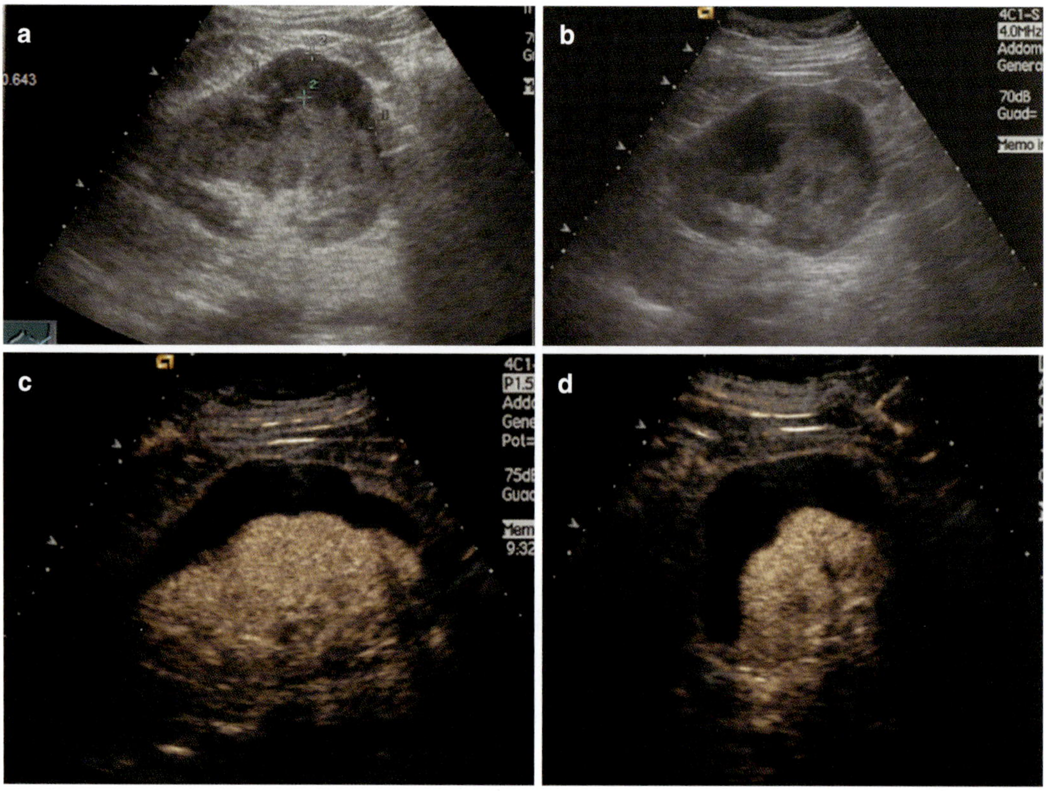

Fig. 24.4 Same patient. Follow-up examination 5 days later. Baseline US (**a**, **b**) shows a slight reduction in hematoma thickness (about 6 cm), that is much better seen with CEUS (**c**, **d**)

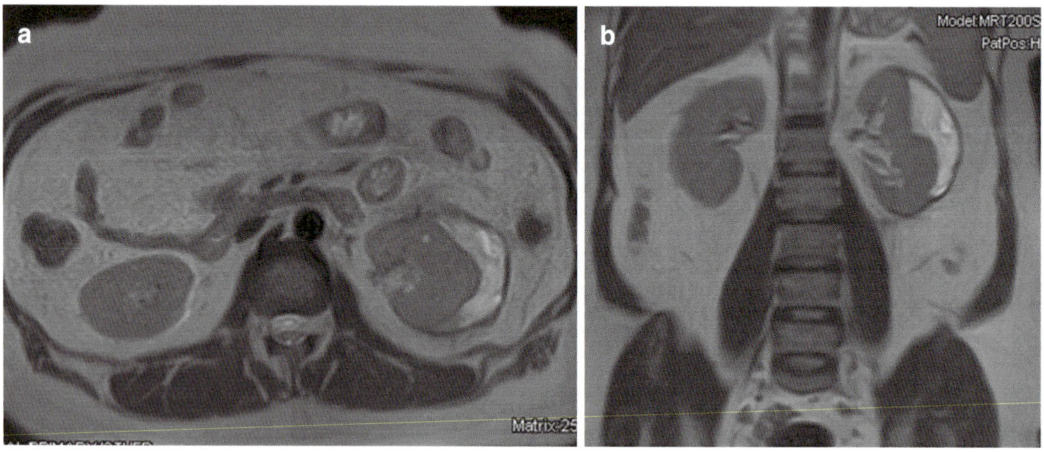

Fig. 24.5 Same patient. Follow-up magnetic resonance imaging (MRI) 1.5 months later: Compared to previous controls, there is a further significant reduction in the subcapsular hematoma thickness of the left kidney. HASTE T_2-weighted sequences axial (**a**) and coronal (**b**); fat-sat VIBE T_1-weighted sagittal scan (**c**). The hematoma appears hyperintense with some small hyperintense areas inside resulting from the different stages of the degradation of hemoglobin

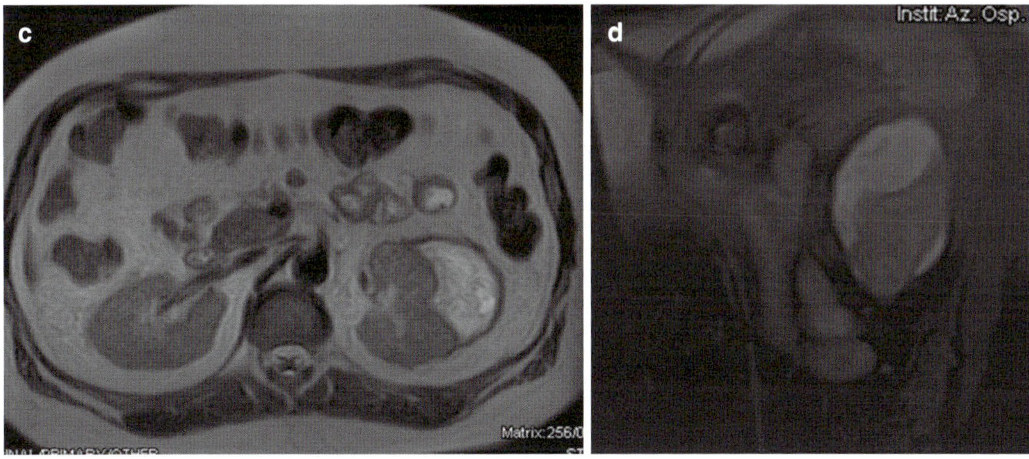

Fig. 24.5 (continued)

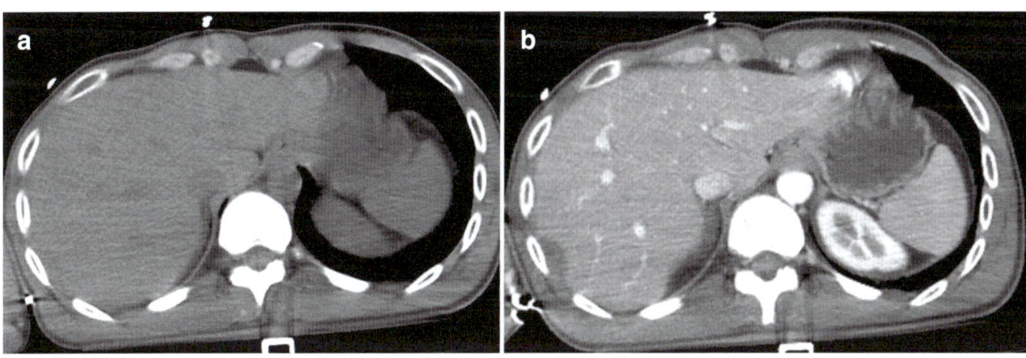

Fig. 24.6 Male. Car accident. Subcapsular hepatic hematoma. (**a**) Nonenhanced CT shows a slightly hyperdense subcapsular hepatic area. (**b**) Contrast-enhanced CT depicts well the same zone as a subcapsular hepatic hematoma

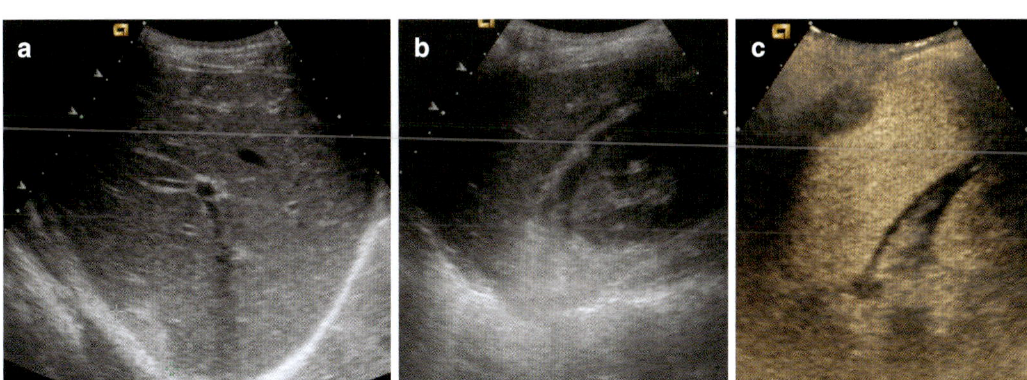

Fig. 24.7 Follow-up examinations with US and CEUS. (**a**, **b**) Baseline US shows a hyperechoic subcapsular lenticular area. (**c**) CEUS depicts the subcapsular hematoma well. Free fluid in the Morrison space is shown well on both US and CEUS

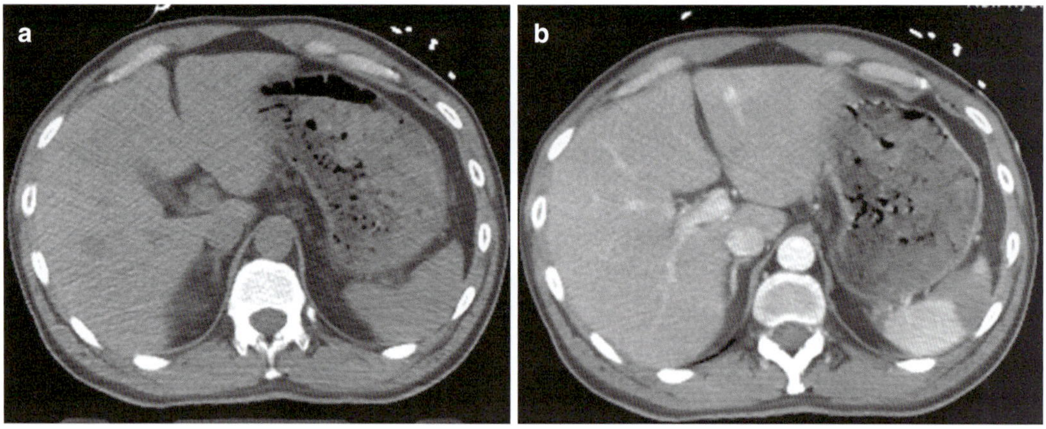

Fig. 24.8 Deep splenic hematoma, not appreciable in nonenhanced CT (**a**), is well defined in contrast-enhanced CT (**b**)

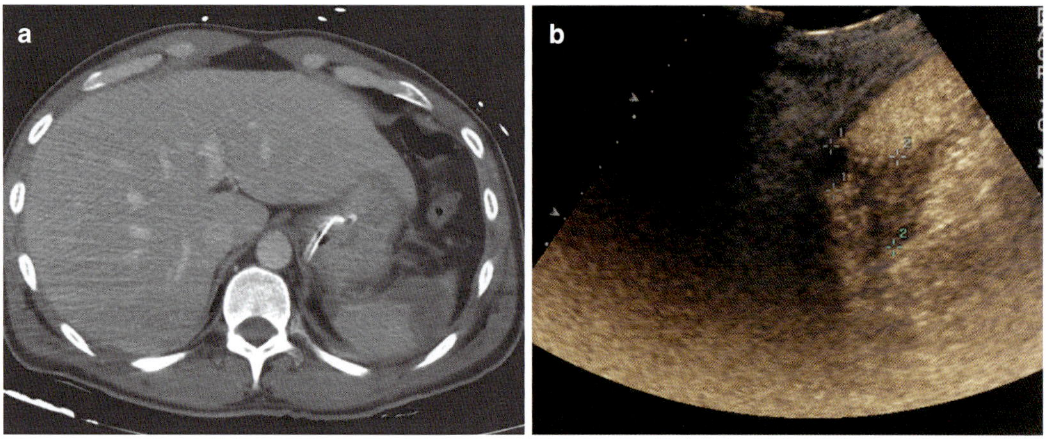

Fig. 24.9 Follow-up 3 days later. Contrast-enhanced CT (**a**) and CEUS (**b**) depict well a laceration area of the lower spleen pole, contacting the splenic capsule

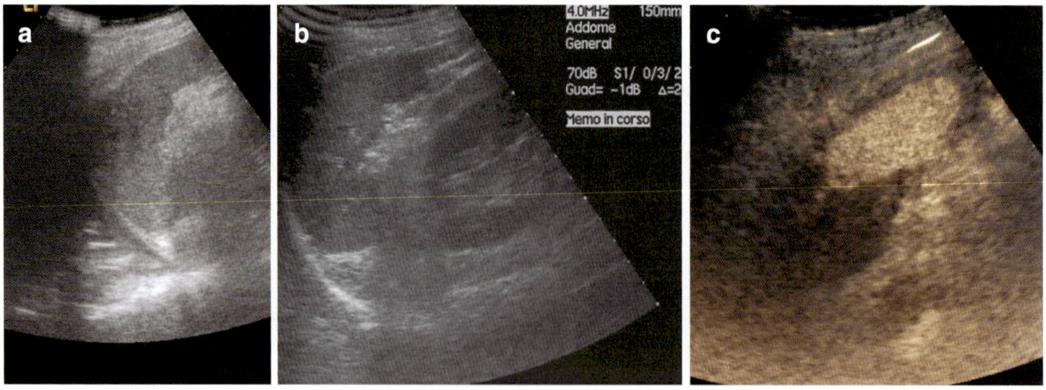

Fig. 24.10 Follow-up examinations, 1 week later. At the US baseline (**a**, **b**), the spleen seems normal. With CEUS (**c**), the persistence of splenic injury is evident

(c) Laceration appears as a hypoechoic linear parenchymal lesion or as a branched lesion, perpendicularly oriented with respect to the organ surface; it can be associated with capsular discontinuity (Figs. 24.15, 24.16, 24.17, 24.18, 24.19, 24.20, 24.21, 24.22, 24.23, 24.24, 24.25, 24.26, and -24.27).

(d) Focal hyperechoic spots within the lesion represent the presence of microbubbles of contrast medium and indicate active intralesional bleeding. If the microbubbles are arranged along the lacerated organ, the resultant outline is identified as a sign of intraperitoneal or retroperitoneal active bleeding.

Evidence of intralesional hyperechoic spots within the lesion or passage of microbubbles outside a lacerated organ is interpreted as a sign of active bleeding [14, 15, 26, 27]. CEUS also improves the already good ability of baseline ultrasound to detect even small amounts of free fluid [26, 28] (Fig. 24.28).

All trauma patients should undergo, first, baseline US, and next, CEUS examination. Patients positive for traumatic lesions of the abdominal organs must undergo CE-CT to better characterize the staging and the severity of these lesions. In fact, CT remains the most accurate technique in the definition of vascular complications, including active bleeding, pseudo-aneurysms, or arteriovenous fistulas, which represent the major predictors of failure of nonsurgical treatment [29, 30] (Figs. 24.29, 24.30, 24.31, 24.32, 24.33, and 24.34).

For urinary tract study, CT protocol includes a phase at 80 s after contrast material injection (late cortical or early homogeneous nephrographic phase) and an excretory phase at 5 min or more after contrast material administration.

Early complications (urinary extravasation and urinoma formation, delayed bleeding, arteriovenous fistula, pseudo-aneurysm) can occur within 4 weeks of injury. These complications are usually a consequence of deep solid organ laceration [31].

Similar to what happens in the brain parenchyma, the evolution of hematomas is known; in particular, it is defined as a hyperacute phase between 0 and 3 h after a traumatic event; an acute phase between 4 h and 3 days; a subacute phase between 4 days and 4 weeks; and a chronic phase after 1 month.

MRI allows also a temporal evaluation of lesions. On MRI images the hematoma appearance changes depending on two factors: the state

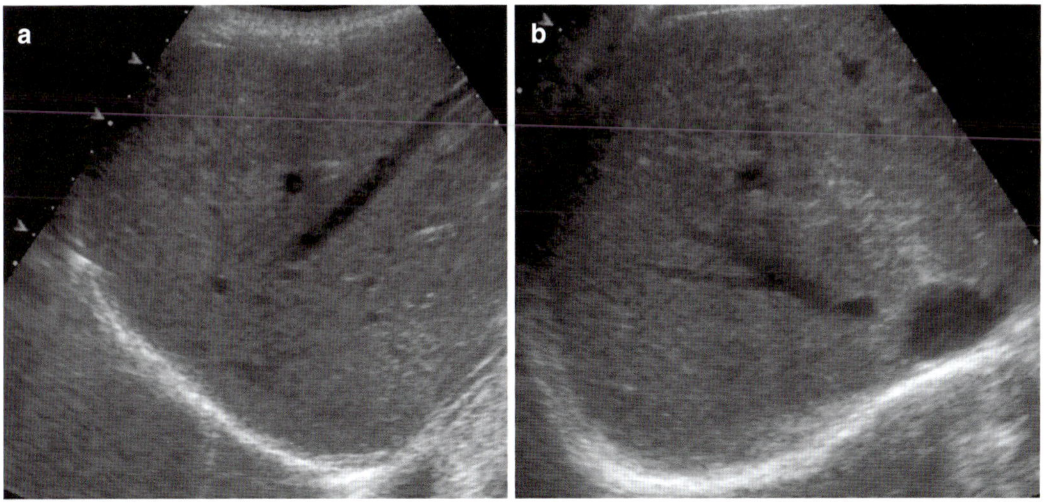

Fig. 24.11 A 16-year-old girl who fell from a scooter (**a**, **b**). Baseline US shows a fuzzy hyper-echogenic area at the VIII and V liver segments

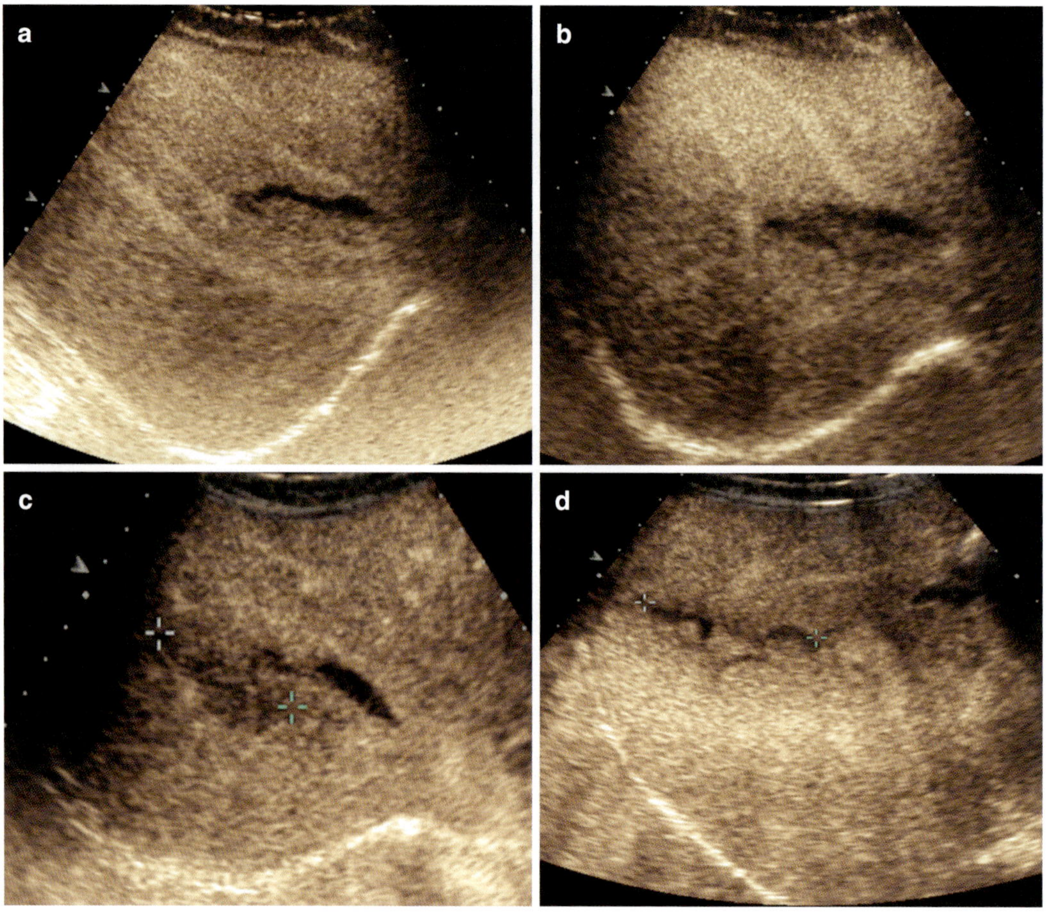

Fig. 24.12 CEUS (**a**–**d**) appreciates several lacero-contusive areas surrounded by nonhomogeneous parenchyma; these areas are poorly defined

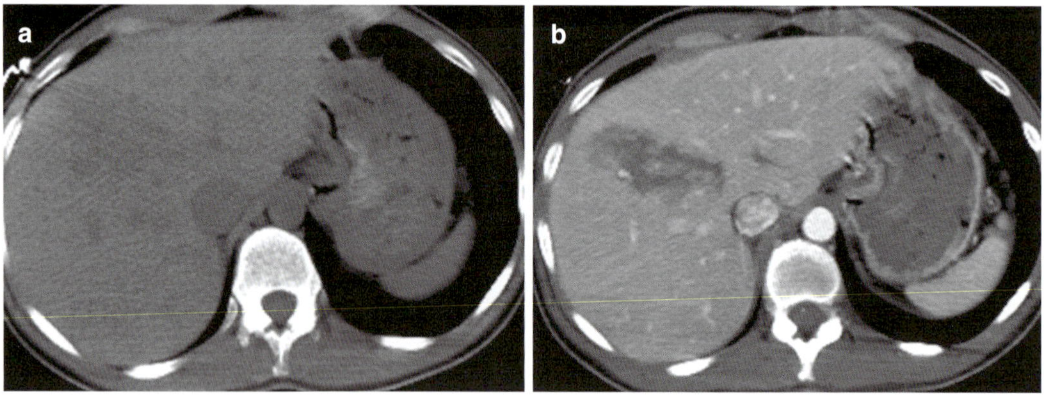

Fig. 24.13 Contrast-enhanced CT (**a**–**d**) confirms the lesions demonstrated by CEUS

Fig. 24.13 (continued)

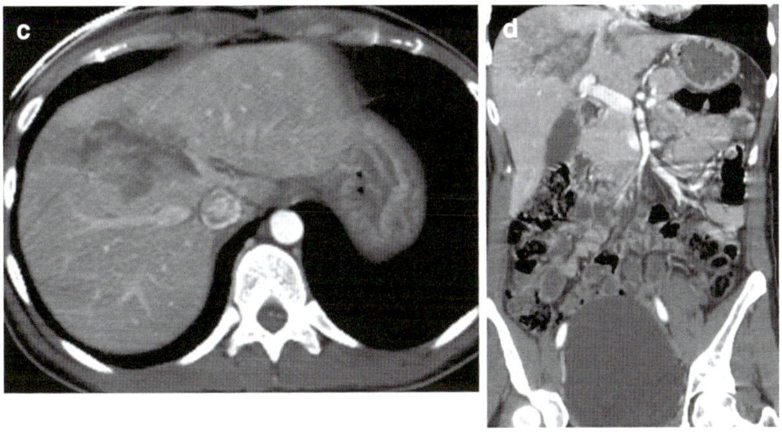

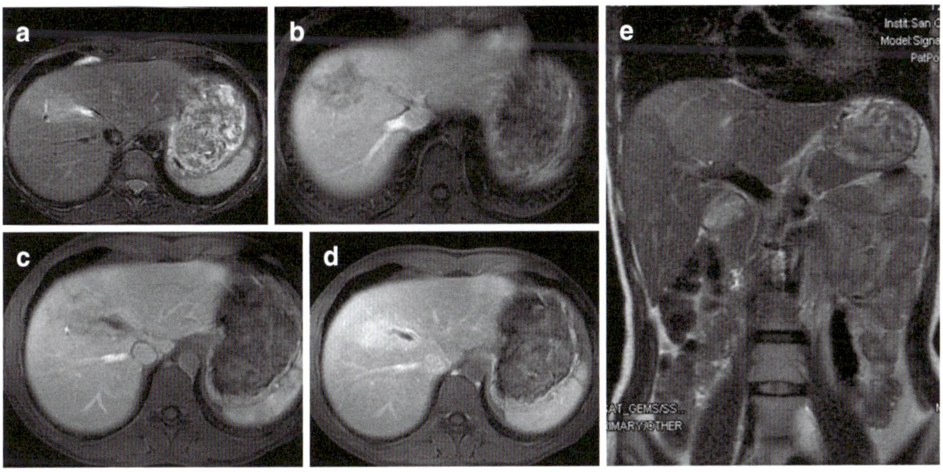

Fig. 24.14 Follow-up with MRI 20 days later (**a**–**e**). The lesion described at CEUS and CT at the VIII–V liver segment appears dimensionally reduced, and it is associated with an adjacent area of altered perfusion

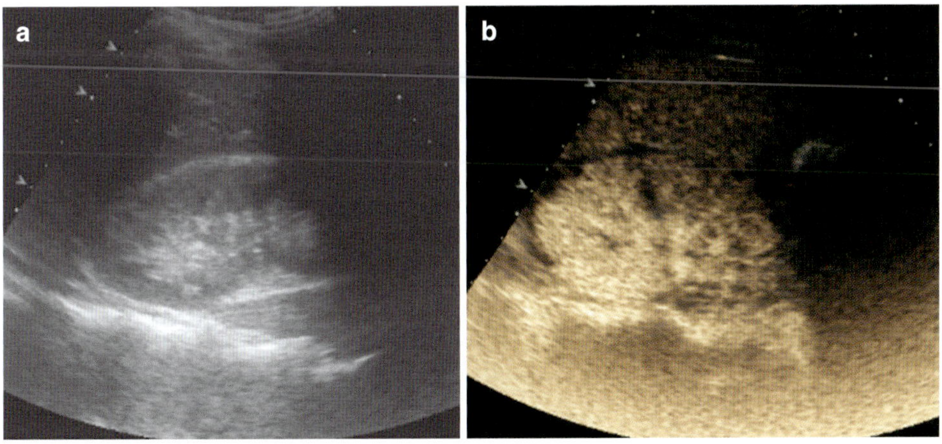

Fig. 24.15 Trauma on the right flank, double traumatic lesion of the right kidney. (**a**) Baseline US is negative for traumatic kidney lesions. (**b**) CEUS shows well a traumatic lesion of the right kidney and a thin fluid collection surrounding the kidney

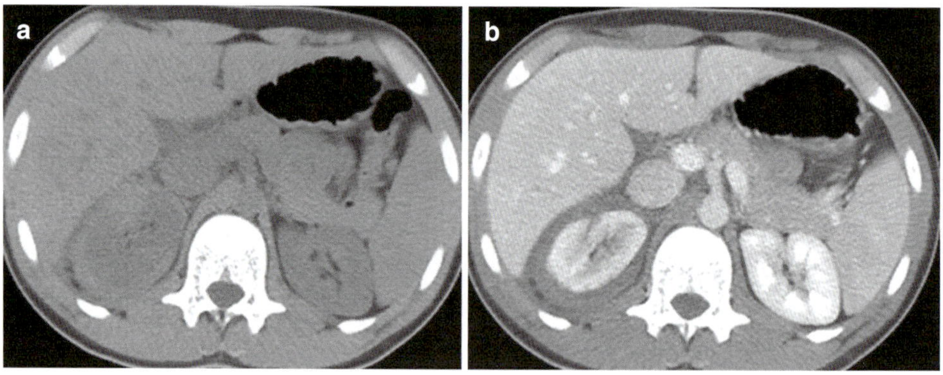

Fig. 24.16 CT (**a**, **b**) confirms right renal parenchymal lesion with peri-renal fluid collection

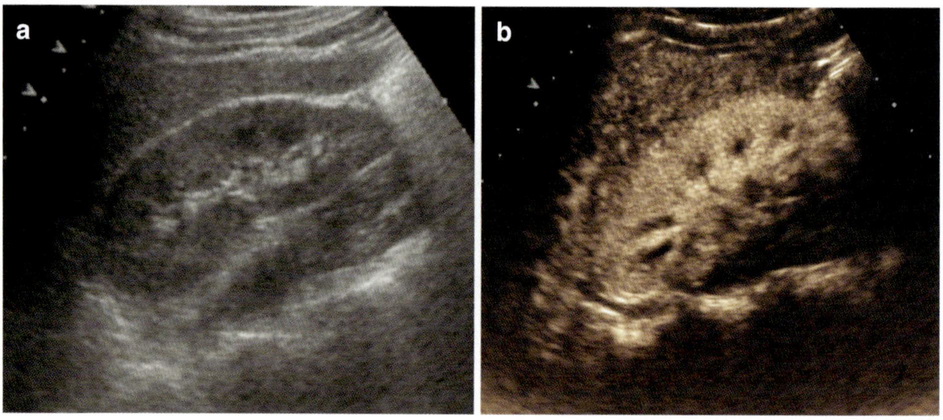

Fig. 24.17 Follow-up examination 1 month later. (**a**) US shows a marked improvement in the parenchymal lesion and the complete disappearance of peri-renal fluid. (**b**) CEUS best depicts both data

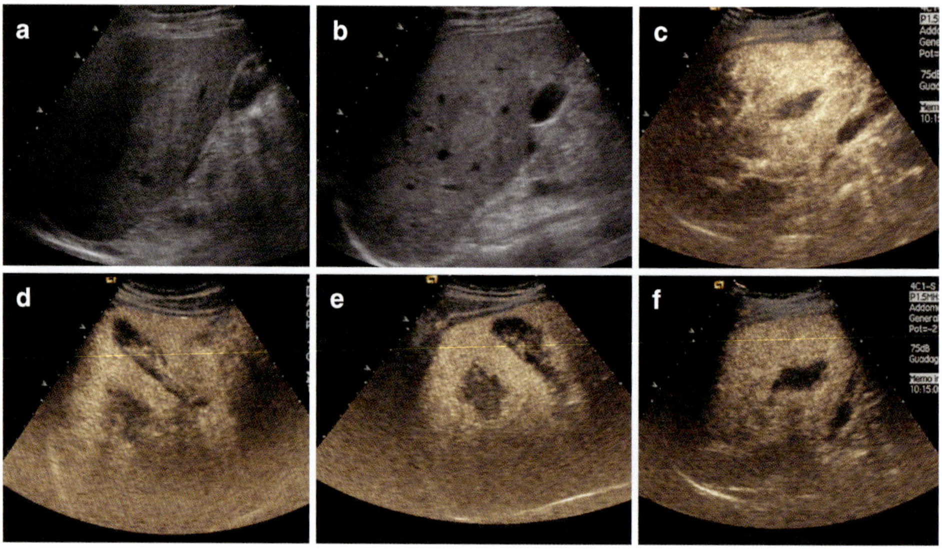

Fig. 24.18 (**a**, **b**) Baseline US shows only a diffuse hyper-echogenicity affecting the right lobe. (**c–f**) CEUS depicts well a large irregular lacerative lesion of the right lobe of the liver, reaching the capsular surface

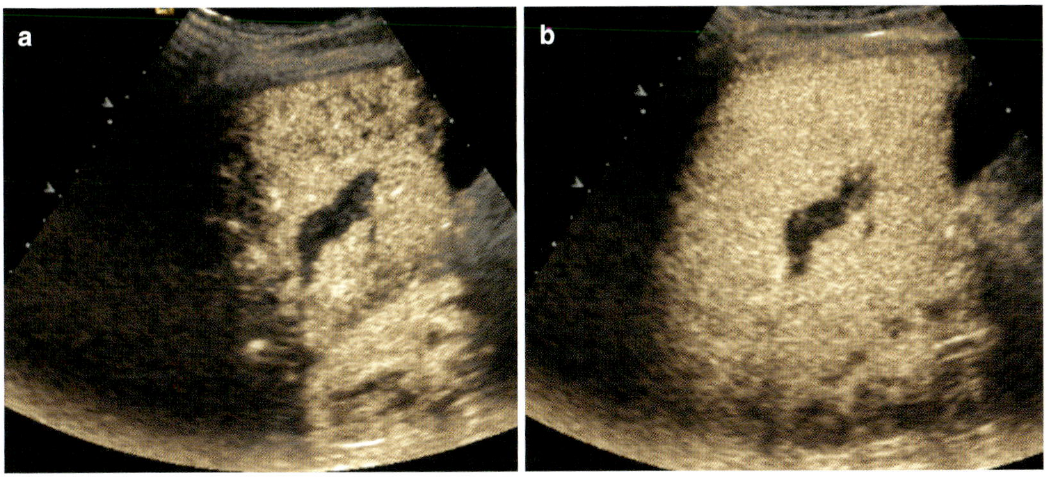

Fig. 24.19 Follow-up with CEUS, 5 days later (**a**, **b**). Lesion appears considerably reduced in size

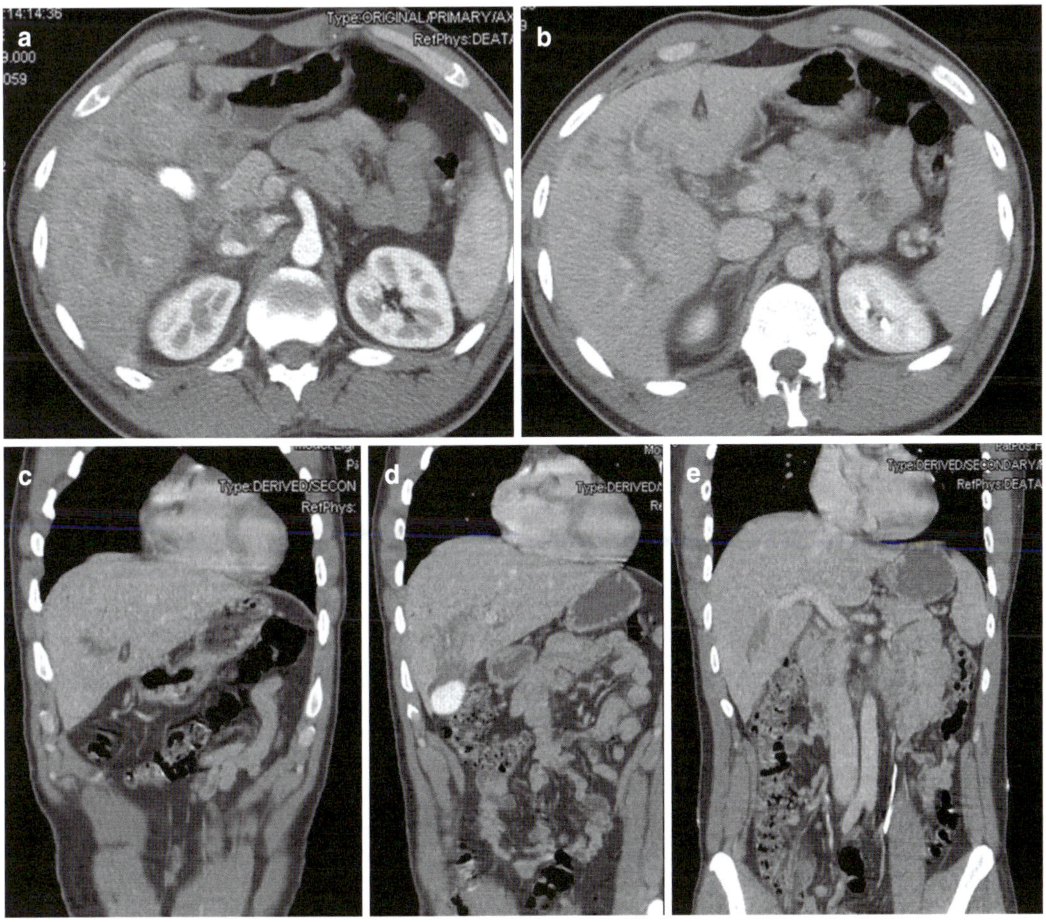

Fig. 24.20 Contrast-enhanced CT (**a**–**e**) confirms the size of the injuries depicted by CEUS

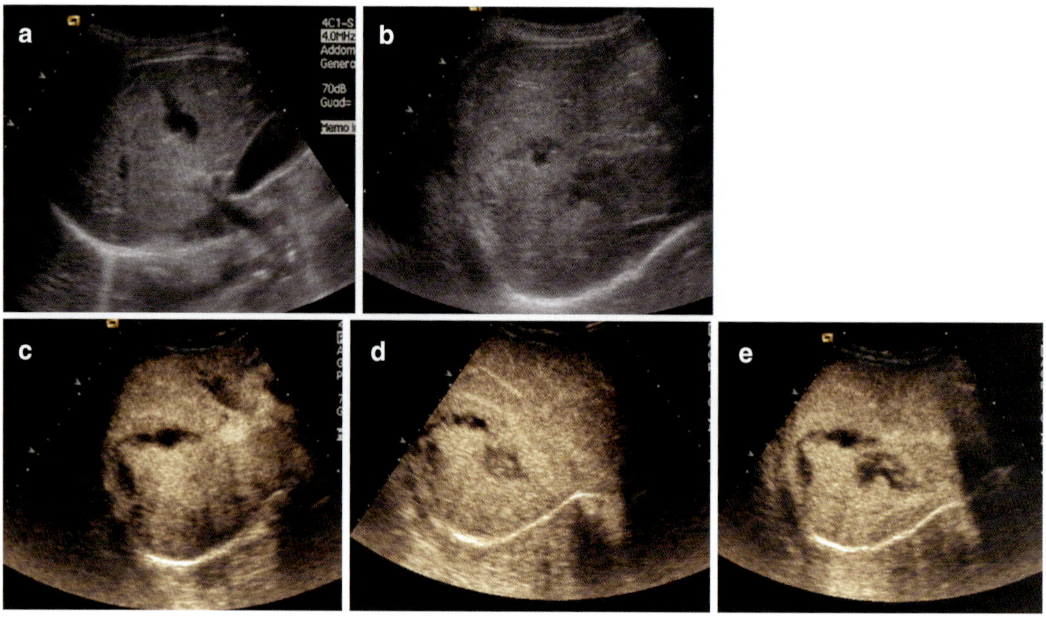

Fig. 24.21 Hepatic laceration. (**a**, **b**) Baseline US shows a parenchymal laceration of the right lobe that reaches the capsule. (**c**–**e**) CEUS better depicts the morphology and size of the laceration

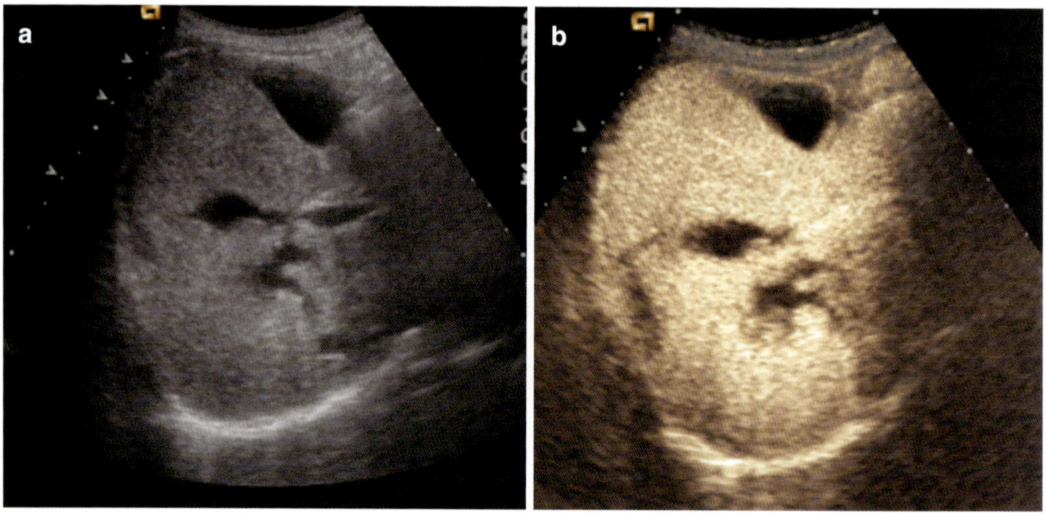

Fig. 24.22 Follow-up with US and CEUS after 2 and 6 days. (**a**, **b**) After 2 days, US baseline and CEUS imaging are essentially unchanged. (**c**, **d**) After 6 days, however, the lesion is better circumscribed than on the previous examination and the surrounding parenchyma is more regularly perfused

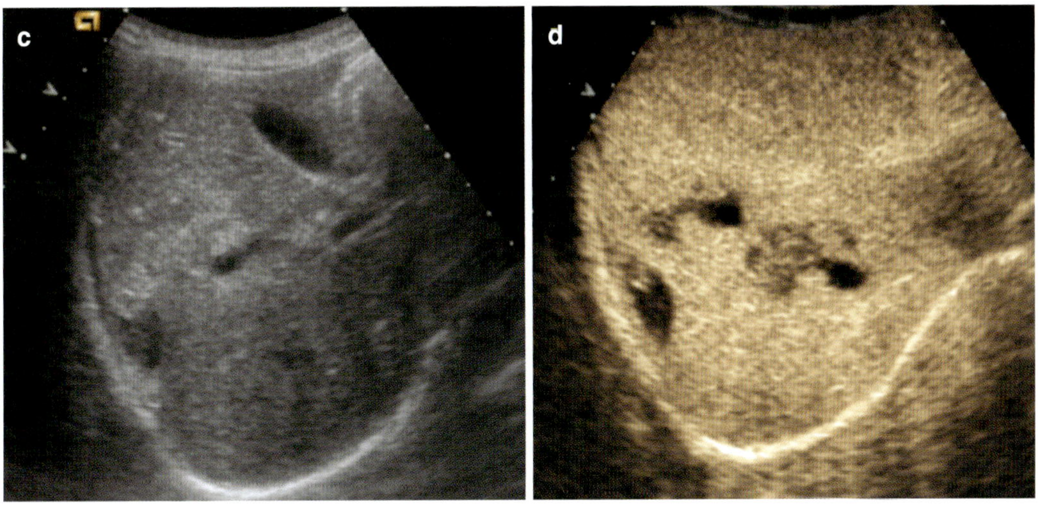

Fig. 24.22 (continued)

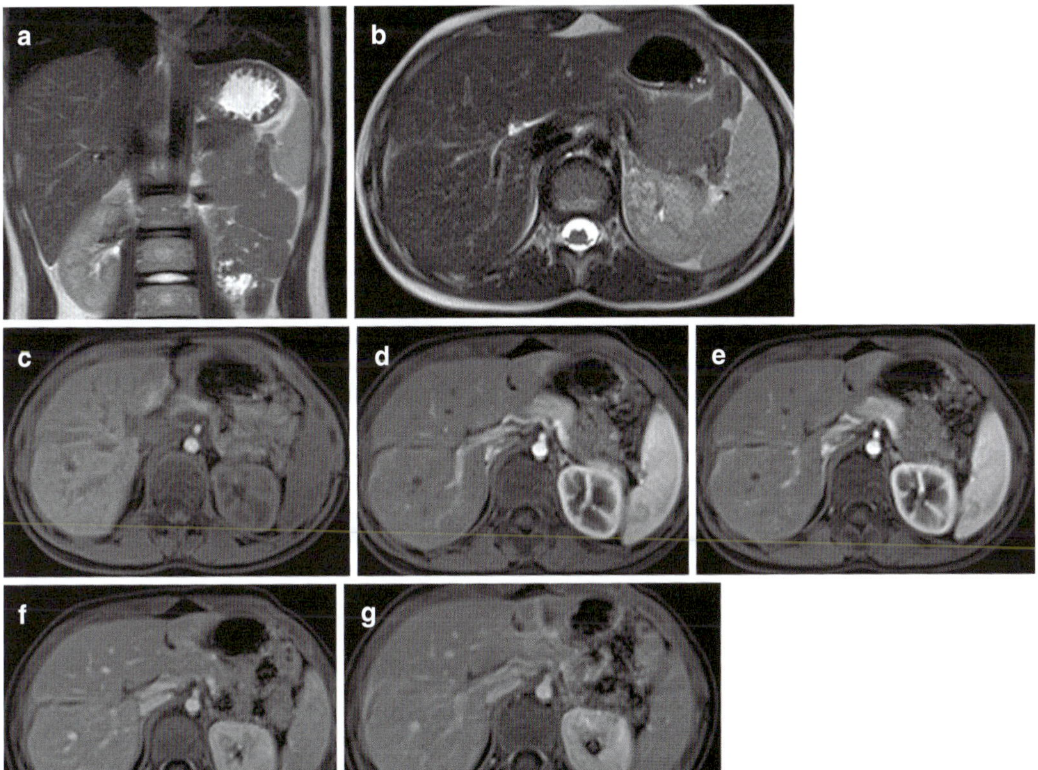

Fig. 24.23 Follow-up with MRI after 1 month. In HASTE T_2-weighted images (**a**, **b**) and VIBE T_1-weighted images (**c**–**g**) after contrast media administration, the results of the right lobe laceration are still apparent, with persistent linear parenchymal hypointensity, reaching the capsule, that appears thickened. There is still a thin, perihepatic fluid collection, best seen in T_2 images

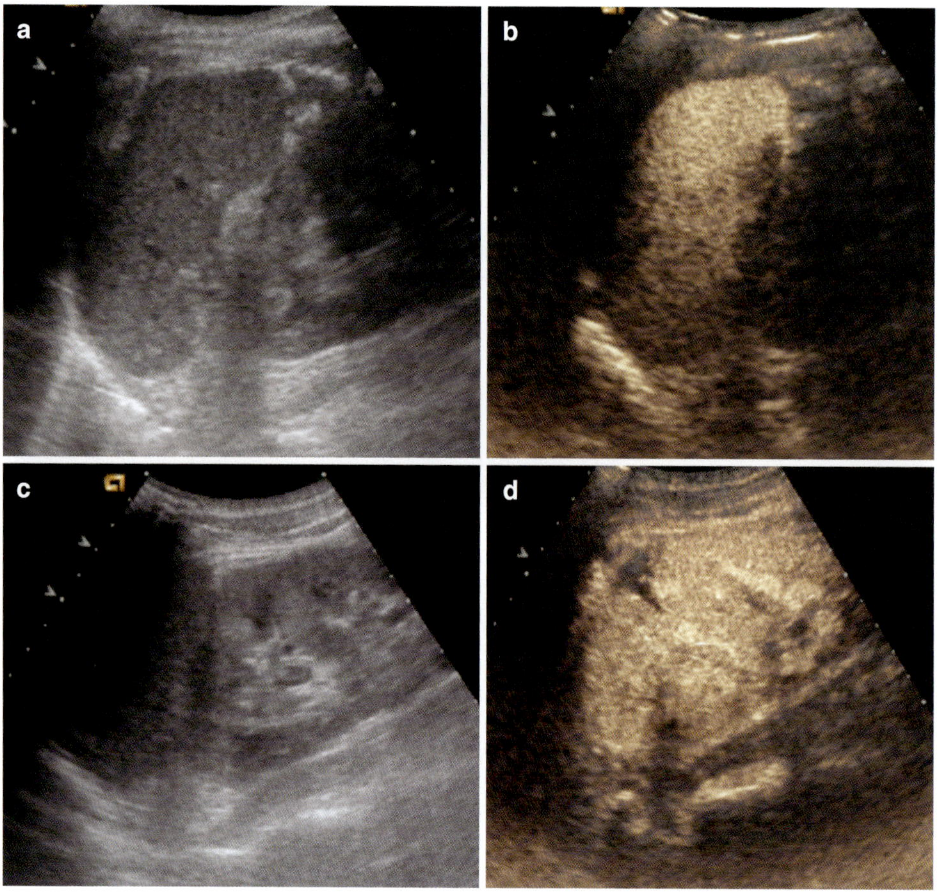

Fig. 24.24 Car accident (**a**–**d**). Splenic laceration and small laceration of the upper left kidney. Baseline US (**a**, **c**) shows slight hyper-echogenicity of the spleen and of the upper lobe of the kidney. CEUS (**b**, **d**) depicts well a small splenic laceration of the lower splenic pole and a hypo-echoic area of the upper pole of the left kidney

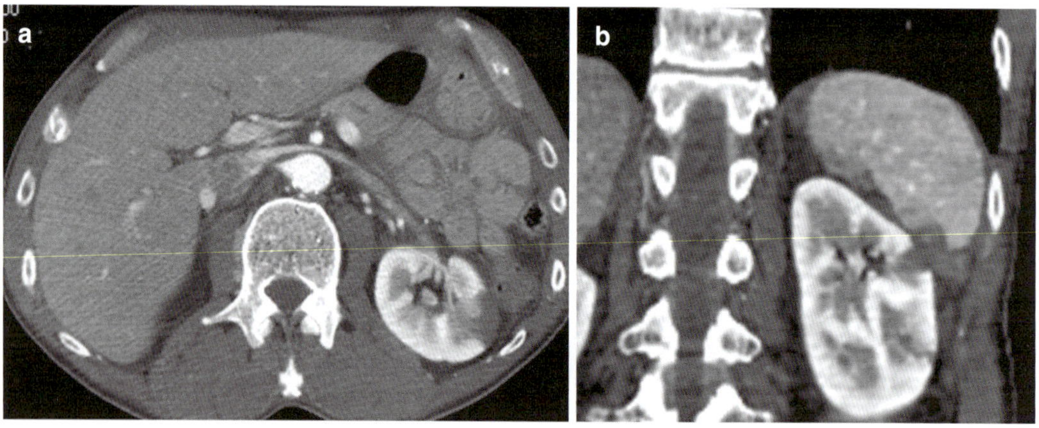

Fig. 24.25 CT confirms CEUS findings. (**a**, **b**) Axial and coronal enhanced CT images confirm well the laceration of the upper pole of the kidney emerging to the renal surface. (**c**, **d**) Axial and sagittal enhanced CT images define better the laceration of the lower pole of the spleen emerging from the capsule surface with a thin associated fluid collection

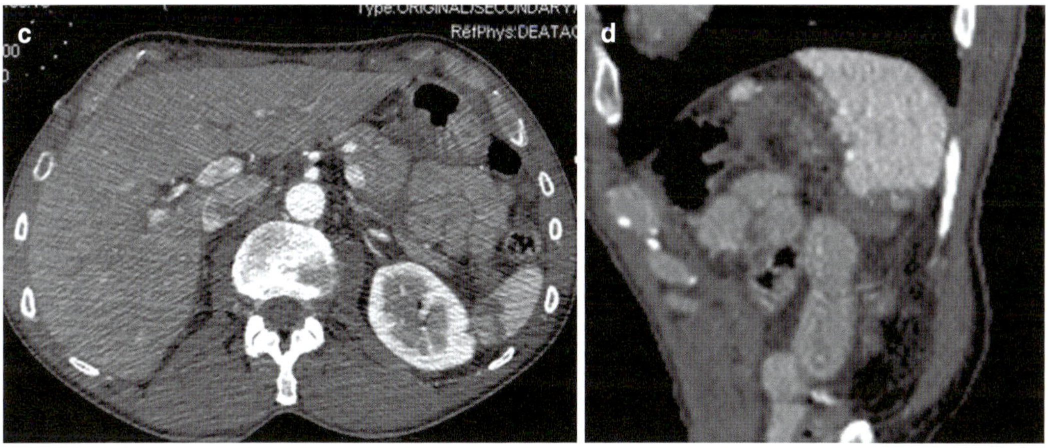

Fig. 24.25 (continued)

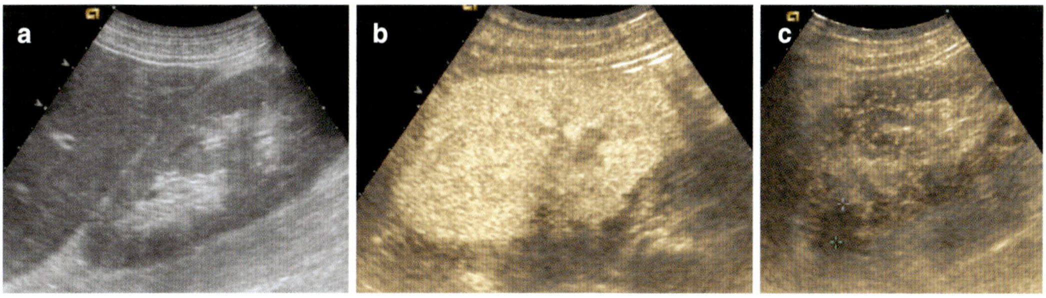

Fig. 24.26 Follow-up after 5 days. (**a**) Baseline US is negative for traumatic lesions. (**b**, **c**) CEUS shows a small laceration of the lower pole of the spleen without peri-splenic fluid and depicts the laceration of the upper pole of the kidney (about 15 mm)

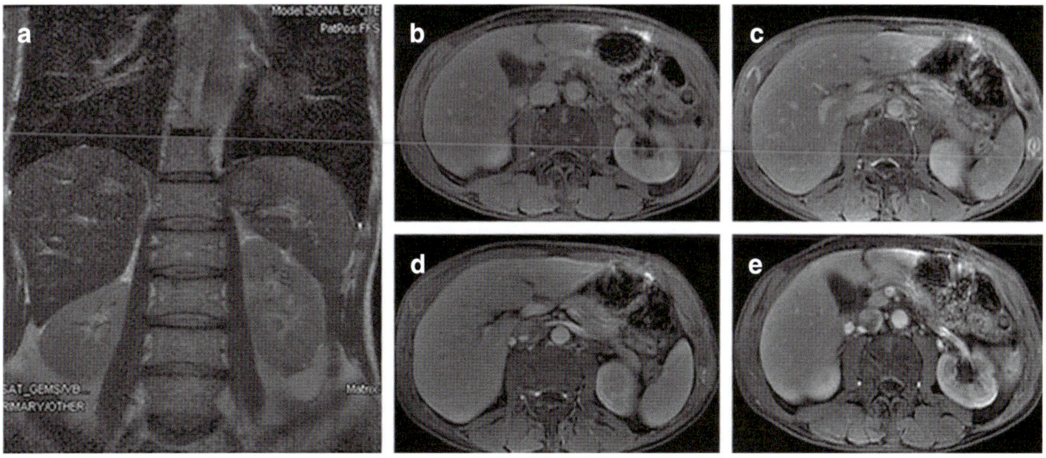

Fig. 24.27 (**a**–**e**) VIBE T_1-weighted image after contrast media administration. MRI follow-up after 1 month shows complete resolution of the splenic lesion; on the superior pole of the kidney a very small hypointense area remains, referred to scar tissue

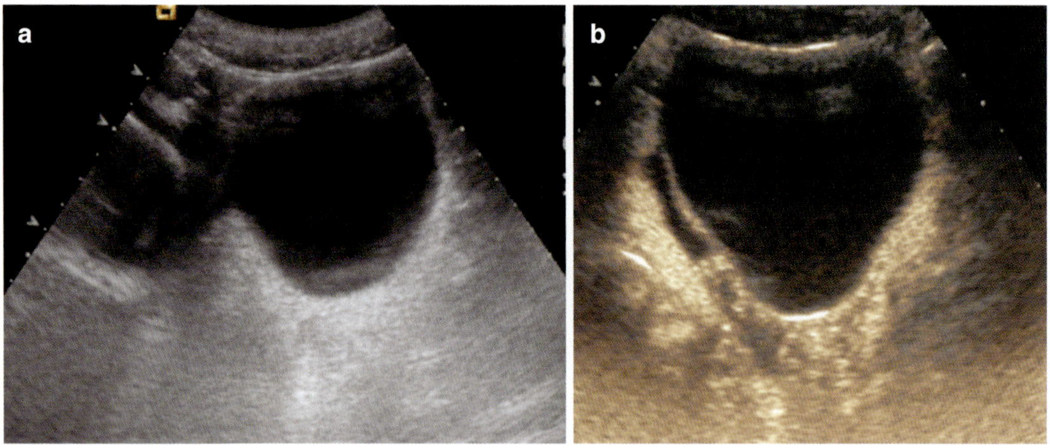

Fig. 24.28 Small amount of free fluid in trauma patient. (**a**) Baseline US does not show the small amount of free fluid that is easily depicted by CEUS (**b**)

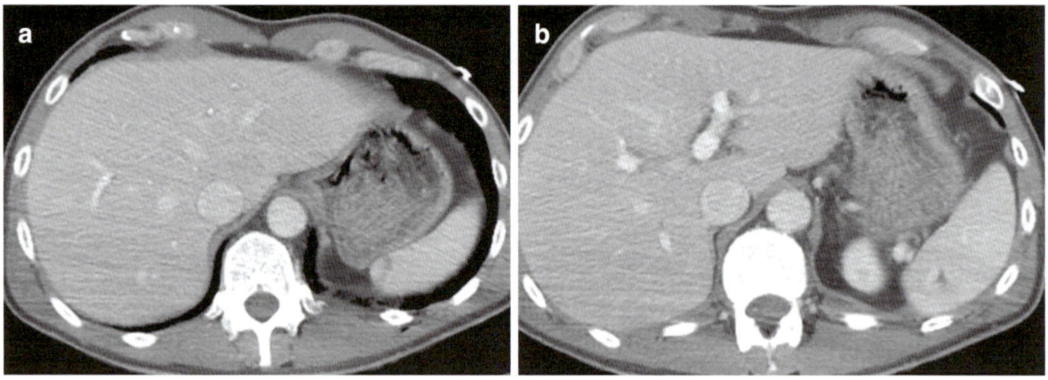

Fig. 24.29 (**a**, **b**) First contrast-enhanced CT on arrival at emergency room. At the level of the upper pole and the middle of the spleen there are some ipodense areas, diagnosed as parenchymal lacerations; currently, no evidence of subcapsular or perisplenic hematoma is seen

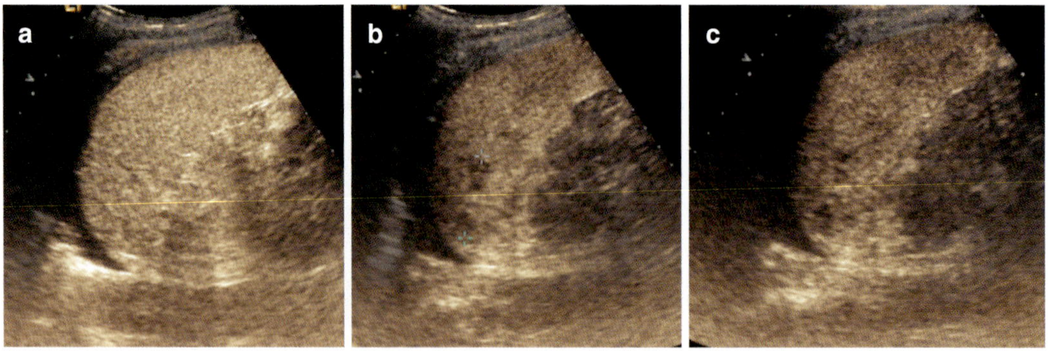

Fig. 24.30 (**a**–**c**) CEUS performed the following day confirms the heterogeneous areas of the upper pole and middle of the spleen, referring to the lacerations already documented in the previous CT examination. CEUS also delineates a subtle subcapsular hematoma

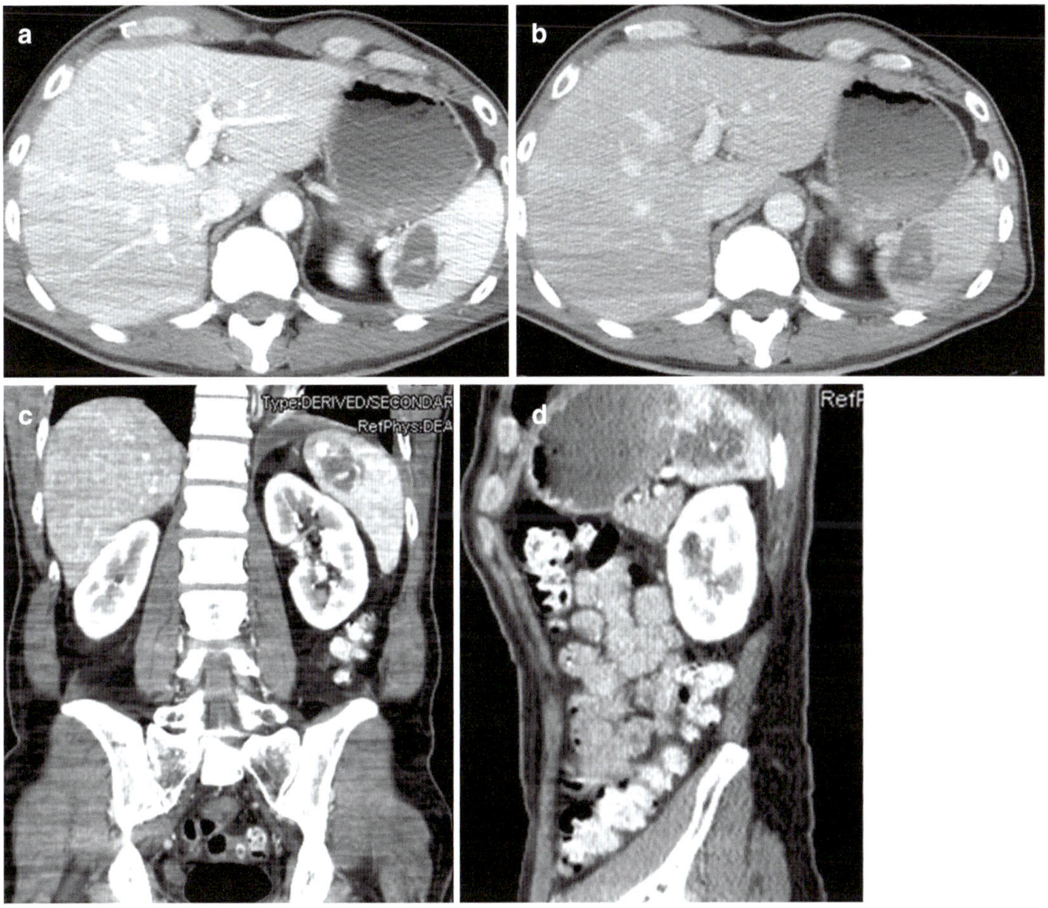

Fig. 24.31 (**a–d**) At CT follow-up after 5 days, splenic lesions are mutated and progressed. The large traumatic lesion that affects the upper pole and the middle part of the spleen is confirmed. At CT exam at the upper spleen pole a large vascular structure is seen. In the enhanced scan there is no evidence of active internal bleeding, but the finding is referred with posttraumatic arteriovenous fistula

of hemoglobin oxygenation and the state of the red blood cell membranes.

Therefore, in the follow-up MRI examination of an injured abdominal solid organ, the hematoma appears iso-intense or hypo-intense on T_1-weighted and hyper-intense on T_2-weighted images during the hyperacute phase (<3 h), iso-intense in T_1-weighted and hypo-intense at the center in T_2-weighted images and hyper-intense at the periphery in the acute stage (<3 days), hyper-intense in T_1 and in T_2 in the subacute phase (<4 weeks), and extremely variable (hyper-, hypo-, or iso-intense) in the chronic phase.

Liver and spleen injuries are considered healed when a homogeneous signal to the parenchyma at both CEUS and MRI examination and the regular distribution of contrast medium during contrast-enhanced examination are seen. These findings can be confirmed by the laboratory parameters.

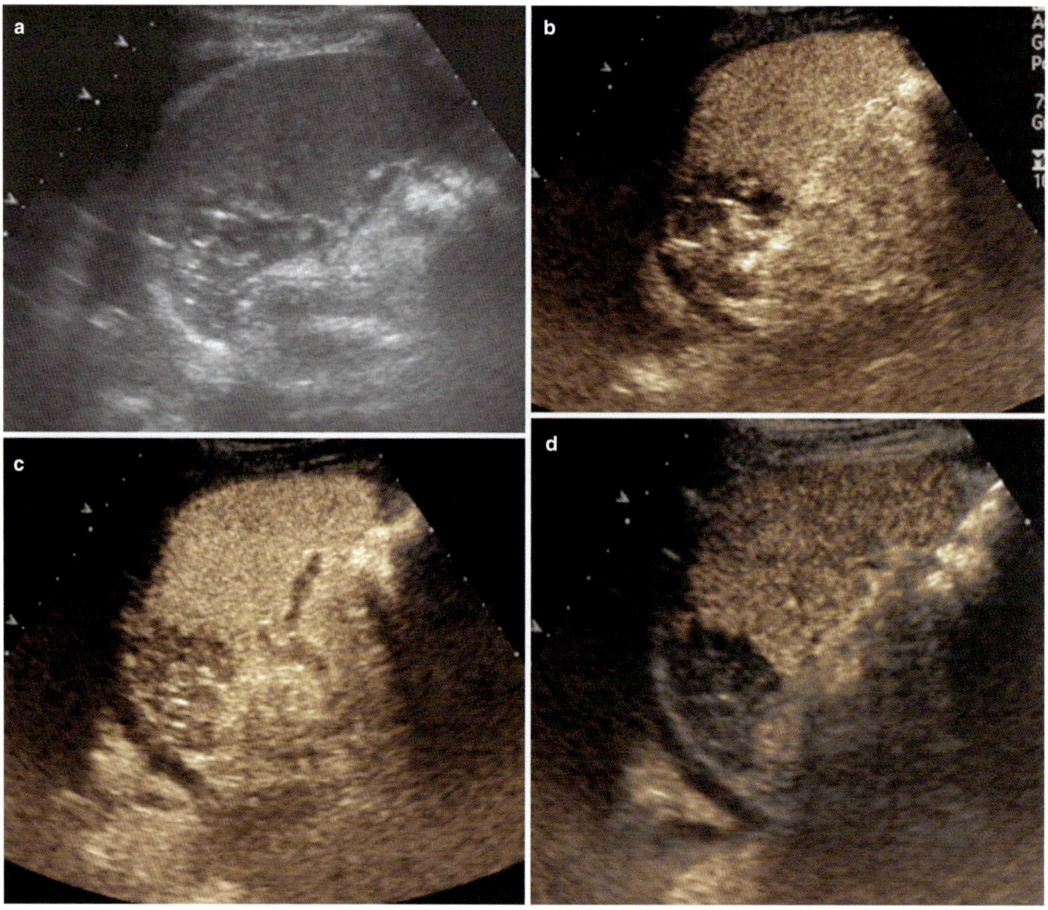

Fig. 24.32 (**a–d**) The following day, the patient undergoes embolization of the spleen. The subsequent US (**a**) and CEUS (**b–d**) follow-up show well the appearance of a hypo-echoic area at the upper pole of the spleen, relative to the ischemic parenchyma after the embolization

24.4 Advantages

Sensitivity and specificity values for identifying abdominal solid organ injuries are 70.2% and 59.2% for US, and 96.4% and 98% for CEUS [3], respectively; regarding the corresponding sensitivity and specificity of MRI, there are still no reliable data reported in the literature.

Because CEUS shows very good correlation with CE-MDCT in lesion staging, to avoid excessive exposure to ionizing radiation and to the contrast medium with possible adverse reactions, it can be considered a valuable tool, especially in the follow-up of blunt abdominal trauma.

Furthermore, CEUS can be performed quickly at the patient's bedside, as the US scanner is portable; moreover, CEUS shows a very low rate of adverse reactions, and, finally, no sedation is needed to perform the CEUS examination. It also does not require fasting or preliminary laboratory findings, it has no contraindications, and the injection of contrast medium is repeatable.

However, CEUS does not replace CT examination, which is more panoramic and standardized, but it can reduces the number of CT scans during the follow-up of patients with a known abdominal injury.

Moreover, MRI, which has a wide panoramic range and is less operator dependent, can be

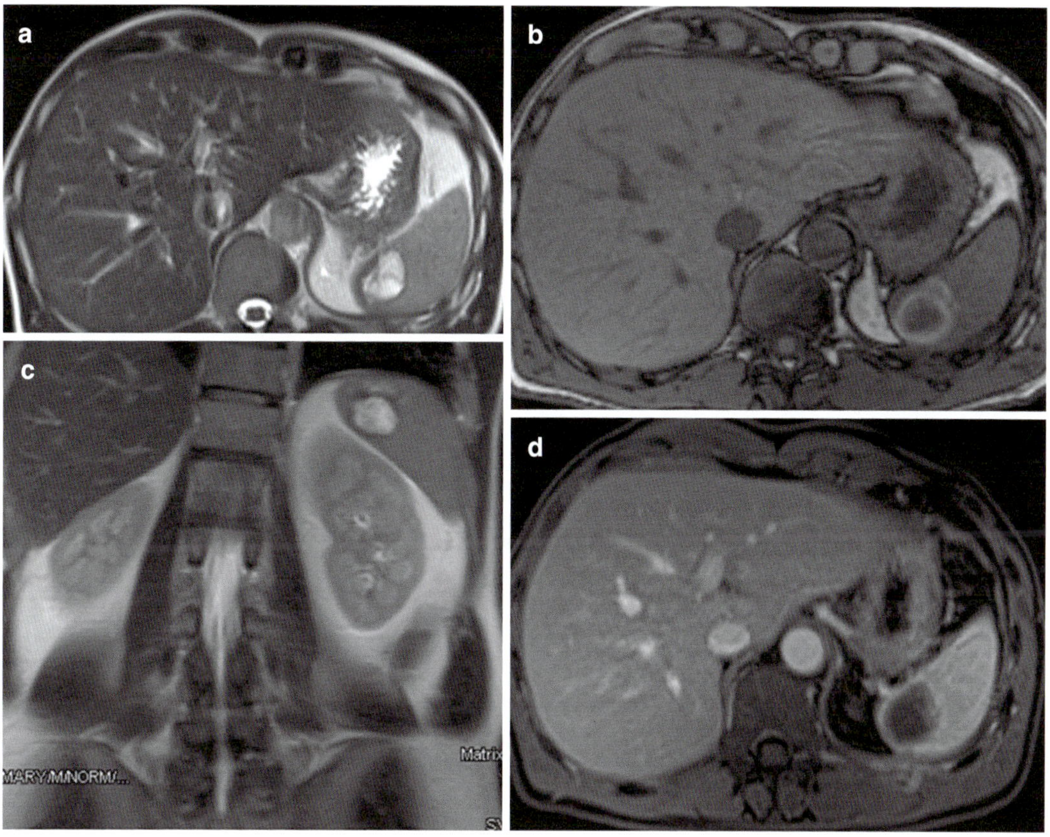

Fig. 24.33 (**a–d**) Same patient. Follow-up with MRI after 1 month. (**a**, **c**) HASTE T_2-weighted axial and coronal sequences. (**b**) T_1 out-of-phase. (**d**) VIBE T_1-weighted image after contrast media administration. In the upper splenic pole a triangular area is confirmed that is hyperintense in T_2-weighted sequences, hypointense in T_1-weighted sequence, with suppression of the signal of the adipose tissue, as an ischemic area

considered a viable alternative to CEUS, especially in the evaluation of possible vascular complications (such as pseudo-aneurysms) (Figs. 24.29, 24.30, 24.31, 24.32, 24.33, and 24.34), intraparenchymal complications (abscesses, bilomas), and lesions of the urinary tract.

24.5 Limits

CEUS also has limitations, however, because it cannot detect lesions that are too small and certain types of injuries, such as diaphragmatic ruptures and bowel and mesenteric injuries, because the view is less panoramic; there is difficulty in examining large patients; and finally, it is operator dependent [32].

Furthermore, the US contrast agent has an intravascular distribution and thus is not suitable for demonstrating extravasation in the renal collecting system (urinomas) because it is not excreted by the kidney [33].

It is not always possible to detect early or late active bleeding; also, some other complications such as abscesses, bilomas, vascular complications, and intestinal damage are difficult to detect and characterize; then, we need to perform a CE-CT or MRI.

MRI also has limits, such as the long examination time, the need to have the cooperation of patients to follow breath-hold commands during image acquisition, the need to transport these patients to the MRI room, and the impossibility of use in cases with a pacemaker or cochlear implants and for patients with claustrophobia.

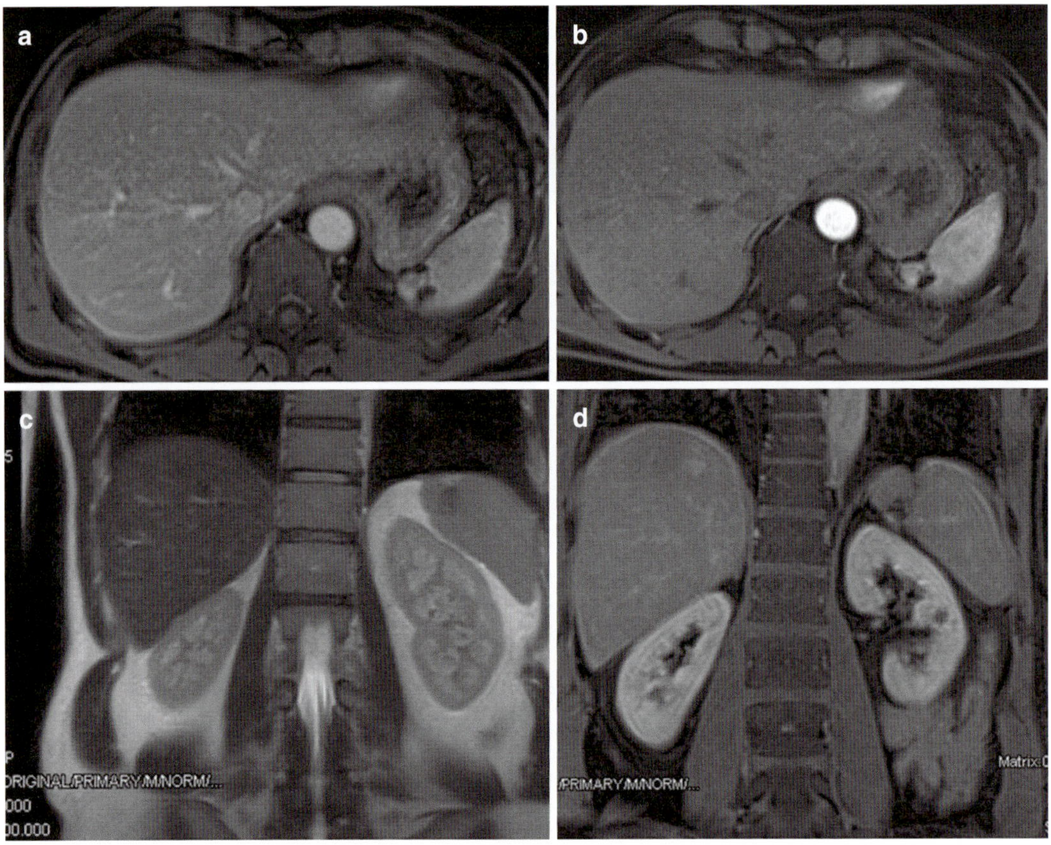

Fig. 24.34 (**a–d**) Follow-up with MRI after 18 months. MRI images demonstrate a reduction of the size of the triangular ischemic area of the upper splenic pole, which appears hypointense in T_1- and T_2-weighted sequences, and in T_1-weighted enhanced images, and refers to a fibrosis area. An associated retraction of the splenic capsule profile is well depicted on MRI images

24.5.1 Take-Home Points

Given the high levels of sensitivity and specificity shown by CEUS in the follow-up of polytrauma patients, or those with minor traumatic lesions, the possibility of replacing CE-MDCT with CEUS is now being considered in these cases, especially to avoid excessive exposure to ionizing radiation. The use of CT in minor trauma is inappropriate, in fact, because of its high cost and unjustified exposure to ionizing radiation in young people and pediatric patients. CEUS allows an accurate definition of the size and the margins of the lesion, the extension to the capsule, and, most importantly, often can depict the presence of vascular injuries.

To date significant cases of reaction to contrast medium have not been reported. Caution must be taken for a patient with heart disease, however, because rare cases of reaction to contrast medium in cases of overdose are known among such patients.

The evaluation with CEUS does not take much time. A close follow-up performed using CEUS is also less expensive than when using CE-CT.

In patients undergoing conservative treatment, CEUS is the procedure most frequentlyperformed for monitoring known traumatic lesions, especially for children and young women; MRI can be used in the long-term follow-up (at 1 month) and until complete resolution of abdominal lesions.

Thus, the use of CEUS can be considered the ideal imaging modality in monitoring all hemodynamically stable patients treated conservatively, especially in consideration of reducing the number of follow-up CT scans, particularly in young patients.

References

1. Parks RW, Chrysos E, Diamone T. Management of liver trauma. Br J Surg. 1999;86:1121–35.
2. Uranus S, Pfeifer J. Nonoperative treatment of blunt splenic injury. World J Surg. 2001;25:1405–7.
3. Valentino M, Ansaloni L, Catena F, et al. Contrast-enhanced ultrasonography in blunt abdominal trauma: considerations after 5 years of experience. Radiol Med. 2009;114:1080–93.
4. Miele V, Buffa V, Stasolla A, et al. Contrast enhanced ultrasound with second generation contrast agent in traumatic liver lesions. Radiol Med. 2004;108:82–91.
5. Regine G, Atzori M, Miele V, et al. Second-generation sonographic contrast agents in the evaluation of renal trauma. Radiol Med. 2007;112:581–7.
6. Pinto F, Miele V, Scaglione M, Pinto A. The use of contrast-enhanced ultrasound in blunt abdominal trauma: advantages and limitations. Acta Radiol. 2014;55:776–84. doi:10.1177/0284185113505517.
7. Pinto F, Valentino M, Romanini L, Basilico R, Miele V. The role of CEUS in the assessment of haemodynamically stable patients with blunt abdominal trauma. Radiol Med. 2015;120:3–11. doi:10.1007/s11547-014-0455-3.
8. Albrecth T, Blombley M, Bolondi L. Guidelines for the use of contrast agents in ultrasound. Ultraschall Med. 2004;25:249–56.
9. Miele V, Piccolo CL, Sessa B, Trinci M, Galluzzo M. Comparison between MRI and CEUS in the follow-up of patients with blunt abdominal trauma managed conservatively. Radiol Med. 2016;121:27–37.
10. Gruessner R, Mentges B, Duber CH. Sonography versus peritoneal lavage in blunt abdominal trauma. J Trauma. 1989;29:242–4.
11. McKenney M, Lentz K, Nunez D. Can ultrasound replace diagnostic peritoneal lavage in the assessment of blunt trauma? J Trauma. 1994;37:439–41.
12. Körner M, Krotz MM, Degenhart C, et al. Current role of emergency US in patients with major trauma. Radiographics. 2008;28:225–44.
13. Poletti P-A, Wintermark M, Schnyder P. Traumatic injuries: role of imaging in the management of polytrauma victim (conservative expectation). Eur Radiol. 2002;12:969–78.
14. Sessa B, Trinci M, Ianniello S, et al. Blunt abdominal trauma: role of contrast-enhanced ultrasound (CEUS) in the detection and staging of abdominal traumatic lesions compared to US and CE-MDCT. Radiol Med. 2015;120:180–9.
15. Valentino M, Serra PP, et al. Blunt abdominal trauma: diagnostic performance of contrast enhanced US in children. Initial experience. Radiology. 2008;246:903–9.
16. Brown MA, Casola G, Sirlin CB, et al. Blunt abdominal trauma: screening US in 2,693 patients. Radiology. 2001;218:352–8.
17. Miele V, Piccolo CL, Trinci M, et al. Diagnostic imaging of blunt abdominal trauma in pediatric patients. Radiol Med. 2016;121:409–30. doi:10.1007/s11547-016-0637-2. Epub 2016 Apr 13
18. Sidhu PS, Cantisani V, Deganello A, et al. Role of contrast-enhanced ultrasound (CEUS) in paediatric practice: an EFSUMB position statement. Ultraschall Med. 2017;38:33–43. PMID: 27414980. doi:10.1055/s-0042-110394.
19. Miele V, Di Giampietro I, Ianniello S, et al. Diagnostic imaging in pediatric polytrauma management. Radiol Med. 2015;120:33–49. doi:10.1007/s11547-014-0469-x. Epub 2014 Nov 7
20. Minarik L, Slim M, Rachlin S. Diagnostic imaging in the follow-up of nonoperative management of splenic trauma in children. Pediatr Surg Int. 2002;18(5-6):429–31.
21. Menichini G, Sessa B, Trinci M, et al. Accuracy of contrast-enhanced ultrasound (CEUS) in the identification and characterization of traumatic solid organ lesions in children: a retrospective comparison with baseline US and CE-MDCT. Radiol Med. 2015;120:989–1001.
22. Freshman SP, Wisner DH, Battistella FD. Secondary survey following blunt trauma: a new role for abdominal CT scan. J Trauma. 1993;34(3):337–40.
23. Cuff RF, Cogbill TH, Lambert PJ. Nonoperative management of blunt liver trauma: the value of follow-up abdominal computed tomography scans. Am Surg. 2000;66:332–6.
24. Manetta R, Pistoia ML, Bultrini C, et al. Ultrasound enhanced with sulphur-hexafluoride-filled microbubbles agent (SonoVue) in the follow-up of mild liver and spleen trauma. Radiol Med. 2009;114:771–9.
25. Catalano O, Lobianco R, Sandomenico F, et al. Real-time, contrast-enhanced sonographic imaging in emergency radiology. Radiol Med. 2004;108:454–69.
26. Poletti PA, Kinkel K, Vermeulen B, et al. Blunt abdominal trauma: should US be used to detect both free fluid and organ injuries? Radiology. 2003;227:95–103.
27. Wilson SR, Burns PN. Microbubble-enhanced US in body imaging: what role? Radiology. 2010;257(1):24–39.
28. Oldenburg A, Hohmann J, Skrok J. Imaging of paediatric splenic injury with contrast-enhanced ultrasonography. Pediatr Radiol. 2004;34(4):351–4.
29. Federle MP, Courcoulas AP, Powell M, et al. Blunt splenic injury in adults: clinical and CT criteria for management, with emphasis on active extravasation. Radiology. 1998;206:137–42.

30. Gavant ML, Schurr M, Flick PA, et al. Predicting clinical outcome of nonsurgical management of blunt splenic injury: using CT to reveal abnormalities of splenic vasculature. AJR Am J Roentgenol. 1997;168:207–12.
31. Kawashima A, Sandler CM, Corl FM, et al. Imaging of renal trauma: a comprehensive review. Radiographics. 2001;21:557–74.
32. Sirlin CB, Brown MA, Deutsch R, et al. Screening US for blunt abdominal trauma: objective predictors of false-negative findings and missed injuries. Radiology. 2003;229:766–74.
33. Miele V, Piccolo CL, Galluzzo M, et al. Contrast enhanced ultrasound (CEUS) in blunt abdominal trauma. Br J Radiol. 2016;89(1061):20150823. doi:10.1259/bjr.20150823 Epub 2016 Jan 8.

Injuries of the Limbs in Polytrauma: Upper and Lower Limbs

25

Anna Maria Ierardi, Filippo Pesapane, Natalie Lucchina, Andrea Coppola, Filippo Piacentino, Andrea Sacrini, Salvatore Alessio Angileri, and Gianpaolo Carrafiello

25.1 Introduction

Polytrauma is a significant cause of mortality and morbidity throughout the world and predominantly affects the young population [1].

There has been a growing role for both diagnostic and Interventional Radiology (IR) in all types of traumas; imaging becomes an integral part of the multidisciplinary approach to modern trauma care: a polytraumatic patient should not be considered as a "vascular" patient, an "orthopedic" patient, or a "plastics" patient but a multipathologic patient requiring a multidisciplinary approach [1].

Classically, vascular injury mechanisms are divided into penetrating or blunt. In blunt trauma, tissue injury is produced by local compression, rapid deceleration, and the resulting shear forces. In penetrating trauma, the injury is produced by crushing and separation of tissues along the path of the penetrating object with the resulting concussive shockwave [1].

Understanding the biomechanics of specific injuries is important in determining the potential for vascular injury and the subsequent hemodynamic consequences of these injuries.

Extremity injuries are the second most common traumatic injuries after head injuries [2] up to 80% of all cases of vascular trauma; most of these injuries involve arteries and veins of the lower extremities. High-velocity weapons (70–80%) account for most of these injuries, followed by stab wounds (10–15%) and blunt trauma (5–10%) [1]. In a large series of penetrating civilian vascular injuries, arterial injuries were caused by gunshot wounds in 64%, knife wounds in 24%, and shotgun blasts in 12% [3].

Peripheral injuries are usually not immediately lethal, whether due to penetrating or blunt injuries, like trauma to torso and head and neck regions [4].

This chapter focuses on injuries of the limbs in polytraumatic patient and the decision processes associated with the workup and the endovascular interventions (EVIs) of these injuries.

25.2 Clinical Aspects and Imaging

Acute limb vascular injuries should be suspected in presence of an open fracture, distal tibia or tibial shaft fractures, fractures of the thoracic outlet, multiple and/or complexed fractures in one extremity, and/or an isolated proximal third.

A.M. Ierardi (✉) • F. Pesapane • A. Sacrini
S.A. Angileri • G. Carrafiello
Diagnostic and Interventional Radiology Department, San Paolo Hospital, University of Milan, Via A. di Rudinì 8, 20142 Milan, Italy
e-mail: amierardi@yahoo.it

N. Lucchina • A. Coppola • F. Piacentino
Unit of Radiology, Insubria University, Viale Borri 57, 21100 Varese, Italy

V. Miele, M. Trinci (eds.), *Diagnostic Imaging in Polytrauma Patients*, https://doi.org/10.1007/978-3-319-62054-1_25

Monazzam et al., in a series of 275 patients, demonstrated that only 6% of the cases requires treatment, and all of them had strong clinical sign as diminished or absent distal pulses on presentation, so they suggest to not routinely use CT angiography (CTA) to evaluate lower extremity injuries unless at least one clinical sign is present [5].

The physical examination represents the first step, because it permits to triage the patients to emergency treatment, imaging, or observation.

The "hard signs" of an extremity arterial injury include loss of distal pulses, an expanding or pulsatile hematoma, a thrill or bruit, pulsatile bleeding, and limb ischemia. "Soft signs" include pallor or a change in color, coolness to the touch, a stable hematoma, a neurological deficit in an anatomically adjacent nerve, unexplained hypotension, and non-pulsatile bleeding (Table 25.1).

There is growing evidence that most of these injuries heal spontaneously or stabilize without further compromising the distal circulation and perfusion [6].

Vascular injuries may be initially undiagnosed in hemodynamically stable patients, so a detailed clinical history including the mechanism of the trauma is important. Factors that can jeopardize diagnosis of acute vascular injuries usually are the presence of distraction injuries, lack of correlation with clinical presentation, radiologist experience, or inadequate CT scan protocol [7].

Subclinical vascular injuries with intact distal perfusion may be observed with serial monitoring, antiplatelet therapy or systemic anticoagulation, and repeat noninvasive imaging [8].

Table 25.1 Hard and soft signs of vascular injury

Hard signs	Soft signs
Shock	Non-pulsatile bleeding
Pulsatile bleeding	Stable hematoma
Bruit or thrill over the wound(s)	Nerve injury
Expanding or pulsatile hematoma	Unequal blood pressures
Absent palpable pulses distally	Proximity of injury tract
Limb ischemia	Distal ischemic manifestations (pain, pallor; paralysis, paresthesias, poikilothermy)

Subclinical vascular defects have been defined as those exhibiting the following characteristics:

1. Low-velocity injury
2. Minimal (<5 mm) arterial wall disruption for intimal defects and pseudoaneurysm (PSA)
3. Adherent or downstream protrusion of intimal flaps
4. Intact distal circulation
5. No active hemorrhage

The liberal use of imaging in the presence of any hard sign to confirm or exclude vascular injury is recommended [4].

Most hard signs in this setting (as much as 87%) are not due to vascular injury, but rather to soft tissue and bone bleeding, traction of intact arteries with pulse loss, or compartment syndrome [9].

If significant vascular injuries (such as occlusion, extravasation, or transection) are excluded, the treatment of soft tissue and skeletal injuries may proceed. How reperfusion is achieved depends on the patient's hemodynamic status, physiologic parameters, skeletal stability, wound characteristics, and resource availability [10].

Vascular imaging is mandatory when expectant management is chosen, but resolution can be seen in 85–90% of these lesions with no operative intervention [11].

Doppler Ultrasound (DUS) has shown an overall accuracy of 98% for diagnosing vascular injury, but it requires time and high experience [1].

DUS provides additional information on clinical examination but there is not consensus in the literature about its importance in the diagnostic management in the injuries of the limbs in trauma patient. DUS can be obtained rapidly and used to detect occlusion, intimal flaps, and luminal defects [12].

For the lower limbs evaluation a DUS assessment should be done also to confirm the absence of pedal pulses and to perform an ankle-brachial index (ABI) when possible. In emergency traumatic setting, an ABI is useful for the evaluation of a patient who is at increased risk for lower extremity arterial injury: an ABI < 0.90 suggests a need for further vascular imaging, whereas an

ABI > 0.90 decreases the likelihood of an arterial injury, and the patient may be observed with serial ABI assessments or may undergo a vascular study on a delayed basis [13].

DUS has some diagnostic limitations in locating the exact point of artery cutoff point and the traumatized area. Moreover, the DUS evaluation of the vascular limbs injuries, especially in trauma patients, requires high level of expertise; it is highly operator dependent and can be time-consuming [14].

Large retrospective reviews have shown that Computed Tomography Angiography (CTA) significantly increases the probability of survival in polytrauma patients [15].

It has the added advantage of simultaneously being able to assess extensive body areas as well as demonstrating associated soft tissue and bony injuries.

CTA has dramatically improved over the last few years and has overtaken catheter angiography as the initial first choice diagnostic tool in the trauma patients [4].

While traditional angiography has been the gold standard and affords opportunity for intervention, the ability to rapidly acquire high-specificity diagnostic imaging with spiral CTA has been a game changer as a rapid screening test and plays a major role in the management of multi-trauma patients.

Digital Subtraction Angiography (DSA) is the diagnostic standard for vascular injury and allows for therapeutic intervention [16].

CTA has a sensitivity of 90–95% and specificity of between 98% and 100% for the detection of upper and lower limbs arterial injuries [16]. CTA may be limited by poor arterial opacification, motion artifact, streak artifact from adjacent metallic fragments, or slowing of flow beyond injured sites [16]. CTA has nowadays replaced catheter angiography as the primary imaging technique to evaluate patients with suspected acute vascular injuries [7, 10, 17]. Nevertheless, some investigators still recommend DSA as the primary imaging test, particularly in patients with finding of metallic fragments or shrapnel on conventional imaging to avoid technical artifacts which may render affected vascular segments non-diagnostic on cross-sectional images [18]. However, in this set, DSA requires an highly trained team readily available at the time of patient admission, it is costly and it is not free from the possibility of serious complications due to catheter insertion, especially in an artery with local hematoma formation, vessel thrombosis and, in more severe cases, post-angiography dissection, embolization and pseudoaneurysm formation [19–21].

CTA pledge the acquisition of three-dimensional images with submillimetric spatial resolution of the entire body, from head to foot in only a few seconds with a single contrast bolus, and state-of-the-art workstations allow Multiplanar Reformations (MPR), Maximum Intensity Projection (MIP), and Volume Rendering (VR) reconstructions [10, 21–24].

It is of fundamental importance the appropriate selection of scan parameters and CT protocols. It is consolidated knowledge that acquiring images in arterial phase improves the detection of arterial injures, AVF, and PSA while the venous phase is essential to detect venous injuries and to differentiate contained vascular injures from actively bleeding lesions. Therefore, both phases should be routinely included in the whole-body CT evaluation of patients with deceleration injury [17].

All studies should be performed with multiphasic, high-resolution protocol, slice thickness and reconstruction interval value of about 1 mm, before and after administration of intravenous, highly concentrated contrast media (350–400 mgI/mL, with a 3.5–5 ml/s infusion rate, followed by a 25–50 ml bolus of isotonic saline at the same flow rate). The field of view (FOV) should be the smallest including both limbs, to minimize the isotropic voxels and to allow evaluation of symmetry of contrast material arrival time and symmetry of flow. The scan coverage should include both the proximal and distal joints to the region of suspected injury. All study should be performed under the supervision of a radiologist, to evaluate any need of additional late phases. An automated bolus tracking, with region of interest placed at the diaphragmatic aorta (for whole-body scanning) at an attenuation threshold of 100HU, is suggested to time the beginning of the arterial phase, in order to avoid poor timing of the contrast material bolus or bolus outrun [10, 17, 21]. Three-dimensional multiplanar reconstructions and maximum intensity projection should be routinely performed to facilitate recognizing the vessel anatomy and look for possible injuries [10, 17, 21].

Many different vascular injuries can be detected. *Active arterial hemorrhage or extravasation* can be defined as extravascular contrast media leakage, recognized as hyperattenuating regions with density similar to that of the arteries. *Dissection* is the evidence of an intraluminal flap with intramural extension of intravenous contrast material. *Arteriovenous fistula* formation is a communication between an artery and an adjacent vein, with premature venous enhancement. *Pseudoaneurysm* is a well-contained accumulation of contrast material-enhanced blood beyond the confines of the arterial wall. *Narrowing* of an artery is an abrupt change in caliber of the vessel within the area of traumatic injury with maintained patency while *occlusion* of an artery is an abrupt complete termination of an artery. *Vessel transection* is seen as an abnormality in the vessel contour due to full thickness laceration with free contrast extravasation detectable in the arterial phase [10, 17].

Hemodynamic instability in limbs injuries is more often associated with Penetrating Extremity Trauma (PET) or exposed fractures. In a 14 patient series who died from isolated limb PET, 70% occurred to the lower extremity and 86% were proximal to the elbow and knee [25].

A patient in shock with PET belong in the operating room and no diagnostic studies, except X-rays of the chest, pelvis and the involved extremity are indicated. If there is no inspective evidence that an arterial injury is present but clinical evidence is still strongly suggesting so, DUS, MDCT or DSA can be obtained [8, 14, 26, 27].

25.3 Upper Limb Injuries

Upper extremity trauma patients generally have a lower injury severity score, lower amputation rate, and lower overall mortality when compared to lower extremity injured patients [28].

Upper extremity injuries are more frequently caused by a penetrating mechanism than blunt etiologies. They are usually associated with lower-velocity missiles and a smaller region of injury than lower extremity injuries [28].

Although much of the current state-of-the-art information is the result of wartime observations, the incidence of civilian extremity vascular trauma is significant. It is estimated that subclavian and axillary artery injuries constitute 5–10% of artery trauma in the European and US civilians [29]. Structures concomitantly involved include the brachial plexus, aerodigestive tract, sympathetic chain, and spinal cord [30].

Axillary artery injuries are very similar to subclavian injuries. High axillary injuries may be difficult to expose and gain proximal control for open operative repair. Both supraclavicular and infraclavicular incision may be necessary to achieve adequate control of the vessel for open repair. Moreover, the proximity to the brachial plexus must also be considered [31–33].

Modern IR techniques offer some promises for both adjuvant care with balloon tamponade and definitive treatment by covered stent placement [4].

New advances in vascular techniques and endovascular care have resulted in outstanding success with limb salvage; the coexisting orthopedic, neurologic, and soft tissue injuries most likely determine the outcome [34].

Associated nonvascular injuries usually are associated with consequent disability and functional outcomes [28]. It is essential to have an early multidisciplinary approach to these patients and to define with appropriate scores functional, orthopedic, and vascular lesions [34]. The Multidisciplinary Team (MT) should include surgeon, interventional radiologist, orthopedic, plastic surgeon, hand surgeon, and neurosurgeon.

Excluding ischemia, acute limb loss is frequently from overwhelming and uncontrolled secondary infection so adequate debridement of nonviable tissue and appropriate coverage of vascular and orthopedic repair is essential [11]. Unstable fractures may require stabilization before repair such that ultimate reduction does not strain the vascular repair. Also in this case, communication and intraoperative collaboration between orthopedic surgeon, interventional radiologist, and vascular surgeon should be essential [1].

25.4 Forearm Vessels

Traumatic injuries to the forearm and hand can be penetrating or blunt, which represent 4–36% of upper limb arterial trauma [34]. Because of the close proximity of the vessels and the nerves as they travel in the upper extremities, injuries are rarely just vascular in nature, often complicating not only the presentation but also the long-term outcome. If not treated in a timely fashion and properly, such injuries can lead to loss of function, loss of limb, or even death [35].

Single vessel injury of the forearm can be simply ligated, after making sure that the opposing vessel is intact to the hand and a palmer arch is present [34]. Bedside handheld DUS evaluation of the palmer arch and digital vessels can be performed to confirm viability prior to ligation of the injured vessel. If in-line flow is not present or an incomplete palmer arch is present, primary repair of the injured vessel should be completed [4].

Endovascular approaches and stent graft have no appreciable role in the management of forearm vessel injuries [35].

25.5 Lower Limb Injuries

Patients with lower limb vascular traumas present daily in emergency departments and trauma centers worldwide. According to the National Hospital Ambulatory Medical Care Survey, among approximately 117 million visits to emergency departments in the USA in 2007, 14.6% were for lower extremity injuries [36].

Nowadays, most polytrauma patients will survive, but will not regain their pre-injury level of function; if multiple trauma is survived, lower extremity injuries mainly affect the functional outcome and quality of life in the long term [37].

25.6 Femoral and Popliteal Injuries

Open surgical repair of the femoral vessels at the level of the groin should be undertaken as routine. Primary repair or short saphenous interposition grafts can be used to reconstruct these vessels [1].

The use of covered stent grafts has been described, but long-term patency data is not available [38]. The popliteal artery provides some clinical controversy. It can be a challenging injury to manage. Historically, amputation rates were as high as 20% with injuries in this location [39]. Classic traction injury from posterior knee dislocation can result in injuries ranging anywhere from a small hemodynamically insignificant intimal flaps to critical ischemia and complete transection [1]. In most clinically apparent injuries, open repair is indicated, either by primary repair (stab wounds) or short segmental saphenous vein bypass (blunt injury, gunshot wounds), but there are also the possibility to use covered stent graft repair for trauma and iatrogenic [38, 40].

25.7 Below-Knee Popliteal, Tibial, and Foot Injuries

As with the upper extremity, injury to one terminal vessel in the lower limb can be dealt with by simple ligation. Injury at the level of the tibioperoneal trunk should prompt open surgical reconstruction. Injury to all three tibial arteries should prompt open operative repair of at least two arteries to avoid a potential risk for future amputation [41]. Currently endovascular techniques have not played a major role in the management of tibial arteries injuries.

25.8 The Role of Interventional Radiology in Polytrauma Extremity

In the last two decades, IR shifted the management of vascular disease from traditional open surgery to complex endovascular interventions (EVIs) [4].

On the basis of CTA findings and with the cooperation and support of the other members of the MT team, the interventional radiologist must be increasingly prepared to provide prompt, efficient, and high-quality service [7].

The primary principle in treating acute traumatic arterial injuries is to avoid prolonged ischemia. This reduces the risk of irreversible ischemia and morbidity associated with ischemia reperfusion [42].

Endovascular techniques have the advantages of avoiding general anesthesia, rapid recovery time, lower costs, less tissue trauma in cases of previous soft tissue or bone injuries, and lower chances of infection when there are associated bone fractures; also, there is less risk of collateral flow damage during surgical exposure [43].

Becker et al. [44] were the first to use a stent graft in the management of a penetrating subclavian injury resulting from catheterization.

A systematic review of axillo-subclavian injuries from DuBose et al. found that results of endovascular repair were promising, with an initial success of endovascular stent placement in 96.9% of patients. No mortalities related to endovascular intervention were reported. New neurologic deficits after the use of endovascular modalities were reported in only one patient over 160 treated with endovascular approach [45]. Endovascular management of axillo-subclavian injuries is less technically challenging than open access and has the potential to reduce injury to the surrounding brachial plexus [46].

In all types of EVIs, the basic concepts of catheter-directed treatment of a vascular lesion include access to the vascular tree at a remote site, crossing the offending lesion with a wire, and delivering a device that will allow correction of the lesion [1].

Transcatheter treatments include balloon occlusion, embolization, and endovascular repair with insertion of stent grafts which will be discussed in the following parts. An appreciation of the collateral circulation to the distal extremity is necessary to evaluate the best strategy of treatment and consequently the success and the safety [47].

An integrated endovascular and open approach for the management of polytraumatic patients is sometimes required [1].

The operating room (OR) may only have portable equipment; a dedicated hybrid room may have a fixed fluoroscopy unit [48].

Uncontrolled hemorrhage and hemodynamic instability have long been considered an absolute contraindication to EVIs but hybrid ORs with endovascular capabilities may permit more liberal use of endovascular techniques in the OR in the event that immediate surgical access is necessary [48].

The inability to use heparin is also an important consideration, but not an absolute contraindication because most open repairs would have the same limitation [49].

Skilled team is mandatory to approach an acutely traumatic patient and unnecessary delays may allow the lethal triad of hypothermia, coagulopathy, and acidosis leading uncontrolled hemorrhage and death [50].

25.9 Balloon Occlusion

Inflation of an angioplasty balloon proximal to a major arterial injury may temporarily stop or reduce life-threatening hemorrhage to allow time and thereby stabilize the patient while more definitive treatment such as surgical or endovascular repair is being arranged [51].

25.10 Embolization

Embolization is a largely used technique in IR in arresting life-threatening hemorrhage in all areas of the body. In particular, it is very effective in treating hemorrhage within the peripheral system in small and medium sized arteries where preservation is not critical [4]. The same principles apply as observed in the rest of the body with most of the embolization agents requiring a relatively intact coagulation cascade with embolization being ideally performed before severe coagulopathy develops [47]. Prompt, effective,

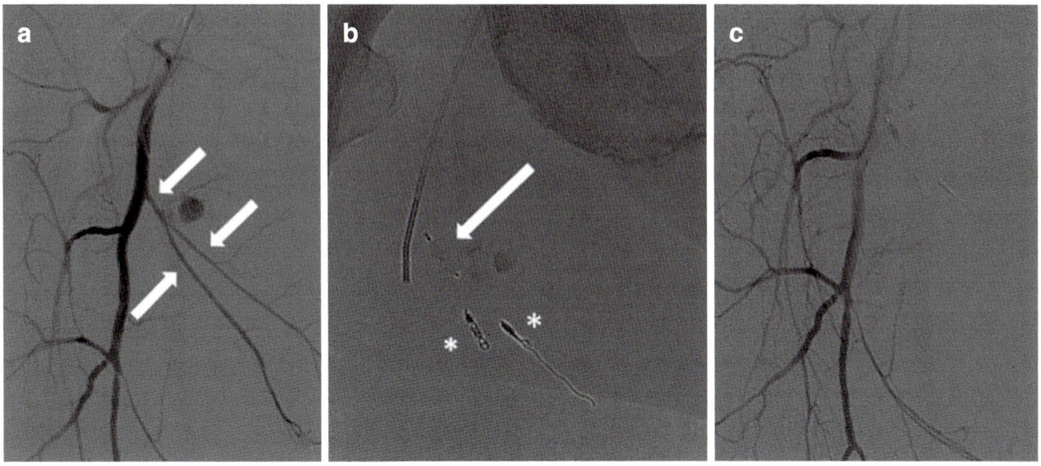

Fig. 25.1 First angiogram reveals pseudoaneurysm of a branch of profunda femoral artery: arrows indicate branches to embolize to avoid refilling of the PSA from collaterals (**a**); figure demonstrates coils (*asterisk*) in the branches and a vascular plug at the origin of the afferent vessel to the PSA (*arrow*) (**b**); final angiogram reveals complete exclusion of the PSA (**c**)

and safe embolization requires skill and knowledge of the available equipment, arterial anatomy, role of collateral arterial flow, and risks. A clear understanding of the target vessel is critical, especially if it contains extensive collateral supply (e.g., via muscular branches) as these can provide distal flow and supply to the bleeding vessel and therefore result in continued bleeding if they are not also embolized. Therefore routinely both the proximal and distal segments of the artery, in relation to the site of injury, are embolized to prevent this from happening [47] (Fig. 25.1a–c).

The choice of embolic agent will vary based on the site and nature of the injury, the desire to preserve collateral flow, and operator preference [52]. Some liquid agents such as *N*-butyl cyanoacrylate (NBCA) and ethylene vinyl alcohol copolymer (Onyx) have been used in the treatment of selected traumatic injuries especially in patients with coagulopathy [53].

The clinical condition of the patient usually determines how selective a distal embolization is performed. In the stable patient, a more superselective technique is usually undertaken, whereas in a patient who is more unstable or has massive bleeding a more nonselective proximal embolization technique is used as the main aim is the cessation of hemorrhage in a more timely manner [47].

The two specific potential complications of embolization in the peripheral vascular system are: (1) inadvertent distal infarction of nonexpendable vessels and (2) continued bleeding distal to the point of embolization secondary to collateral flow [4].

Embolization requires skilled operators, specialized in EVI and should be available in short time.

25.11 Stent Grafts and Balloon Inflations

Stent grafts can provide life- and limb-saving when applied to the treatment of vessel injuries (Fig. 25.2a–d).

Stent grafts are available in several varieties and sizes (both lengths and diameters) from multiple manufacturers and may be either self-

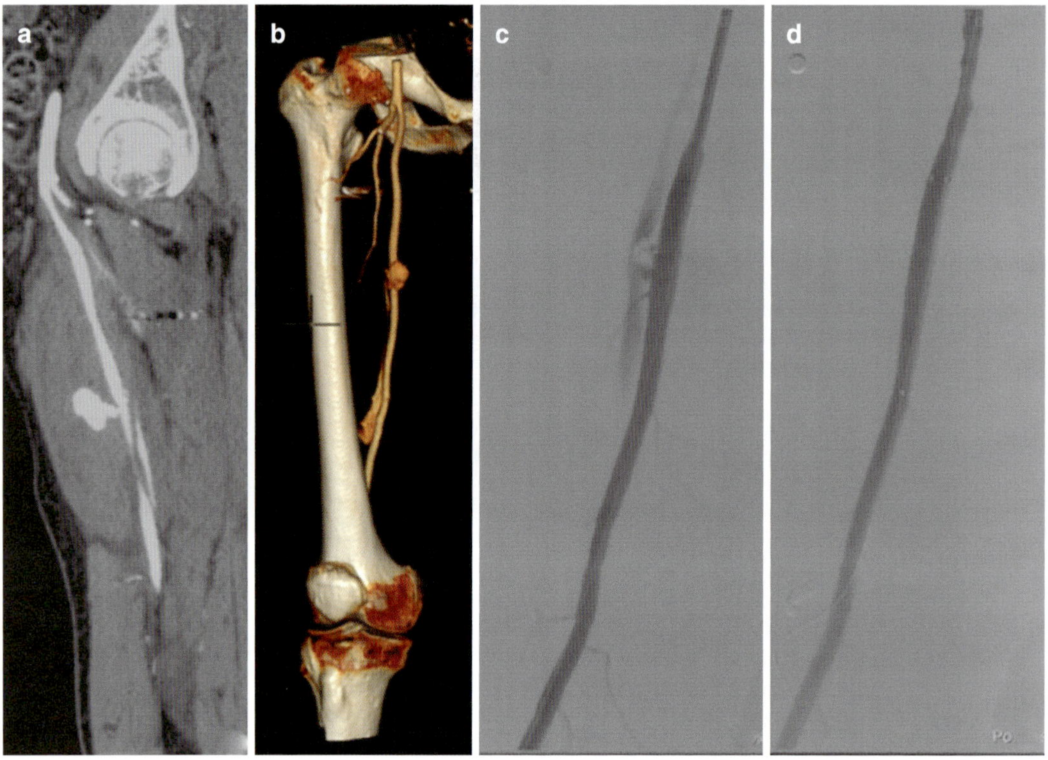

Fig. 25.2 PSA and dissection of superficial femoral artery caused by a gunshot (**a**); VR reconstruction confirmed findings (**b**); angiogram reveals findings of CTA and a high flow arteriovenous fistula (**c**); final angiogram performed after deployment of a covered stent (**d**)

expanding or balloon expandable. Stent grafts are covered with material such as polytetrafluoroethylene (PTFE); stent grafts covers the neck of the PSA or the nidus of the AVF while maintaining the patency of the vessel [4].

Dissection and occluding intimal flap could be treated with prolonged and repeated balloon inflations. This procedure is preferred in young patients; implantation of a bare stent is mandatory when inflation is inconclusive, and direct stent placement is safer in long occlusions to avoid distal embolism [54].

Ideally, deployment of covered or uncovered stents requires proximal and distal landing zones of 2 cm of normal vessel to ensure an adequate seal to prevent a type I endoleak [54].

Potential complications of stent placement include stent occlusion, loss of vessel branches after stent placement, deformation, and kinking, although newer stent grafts have greater flexibility (Fig. 25.3a–g). Although rarely, covered stents have also the potential of getting infected in case of bacteremia and sepsis [47].

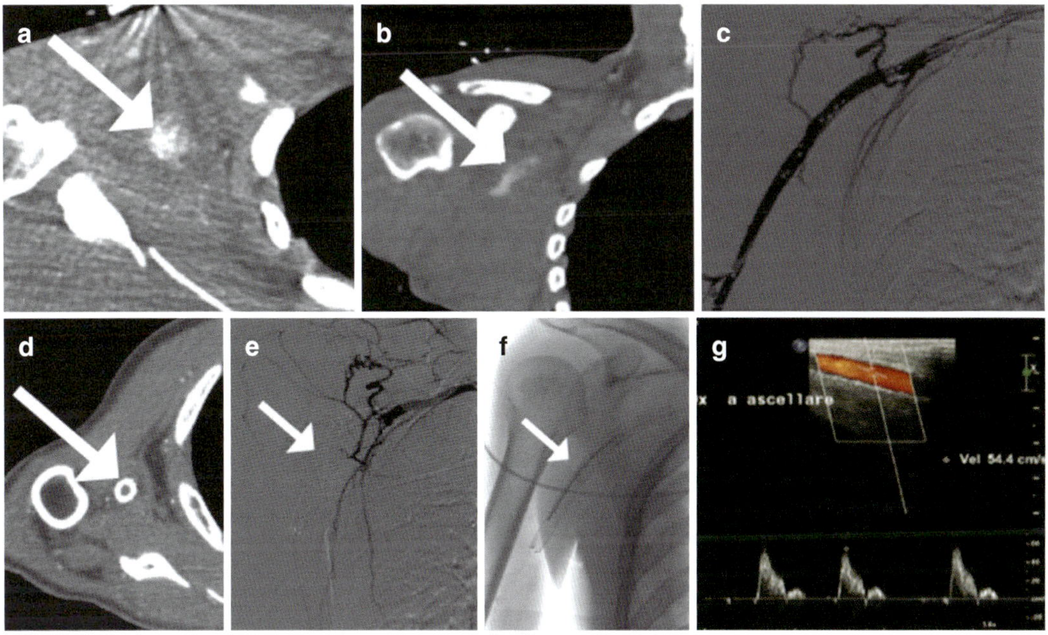

Fig. 25.3 CTA (axial (**a**) and coronal (**b**) views) reveals an active bleeding (*arrow*) resulting by a transection of axillary artery; angiogram performed after deployment of three imbricated covered stents (**c**); 6 months later, CTA reveals occluded stents (*arrow*) and ischemia of the right arm (**d**); angiogram confirms (**e**) CT finding, therefore a catheter for fibrinolysis was deployed (**f**); DUS performed during follow-up confirms patency of the artery (**g**)

25.12 Follow-Up of Patients Treated with EVIs

Follow-up of the traumatic patients treated with EVIs is notoriously poor [55]. Diligent prospective surveillance, including clinical examinations, DUS studies and ensuring continued antiplatelet therapy, is recommended to maximize durability and reduce long-term failure of EVIs [56].

IR also has an important role in the treatment of thromboembolic episodes in this group of patients who are at higher risk due to immobility.

There are currently several different available methods in dealing with prophylaxis of pulmonary embolism (PE) including the use of low dose heparin, low molecular weight heparin and gradient compression stockings. Despite this array of methods, venous thrombotic complications including PE may still occur [57].

Inferior vena caval (IVC) filter role in the prophylaxis of PE is controversial [58]. The use of retrieval filters has helped to reduce or eliminate many of the long-term complications associated with permanent IVC filters like the thrombosis or migration of the IVC filter itself. However, there is no sufficient evidence based on the actual literature about the use of retrievable IVC filters in traumatic patients [59].

Conclusions

Both diagnostic and IR have an essential role in the management of trauma patients with limbs injuries and play a key part in the MT approach to the patients with limbs injuries.

Current literature suggests that IR has much to offer in the treatment of traumatic injuries of the limbs and this role may expand in time due to desire for organ preservation and avoidance of surgery as well as due to improvements in trans-catheter equipment. IR procedures allow rapid control of hemorrhage and repair of vessels that are surgically difficult to access.

Longer-term follow-up is required and the natural history of these interventions in young patients has to be better defined.

References

1. Dua A, Desai SS, Holcomb JB, Burgess AR, Freischlag JA. Clinical review of vascular trauma. Berlin: Springer; 2014.
2. Kaewlai R, Avery LL, Asrani AV, et al. Multidetector CT of carpal injuries: anatomy, fractures, and fracture-dislocations. Radiographics. 2008;28(6):1771–84.
3. Pasch AR, Bishara RA, Lim LT, et al. Optimal limb salvage in penetrating civilian vascular trauma. J Vasc Surg. 1986;3(2):189–95.
4. Murthy R, Hastings GS, Richard HM, Levitin A. Angiography and endovascular intervention for vascular trauma to the extremities. Semin Intervent Radiol. 2003;20(2):081–8.
5. Monazzam S, Goodell PB, Salcedo ES, Nelson SH, Wolinsky PR. When are CT angiograms indicated for patients with lower extremity fractures? A review of 275 extremities. J Trauma Acute Care Surg. 2017;82(1):133–7.
6. Frykberg ER, Vines FS, Alexander RH. The natural history of clinically occult arterial injuries: a prospective evaluation. J Trauma. 1989;29(5):577–83.
7. Uyeda JW, Anderson SW, Sakai O, Soto JA. CT angiography in trauma. Radiol Clin N Am. 2010;48(2):423–38. ix–x
8. Wallin D, Yaghoubian A, Rosing D, et al. Computed tomographic angiography as the primary diagnostic modality in penetrating lower extremity vascular injuries: a level I trauma experience. Ann Vasc Surg. 2011;25(5):620–3.
9. Fox N, Rajani RR, Bokhari F, et al. Evaluation and management of penetrating lower extremity arterial trauma: an Eastern Association for the Surgery of Trauma practice management guideline. J Trauma Acute Care Surg. 2012;73(5 Suppl 4):S315–20.
10. Foster BR, Anderson SW, Uyeda JW, Brooks JG, Soto JA. Integration of 64-detector lower extremity CT angiography into whole-body trauma imaging: feasibility and early experience. Radiology. 2011;261(3):787–95.
11. Frykberg ER. Advances in the diagnosis and treatment of extremity vascular trauma. Surg Clin North Am. 1995;75(2):207–23.
12. Pezeshki Rad M, Mohammadifard M, Ravari H, et al. Comparing color Doppler ultrasonography and angiography to assess traumatic arterial injuries of the extremities. Iran J Radiol. 2015;12(1):e14258.
13. Johansen K, Lynch K, Paun M, Copass M. Non-invasive vascular tests reliably exclude occult arterial trauma in injured extremities. J Trauma. 1991;31(4):515–9. discussion 519–522
14. Feliciano DV, Moore FA, Moore EE, et al. Evaluation and management of peripheral vascular injury. Part 1. Western Trauma Association/critical decisions in trauma. J Trauma. 2011;70(6):1551–6.
15. Huber-Wagner S, Lefering R, Qvick LM, et al. Effect of whole-body CT during trauma resuscitation on survival: a retrospective, multicentre study. Lancet. 2009;373(9673):1455–61.
16. Miller-Thomas MM, West OC, Cohen AM. Diagnosing traumatic arterial injury in the extremities with CT angiography: pearls and pitfalls. Radiographics. 2005;25(Suppl 1):S133–42.
17. Iacobellis F, Ierardi AM, Mazzei MA, et al. Dual-phase CT for the assessment of acute vascular injuries in high-energy blunt trauma: the imaging findings and management implications. Br J Radiol. 2016;89(1061):20150952.
18. Shah N, Anderson SW, Vu M, et al. Extremity CT angiography: application to trauma using 64-MDCT. Emerg Radiol. 2009;16(6):425–32.
19. O'Moore PV, Denham JS, Steinberg FL. The complications of angiography: a prospective study. Radiology. 1988;169:317.
20. Egglin TK, O'Moore PV, Feinstein AR, Waltman AC. Complications of peripheral arteriography: a new system to identify patients at increased risk. J Vasc Surg. 1995;22(6):787–94.
21. Adibi A, Krishnam MS, Dissanayake S, et al. Computed tomography angiography of lower extremities in the emergency room for evaluation of patients with gunshot wounds. Eur Radiol. 2014;24(7):1586–93.
22. Hiatt MD, Fleischmann D, Hellinger JC, Rubin GD. Angiographic imaging of the lower extremities with multidetector CT. Radiol Clin N Am. 2005;43(6):1119–27. ix
23. Willmann JK, Wildermuth S. Multidetector-row CT angiography of upper- and lower-extremity peripheral arteries. Eur Radiol. 2005;15(Suppl 4):D3–9.
24. Anderson SW, Lucey BC, Varghese JC, Soto JA. Sixty-four multi-detector row computed tomography in multitrauma patient imaging: early experience. Curr Probl Diagn Radiol. 2006;35(5):188–98.
25. Dorlac WC, DeBakey ME, Holcomb JB, et al. Mortality from isolated civilian penetrating extremity injury. J Trauma. 2005;59(1):217–22.

26. Bynoe RP, Miles WS, Bell RM, et al. Noninvasive diagnosis of vascular trauma by duplex ultrasonography. J Vasc Surg. 1991;14(3):346–52.
27. Patterson BO, Holt PJ, Cleanthis M, et al. Imaging vascular trauma. Br J Surg. 2012;99(4):494–505.
28. Tan TW, Joglar FL, Hamburg NM, et al. Limb outcome and mortality in lower and upper extremity arterial injury: a comparison using the National Trauma Data Bank. Vasc Endovasc Surg. 2011;45(7):592–7.
29. Hyre CE, Cikrit DF, Lalka SG, Sawchuk AP, Dalsing MC. Aggressive management of vascular injuries of the thoracic outlet. J Vasc Surg. 1998;27(5):880–4. discussion 884–885
30. Abouljoud MS, Obeid FN, Horst HM, et al. Arterial injuries of the thoracic outlet: a ten-year experience. Am Surg. 1993;59(9):590–5.
31. Castelli P, Caronno R, Piffaretti G, et al. Endovascular repair of traumatic injuries of the subclavian and axillary arteries. Injury. 2005;36(6):778–82.
32. Joo JY, Ahn JY, Chung YS, et al. Therapeutic endovascular treatments for traumatic carotid artery injuries. J Trauma. 2005;58(6):1159–66.
33. Xenos ES, Freeman M, Stevens S, et al. Covered stents for injuries of subclavian and axillary arteries. J Vasc Surg. 2003;38(3):451–4.
34. Klocker J, Falkensammer J, Pellegrini L, et al. Repair of arterial injury after blunt trauma in the upper extremity - immediate and long-term outcome. Eur J Vasc Endovasc Surg. 2010;39(2):160–4.
35. Joshi V, Harding GE, Bottoni DA, Lovell MB, Forbes TL. Determination of functional outcome following upper extremity arterial trauma. Vasc Endovasc Surg. 2007;41(2):111–4.
36. Niska R, Bhuiya F, Xu J. National Hospital Ambulatory Medical Care Survey: 2007 emergency department summary. Natl Health Stat Report 2010;(26):1–31.
37. Stalp M, Koch C, Ruchholtz S, et al. Standardized outcome evaluation after blunt multiple injuries by scoring systems: a clinical follow-up investigation 2 years after injury. J Trauma. 2002;52(6):1160–8.
38. Kovacs F, Pollock JG, DeNunzio M. Endovascular stent graft repair of iatrogenic popliteal artery injuries--a report of 2 cases. Vasc Endovasc Surg. 2012;46(3):269–72.
39. Wagner WH, Yellin AE, Weaver FA, Stain SC, Siegel AE. Acute treatment of penetrating popliteal artery trauma: the importance of soft tissue injury. Ann Vasc Surg. 1994;8(6):557–65.
40. Goltz JP, Basturk P, Hoppe H, Triller J, Kickuth R. Emergency and elective implantation of covered stent systems in iatrogenic arterial injuries. Rofo. 2011;183(7):618–30.
41. Shah DM, Corson JD, Karmody AM, Fortune JB, Leather RP. Optimal management of tibial arterial trauma. J Trauma. 1988;28(2):228–34.
42. Zhong S, Zhang X, Chen Z, et al. Endovascular repair of blunt popliteal arterial injuries. Korean J Radiol. 2016;17(5):789–96.
43. Lopera JE, Suri R, Cura M, Kroma G, El-Merhi F. Crural artery traumatic injuries: treatment with embolization. Cardiovasc Intervent Radiol. 2008;31(3):550–7.
44. Becker GJ, Benenati JF, Zemel G, et al. Percutaneous placement of a balloon-expandable intraluminal graft for life-threatening subclavian arterial hemorrhage. J Vasc Interv Radiol. 1991;2(2):225–9.
45. DuBose JJ, Rajani R, Gilani R, et al. Endovascular management of axillo-subclavian arterial injury: a review of published experience. Injury. 2012;43(11):1785–92.
46. Scott AR, Gilani R, Tapia NM, et al. Endovascular management of traumatic peripheral arterial injuries. J Surg Res. 2015;199(2):557–63.
47. Lopera JE. Embolization in trauma: principles and techniques. Semin Intervent Radiol. 2010;27(1):14–28.
48. G Cornalba FM, AM Ierardi, G Carrafiello. Equipment and logistic organization for endovascular procedures (OR vs. hybrid room)" in Endovascular techniques in the managment of aortic and peripheral arterial disease. Minerva Medica. 2015. https://www.minervamedica.it/it/preview.php?pdf=L10031.
49. Resnick SB, Resnick SH, Weintraub JL, Kothary N. Heparin in interventional radiology: a therapy in evolution. Semin Intervent Radiol. 2005;22(2):95–107.
50. Ierardi AM, Piacentino F, Fontana F, et al. The role of endovascular treatment of pelvic fracture bleeding in emergency settings. Eur Radiol. 2015;25(7):1854–64.
51. Doody O, Given MF, Lyon SM. Extremities--indications and techniques for treatment of extremity vascular injuries. Injury. 2008;39(11):1295–303.
52. Gould JE, Vedantham S. The role of interventional radiology in trauma. Semin Intervent Radiol. 2006;23(3):270–8.
53. Ierardi AM, Xhepa G, Duka E, et al. Ethylene-vinyl alcohol polymer trans-arterial embolization in emergency peripheral active bleeding: initial experience. Int Angiol. 2015;34(6 Suppl 1):28–35.
54. Carrafiello G, Lagana D, Mangini M, et al. Percutaneous treatment of traumatic upper-extremity arterial injuries: a single-center experience. J Vasc Interv Radiol. 2011;22(1):34–9.
55. Johnson CA. Endovascular management of peripheral vascular trauma. Semin Intervent Radiol. 2010;27(1):38–43.
56. Reuben BC, Whitten MG, Sarfati M, Kraiss LW. Increasing use of endovascular therapy in acute arterial injuries: analysis of the National Trauma Data Bank. J Vasc Surg. 2007;46(6):1222–6.
57. Thorneycroft IH, Goldzieher JW. Venous thromboembolism. A review. J Reprod Med. 2003;48(11 Suppl):911–20.
58. Aryafar H, Kinney TB. Optional inferior vena cava filters in the trauma patient. Semin Intervent Radiol. 2010;27(1):68–80.
59. Johnson ON 3rd, Gillespie DL, Aidinian G, et al. The use of retrievable inferior vena cava filters in severely injured military trauma patients. J Vasc Surg. 2009;49(2):410–6. discussion 416

Printed by Printforce, the Netherlands